OPHTHALMOLOGY
for Undergraduates

OPHTHALMOLOGY
for
Undergraduates

PS Girija Devi MS DO DNB
Director
Regional Institute of Ophthalmology
Thiruvananthapuram, Kerala, India

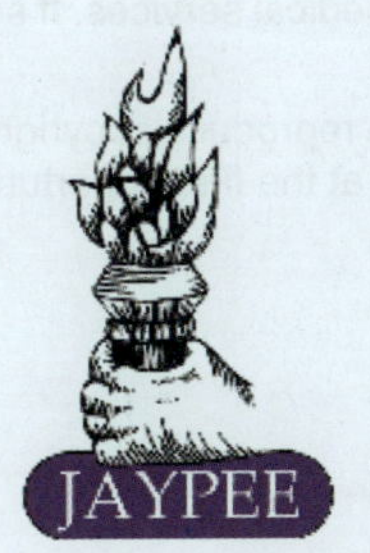

JAYPEE *The Health Sciences Publisher*
New Delhi | London | Philadelphia | Panama

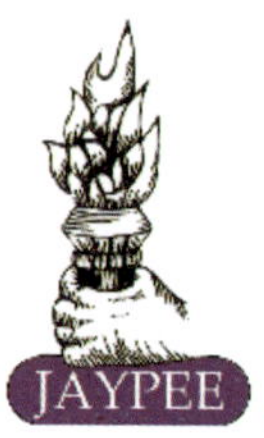

Jaypee Brothers Medical Publishers (P) Ltd

Headquarters

Jaypee Brothers Medical Publishers (P) Ltd
4838/24, Ansari Road, Daryaganj
New Delhi 110 002, India
Phone: +91-11-43574357
Fax: +91-11-43574314
Email: jaypee@jaypeebrothers.com

Overseas Offices

J.P. Medical Ltd
83 Victoria Street, London
SW1H 0HW (UK)
Phone: +44 20 3170 8910
Fax: +44 (0)20 3008 6180
Email: info@jpmedpub.com

Jaypee-Highlights Medical Publishers Inc
City of Knowledge, Bld. 237, Clayton
Panama City, Panama
Phone: +1 507-301-0496
Fax: +1 507-301-0499
Email: cservice@jphmedical.com

Jaypee Medical Inc
The Bourse
111 South Independence Mall East
Suite 835, Philadelphia, PA 19106, USA
Phone: +1 267-519-9789
Email: jpmed.us@gmail.com

Jaypee Brothers Medical Publishers (P) Ltd
17/1-B Babar Road, Block-B, Shaymali
Mohammadpur, Dhaka-1207
Bangladesh
Mobile: +08801912003485
Email: jaypeedhaka@gmail.com

Jaypee Brothers Medical Publishers (P) Ltd
Bhotahity, Kathmandu, Nepal
Phone +977-9741283608
Email: kathmandu@jaypeebrothers.com

Website: www.jaypeebrothers.com
Website: www.jaypeedigital.com

Inquiries for bulk sales may be solicited at: jaypee@jaypeebrothers.com

Ophthalmology for Undergraduates

First Edition: ***2015***

ISBN 973-93-5152-582-0

Printed at Sanat Printers, Kundli

Dedicated to

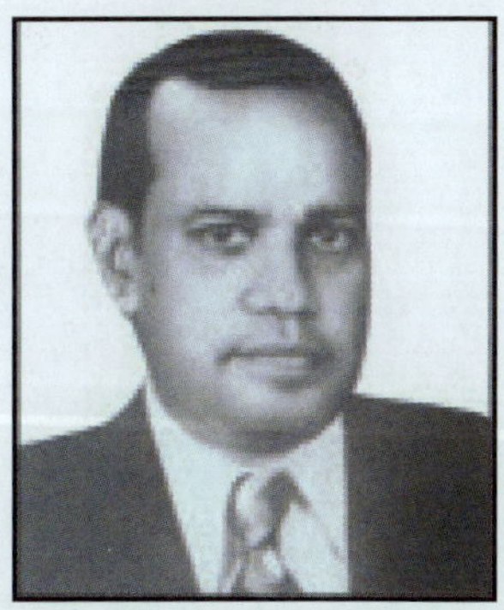

Late Dr ***TA Joseph****, my guru*
and
All my teachers, patients and students
who taught me what little I know

Contributors

Anitha Balachandran
MBBS MS DO DNB
Associate Professor
Regional Institute of Ophthalmology
Thiruvananthapuram, Kerala, India
Anatomy and Physiology of Extraocular Muscles, Strabismus

Anuja Sathar
MBBS MS DO DNB
Assistant Professor
Regional Institute of Ophthalmology
Thiruvananthapuram, Kerala, India
Nystagmus, Migraine, Diseases of the Optic Nerve

Biju John
MS DNB FRCS
Associate Professor
Regional Institute of Ophthalmology
Thiruvananthapuram, Kerala, India
Retina

Jasmin LB
MBBS MS DO
Assistant Professor
Regional Institute of Ophthalmology
Thiruvananthapuram, Kerala, India
Ocular Trauma

Kanchana
MBBS MS DO
Professor
Regional Institute of Ophthalmology
Thiruvananthapuram, Kerala, India
Uvea

Lakshmi G
MBBS MD (Physiology)
Associate Professor
Department of Physiology
Medical College, Thiruvananthapuram
Thiruvananthapuram, Kerala, India
Physiology of the Eye

Lekshmi H
MBBS MS DO
Senior Resident
Regional Institute of Ophthalmology
Thiruvananthapuram, Kerala, India
Sclera

Lekshmi P Moorthi
MBBS DNB
Senior Resident
Regional Institute of Ophthalmology
Thiruvananthapuram, Kerala, India
Lids

Mahadevan
MBBS DO MS
Former Professor
Regional Institute of Ophthalmology
Senior Consultant
Vasan Eye Care Hospital
Thiruvananthapuram, Kerala, India
Retina

Pappa P
MBBS MS DO DNB
Assistant Professor
Regional Institute of Ophthalmology
Thiruvananthapuram, Kerala, India
Retina

Rajeevan P
MBBS DO DNB MPhil
Associate Professor
Regional Institute of Ophthalmology
Thiruvananthapuram, Kerala, India
Low Vision Aids, Causes of Blindness, National Program for Control of Blindness

Sahasranamam
MBBS MS DO
Professor
Regional Institute of Ophthalmology
Thiruvananthapuram, Kerala, India
Lacrimal Apparatus

Sheeba CS
MBBS DO MS
Associate Professor
Regional Institute of Ophthalmology
Thiruvananthapuram, Kerala, India
Low Vision Aids

Sija S
MS DO
Sr Resident
Regional Institute of Ophthalmology
Thiruvananthapuram, Kerala, India
Orbit

Simon George
MBBS DNB FRCS MNAMS
Associate Professor
Regional Institute of Ophthalmology
Thiruvananthapuram, Kerala, India
Vision 2020, National Program for Control of Blindness

Sunil
MBBS MS DNB FICO FRCS
Assistant Professor
Regional Institute of Ophthalmology
Thiruvananthapuram, Kerala, India
Ocular Pharmacology, Clinical Examination of the Eye

Susan Philip
MBBS DO DNB
Associate Professor
Regional Institute of Ophthalmology
Thiruvananthapuram, Kerala, India
Glaucoma

Susan Thomas
MBBS MS
Assistant Professor
Regional Institute of Ophthalmology
Thiruvananthapuram, Kerala, India
Ophthalmic Microsurgical Instruments

Thomas George T
MBBS DOMS MS
Associate Professor
Regional Institute of Ophthalmology
Thiruvananthapuram, Kerala, India
Glaucoma, Glaucoma Surgery

Umesan KG
DO MD (Anatomy)
Assistant Professor
Department of Anatomy
TD Medical College
Alappuzha, Kerala, India
Anatomy of the Eyeball, Development of the Eye

Preface

Eyes are the windows through which we see the world around us. Not only that, by looking into a person's eyes, we can gather a lot of information about his general health and the various medical problems he may be having. So, a basic knowledge in ophthalmology is essential for general practitioners and physicians. This book is meant not only as a textbook for undergraduate students but also we have tried to make it a book useful for them in their future practice.

Recently, there is an unfortunate trend to consider that eye care is the responsibility of an ophthalmologist and the optometrist alone, and any knowledge in even basic things in ophthalmology is unnecessary for a general practitioner or a physician. The sole purpose of studying ophthalmology at the undergraduate level is to get through the examination. The end result is that the doctors at the primary care level are not competent to handle even the most basic things like identifying and removing a corneal foreign body or to decide on when to refer a diabetic patient for evaluation for diabetic retinopathy. What they often do is to send all patients with any eye problem to the refractionist or optometrist working with them. And in no other specialty in modern medicine this sort of affairs takes place. This unfortunate practice is to be discouraged and the primary care in any eye problem should be the responsibility of the general practitioner and they should have the basic knowledge to handle them. This book is written with this aim in mind.

We have tried to include as many pictures as possible so as to make the subject interesting and also any future reference easy. Some multiple choice questions (MCQs) are also included to help in postgraduate entrance examination.

We hope that both students as well as teachers will find this book useful.

PS Girija Devi

Acknowledgments

I would like to express my sincere gratitude to all my colleagues and residents who had worked hard to bring this book to its final shape. A special word of gratitude to Dr Lekshmi P Moorthi and Dr Lekshmi H, Senior Residents of my department who have put in several hours of hard work to compile all the pictures included in this book and to bring this book to the final form. My office staff had put in extra effort to convert all the handwritten material to computer format; I greatly appreciate their sincere hard work and I am thankful to them.

Finally, I thank Shri Jitendar P Vij (Group Chairman), Mr Ankit Vij (Group President), Mr Tarun Duneja (Director-Publishing) and all staff of Bengaluru Branch of M/s Jaypee Brothers Medical Publishers (P) Ltd, New Delhi, India, for their encouragement and support, which made this book possible.

Contents

Section 1 An atomy and Physiology of the Eye

SECTION 1

Anatomy and Physiology of the Eye

Development of the Eye

1

Girija Devi PS, Umesan KG

The eye develops from:

1. The neural ectoderm: This part gives rise to the retina and accessory pigmented structures as well as the fibers of the optic nerve.
2. Surface ectoderm: It forms the lens, corneal and conjunctival epithelium; and also the tarsal and lacrimal glands.
3. The neural crest mesenchyme: This part differentiates to form the fibrous coats of the eye, choroid, vitreous and tissues in the anterior segment of the eye.

STAGES OF DEVELOPMENT

The development has three stages, which are as follows:

1. Optic sulcus.
2. Optic vesicle.
3. Optic cup.

Optic Sulcus

Optic sulcus first appears as a thickening on the diencephalic neural fold called optic sulcus. This occurs by about 29 days postovulation. The optic sulcus appears as transverse sulcus on either side of the cranial end of the neural crest. By the 30th day, the walls of diencephalons evaginate around the optic sulcus and this leads to the formation of the optic vesicle by the 32nd day. The vesicle becomes surrounded by the cranial mesenchyme and cells of neural crest origin.

Optic Vesicle

Optic vesicle shows three distinct parts:

1. Optic stalk attaches the vesicle to the diencephalon.
2. A flat disk of thickened epithelium close to the surface epithelium, this differentiates into the neural retina.
3. A layer of epithelial cells lying between the optic stalk and the flat disk of thickened epithelium, which differentiates into the future pigment epithelium of retina.

Optic Cup

Optic vesicle undergoes invagination in its lateral part. The invagination results in the formation of the optic cup (Fig. 1.1) with an inner wall and an outer wall. The inner layer becomes the sensory retina and the outer layer forms the retinal pigmented epithelium. The lumen of the original vesicle gets converted to the potential space between the sensory retina and the pigment layer.

DEVELOPMENT OF DIFFERENT PARTS OF EYE

Choroid Fissure/Optic Fissure

Ventral part of the optic vesicle and the lateral part of the optic stalk invaginate to form the choroid fissure (Figs 1.2A and B). At about the 5th week of intrauterine life (IUL), the hyaloid artery grows into this fissure. Apoptosis at the margins of the optic fissure gradually leads to closure of the fissure.

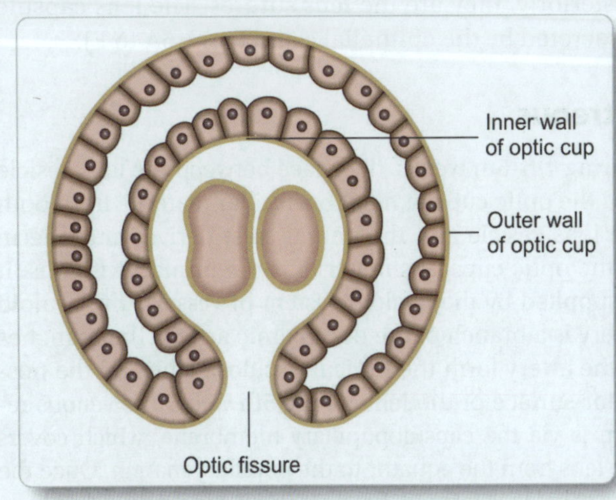

FIGURE 1.1: Development of optic cup and optic fissure

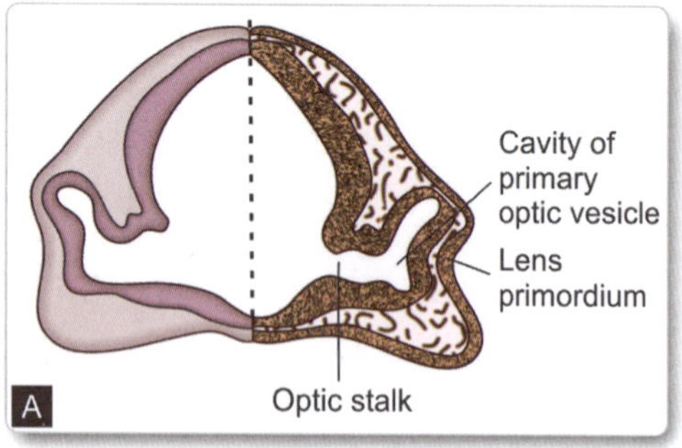

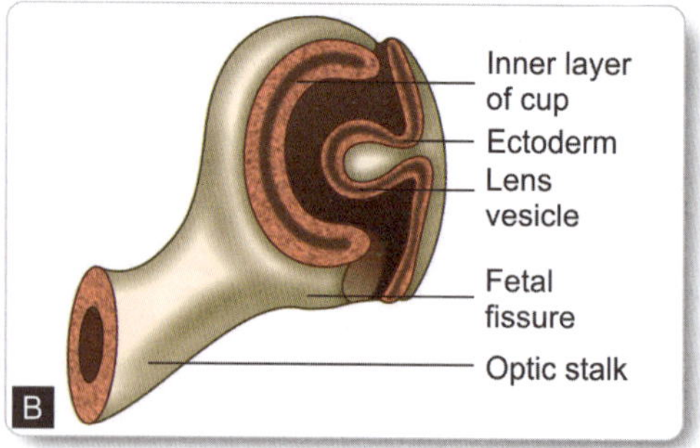

FIGURES 1.2A and B: Transverse section of forebrain of a 5 mm embryo showing the optic vesicle and lens primordium. **A.** Optic primordium; **B.** Optic fissure.

Lens Placode

Due to induction by the optic vesicle, the surface ectoderm overlying the optic vesicle thickens and forms the lens placode by the 33rd day (Fig. 1.3). By the 35th day, the lens placode invaginates to form a pit. The invaginated ectoderm gradually detaches from the surface ectoderm to form the lens vesicle. The surface ectoderm at the site of detachment regrows and forms the corneal epithelium.

Lens

Lens vesicle migrates toward the optic cup. The cubical cells from its posterior wall elongate to form the primary lens fibers, thus producing the embryonic nucleus (Figs 1.4A and B). Cells at the equator of the vesicle elongate to form the secondary lens fibers. They are added around the embryonic nucleus to get the fetal nucleus. The elongating lamina of lens fibers form a Y-shaped junction anteriorly and a λ-shaped junction posteriorly, they are the lens sutures. The lens capsule is secreted by the epithelial cells (Figs 1.5A to E).

Vitreous

During 4th–5th weeks, the space between the lens vesicle and the optic cup get filled by fibrillar material from both the lens vesicle and the neural crest derived mesoderm in the optic cup. This material is the primary vitreous. It is supplied by the hyaloid system of vessels. The hyaloid artery is a branch of the ophthalmic artery. The branches of the artery form the tunica vasculosa lentis on the posterior surface of the lens by the 5th week. The venous return is via the capsulopupillary membrane, which covers the lens from the equator to the pupillary margin. Once the lens capsule is formed, further vitreous is produced only by the neuroectoderm of the optic cup. This constitutes the secondary vitreous. A passage develops for the hyaloid vessels between the primary vitreous and secondary vitreous by the 4th month, the tunica vasculosa lentis regresses and the hyaloid artery atrophies. Remnants on the posterior lens capsule form the Mittendorf's dots.

The tertiary vitreous is formed from the neuroectoderm of the ciliary region at the 12th week. The zonules develop from the tertiary vitreous. The outermost layers of the vitreous body condense to form the hyaloid membrane.

Retina

Inner and outer layers of the bilaminar optic cup give rise to the retinal layers (refer Fig. 1.5D). They are separated by the cavity of the optic cup, which becomes the intraretinal space. The outer layer of cubical cells becomes the retinal pigment epithelium. The inner layer multiplies to get three to four layers of cells by mitosis by the 26th day. The outermost layer is called the germinative or ependymal layer. It gets attached to the pigment layer and forms the outer segments of rod and cones by the 4th month. The inner marginal layer forms the nerve fiber layer. During the retinal differentiation, ganglion cells and Muller's cells

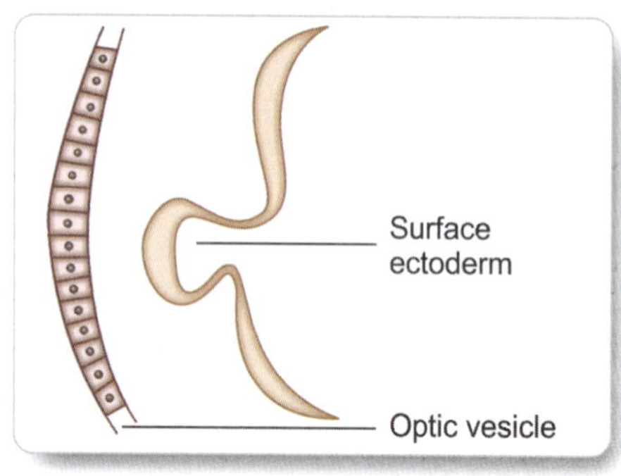

FIGURE 1.3: Development of lens placode

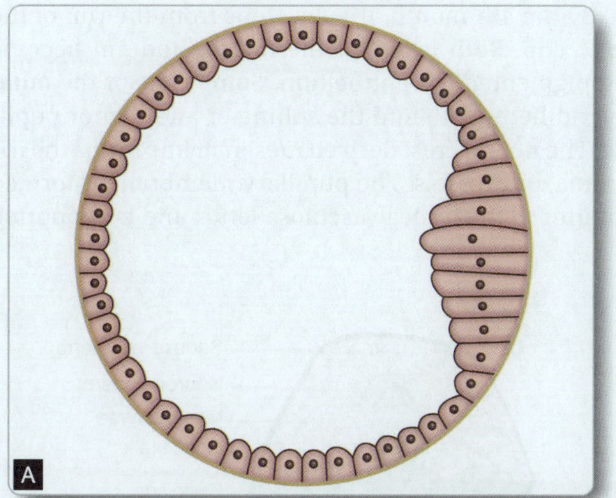

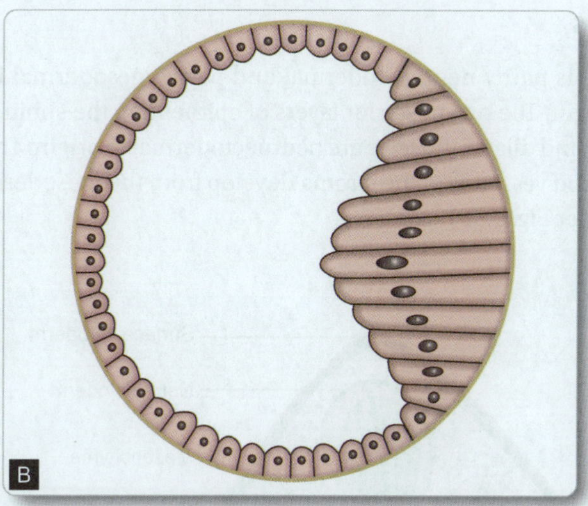

FIGURES 1.4A and B: Lens vesicle. **A.** Elongating posterior lens cells; **B.** Formation of lens fibers.

develop very early. The transient layer of Chievitz forms the inner plexiform layer by the 10th week. Rods are formed by 22nd week. Bipolar cells and horizontal cells develop by the 25th week. The fovea centralis is fully developed by the 7th month. The ora serrata is developed by the 6th month.

At first, the retina and the optic nerve are avascular since the hyaloid system blood vessel supplies only the vitreous and the lens. Blood vessels of retina grow from the hyaloid vessels from the 4th month of IUL. They reach full growth by the 3rd month after birth. The hyaloid system regresses and the portion within the optic nerve remains as the central retinal artery.

Optic Nerve

Closure of the optic (choroid) fissure causes the optic stalk to become a double walled tube, which connects the cavity of the diencephalon with the primary optic vesicle. The cavity of the tube gets filled by the growth of axons from ganglion cells (refer Fig. 1.5E). These axons grow toward the brain and reach it by the 6th week of IUL. The nerve sheaths are formed from the neural crest cells around the optic stalk. Crossing of nasal fibers at the optic chiasma occurs at 9th week. Myelination of optic nerve fibers starts from the distal end at 7th month of IUL and proceeds toward the optic disk. It stops at the level of lamina cribrosa.

Bergmeister's Papilla

Bergmeister's papilla is a projection due to glial proliferation at the site of entry of hyaloid vessels into the vitreous. Later this glia disappears due to apoptosis. This leads to the formation of the optic cup.

Uveal Tract

Neuroectoderm, neural crest derived mesenchyme and vascular channels together form the uveal tract. Condensation of neural crest cells around the optic cup forms the mesenchyme where blood spaces appear. Vessels close to RPE form the choriocapillaris during 4th–5th week. Cytoplasmic processes extending into the lumen is a feature of the endothelium of these vessels. Pericytes appear by the 6th week. Basal lamina is formed by the 6th week. By the 3rd–5th month of IUL, the outer large vessel layer of Haller's and Sattler's layer appear. The veins drain to the vortex veins. The choroidal stroma is formed from fibroblasts, collagen fibrils, elastic fibers and melanocytes of neural crest origin. The inner layer of collagen condenses to form the Bruch's membrane by the 3rd month.

Ciliary Body

Ciliary body develops from the growing rim of the optic cup. The part of the cup that extends beyond the lens is called pars caeca and the part behind is pars optica. The pars caeca, by the 3rd month shows about 75% longitudinal folds. These folds are invaded by a vascular mesenchyme by the 4th month and form the ciliary processes. The double membrane of the optic cup forms the ciliary epithelium lining these folds. By the 12th week, ciliary muscle differentiates from the mesenchyme. Ciliary zonules develop by the 7th month. The outer layer of the ciliary epithelium becomes pigmented.

Iris

Iris is partly neuroectodermal and partly mesodermal in origin. The two posterior layers of epithelium, the sphincter and dilator muscles are neuroectodermal in origin. The blood vessels and the stroma develop from the mesoderm (refer Fig. 1.5E).

By the 4th month, iris develops from the rim of the optic cup. Both layers of the neuroectoderm become the pigmented iris epithelium. Some cells of the outer layer differentiate into the sphincter and dilator pupillae. The neural crest derived mesenchyme forms the iris stroma and vessels. The pupillary membrane is formed anterior to the tunica vasculosa lentis and is supported

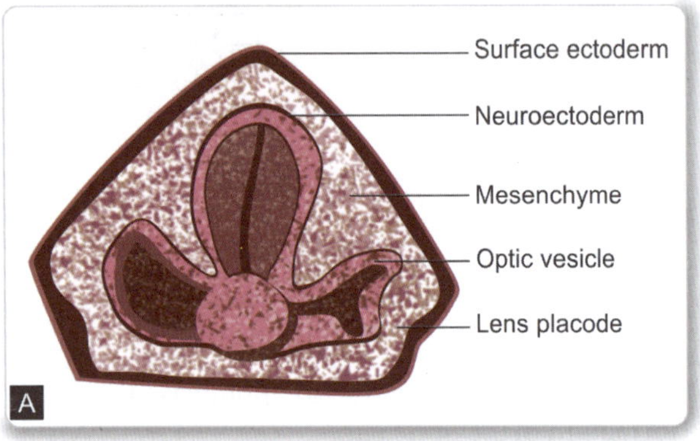

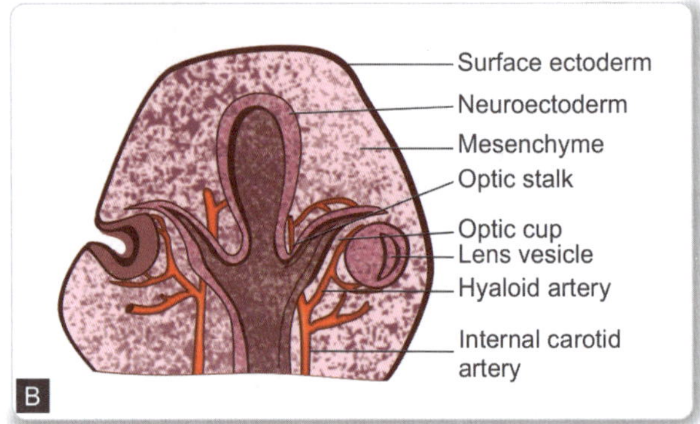

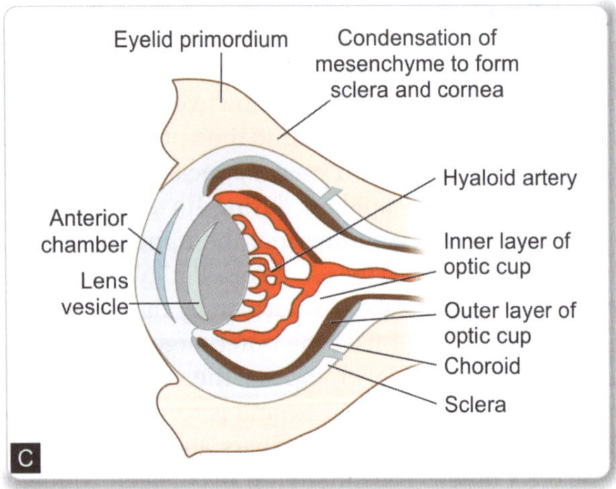

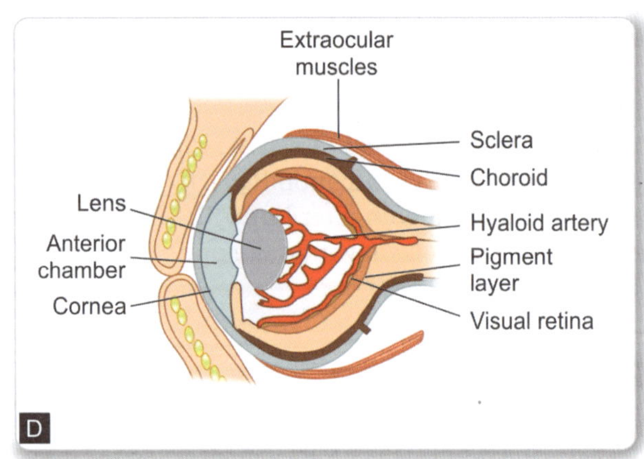

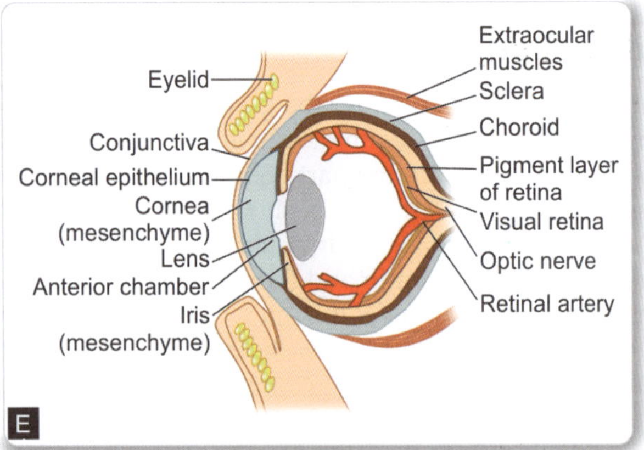

FIGURES 1.5A to E: Stages of development of human eye. **A.** Layers of eye in developmental stage; **B.** Formation of optic stalk and optic cup; **C.** Differentiation of choroid, sclera and cornea; **D.** Formation of lens and visual retina; **E.** Differentiation into eyelid, conjunctiva, iris and other features of a developed eye.

by the long posterior ciliary arteries and the annular vessel at the anterior margin of the optic cup. During the 6th month the pupillary portion of tunica vasculosa gets regressed and the remnants are phagocytized. By the 9th month the pupillary membrane disappears leaving a ring of vessels around the sphincter. This region becomes the collarette.

Cornea

The mesoderm between the surface ectoderm and the lens vesicle splits into two. The anterior part becomes the corneal stroma and the posterior part becomes the iridopupillary membrane. The cavity between the two, lined by mesothelium becomes the anterior chamber. The corneal endothelium formed from neural crest cells by the 5th week. The Bowman's membrane is formed by about the 16th week. The corneal epithelium is differentiated from the surface ectoderm by the 5th month of IUL (refer Figs 1.5D and E).

Sclera

Anterior part of sclera is formed from the neural crest derived mesenchyme around the optic cup. The caudal part is from the paraxial mesoderm (refer Figs 1.5C to E).

Eyelids

The upper lid is formed from the frontonasal process and the lower lid is from the maxillary process. The surface ectoderm of the corresponding process develops into the eyelid skin externally and the conjunctiva internally. The lids are kept closed between the 10th week and 5th month. Eyelids are totally separated by the 8th month (refer Fig. 1.5E).

Tarsal Glands

Ectodermal cells grow into the lid mesoderm as cords by the 10th week. Later they canalize to form the tarsal glands.

Lacrimal Glands

By the 8th week, epithelial cords grow upwards from the superolateral aspect of the conjunctival sac with the formation of the levator palpebrae superioris, the gland is divided into the orbital part and palpebral part. The gland starts secreting only by the 3rd month after birth. Conjunctival glands are formed as early as the 6th month of IUL.

Lacrimal Pathway

The ectoderm in the groove between the lateral nasal and maxillary process gets buried to form a solid cord of cells. Upper part of this canalizes at 3rd month to form the lacrimal sac. It grows upward the lids to form the canaliculi. The caudal part of the epithelial cord develops into the nasolacrimal duct at about the 6th month.

Anatomy of Eyelids

2

Girija Devi PS

Eyelids are also called palpebrae. They are necessary for protection against mechanical and physical injury, and excess light. They keep the cornea moist and are essential for distribution and drainage of the tears restoring the tear film with each blink.

The upper eyelid passes over the superior orbital margin to the eyebrow. The lower eyelid is limited by the nasojugal and malar sulci, where the skin is fixed to the periosteum. At the nasojugal sulcus, connective tissue separates the orbicularis oculi from levator labii superioris (Fig. 2.1).

The upper eyelid overlaps the cornea for 2 mm in forward gaze and the lower eyelid is just below the cornea. The opened eyelids enclose the elliptical palpebral fissure. The palpebral fissure is 30 mm long and 15 mm high.

CANTHI OR ANGLES

Lateral canthus measures about 40° and is at about 1 cm from the frontozygomatic suture. Small furrows (crow's feet) grow around the lateral angle skin on aging. The medial canthus is wider and ends medial at a ridge produced by the medical palpebral ligament.

The medial canthus is separated from the globe by the lacus lacrimalis, a pool of tears. The lacrimal caruncle is a fold of conjunctiva containing modified sweat glands, sebaceous glands and fine hairs.

Lateral to the caruncle is a pink fold of conjunctiva, the plica semilunaris, representing the nictitating membrane of lower animals (third eyelid). It may contain non-striated muscle.

The lacrimal papilla is seen opposite to the plica in each lid margin. It bears the punctum lacrimale, which conveys tears into the lacrimal canaliculi. The punctum divides the eyelid margin into a medial lacrimal part and a lateral ciliary part. The palpebral margin is narrow in children and is about 2 mm in the adult. The rounded anterior (ciliary) border shows eyelashes in 2–3 rows. The cilia last for 5 months and are replaced within about 2 months. The cilia have no erector muscle. They are darker than other hairs.

The posterior border is sharp and is opposed to the surface of the eyeball. The tarsal glands open anterior to this border. Between the tarsal glands orifices and the cilia is a narrow gray line, which indicates the avascular plane of the eyelid (refer Fig. 2.1).

STRUCTURE OF EYELID

Skin

Skin of eyelids is less than 1 mm thick, very transparent and elastic. There is a superior tarsal sulcus corresponding to upper tarsal border where the levator palpebrae superioris is attached. The lower tarsal sulcus is poorly developed on the medial part of the eyelid, the skin smoother with minimum hairs and is oily due to unicellular sebaceous glands in epidermis. The mucocutaneous junction behind the joining of the tarsal glands represents the anterior limit of the marginal strip of tear film. Melanocytes in perivascular connective tissue and hair follicles are mobile, and this is responsible for the color changes in the eyelids.

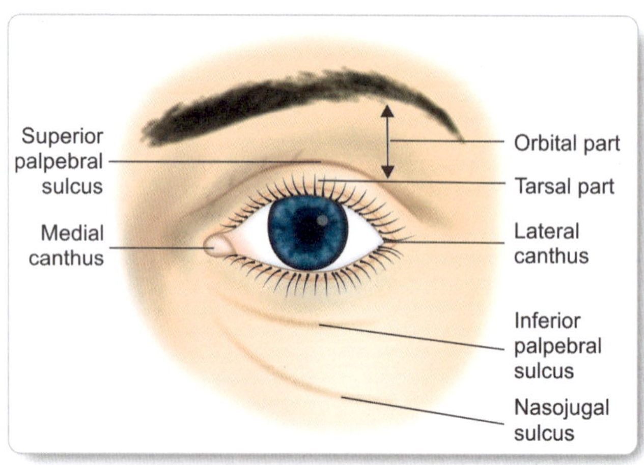

FIGURE 2.1: Surface anatomy of eyelid

Subcutaneous Areolar Tissue

Subcutaneous areolar tissue is loose and there is no adipose tissue in it. It is absent near the ciliary margin and palpebral sulci, and at the canthi. Elsewhere it permits the skin to move over the muscle.

Palpebral Part of the Orbicularis Oculi

Palpebral part of the orbicularis oculi consists of striated muscle fibers, which encircle the palpebral fissure, overlapping each other. Muscle of Riolan has its ciliary part at the lid margin. It is traversed by ciliary follicles, glands of Moll and meibomian ducts (Fig. 2.2).

Submuscular Areolar Tissue

Submuscular areolar tissue is continuous superiorly with the subaponeurotic layer of the scalp forming a tract for pus and blood to enter the upper lid from scalp. When an incision is made through gray line, the eyelid may be split into anterior and posterior layers along the plane. It is traversed by the palpebral nerves. So, local anesthetic to eyelid must be injected in the plane between orbicularis and tarsal plate.

In the upper eyelid, the space is divided by fibers of the levator into a preseptal space and a pretarsal space. Preseptal space superiorly contains the preseptal fat pad, which separates preseptal space from the dangerous area of scalp.

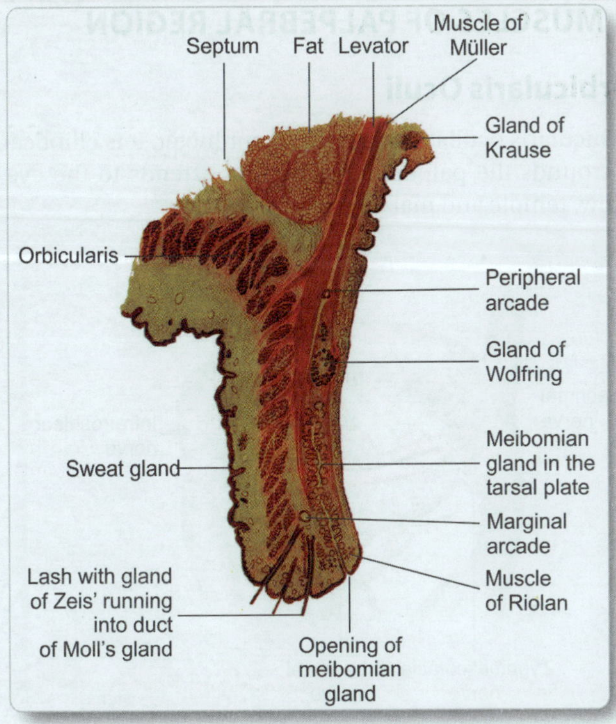

FIGURE 2.2: Cross section of eyelid

The pretarsal space encloses the peripheral anterior arcade of the eyelid and is limited above by the origin of the superior tarsal muscle from levator tendon.

Tarsal Plates

Thickened central part of the fibrous layer of the eyelid forms the tarsal plates and the peripheral part forms the septum orbitale. The tarsal plates maintain the shape and texture of the eyelids. They are made up of dense collagen and elastic tissues. Both tarsal plates are about 2.5 mm long and 1 mm thick. The upper one is crescentic and is of 11 mm height, while the lower tarsus is only 5 mm in height.

The posterior surface of tarsus is concave and is adherent to the conjunctiva. The free border lies at the eyelid margin. The palpebral muscles are attached to the upper and lower borders of the respective tarsal plates. The attached borders of the plates are connected to the orbital margin by the orbital septum. The medial and lateral ends of the tarsal plates are attached to the orbital margins by the medial and lateral palpebral ligaments respectively.

Medial Palpebral Ligament

Medial palpebral ligament is a triangular band, which is attached to the anterior lacrimal crest. It divides at the lacrimal crest into anterior and posterior bands. The posterior band blends with the lacrimal fascia. The anterior part crosses the lacrimal fossa and blends with the tarsal plates forming a band to each eyelid. These bands enclose the caruncle and contain the canaliculi.

Lateral Palpebral Ligament

Lateral palpebral ligament is behind the lateral palpebral raphe, attached to the Whitnall's tubercle about 1 cm inferior to the frontozygomatic suture. It is thinner and less conspicuous than the medial ligament. Anterior to it are the preciliary fibers of orbicularis oculi; posterior to it is the lateral check ligament and a lobule of the lacrimal gland. The upper border is united with the inferior oblique and inferior rectus.

Orbital Septum

Orbital septum is also called palpebral fascia; it is attached to the arcus marginalis where the periorbita continues as the extraorbital periosteum. It is continuous with tarsal plates, pierced by the levator in upper eyelid and a slip form inferior rectus in the lower eyelid (Fig. 2.3).

It may be considered as the deep fascia of the palpebral part of the orbicularis.

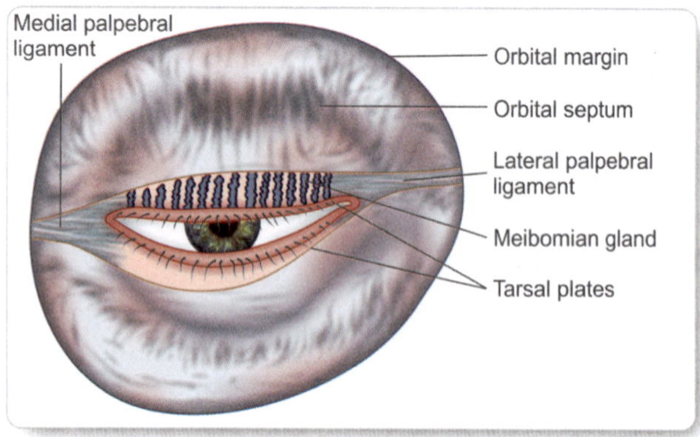

FIGURE 2.3: Orbital septum

Laterally, the septum is anterior to the lateral palpebral ligament. Medially, it is behind the pars lacrimalis of orbicularis.

Non-striated Muscles of the Eyelids

Muller's muscle is composed of non-striated, vertical fibers derived from the levator muscle in upper eyelid and the inferior rectus in the lower eyelid; and is attached to the margin of the corresponding tarsal plates. Non-striated muscle is also seen across the inferior orbital fissure (orbitalis) and within the fascia bulbi. Morphologically it is the retractor bulbi of lower animals.

GLANDS IN EYELID

1. Cutaneous glands.
2. Conjunctival glands.
3. Tarsal glands: Meibomian, Zeis' and Moll's glands.

Tarsal Glands

Meibomian Glands

Meibomian glands are long sebaceous glands, not connected to hairs, lying within the tarsal plates. There are about 25 glands in the upper eyelid and 20 in the lower eyelid. They have a central duct receiving 10–15 sebaceous acini. The duct opens anterior to the mucocutaneous junction. The orifice is keratinized.

Ciliary Glands of Moll

Ciliary glands of Moll are modified sweat glands; 5–2 mm long and are more seen in the lower eyelid. They are simple tubular, starting as a spiral showing a fundus, body, ampulla and neck. The duct enters the epidermis and opens between cilia into a ciliary follicle or into a Zeis' gland duct.

Sebaceous Glands of Zeis'

Sebaceous glands of Zeis' are pair of glands opening into each ciliary follicle. Each gland has about three acini with cubical cells, which multiply, degenerate and secrete into the duct.

INNERVATION OF EYELID

Sensory Innervation

Upper Eyelid

1. Supraorbital.
2. Supratrochlear.
3. Infratrochlear.
4. Lacrimal branch of ophthalmic.

Lower Eyelid

1. Infraorbital.
2. Lacrimal.
3. Infratrochlear.

Sensory nerves pass between the orbicularis and the tarsal plate (Fig. 2.4).

MUSCLES OF PALPEBRAL REGION

Orbicularis Oculi

Orbicularis oculi is the palpebral sphincter. It is elliptical, surrounds the palpebral fissure and extends to the eyebrow, temple and malar region.

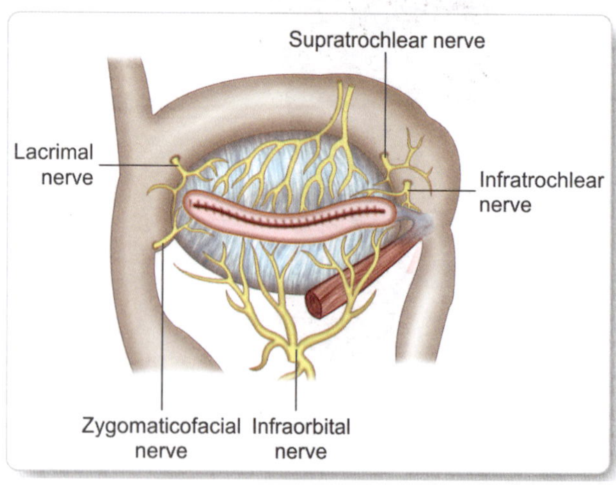

FIGURE 2.4: Nerve supply of eyelid

Palpebral Part

Palpebral part is contained in the eyelids and is divided as the pretarsal and preseptal layers. The fibers originate from the medial palpebral ligament and the adjacent bone, form half ellipses across the eyelids. The fibers form a lateral palpebral raphe outer to the lateral canthus, which is reinforced by fibers of the orbital septum.

Orbital Part

Origin

- Superior orbital margin medial to the notch
- Maxillary process of frontal bone
- Frontal process of maxilla
- Medial palpebral ligament
- Inferior orbital margin medial to infraorbital foramen.

Orbital part of orbicularis fibers form concentric loops. It has four parts:

1. The peripheral fibers attached to the skin are the musculus superciliaris. They depress the medial ends of the eyebrow.
2. Musculus malaris is formed by the most medial and lateral fibers attached to malar skin.
3. The pars ciliaris/muscle of Riolan is at the eyelid margin. The Moll's glands are placed between it and the palpebral part.
4. Tensor tarsi/pars lacrimalis, also called Horner's muscle, consists of a thin layer of muscle fibers posterior to the lacrimal sac attaching to the upper part of the posterior lacrimal crest and the lacrimal fascia. It divides into two slips around the canaliculi and gets fused to the pretarsal and ciliary parts of orbicularis oculi (Table 2.1).

TABLE 2.1: Parts of orbicularis

Orbicularis	Oculi
Palpebral part	Orbital part
Pretarsal and preseptal	Musculus superciliaris Musculus malaris Pars ciliaris Pars lacrimalis

Actions

Palpebral part causes gentle eyelid closure, usually involuntary as in blinking.

The orbital part causes tight eyelid closure giving protection. It draws the skin of forehead, temple and cheek medially, causing crow's feet, i.e. radial furrows at the lateral canthus. It also causes depression of the eyebrow to cut excess light from above. The palpebral part is antagonized by levator palpebrae and the orbital part by occipito frontalis.

Nerve Supply of Eyelid

1. Upper half: From temporal branches of facial nerve.
2. Lower half: Upper zygomatic branches (Fig. 2.6).

Blood Supply of Eyelid

Blood supply of eyelid is from the ophthalmic and lacrimal arteries by their medial and lateral palpebral branches. The medial palpebral artery anastomoses with the lateral palpebral artery to form the tarsal arcades, which lie between the orbicularis and the tarsal plate close to the eyelid margin. In the upper eyelid there is a second arterial arcade formed from the superior branch of the medial palpebral situated in front of the upper border of the tarsal plate. The veins are arranged as a pretarsal and post-tarsal plexus, and they drain into the superior ophthalmic vein and the veins of the forehead and temple (Fig. 2.5).

CONJUNCTIVA

Conjunctiva is the anatomical structure, which joins the eyeball to the eyelids, forms the fornices where it is reflected onto the sclera from the eyelids. At the limbus, it continues as the corneal epithelium.

The conjunctival sac is open at the palpebral fissure. Normally it holds 7 μL of lacrimal fluid.

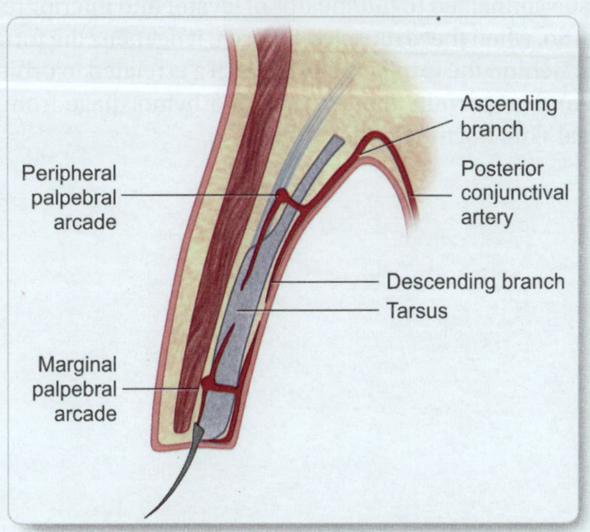

FIGURE 2.5: Blood supply of eyelid

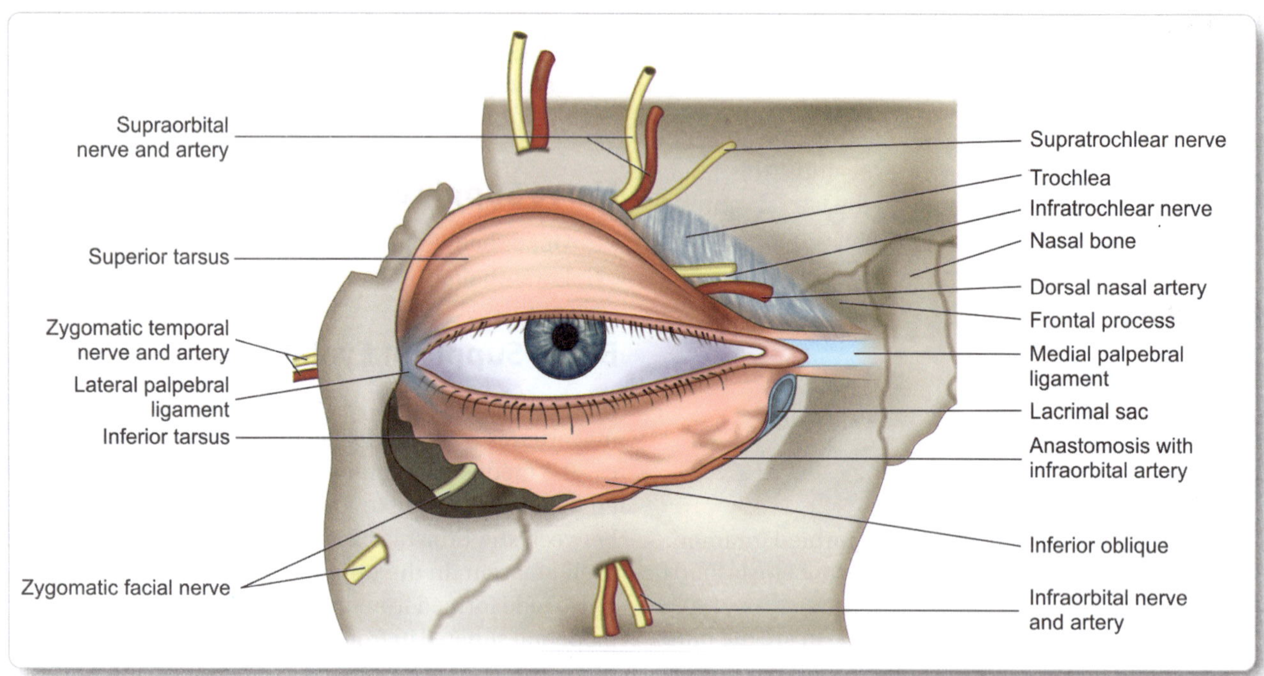

FIGURE 2.6: Relationship of the structures of the eyelid, and the nerves and arteries

Palpebral conjunctiva is thin and translucent, spreading over the inner aspect of the eyelid. It is firmly fixed to the tarsal plate, while the rest is freely mobile and thrown into folds with eyelid movements.

Conjunctival Fornix

Superior fornix lies 10 mm from limbus and the inferior lies 8 mm. The forniceal conjunctiva is related to areolar tissue connected to the sheaths of levator and inferior rectus. So, when these muscles contract, it deepens the fornices. Behind the fornix, the conjunctiva is related to orbital fat and so permits the advance of a hemorrhage from a basal skull fracture to the limbus.

Incisions at superior fornix lead to a plane between levator and superior rectus. In the inferior fornix, it leads to a plane between the inferior palpebral and inferior rectus muscles. The forniceal conjunctiva contains Krause's glands, Muller's muscle and a venous plexus.

Bulbar Conjunctiva

Bulbar conjunctiva is thin and translucent, and is attached to sclera by areolar tissue. The loose episcleral tissue under the bulbar conjunctiva holds anterior ciliary arteries, pericorneal plexus of vessels and tendons of recti. The conjunctiva, the Tenon's capsule and sclera are adherent at 3 mm from limbus and forms the limbal conjunctiva.

Anatomy of the Orbit

3

Girija Devi PS

DIMENSIONS

Orbits are bony cavities that contain the globes, extraocular muscles, nerves, fat and blood vessels. Each bony orbit is pear shaped, tapering posteriorly to the apex and the optic canal (Figs 3.1A and B).

The bony orbit has a volume of approximately 30 mL. The adult orbital margin is approximately rectangular with a horizontal dimension of 40 mm and a vertical dimension of 32 mm. The widest dimension of the orbit is 1 cm behind the anterior orbital rim. The medial walls are separated by 25 mm in the average adult and are roughly parallel. The adult lateral orbital walls are angled 90° from each other or 45° in the anteroposterior direction (Fig. 3.2).

The intraorbital optic nerve measures 24 mm on the average between the back of the globe and the entrance into the optic foramen, but the distance between these structures is only 18 mm. This 6 mm of slack in the optic nerve allows free eye movement and affords a margin of safety in proptosis.

ORBITAL MARGIN

Lateral Orbital Margin

Zygomatic bone forms the lateral orbital margin. It serves as an orbital protector or 'facial buttress' that can withstand significant trauma without fracturing. When fractured, steps may be palpable inferiorly at the zygomaticomaxillary suture and superolaterally at the zygomaticofrontal suture. The frontal bone comprises the superior orbital margin. In most skulls, the medial superior rim is indented by a supraorbital notch where the supraorbital artery and nerve pass to the forehead. In some skulls, the frontal bone covers these structures, forming a foramen.

Medial Orbital Margin

Medial orbital margin is formed by the maxillary bone rising to meet the maxillary process of the frontal bone. The lacrimal sac fossa indents the bone and forms anterior (maxillary bone) and posterior (lacrimal bone) lacrimal crests (Figs 3.3A and B).

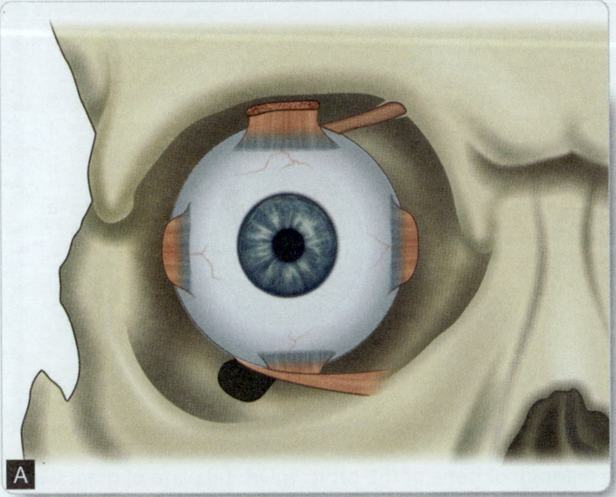

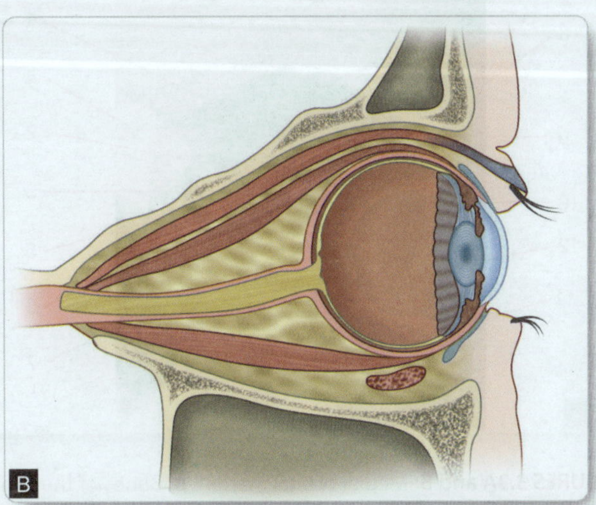

FIGURES 3.1A and B: Bony orbit and its relation to eyeball and extraocular muscle. **A.** Anterior orbit anatomy; **B.** Bony orbit of eye.

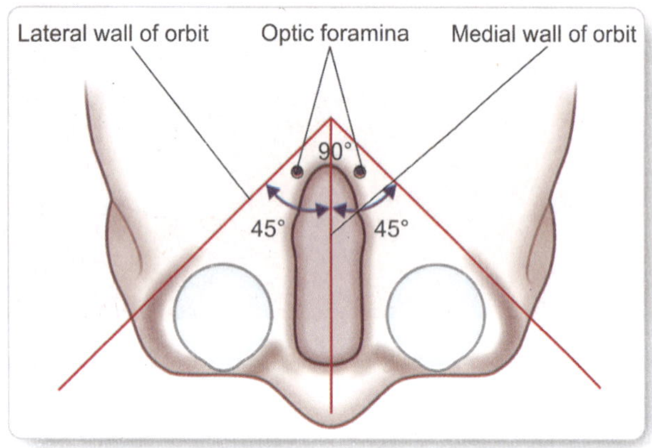

FIGURE 3.2: Relationship of orbital bony walls to the eyeball

ORBITAL WALLS

Orbital walls are embryologically derived from neural crest cells. Ossification of the orbital walls is completed by birth except at the orbital apex.

The walls are made up of seven bones (Fig. 3.4). The roof consists of the sphenoid and frontal bone, the lateral wall consists of sphenoid and zygomatic bones, the floor consists of the maxilla, the palatine and zygomatic bones; and the medial wall consists of the sphenoid, maxilla, ethmoid and lacrimal bones.

Roof of Orbit

Roof of orbit composed of the frontal bone and the lesser wing of the sphenoid (refer Fig. 3.4).

It includes these important landmarks—the lacrimal gland, fossa, which contains the orbital lobe of the lacrimal gland, fossa for the trochlea of the superior oblique tendon located 5 mm behind the superior nasal orbital rim and supraorbital notch or foramen, which transmits the supraorbital vessels and branch of the frontal nerve (refer Fig. 3.2). Roof of the orbit is located adjacent to anterior cranial fossa and frontal sinus.

Lateral Wall of Orbit

Lateral wall composed of the zygomatic bone and the greater wing of the sphenoid and it is separated from the lesser wing portion of the orbital roof by the superior orbital fissure.

Lateral wall includes these important landmarks; the lateral orbital tubercle of Whitnall, which has multiple attachments such as the lateral canthal tendon, the lateral horn of the levator aponeurosis, the check ligament of the lateral rectus. Lockwood's ligament (the suspensory ligament of the globe) and Whitnall's ligament, and the frontozygomatic suture located 1 cm above the tubercle.

Lateral wall is located adjacent to the middle cranial fossa and the temporal fossa. It commonly extends anteriorly to the equator of the globe; protect the posterior half of the eye, while still allowing wide peripheral vision. It is the thickest and strongest of the orbital walls.

Medial Wall of Orbit

Medial wall of orbit is composed of the ethmoid, lacrimal, maxillary and sphenoid bones (Fig. 3.5).

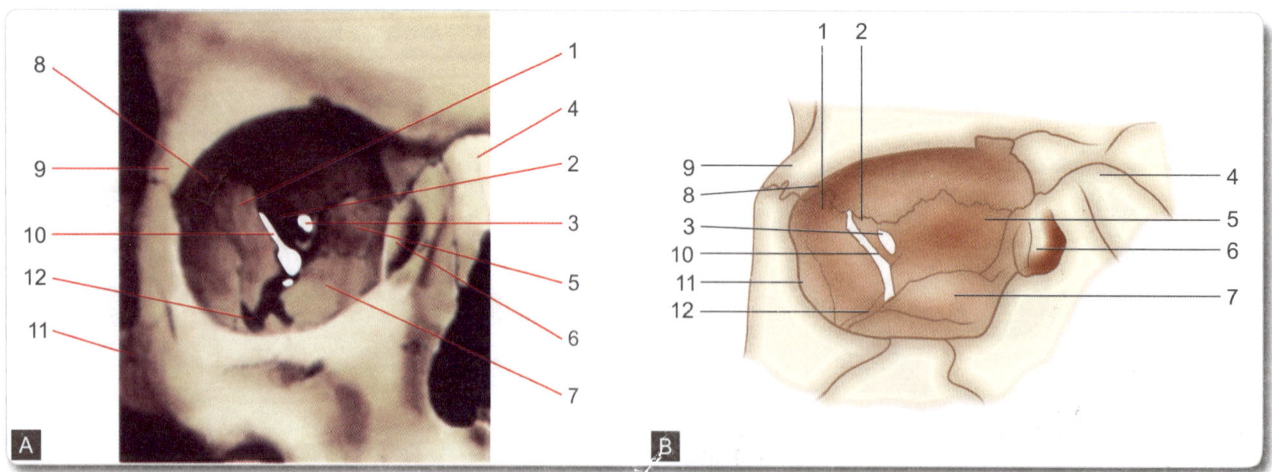

FIGURES 3.3A and B: Medial orbital margin. A. Bones of the orbit; B. Line diagram of bone of the orbit. 1. Orbital plate of great wing of sphenoid; 2. Lesser wing of sphenoid; 3. Optic foramen; 4. Nasal bone; 5. Ethmoid; 6. Lacrimal bone and fossa; 7. Orbital plate of maxilla; 8. Fossa for lacrimal gland; 9. Zygomatic process; 10. Superior orbital fissure; 11. Zygomatic bone; 12. Inferior orbital fissure.

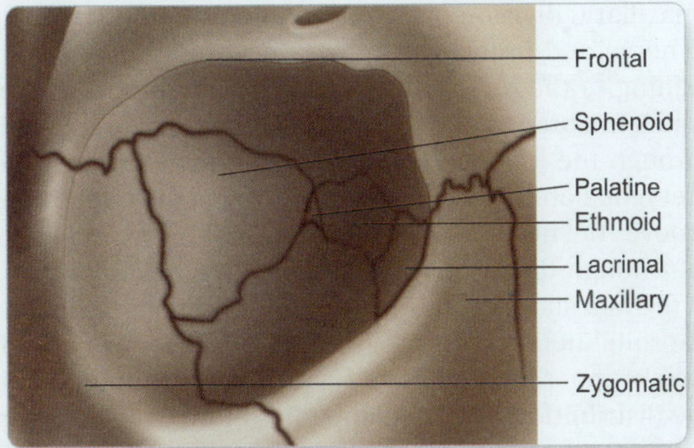

FIGURE 3.4: Roof of eye orbital wall

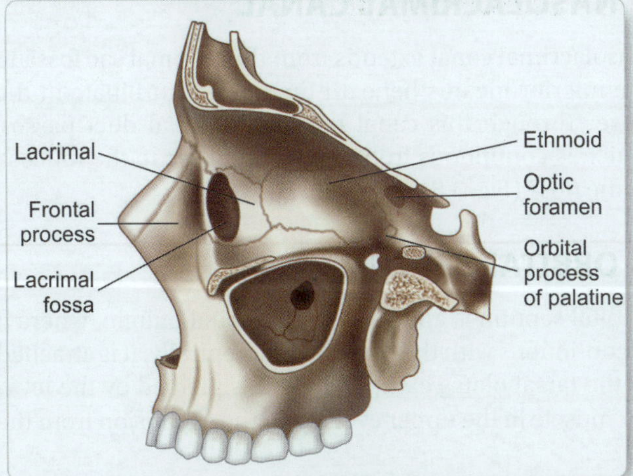

FIGURE 3.5: Medial wall of orbit

It includes important landmarks such as the frontoethmoidal suture, which marks approximately the level of the cribriform plate, the roof of the ethmoids and the floor of the anterior cranial fossa. Medial wall is located adjacent to the ethmoid and sphenoid sinuses, and nasal cavity. The thinnest walls of the orbit are the lamina papyracea, which covers the ethmoid sinuses along the medial wall and the maxillary bone, particularly in its posteromedial portion. The many bulla of ethmoid pneumatization can be seen as the honeycomb pattern beneath the ethmoidal orbital plate. This supportive structure in part explains, why the medial wall fractures less often than the thicker orbital floor. In children, infections of the ethmoid sinuses commonly extend through the lamina papyracea as a result of dehiscences or valveless venous channels to cause orbital cellulitis and proptosis.

Important to the orbital surgeon are the anterior and posterior ethmoidal foramina, conveying branches of the ophthalmic artery and the nasociliary nerve. They are located at the frontoethmoidal suture 20 mm and 35 mm posterior to the anterior lacrimal crest, respectively. It is important to remember the location of these foramina when the surgeon gives an anterior ethmoidal nerve block for local anesthesia during medial orbitotomy.

Floor of Orbit

Floor of orbit is composed of the maxillary, palatine and zygomatic bones (Fig. 3.6).

It forms the roof of the maxillary sinus, does not extend to the orbital apex, but instead ends at the pterygopalatine fossa and hence, it is the shortest of the orbital walls. Floor of the orbit includes important landmarks such as the infraorbital groove and canal, which transmits the infraorbital foramen situated immediately below the orbital margin. But as the face grows into adult size, the foramen migrates 6 mm below the margin. The floor remains strong laterally to the infraorbital nerve, but becomes thin medially with maxillary sinus expansion. This unsupported dome of maxillary sinus is where the floor usually fractures with trauma.

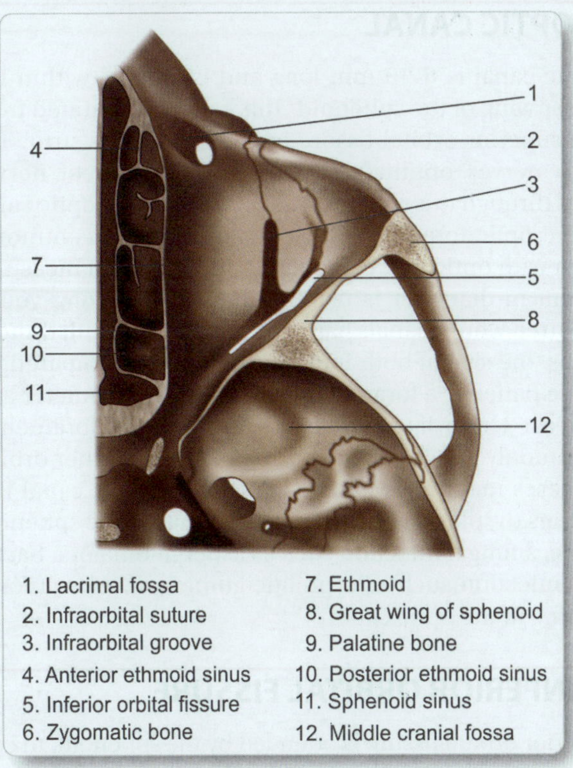

FIGURE 3.6: Floor of orbit

Orbital Apex

Orbital apex contains a plethora of vital structures. A large number of arteries, veins and nerves pass through several significant foramina and fissures.

SUPERIOR ORBITAL FISSURE

Superior orbital fissure separates the greater and lesser wings of the sphenoid. Although the shape of the superior orbital fissure is variable, the superior portion is usually narrower where the lacrimal, frontal and trochlear nerves pass (Fig. 3.7). Other structures passing through the superior orbital fissure include the superior and inferior divisions of the III cranial nerve, the VI cranial nerve and the nasociliary branch of the ophthalmic trigeminal nerve. Most of the venous drainage from the orbit passes through this fissure by way of the superior ophthalmic vein to the cavernous sinus.

Radiographic enlargement of superior orbital fissure may accompany pathologic processes such as aneurysm, meningioma, chordoma, pituitary adenoma or tumors of the orbital apex. The Tolosa-Hunt syndrome (painful ophthalmoplegia) results when idiopathic inflammation affects the superior orbital fissure.

OPTIC CANAL

Optic canal is 8–10 mm long and is located within the lesser wing of the sphenoid. This canal is separated from the superior orbital fissure by the bony optic strut. The optic nerves, ophthalmic artery and sympathetic nerves pass through this canal. The orbital end of the optic canal is the optic foramen, whose enlargement is commonly seen with optic nerve gliomas. A foramen that measures 7 mm in diameter is usually abnormal. Among young children whose canals have not yet reached adult dimensions, the size of both foramina should be compared. In these patients, a foramen that is 6.5 mm in diameter and at least 1 mm larger than the contralateral foramen is commonly considered abnormal. A host of other orbital diseases may cause enlargement of the optic canal like fibrous dysplasia and ossifying fibromas of the sphenoid bone, a fungal infection such as aspergilloma or a bacterial infection such as syphilitic gumma or tuberculoma setting in the optic canal.

INFERIOR ORBITAL FISSURE

Inferior orbital fissure is bounded by the sphenoid, maxillary and palatine bones, and lies between the lateral orbital wall and the orbital floor. It transmits the second (maxillary) division of the V cranial nerve, the zygomatic nerve and branches of the inferior ophthalmic vein leading to the pterygoid plexus. The infraorbital nerve, which is a branch of the maxillary nerve, leaves the skull through the foramen rotundum and travel through the pterygopalatine fossa to enter the orbit at the infraorbital groove. The nerve travels anteriorly in the floor of the orbit through the infraorbital canal, emerging on the face of the maxilla 1 cm below the inferior orbital rim. The infraorbital nerve carries sensation from the lower eyelid, cheek, upper lip, upper teeth and gingiva. Numbness in the distribution often accompanies blowout fractures of the orbital floor.

NASOLACRIMAL CANAL

Nasolacrimal canal extends from the lacrimal sac fossa to the inferior meatus beneath the inferior turbinate in the nose. Through this canal the nasolacrimal duct passes, which is continuous from the lacrimal sac to the mucosa of the nose (Fig. 3.8).

ORBITAL SEPTUM

Orbital septum is attached to the orbital margin, where it is continuous with the periosteum. Centrally, it is attached to the tarsal plates except where it is pierced by the levator muscle in the upper eyelid and the expansion from the

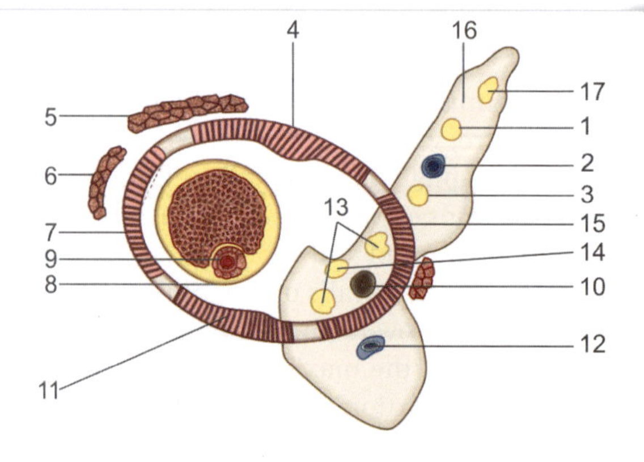

1. Frontal nerve
2. Superior ophthalmic vein
3. Trochlear nerve
4. Superior rectus
5. Levator palpebrae superioris
6. Superior oblique
7. Medial rectus
8. Optic nerve
9. Ophthalmic artery
10. Nasociliary nerve
11. Inferior rectus
12. Inferior ophthalmic vein
13. Oculomotor nerves
14. Abducens nerve
15. Lateral rectus
16. Superior orbital fissure
17. Lacrimal nerve

FIGURE 3.7: Superior orbital fissure and its contents

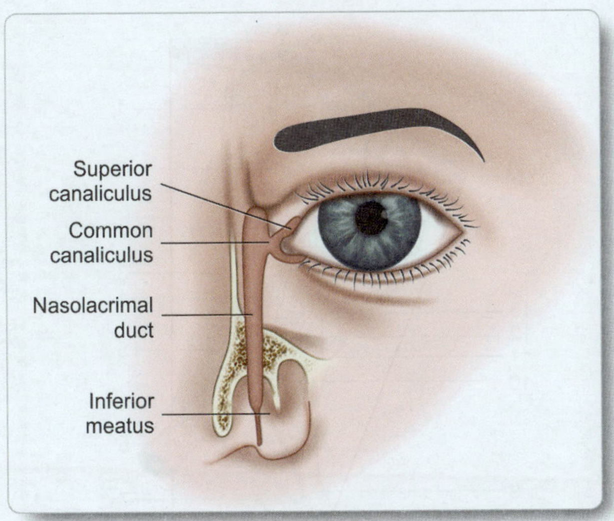

FIGURE 3.8: Nasolacrimal canal

inferior rectus in the lower eyelid. It is thicker and stronger on the upper lid than the lower lid and on the lateral than the medial side. Immediately posterior to the septum, the preaponeurotic fat is encountered (Fig. 3.9).

ORBITAL FAT

Orbital structures are surrounded by orbital fat, which provides a resilient cushion and supports the globe.

As the fascial layers in the orbit thin with age, the orbital fat sometimes prolapses through the weakened orbital septum into the eyelids. The orbital fat can be site of an orbital abscess that leads to fat liquefaction. All types of chronic granulomatous disease, either infectious or non-infectious such as Wegener's granulomatosis may involve the orbital fat.

In the anterior portion of the orbit, the rectus muscles are connected by a membrane known as the intermuscular septum. When viewed in the coronal plane, this membrane forms a ring that divides the orbital fat into the intraconal fat (peripheral surgical space). These anatomical designations are helpful for describing the location of an orbital mass.

EXTRAOCULAR MUSCLES AND ANNULUS OF ZINN

Described later (refer chapter 5 'Anatomy and Physiology of Extraocular Muscles').

VASCULATURE OF ORBIT AND EYE

Blood supply to the orbit arises primarily from the ophthalmic artery, which is a branch of the internal carotid artery. Smaller contributions come from the external carotid artery via the internal maxillary artery and the facial artery. The ophthalmic artery travels underneath the intracranial optic nerve through the dura mater along the optic canal to enter the orbit (Fig. 3.10).

The major branches of the ophthalmic artery are:

- Branches to the extraocular muscles
- Central retinal artery (to the optic nerve and retina)
- Posterior ciliary arteries (two long ciliary arteries to the anterior segment and short ciliary arteries to the choroids).

Terminal branches of the ophthalmic artery travel anteriorly and form rich anastomoses with branches of the external carotid in the face and periorbital region (Fig. 3.11).

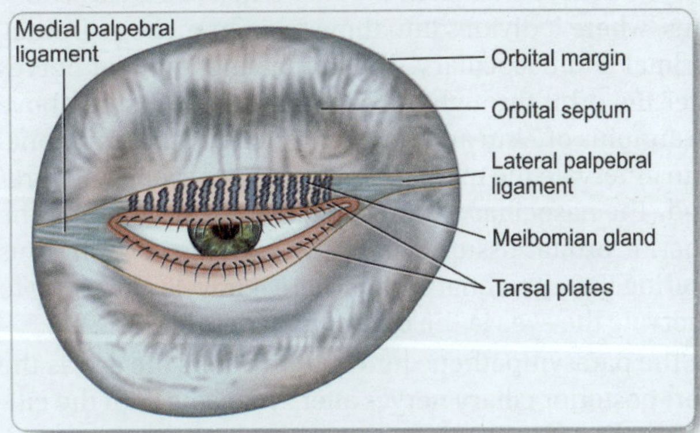

FIGURE 3.9: Orbital septum

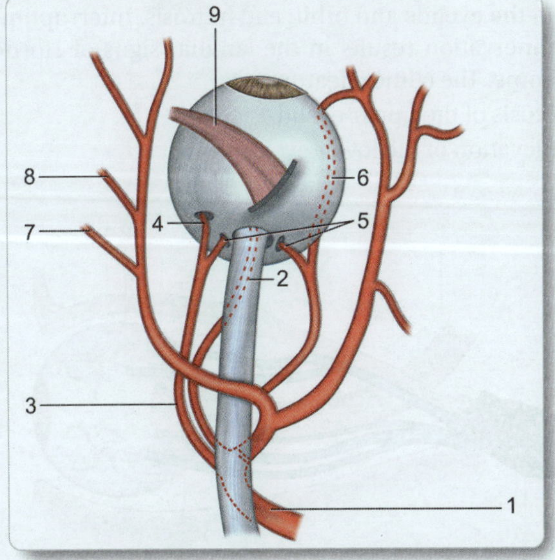

FIGURE 3.10: Orbital vascular anatomy. **1.** Ophthalmic artery; **2.** Central retinal artery; **3.** Ciliary artery; **4.** Long posterior ciliary artery; **5.** Short posterior ciliary arteries; **6.** Posterior ciliary artery in suprachoroidal space; **7.** Posterior ethmoidal artery; **8.** Anterior ethmoidal artery; **9.** Superior oblique muscle.

Blood in the choroid circulates through the choriocapillaris and larger vessels of the choroid to drain into the 4–6 vortex veins. These emerge just posterior to the equator in quadrants. The superotemporal and superonasal vortex veins will drain into the superior ophthalmic vein. The inferonasal and inferotemporal vortex veins will drain into the inferior ophthalmic vein. These vessels will eventually exit via the cavernous sinus.

NERVES

Sensory innervation to the periorbital area is provided by the ophthalmic and maxillary divisions of the V cranial nerve. The ophthalmic division of the V nerve travels anteriorly from the ganglion in the lateral wall of the cavernous sinus, where it divides into three main branches—frontal, lacrimal and nasociliary. The frontal and lacrimal nerves enter the orbit through the superior orbital fissure above the annulus of Zinn and travel anteriorly in the extraconal fat to innervate the medial canthus, upper eyelid and forehead. The nasociliary branch enters the orbit through the superior orbital fissure within the annulus of Zinn, thus entering the intraconal space where it travels anteriorly to innervate the eye via the ciliary branches (Fig. 3.12).

The parasympathetic innervation enters the eye as the short posterior ciliary nerves after synapsing with the ciliary ganglion (Fig. 3.13).

The sympathetic innervation to the orbit provides pupillary dilatation, vasoconstriction, smooth muscle function of the eyelids and orbit, and hidrosis. Interruption of this innervation results in the familiar signs of Horner's syndrome. The clinical features are:

1. Ptosis of the upper eyelid.
2. Elevation of the lower eyelid.

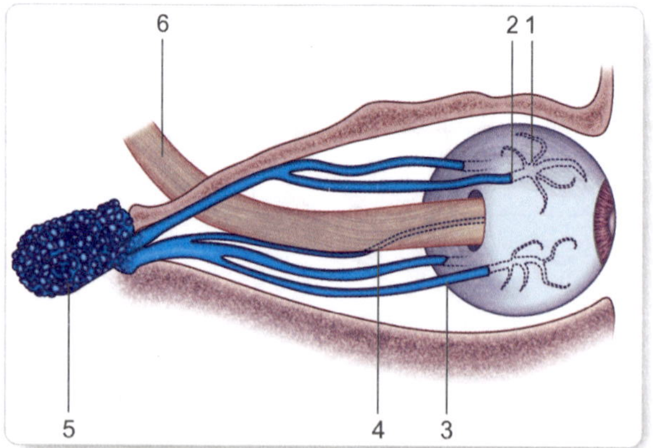

FIGURE 3.11: Blood circulation in choroid of eye. **1.** Vortex vein; **2.** Site of emergence from eye; **3.** Inferior vortex vein; **4.** Central retinal vein; **5.** Cavernous sinus; **6.** Optic nerve.

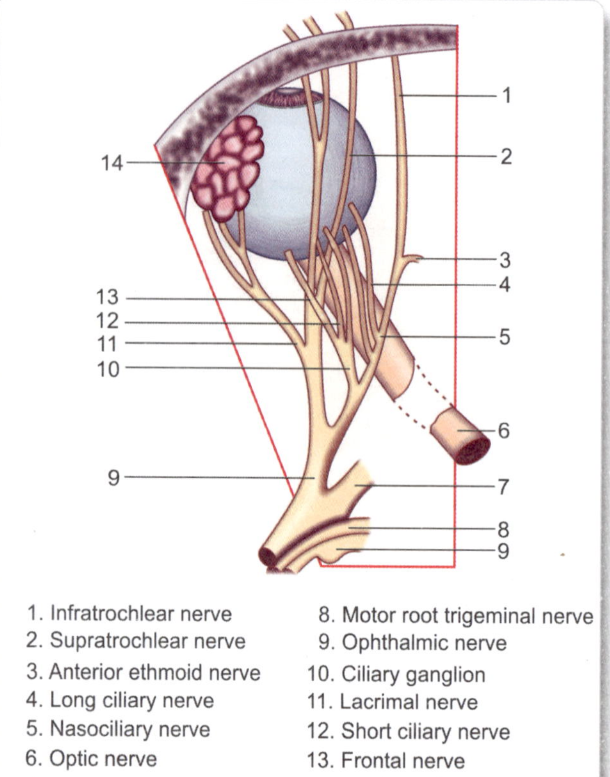

1. Infratrochlear nerve
2. Supratrochlear nerve
3. Anterior ethmoid nerve
4. Long ciliary nerve
5. Nasociliary nerve
6. Optic nerve
7. Maxillary nerve
8. Motor root trigeminal nerve
9. Ophthalmic nerve
10. Ciliary ganglion
11. Lacrimal nerve
12. Short ciliary nerve
13. Frontal nerve
14. Lacrimal gland

FIGURE 3.12: Nerve supply of orbit

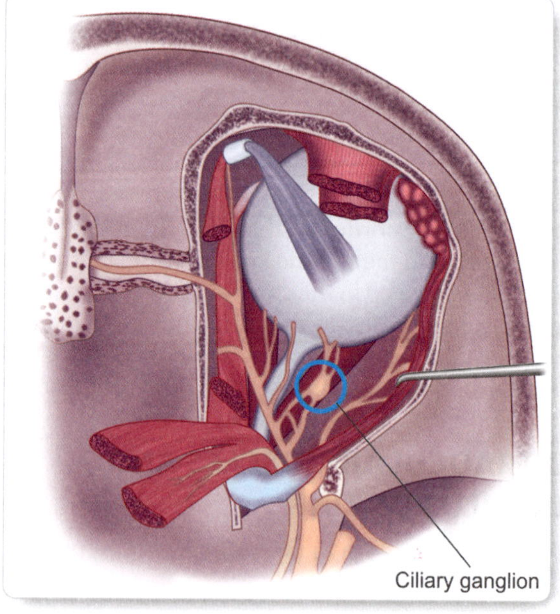

FIGURE 3.13: Parasympathetic innervation of orbit

3. Miosis.
4. Anhidrosis and vasodilatation.

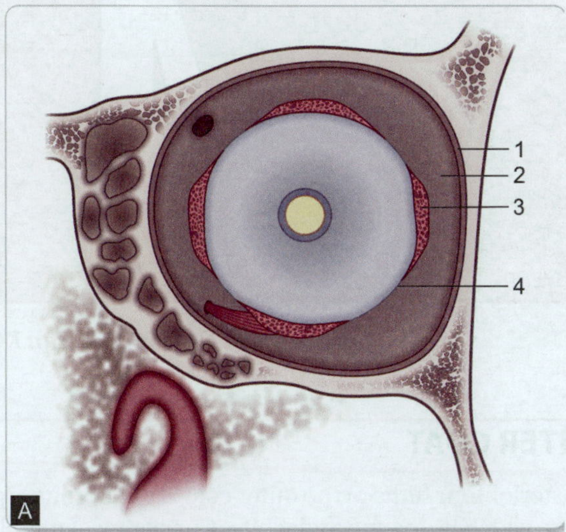

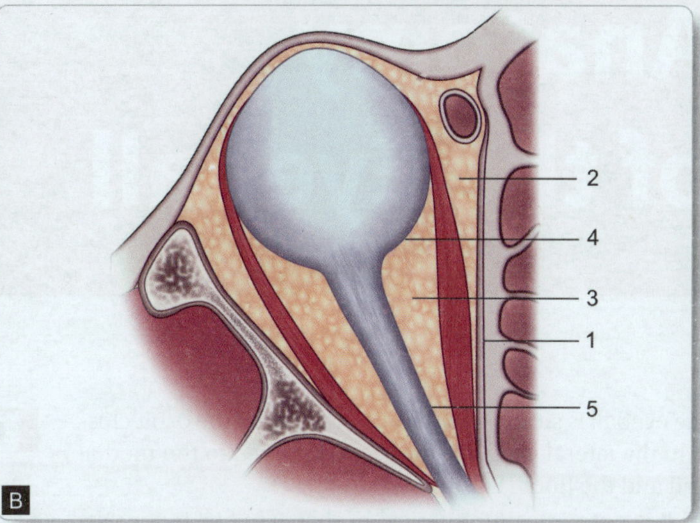

FIGURES 3.14A and B: Anatomy of orbit spaces. **A.** Spaces of the orbit; **B.** Surgical spaces of orbit. **1.** Subperiosteal space; **2.** Peripheral orbital space; **3.** Intraconal space; **4.** Sub-Tenon's space; **5.** Subarachnoid surgical space.

Motor innervation to the extraocular muscles is by III, IV and VI cranial nerves.

The muscles of facial expression including the orbicularis oculi, procerus, corrugator superciliaris and frontalis muscle receive their motor supply via branches of VII cranial nerve.

Surgical Spaces of the Orbit

1. Subperiosteal space.
2. Peripheral orbital space.
3. Intraconal space.
4. Sub-Tenon's space (Figs 3.14A and B).

Subperiosteal Space

Subperiosteal space is the potential space between the orbital bony walls and the periosteum. Pus can collected in this space from the paranasal sinuses, especially the frontal or ethmoid sinus infections.

Peripheral Orbital Space

Peripheral orbital space or extraconal space is the space between the periosteum and the extraocular muscles with their connecting fascia. Tumors or abscesses in this space will cause eccentric proptosis.

Intraconal Space

Intraconal space is the space within the muscle cone. Tumors or any pathology in this space will cause axial proptosis. Since the optic nerve is within this space, tumors in this space can affect vision early in its course.

Sub-Tenon's Space

Sub-Tenon's space is the potential space between the eyeball and the Tenon's capsule. Inflammation or spread of infection into this space from the eye leads to marked chemosis and minimal axial proptosis. So, from the clinical signs we can have an idea where the lesion is situated within the orbital cavity.

Anatomy of the Eyeball

4

Girija Devi PS, Umesan KG

The eyeball is situated in the anterior part of the orbit closer to the lateral wall and the roof compared to the medial wall and the floor (Fig. 4.1).

It is not perfectly spherical in shape; in fact it consists of parts of two spheres joined together. The anterior segment, namely the cornea, forms part of a smaller sphere with a radius of curvature of 8 mm and the posterior segment, the sclera, forms part of a larger sphere with radius of curvature of 12 mm (Fig. 4.2).

The walls of the eyeball enclose the transparent media through which light rays passes—the aqueous, lens and the vitreous. The wall of the globe consists of three layers, outermost coat consists of the sclera and the cornea, middle coat is the uveal tract and innermost coat is the retina (Fig. 4.3).

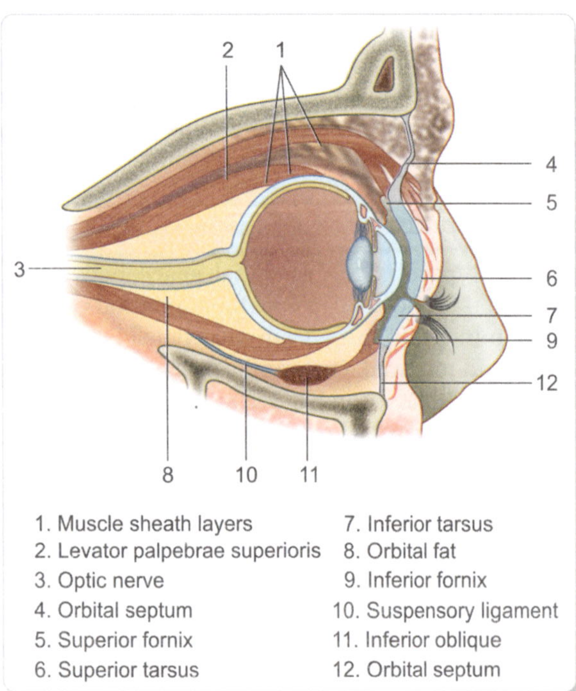

FIGURE 4.1: Cross section of eyeball and its relation to orbital structures

OUTER COAT

The posterior four fifths of the outer coat is the fibrous layer sclera, which is opaque and white. Consisting of mainly fibrous tissue it is rigid and white, and it gives support and shape to the eyeball. It transmits all the blood vessels and the nerves from the orbit to the inner layers of the eyeball. The anterior one fifth of the outer coat is formed by the transparent cornea, and the junction between the sclera and cornea is the limbus.

Sclera

The sclera forms part of a sphere 22 mm in diameter. It is thicker posteriorly (about 1 mm), becomes thinner toward the cornea and it is thinnest at the insertion of the muscles. It becomes a fenestrated membrane called the lamina cribrosa at the site of attachment of the optic nerve. Through the holes of the lamina cribrosa the axons of the ganglion cells of the retina pass to form the optic nerve.

The sclera consists of dense bundles of collagen fibers arranged parallel to the surface, but cross each other in all directions, divide and then reunite. It contains no elastic fibers and the fibroblasts are similar to that of cornea, but have irregular nuclei. The sclera is relatively avascular and the vessels it contains are mostly in transit.

Episcleral Tissue

The episcleral tissue is the loose connective and elastic tissue that connects the sclera to the conjunctiva anteriorly. It is continuous with the loose tissue of Tenon's space. The episcleral tissue is thick anteriorly in front of the insertion of the muscles, but thinner behind.

Canal of Schlemm

The canal of Schlemm (refer Fig. 4.3) is a circular venous channel situated in the sclera at the sclerocorneal junction.

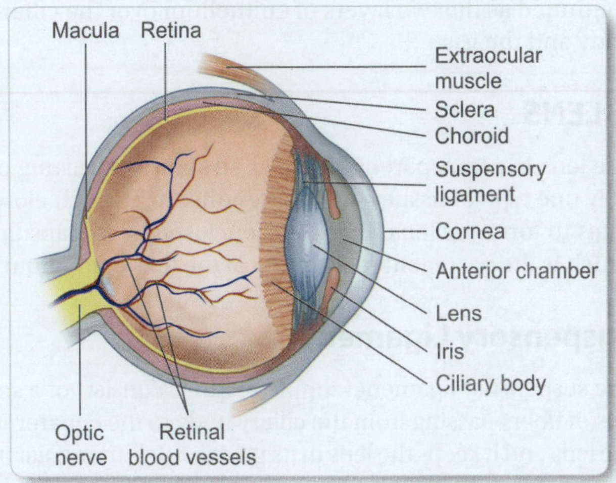

FIGURE 4.2: Cross section of eyeball

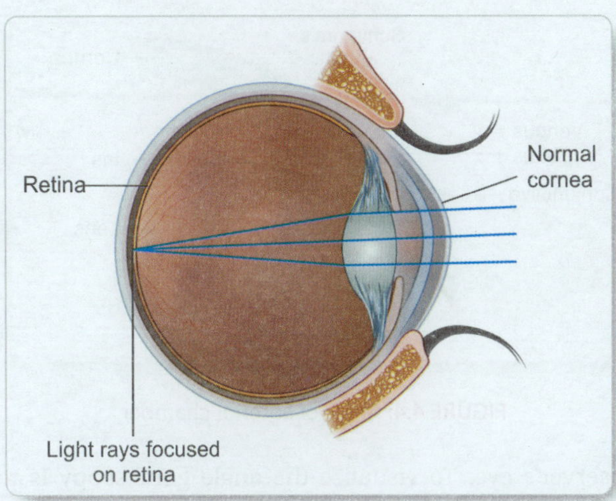

FIGURE 4.3: Focusing of light rays on retina

The inner wall of the canal of Schlemm is adjacent to the trabecular meshwork and the outer wall is bounded by the sclera spur. It is lined by endothelium and about 0.5 mm across in size. The loose trabecular meshwork is placed between the canal of Schlemm and the angle of the anterior chamber (AC). The aqueous from the AC drains into the canal of Schlemm through the trabecular meshwork. The collector channels leave the canal of Schlemm at various points and join the intrascleral venous plexus. The aqueous veins are some larger drainage channels, which join the venous plexus only after leaving the sclera.

Cornea

The cornea, which forms the anterior one fifth of the outer coat, is transparent. It is about 12 mm in the horizontal meridian and 11 mm in the vertical meridian. It consists of five layers:

1. Surface epithelium.
2. Bowman's membrane.
3. Stroma.
4. Descemet's membrane.
5. Endothelium.

The parallel arrangement of the stromal lamellae, the avascularity, lack of myelination of the corneal nerves and the relative dehydrated state maintained by the endothelial pump are the important factors contributing to the transparency of the cornea.

The avascular cornea receives its nutrition from the aqueous and the limbal capillaries, and oxygen from the atmosphere. The nerve supply is by the ophthalmic division of the trigeminal nerve via the ciliary nerves.

TENON'S CAPSULE (FASCIA BULBI)

Tenon's capsule is a thin fibrous membrane, which covers the eyeball from the cornea up to the optic nerve. Its inner aspect is connected to the sclera by fine trabeculae. Its posterior surface is closely connected to the orbital fat. Anteriorly it is thin and connected to the conjunctiva by loose connective tissue and posteriorly it becomes continuous with the dural sheath of the optic nerve. In the lower part, it is thickened to form a hammock or sling on which the eyeball rests—the suspensory ligament of Lockwood. It is pierced by the blood vessels and nerves of the eye as well as the muscles. Where the muscles pierce the fascia, it gives tubular reflections on to the muscles. These expansions act as check ligaments of the muscles.

Tenon's capsule forms an articular socket in which the eye moves. Since the Tenon's capsule is attached to the muscles, only slight movements take place between it and the eyeball and in large movements, the eye and its fascia move together in the orbital fat.

Anterior Chamber

Anterior chamber is the space between the cornea in front and the iris-lens diaphragm behind. It is filled with aqueous humor secreted by the ciliary processes, which reaches the AC through the pupil. It is about 2.5 mm in depth in the center.

Angle of the Anterior Chamber

The angle of the AC (Fig. 4.4) is the recess in the periphery of the AC. It is normally not visible since light rays from the angle undergo total internal reflection and do not reach the

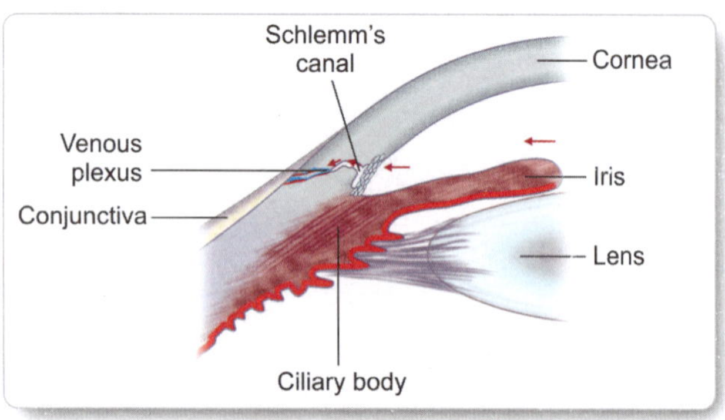

FIGURE 4.4: Angle of anterior chamber

observer's eye. To visualize the angle gonioscopy is required. The angle is bounded by the corneoscleral junction in front, and the ciliary body and the root of the iris behind. The trabecular meshwork is situated between the angle and the Schlemm's canal at the corneoscleral junction. Aqueous drains out of the eye at the angle of AC through the trabecular meshwork. This is an anatomically important part of the eye since any abnormalities in the structure of the angle can interfere with aqueous drainage and produce an increase in the intraocular pressure.

Posterior Chamber

Posterior chamber is the space between the iris in front, and the lens and the suspensory ligament behind. The aqueous is secreted into the posterior chamber by the ciliary processes.

All the structures up to the lens and the suspensory ligament are considered to be the anterior segment of the eye. The structures behind constitute the posterior segment of the eye.

MIDDLE COAT

The middle coat consists of the choroid, ciliary body and the iris. It is the vascular coat of the eye. The choroid extends from the optic disk to the ora serrata. It consists of mainly blood vessels with a loose stroma of collagen tissue with some melanocytes. The ciliary body extends from the ora up to the angle of AC. It is triangular in cross section. The posterior part is smooth (pars plana) and the anterior part has ridges formed by the ciliary processes (pars plicata). The iris is the most anterior part, which forms a circular diaphragm with a central opening called pupil.

INNERMOST COAT OR THE NERVOUS LAYER

The innermost coat is formed by the retina. It extends from the optic disk to the ora serrata. Beyond the ora it is continued as the two layers of epithelium over the ciliary body and the iris.

LENS

The lens is a transparent biconvex structure consisting of only one type of tissue—the lens epithelium, which elongates to form the lens fibers. It is enclosed by its capsule, which is the basement membrane of the lens epithelium.

Suspensory Ligament

The suspensory ligament (zonule of Zinn) consists of a series of fibers passing from the ciliary body to the equator of the lens and it keeps the lens in its position. It is triangular in cross section. The lens and the suspensory ligament divide the eye into an anterior compartment containing aqueous and a posterior compartment containing vitreous.

Vitreous

Vitreous is a transparent gel filling the space behind the iris lens diaphragm filling the posterior four fifths of the eyeball. It is firmly anchored to the vitreous base—a 4 mm broad zone including the most anterior part of the ora and the posterior 2 mm of the ciliary body. It has attachment to the edge of the optic disk and at the macula, and also along the retinal vessels. There is firm anchorage of the vitreous to the posterior lens capsule in childhood, but this attachment weakens as age advances.

The detailed anatomy of the various parts of the eyeball is given Section 4, Diseases of the Eye describing the diseases of these structures.

Blood Supply

The blood supply is from the ophthalmic artery and the venous drainage is to the cavernous sinus through the superior and inferior ophthalmic veins (Fig. 4.5).

Sclera

Sclera is relatively avascular. It is supplied by small branches from the short ciliary arteries as they pass through it.

Retina

Retina receives the blood supply through the central retinal artery. The layers up to the outer plexiform layer receive nutrition from the choriocapillaris by diffusion and the remaining layers are supplied by the central retinal artery. The venous drainage is through the central retinal vein to the cavernous sinus via the ophthalmic vein.

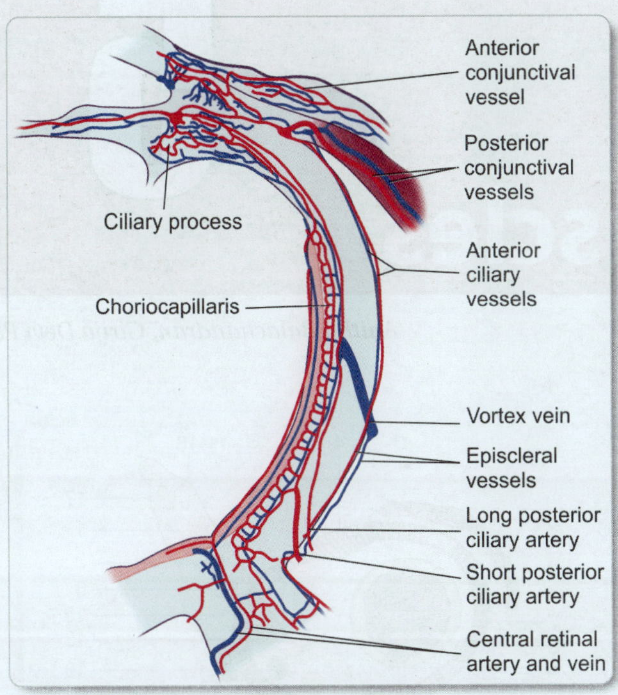

FIGURE 4.5: Blood supply of eyeball

Uveal Tract

The blood supply is from three sources. They are as follows.

Short Posterior Ciliary Arteries

The short posterior ciliary arteries are about 20 in number and they pierce the sclera around the optic nerve and pass forward to supply the choroid and the sclera.

Long Posterior Ciliary Arteries

The two long posterior ciliary arteries pierce the sclera a little more anteriorly in the horizontal meridian on the nasal and temporal side and pass forwards between the sclera and the choroid to reach the ciliary body. Here it bends and runs circumferentially and break into branches, which anastomoses with the branches from the other side to form the circulus arteriosus iridis major. This is situated at the base of the iris and supply the iris and ciliary body. Branches from the circulus arteriosus iridis major run radially into the iris and form another circular anastomosis behind the pupil—the circulus arteriosus iridis minor.

Anterior Ciliary Arteries

The anterior ciliary arteries, arising from the muscular branches of the ophthalmic artery, pierce the sclera 5–6 mm behind the limbus and they supply the conjunctiva, sclera and anterior uvea. The venous drainage is by three groups of veins:

1. The short posterior ciliary veins.
2. The vena vorticosa.
3. The anterior ciliary veins.

The veins do not correspond to the arteries. The short posterior ciliary veins are small vessels, which drain the sclera alone and do not receive any blood from the choroid. The veins from the uveal tract converge to four points behind the equator to form the four vortex veins, which drain to the cavernous sinus via the ophthalmic veins. The anterior ciliary veins are small vessels, which receive blood from the outer aspect of the ciliary muscles alone. All the remaining drainage is through the vortex veins.

Anatomy and Physiology of Extraocular Muscles

5

Anitha Balachandran, Girija Devi PS

ANATOMY AND PHYSIOLOGY

There are six extraocular muscles in each eye of which four are rectus muscles or straight muscles and two are oblique muscles. The rectus muscles are:

1. Superior rectus.
2. Inferior rectus.
3. Medial rectus.
4. Lateral rectus.

The oblique muscles are:

5. Superior oblique.
6. Inferior oblique.

The four recti originate from annulus of Zinn, which is a tendinous ring surrounding the optic nerve at the apex of orbit (Fig. 5.1). The muscles are approximately 40 mm long and become tendinous for the last 4–5 mm from their insertion. Each muscle is inserted on the sclera, anterior to the equator. The medial rectus insertion is 5–5.5 mm from limbus that of inferior rectus 6.5 mm, lateral rectus about 7 mm and superior rectus 7.7 mm (Fig. 5.2).

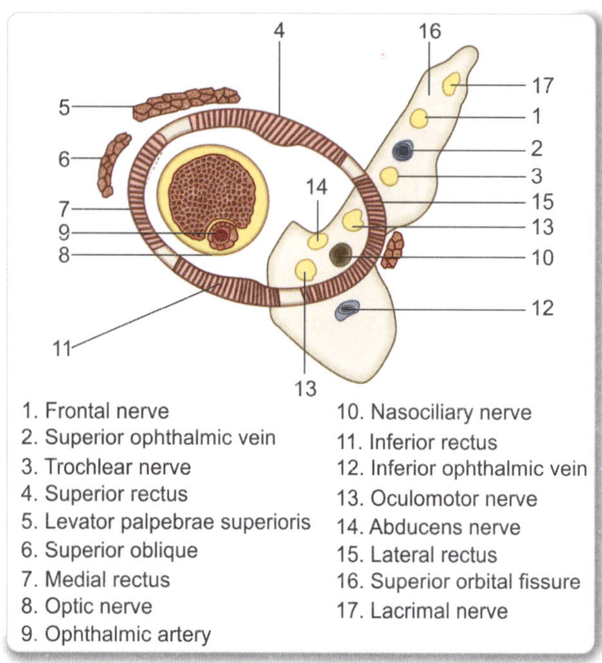

FIGURE 5.1: Annulus of Zinn and the neighboring structures

Oblique Muscles

The superior oblique arises from the annulus of Zinn just above the origin of superior rectus muscle, runs forward to the cartilaginous ring trochlea attached to the superior and nasal angle of orbit. Here it is reflected downwards, outwards and posteriorly, passes under the superior rectus muscle and is inserted into the upper and outer part of sclera behind the equator.

The inferior oblique is the only muscle not arising from the apex of orbit, it originates from the floor of orbit near the inner end of inferior orbital margin and then passes outwards below the inferior rectus muscle and is inserted into the outer part of the sclera behind the equator and underneath lateral rectus muscle.

The reflected tendons of superior oblique and inferior oblique muscles make an angle of 51° with anteroposterior meridians. The extraocular muscles are ensheathed by the fascia of orbit, which covers the sclera as Tenon's capsule. The facial sheaths send prolongations to the orbital walls, which are known as check ligaments because they check the movements of eyeball.

Nerve Supply of Extraocular Muscles

Superior oblique by the VI cranial nerve (Fig. 5.3). Lateral rectus by the VI cranial nerve. Superior, inferior and medial rectus and inferior oblique by III cranial nerve.

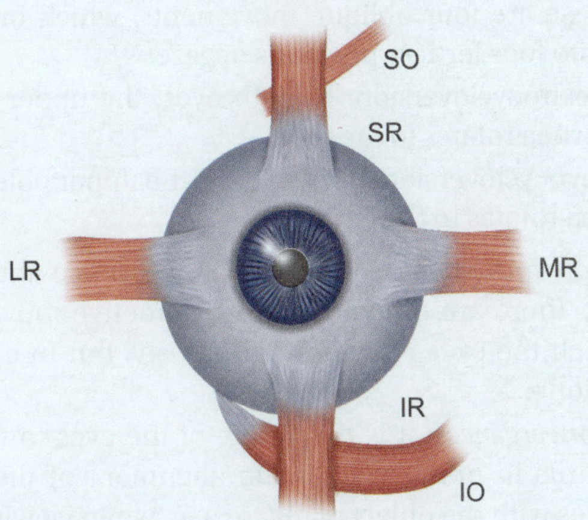

FIGURE 5.2: Insertions of extraocular muscles (IO, inferior oblique; IR, inferior rectus; LR, lateral rectus; MR, medial rectus; SO, superior oblique; SR, superior rectus).

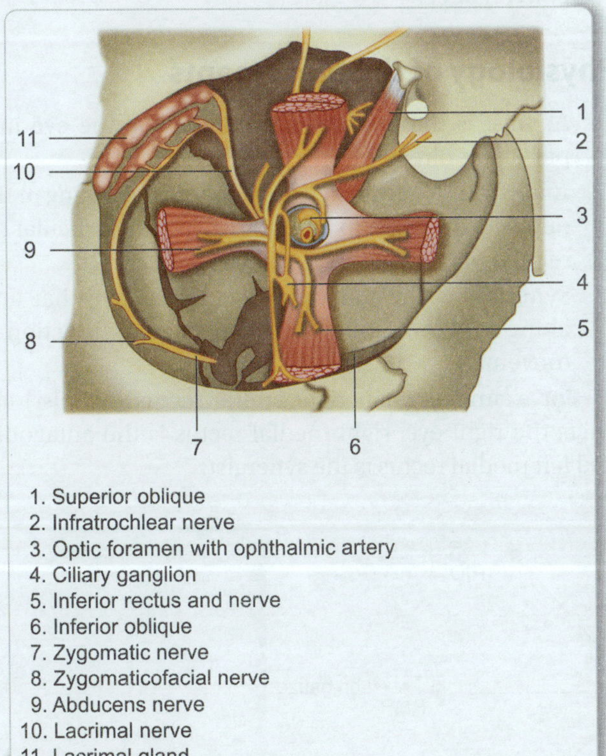

FIGURE 5.3: Origin of the extraocular muscles and their nerve supply

Blood Supply

Blood supply by the muscular branches of ophthalmic artery.

Actions of Extraocular Muscles

Extraocular muscles rotate the eye around a center of rotation situated at a horizontal plane approximately 12–13 mm behind cornea (Table 5.1).

TABLE 5.1: Actions of extraocular muscles

Muscle	Primary action	Secondary action
Medial rectus	Adduction	–
Lateral rectus	Abduction	–
Superior rectus	Elevation, adduction	Intorsion
Inferior rectus	Depression, adduction	Extortion
Superior oblique	Intorsion, abduction	Depression
Inferior oblique	Extortion, abduction	Elevation

Three types of movements are possible:

1. Rotation around the vertical axis to move the eye laterally or medially.
2. Rotation around the horizontal axis to move the eye upwards and downwards.
3. Rotation around the anteroposterior axis to create the movement of torsion. This is of two types, intorsion—upper pole of cornea rotates nasally, extorsion—when the upper pole of cornea moves temporally.

The action of a muscle when the eye is in primary position (looking straight) is termed primary action. All other actions depending upon various other positions of the eye are termed secondary actions. The field of action of a muscle is that direction in which its primary action is the greatest.

Actions of Horizontal Rectus Muscles

The lateral rectus muscle has sole function of moving eye laterally, while medial rectus has sole function of moving eye medially.

Actions of Superior and Inferior Recti

The superior and inferior recti involve torsion owing to obliquity of their course. They form an angle of 23° with the optical axis. Thus, when superior rectus contracts with eye in primary position it pulls the eye upwards, inwards and also intorts it. Similarly, inferior rectus pulls the eye downwards, inwards and extorts it.

Actions of Oblique

The oblique are inserted behind the equator and form an angle of 51° with the optical axis with the eye in primary position. When the superior oblique contracts with the globe in primary position, the primary action is intorsion, but it also rotates the eye downwards and outward. The inferior oblique primarily causes extortion, but it also rotates the eye upwards and outwards.

Eye Movements

Monocular

Ductions: These are the movements of each eye tested separately. They consist of:

1. Adduction: Rotating eye medially.
2. Abduction: Rotating eye laterally.
3. Sursumduction: Elevation.
4. Deorsumduction: Depression.
5. Incycloduction: Intorsion.
6. Excycloduction: Extorsion.

Binocular

Conjugate movements (versions): These are the movements of both eyes together and their parallelism is maintained:

1. Dextroversion: Right gaze.
2. Levoversion: Left gaze.
3. Deorsum version: Down gaze.
4. Sursum version: Up gaze.

These four movements bring the eyes into four secondary positions of gaze:

1. Dextroelevation: Up and right gaze.
2. Dextrodepression: Down and right gaze.
3. Levoelevation: Up and left gaze.
4. Levodepression: Down and left gaze.

These are four oblique movements, which bring the eyes into four tertiary positions of gaze:

1. Dextrocycloversion: In both eyes; the upper pole of cornea rotates to the right.
2. Levocycloversion: In both eyes; the upper pole of cornea rotates to the left.

Disjugate movements (vergence): Convergence and divergence. There are binocular, but disjunctive movements in which the eyes move synchronously, but in opposite directions:

1. *Convergences:* It is the ability of the eyes to turn inwards in order to maintain alignment of the visual axes with the object of regard, e.g. when viewing near objects.
2. *Divergence:* It is the ability of eyes to turn outwards from a convergent position. There is evidence that this is an active process and not just relaxation of convergence.

Physiology of the Movements

1. Agonist is the primary muscle moving the eye in a particular direction.
2. Antagonist is the muscle in the same eye acting in the opposite direction to the agonist, in that particular direction of movement.
3. Synergist is the muscle in the other eye that acts along with the agonist in that particular direction of movement.

For example, when right lateral rectus (agonist) abducts the right eye, right medial rectus is the antagonist and left medial rectus is the synergist.

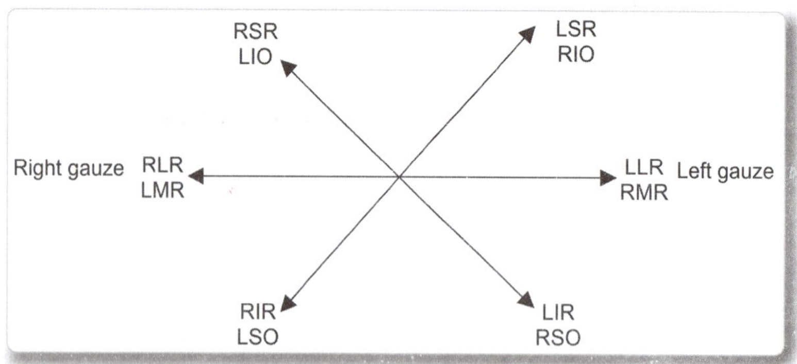

FIGURE 5.4: Cardinal positions and muscles acting together (yolk muscles) (LIO, left inferior oblique; LIR, left inferior rectus; LLR, left lateral rectus; LMR, left medial rectus; LSO, left superior oblique; LSR, left superior rectus; RIO, right inferior oblique; RIR, right inferior rectus; RLR, right lateral rectus; RMR, right medial rectus; RSO, right superior oblique; RSR, right superior rectus).

Sherrington's Law of Reciprocal Innervation

Sherrington's law states that to produce a given movement the contraction of an agonist muscle is associated with a reciprocal decrease in innervation of its antagonist. For example, in turning the eye in right gaze, right lateral rectus and left medial rectus muscles contract, while the right medial rectus and left lateral rectus muscles relax.

Hering's Law of Equal Innervation

When the eyes are moving into cardinal positions of gaze, a muscle from one eye is paired with one of other eye. These paired muscles are called yolk muscles. In dextroversion (right gaze) the right lateral rectus and the left medial rectus muscle acts as yolk muscle (Fig. 5.4).

Hering's law states that in any conjugate movement of the eye, yolk muscle receive simultaneous and equal innervation.

Physiology of Eye

6

Girija Devi PS, Lakshmi G

CORNEAL TRANSPARENCY

A high degree of corneal transparency is of utmost importance for the formation of a clear and sharp retinal image. Anatomical and physiological factors play an important role in maintenance of corneal transparency.

Anatomical Factors

1. Regular and uniform arrangement of the epithelial cells that have a homogeneous refractive index is very important for corneal transparency. Any microscopic irregularities will be corrected by the precorneal tear film.
2. Absence of blood vessels in cornea and non-myelination of corneal nerve fibers. The corneal nerves lose their myelin sheaths within 1-2 mm from limbus. Cornea is avascular except for the capillaries in limbal margin.
3. Stroma is composed of regularly arranged collagen fibrils of equal size set in a clear ground substance. The regularity of the arrangement of fibrils is very important for corneal transparency.

Physiological Factors

The relative dehydrated state of the cornea is important for maintaining the transparency. This is made possible by:

1. Barrier functions of limiting layers epithelium and endothelium. It is affected by tight cell membrane interdigitations between adjacent cells and desmosomes. These create barriers to diffusion of electrolytes and water thereby preventing corneal hydration and edema.
2. Pump function of endothelium. Some fluid enters the corneal stroma across the limbus and constant removal of this fluid is essential to maintain corneal deturgescence. This takes place by the endothelial pump, which actively pumps out Na^+ and water follows passively. The mitochondria that populate the cytoplasm provide the ATP that is necessary to maintain pump function.

   In addition, epithelium also pumps out Na^+ actively. Whatever is the pump mechanism, the ions are actively pumped out and water follows passively.

   Endothelium is more important than epithelium in maintaining corneal deturgescence and the HCO_3^- transportation is more important than Na^+ and K^+ active transport in maintaining corneal transparency. So in conditions where there is a decrease in endothelial cell count the cornea imbibes water and becomes edematous and hazy.
3. Evaporation of tears from the corneal surface results in hypertonicity of the tear film. As a result, osmotic extraction of the fluid from corneal stroma occurs causing 4% corneal thinning. This is not of much importance in maintaining corneal deturgescence as the fluid lost is readily replaced by aqueous.

PHYSIOLOGY OF TEAR FILM

Tear film is a thin fluid layer covering the cornea and conjunctiva. This fluid layer is maintained by secretary, distributive and excretory functions of lacrimal apparatus. Tear film is highly necessary for maintenance of corneal transparency (Fig. 6.1).

Functions of Tear Film

1. This layer smooths out the slight irregularities on corneal epithelial surface and provides a smooth optical surface for refraction.
2. Tear film serves as a source of oxygen (nutrition) to cornea.
3. Also acts as a lubricant between lids and corneal surface.

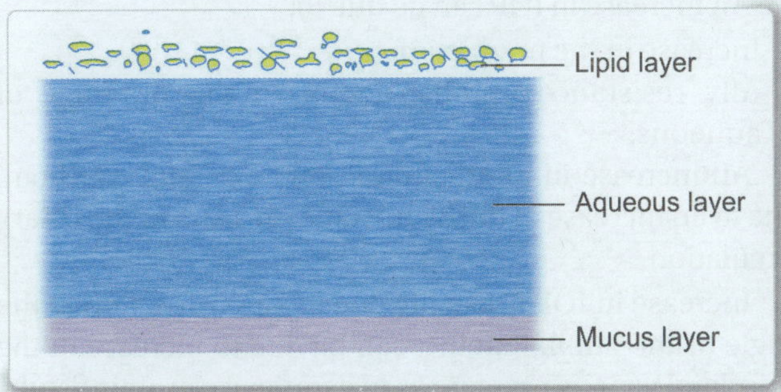

FIGURE 6.1: Precorneal tear film

4. Serves to regulate the hydration of cornea by developing an osmotic gradient by means of changes in the tonicity of the film secondary to evaporation (explained in maintenance of corneal transparency).
5. Tears contain antibacterial agents such as lysozyme, Betalysin and lactoferrin, which protect the eye from infections.
6. Flushing action of tears washes away cellular debris and foreign bodies.

Summary

Maintenance of normal corneal thickness (deturgescence) and transparency is by:

- Barrier function of epithelium and endothelium
- Active metabolic pump of corneal endothelium.

Constitution of Tear Film

Thickness of tear film is 7–10 microns. The tear film is constituted in three layers:

1. Outer lipid layer secreted by meibomian glands, with a small contribution from glands of Zeis and Moll.
2. Middle aqueous layer secreted by the lacrimal glands (95%) and accessory glands of Krause and Wolfring. This makes upto 90% of tear film thickness.
3. Innermost mucin layer secreted by the goblet cells of the conjunctiva onto the ocular surface. This layer rests on the underlying corneal and conjunctival epithelium.

Drainage of Tears

About 25% of tears are lost by evaporation and 75% is pumped into nasal cavity. Tears are secreted by the lacrimal glands into the upper and outer part of the globe, spreads over the globe by lid movements and then by capillary action move toward the puncta and vertical part of canaliculi. Blinking movements of lids and contraction of orbicularis muscle during blink movements drive the tear fluid into the lacrimal sac. When the orbicularis relaxes the sac collapses and drives the tears collected in the sac into the nasolacrimal duct, and nose.

PHYSIOLOGY OF AQUEOUS

Aqueous humor is the clear, optically transparent fluid filling anterior and posterior chamber of the eye. It serves a metabolic function to the a vascular cornea and lens.

Formation of Aqueous Humor

Aqueous humor is formed by the non-pigmented epithelium of the ciliary body by active secretion and ultrafiltration. Active secretion accounts for about 75% of aqueous formation. It takes place by the Na^+- K^+-ATPase pump, which secretes Na^+ into the posterior chamber and diffusion of water follows.

Passive secretion occurs by ultrafiltration and diffusion and is dependent on capillary hydrostatic pressure and osmotic pressure of blood. Here water and a water soluble substance from the plasma go into the posterior chamber.

Aqueous Outflow

From the eyeball 90% of aqueous flows through the trabecular meshwork into the Schlemm's canal and is then drained by the episcleral veins.

Uveoscleral outflow accounts for the remaining 10%. Here the aqueous passes across the face of the ciliary body into the suprachoroidal space and is drained by venous circulation in ciliary body, choroid and sclera.

Intraocular pressure (IOP) is determined by a balance between the rate of aqueous secretion and outflow. The outflow in turn is dependent on the resistance in the outflow channels (trabecular meshwork mainly) and the episcleral venous pressure (Table 6.1).

Aqueous that is secreted into the posterior chamber by the non-pigmented epithelium of the ciliary body passes into the anterior chamber (AC) through the pupil. Then it is drained out of the anterior chamber through the

TABLE 6.1: Aqueous inflow vs aqueous outflow

Aqueous inflow	Aqueous outflow
Active secretion (75%)	Through trabecular meshwork (90%)
Passive diffusion	Uveoscleral outflow via ciliary body to suprachoroidal space (10%)

trabecular meshwork mainly and a small amount escapes from AC by uveoscleral outflow. The aqueous drains through the trabecular meshwork into the circular venous channel called Schlemm's canal. From the Schlemm's canal into the episcleral veins either directly through collector channels or aqueous veins (Fig. 6.2).

Maintenance of Intraocular Pressure

The IOP is decided by the balance between the aqueous production at the ciliary body and the drainage at the angles.

The normal IOP is considered to be between 15 and 20 mm Hg. This is a value obtained by statistical analysis from the values obtained by recording the IOP from thousands of people with normal healthy eyes. But there is great individual variation in this. The normal IOP for a particular eye is that pressure that eye can withstand without any damage to the optic disk or nerve fiber layer. In the majority of normal persons this value is between 15 and 20 mm Hg. But there is a small group of people who can withstand higher pressures for long periods without any structural or functional damage to the optic nerve head. Similarly, there is a small group of people who cannot tolerate even an IOP within this normal range and develop glaucomatous damage.

So, the IOP can be considered to be normal or abnormal only by correlating it with the condition of the optic disk and presence or absence of any field defects.

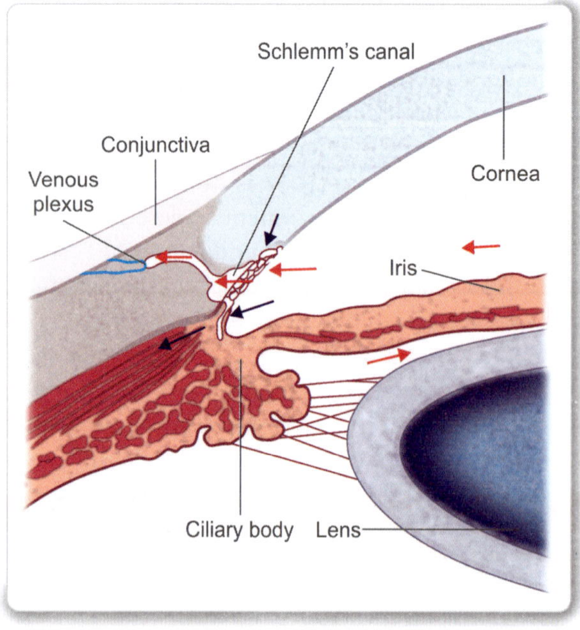

FIGURE 6.2: Circulation of aqueous

An increase in IOP can be due to:

- Increase in the production
- Any resistance or obstruction to the drainage of aqueous.

An increase in production is very rare and transient, due to an increase in the hydrostatic pressure in the ciliary circulation.

Increase in IOP is usually due to an obstruction at the angle or the pupil. Rarely it can be due to increase in the episcleral venous pressure as in caroticocavernous fistula.

PHYSIOLOGY OF VISION

Vision is the most important of special senses. Most of the information is brought to brain by eyes.

Visible spectrum of light is 400–700 nm. Light coming from external objects are brought to a focus on retina by refraction through the transparent layers of eyeball (cornea and lens). In the retina are situated the photoreceptors, which are sensitive to light. The light falling on the retina initiates certain photochemical changes, which in turn trigger off a series of biochemical changes. These biochemical changes lead to generation of an electrical change. These electrical changes stimulate the bipolar and amacrine cells and the impulse reaches the ganglion cell layer. The nerve impulse then passes along the axons of ganglion cells (axons of ganglion cells form the optic nerve) to the optic chiasma. From the chiasma the impulses pass via the optic tract to lateral geniculate body (LGB). From the lateral geniculate body the impulses travel along the optic radiation to the occipital cortex where the center for vision is located and visual perception occurs. Thus the physiology of vision is in three steps.

Phototransduction

Phototransduction is the process of conversion of the light energy that falls on the retina to nerve impulse. There is a series of photochemical and biochemical reactions, which bring about electrical changes that get converted to nerve impulses in the photoreceptor cells (Fig. 6.3).

Transmission

The electrical impulses in the photoreceptors get converted into nerve impulse once the ganglion cell layer is stimulated. The nerve impulses pass along the optic nerve to LGB then to occipital cortex (Fig. 6.4).

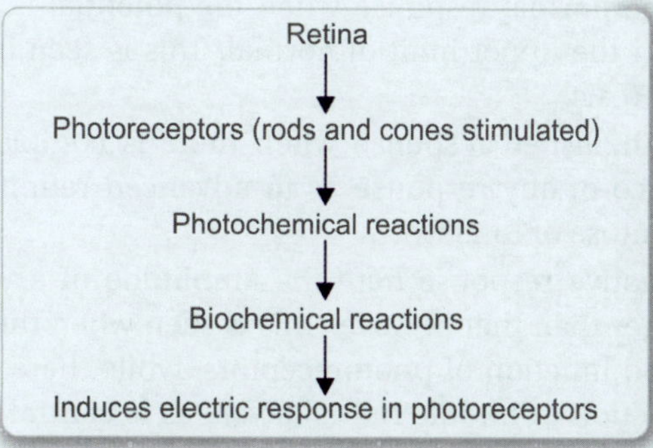

FIGURE 6.3: Light fall on retina

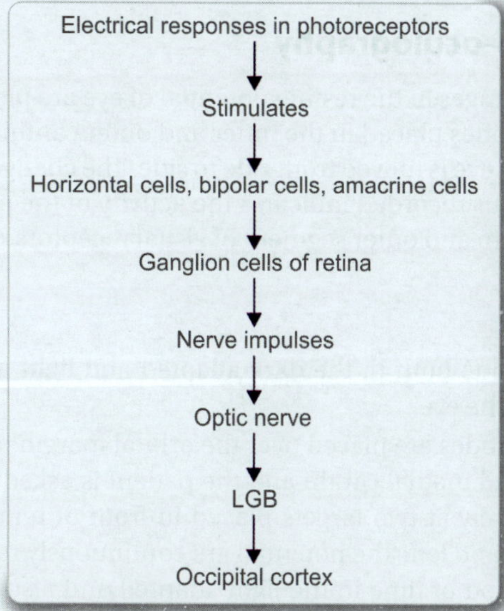

FIGURE 6.4: Transmission

Visual Perception

Visual perception takes place in the visual cortex in the occipital lobe. It is a complex process involving the fusion of two retinal images formed in the two eyes together to a single image and also three types of visual perceptions light sense, form sense and color sense. Photochemical changes include:

1. Pigment bleaching.
2. Pigment regeneration.

Pigment Bleaching

Pigment present in rods is rhodopsin and that in cones is iodopsin. When light falls on rods, the photochemical reaction is started by the energy present in photons of light, which are absorbed by the rhodopsin. The rhodopsin cycle is shown in Figure 6.5.

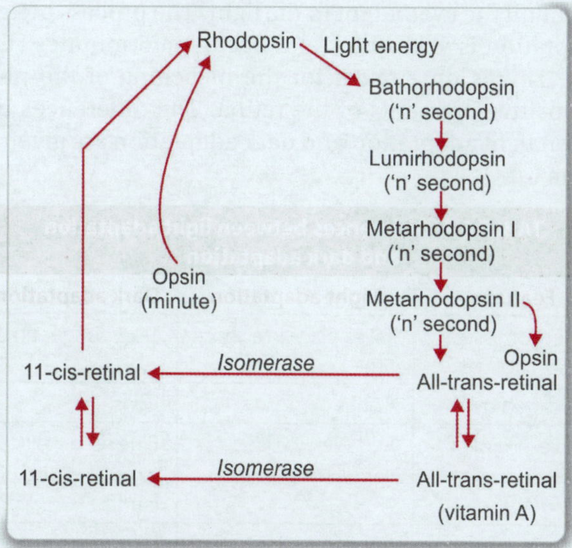

FIGURE 6.5: Rhodopsin cycle

Dark Adaptation

When a person goes from a bright light to a dimly lighted room, it takes some time for him/her to see the objects around him/her clearly. This is called dark adaptation. It is the time taken for the regeneration of bleached retinal pigments in the cones.

After 10–15 minutes the luminous energy required to see an object decrease by 1,000–10,000 folds and this is attributed to regeneration of rhodopsin in the rods. A fully dark adapted retina is 10,000 times more sensitive to light than the earlier light adapted one.

Delayed dark adaptation occurs in the diseases of rod (retinitis pigmentosa) and in vitamin A deficiency.

Light Adaptation

When a person passes from a darkroom to a brightly lighted one, the light seems intensely and uncomfortably

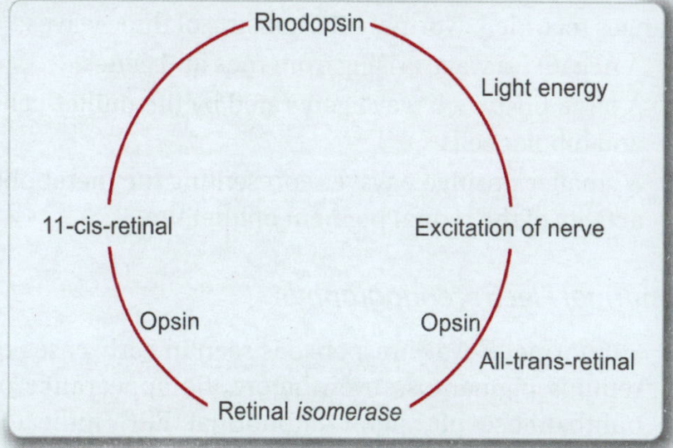

FIGURE 6.6: Light-induced changes in rhodopsin

bright till the eyes adapt to the light. The process of light adaptation is very quick and occurs in 5 minutes (Fig. 6.6). This is time taken for the bleaching of the photosensitive pigments of the retina. The differences between light adaptation and dark adaptation are given in Table 6.2.

TABLE 6.2: Differences between light adaptation and dark adaptation

Features	Light adaptation	Dark adaptation
Direction	Takes place in a short time	Takes longer time
Mediated by	Cones	Rods
Wave length of light	Red seen well (larger wave length)	Blue seen well (smaller wave length)
Pupil	Constricted	Dilated

ELECTROPHYSIOLOGICAL TEST

Electroretinography (ERG), electro-oculography (EOG) and visually evoked potential (VEP). These are electrophysiological tests that help in assessing and evaluating retinal functions.

Electroretinography

Electroretinography is the recording of the electrical changes that occur to the resting potential of the eye when the retina in dark adapted state is stimulated by a flash of light (Figs 6.7A and B).

Method

In the dark adapted eye, active electrode fixed to contact lens is placed on the cornea and a reference electrode is placed on forehead. The retina is stimulated and electrical changes recorded. Normal ERG consists of three waves:

1. A negative a wave arising from rods and cones.
2. A large positive b wave generated by the muller cells and bipolar cells.
3. A smaller positive c wave representing the metabolic activity of the retinal pigment epithelium.

Abnormal Electroretinography

1. Subnormal b-wave response is seen in early cases of retinitis pigmentosa even before the appearance of ophthalmoscopic signs. Subnormal ERG indicates that a large area of retina is not functioning.
2. Supernormal response when the potential is higher than the upper limit of normal. This is seen in early sclerosis.
3. Extinguished response when there is complete absence of any response as in advanced retinitis pigmentosa or total RD.
4. Negative response here the amplitude of a wave is larger than that of wave. This is seen when there is a good function of photoreceptors, while there is dysfunction of middle retinal layers as is central retinal artery occlusion, proliferative diabetic retinopathy and congenital retinoschisis.

Electro-oculography

Here, changes in the resting potential of eye are picked up by electrodes placed in the inner and outer canthi of eyes when the eye is moved from side to side. The change in potential thus recorded indicates the activity of the pigment epithelium and outer segment of visual receptors.

Method

Test is done both in the dark adapted and light adapted states of the eye.

Electrodes are placed over the orbital margin near the lateral and medial canthi and the patient is asked to look alternatively at two targets placed in front of him/her to the right and left. The potential are continuously recorded for a period of time in the light adapted and also in dark adapted states of the eye.

The ratio of the light peak to dark trough is called Arden ratio. The value of 185 is normal.

Visually Evoked Response

Visually evoked response (VER) is an investigation done in patients in whom retina is found to be normal (ERG and EOG normal), but visual function is abnormal. The VER detects functional loss in visual pathway from retina to visual cortex. The VER is the electrical activity produced in the visual cortex in response to stimulation of the retina either by a pattern or by a flash of light (Fig. 6.8).

Method

Refractive errors should be corrected before the test as they may interfere with the result. The retina is stimulated either by a flash of light (flash VER) or by using a pattern reversal stimuli such as a checker board in which the black squares go white and then return back to black.

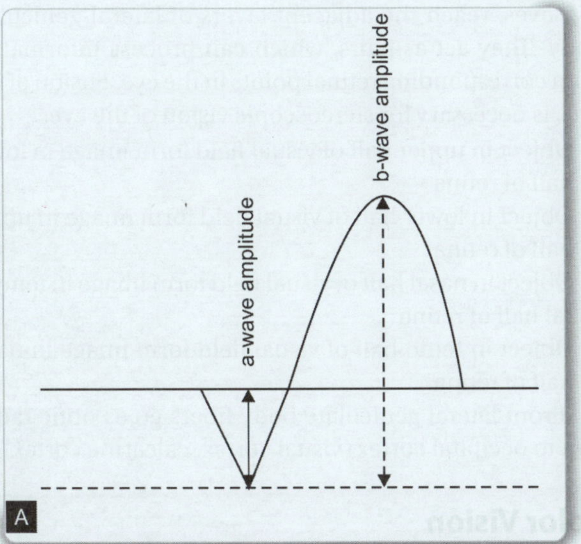

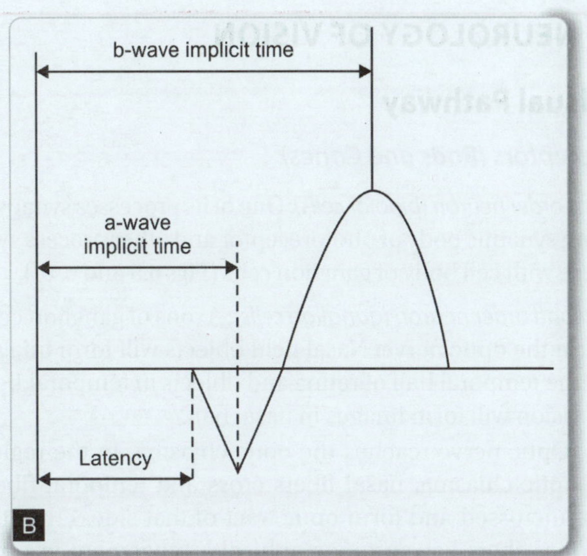

FIGURES 6.7A and B: Normal electroretinography. **A.** Shows height of a- and b-waves; **B.** Shows the latent period.

The recording of VER is done by scalp electrodes placed over the occipital cortex. The VER is nothing, but the electroencephalogram (EEG) changes in occipital cortex brought about by stimulation of retina either by a flash of light on by a pattern.

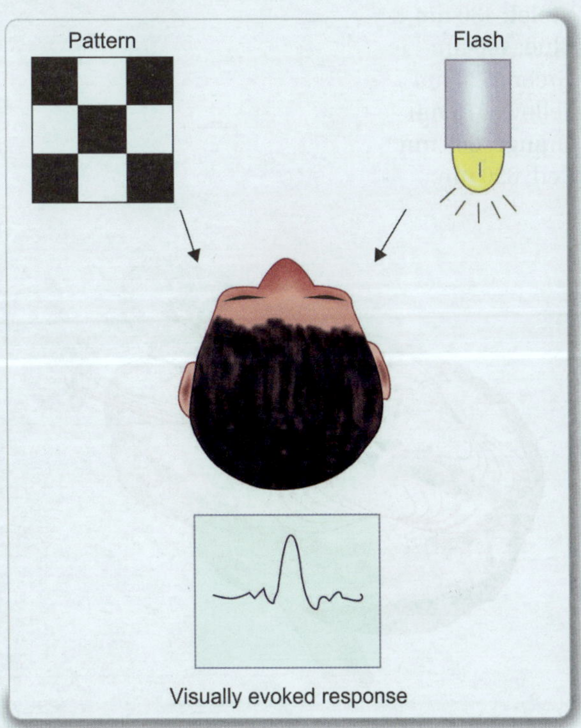

FIGURE 6.8: Recording of visually evoked response

Flash Visually Evoked Response

Retina is stimulated by intense flash light and EEG changes in occipital cortex are recorded.

Uses: This is only a rough test and has only the following uses:

1. Assess the visual pathway in mentally retarded and aphasic patients.
2. Distinguish between organic and psychological blindness, i.e. between organic eye disease and malingering.
3. To assess visual potentials in opaque media.

Pattern Reversal Visually Evoked Response

Pattern reversal VER is a fovea specific response and may give a rough estimate of visual acuity.

Interpretation

Latency

Latency is the time interval between the stimulus and the onset of cortical response.

Amplitude of VER is the amplitude of the waves in VER. Latency is more informative than amplitude. Latency is the time interval from stimulus presentation to onset of ERG changes in visual cortex. In optic nerve diseases and in lesions affecting the conduction of nerve impulse along the visual pathway, there is a decrease in amplitude of waves and increase in latent period. The latent period is more important than amplitude. Other diseases, which can be recognized by VER are refractive error, amblyopia, color blindness (using colored stimuli), etc.

NEUROLOGY OF VISION

Visual Pathway

Receptors (Rods and Cones)

First order neuron (bipolar cells): One of its processes synapses with synaptic body of photoreceptor and other process synapse with cell body of ganglion cells (Figs 6.9 and 6.10).

Second order neuron (ganglion cells): Axons of ganglion cells form the optic nerve. Nasal field objects will form images in the temporal half of retina and objects in temporal field of vision will form images in nasal half.

Optic nerve reaches the optic chiasma. In the region of optic chiasma, nasal fibers cross and temporal fibers go uncrossed and form optic tract of that side. From the retina, fibers have a topographical arrangement in optic nerve, so that fibers from upper half of retina will lie above, fibers from lower half of retina lie below, medial fibers on medial side and lateral fibers laterally.

Third order neuron: In lateral geniculate body.

In optic tract—fibers from upper half of retina are seen medially and end in medial part of lateral geniculate body.

Fibers from lower half of retina are seen laterally and end in lateral part of lateral geniculate body.

Lateral geniculate body has 6 layers. Layers 2, 3 and 5 receive the temporal fibers from same eye and 1, 4 and 6 receive crossed fibers (nasal fibers from opposite side).

Lateral geniculate body receives the fibers, which bring impulses from the corresponding retinal points of 2 eyes, reach the adjacent layers of lateral geniculate body. They act as pairs, which can process information from corresponding retinal points in the eye. Fusion of images is necessary for stereoscopic vision of the eye:

- Object in upper half of visual field form image in lower half of retina
- Object in lower half of visual field form image in upper half of retina
- Object in nasal half of visual field form image in temporal half of retina
- Object in temp half of visual field form image in nasal half of retina.

From lateral geniculate body fibers go as optic radiation to occipital cortex (visual cortex, calcarine cortex).

Color Vision

Color vision is the ability of the eye to discriminate between different colors. Color is a purely sensory phenomenon that is brought about by stimulation of retina by lights of different wavelength. Color vision is a function of cones and hence, better appreciated in photopic vision (i.e. vision in bright light) than in scotopic vision (vision in dim light, which is a function of rods). The visible spectral colors include:

- Violet: 430 nm
- Blue: 460 nm
- Green: 520 nm
- Yellow: 575 nm
- Orange: 600 nm
- Red: 650 nm.

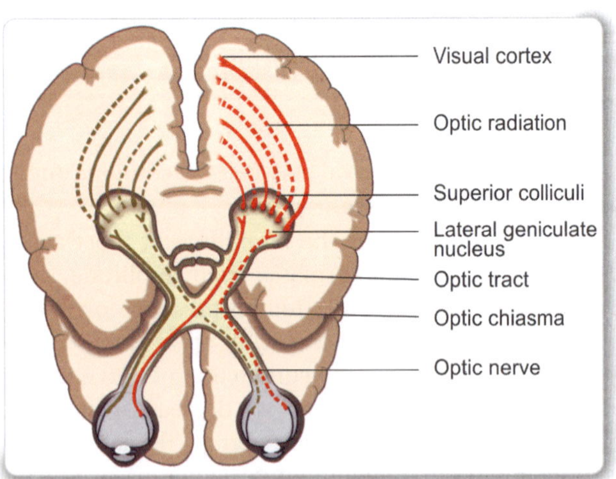

FIGURE 6.9: Primary visual area—area 17

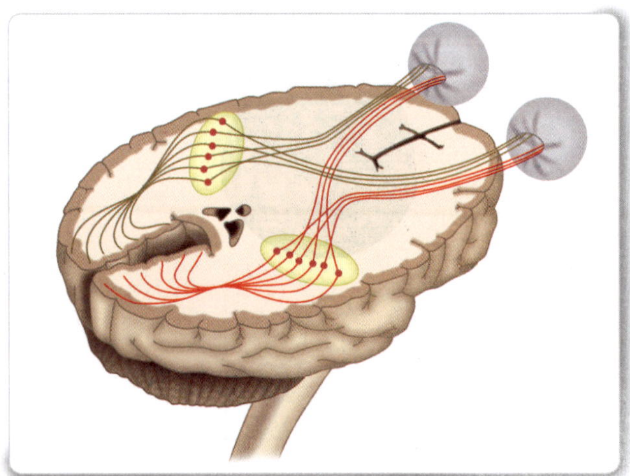

FIGURE 6.10: Visual pathway

THEORIES OF COLOR VISION

Young-Helmholtz-Maxwell Theory or Trichromatic Theory

Trichromatic theory for color vision was originally formulated by Young and then modified by Helmholtz. This theory postulates that there are three primary colors and three types of cones. Each type of cone is maximally sensitive to one of the three primary colors and any given color is a mixture of the primary colors in different proportions. The accuracy of this theory has been proved by the identification of the three different types of pigments in the three different types of cones having different description spectrum.

Red Sensitive Cones

Red sensitive cones contain the pigment erythrolabe. This pigment is sensitive to rays of long-wavelength 560–650 nm, senses colors in yellow and red spectrum.

Green Sensitive Cones

Green sensitive cones contain the pigment chlorolabe, which is sensitive to light of medium-wavelength with the peak absorption of light of 535 nm wavelength.

Blue Sensitive Cones

Blue sensitive cones with the pigment cyanolabe, which is sensitive to light of short-wavelength blue-violet range and maximally absorbs light of 440 nm.

Thus, the Young-Helmholtz-Maxwell theory concludes that blue, green and red are the primary colors, but the cones can stimulated by a varying range of light waves.

Opponent Color Theory of Hering

Opponent color theory states that some colors, such as red versus green and yellow versus blue are mutually exclusive. Mixing lights of such colors do not produce a composite sensation and there is no color as reddish green, such a phenomenon cannot be explained by trichromatic theory alone. The two theories are correct as:

1. Color vision is trichromatic at the level of photoreceptors.
2. Opponent theory occurs at the level of ganglion cells onwards.

BINOCULAR SINGLE VISION

When a normal person fixes the gaze on an object, the image is formed in the retina of both eyes (two images are formed), but the individual perceives only a single image. The two images are slightly dissimilar, i.e. the right eye sees more of the right side of an object, while the left eye sees more of the left side. This ability to fuse the two slightly dissimilar images to form a single mental picture is called binocular single vision (BSV).

Prerequisites for Development of Binocular Single Vision

1. Vision should be fairly good in both eyes.
2. Visual axes should be parallel.
3. Precise coordination of ocular movements in all directions of gaze.
4. Visual pathways should be normal.
5. Visual cortex should be able to fuse the two images from the two eyes and promote BSV.

Corresponding Points of Retina

For BSV one point in one retina should correspond to a point on the other retina. Foveas of both eyes are corresponding points. A point on the nasal side of one retina corresponds to a point on the temporal side of the other eye. But this is not a point-to-point matching. One point in one eye corresponds not only to a similar point on the other eye, but a small area surrounding this point. This is the Panum's area of single vision.

Horopter and Panum's Area

Horopter is an imaginary surface in space all points of which stimulate corresponding points in the retina of the two eyes.

Panum's area of single vision is a zone surrounding the points in the Horopter in which objects are seen singly.

Grades of Binocular Single Vision

Worth classified binocular single vision into three grades (Fig. 6.11).

Simultaneous Perception

Simultaneous perception is the awareness of two dissimilar images presented to both eyes. When the picture of a bird is projected into one eye and that of a cage is projected into the other eye a person with simultaneous perception will see a bird inside a cage.

This is only the basic requirement for BSV. In real life, on viewing moving objects when the body or the head in motion the ability of fusion is essential to maintain BSV.

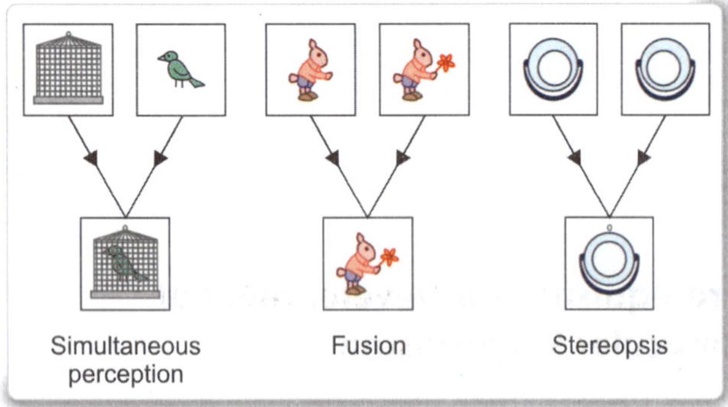

FIGURE 6.11: Grades of binocular single vision

Fusion

Fusion is the blending of slightly different images from the two eyes into a single image, e.g. picture of rabbit with tail is shown to one eye and rabbit with flowers to other eye a person with fusion will see a rabbit with tail and holding flowers.

Stereopsis

Stereopsis is the ability of a person to perceive the third dimension, i.e. the depth, by parallax. This needs at least two objects lying within the Panum's area with horizontal disparity. This can be assessed by slides in synaptophore. The eye achieves this ability by fusing slightly dissimilar objects seen by either eye. The right eye sees more of the right side of an object and the left eye more of the left side of an object and by fusing these two images depth perception is achieved.

Tests for Binocular Single Vision

Various devices, such as synoptophore, Bagolini striated glasses, polarized objects; testing visual fields with red-green glasses, etc. have been used to test BSV. The following are some simple tests.

Worth's Four-dot Test

Patient is made to sit at a distance of 6 m from the Worth's four-dot screen. It has four lights, one red, two green and one white. Put a red glass in front of right eye and a green one in front of left eye (red-green goggles). Ask how many dots the patient can see (Fig. 6.12).

Result: If the patient can see four dots—one red, one green, one fluctuating mixture of red and green indicates normal fusion.

- Five lights indicate diplopia
- Three green indicate right suppression
- Two red indicate left suppression.

Bagolini's Striated Glass

The glasses are placed in front of either eye with the striations perpendicular to each other at 45° and 135° (Figs 6.13A to C).

The patient is asked to focus a small light source kept at a distance of 6 feet (far) or 33 m (near).

Result: These are as follows:

- If the patient sees an oblique cross (X) with the intersection at the center the patient has BSV
- If two lines are seen, which do not intersect diplopia is present
- If only one streak of light is seen there is no simultaneous perception and suppression is present.

Tests for stereopsis are:

- Random-dot tests (RDS); namely the TNO test and Frisby test provide the most definitive evidence of a high grade BSV
- Contour-based tests such as Titmus fly give more reliable evidence of stereopsis, when the BSV is weak or there is abnormal retinal correspondence.

PUPILLARY REFLEXES

Pupil is the circular aperture in the center of the iris and has a diameter of 2–4 mm. Its main functions is to regulate the amount of light entering the eye.

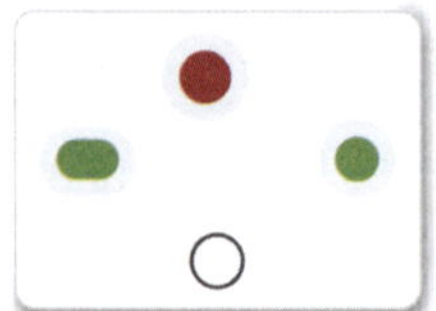

FIGURE 6.12: Worth's four-dot test

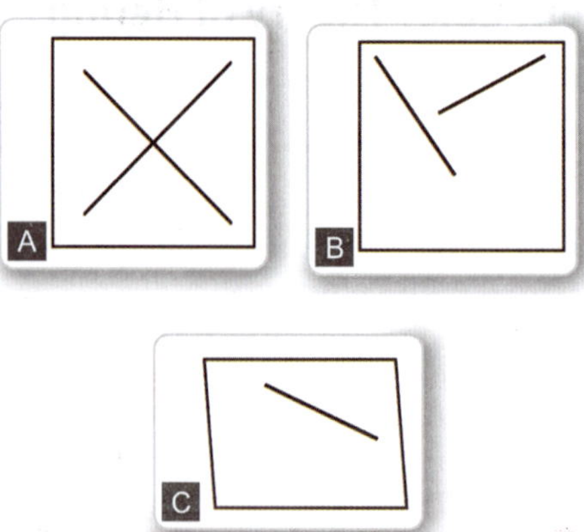

FIGURES 6.13A to C: Bagolini's striated glass test for binocular single vision. **A.** Image in BSV; **B.** Image in diplopia; **C.** Image in suppression.

The iris contains two muscles—the sphincter pupillae, which contracts the pupil when more light enters eyes and dilator pupillae, which dilates the pupil when less light enters eye. The sphincter papillae are supplied by parasympathetic fibers from the EW nucleus through the III nerve. The EW nucleus has connections with the dilator center as well as the frontal and occipital cortex (Figs 6.14A and B).

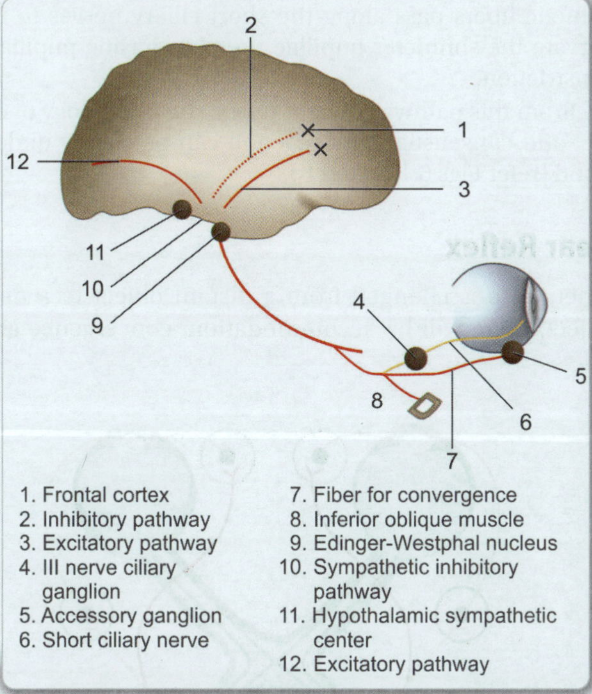

FIGURE 6.14A: Parasympathetic pupillary system

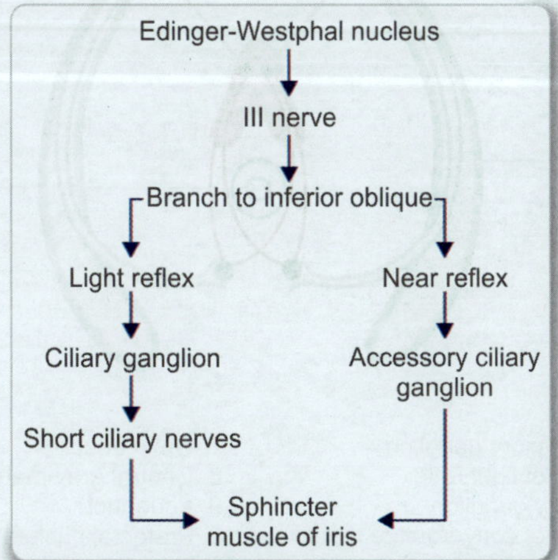

FIGURE 6.14B: Schematic representation of parasympathetic pupillary system

The dilator muscle is supplied by the sympathetic fibers from the cervical sympathetic nerve. The fibers start from the hypothalamus, and pass downwards through the medulla oblongata and the lateral columns of the spinal cord. They come out through the ventral roots of the first three dorsal and last three cervical nerves, and run to the first thoracic ganglion. From here the fibers reach the carotid plexus via the superior cervical ganglion. The fibers run over the semilunar ganglion and pass into the ophthalmic division of the trigeminal nerve. These fibers reach the dilator muscle through the nasociliary nerve and the long ciliary nerves (Figs 6.15A and B).

Anisocoria is the difference in size of the pupil between two eyes. The types of pupillary reflexes are as follows:

- Light reflexes—direct and consensual
- Near reflex
- Psychosensory reflex.

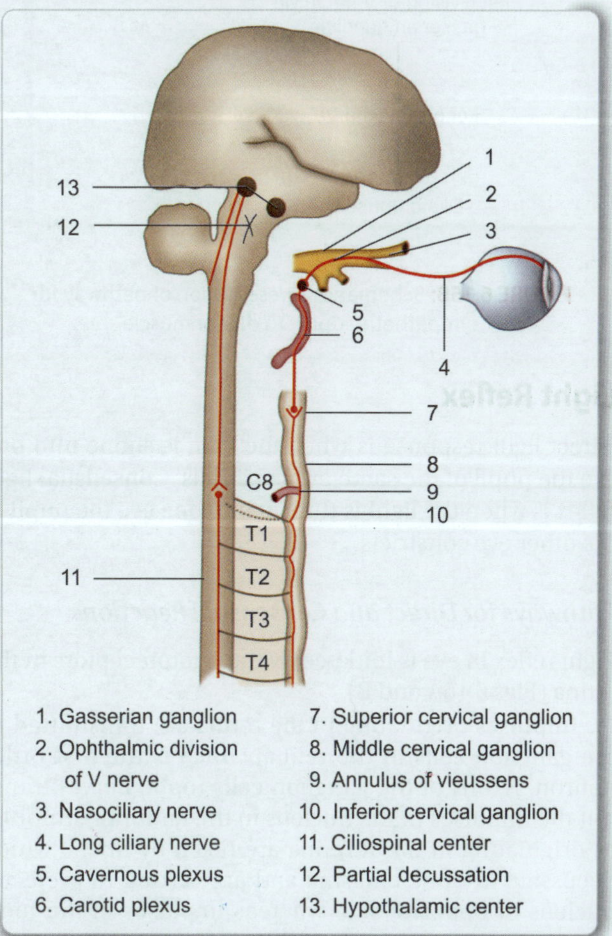

FIGURE 6.15A: Pathway for sympathetic supply to dilator muscle

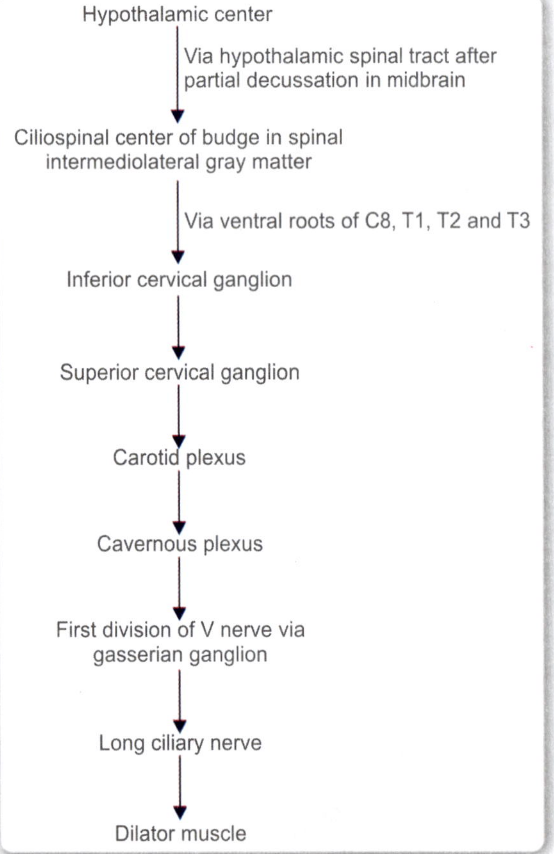

FIGURE 6.15B: Schematic representation of pathway for sympathetic supply to dilator muscle

Light Reflex

Direct light response is when the light is shone into one eye the pupil of the same eye constricts. Consensual light reflex is when the light is thrown into one eye the pupil of the other eye constricts.

Pathways for Direct and Consensual Reactions

Light reflex in eye is initiated by the photoreceptors in the retina (Figs 6.16A and B).

Impulses originating in the retina are transmitted to the ganglion cells in the retina, which is the first order neuron. Axons of the ganglion cells (optic nerve) transmit the impulses to the nucleus in the midbrain. Impulses originating in nasal retina are taken by fibers, which decussate in optic chiasma and are carried to pretectal nucleus of opposite side whereas impulses in the temporal retina are carried by fibers, which pass uncross in the chiasma and are carried to the pretectal nucleus of same side.

Pretectal nucleus is the second nucleus in the reflex pathway. Each pretectal nucleus is connected to both EW nucleus by internuncial fibers. Thus uniocular light stimulation causes bilateral symmetrical pupillary constriction. Damage to these internuncial fibers is responsible for the light near dissociation in neurosyphilis.

The EW nucleus is connected to the ciliary ganglion. The parasympathetic fibers pass through the oculomotor nerve to enter the ciliary ganglion.

From the ciliary ganglion, the postganglion parasympathetic fibers pass along the short ciliary nerves to innervate the sphincter pupillae thereby causing pupillary constriction.

From this pathway of light reflex, the physiology of direct and consensual light reaction can be clearly understood (refer Figs 6.16A and B).

Near Reflex

When gaze is changed from a distant object to a near object, there will be accommodation, convergence and

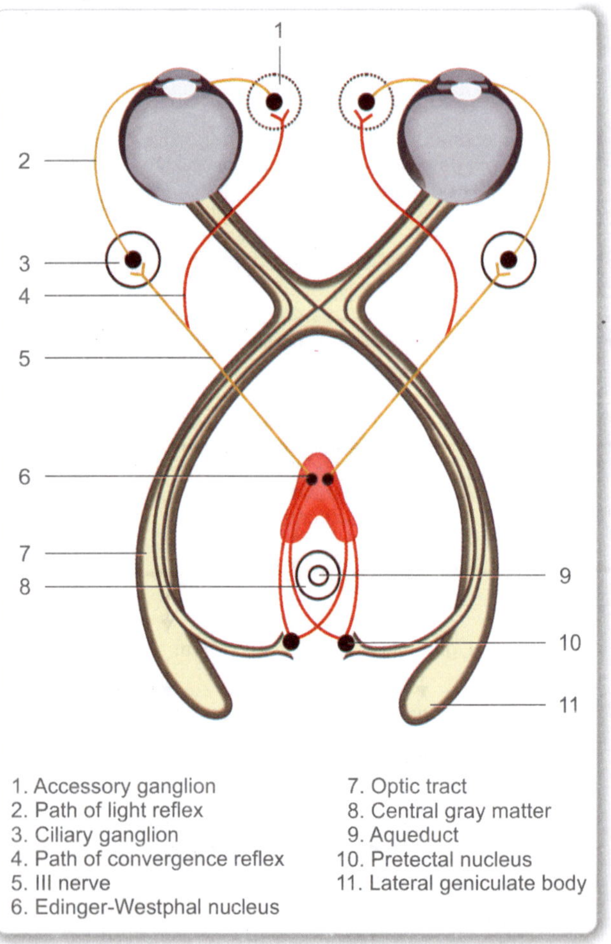

FIGURE 6.16A: Pupillary path for light reflex

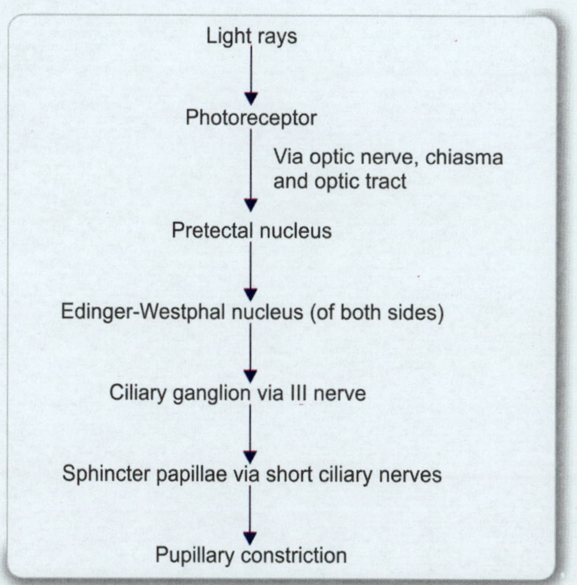

FIGURE 6.16B: Schematic representation of pathway of light reflex

constriction of pupil. This is called near reflex and vision is not essential for this reflex.

Pupil contracts on looking at a near object. When the medial rectus contracts on convergence afferent fibers run via the III nerve to the mesencephalic nucleus of trigeminal nerve. From here it goes to a presumptive convergence center in the tectal or pretectal region. From here it is relayed to the EW nucleus and to the sphincter papillae via the III nerve.

Accommodation (contraction of the ciliary muscles to focus near objects) occur along with convergence. The afferent pathway of accommodation goes along the visual pathway to the visual cortex; striate cortex area 17 and it is relayed to the parastriate area 19. The efferent pathway goes to the EW nucleus via the occipitomesenchepalic tract.

Psychosensory Reflex

The pupil dilates on painful stimuli to any part of the body or by an excitement or strong emotion. The pathway is complex and involves stimulation of the dilator muscle via the cervical sympathetic and a slow inhibition of the sphincter muscle.

SECTION 2

Refraction

Basic Principles of Optics

7

Girija Devi PS

Vision is the function of the eye and for this, eye acts as an optical instrument. To see an external object, the light rays from the object have to be focused on the retina to form a sharp and clear image. To understand the mechanism of vision and the problems associated with this, a basic knowledge of optics is essential.

The light rays, for all practical purposes, can be considered to be traveling in straight lines. The light rays traveling through one medium, e.g. air, undergo three changes when they reach another medium or object.

ABSORPTION, REFLECTION OR REFRACTION

If a light ray strikes an opaque medium, e.g. wood, it is absorbed by that media. If it strikes a reflecting surface like a mirror, the ray is reflected back into the medium through which it was traveling before (Fig. 7.1).

The light ray that is falling on the reflecting surface is called the incident ray and the ray that is reflected back is called the reflected ray. The angle, which the incident ray forms with the perpendicular drawn to the surface is called the angle of incidence and the angle, which the reflected ray forms with the perpendicular drawn at that point is called the angle of reflection. The angle of incidence and the angle of reflection are equal (refer Fig. 7.1).

When the light ray travelling through a medium that substance is called transparent medium, e.g. air, water and glass. When light ray travels through a transparent medium reaches another transparent medium, the speed of travel changes depending on the resistance the second medium offers to the passage of light, compared to the first medium.

If the light ray strikes the second medium perpendicularly, its progress will be slowed down, but there is no deviation of the rays, e.g. a stick dipped into a pond exactly perpendicularly looks straight, but slightly shorter (Fig. 7.2).

If the beam strikes the second medium obliquely, one side of the beam will be striking the surface of the second medium earlier and so it is slowed down earlier compared to the other side. Consequently, the direction of the beam in the second medium will be deviated from the original straight line of travel, e.g. a stick dipped obliquely in a pond of water appears bent at the surface (Fig. 7.3).

The amount of deviation of the light beam depends on three factors:

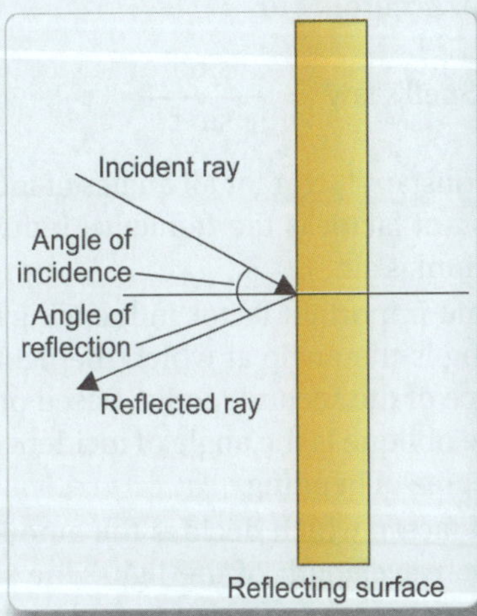

FIGURE 7.1: Reflection

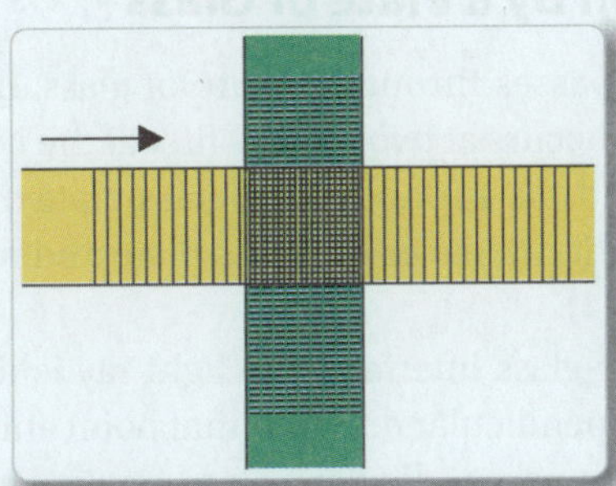

FIGURE 7.2: Light rays striking a transparent medium perpendicularly

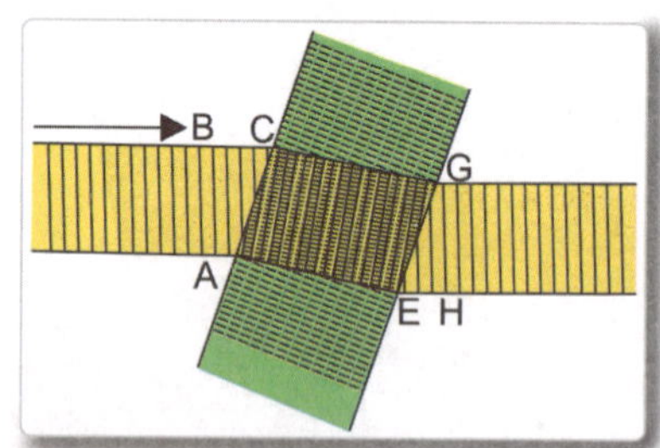

FIGURE 7.3: Light rays striking a transparent medium obliquely

1. The resistance the medium offers to the passage of light is otherwise known as optical density. It varies with different media. The optical density of the universal medium through which light passes, i.e. air, is taken as the standard. The refractive power (i.e. the resistance to the light travel) of a substance in comparison with that of air is called its refractive index. The refractive power of air is taken as 1, water is taken as 1.33, etc.

   The refractive index is calculated from the relationship between the angle of incidence and the angle of refraction. According to:

   $$\text{Snell's law} = \frac{\sin i}{\sin r}$$

   It is a constant factor for all angles of incidence and this constant factor is the refractive index, when the first medium is air.
2. The second important factor influencing the amount of bending is the angle at which the light rays strike the surface of the second media. Based on the Snell's law, more oblique is the angle of incidence; more will be the degree of bending.
3. The third factor, which decides the amount of bending, is the wavelength of the light. The shorter blue light is more bent than the longer red rays.

Refraction by a Plate of Glass

When light passes through a plate of glass, deviation of the light ray occurs at two planes, first at the interface between air and the surface of the glass plate and second, when the light ray leaves the glass plate and re-enters air again (Fig. 7.4).

At the air-glass interface, the light ray is deviated toward the perpendicular drawn at that point and it deviates away from the perpendicular as it re-enters air again. The net effect will be that the incident ray and the emergent ray are parallel (refer Fig. 7.4).

Refraction by a Prism

If the two surfaces of the glass plate meet at a point, a prism will be formed. Here also refraction occurs at the two surfaces in the same manner (Fig. 7.5).

Here the incident ray and the emergent ray appear to meet at some point in the middle of the prism. If we look at an object through a prism, the object will appear deviated toward the apex of the prism because we tend to project an object along the line of the light ray, which strikes our eyes.

Thus, light passing through a prism will be deviated toward the base of the prism and objects seen through a prism will appear displaced toward the apex of prism. This effect of a prism on the direction of light rays is used in the construction of many optical instruments used in ophthalmology and also in the management of squint.

Refraction by a Lens

A lens is an optical medium enclosed by two smooth curved surfaces. Lenses can be biconcave, biconvex, planoconcave, planoconvex or convexo, concave or otherwise called meniscus (Figs 7.6A to E).

The effect of light rays on these various types of lenses is similar to a set of prisms aligned together.

A convex lens can be considered as two prisms placed base to base and thus, can bring two parallel beams of light to a focus on the other side (Fig. 7.7).

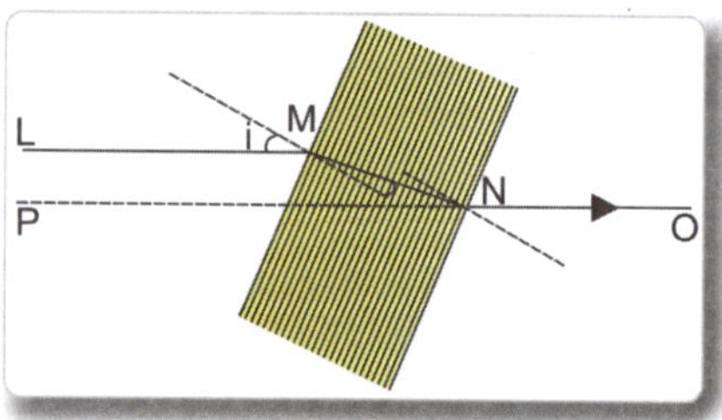

FIGURE 7.4: Refraction by a plate of glass

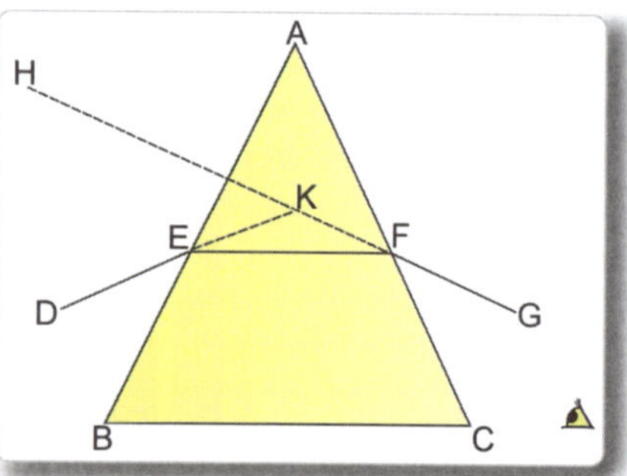

FIGURE 7.5: Refraction by a prism

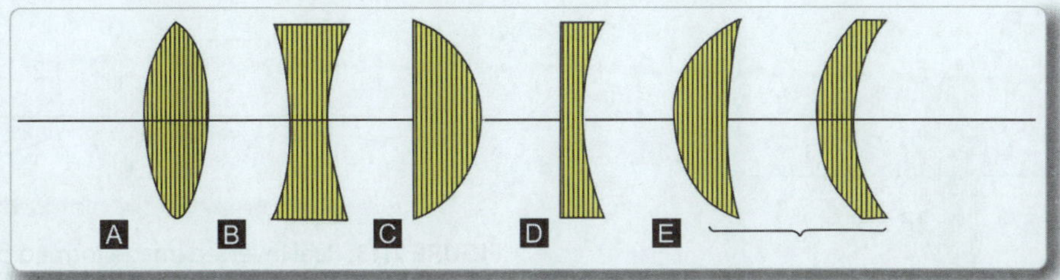

FIGURES 7.6A to E: Types of lenses. **A.** Biconvex; **B.** Biconcave; **C.** Planoconvex; **D.** Planoconcave; **E.** Meniscus lens.

A concave lens can be considered as two prisms placed apex to apex and two parallel beams of light will be made divergent so as to appear to emerge from a point on the same side as the beam of light (Fig. 7.8).

In any type of spherical lens, one or both surfaces form part of the surface of a sphere (Figs 7.9 and 7.10). The center of the sphere of which the surface forms a part is called the center of curvature and the radius of the sphere is called the radius of the curvature.

In any lens there is a small area in the center, which can be considered as a glass plate with parallel sides and hence a beam of light passing through this center will pass through undeviated. This line of the light ray is called the principal axis (Fig. 7.11).

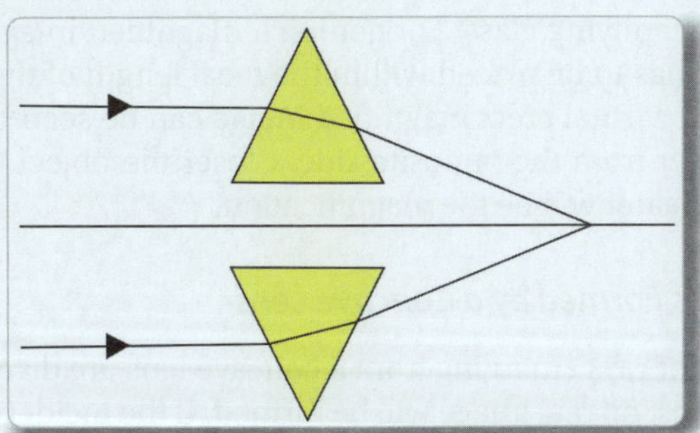

FIGURE 7.7: Refraction by a convex lens

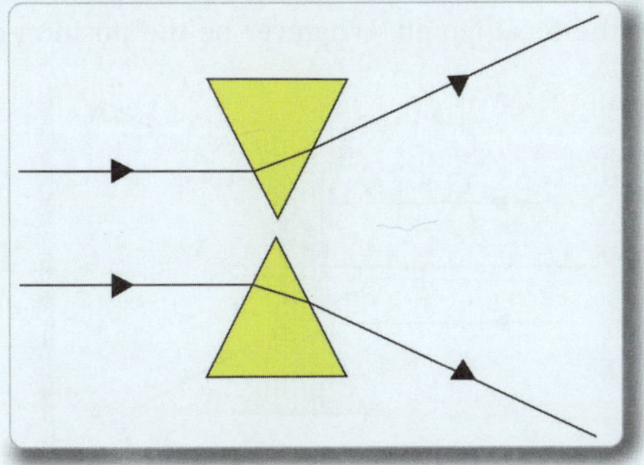

FIGURE 7.8: Refraction by a concave lens

When a light beam strikes a lens obliquely (PQRS), again there is a central beam (Fig. 7.12), which passes through with minimal deviation, but parallel to the original direction of the beam, provided the lens is a thin one. Here again, the point where this beam strikes and then emerge from the lens can be considered as a parallel plate. Such a pathway of the light beam is called the secondary axis of the lens.

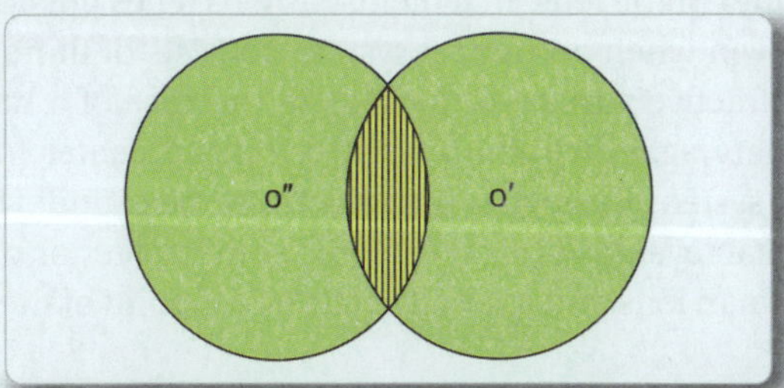

FIGURE 7.9: Center of curvature of a spherical lens

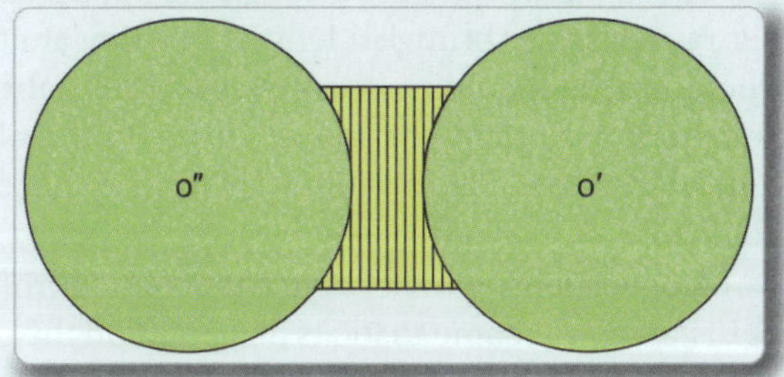

FIGURE 7.10: Center of curvature of a concave lens

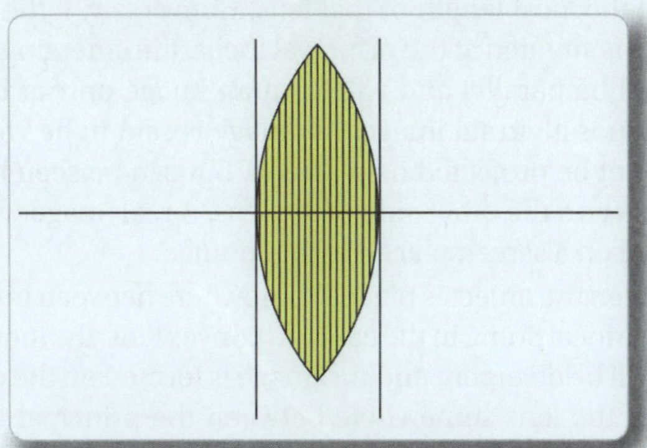

FIGURE 7.11: Principal axis of a lens

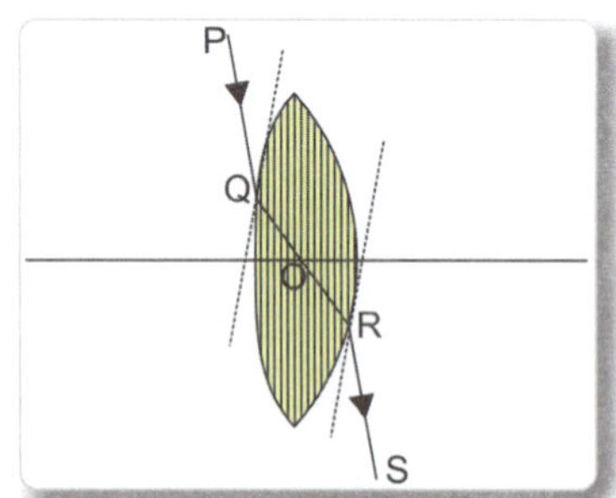

FIGURE 7.12: Optical center of a lens ('O' in the Figure)

There is a point in the center of the optical system of the lens where all the secondary axes meet the principal axis. This is the optical center of the lens (refer Fig. 7.12). All the light rays, which pass through the optical center, can be considered to be undeviated.

The optical center need not always be in the geometrical center of the lens. In a meniscus lens it lies outside the lens. Even when an optical system consists of more than one refractive surface or lens, as in the case of a human eye, there again will be a point or optical center for the whole system through which light rays pass undeviated. In human eye this optical center is at the posterior part of the human lens and it is called the nodal point of the eye.

Images Formed by Convex Lens

Except for the light rays passing through the optical center, all other rays passing through a lens will be deviated and thus, should meet at a point (theoretical). Thus light rays will come to focus at a point and an image of the object 'AB', from which the light rays come, will form at that point 'ba' (Fig. 7.13).

In a biconvex lens, parallel light rays coming from an infinite distance will come to focus at a point on the other side of the lens and this point is called the principal focus and the distance of the principal focus from the lens is called the focal length of that lens. Conversely, if the light source is situated at the principal focus, the emerging light ray will be parallel and will form an image only at infinity. So it is a virtual image. An image is said to be virtual, if cannot be projected on a screen, but can be seen by an observer on the other side of the lens. A real image will be formed on a screen placed at that point.

When the object is placed somewhere between infinity and the focal point, in the case of a convex lens, the incident rays will be divergent and the image is formed on the other side of the lens somewhere between the principal focus and the infinity (Fig. 7.14). Closer the object is to the principal focus, more divergent will be light rays and further

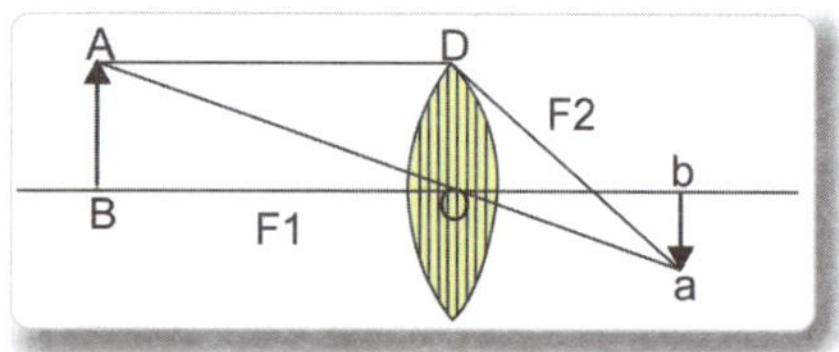

FIGURE 7.13: Real inverted image formed by a convex lens with object beyond focal point

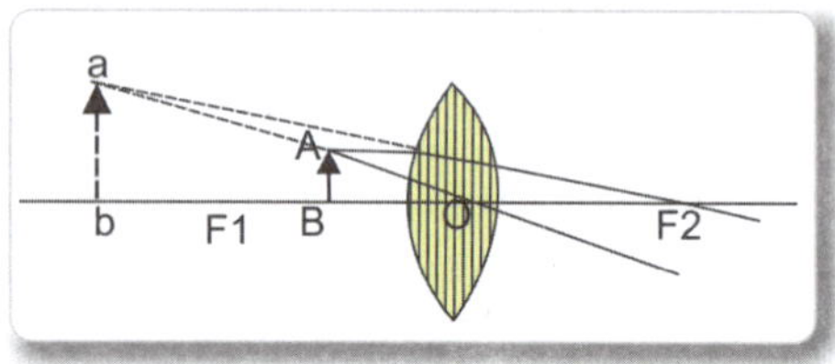

FIGURE 7.14: Virtual magnified image formed by a convex lens with object within focal length

away from the lens will be the image. If the object is at the principal focus; the emerging rays will be parallel and the image will be theoretically formed at infinity. So the image will be virtual.

If the object is placed closer to the lens than the principal focus, the emerging rays will be divergent and a virtual, erect, magnified image is formed on the same side as the object. This is the situation where convex lens act as a magnifying glass. For getting a magnified image, the object has to be placed within the focal length of the lens and the virtual erect magnified image can be seen by the observer from the opposite side. Closer the object to the lens, greater will be the magnification.

Images Formed by a Concave Lens

The light rays emerging from a concave lens are divergent and thus, no real image will be formed. If the incident rays are parallel, they will appear to be diverging from a point on the same side as the incident light and this is the principal focus of the lens. The distance of this point from the lens is the focal length. Whatever be the position of the

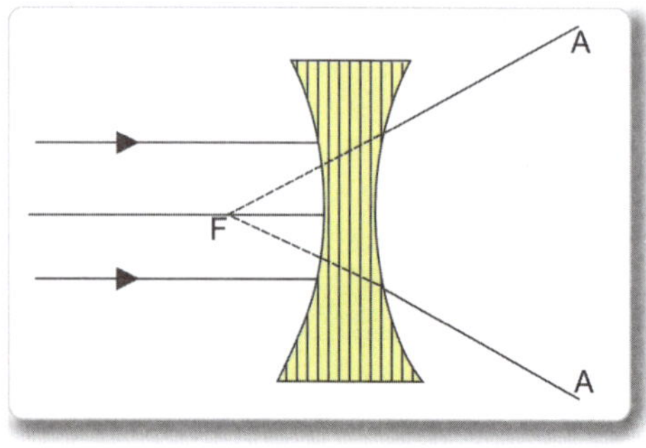

FIGURE 7.15: Image formed by a concave lens

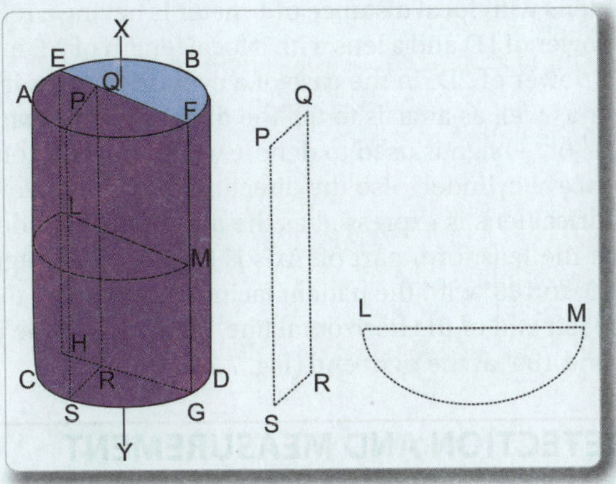

FIGURE 7.16: Convex cylinder

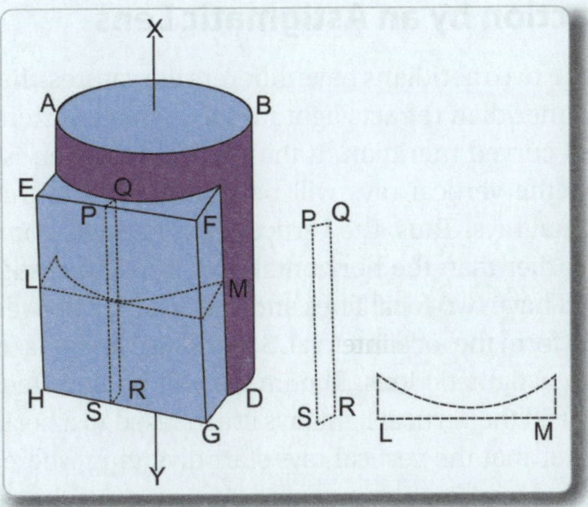

FIGURE 7.17: Concave cylinder

object, with a concave lens, the images is virtual, erect and smaller than the object (Fig. 7.15).

Construction of Images Formed by Lenses

The image formed by any lens or a system of lenses can be constructed by knowing the direction of two rays of light from the object:

1. Light ray, which is parallel to the principal axis and thus passing through the principal focus.
2. Light ray passing through the optical center of the lens and this is undeviated. The image will be formed at the point when these two lines meet (refer Fig. 7.13).

Refraction by a Cylindrical Lenses

Cylindrical lenses are used in ophthalmology for correcting the refractive error called astigmatism.

Cylindrical lenses are called so because they form a part of a cylinder by intersection of a cylinder by a plane in the same direction as the axis of a cylinder (Figs 7.16 and 7.17).

The surface of such a lens is curved only in one direction and in the plane at right angle to the curved surface, it is flat. The axis of a cylindrical lens is the axis of the cylinder of which it forms part. Light rays falling on a cylindrical lens in the direction of its axis are not deviated, since the surface is flat in this plane. The light rays falling to the plane perpendicular to the axis are refracted similar to a spherical lens. So the parallel light rays falling on a cylindrical lens are not focused to a point, but to a line running in the same direction of the axis of the cylinder (Fig. 7.18). Thus, a cylindrical lens has a focal line instead of a focal point.

The image seen by an eye with astigmatic error will form a sharp image in the direction of the axis of the error and

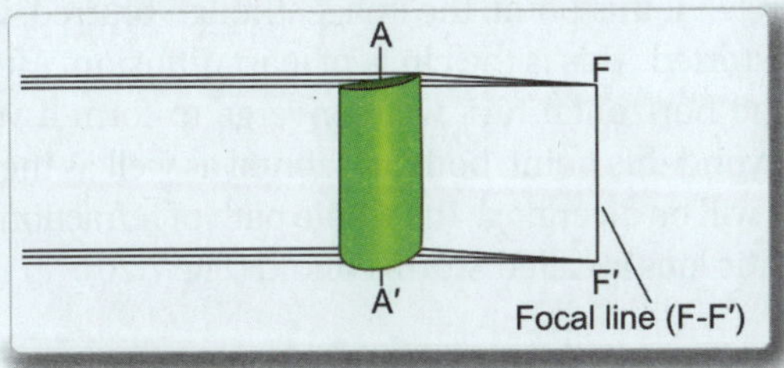

FIGURE 7.18: Focal line of a cylindrical lens

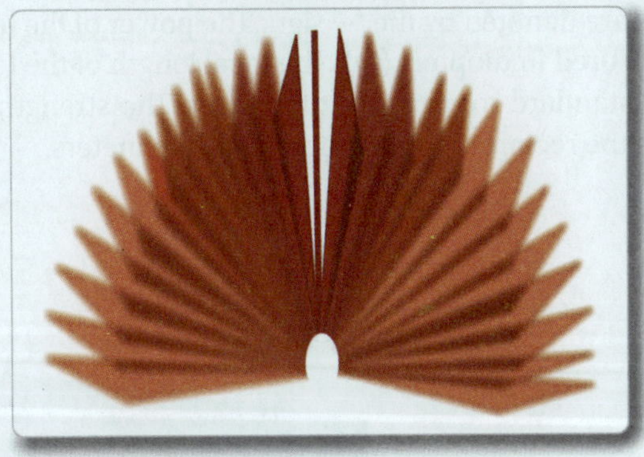

FIGURE 7.19: Astigmatic fan (sharp image in the vertical meridian)

the image will be blurred maximum in the direction at right angle to its axis as depicted by the picture of astigmatic fan (Fig. 7.19). If an eye has no astigmatic error all the lines of an astigmatic will be seen equally sharp and clear.

Astigmatic Lenses

In a cylindrical lens one meridian is curved and the one at right angle has no curvature at all whereas in an astigmatic lens both meridians are curved, but to different powers as in the bowl of a spoon.

Refraction by an Astigmatic Lens

Since the two meridians have different curvatures, the more curved meridian refracts light rays to a greater extent than the less curved meridian. If the vertical meridian is more curved, the vertical rays will be refracted more than the horizontal rays. Thus, the vertical light rays will come to a focus earlier than the horizontal rays. Thus, the astigmatic lens will have two focal lines and the distance between the two will form the focal interval. So no sharp image is formed with an astigmatic lens. The image will be deviated horizontally till the vertical light rays are focused to a horizontal line. After that the vertical rays start diverging whereas the horizontal rays keep converging. At one point the vertical rays will be diverging to the same extent as the horizontal rays are converging. Here the cross section of the beam will be a circle. At this point, the image, though blurred, will be least distorted. This is the circle of least diffusion. After this point the horizontal rays will converge to form a vertical line. Beyond this point, both horizontal as well as the vertical rays will be diverging. The whole path of refraction by an astigmatic lens is called Sturm conoid (Fig. 7.20).

NOTATION OF LENS

Convex lenses are denoted by the '+' sign and concave lenses are denoted by the '–' sign. The power of the lenses is measured in diopters (D). The focal length of the lenses is the standard to measure the power. The strength of a lens is the reciprocal of the focal length in meters.

A lens with focal distance of 1 meter is having a refractive power of 1D and a lens with a focal length of 0.5 meter has a power of 2D. In the case of a cylindrical lens, it has power as well as an axis to tell the direction of curvature. The '+' or '–' sign is used to denote whether it is a convex or concave cylinder. Also the direction of curvature of the cylindrical lens is expressed as the axis of the cylinder of which the lens form part of. Axis is expressed in degrees from 0° to 180° with the patient facing the observer, the 0° to the left end of the horizontal line, 90° below at the bottom and 180° at the right end (Fig. 7.21).

DETECTION AND MEASUREMENT OF LENS

Spherical Lenses

To detect the type of lens, it is held close to the eye and a distant straight object is observed through it. The lens is moved slightly from side to side and the movement of the object through the lens is noted. If the image is moving in the opposite direction to the movement of the lens, it is a convex lens since the image formed by a convex lens is inverted. If the movement is in the same direction as that of the lens, it is a concave lens since the image formed by a concave lens is erect (Fig. 7.22).

The power of the lens is determined by neutralizing it with a lens of the opposite type, e.g. if the lens is a convex lens, a concave lens of a known power, one at a time, is held close together with the lens to be detected and the

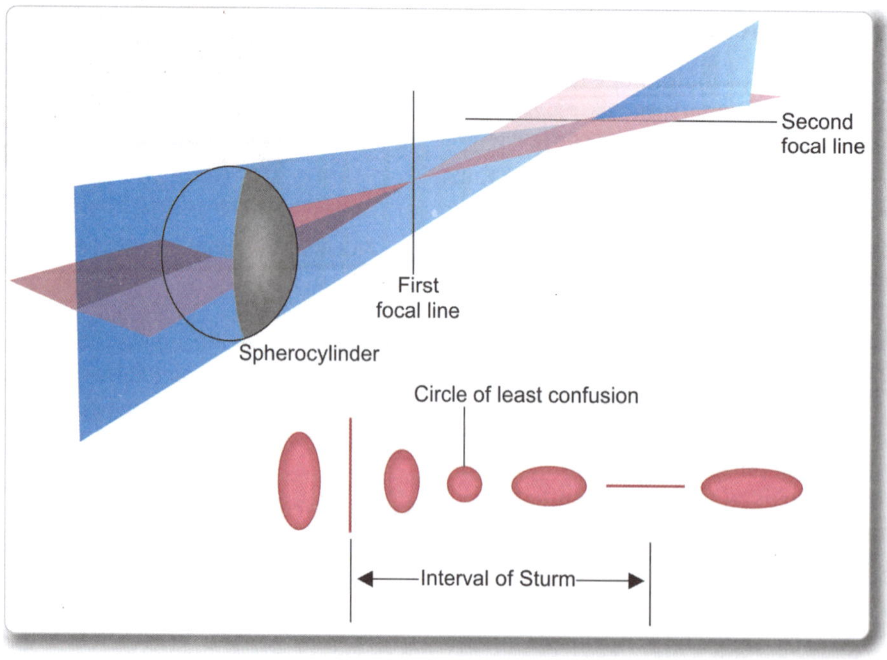

FIGURE 7.20: Sturm conoid

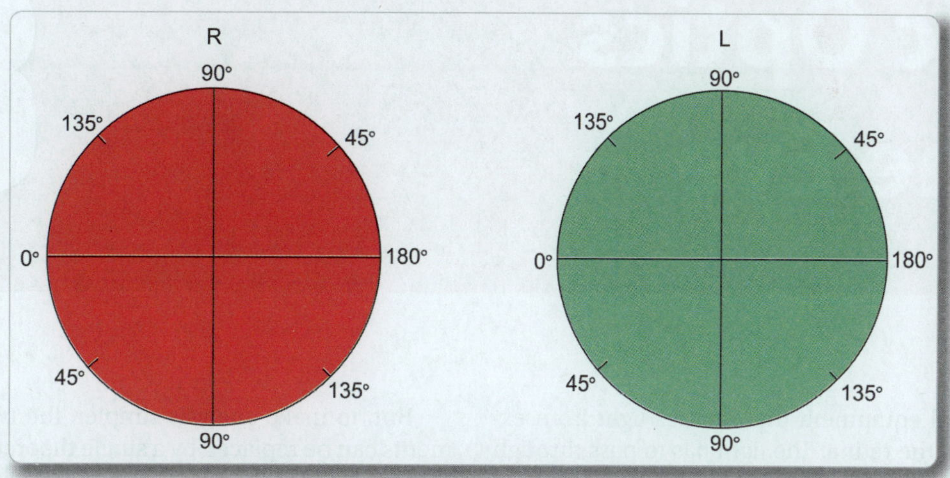

FIGURE 7.21: Axis of cylindrical lenses

combination of lenses is moved and the movement of images through the lens is noted. When the unknown lens is held with the same power lens of the opposite type, no movement of object will be noticed when the combination of lens is moved from side to side. At this point the combination of lenses acts like a plate of glass. Then the power of the lens used for neutralization with the opposite sign will give the power of the lens (e.g. if +2D lens was used for neutralization, the power of the unknown lens is –2D).

Cylindrical Lenses

Cylindrical lenses will be provided as simple cylindrical lens or as spherocylindrical lens for use as spectacles. To know whether the spectacle lens have cylindrical power, hold it close to the eyes and move it side to side and then up and down, while viewing a distant object. If the movement of the object is equal in both directions the lens is a pure spherical lens. If there is movement only in one direction and no movement in the opposite direction it is purely cylindrical lens. If there is movement in both directions, but unequal, then it is a spherocylindrical combination.

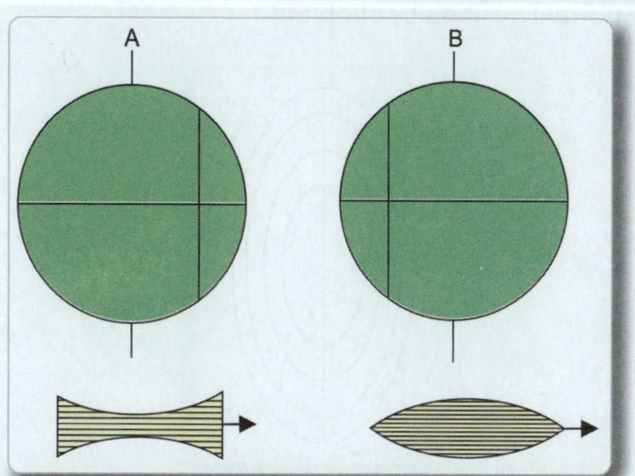

FIGURE 7.22: Detection of the type of lens by displacement of image seen through it

The presence of cylindrical correction in a lens can be detected easily by rotating the lens, while viewing a linear object. If there is a cylinder in the lens, there will be an apparent rotation of the object in the same direction as the rotation of lens, if it is a concave lens and in the opposite direction, if it is a convex lens.

The notation of a cylindrical lens includes the axis of the cylinder as well as power with '+' or '–' sign to denote whether it is concave or convex. This axis is detected by noticing in which direction the displacement of the object seen through the lens is absent (in a pure cylindrical lens) or minimum (in a spherocylindrical combination). The displacement will be maximum in the direction at right angle to the axis. The displacement will be in the same direction, if it is a concave cylinder and in opposite direction, if it is a convex cylinder. Thus, the power as well as the axis of a cylindrical lens are detected and expressed, e.g. +1D cylinder axis 90°.

Detection of Prisms

Many high power lenses may contain prisms also. To detect a prism in a lens, look at a linear object through the lens. If the line seems to be broken and the portion seen through the lens is shifted, it means that a prism is present. Since the line will be deviated toward the apex of the lens, we can know where the apex of the prism is.

Lensometer is the equipment with which we can easily and accurately measure the power of a lens. The axis of a cylinder can also be accurately detected.

Basic Optics of the Eye

8

Girija Devi PS

The eye is optical equipment that focuses light from external objects on the retina. The light has to pass through cornea, anterior chamber, lens and finally the vitreous to reach the retina. All these structures have to be perfectly transparent to form a clear image. Also the light rays have to be accurately focused on the retina. Of these structures, refraction takes place mainly at anterior corneal surface and lenses.

The short radius of curvature (less than 8 mm) of the corneal surface and the big difference in the refractive index between the cornea and air causes maximum refraction at the anterior surface of the cornea, (around 40D–45D).

There is minimal difference in the refractive index of the cornea and aqueous. So no significant deviation of the light rays occurs when it leaves the cornea and enters the aqueous humor.

The remaining refraction occurs in the lens. But the lens cannot be considered as a single refractive medium enclosed by two surfaces. The curvatures of the two surfaces are unequal. The radius of curvature of the anterior surface is about 10 mm, while that of the post surface is about 6 mm. The lens substance can be considered to be made up of several layers, the curvature and the refractive index of each layer increases downwards the center of the lens (Fig. 8.1).

The increase in the refractive index and curvature toward the center of the lens effectively increase the converging power of the lens. The optical power of the lens is about 17D–20D.

Thus, the principal refractive element in the eye is the anterior corneal surface, which has nearly twice the refractive power of the lens. So, ever in an aphakic eye, the light rays form an image, though blurred and out of focus, on the retina.

REDUCED EYE

The human eye is a complex optical system with two refractive surfaces, two principal points and two nodal points.

But, to make analysis simpler, the two refractive elements can be replaced by a single theoretical refractive element placed in the anterior chamber with the same combined effective refractive properties and a single nodal point in the post part of the eye.

Thus, they will be able to convert the complex optical system of the eye into a single refractive surface. Such a schematic eye is called 'reduced eye' (Fig. 8.2). The concept was introduced by Donders. This concept of reduced eye makes it easier to study and understand the various anomalies of refraction and its correction with spectacles.

Retinal Images

With the help of a reduced eye the construction of a retinal image is simple. Since light rays passing through the nodal point are undeviated, the image of an object on the retina can be constructed by drawing straight lines from the two ends of the object passing through the nodal point and reaching the retina (Fig. 8.3).

The image thus formed on the retina will be inverted and smaller in size (since the images are formed by convex lens). This inverted image is reinverted and appreciated in the normal position by our brain.

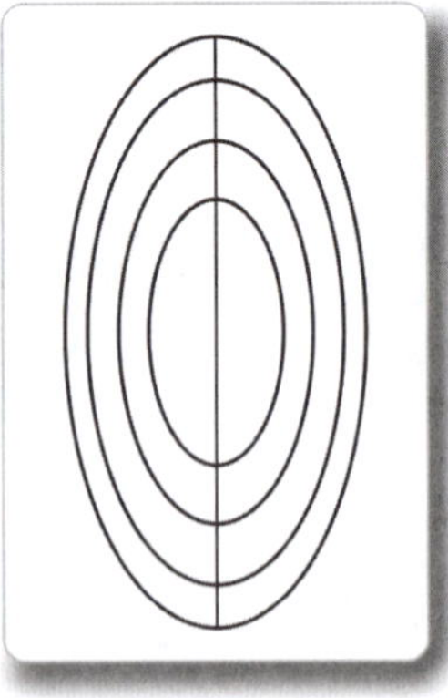

FIGURE 8.1: Curvature and refractive index of each layer of lens increases toward the center

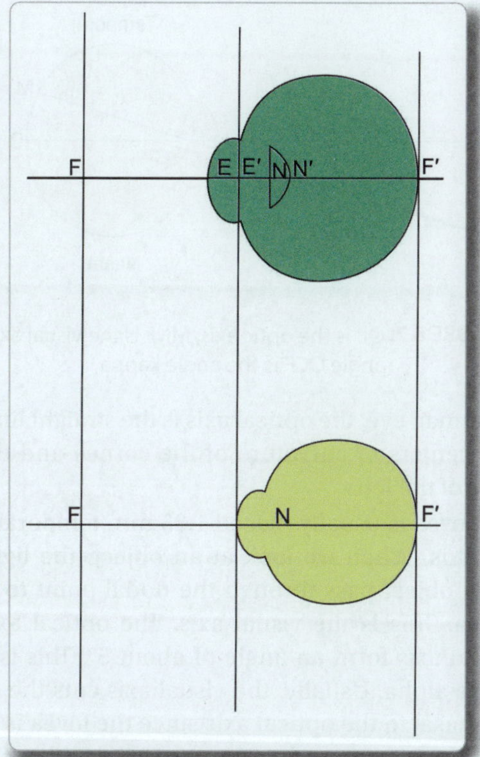

FIGURE 8.2: Reduced eye

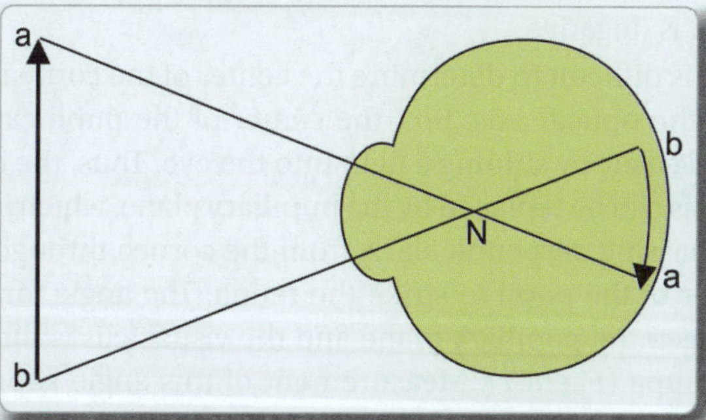

FIGURE 8.3: Images in a reduced eye

PHYSIOLOGICAL OPTICAL DEFECTS

Every lens system has some inherent defects and the human eye is no exception. But, the adaptability of a living tissue keeps these optic defects minimum.

Diffraction of Light

As the light rays travel, the peripheral rays in a beam tend to diverge as if they are falling away due to lack of support. This is called diffraction. This effect is more in a narrow beam like that which passes through a small pupil. The net effect of this divergence is that the beam of light as it gets focused does not form a pinpoint image. Instead, it will be a central disk surrounded by light and dark bands (Fig. 8.4). This phenomenon limits the sharpness of the image formed. Smaller the size of the pupil more will be the effect of diffraction.

Chromatic Aberration

The shorter rays at the blue end of the spectrum are bent more than the longer rays at the red end, when they pass from one medium to another. Thus, the blue rays come to a focus in front of the longer red rays (Fig. 8.5).

Chromatic aberration also reduces the sharpness of the retinal images. Chromatic aberration increases as the size of the pupil increases. But, the human lens with the greater refractive strength of the nucleus effectively decreases chromatic aberration.

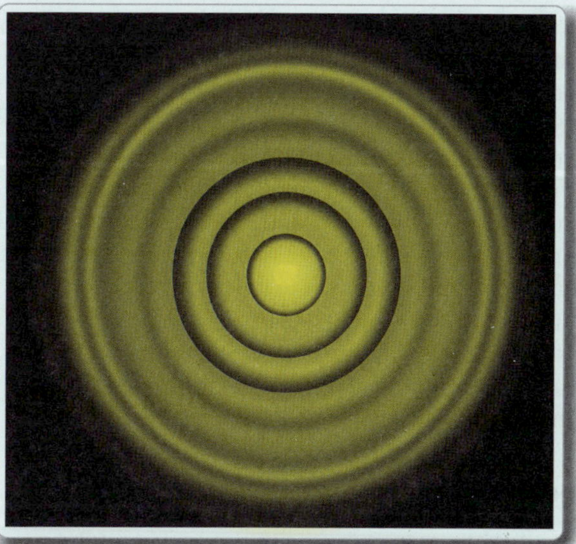

FIGURE 8.4: Image of a point source of light influenced by diffraction of light

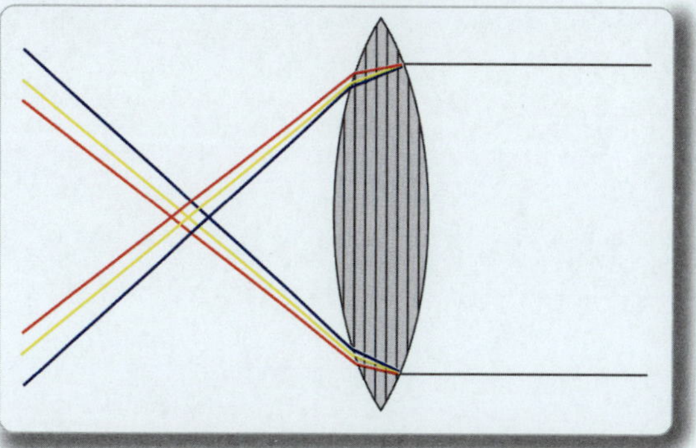

FIGURE 8.5: Chromatic aberration

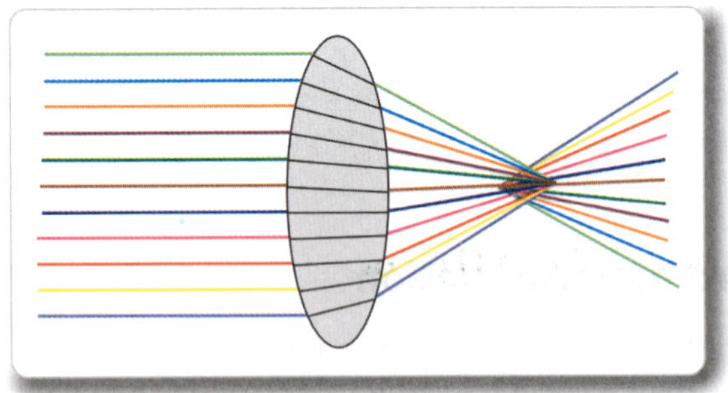

FIGURE 8.6: Spherical aberration

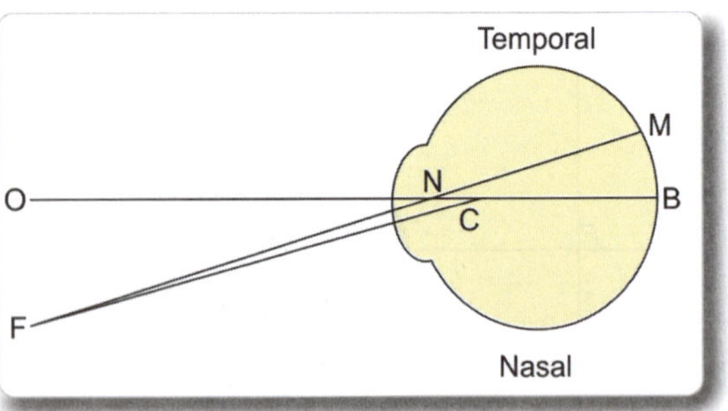

FIGURE 8.7: OB is the optic axis, MNF is the visual axis, angle OCF is the angle kappa

In optical instruments chromatic aberration can be reduced by making lens by combining glasses of different refractive indices. Such lenses are called achromatic lenses.

Spherical Aberration

The central part of a lens has less refractive power compared to the periphery. Thus, the peripheral rays come to a focus earlier than the central rays (Fig. 8.6).

Spherical aberration has no practical significance in the eye since only the central rays reach the retina through the pupil. Even when the pupil is dilated, the effect is insignificant since the cornea is flatter at the periphery. Also, the central parts of the crystalline lens have more effective refractive power compared to the periphery.

In optical instruments, the spherical aberration of the lens is minimized by altering the curvature of the periphery or by combining glasses of different refractive indices to make the lens. Such lens is called aspheric lenses.

Decentering

To form a sharp image the optical centers of the various lenses in the optical system should be in a straight line. In the human eye, the optical axis is the straight line joining the centers of curvature of the cornea and the two surfaces of the lens.

The fovea is usually placed 1.25 mm temporal to the optical axis. When we look at an object, the light rays from the object pass through the nodal point to fall on the fovea. This is the visual axis. The optical axis and the visual axis form an angle of about 5°. This is called the angle alpha. Usually, the visual axis cuts the cornea slightly nasal to the optical axis since the fovea is placed temporally and the angle alpha is designated positive in this situation. If the two axes coincide, the angle is nil or if the visual axis is temporal to the optical axis the angle alpha is negative.

It is difficult to determine the center of the cornea and thus the optical axis. But, the center of the pupil can be noted easily by shining a light into the eye. Thus, the optical axis can be replaced by the pupillary plane, which is the line passing perpendicularly from the cornea through the center of the pupil to strike the retina. The angle formed between the pupillary plane and the visual axis is the angle kappa (Fig. 8.7). Measurement of this angle kappa is important in the evaluation of a case of squint.

Visual Functions and its Evaluation

9

Girija Devi PS

The human eye is often compared to a photographic camera. But, the quality of the images produced by our eyes is far superior to the images produced by the finest camera available. This is made possible by the various abilities our eyes have, which are collectively called visual function.

The various aspects of the visual functions include:

- Visual acuity
- Contrast sensitivity and glare
- Color vision
- Dark adaptation
- Field of vision
- Binocular single vision and depth perception.

All these various aspects have to be in good function for the human eyes to perceive objects of various size, shapes or colors, near or far, moving or stationary and also in various grades of illumination.

VISUAL ACUITY

'Visual acuity' refers to the spatial limit of visual discrimination. It is the single most important measure of the functional integrity of the eye, but not the sole determinant of quality of vision. A person's visual acuity depends not only on the optical system of the eye but also on the proper functioning of the retina, visual pathway and the central nervous system (CNS).

The pinhole test is a simple method to differentiate between visual impairment due to abnormality of the optical system of the eye from other reasons for poor vision. In this test, a disk with a small central hole is held close to the eye and the person is asked to read through the hole. The principle of the pinhole test is that only a single or few light rays from the object are allowed to pass through the hole. This narrow beam will pass through the principal axis of the optical system of the eye. As mentioned earlier, a light ray passing through the principal axis of a lens passes undeviated and this ray will form a clear image on the retina irrespective of the presence of any refractive error. Therefore, if the visual acuity improves with the pinhole, this means that the decrease in visual acuity is due to some refractive error. If there is no improvement in vision with the pinhole, the cause of the defective vision is organic and not related to the abnormalities in the optical system.

Visual acuity estimates the ability of the eye to discriminate between two points and seen them as two separate points and not as a single blurred point. For this to happen, the two points should stimulate two separate cones with an unstimulated cone in between.

The size of the retinal image depends not only on the size of the object, but also its distance from the eye. The farther the object, the smaller will be the retinal image. To see an object clearly, the eye should be able to appreciate the different parts of the object clearly. For this, each part of the object should subtend an angle of 1 minute at the nodal point. This forms the principle of the Snellen's chart used for testing the visual acuity (Fig. 9.1).

Snellen's Chart

Snellen's chart contains a series of letters in diminishing size from above downwards (Fig. 9.2). The letters are constructed in such a manner that each letter subtends an angle of 5 minutes and each individual part of the letter subtends 1 minute at the nodal point, at a particular distance from the eye.

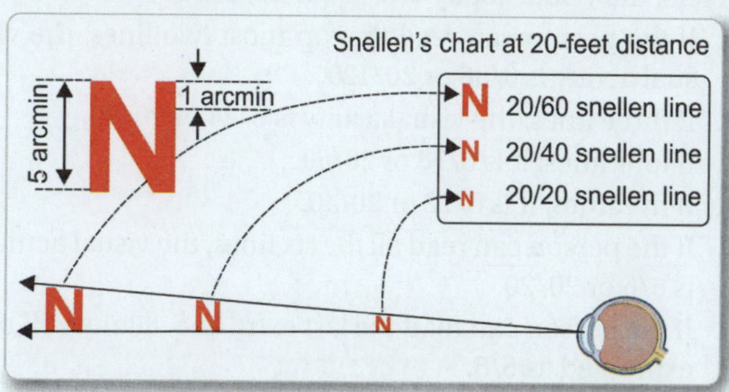

FIGURE 9.1: Principle of a Snellen's chart

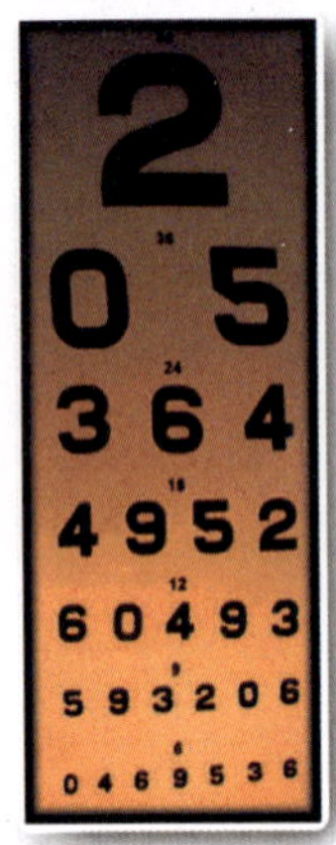

FIGURE 9.2: Snellen's chart

The top most letters subtends an angle of 5 minutes and its individual parts, an angle of 1 minute at a distance of 60 meters (200 feet):

1. The 2nd row at 36 meters (120 feet).
2. The 3rd row at 24 meters (80 feet).
3. The 4th row at 18 meters (60 feet).
4. The 5th row at 12 meters (40 feet).
5. The 6th row at 9 meters (30 feet).
6. The last row at 6 meters (20 feet).

Some chart contains one more row of letters, which a normal person can read only at 5 meters, but some people will be able to read at 6 meters.

The visual acuity is expressed as a fraction. The numerator is the distance at which the person is placed from the chart, which is usually 6 meters (20 feet in countries like America, where the metric system is not followed) and the denominator is the distance at which a person with normal visual acuity will be able to read the last letter, which the person examined is able to read.

A person is normally placed at 6 meters to read the Snellen's chart. If he can read only the topmost letter, since a normal person can read the topmost letter at 60 meters, the visual acuity is 6/60 (or 20/200):

1. If the person can read the top most two lines, the visual acuity is 6/36 or 20/120.
2. If three lines, the visual acuity is 6/24 or 20/80.
3. If four lines, it is 6/18 or 20/60.
4. If five lines, it is 6/12 or 20/40.
5. If the person can read all the six lines, the visual acuity is 6/6 or 20/20.
6. If the person can read the last extra line, acuity will be expressed as 6/5.

If the person examined cannot read even the topmost letter, he/she is gradually brought forward until he/she can read the second row of letters. When he/she reads the first letter, he/she can be asked to go back slowly and tell at which position he/she can still read the first letter. This is done because at the first instance, he/she may not realize where to look or what he/she is expected to see. If he/she can read the first letter at 5 meters vision is recorded as 5/60, if at 4 meters, the visual acuity is 4/60, if at 3 meters the visual acuity is 3/60, if at 2 meters the visual acuity is 2/60 and if only at 1 meter the visual acuity is 1/60.

If the person cannot read the topmost letter even at 1 meter, the examiner can show fingers before his/her eye and ask him/her to count the number of fingers shown. If he can count the fingers shown before his/her face, the vision is recorded as counting fingers close to face (CFCF) or CF at ½ meter, if he/she can count fingers at ½ meter. If the patient is unable to count fingers, the examiner can wave his/her hands before his/her face and see if the patient can appreciate the movement and if he/she can, the vision is recorded as hand movement (HM). If he/she cannot appreciate this movement, he/she may be placed in a darkened room and light is thrown into his/her eyes and asked whether he/she can appreciate the presence of light. The flash light may be switched off and on repeatedly and he/she may be asked to tell when the light is switched on. In this way, the examiner can make sure the patient actually perceives the light and the vision is recorded as perception of light or PL. If even perception of light is not present, the vision is recorded as 'no PL'.

Projection of Light

The test is done when the visual acuity is reduced to HM or PL. The patient is asked to look straight and a narrow beam of light is shown into his eye from the four quadrants and check whether the patient is able to tell, which direction the light is coming from. If he can appreciate this correctly, it is recorded as projection of light accurate or PR+. If it is defective or the patient is not able to tell from which quadrant it is coming, it is recorded by the symbol +/- or -ve and the affected quadrant is also marked. For example, if the patient can appreciate the light, but not the direction of light in the upper temporal quadrant and cannot appreciate the light in the lower temporal quadrant, but the nasal quadrants are normal in RE, it is recorded as shown in Figure 9.3.

Decimal Acuity

The fraction obtained with the Snellen's chart can be expressed as a decimal number and this is known as decimal acuity. Here, the eye with better vision will have a numerically larger number (Table 9.1).

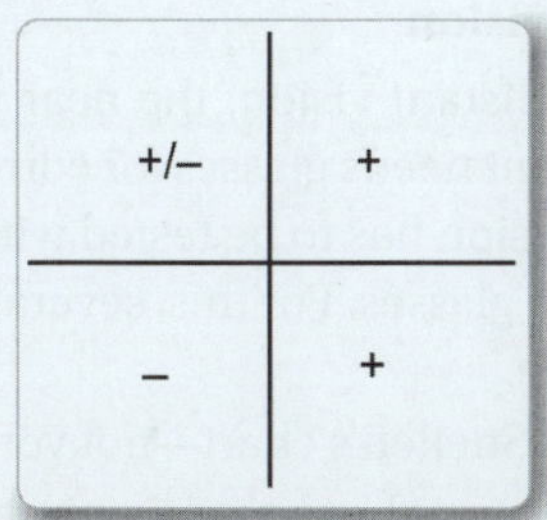

FIGURE 9.3: Projection of light

TABLE 9.1: Comparison of recording of visual acuity by different methods

Snellen's equivalent		Decimal equivalent	LogMAR* equivalent
Meters	Feet		
6/5	20/60	1.20	–0.1
6/6	20/20	1.00	0.00
6/7.5	20/25	0.80	+0.1
6/9	20/30	0.6	+0.2
6/12	20/40	0.50	+0.3
6/15	20/50	0.40	+0.4
6/18.9	20/63	0.32	+0.5
6/24	20/80	0.25	+0.6
6/30	20/100	0.20	+0.7
6/36	20/120	0.17	+0.8
6/37.5	20/125	0.16	+0.8
6/48	20/160	0.13	+0.9
6/60	20/200	0.10	+1.0

*LogMAR, logarithm of the minimum angle of resolution

LogMAR Chart

For research purposes and statistical analysis, the visual acuity is recorded with the logMAR chart. For each letter read, the 'logarithm of the minimum angle of resolution' (logMAR) is added. To get the MAR, the Snellen's visual acuity is inverted and reduced. For example, 6/24 corresponds to a MAR of 4 minutes. LogMAR allows constant geometric progression at each step. In Snellen's chart, the progression of difficulty is not uniform from one line to the next one. In logMAR charts, the lines progress in 0.1 logMAR steps and every letter read by the patient counts as 0.02 of each line. If a patient can read 3 lines in the Snellen's chart, the visual acuity is 6/24 or the MAR is 4 minutes, which corresponds to a logMAR of 0.4. If he/she can read 2 more letters in the next line, every letter will be counted as 0.02 of that line. So his logMAR visual acuity will be $0.4 + (0.02 \times 2) = 0.44$. Thus, special logMAR charts like Modified Bailey-Lovie chart are used to record logMAR visual acuity. The letters in the chart has a constant geometric progression. LogMAR charts help in more accurate recording of any increase or decrease in vision and so are used for recording vision in scientific studies (Fig. 9.4).

Testing Visual Acuity in Illiterate Persons

The test can be done with the Snellen's E chart or Landolt C chart. The patient is asked to tell in which direction each letter is open. Chart with picture of diminishing sizes can also be used. This chart is useful in testing vision in older children who have not yet learnt to read.

Testing Visual Acuity in Children

The testing methods will depend on the age of child.

Infants

Fixation will develop by 6 weeks of age. In young infants of 6 weeks or more, a colorful toy may be held before the baby and moved in various directions and see whether the baby fixes on the toy and maintain fixation when the toy is moved to a different position. This test is done with both eyes open or one eye alone and other eye closed with mother's hand. This simple test will help the examiner to tell whether the vision of the baby is grossly normal.

Optokinetic Nystagmus

In infants, the visual acuity can be tested by the optokinetic nystagmus. It is the slow movement of the eye in pursuit of a moving object and rapid backward movement to take up fixation, when the objects move forward rapidly across the visual field.

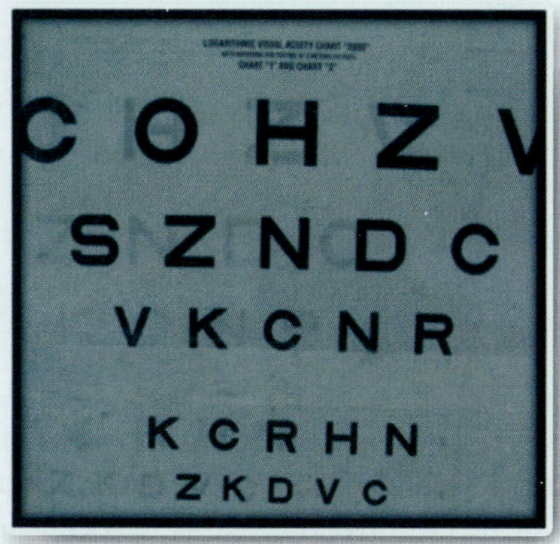

FIGURE 9.4: LogMAR chart

This phenomenon can be used to assess the visual acuity in infants and also in uncooperative or malingering patients. A drum with alternate dark and white stripes is rotated before the eye and the eye is watched for the presence of optokinetic nystagmus. The size of the stripes rotated before the eye is decreased until the end point is reached, i.e. the optokinetic nystagmus ceases. That is the point when the individual stripes become invisible and from the size of the smallest stripes visible, the visual acuity can be assessed.

Worth's Ivory Ball Test

In children between 1 and 2 years, this test is useful. There are five balls of different sizes ranging from ½ to 1½ inch diameter. Child is given the balls to play for some time. After this, with each eye occluded, the balls are thrown one by one starting by the biggest one. The child is encouraged to go after the balls and the smallest ball, the child can see is thus determined and from this, an approximate estimate of the visual acuity can be made.

Sheridan-Gardiner Test

The test can be used in children from 3 to 5 years. The child is given a card containing a few letters. The examiner stands at a distance of 6 meters and shows some letter at various Snellen's test type and size and the child is encouraged to show from the card, which letter the examiner is showing. The child has to identify the letter from the shape. In smaller children of 2–3 years age, a card containing a few pictures can be used in this manner and the examiner shows the picture in varying sizes and the child has to identify the picture. The child can be encouraged to cooperate making this a game played by the mother and the child.

In elder children up to 5-6 years, who have not yet learned to read and write, the Landolt's broken ring test —C or E test can be used and the child has to point out in which direction each letter is 'open'.

Refraction

In children who are uncooperative or mentally challenged, a cycloplegic refraction and fundus examination can be done to rule out refractive error or pathological conditions that can impair vision.

Electrophysiological Tests

In children who show no obvious pathological changes or refractive error especially in mentally challenged children, electrophysiological tests like visual evoked potential (VEP) or electrophysiological (ERG) can be done to rule out any gross impairment of vision.

Testing for near vision

After testing the distant vision, the near vision has to be tested. If the patient needs glasses for correction of distant vision, the near vision has to be tested without the glasses as well as with the glasses. For this, several near vision test types are available.

1. Miniaturized Snellen's chart—not very popular.
2. Jaeger's test type—the near vision is recorded as J1, J2, etc. not very widely used.
3. Faculty's notation, the most widely used and standardized by the faculty of ophthalmologists of Great Britain in 1952. In this, near vision is recorded by the letter 'N' followed by number indicating the test type. N5 is the normal near vision, followed by N8, N10, N12, N18, N36 showing decreased near vision graded in severity (Fig. 9.5).

CONTRAST SENSITIVITY AND GLARE

The test is an assessment of the quality of vision. The Snellen's visual acuity test is a high contrast test—dark letters in an illuminated bright background. In real life situation, such contrast between the object of our interest and the surroundings is rarely seen. Often the difference between the object and its surroundings will be minimal, e.g. a white paper on a table covered with a white tablecloth. So, the quality of vision depends to a large extent on the contrast sensitivity. In spite of a normal visual acuity of 6/6, the contrast sensitivity can be poor in many situations, e.g. early cataract, nuclear sclerosis of advance age, early glaucoma, etc.

To see an object clearly and separately from its surroundings, it should differ from its surroundings in luminance, color, texture, motion or binocular disparity. Various tests called contrast sensitivity tests are used to assess how far these differences should be present for a particular person to identify objects clearly.

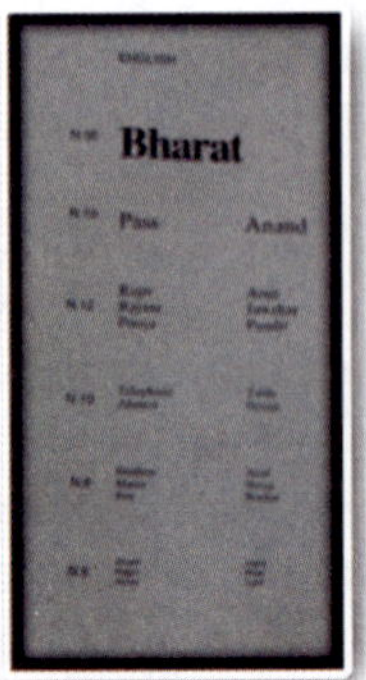

FIGURE 9.5: Near vision chart

Contrast sensitivity gratings or letter contrast sensitivity test are commonly used for testing contrast sensitivity. In Cambridge contrast sensitivity gratings, gratings of decreasing contrast on a blank card is shown to the patient till he cannot see the gratings and can appreciate the card alone.

The Pelli-Robson (Fig. 9.6), Hamilton-Veale contrast sensitivity test, Regan chart, etc. use letter of diminishing contrast down the chart and the patient is asked to read the letters from the chart placed at 1 meter from the patient.

These contrast sensitivity tests compliment the Snellen's visual acuity tests and help to assess the quality of vision.

Glare Susceptibility

The ability to see objects clearly separated from its background may fall considerably in high glare situations such as driving at night or walking on the beach on midday. This is caused by scattering of the light within the eye, thus diminishing the clarity of the retinal image formed. This can happen in normal lighting also, if the person has early cataract, corneal opacities, hypopigmented eyes as in albinism, irrespective of the age of the person. It occurs to some extent as age advances due to the increase in refractive index of the lens with age.

Glare susceptibility is defined as visual acuity with no glare source divided by visual acuity, in the presence of a standard light source measured by glare susceptibility ratio.

COLOR VISION

Color vision is the ability to differentiate and appreciate different wavelengths of light. There are three main characteristics of color vision—hue, saturation and brightness. A hue is a function of the wavelength and depends on the predominant wavelength of the incoming light. It is the color of the object. Saturation refers to the richness of the hue and brightness is a subjective sensation produced by a given luminance.

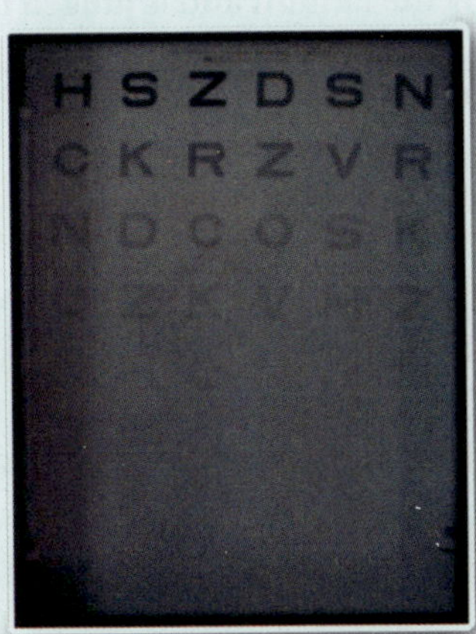

FIGURE 9.6: Pelli-Robson contrast sensitivity chart

Factors Influencing Color Vision

Three types of cones have been identified—long-wavelength-sensitive cones (LWL cones), middle-wavelength sensitive cones (MWL cones) and short-wavelength-sensitive cones (SWL cones). The LWL cones are best stimulated by red light, MWL cones by green light and SWL cones by blue light. The central 30° field, which has the maximum number of cones, has the maximum ability for color perception. The LWL cones are absent in the center of the fovea and hence it is blue blind. Far peripheral retina has negligible color discrimination ability and images from this area are appreciated as various shades of gray.

Illumination affects color vision. Color vision is best in photopic vision where the illumination is good and cones function maximum. It is defective in mesopic vision and absent in scotopic vision where vision solely depends on the rods.

As age advances the human lens absorbs shorter wavelength and this will affect the color discrimination ability.

Anomalies of Color Vision

Color vision deficiency can be congenital or acquired (Table 9.2).

TABLE 9.2: Congenital/Acquired color deficiency

Congenital	Acquired
Hereditary	Not hereditary
Red-green deficiency	Blue-yellow is more affected
Since X-linked inheritance, males are more affected	Not related to gender
Patients are usually unaware of the problem and tests are needed to detect it	Patients may be aware of the deficiency and will have difficulty in identifying colors
Both eyes are symmetrically affected	May be asymmetrical
Easily identified by standard tests	More subtle and difficult to diagnose
Visual acuity will be normal and no history of any disease or trauma of the eye	Visual acuity may be affected by the primary problem—disease or trauma affecting the eye

Congenital Color Deficiency

Congenital color deficiency is usually X-linked and hence affects mostly men. Congenitally color deficient persons are unaware of their deficiency and go through life identifying colors based on their luminosity and other aspects, which they pick up from experience since childhood. Confusions in identifying colors occur when confusing wavelengths are simultaneously presented as at the time of testing for color deficiency. Color blindness makes people unsuitable for many jobs as in the military and police force. Good color vision is important for tasks like color matching and coding and is essential for students of arts, chemistry, geography and geology. Children should be tested for color vision early in life so that they can plan their career accordingly and avoid future disappointments when they want to take up a particular profession and find that they are unsuitable on testing color vision.

Acquired Color Deficiency

Acquired color deficiency is usually due to diseases of the retina or optic nerve. Lesions of the outer layers of the retina generally give rise to blue-yellow defect and lesions of inner layers of the retina and optic nerve result in red-green defects, but exceptions can happen. Some patients with involvement of cerebral cortex can also develop color deficiency.

Causes of acquired color deficiency:
- Primary glaucoma
- Diabetic retinopathy
- Age-related macular degeneration
- Degenerative myopia
- Retinitis pigmentosa
- Siderosis bulbi
- Chorioretinitis
- Optic nerve disorders, optic atrophy, toxic amblyopia
- After panretinal photocoagulation.

Nomenclature of Color Vision

Color vision abnormalities are expressed in a specific terminology. The Greek words for first, second and third (protos, deuteros and tritos) are substituted for red, green and blue. The suffix added indicates the severity of the defect. Suffix for partial defect is anomaly and complete defect is anopia.

Incidence

Congenital types of defective color vision occur in 8% of male population:
- Protanopes (insensitive to red)—1%
- Protanomalous—1%
- Deuteranopes (insensitive to green)—1%
- Deuteranomalous—5%
- Tritanomalous and trianopes (insensitive to blue)—0.01%.

Tests for Color Vision

Pseudoisochromatic Plates

Pseudoisochromatic plates are color confusion tests. A figure or a letter made of dots of one color is placed in a background of dots of another color. The color of the figure and the background are isochromatic to a color deficient person and they find it impossible to identify the figure.

Ishihara Pseudoisochromatic Plates

Ishihara pseudoisochromatic plates are most widely used (Fig. 9.7). It is a screening test used to identify congenital red-green deficiency.

Hardy, Rand Rittler Plates

Hardy, Rand Rittler (HRR) plates are another type of pseudoisochromatic plate test useful for detecting tritan (blue-yellow) defects. So, it is more useful for detecting acquired color deficiencies. American Optical Company plates and the Dvorine are widely used screening tests for protan and deutan defects.

Farnsworth Munsell 100 Hue Test

Farnsworth Munsell 100 Hue test consists of colored chips, which the tested person has to arrange in a color sequence. The chips have similar brightness and saturation, but differ from one another. Color deficient people may err in arranging the chips. This test will show the type of defect, but not its severity.

Lantern Tests

There are different types of lantern tests used in different countries mainly for occupational purpose, as by marine and aviation authorities. The subject names the various colors shown by the lantern and is judged by the matches he makes.

Edridge-Green lantern test used in US for testing coastal guards is useful when used by an expert though many lanterns are useless.

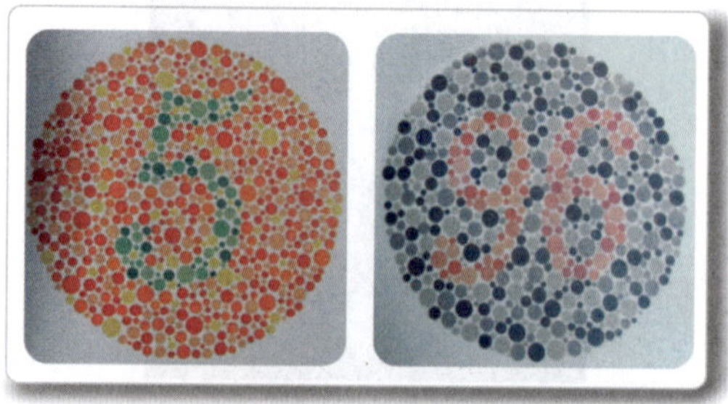

FIGURE 9.7: Ishihara's color vision plates

Holmgren Wools

The candidate is required to match the colored wool and is judged by the mistakes that he makes. This test is not accurate and not used now in clinical practice.

Anomaloscopes

Anomaloscopes are expensive tests that help in making a definite diagnosis and also to measure the extent of the defect.

In Nagel's anomaloscopes, the patient is asked to match a mixture of red and green light with yellow. The instrument has a prism that splits a white light to various colors and these colors are viewed through a telescope. The person tested sees a circle of light divided into two halves. The lower half is yellow and he has to match it with a mixture of red and green light in the upper half. There are controlling knobs to alter the ratio of the two colors to get a match. It is useful to distinguish dichromatic vision from anomalous trichromatic color vision by measuring the ratio of green and red light used.

Color perimetry: It may be used mainly for acquired color defects, such as in cases of alcohol optic neuropathy and retrobulbar neuritis. It will be found that blue and yellow colors are recognized as such, but not red and green. Acquired defects in color vision may be seen in diseases of the retina and also optic nerve/tract.

Electroretinography: It is possible to observe separately the photopic and scotopic components of ERG and thus detect color vision abnormalities.

FIELD OF VISION

The normal field of vision (Fig. 9.8) for white light extends 60° upwards, 70° downwards and 90° outwards. The extent of the fields depends on the color of the testing object, illumination, the contrast of the test object with the surrounding and the state of adaptation of the eye. The fields will be smaller in extent for colored objects, smaller objects, in dim illumination, in low contrast conditions and in dark adapted state.

There is a non-seeing area within the field of vision corresponding to the optic disk called the blind spot.

Binocular field of vision: It is the total visual field of both eyes together. It has a large central area common to both eyes and a temporal uniocular area, which corresponds to the eye of that side alone. The blind spot of one eye will be covered by the seeing area of the other eye.

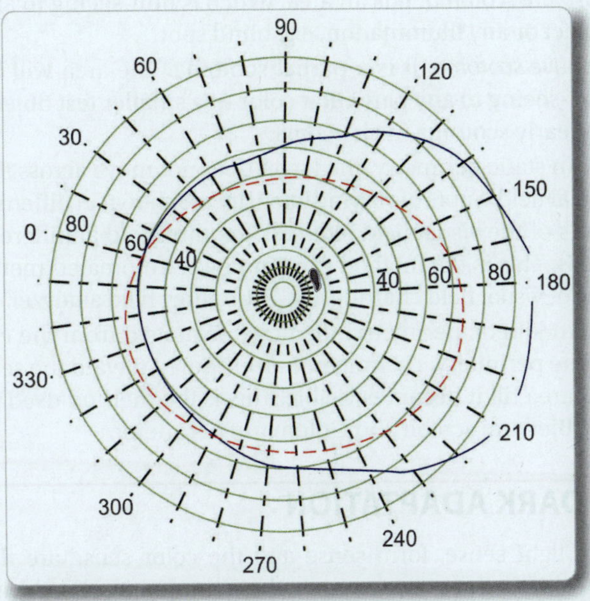

FIGURE 9.8: Field of vision

Traquir's hill of vision: The sensitivity of the eye is maximum at the macula and it decrease toward the periphery. This is represented by Traquir's hill of vision (Fig. 9.9).

Contraction of the field: It denotes that there is a diminution of the field in some area.

Scotoma: A non-seeing area surrounded by seeing area. The blind spot is the commonest scotoma.

Perimetry: It denotes a technique to examine and quantify the visual field using targets of various sizes or color. It can be of two types—static or kinetic perimetry.

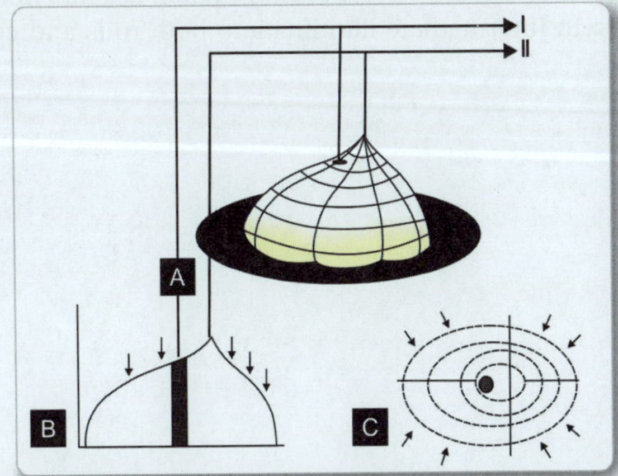

FIGURE 9.9: Traquir's hill of vision I—blind spot, II—fovea (3-dimensional representation of field of vision as an island in a sea of darkness, 2-dimensional representation as a hill of vision and as a unidimensional plot).

Absolute scotoma: It is an area, which is non-seeing to any object or any illumination, e.g. blind spot.

Relative scotoma: It is a partial scotoma. The area will be non-seeing to any particular color or a smaller test object, e.g. early scotoma in glaucoma.

In static perimetry, the target does not move across the visual field. Spots of varying intensity are shown in different parts of the visual field to assess the threshold at different areas. This is the method used in newer automated methods of visual field charting, e.g. Humphrey field analyzer.

In kinetic perimetry, the target is moved from the extreme periphery, i.e. from non-seeing area toward the seeing area till it becomes visible. This is the method used in the Bjerrum screen and Goldmann perimeter.

DARK ADAPTATION

The light sense, form sense and the color sense are the three sensations elicited when the retina is stimulated with light. Light sense is the ability to appreciate light and also its variations in intensity. The minimum intensity of the light, which an eye can perceive is called light minimum.

The light minimum depends on the amount of light that has been falling in the retina before. This is called light adaptation.

In normal light (luminance level 1–106 cd/m^2), the vision is the function of the cones and it is called photopic vision. Maximum visual acuity and good color vision are features of photopic vision. In dim illumination, rods take up the visual functions. This is called scotopic vision. Low vision acuity and poor color discrimination are features of scotopic vision, since color discrimination is a function of cones. In intermediate illumination, both rods and cons take part in the visual functions and it is called mesopic vision. Mesopic vision is characterized by inaccurate visual acuity and color discrimination. In scotopic vision, all colors appear dark or various shades of gray.

When we go from bright light into a poorly-illuminated room, it takes some time for us to see clearly. This is the time taken for dark adaptation, i.e. the time taken for change over from the cones to rods. In conditions, which affect the rods like vitamin A deficiency, retinitis pigmentosa, dark adaptation is impaired and the person will have difficulty in seeing in dim light.

Dark Adaptometry

This test is done to distinguish between genuine night blindness due to retinal diseases from the benign complaints of poor night vision.

After dilatation, the person to be tested is placed with the head at an internally illuminated bowl. Light is shown and its brightness is increased till it becomes visible. After this, the light will be gradually decreased till it becomes invisible. This cycle is repeated for 30 minutes for either eye.

Dark Adaptation Curve

The dark adaptation curve shows two phases. The 1st phase corresponds to the adaptation of the cones, which is a small curve. It bends at a point and the 2nd phase corresponds to adaptation by the rods and it reaches a plateau after 20 minutes.

In doubtful case, the electrophysiological tests, EOG, VEP will confirm or exclude any pathological cause for defective dark adaptation.

Refractive Errors

10

Girija Devi PS

If the parallel light rays striking an eye are refracted so as to converge upon the retina to form a clear image in the eye in a state of rest, i.e. the accommodation is not acting; the condition is called 'emmetropia' (Fig. 10.1). This is an eye with no refractive error.

The opposite condition where the parallel light rays are not brought to a focus on the retina when the eye is at rest is called 'ametropia'. Such an eye has a refractive error.

If the two eyes are focusing the light rays unequally, such condition is called 'anisometropia'.

TYPES OF REFRACTIVE ERRORS

Refractive errors are of three types:

1. Hypermetropia: The principal focus of the eye is behind the retina and consequently the parallel light rays come to a focus to form an image behind the retina (Fig. 10.2) when the eye is at rest.
2. Myopia: Here, the principal focus of the eye is in front of the retina and consequently, the parallel light rays come to a focus to form an image in front of the retina, when the eye is at rest.

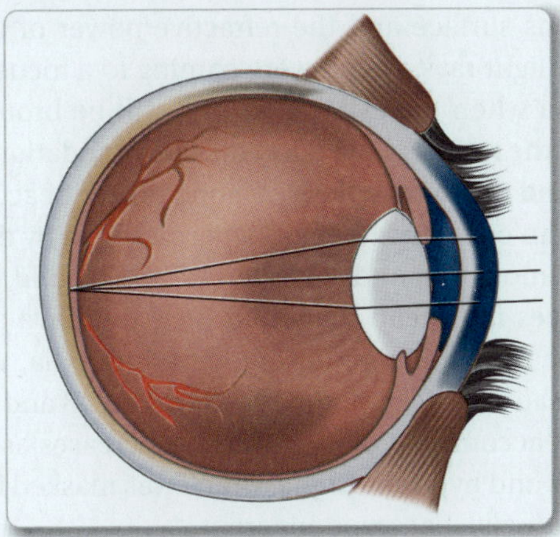

FIGURE 10.1: Emmetropia

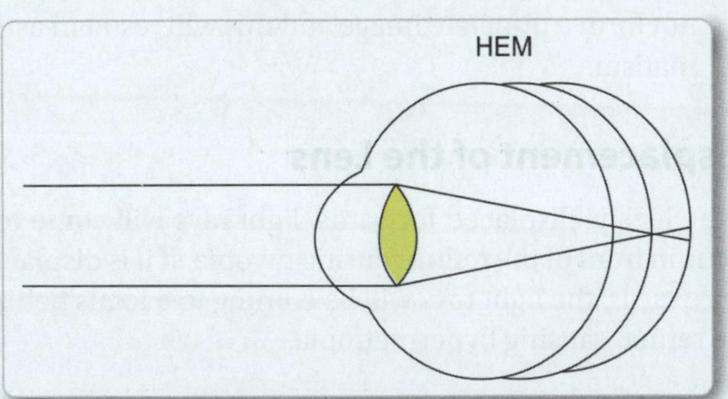

FIGURE 10.2: Focusing of light rays in hypermetropia, emmetropia and myopia (HEM)

3. Astigmatism: Here, the refractive power varies in different meridians, so that the light rays are not brought to focus at a single point.

CAUSES OF REFRACTIVE ERRORS

Abnormal Anteroposterior Dimensions of the Eye

Abnormal dimensions of the eye are the most common cause for refractive errors. If it is too short (a small eye) axial hypermetropia will result. If it is too long, axial myopia will be the result since; the retina will be far away from the optical system of the eye.

Abnormalities of the Refractive Surfaces

If the radius curvature of the lens or the corneal surfaces is too small, curvature hypermetropia will result. If it is too long it will be a condition of curvature myopia. If the curvature varies in different meridian, it will give rise to astigmatism.

Abnormalities of the Refractive Index

If the refractive index of the lens is too low, this will result in index hypermetropia. If it is too high this will result in index myopia. If the refractive index varies in different meridians, this will give rise to index astigmatism.

Abnormalities in the refractive index of the cornea are insignificant.

Obliquity of Elements of the Optical System

1. Lenticular obliquity: If the lens is tilted as in subluxation, astigmatism will be the result.
2. Retinal obliquity: If the posterior pole of the eye is distorted as in posterior staphyloma, the light rays cannot form a punctate image and this will result in astigmatism.

Displacement of the Lens

If the lens is displaced forwards, light rays will come to a focus in front of the retina causing myopia. If it is displaced backwards, the light rays will be coming to a focus behind the retina, causing hypermetropia.

HYPERMETROPIA

Definition

'Hypermetropia' is that form of refractive error where the parallel light rays are brought to a focus behind the retina when the eye is at rest (Fig. 10.3A).

This is the commonest cause of refractive error because it is physiological in little children due to the smallness of their eyes.

Causes

Axial Hypermetropia

Axial hypermetropia is due to decrease in the axial length of the eye. As mentioned before, it is physiological in children. At birth all eyes have 2.5D–3D hypermetropia, which slowly decreases as the child grows and the anteroposterior length of the eye increases. Gradually, the eye reaches emmetropia. In some cases the axial length continues to increase even beyond this and the child goes in for myopia.

Pathological shortening of the axial length of the eye can occur, if there is edema of the posterior pole as in central serous retinopathy, in retinal detachment or if the posterior pole is pushed inwards by orbital tumors or any mass lesion behind the eye. About 1 mm decrease in the anteroposterior dimension can cause 3D of hypermetropia.

Curvature Hypermetropia

Curvature hypermetropia happens when the curvature of the cornea or the lens is less than normal. Cornea is usually the involved tissue as 1 mm increase in radius of curvature can cause 6Ds of hypermetropia.

Index Hypermetropia

Index hypermetropia happens due to decrease in the refractive index of the lens. This is the cause of hypermetropia, which is physiological in old age. As more and more lens fibers are added to the cortex as the age advances, the refractive index of the cortex also increases and approximates that of the nucleus. Thus, the lens starts functioning as a single lens of uniform refractive index unlike the lens of a young person, which acts like a series of lenses with progressively increase in refractive index toward the central portion and consequently increased converging power. Thus, the refractive power of the lens progressively decreases as age advances and results in hypermetropia, which is physiological in old age.

When the blood sugar rapidly falls as uncontrolled diabetes gets quickly controlled, there is a decrease in the refractive power of the lens and a temporary phase of hypermetropia occurs.

Backward displacement of the lens as a congenital anomaly or by trauma can result in hypermetropia. Absence of the lens otherwise called aphakia, results in a high degree of hypermetropia.

Effect of Accommodation on Hypermetropia

When the ciliary muscle contracts during accommodation this relaxes the zonules and increases the curvature of the lens surface and the refractive power of the lens. Thus the light rays, which were coming to a focus behind the retina when the eye was at rest, will be brought to a focus on the retina by the effort of accommodation. Young people and children, who have good power of accommodation, can compensate their hypermetropia by the effort of accommodation and see clearly. Thus, a child with 6/6 vision does not mean that child does not have a refractive error. They may be having hypermetropia, which is compensated by accommodation (Figs 10.3B and C). This power of accommodation gradually decreases as the age advances and hypermetropia, which was masked in childhood gradually, becomes apparent.

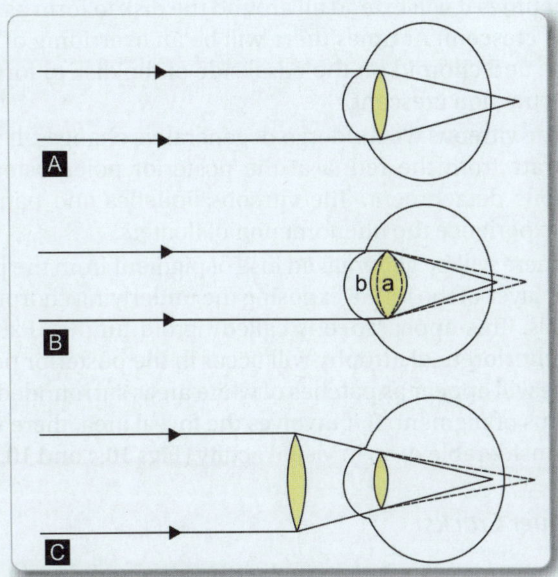

FIGURES 10.3A to C: A. Hypermetropia; B. Getting corrected by accommodation; C. Getting corrected with suitable convex lenses.

Clinical Features

Symptoms

Accommodative asthenopia

Hypermetropes especially the young adults or children, who have good accommodative power, will be constantly using their power of accommodation to overcome the effect of hypermetropia and to see distant objects clearly. To see near objects clearly they require additional effort of accommodation. This continuous and excessive action of the ciliary muscles produces symptoms of eye strain or accommodative asthenopia. These symptoms are more after some near work like reading or toward the evening when they are tired. There will be headache and the eye will feel hot, dry and tired. The ciliary muscle will fail to continue their sustained action and relaxes and the patients will find letters blurred and reading difficult. Or the ciliary muscles may go into spasm—'the spasm of accommodation' and the distant objects all look blurred after reading for some time.

Thus, hypermetropia is one of the commonest ophthalmic causes for headache and eyestrain and a recording of normal vision (6/6) in these people does not exclude a refractive error.

Convergent squint

The action of accommodation and convergence are interrelated and the constant efforts of accommodation lead to excessive convergence and thus the development of convergent squint in children. So, full cycloplegic refraction is absolutely essential in all children with convergent squint. If hypermetropia is the reason for their convergent squint, correction of the refractive error with suitable spectacles will correct the convergent squint also.

Earlier onset of presbyopia

Since hypermetropes need more accommodative power for near work, the gradual receding of near point with age will create problems for near work earlier than in normal people. So, presbyopia will have an earlier onset in these patients and they will require glasses for reading at an earlier age than normal.

Signs

Hypermetropic eyes are smaller eyes than normal since the decrease in anteroposterior dimension of the eyeball is the commonest cause for hypermetropia. So, the optic disk will be smaller than normal. This will cause an overcrowding of the nerve fibers at the optic disk. This will cause an appearance of blurring of the disk margins—an appearance resembling papillitis. This condition is called 'pseudoneuritis'.

Since the eye is small, the anterior chamber (AC) is shallow and the angle of AC is narrower than normal. So, these patients are more prone for the development of angle-closure glaucoma.

Treatment

Hypermetropia is physiological in children and requires correction with convex glasses if:

1. They are experiencing symptoms of eyestrain.
2. If the power is large, to ease the effort of accommodation, even if there are no definite symptoms of eye strain.
3. Full and constant correction in children with convergent squint.

Adults require suitable spectacle correction for comfortable distant vision. They may require additional power for near work also at an earlier age than normal.

MYOPIA

Definition

Myopia is that form of refractive error where parallel rays of light come to a focus in front of the sentient layer of the retina when the eye is at rest.

Causes

The majority of cases are due to an increase in the anteroposterior dimension of the eyeball—axial myopia.

Curvature myopia due to an increase in the curvature of the cornea or lens surface is rare and it is often associated with some irregularity of the surface leading to an associated astigmatism also.

Marked degrees of increases in curvature of the lens surface can occur in condition of anterior or posterior lenticonus. Such an increase in curvature can occur when the suspensory ligaments are relaxed as in spasm of accommodation or when they are torn as in subluxation or dislocation of the lens.

Index myopia occurs in nuclear cataract or when the blood sugar level is high due to changes in the refractive index of the lens.

Types

Developmental Myopia

The child is born with a large eye. Here, the myopia does not progress much as the child grows and it is not usually associated with any degenerative changes in the eye.

Simple Myopia

In this condition, there is over shooting of the correction of hypermetropia as the child grows. Instead of stopping at emmetropia, it will progress to the development of myopia.

Here, the power is usually less than -6D or -7D. Myopia develops in young children or adolescents and does not increase beyond the age of 25 years when the growth of the body is finished. It is not associated with any degenerative changes in the eye.

Pathological Myopia

Manifests in early childhood and progresses rapidly and may continue even after the growth of the body stops. Power exceeds -6D and it is associated with degenerative changes in the eye.

Degenerative changes in pathological myopia: Stretching and elongation of the eyeball is confined to the posterior half of the eye. The anterior half of the globe is relatively of normal size. The entire eye appears large and prominent. The AC will be deep.

Myopic Crescent

Myopic crescent is due to the stretching and elongation of the eyeball, the retina and choroid does not reach up to the edge of the optic disk on the temporal side exposing the underlying sclera. This crescentic white area seen in the temporal side of the disk is called 'temporal crescent'. Sometimes it will extend all around the disk to form as annular crescent. At times there will be an overriding of the retina and choroid on the nasal side of the disk to form a supertraction crescent.

The vitreous will undergo degenerative changes. It will separate from the retina at the posterior pole-posterior vitreous detachment. The vitreous liquefies and patient will experience the phenomenon of floaters.

There will be generalized lose of pigment from the pigment layer of the retina exposing the underlying choroidal vessels. This appearance is called tigroid fundus. Extensive chorioretinal atrophy will occur in the posterior pole. These will appear as patches of white areas surrounded by clumps of pigment. If it involves the foveal area, there will be considerable drop in visual acuity (Figs 10.4 and 10.5).

Lacquer Cracks

Lacquer cracks are breaks in the Bruch's membrane in the posterior pole; seem as irregular branching white line.

Choroidal Neovascular Membrane

Choroidal neovascular membrane (CNM) may grow into the retina through these breaks in Bruch's membrane leading to exudation and hemorrhage into the retina. But they are often self-limiting and not associated with much fibrovascular scarring as in age-related macular degeneration (ARMD).

Forster-Fuch's Spot

Forster-Fuch's spot are raised circular pigmented lesion at the macula that appears following a macular hemorrhage.

Posterior Staphyloma

A thinning and protrusion backwards of the sclera may occur at the posterior pole leading to distortion of the overlying retina and loss of central vision.

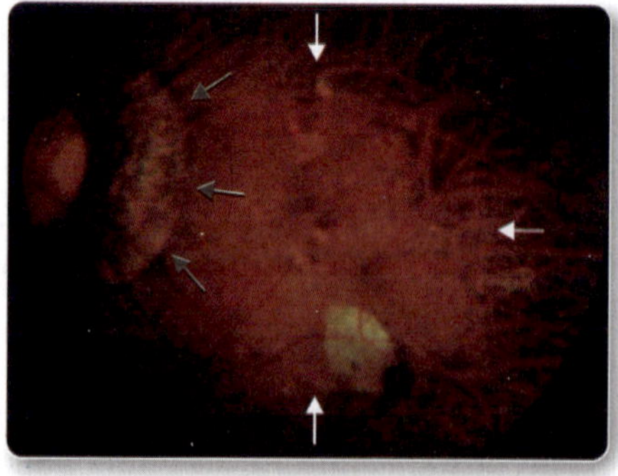

FIGURE 10.4: Myopic chorioretinal degeneration—temporal crescent (black arrows) and chorioretinal degeneration (white arrows)

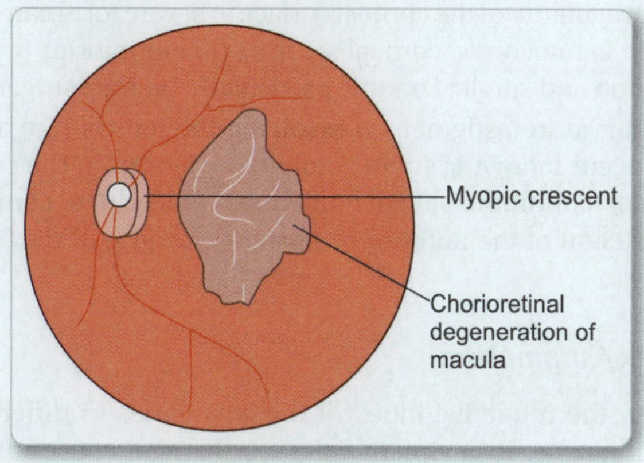

FIGURE 10.5: Myopic chorioretinal degeneration—diagrammatic representation

Peripheral Retinal Degeneration

Pathological myopia is associated with peripheral retinal degenerations like lattice degeneration. This will lead to peripheral retinal holes and subsequent retinal detachment.

Due to these various degenerative changes, people with pathological myopia are at a high risk of loss of vision as age advances.

Clinical Features

In myopia, the parallel light rays from distant objects are brought to a focus in front of the retina. But, the divergent rays from nearer objects will be brought to a focus on the retina (Figs 10.6A and B).

So, myopes can see nearer objects clearly even though distant objects appear blurred. Higher the myopia, the nearer the objects have to be brought to see them clearly. This clear near vision is achieved with little or no effort of accommodation. So, the main symptom in myopia is defective distant vision.

They usually do not have symptoms of eyestrain because little effort of accommodation is used to see clearly. But, people with high errors have to hold looks close to the eye to read. This excessive convergence with little accommodation will disturb the normal relationship between accommodation and convergence. The eyes tend to abandon the efforts for convergence and one eye will diverge, while the other eye takes up fixation. So, uncorrected myopia can be associated with unilateral or alternating divergent squint.

Treatment

Spectacles

Concave lenses will make the parallel light rays divergent, so that they can be brought to a focus on the retina (Figs 10.7A and B).

So, appropriate concave lenses should be prescribed to correct the refractive error.

As the child grows, the eyeball continues to enlarge and myopia increases. So, regular checkup at 6 month to 1 year intervals and change of spectacles are required till the power becomes steady. This usually happen at 20–25 years of age in simple myopia, but may continue to progress in pathological myopia.

Contact Lens

The advantage of contact lens over spectacles is better peripheral vision and normal-sized images, since the lens is placed closer to the eyeball. Concave lenses cause decrease in size of the images, more the effect higher the power of lenses. The disadvantage of contact lenses is the higher risk of corneal infection, if proper cleaning precautions of the lenses are not followed, since the lens is remaining in contact with the cornea (Table 10.1).

Refractive Surgeries

Refractive surgeries alter the curvature of the cornea and bring the light rays to a focus on the retina. For example, laser-assisted in situ keratomileusis (LASIK).

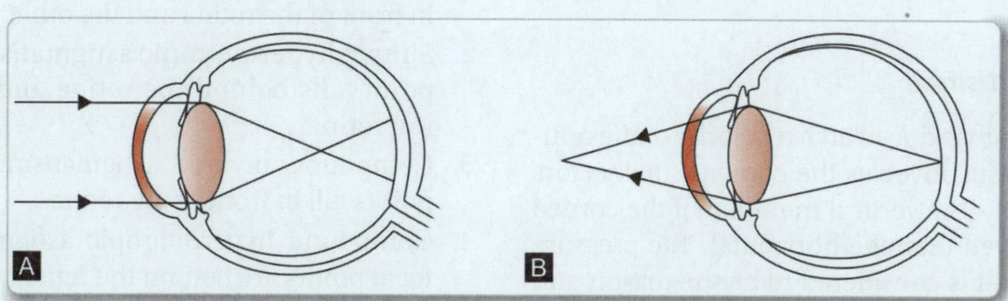

FIGURES 10.6A and B: Focusing of parallel light rays. **A.** In front of retina; **B.** Divergent light rays on the retina in myopia.

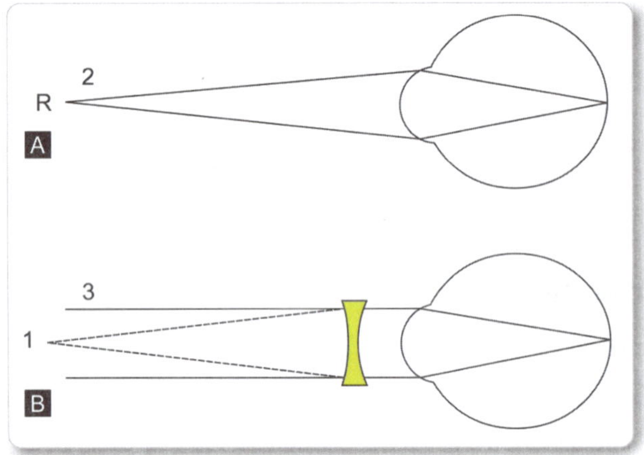

FIGURES 10.7A and B: In myopia. A. Diverging; B. Parallel rays made divergent with concave lenses are focused on retina.

TABLE 10.1: Differences between myopia corrected with spectacles and contact lenses

Myopia corrected with spectacles	Myopia corrected with contact lenses
Smaller the images higher the power	Normal-sized images
Restriction of peripheral visual fields	No restriction of visual fields
Less difficulty in adjusting to wearing spectacles	Insertion and removal of contact lenses need some practice
Less chance of any corneal infection	More chance for corneal infections, if proper cleaning of lenses not followed

ASTIGMATISM

Definition

Astigmatism is that condition of refraction wherein a beam of light cannot form a punctate image on the retina. This type of ametropia is caused by unequal refraction of light in different meridians of the optical system of the eye.

Causes

Curvature Astigmatism

Curvature astigmatism is due to an irregularity of the optical surface. This mostly involves the cornea. Small errors are universal. Usually, the vertical meridian of the cornea is slightly more curved than the horizontal. The pressure from the upper eyelid is considered to be the reason and this small amount of astigmatism (about 0.25D) can be considered physiological.

Irregularity of the corneal surface in severe form can occur in keratoconus, corneal scarring due to injuries or ulceration and surgical trauma particularly cataract surgery.

Curvature astigmatism involving the lens is rare and can occur following subluxation of the lens or in the congenital condition called lenticonus, wherein a conical protrusion of the anterior or posterior surface of the lens occurs.

Index Astigmatism

When the refractive index of the lens varies in different meridians as in incipient cataract, this can cause index astigmatism.

Decentering

If the principal axes of the various refractive surfaces are not in a straight line, this can cause astigmatism. This can occur in subluxation of the lens.

Types

Where the change in the curve occurs in a gradual fashion and the two principal meridians of least and greatest curvature are at right angles it is called regular astigmatism.

Usually, these two meridians are vertical and horizontal. If the two meridians are at right angles, but they are not vertical and horizontal, it is called oblique astigmatism. If the two principal axes are not at right angles it is called bi-oblique astigmatism.

If the curvature is irregular and does not follow any pattern, it is called irregular astigmatism.

The common physiological type of astigmatism where the vertical meridian is more curved than the horizontal, it is called direct astigmatism or astigmatism with the rule. The opposite condition where the horizontal meridian is more curved is called indirect astigmatism or astigmatism against the rule.

Depending on the relationship between the focal points and the retina, regular astigmatism can be clarified as:

1. Simple myopic astigmatism: Here, one focal point falls in front of the retina and the other one on the retina.
2. Simple hypermetropic astigmatism: Here, one focal point falls behind the retina and the other one on the retina.
3. Compound myopic astigmatism: Here, both focal points fall in front of the retina.
4. Compound hypermetropic astigmatism: Here, both focal points are behind the retina.
5. Mixed astigmatism: Here, one focal point is behind the retina and the other one is in front of the retina.

Sx **Symptoms**

Here, the eye is unable to bring the light rays to a focus from distant as well as near objects. The eye constantly tries to focus one of the focal lines—the vertical focal line is usually preferred. During near work, constant efforts of accommodation are made to bring objects to a sharp focus especially in hypermetropic astigmatism. This usually happens in small errors. In large errors the focal points will be so far away that the eye abandons all efforts to focus the image. So, small errors of astigmatism will produce marked eyestrain whereas in large errors the only complaint will be defective vision. There will be complaints of distortion of images—circles will appear oval, rectangles appear as trapezoid and lights appear to tail off. People tend to squeeze the lids together to make stenopaic slits, so that one meridian is cut off and objects appear more distinct. In oblique astigmatism, the head is kept tilted to one side to reduce distortion.

Treatment

Spectacles

Even small errors need correction with suitable cylindrical spectacles, so that the patient will have symptom-free clear vision. Careful refraction is needed to determine the axis of the cylindrical lenses and the fitting of the lenses have to be in the correct position because even a 5° difference in the position of the axis of the cylindrical lenses will result in continuing complaints of eyestrain.

Contact Lens

Soft contact lenses are not useful, since they mold on to the corneal contour and the astigmatic error will persist. Rigid gas permeable lens are useful in moderate degree of astigmatism. In high errors, special toric lenses (lenses with cylindrical curvature on its surface) are needed to correct the distortion.

Refractive surgeries like LASIK can be done to correct larger errors. When people with larger astigmatic error undergo cataract surgery special intraocular lenses (IOLs) will toric correction (toric IOLs) can be used to correct the astigmatism also.

In severe keratoconus cases if the toric lenses are not giving satisfactory correction or if they are not tolerated, keratoplasty is indicated for correcting the error.

The rare congenital condition called lenticonus will also require removal of the lens and IOL implantation to correct the visual disability.

ANISOMETROPIA

Anisometropia is the condition in which the refraction of the two eyes is unequal. Any type of combination can occur—hypermetropia in one eye and myopia or astigmatism in the other eye or both eyes may be having the same error, but marked disparity in power between the eyes.

Effects

If one eye has normal or near normal visual acuity and the other has marked refractive error and this is left uncorrected, the blurred image from the eye with gross refractive error will be suppressed by the brain. If this is not detected and corrected in early childhood itself, i.e. before 8–9 years, the more ametropic eye develops amblyopia and it will become impossible to improve its vision even with suitable spectacles. This often happens because the child will rarely experience any visual problem, since he has good vision in one eye and a unilateral refractive error will be picked up only in an ophthalmic check up.

The differences in the refractive error will produce a difference in the size of the image—aniseikonia. The concave lens will produce a decrease in the size of the image and a convex lens an increase in the size of the image. So, a difference of more than 5D in the power of the spectacle between the two eyes is rarely tolerated and will lead to diplopia.

If one eye is myopic and the other hypermetropic or emmetropic, the myopic eye will be used for near vision and the other eye for distant vision and this can lead to development of alternating squint.

Anisometropia can influence the development of unilateral squint also; often the deviating eye will be having ametropia.

Management

Anisometropia has to be detected in early childhood itself and corrected to prevent amblyopia. In an infant, this can be done by the mother herself. Occlude one eye with mother's hand and then the other eye, while the baby is playing. If the child sits passively when one eye is occluded, but protests and tries to pull away mother's hand when the other eye is occluded, this mean the first eye is having poor vision.

All children should be screened for any refractive error in the preschool age itself and suitable spectacle correction should be given and if there is anisometropia parents should be instructed to make sure that the children wear the spectacles constantly. If there is marked anisometropia and some amblyopia in the eye with high error, intermittent occlusion for the better eye should be given. Occluder is worn over the better eye and the child is asked to do some near work like reading, drawing pictures, etc. with the amblyopic eye alone. Thus, the brain will be forced to use the amblyopic eye and it is stimulated to overcome the amblyopia and to improve its visual acuity.

If the error is large and it is difficult to tolerate spectacles, contact lens can be given. The contact lens being closer to the eye produces minimal change in the size of the image and hence will be better tolerated in anisometropia than spectacles.

Refractive surgeries like LASIK are another solution, if contact lenses are not tolerated, when the person becomes older and the refractive error becomes stable.

AMBLYOPIA

Amblyopia is a condition of reduced visual acuity in the absence of any structural abnormality in the eye or visual pathway to account for the poor vision.

Etiology

At the time of birth, the retina, the visual pathway and the visual functions are quiet immature. The proper development of visual function depends on proper stimulation of the retina with clear image. The critical age during which the vision develops is up to 3 years. The reciprocal is also true, if there is any interference with the formation of clear image on the retina during this critical period of development of visual function, vision will be affected in spite of proper anatomical development of the retina and the visual pathway. This will result in the condition called amblyopia. The effect will be more, if one eye is normal and the image formed on the other eye is of subnormal quality. In this situation, there will be active suppression of the impulses from that eye with preference for the eye with normal image.

Even if amblyopia develops in this early age up to 3 years; this amblyopia can be reverted by specific treatment after correction of the cause for improper visual stimulation. This is possible to some extent up to the age of 8–9 years. After this age, it is rarely possible to improve vision in the amblyopic eye.

Causes

Strabismic Amblyopia

Strabismic amblyopia is due to unilateral squint. In the squinting eye, the image of the object of interest will be falling in some part of retina other than the macula and the image of another object will be falling on the macula. The attempt to fuse the dissimilar images will lead to suppression of the impulse from the squinting eye and the development of amblyopia.

Anisometropic Amblyopia

Anisometropic amblyopia is due to difference in the refraction between the two eyes. There will be differences in the size of the images also, even if the refractive error is corrected with spectacles. This will lead to amblyopia of the eye with poorer vision.

Stimulus Deprivation Amblyopia

If there is unilateral cataract or corneal opacity or ptosis covering the pupil, this will lead to form deprivations of the affected eye and consequently amblyopia.

Isoametropic Amblyopia

Isoametropic amblyopia occurs in high refractive error due to vision deprivation. It is bilateral.

Meridional Amblyopia

Meridional amblyopia occurs in astigmatism. It can be unilateral or bilateral and results from vision deprivation in one meridian.

Diagnosis

Diagnosis is by excluding any organic cause for the decrease in vision and also by the presence of any abnormality that can lead to amblyopia, e.g. unilateral squint, unilateral refractive error or anisometropia.

We can confirm the cause of defective vision as amblyopia by some special tests.

Crowding Phenomenon

If vision is tested with a chart with a single letter in each line the visual acuity will be better in amblyopia compared to a standard Snellen's chart with a row of letters in each line. A difference in visual acuity of two or more lines is significant.

Treatment

Correction of the Cause of Amblyopia

The reason for amblyopia has to be investigated and corrected in early childhood itself before 8–9 years—by giving spectacles, by squint surgery, cataract surgery, etc. Otherwise, the vision loss will be permanent.

Stimulation of the Amblyopic Eye

Along with the correction of the cause for amblyopia, the brain should be encouraged to use the amblyopic or lazy eye by occlusion of the normal eye. If the child is not cooperative for occlusion, penalization is the method that can be adopted. Here, vision in the normal eye is blurred using atropine or other shorter acting mydriatic-cycloplegic, so that the child is forced to use the amblyopic eye.

Objective Method of Refraction

11

Girija Devi PS

RETINOSCOPY

Retinoscopy is the standard technique for assessing the refraction of an eye.

Principle

Retinoscopy is done with a reflecting mirror with a central hole through which the examiner can look or a 'streak retinoscope' can be used. A reflecting mirror reflexes a circular beam of light from a source of light and the streak retinoscope produces a streak of light. The light from the mirror or retinoscope is shown into the patient's eye. This light will illuminate a portion of the retina. The light reflected back would produce an illuminated portion of the pupil. This reflex at the pupil can be seen by the examiner through the central hole in the mirror or the retinoscope. The lenses are tilted gently from side-to-side in the vertical and horizontal meridian and see whether the reflex moves with the mirror 'with movement' or against the movement of the mirror 'against movement'. 'With movement' means, the image is formed between the patient and the examiner. If the image is formed outside the area, i.e. behind the patient's retina or behind the examiner, an 'against movement' is seen.

When the far point of the patient's eye corresponds to the examiner's nodal point, i.e. the image is formed at the nodal point of the examiner; it is called the neutral point or point of reversal.

Neutralization Point

The neutralization point is detected by placing lenses before the patient's eye and repeating the movements of the mirror. If 'with movements' are obtained '+' lens are placed before the patient eye and '–' lens, if the movement is against that of the mirror. At the point of neutralization, the pupil will be completely illuminated or completely dark. Beyond this point, if higher power lenses are placed, the movement of the reflex is reversed.

If the patient and examiner are seated 1 meter apart at the point of reversal, the patient is –1D myopic. If 2 meter apart, it is –2D myopic and if 2/3 meter apart, the patient have –1.5 D myopic at the point of neutralization. When this power is added to the power of lens placed before the patients eye, this will give the refractive power of the patient at that meridian, i.e. if +2D lens was placed before the patient's eye and the patient and the examiner were seated 1 meter apart, the power is +2D + (–1D) = +1D (Fig. 11.1).

Similarly, the neutralization point is found out in the opposite meridian and the retinoscopy reading is expressed as shown in Figure 11.1 as the power in the horizontal and vertical meridian. If there is oblique astigmatism, the movement of the reflex will not be in the same direction as the tilt of the mirror and from the deviation, the axis of astigmatism can be found out. This is much easier if a streak retinoscope is used instead of a reflecting mirror.

Dilation of the pupil makes it easier to visualize the reflex (Figs 11.2A to C). If a cycloplegic like atropine, homatropine or cyclopentolate is used for dilation of the pupil, adjustment in the reading has to be made for the cycloplegic power of the drug used.

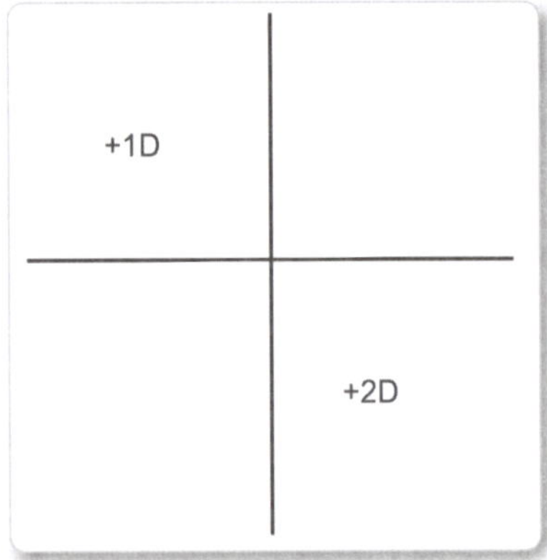

FIGURE 11.1: Retinoscopic reading

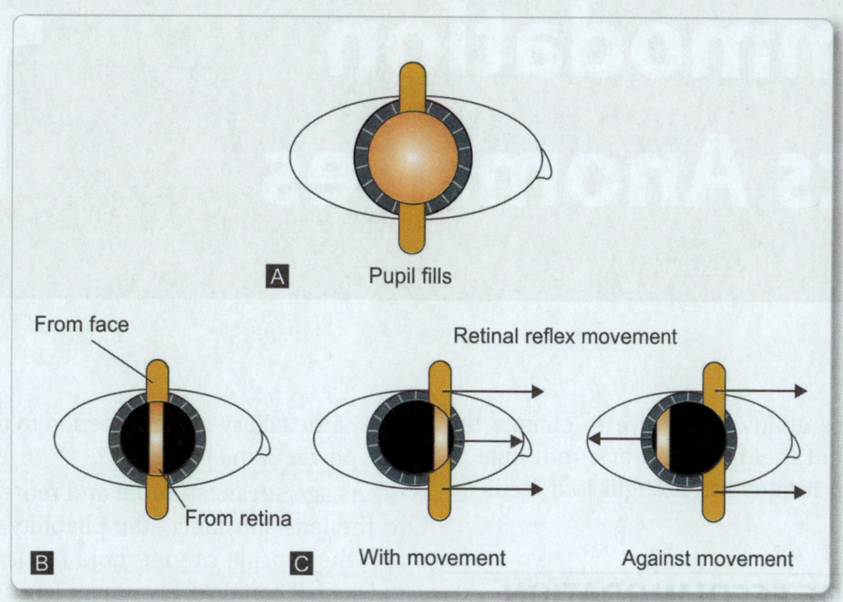

FIGURES 11.2A to C: Principle of retinoscopy. A. Neutralization; B. Streak reflex; C. Retinal reflex movement.

Autorefractometry

Autorefractometry is an automated method to calculate the refractive error. It cannot give an accurate reading, but only an approximate value. Subsequent trial with lens will give the accurate power and autorefractometry will make the trial of lens easier and quicker, especially in illiterate persons and children.

Cycloplegic Refraction—When it is Needed?

If tropicamide is used, which has insignificant cycloplegic effect, no correction for cycloplegia is needed. In children, who have good power of accommodation, the full extent of hypermetropia and hypermetropic astigmatism will be revealed only when the ciliary muscle action is excluded by cycloplegic drugs. In all children with defective vision, cycloplegic refraction has to be done since they have good power of accommodation, which can mask the true extent of refractive error in hypermetropia and hypermetropic astigmatism. In children below 7–8 years owing to the long duration of action of atropine (2–3 weeks), cyclopentolate is often the drug used. In older children, homatropine or cyclopentolate is used. As the child grows and the size of the eyeball increases, the refractive error will also get modified. The hypermetropia will decrease and myopia will increase. The astigmatic error may also progress or recede depending on whether it is hypermetropic or myopic, but to a lesser degree compared to a spherical error. So, the subsequent follow-up of children with hypermetropia or hypermetropic astigmatism require cycloplegic refraction. Since myopia is not influenced by accommodation, the myopic children do not require cycloplegic refraction after the initial assessment. Undilated or dry retinoscopy with a streak retinoscope is sufficient in such children. Adults above 35–40 years, who have minimal accommodation power, usually do not require cycloplegic refraction.

Postmydriatic Test

The refraction done with cycloplegia and mydriasis is unphysiological. Dilatation of the pupil and cycloplegia reveal the spherical and peripheral aberrations of the optical system of the eyes, which are masked in normal stage of pupil and tone of the ciliary muscles. So the refractive error detected by retinoscopy will be modified in real-life situation. So, a trial of lenses has to be done after dilation and cycloplegia wear off and the eye comes back to the normal physiological condition. Small modifications from the refractive state revealed by the retinoscopy have to be made and the spectacle, which is most acceptable to the patient, will be prescribed.

The postmydriatic test (PMT) is done after 3 weeks if atropine is used, after 3 days if homatropine is used and after 2 days if it is cyclopentolate.

Accommodation and its Anomalies

12

Girija Devi PS

Accommodation is the ability of the eye to change the focus of the eye, so that the divergent rays from objects nearer to the eye than infinity are brought to a focus on the retina (Fig. 12.1).

MECHANISM OF ACCOMMODATION

Accommodation is brought about by the contraction of the ciliary muscle. This contraction makes the circle formed by the ciliary muscle, smaller. This relaxes the suspensory ligament, which is normally in a state of tension in the unaccommodated state. The capsule of the lens is naturally elastic and with the release of the pull from the suspensory ligament, the elastic capsule acts on the lens substance and molds it into a more spherical state. The change in the curvature of the lens affects the anterior surface more than the posterior one. In the unaccommodated state, the radius of curvature of the anterior surface is 10 mm. When fully accommodated, it is reduced to 6 mm. This increase in the refractive power of the lens brings the divergent rays from nearer objects also into focus on the retina (Fig. 12.2).

Thus, the act of accommodation has two components:

1. Physical accommodation: It is the actual physical deformation of the lens and expressed in diopters. If the converging power of the lens increases by 1D, the eye is said to have exerted 1D of accommodation.
2. Physiological accommodation: It is the actual contractile power of the ciliary muscle. It is expressed by the unit of myodiopter and it is the contractile power of the ciliary muscle needed to increase the refractive power of the lens by 1D.

As age advances, more and more lens fibers are added to the lens substance, the pliability of the lens decreases and the capsule cannot mold the lens to the same extent to which it can do in a younger lens. Thus, the power of accommodation decreases and results in the condition called presbyopia. Change is mostly in the physical accommodation. Change in the physiological accommodation, i.e. in the contractile power of the ciliary muscle is minimal, but in conditions of debility as when recovering from some serious illness, the physiological accommodation can fail and can result in temporary weakness of accommodation. This can recover fully when the general condition improves.

Presbyopia

Presbyopia is the condition of natural decrease in accommodation with age. Presbyopia is not a refractive error, but a physiological change in accommodation with age.

Amplitude and Range of Accommodation

The farthest distance at which an eye can see clearly is called the far point of accommodation. In an emmetropic eye, this point is at infinity. The nearest point at which a person can see objects clearly, exerting maximum accommodation is called near point of accommodation.

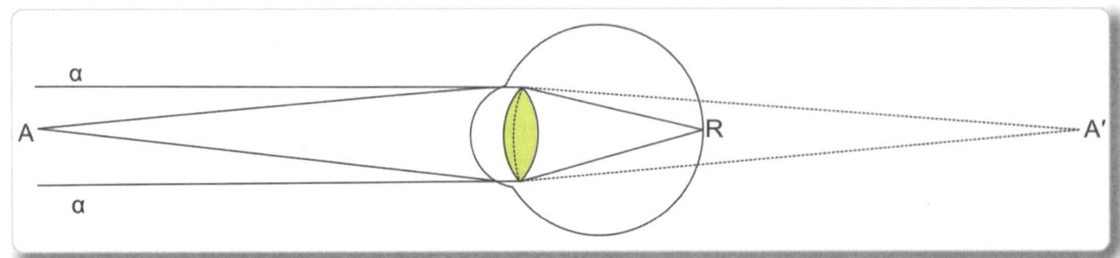

FIGURE 12.1: Diverging light rays from point A come to a focus behind the retina at A′ in the unaccommodated state. On increasing the curvature of the lens by the effort of accommodation, light rays get focused on retina.

The difference between the refractivity of the two eyes when at rest and when fully accommodated gives the amplitude of accommodation. In an emmetropic person, the far point is at infinity and the near point is at 10 cm in the eye of a 20-year-old person. So, the amplitude of accommodation is large.

Hypermetropic Eye

If one follows the pathway of light rays, the parallel light rays from a distant object come to a focus behind the eye and the person has to exert the power of accommodation equivalent to his/her hypermetropia to see distant objects clearly. If he/she has hypermetropia of 2D, the far point is ½ meter, i.e. 50 cm behind the eye; he/she has to exert 2D of accommodation to see distant objects clearly. Since a hypermetropic person has to exert accommodative power to bring the far point on the retina, he/she is at a disadvantage compared to an emmetropic. To see nearer objects clearly, person has to exert accommodative power equivalent to the refractive power + accommodation effort to bring the divergent rays from nearer object to focus on the retina. So, depending on his/her degree of hypermetropia, the demands he/she places on his/her ciliary muscles is higher and his/her near point will naturally be farther from the eye compared to an emmetrope (Figs 12.3A to C).

For a myopic eye, the far point is at a definite distance in front of the eye, depending on the degree of myopia. If he/she has myopia of 2D, the far point is ½ meter, i.e. 50 cm in front of the eye.

In a myopic, even though he/she cannot see distant objects clearly, he/she can see near objects clearly without exerting any effort of accommodation. The divergent rays from a nearer object will be focused on the retina without exerting any accommodative effort, which is an added advantage. The near point at which he/she can see clearly will be closer to the eye compared to an emmetropic, again depending on the degree of myopia (Figs 12.4A to C).

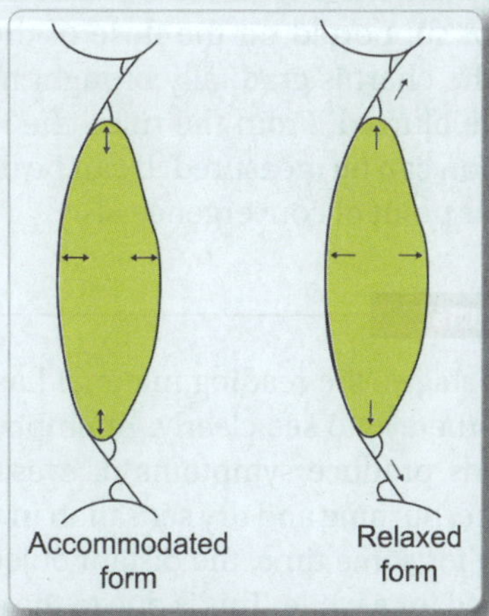

FIGURE 12.2: Effect of contraction of ciliary muscle on suspensory ligament and lens

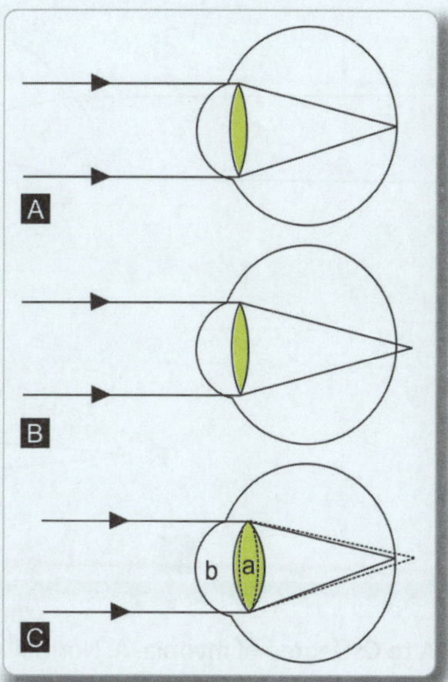

FIGURES 12.3A to C: Emmetropia. **A.** Normal emmetropic eye; **B.** Hypermetropic eye; **C.** Hypermetropia overcome by effort of accommodation.

So, a myope, in the presbyopic age with his/her glasses off, will be able to read small print, which an emmetrope of his/her age will not be able to read. The extent to which this is possible will depend on the degree of myopia. If the myopia is 3D or more, theoretically he/she will never experience presbyopia. But in higher degrees of myopia, the near point will be very close to the eye and comfortable reading will be difficult due to the excessive convergence required. A myope with his/her glasses will be having his/her near point farther from the eye comparable to an emmetrope of his/her age, and will require presbyopic correction added to his/her distant correction as bifocals, to read clearly through his/her glasses.

Normal Changes in Accommodation with Age

Emmetropia

In a child, the near point is at 7 cm from the eye and the amplitude of accommodation is 14D. As age increases and newer lens fibers are added to the substance of the lens, the near point gradually recedes and the amplitude of accommodation decreases. Around 25 years of age, the near point is at 14 cm and the amplitude of accommodation is 7D. Since a normal person usually holds the reading material at

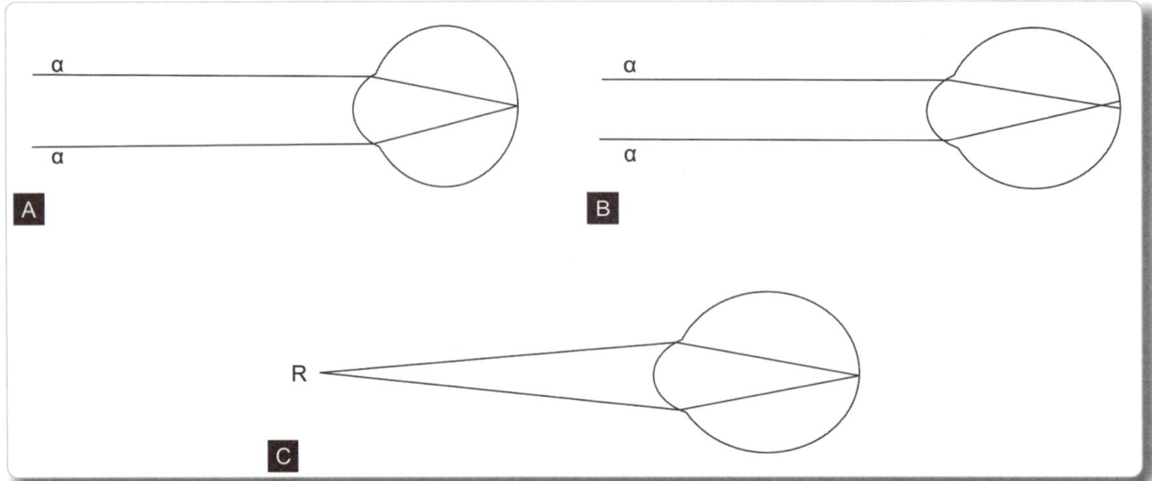

FIGURES 12.4A to C: Degree of myopia. **A.** Normal emmetropic eye; **B.** Myopic eye where parallel rays from far objects focused in front of retina; **C.** In myopic eye light rays from near objects get focused on retina.

a distance of 30 cm from the eye, this is a comfortable situation. But the near point continues to recede and the amplitude of accommodation to decrease. At 40–45 years of age, the near point reaches 30 cm, the usual distance of holding reading material. In this situation to see small print clearly, the person will have to exert his/her full power of accommodation. For comfortable reading continuously, one third of the power of accommodation has to be kept in reserve. So at this age, the accommodation has to be supplemented with +1D convex lens for comfortable reading.

As age increases, accommodation power decreases further and the power of the reading glass have to be increased further. At the age of 60, usually +3D glasses are needed for near vision and further addition is usually not required as age advances.

Hypermetropia

Hypermetropia persons have their near point farther away compared to an emmetrope and they have to exert an additional accommodative power equivalent to their refractive power to see distant objects clearly. So, symptoms of presbyopia will appear earlier in a hypermetropia.

Myopia

Myopic persons can see near objects clearly without exerting any accommodative effort and their near point is nearer to the eye compared to an emmetrope. So, symptoms of presbyopia appear later and if the refractive power is –3D or more, symptoms of presbyopia will never appear. The person can read comfortably without any near vision correction all through his/her life.

But in hypermetropia and myopia, the situation becomes almost similar to that on an emmetropic, once the refractive error is corrected with spectacle. So, a myopic person of 45 years or more, have to take off his/her glass to read small print or add near vision correction to his/her spectacle power and use bifocals.

The presbyopia is a relative term related to the age of the person, refractive power and whether using glasses for correction of refractive error, etc.

Measurement

The near point of accommodation can be measured with royal air force (RAF) rule (Figs 12.5A and B).

This equipment has a near vision chart mounted on a ruler. It is kept supported on the nose of the person examined and the chart is gradually brought nearer till the letters become blurred. From the ruler, the near point of accommodation can be measured. It can be used for measuring the near point of convergence also.

Sx Symptoms

In the initial stages, the reading material has to be held farther from the eye to see clearly. Attempts to read for longer periods produce symptoms of eyestrain, headache, eye ache, burning and dry sensation in the eye, etc. After reading for some time, the distant objects may appear as blurred for a while. This is due to the ciliary muscles going into spasm and artificially inducing myopia. As age advances all near work becomes impossible.

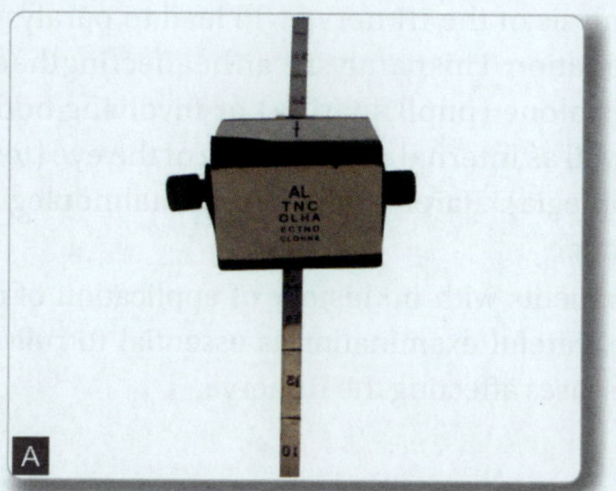

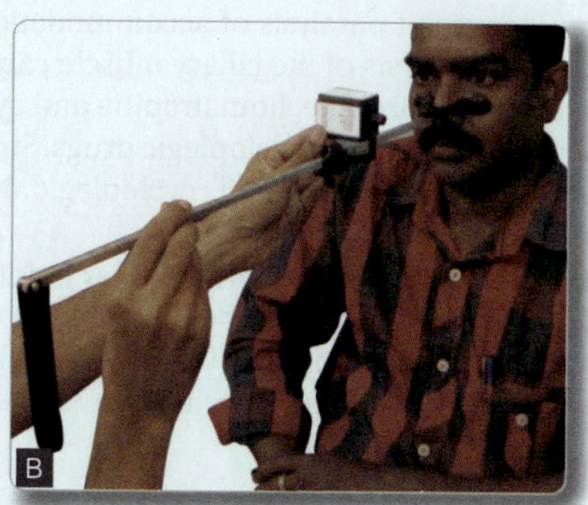

FIGURES 12.5A and B: Royal air force (RAF) rule and measuring near point

Treatment

Suitable spherical lenses can be used for near work as simple reading glasses. People who have refractive errors have to wear bifocals with the near vision correction added to the distant vision power in the reading segment. For example, for a hypermetropia needing +2D for distant vision and +1D for near vision, the power of the spectacle will be +2D in the upper segment and +3D in the bifocal segment for near work. For a myopia of -2D requiring +1D for near work, the power of the spectacles will be -2D in the upper segment for distant vision and -1D for the near vision segment.

Other Methods for Presbyopic Correction

- Presbyopic contact lenses
- Presbyopic laser-assisted in situ keratomileusis lasik (LASIK)
- Multifocal intraocular lenses (IOLs) when patients undergo cataract surgery.

Second sight: When a presbyopic person develop nuclear cataract, the increase in the refractive index of the nucleus will compensate for the presbyopia and he may start seeing nearer objects better, even though the distant vision is now blurred. He may find that he can read small print without spectacles, which he was not able to do earlier. This is called second sight. This is usually a temporary phenomenon and as cataract progresses further, the advantage of better near vision will also fail.

Anomalies of Accommodation

Spasm of accommodation: In this condition, the ciliary muscle goes into sustained contraction, which produces pseudomyopia. The distant objects appear blurred, while near vision remains normal. This can occur in uncorrected presbyopia and uncorrected hypermetropia.

Uncorrected presbyopia: The excessive use of the ciliary muscles for clear vision leads to the muscle going into spasm. The distant objects appear blurred often reading for some time.

Uncorrected hypermetropia: In this condition also, excessive use of the ciliary muscle make it go into spasm. The refraction without cycloplegia will appear as myopia—due to sustained contraction of the ciliary muscle. Prescription of this myopic glass correction will only worsen the symptoms. When refraction is done with Atropine, which produces full cycloplegia, the true refractive error—hypermetropia will be revealed. Prescription of this hypermetropic correction will relieve the symptoms.

Use of miotics: Use of Pilocarpine or stronger miotics as Eserine will lead to spasm of the ciliary muscles leading to blurring of vision.

Insufficiency of Accommodation

In this condition, the accommodative power is below the level of what is expected for a normal person of that age. It can occur in conditions of general debility—as in some serious systemic diseases, malnutrition, anemia, etc. It is occurring as a part of general muscular fatigue.

In open-angle glaucoma, rapid decrease in accommodative power and consequently frequent change of glasses for near work can be an early symptom.

Paralysis of Accommodation

Paralysis of accommodation can occur as part of some diseases of central nervous system (CNS) as encephalitis lethargica, CNS syphilis, herpes zoster botulinum toxicity, etc. A weakness of accommodation can occur in Adie's myotonic pupil.

Common cause of paralysis of accommodation is the effect of drugs. Paralysis of the ciliary muscle can be produced by drugs like atropine, homatropine and cyclopentolate. Such drugs are called cycloplegic drugs. Since, they also cause dilatation of the pupil, cycloplegic drugs are mydriatics also.

In paralysis of accommodation, the near point recedes and reading and other work will be difficult. If it is due to the effect of drugs, the condition will revert back to normal, once the effect of the drugs wears off.

Paralysis of the III nerve will lead to paralysis of accommodation. This paralysis can be affecting the external muscles alone (pupil sparing) or involving both external as well as internal musculature of the eye (total ophthalmoplegia). Rarely internal ophthalmoplegia alone can occur.

In patients with no history of application of drugs in the eye, careful examination is essential to rule out any CNS diseases affecting the III nerve.

SECTION 3

Examination of the Eye

Clinical Examination of the Eye

13

Girija Devi PS, Sunil

Proper and careful elicitation of the history of illness and systematic examination are essential for proper diagnosis of any disease.

HISTORY TAKING

Important symptoms in eye diseases are:

- Defective vision
- Pain
- Redness of the eye
- Discharge and/or watering
- Photophobia
- Itching, irritation, foreign body sensation, etc.
- Protrusion/prominence of the eye
- Deviation of the eyes
- Rare symptoms are double vision, leukocoria or white pupil, distortion of images, black spots before the eye, a defect in the field of vision, etc.

Since the posterior segment of the eye consisting of retina, choroid and vitreous does not have sensory nerve supply, diseases affecting these parts produce symptoms, which are solely visual (defective vision, distortion of the images, black spots before the eye, etc.). Diseases of the anterior segment (structures up to the ciliary body) are associated with pain, redness, watering, etc.

Defective Vision

Defective vision can be:

- Painless and progressive
- Sudden and painless reduction
- Sudden painful reduction in vision.

Painless Progressive Reduction in Vision

Painless progressive reduction in vision is commonly due to:

- Cataract (most common)
- Open angle glaucoma
- Diabetic retinopathy (increasing in prevalence now)
- Age-related macular degeneration
- Corneal dystrophy
- Retinitis pigmentosa
- Hereditary macular degeneration
- Compressive optic neuropathy
- Refractive errors: They are the most common cause for defective vision. The decrease in vision shows only minimal progression mainly in the growing period of life. Unlike other causes for defective vision, they can be corrected with suitable spectacles.

Sudden Painless Reduction in Vision

Sudden painless reduction in vision can be unilateral or bilateral. Causes for unilateral loss are:

- Retinal detachment
- Vitreous hemorrhage
- Optic neuritis
- Central retinal artery occlusion
- Ischemic central retinal vein occlusion
- Exudative type of macular degeneration
- Retinal hemorrhage at macula.

Causes for bilateral loss of vision of sudden onset are:

- Methyl alcohol poisoning and other toxic optic neuropathies
- Bilateral cortical infarction
- Bilateral optic neuritis
- Diabetic retinopathy
- Malignant hypertension.

Sudden Painful Reduction in Vision

Sudden painful reduction in vision is due to:

- Acute congestive glaucoma
- Severe anterior uveitis
- Severe trauma to the eye
- Corneal ulcer
- Endophthalmitis.

DISEASES OF THE ANTERIOR SEGMENT

Pain

Pain in and around the eyes is present in anterior segment problems like:

- Acute congestive glaucoma
- Anterior uveitis
- Corneal ulcers
- Orbital cellulitis
- Scleritis.

Optic neuritis produces a mild pain mainly on ocular movements.

Redness of the Eye

Redness of the eye is seen in the following cases:

- Conjunctivitis
- Corneal problems like epithelial defects, keratitis, etc.
- Iridocyclitis
- Acute congestive glaucoma
- Neovascular glaucoma
- Scleritis
- Episcleritis.

Redness is an important symptom in diseases of the anterior segment. Associated symptoms and the nature of congestion on clinical examination will give important clues as to the diagnosis as follows:

1. Redness with some watering alone and no pain or defective vision usually denotes a viral or irritant conjunctivitis.
2. A similar situation of redness, but no pain or defective vision, but the discharge is mucoid or mucopurulent means a bacterial conjunctivitis.
3. Redness with some watering and itching, but no visual problems, pain or discharge denotes an allergic etiology.
4. If there is an associated irritation or foreign body sensation and some drop in vision and pain, a corneal problem should be suspected.
5. If the redness is associated with variable pain along the distribution of the trigeminal nerve (trigeminal neuralgia) and some drop in vision.
6. Iridocyclitis or acute congestive glaucoma may be the reason.
7. Redness in episcleritis and scleritis will be associated with tenderness and there will be no watering or discharge.

Discharge and/or Watering

Watering of the eye will be seen in irritant, allergic conjunctivitis, viral conjunctivitis, keratitis, corneal abrasions, iridocyclitis and acute congestive attacks.

Mucoid or mucopurulent discharge is seen in infections other than viral such as bacterial conjunctivitis or corneal ulcers.

Photophobia

Photophobia symptom is seen when there is irritation of the trigeminal nerve endings as in corneal abrasions or corneal ulcerations and irocyclitis. It is an abnormal sensitivity and discomfort to normal ambient light.

Glare

Photophobia has to be differentiated from 'glare', which is an excessive awareness of light.

Causes

Either excessive light is reaching the retina as in aniridia (absence of iris), dilation of the pupil with mydriatics (commonest cause) or ocular albinism. Glare can be produced by irregular scattering of light in posterior subcapsular cataract.

Itching, Irritation and Foreign Body Sensation

Itching and irritation symptoms are caused by allergic or irritant conjunctivitis and dry eye syndrome.

Protrusion or Prominence of the Eye

Acute proptosis is seen in orbital hemorrhage, orbital cellulitis or orbital emphysema following trauma. Chronic protrusion or prominence of the eye is seen in the following cases:

- Thyroid ophthalmopathy (most common cause for both unilateral and bilateral proptosis)
- Pseudotumor of the orbit
- Advanced retinoblastoma
- Optic nerve glioma (usually in children)
- Optic nerve sheath meningioma (usually in middle age women)
- Cavernous hemangioma (usually in middle age women)
- Capillary hemangiomas (in children)
- Orbital metastasis.

Pseudoproptosis means there is prominence of the eyeball, but there is no true protrusion of the eye as in high myopia and buphthalmos.

Rare Symptoms

Rare symptoms are as follows:

- Double vision
- Leukocoria or white reflex
- Distortion of images
- Black spots before the eye
- A defect in the field of vision.

Double Vision or Diplopia

Double vision or diplopia can be monocular or binocular. Binocular diplopia is caused by a paralytic squint leading to an ocular muscle imbalance. The image of the object of interest is falling on the fovea in one eye only, while in the deviating eye the image is falling on some point other than the fovea and the image of some other object will be falling on the fovea. This leads to binocular diplopia and the diplopia disappears on closing one eye. Uniocular diplopia can rarely occur in situations like large iridodialysis or early cataract.

Leukocoria or White Reflex

Leukocoria or white reflex from the pupil is typically seen in retinoblastoma.

Metamorphopsia

Distortion of images is seen in distortion of the macula with edema fluid as in central serous retinopathy, age-related macular degeneration or diabetic maculopathy. Straight lines will look bent and objects may appear larger than normal (macropsia) or appear smaller than normal (micropsia).

Black Spots or Floaters

Black spots or floaters are seen when there is any vitreous degeneration (as in old age or myopia) or exudation or bleeding into the vitreous (as in chorioretinitis or vitreous hemorrhage).

Defects in the Field of Vision

Defects in the field of vision are seen in retinal detachment. Compressive optic neuropathy or central nervous system (CNS) lesions along the visual pathway can cause similar symptoms.

Colored Halos

Colored halos are rainbow-like rings seen around a bright light source like a lighted bulb and more clearly seen at night. They can occur in conjunctivitis, narrow angle glaucoma and immature cataract. Colored halos in conjunctivitis are caused by flakes of mucus on the cornea and disappear on blinking. In narrow angle glaucoma they occur when there is an acute rise in intraocular pressure (IOP) as in prodromal attacks. These colored halos in glaucoma are usually associated with some decrease in vision and headache and relieved by rest or sleeping. The corneal edema caused by the raised IOP results in scattering of light and this is the reason for the colored halos in narrow angle glaucoma. In immature cataracts colored halos occur in the stage of lamellar separation when the fluid vacuoles in the lens cause the scattering of light. Unlike narrow angle glaucoma the halos in cataract will be constantly present and not associated with headache or rise in IOP. These colored halos of cataract disappear when the stage of lamellar separation is over.

Scintillating Scotoma

Scintillating scotoma occurs as prodromal symptoms of an attack of migraine. They can take various forms. They can appear as black spots or even as hemianopic field defects. These black areas will show flickering spots or lightning-like rays (fortification spectra) or colored halos surrounding them. These visual disturbances will disappear within an hour followed by headache.

Chromatopsia

Chromatopsia (colored vision) occur after cataract surgery or a vitreous bleed. A nuclear cataract will be absorbing blue or red rays excessively and the eye gets adjusted to this. Once the cataract is removed by surgery normal amount of blue or red light will be reaching the retina and the retina shows an increased sensitivity to these rays and patient experiences that all objects are colored blue or red. This will disappear within a few weeks.

Amaurosis Fugax

Amaurosis fugax is a temporary blackout usually unilateral, if the cause is a retinal condition. The cause is transient blockage of circulation to the retina. It can be due to atheromatous plaques or fibrin plaques in valvular diseases causing a temporary blockage of circulation. It can occur as a prodromal symptom of central retinal artery occlusion, optic neuritis and venous stasis retinopathy.

It can rarely be bilateral when the cause is cortical, e.g. uremic amaurosis in nephropathy or eclampsia. The cause in these cases is toxic damage to the brain and usually recovers in 24–48 hours.

Gaze-evoked Amaurosis

Gaze-evoked amaurosis can occur in optic sheath meningioma on looking in a particular direction possibly due to compression of the optic nerve or its blood supply on looking in that direction.

Night Blindness

Night blindness is actually defective vision in dim light. Commonest causes are retinitis pigmentosa, vitamin A deficiency and congenital condition called congenital stationary night blindness.

Functional Visual Loss

Functional visual loss can be:

1. Malingering: Where the person is intentionally feigning blindness for gaining some monetary benefits like insurance claims or in the case of children to avoid school or to gain attention of relatives.
2. Hysterical: Wherein it is a subconscious expression of signs and symptoms of non-organic defective vision. Careful observation and sometimes the help of a psychiatrist may be required to differentiate these two situations:
   a. If it is a case of malingering, the person will be behaving normally when he/she feels that nobody is watching him/her.
   b. The visual disability exhibited by a hysterical person will be fluctuating and usually there will be other evidences of hysterical behavior.

Some tests are sometimes required to differentiate malingering from genuine visual loss.

Bilateral Visual Loss

Pupillary reflexes: If it is malingering, the pupillary reflexes will be normal.

Menace reflex: Reflex closure of the eyes will occur on bringing the hands or some object quickly toward the face. Menace reflex will not be present, if the person is genuinely blind.

Optokinetic reflex: It can be elicited, if it is malingering. This reflex is elicited by rotating a drum with alternate black and white stripes on it. But an intelligent person may fix on some object beyond the optokinetic drum and can confuse the picture.

It is difficult to detect malingering if the person is feigning partial loss of vision of both eyes. In such cases visually evoked potentials (VEP) has to be tested to detect malingering.

Unilateral Cases of Malingering

Certain tests will help to reveal malingering, which are as given below:

1. Look for any relative afferent pupillary defect (RAPD). Presence of a RAPD is against malingering.
2. Place a low power lens like 0.25 or 0.5 before the 'blind' eye and a high power lens like +10D lens before the 'normal eye'. If he/she can still read the vision chart, it means he/she is reading with so called blind eye and malingering is proved.
3. Place a prism with base downwards before the 'blind' eye and ask to look at a light. If he/she admits seeing two lights, malingering is proved. This is because human eye has limited ability to fuse vertically displaced images.
4. Place a 5D or 10D prism before the 'blind' eye with the base outwards. If the eye moves inwards, this means that eye is trying to eliminate diplopia and hence it has good vision. Malingering is proved.

INSTRUMENTS USED IN THE CLINICAL EXAMINATION OF THE EYE

Instruments used in the clinical examination of the eye are usually torchlight and slit lamp for anterior segment examination. Schiotz tonometer and applanation tonometer are used for IOP estimation. Direct ophthalmoscope, 90D lens and indirect ophthalmoscope are the instruments used for fundus examination. The various signs are elicited in an order as follows.

Head Posture

Clinical examination is commenced with 'head posture' of the patient. Head posture can be normal or abnormal. Abnormal head postures are usually seen in III, IV and VI cranial nerve palsies or in restrictive muscle disease. In any cranial nerve palsy, eye will be rotated in the direction of action of the paralyzed muscle. This posture is attained to avoid diplopia. For example, in right VI nerve palsy head will be horizontally rotated (head turn) to the right side. In vertical muscle palsy not only there is head turn, but there is head tilt and chin elevation or depression. For example, in left superior oblique palsy there will be right head turn, right head tilt and chin depression.

Position of the Eyes

Next thing to look for is whether eye is 'orthophoric or orthotropic', i.e. whether eye is straight ahead or not. When we shine a torchlight into the eye, a reflex of the light is falling on the center of the pupil in both eyes when the eye is orthophoric. 'Esotropia' means convergent squint (eye is deviated medially). 'Exotropia' means divergent squint (eye is deviated laterally) (Fig. 13.1).

Lids

Next is examination of the lids. In the lids we should look for any ptosis (drooping of upper lid). Normally upper lid covers the cornea by 2 mm. If it covers the cornea by an extra 1 mm it is mild ptosis, 2–4 mm is moderate ptosis and 4 mm or more is severe ptosis (Fig. 13.2).

We should also look for any lid scar, brow scar, loss of eyelashes (madorosis) or poliosis (white eyelashes). Loss of eyelashes is seen in leprosy and white eyelashes are seen in Vogt-Koyanagi-Harada disease. Any abnormality in the position of the lid margin should also be checked. A rolling in of the lid margin is called entropion (Fig. 13.3) and a rolling out or eversion of the lid margin is called ectropion (Figs 13.4 to 13.6). Any swelling of the lid is also evaluated as to their size and shape, tenderness, fixity to the underlying tissues and vascularity (Fig. 13.7).

Lacrimal Apparatus

The palpebral portion of the lacrimal gland will be visible on everting the upper lid and the patient will look downwards and medially. Enlargement of the lacrimal gland can occur in several conditions such as mumps, Mikulicz's syndrome, etc.

An enlargement of the orbital portion of the lacrimal gland will cause eccentric proptosis with the eyeball displaced downwards and medially.

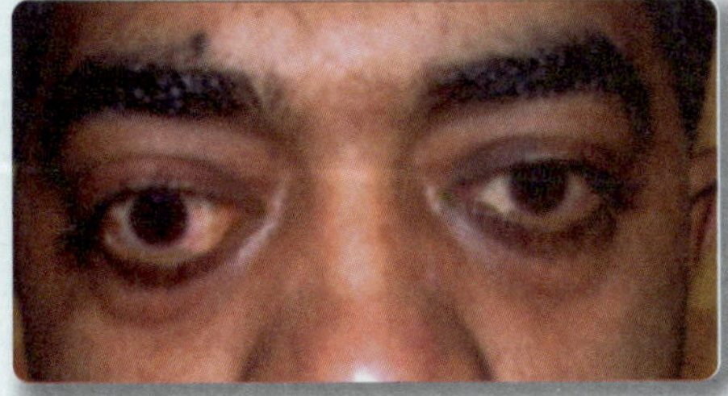

FIGURE 13.1: Right eye proptosed and divergent

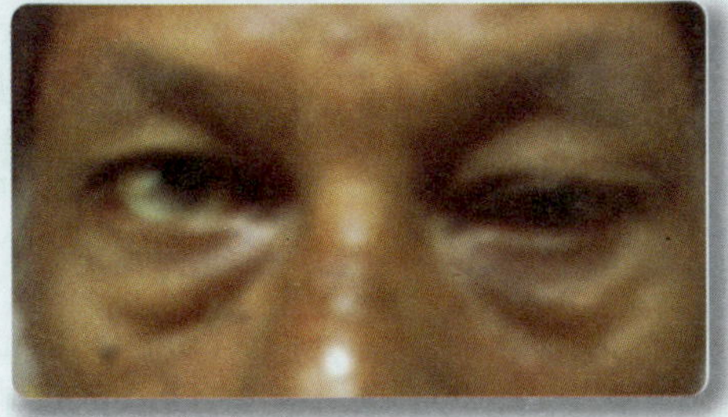

FIGURE 13.2: Ptosis in left eye

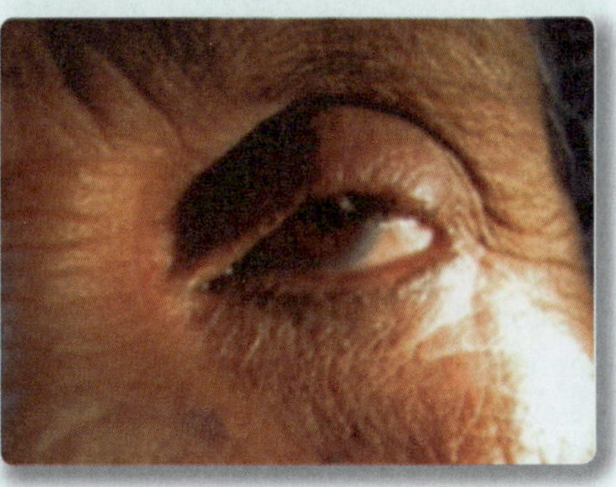

FIGURE 13.3: Entropion with trichiasis

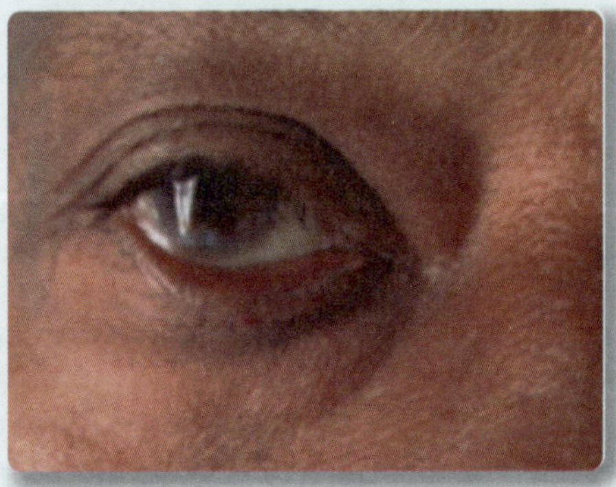

FIGURE 13.4: Ectropion of lower lid

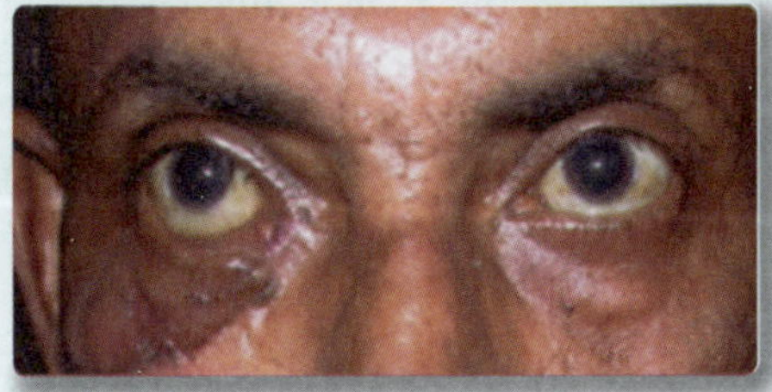

FIGURE 13.5: Cicatricial ectropion

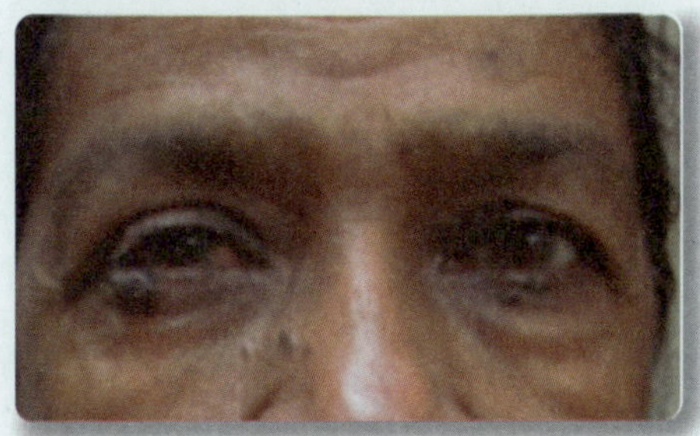

FIGURE 13.6: Pigmented growths on both lower lids

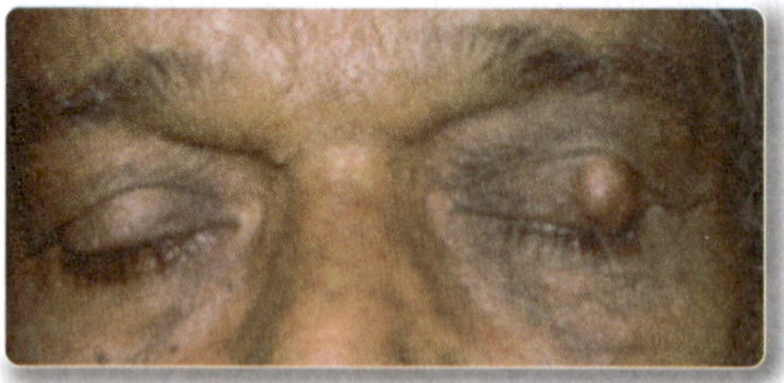

FIGURE 13.7: Meibomian carcinoma, which mimics a chalazion

The lower punctum should be in contact with the eyeball and become visible only by pulling the lid down. If the punctum is visible without pulling the lid down, it means there is eversion of the punctum and can cause epiphora.

Enlargement of the lacrimal sac with retention of tears will form a swelling near the medial canthus in chronic dacryocystitis. Any swelling of the lacrimal sac will appear below the medial palpebral ligament (Fig. 13.8). Any swelling extending above the medial palpebral ligament cannot be a lacrimal pathology. The medial palpebral ligament can be identified by stretching the lids toward the lateral canthus with fingers when the medial palpebral ligament will become prominent.

Conjunctiva

Examination of the conjunctiva includes examination of the inferior and superior palpebral conjunctiva, bulbar conjunctiva as well as the fornices. Pull down the lower lid and look at the inferior palpebral conjunctiva for any congestion or inflammation of the meibomian glands or any foreign body. Then look at the interpalpebral conjunctiva for any pinguecula, pterygium limbal nodule, etc. If there is any congestion of the conjunctiva, see whether it is circumcorneal congestion or conjunctival congestion. Circumcorneal congestion is seen around the limbus where the fine ciliary vessels are engorged to give a pink zone around the cornea. In typical conjunctival congestion where the conjunctival vessels are engorged, the congestion will be more toward the fornices and the conjunctiva around the limbus will be less affected. Moreover, in conjunctival congestion the individual vessels can be made out clearly branching in an irregular fashion (Figs 13.9 to 13.12). Circumcorneal (ciliary congestion) is seen in diseases like corneal ulcer, uveitis or when there is an acute rise in IOP as in acute angle-closure glaucoma.

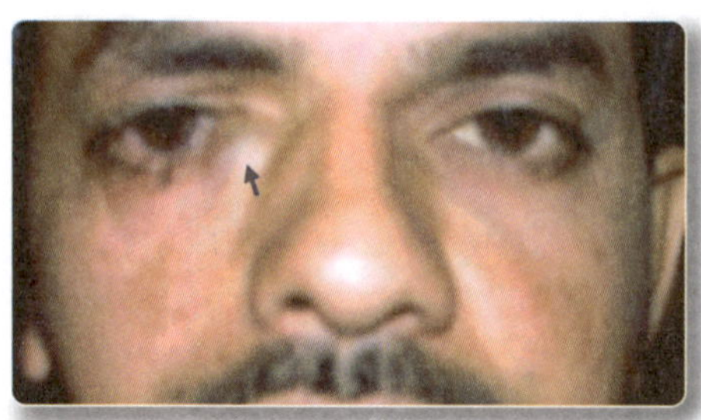

FIGURE 13.8: Swelling of the lacrimal sac

Any swelling of the conjunctiva has to be evaluated for their size, tenderness, type of vascularization (superficial or deep) and fixity to the sclera.

Examination of the upper palpebral conjunctiva requires eversion of the upper lid. Ask the patient to look down and pull the lashes with fingers of one hand, while exerting firm pressure at the upper tarsal border with the index finger of the other hand or a pencil and then roll the lid upwards. The upper tarsal conjunctiva up to the upper tarsal border will be exposed. Inspect the upper palpebral conjunctiva for foreign bodies, papillae, follicles, etc. Papillae are glomeruli-like tuft of capillaries under the conjunctiva, while follicles are aggregation of lymphocytes, which appear as pale tiny protrusions.

Lower fornix is easily visible by pulling the lower lid down, but examination of the upper fornix needs double eversion of the lid. For this, conjunctival sac has to be anesthetized with topical local anesthetic drops. Patient should be relaxed and comfortable and not squeezing the lids. Lying down, relaxed lid is first everted once by pulling the lashes. The exposed upper border of the upper tarsal conjunctiva is gently grasped with a forceps or pulled with a lid retractor, while the patient keeps looking down. The upper lid will be everted once again and the upper fornix will become visible. This double eversion of the lid is important when a foreign body at the upper fornix is suspected.

Sclera

Next is examination of the sclera. Look for any deep congestion, which is usually localized. Deep scleral or episcleral congestion is seen as a purplish-red zone where the individual vessels are not made out. This may be either scleritis or episcleritis. In scleritis, the congestion will be more and there will be more tenderness. To differentiate between these two conditions, ask the patient to close the eyelids and press the area of congestion. In scleritis, patient will try to withdraw the head because of the severe tenderness. In episcleritis, the patient will tell there is tenderness in the area of pressure (he/she will not withdraw the head as in scleritis) (Fig. 13.13).

A scleral staphyloma is seen as a bluish bulging of the sclera. It can be an intercalary, ciliary, equatorial or posterior staphyloma depending on its situation (Fig. 13.14).

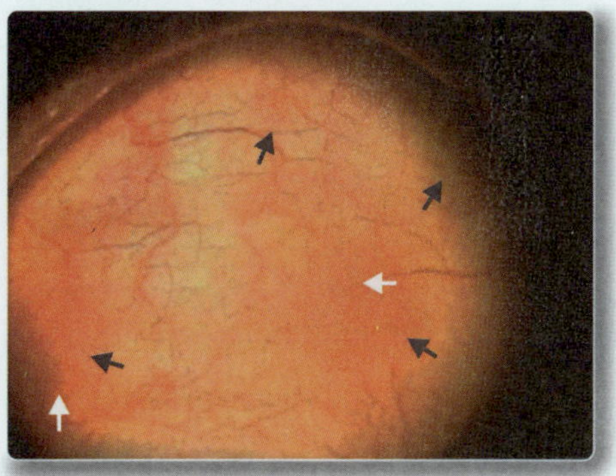

FIGURE 13.9: Superficial congestion (black arrows) and deep congestion (white arrows)

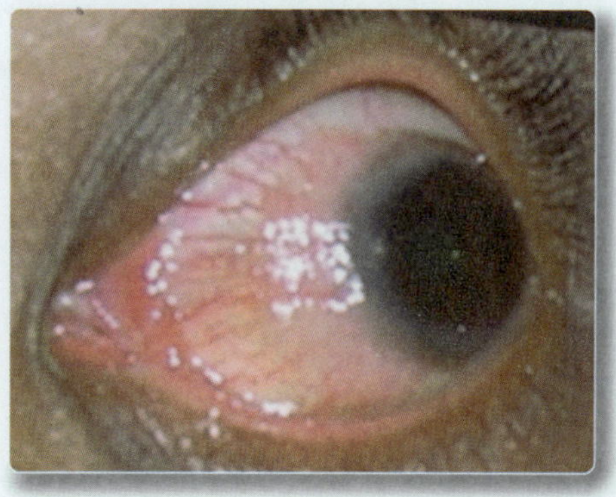

FIGURE 13.10: Circumcorneal congestion

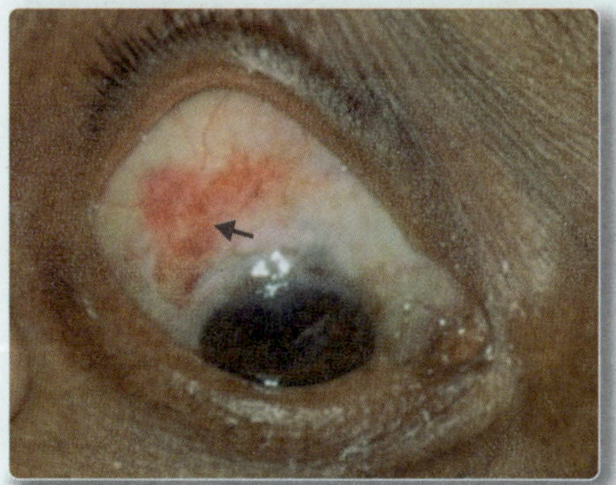

FIGURE 13.11: Subconjunctival hemorrhage

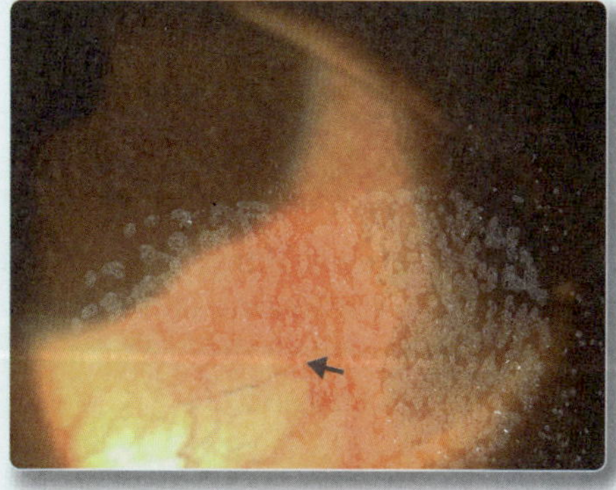

FIGURE 13.12: Swelling at the limbus with deep congestion and feeder vessel (black arrow)

Cornea

Look for the size, the shape, any loss of transparency, any vascularization, superficial or deep and check the corneal sensation.

An increase in the size of the cornea is seen in megalocornea (Fig. 13.15) and buphthalmos (Fig. 13.16). A decrease in the size of the cornea is seen in the congenital conditions such as microcornea or microphthalmos.

A conical protrusion of the cornea is seen in keratoconus (Fig. 13.17) and a globular protrusion in keratoglobus. An acquired protrusion of the cornea can occur in keratectasia or anterior staphyloma. Keratectasia is a simple protrusion of the cornea caused by a structural weakness due to disease or injury. An anterior staphyloma is an ectatic scar of the cornea to which the iris tissue is adherent. Look for arcus senilis, any corneal opacity, corneal infiltrate, corneal ulcer or corneal edema, which can affect the transparency of the cornea.

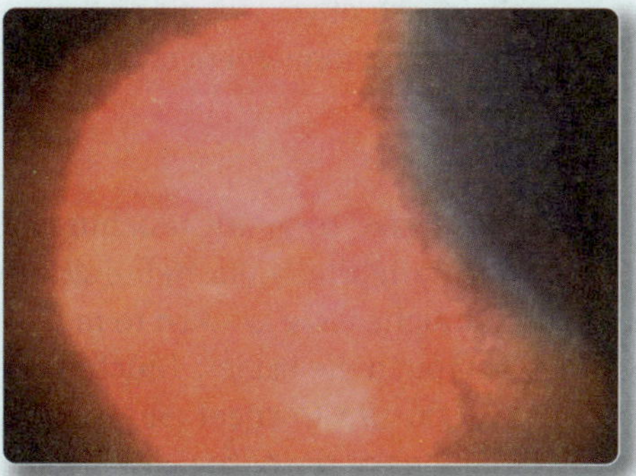

FIGURE 13.13: Scleritis

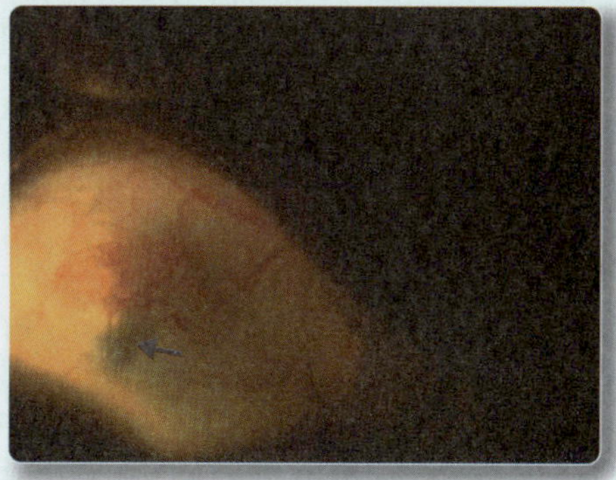

FIGURE 13.14: Scleral staphyloma

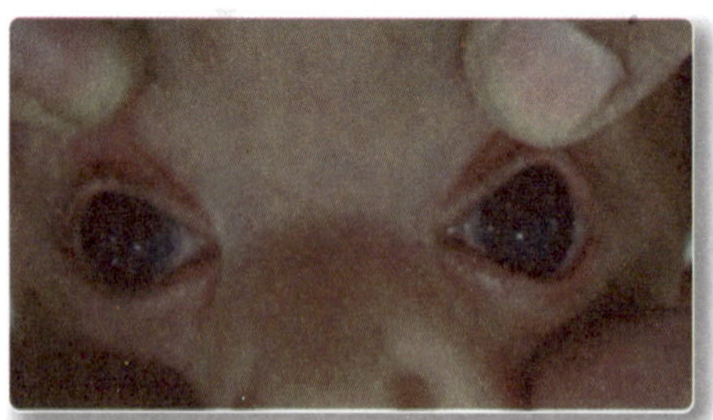

FIGURE 13.15: Megalocornea

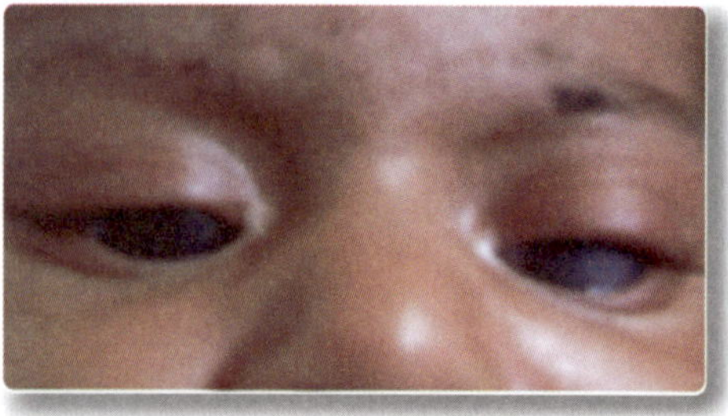

FIGURE 13.16: Buphthalmos

Arcus Senilis

Arcus senilis is seen as a white ring in the corneal periphery with a 1 mm clear corneal tissue between the opacity and the limbus. This is an age-related physiological change seen in the elderly and has no practical significance.

Corneal Epithelial

Corneal epithelial defects can be identified by looking carefully at the corneal reflex. If there is an epithelial defect that area shows an irregularity of the corneal reflex. After staining it with fluorescein dye the area denuded of epithelium will take a green stain.

Corneal Edema

The cornea will have a hazy appearance like a glass on which steam has deposited and the surface may show tiny elevations due to collection of fluid under the epithelium (bullous keratopathy).

Corneal Ulcer

Corneal ulcer can be differentiated from a corneal opacity by the break in the surface epithelium with slough or whitish infiltrate underneath. Being an active inflammatory condition, a corneal ulcer shows symptoms and signs of inflammation like redness, watering, photophobia, etc. A corneal opacity is not associated with signs or symptoms of inflammation. Also the surface will usually be smooth with intact epithelium and it will not be taking any staining with fluorescein (Figs 13.18A and B).

Avascular Cornea

Normally cornea is avascular. Any blood vessels in the cornea are abnormal. Superficial vessels are bright red in color and individual vessels can be clearly made out branching in an irregular fashion. Deep vessels appear as purplish in color (since they are seen through overlying stroma).

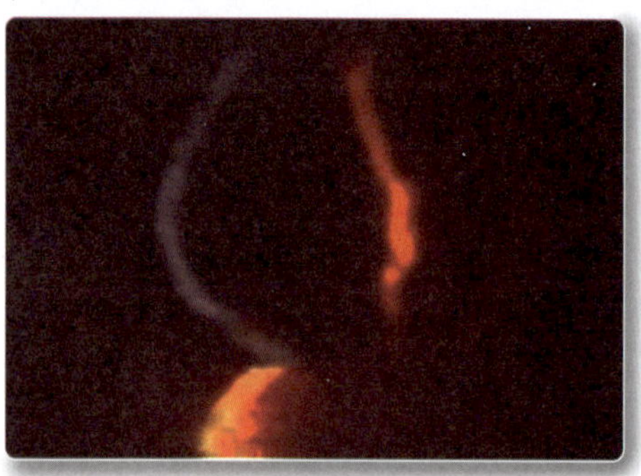

FIGURE 13.17: Keratoconus

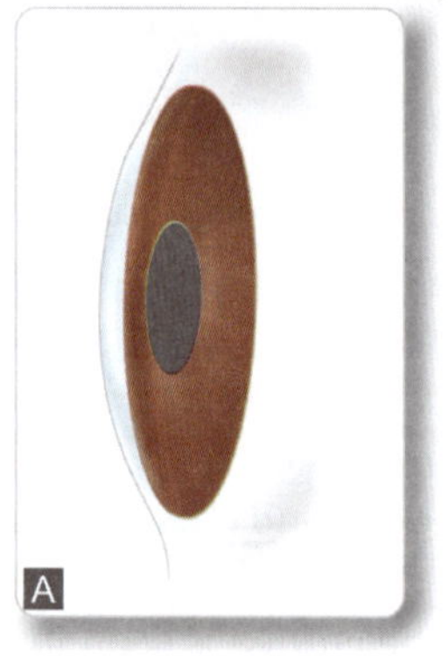

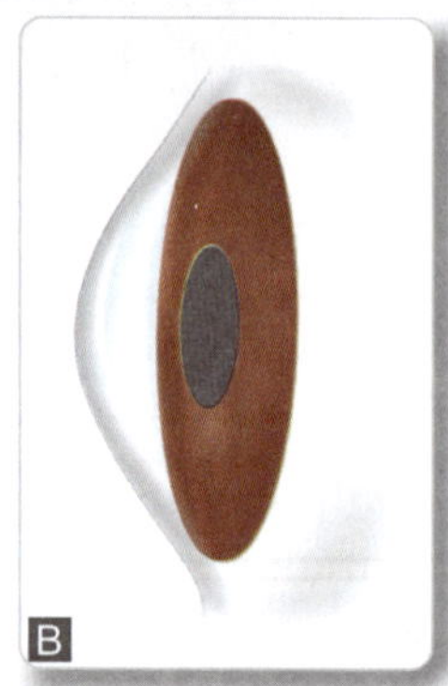

FIGURES 13.18A and B: Changes in corneal curvature. **A.** Normal cornea; **B.** Keratoconus.

It is difficult to make out the individual vessels and they appear as a parallel leash of vessels, since their growth is restricted by the parallel arrangement of corneal lamellae.

Corneal Sensation

Corneal sensation is tested by gently touching the cornea with a tiny wisp of cotton brought from the side, while the patient is looking straight. Care is taken to make sure that the cotton does not touch the lashes. Touching the lashes can cause a brisk lid closure. Corneal sensation will be deficient in viral infections of the cornea and lesions affecting the trigeminal (Fig. 13.19).

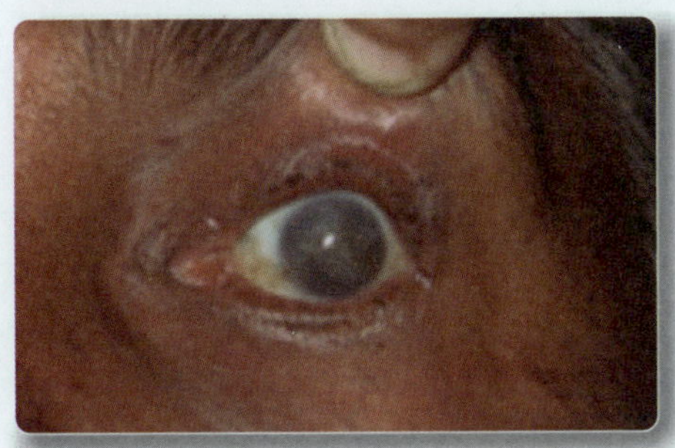

FIGURE 13.19: Corneal opacity

Back Surface of the Cornea

Back surface of the cornea should also be looked for keratic precipitates in uveitis. They can be made out only with the help of a slit lamp.

Anterior Chamber

Look for the depth of the anterior chamber, any irregularity in its depth and any abnormal contents. Normal depth of the anterior chamber is 2.5 mm in the center. Anterior chamber is normally shallow in extremes of age. A shallow anterior chamber is seen in narrow angle glaucoma and anterior subluxation of the lens. A deep AC is seen in iridocyclitis, aphakia and posterior dislocation of lens and in iridocyclitis with posterior synechiae. In iris bombe, the AC will be funnel shaped deep in the center and extremely shallow in the periphery. An irregular depth is seen in subluxation of the lens or ciliary body tumors pushing from behind.

The abnormal contents can be pus (hypopyon) as shown in Figures 13.20A to C, blood (hyphema) as shown in Figures 13.21A to C pigments (black hypopyon) or tumor cells (pseudohypopyon).

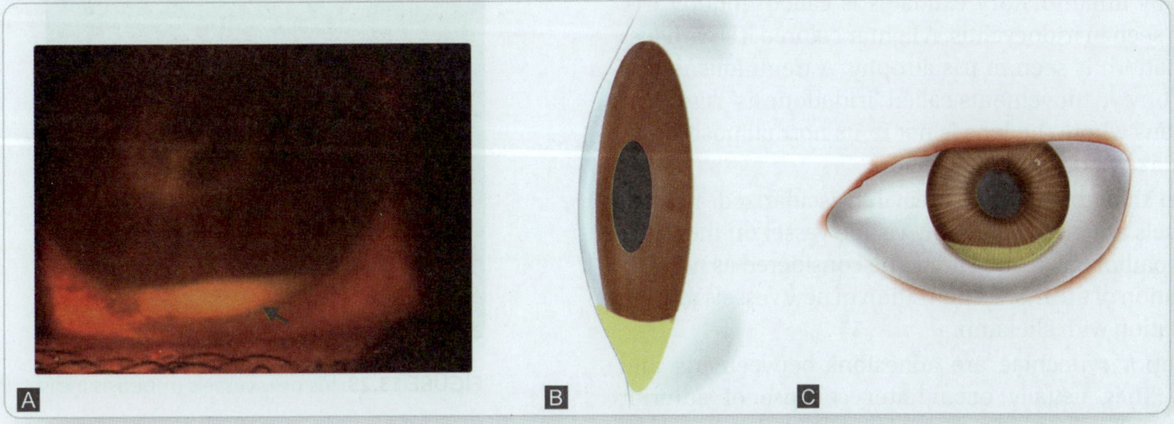

FIGURES 13.20A to C: Hypopyon. **A.** Photograph of hypopyon uveitis with exudates in the papillary area and pus filling the lower part of anterior chamber (black arrow); **B and C.** Diagrammatic representation of hypopyon.

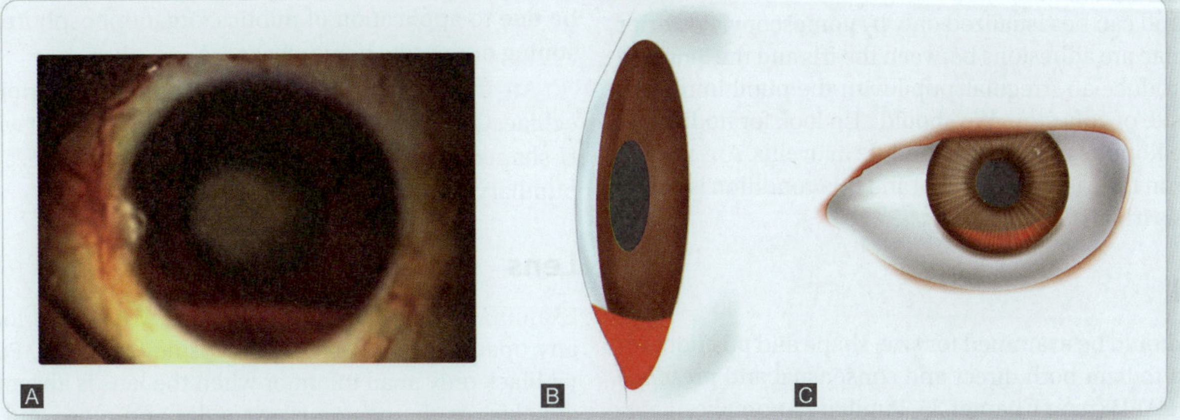

FIGURES 13.21A to C: Hyphema. **A.** Photograph of hyphema; **B and C.** Diagrammatic representation of hyphema.

Anterior chamber should be examined under the slit lamp for cells and flare. It is examined with a slit beam of size 2 × 1 mm under higher illumination and magnification.

Iris

Next is examination of the iris. Note the color of the iris, iris pattern, any nodules or new vessels on the iris surface or for the presence of any anterior or posterior synechiae (Fig. 13.22).

The color of the iris depends on the racial characteristics. It can be blue in Caucasians, while dark brown in Asians and Africans. A difference in the color between the two eyes is called 'heterochromia iridum.' It can occur in 'heterochromic cyclitis of Fuchs.' A difference in the color in different parts of the same iris is called 'heterochromia iridis.'

The iris surface shows a characteristic pattern with many crypts and the collarette. An indistinct iris pattern caused by inflammatory exudates is called 'muddy iris' and it is seen in iridocyclitis. A lighter colored iris with loss of iris pattern is seen in iris atrophy. A tremulousness of the iris on eye movements called 'iridodonesis' is seen in conditions where the lens is not in its normal position as in aphakia or posterior dislocation.

Even though the iris is heavily vascularized, normal iris vessels are not visible. Any visible vessel on the iris is usually pathological and should be considered as neovascularization of the iris. Visualization of new vessels require examination with slit lamp.

Anterior synechiae are adhesions between iris and cornea. They usually occur after collapse of anterior chamber following perforation of a corneal ulcer or a penetrating injury involving the cornea. Toward the anterior synechiae the anterior chamber becomes shallow and the corneal opacity will show pigmentation. Peripheral anterior synechiae occur in the angle in narrow angle glaucoma and can be visualized only by gonioscopy. Posterior synechiae are adhesions between the iris and the lens and they produce an irregular pupil with the pupil immobile at the site of adhesion. We should also look for nodules in iris like Koppe's or Busacca's nodule in uveitis. Any vessels visible on the iris are abnormal and this condition is called rubeosis iridis (Fig. 13.23).

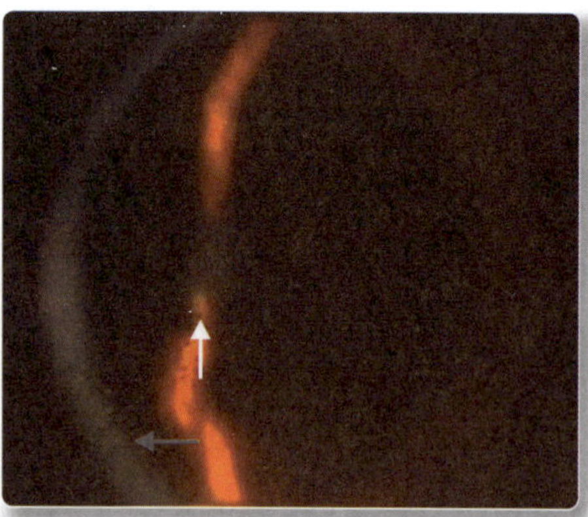

FIGURE 13.22: Keratic precipitates (KPs) (black arrow) and irregular pupil (white arrow) due to posterior synechiae

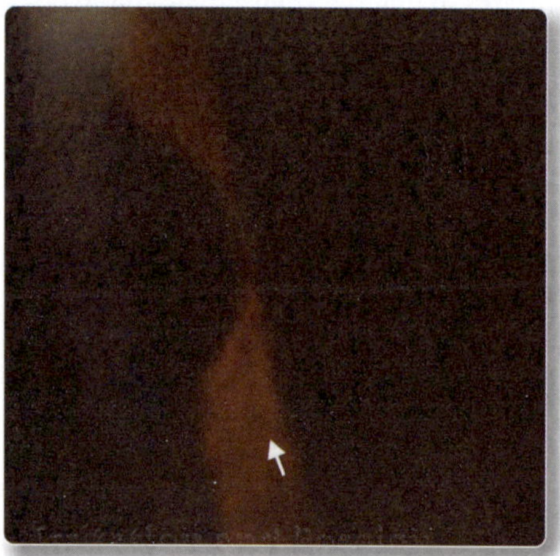

FIGURE 13.23: Iris new vessels (rubeosis iridis)

Pupil

Pupil should be examined for size, shape and position, reactions to light both direct and consensual and presence of any RAPD (refer Chapter 35 'Pupillary Anomalies').

Normally, the pupil is 3–4 mm in size, round in shape and central in position. Pupil will be smaller in babies and old people (senile miosis). A large pupil is usually due to the application of mydriatics. A large pupil can occur in over excited state (due to over action of the sympathetic), III nerve palsy and Horner's syndrome. A small pupil can be due to application of miotics, organophosphorus poisoning or pontine hemorrhage.

An irregular pupil is usually due to posterior synechiae. Coloboma of the iris is a congenital defect where a U-shaped defect is seen in the inferomedial aspect of the pupillary margin.

Lens

Examination of the lens is done next. We should look for any opacity in the lens or its capsule (cataract). Pupil is jet black only in an infant or when the lens is absent as in aphakia. As the person grows older and more and more lens fibers are added, the scattering of light from the lens increases and normally the clear lens will have a gray tint.

This normal appearance of the lens can be differentiated from an early lenticular opacity by examination of the lens after dilatation of the pupil with a slit lamp or by distant direct ophthalmoscopy. With the slit lamp the cataract will appear as gray zones and we can make out the type of cataract; whether cortical, nuclear or posterior subcapsular. In distant direct ophthalmoscopy where the fundus is observed with the direct ophthalmoscope at a distance of 22 cm, the lenticular opacity will be seen as a dark area standing out prominently in the red glow from the fundus. But any opacity in the media, in the cornea, aqueous or vitreous can cause a similar picture. The level of the medial opacity can be determined by noting the parallactic displacement of the opacity on movements of the eye, while the fundus is observed with the direct ophthalmoscope. If the opacity is in the pupillary plane there will not be any movement of the opacity on movement of the eye. Opacities anterior to the pupillary plane will move in the same direction as the movement of the eye, while those behind will move in the opposite direction. The movement will be more, if the opacity is farther from the pupillary plane. If the lens is totally opaque, no red glow will be seen and the pupil will appear as totally dark.

Look for whether the cataract is cortical or nuclear (refer Chapter 18, 'Lens'). In aphakia, the pupil will be jet black in color. Also the anterior chamber will be deep and the iris will show iridodonesis.

A tremulousness of the lens 'phacodonesis' is seen on moving the eyes in subluxation of the lens. In this situation the AC will be irregular in depth—shallow in some areas and deep in some other areas. In gross displacement the edge of the lens may cross the pupil and the pupil will be partly phakic and partly aphakic.

Fundus Examination

Fundus examination (Figs 13.24A to D) is done with direct ophthalmoscope, 90D lens or indirect ophthalmoscope. (refer Chapter 20, 'Retina').

BASIC INVESTIGATIONS

Checking Visual Acuity

Visual acuity of both eyes should be checked separately after occluding the other eye. In people wearing glasses, vision with glasses as well as unaided visual acuity should be assessed. In people with defective vision, vision with pinhole should be checked to determine the presence of refractive error (refer visual functions of the eye).

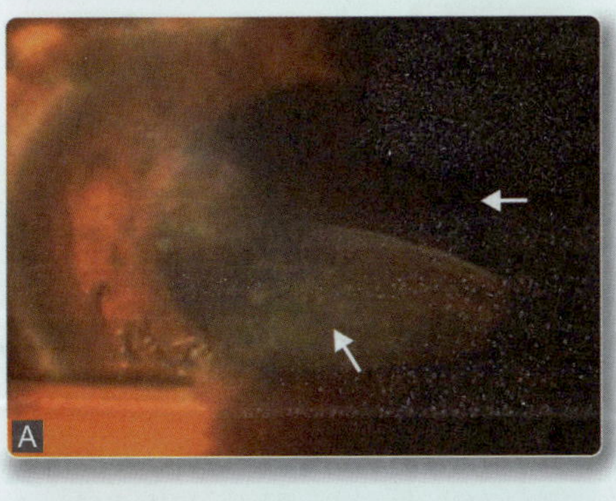

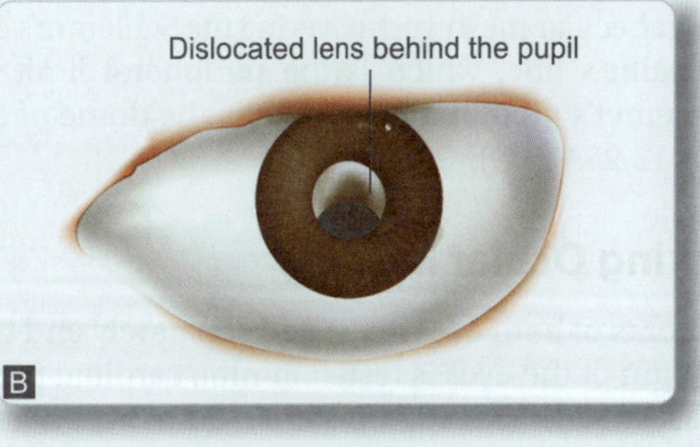

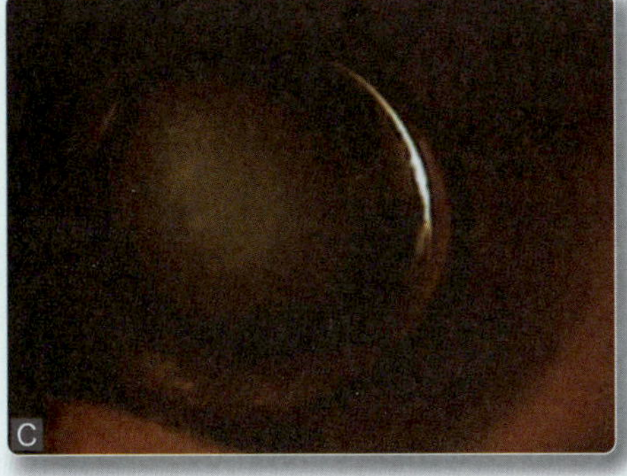

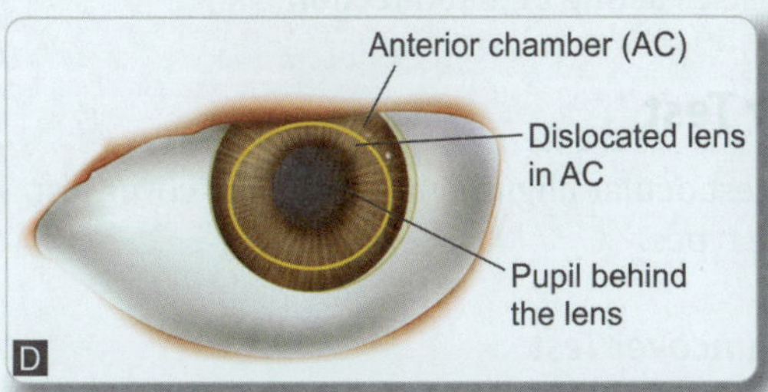

FIGURES 13.24A to D: Displacement of the lens. **A.** Posterior dislocation of lens aphakic portion of pupil (white arrow); **B.** Diagrammatic representation of posterior dislocation of lens; **C.** Anterior dislocation; **D.** Diagrammatic representation of anterior dislocation of lens.

Checking the Intraocular Pressure

Intraocular pressure can be estimated roughly without any instruments by digital tonometry or with Schiotz tonometer or with applanation tonometer.

Digital Tonometry

Digital tonometry is a simple method to detect gross increase or decrease in IOP. Patient is asked to look downwards and tip of both index fingers of the examiner are placed on the upper lid above the tarsal plate. Firm pressure is applied with one finger, while the fluctuation felt at the tip of the other finger denotes the IOP. Details of the methods of checking IOP with various equipments like Schiotz indentation tonometry, applanation tonometry and non-contact tonometry are described with glaucoma.

Gonioscopy

Gonioscopy is the technique to visualize the angle of the anterior chamber. Normally, the scleral ridge at the limbus blocks the view of the angle. A gonioscope is a corneal contact lens with a mirror fitted at an angle of 45°. This mirror reflects the light rays from the angle to reach the observer's eye and the image is viewed with a slit lamp. The structures visualized from behind forward are:

- The peripheral iris
- The ciliary band
- The trabecular meshwork covering the Schlemm's canal
- Schwalbe's line, which is the peripheral limit of the Descemet's membrane and finally the dome of cornea (Figs 13.25A to C).

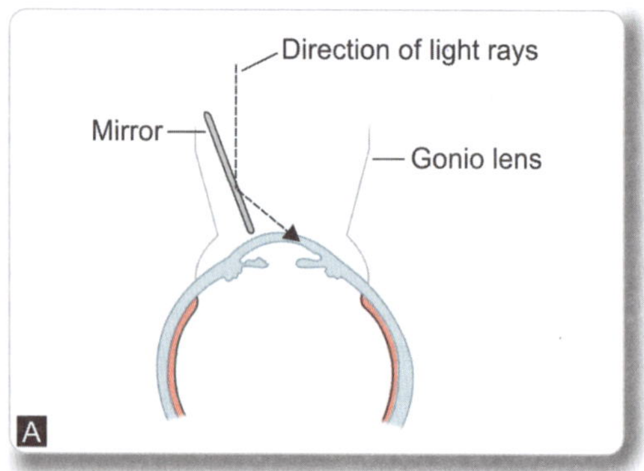

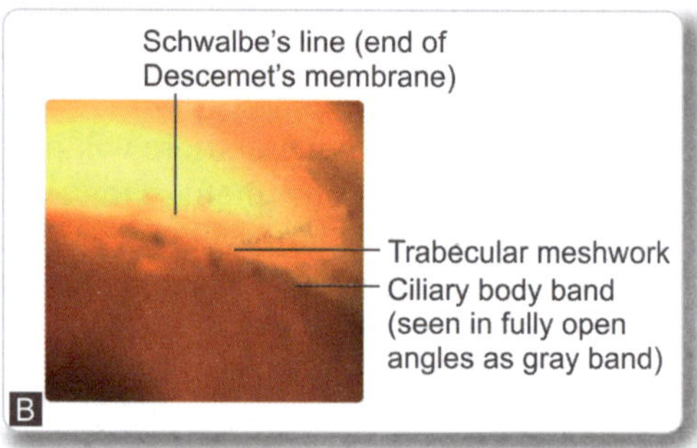

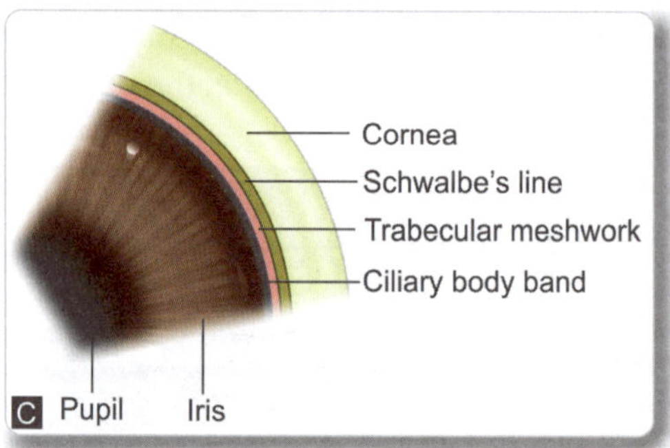

FIGURES 13.25A to C: Gonioscopy. **A.** Genio lens of the eye and the direction of the light rays; **B.** Structures in angle of AC; **C.** Structure in angle (a diagrammatic representation).

Checking Ocular Motility

Movements of both eyes are tested separately and together. Position of the eyes is tested in nine cardinal positions such as straight ahead, upwards, downwards, straight left, straight right, obliquely in right upwards, right downwards, left upwards and left downwards directions. Any limitation in movement means weakness or paralysis of the muscles acting in that direction.

Cover Test

Cover test ocular alignment is tested by cover test. This is of three types.

Cover-uncover Test

Cover-uncover test will reveal any manifest squint. Patient is asked to maintain fixation on a distant or a near object. One eye is occluded and the cover is removed, while losely watching the uncovered eye. If the eye shows a movement when the occluder is removed, that eye is having a manifest squint.

Alternate Cover Test

In alternate cover test the occluder is placed alternatively before either eye, while the patient is maintaining steady fixation on a distant or near object. Any movement of the occluded eye on removal of the occluder is noticed. If eye is showing a movement to take up fixation on removal of the occluder that means the eye was deviating under cover when the stimulus to maintain ocular alignment was temporally suspended by occlusion. This means that person has a latent squint.

Simultaneous Prism and Cover Test

In simultaneous prism cover-uncover test of the fixing eye is combined with the placement of prisms of progressively increasing power in front of the deviating eye till no movements of the eye is noticed. The power of the prism gives the degree of squint.

Hirschberg's Corneal Reflex Test

Hirschberg's corneal reflex test is used in uncooperative patients and also in patients who cannot maintain fixation due to poor vision. A light from a torch is thrown into the eyes and the position of the corneal reflex is noted. If the reflex is at the pupillary margin, that eye has 15° squint, if the reflex is between the pupillary margin and the limbus, it is 30° and if the reflex is falling at the limbus, it is 45° of squint (Figs 13.26A to C).

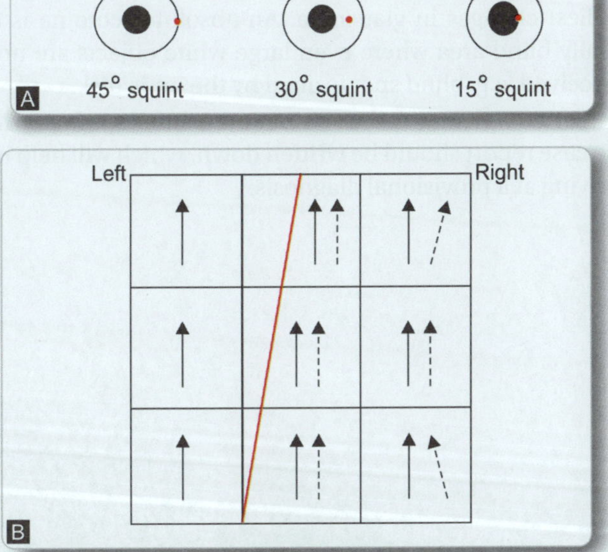

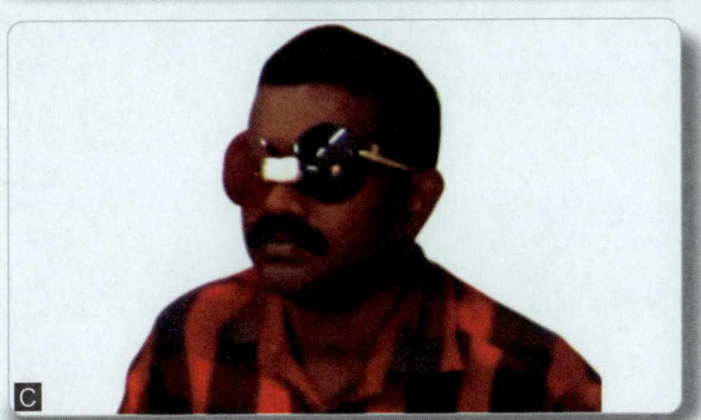

FIGURES 13.26A to C: Hirschberg's corneal reflex test. **A.** Hirschberg's test (red dot denotes the corneal reflex); **B.** Diplopia charting in right lateral rectus palsy; **C.** Patient wearing red-green goggles for diplopia charting.

Diplopia Charting

Diplopia charting test is done in patients who complain of binocular diplopia. A red-green goggle is used for this test. The red is placed before the right eye and the green before the left eye. The patient is asked to keep the eye steady and a torchlight is thrown into the eye through a stenopaic slit from nine cardinal points of the binocular visual field from a distance of 4th feet. The right eye will be seeing a red streak and the left eye a green streak. In areas where there is no diplopia the red and green slits will be superimposed. In the area of action of the paralysed muscle the two images will be seen separately, i.e. diplopia is present. If the image of the right eye is seen on the right side and that of the left eye is seen on the left side it is uncrossed or homonymous diplopia. If the two images cross each other it is crossed diplopia. The images of both eyes in the nine cardinal positions are marked on a diplopia chart (refer Figs 13.26B and C).

Field of Vision

Several computerized perimeters are available for testing the field of vision. A simple method without any equipment is the confrontation test.

Method

The patient and the examiner sit at a distance of 2 feet with their eyes at the same level. The patient closes left eye and looks at the examiner's right eye. The examiner closes right eye. The examiner keeps the hand outstretched midway between them and brings it slowly from the periphery toward the center from above and below, from the right and the left. The patient is asked to tell when he starts seeing the movement of the hand in all the four directions. The test is repeated with the other eye also. The examiner also tries to see the movements of his hand and compares this with that of the patient. Assuming that the examiner's field of vision is normal, it is possible to make an approximate estimate as to whether there is any restriction of the visual fields of the patient. If any defect is suspected detailed evaluation using perimeters is essential.

Normal Extent of the Visual Field

The normal extent of the visual field depends on the color and the size of the target as well as the illumination (Fig. 13.27). The extent of the visual field with a 5 mm white object in good illumination is 60° upwards, 90° outwards, 70° downwards and 60° inwards.

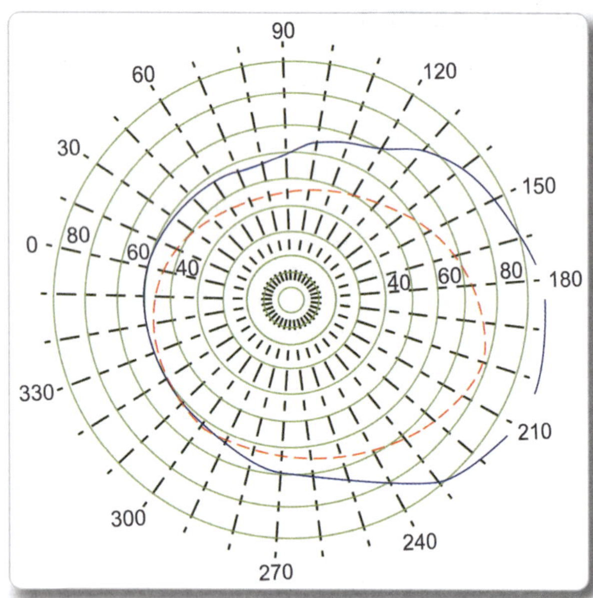

FIGURE 13.27: Normal visual field

Binocular Field of Vision

The binocular field of vision is the extent of the visual fields of both eyes together. It has a large central area common to both eyes and a monocular field on either side temporally. The binocular field of vision extends to 180° outwards, 60° upwards and 70° downwards.

The field of vision for colored objects is lesser than that of white objects, the fields for red and green is more restricted than that of blue and yellow.

Contraction of the Visual Fields

Contraction of the visual fields means the extent of the visual fields is less compared to that of a normal person.

Scotoma

Scotoma is a blind area within a visual field. The blind spot is a normally occurring scotoma in the visual fields of all people corresponding to the optic disk. A relative scotoma is a partially blind area where small objects or colored objects are not visualized. Relative scotomas are one of the earliest changes in glaucoma. An absolute scotoma is a totally blind area where even large white objects are not perceived, e.g. blind spot formed by the optic disk.

On completing the examination a brief summary of the case report should be written down, which will help in arriving at a provisional diagnosis.

SECTION 4

Diseases of the Eye

Conjunctiva

14

Girija Devi PS

Conjunctiva is the transparent mucous membrane covering the ocular surface. It extends from the anterior edge of lid margin where it becomes continuous with the skin of the lids, up to the corneoconjunctival junction (limbus) where it continues as the corneal epithelium. When the lids are closed along with the corneal surface, it becomes a closed space called conjunctival sac.

PARTS OF THE CONJUNCTIVA

The part lining the lid margin is a transitional zone between the skin and conjunctiva and it is called intermarginal strip. The part lining the inner aspect of the lids is called palpebral conjunctiva. The portion covering the eyeball is called bulbar conjunctiva. The junction between the palpebral and bulbar conjunctiva is called fornix. The junction between the bulbar conjunctiva and the cornea is the limbus. The superior fornix is deeply placed and visible only by double exerting the lids. The inferior fornix becomes easily visible by pulling the lower lid down.

ANATOMY

Conjunctiva has three layers.

Epithelium

At the intermarginal strip, it is a transitional zone of stratified epithelium with gradual change of epithelium of the skin to that of conjunctiva. On the palpebral conjunctiva, it is a two cell-layered epithelium. From the fornices to the limbus, the number of layers gradually increases and becomes a stratified epithelium at the limbus.

Adenoid Layer

Adenoid layer is a loose layer of connective tissue containing leukocytes under the epithelium.

Fibrous Layer

Below the adenoid layer comes the fibrous layer containing blood vessels. It becomes denser toward the deeper zones and become continuous with the episcleral tissues with no definite demarcation between the two layers.

The palpebral conjunctiva is firmly adhered to the tarsal conjunctiva. The bulbar conjunctiva is freely movable over the eyeball except at the limbus. Any lesion confined to the conjunctiva moves when the bulbar conjunctiva is moved by firm pressure applied by a finger through the lids.

Conjunctival vessels also move with the conjunctiva when it is moved over the sclera in this manner.

COLOR OF CONJUNCTIVA

Conjunctiva is perfectly transparent only in infants. Continuous exposure to various irritants like ultraviolet (UV) light, dust, etc. gradually lead to change in color and clarity and also leads to various degenerative changes. These normal variations in color and texture have to be differentiated from pathological changes.

BACTERIOLOGY

Conjunctival sac can never be totally free from organism, owing to its exposed position. But organisms rarely survive and proliferate there because:

1. The organisms are continuously washed away with the tears.
2. Conjunctival sac has a lower temperature compared to the body temperature, owing to continuous evaporation of the tears and low vascularity. This does not support multiplication of organisms.
3. Tears contain bacteriostatic enzymes called lysozyme and lactoferrin.

NORMAL FLORA OF CONJUNCTIVAL SAC

Non-pathogenic organisms like *Corynebacterium xerosis (C. xerosis), Staphylococcus epidermidis,* non-pathogenic streptococci, *Micrococcus,* etc.

HEALING OF CONJUNCTIVAL WOUNDS

Healing is rapid even in large wounds, if it is uncomplicated by infection and prolapse of subconjunctival tissues. A loosened conjunctival flap will adhere to the underlying episcleral tissue in 1 hour and the epithelium will cover the defects by an epithelial slide as well as by mitotic multiplication of cells. Even large areas of sclera denuded of conjunctiva will get epithelized in this way within a few days. Scars are hardly visible on the conjunctiva unless a prolapse of subconjunctival tissue has occurred through the wound.

PATHOLOGICAL CHANGES IN THE CONJUNCTIVA

Red Eye

Red eye is the commonest manifestation of any pathological process involving the anterior segment of the eye. It is important to differentiate among:

1. Superficial conjunctival congestion occurring in conjunctival diseases (Fig. 14.1).
2. Circumcorneal or ciliary congestion (Figs 14.2A and B), which denotes a serious problem like:
   a. An infection or inflammation of the cornea.
   b. Inflammation of anterior uveal tissue, or
   c. Any sudden rise in intraocular pressure (IOP).

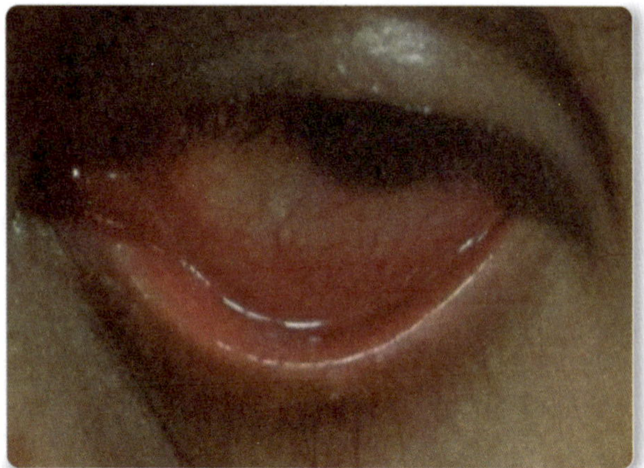

FIGURE 14.1: Conjunctival congestion

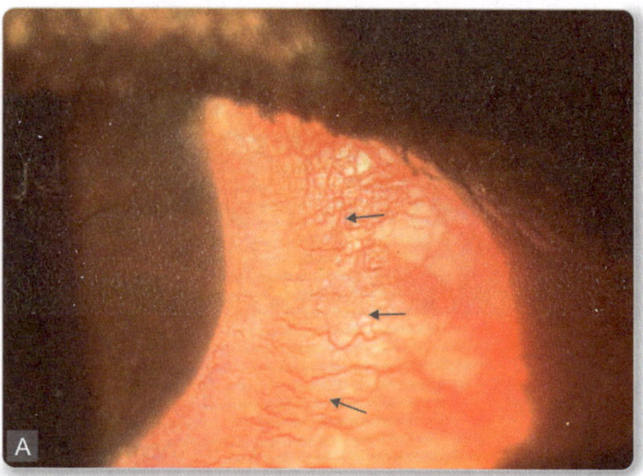

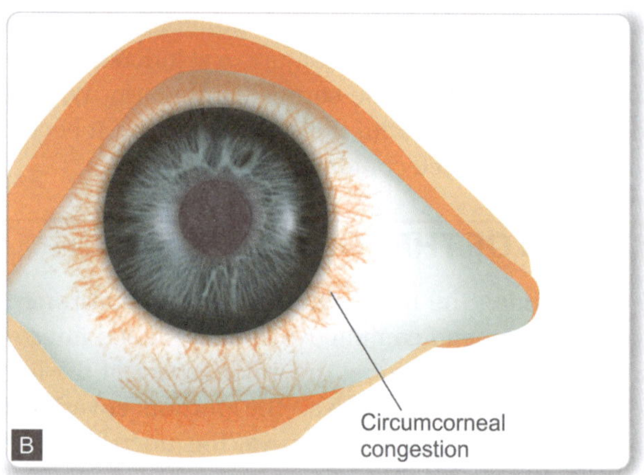

FIGURES 14.2A and B: Circumcorneal congestion. **A.** Photograph; **B.** Diagrammatic representation.

The differences between superficial conjunctival congestion and ciliary congestion are given in Table 14.1.

3. An engorgement of the vessels (Fig. 14.3). This may be:
   a. An anatomical variation.
   b. Due to mechanical obstruction of the circulation as in caroticocavernous fistula or tumor at the apex of the orbit.

Here the veins and venules are dilated and tortuous, but the capillaries are little affected. So, in between the dilated vessels, the conjunctiva appears normal.

Subconjunctival Hemorrhage

Bleeding from the conjunctival vessels appear as bright red sheet of blood in the subconjunctival space. The individual vessels cannot be made out in this area of blood. If there is a pinguecula in the area of subconjunctival hemorrhage (SCH), then it usually does not stand prominently (Fig. 14.4).

TABLE 14.1: Differences between superficial conjunctive congestion and ciliary congestion

Superficial conjunctival congestion	Ciliary congestion
Most intense at the fornix and least toward limbus	Most intense at the limbus, close to the limbus
Conjunctival vessels are bright red and branching irregularly	The deep ciliary vessels appear purple and are radially arranged as fine vessels around the limbus
Conjunctival vessels move with the conjunctiva when it is moved with finger pressure through lower lid	The ciliary vessels are unaffected
The blood flow is from the fornix toward the limbus	In the deeper vessels, the blood flow is from limbus toward fornix
If they are emptied by finger pressure, they slowly fill from fornix toward limbus	If they are emptied, they fill immediately from limbus toward fornix

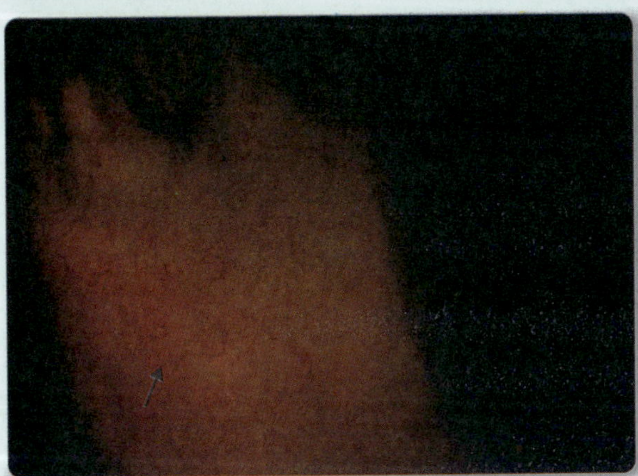

FIGURES 14.3: Engorged conjunctival vessels

Causes

1. Trauma:
   a. Local trauma: It is the commonest cause. Direct injury to the conjunctiva can lead to rupture of blood vessels and spread of blood under the conjunctiva.
   b. Fracture of orbital bones: This can lead to spread of blood under the conjunctiva. The blood usually appears 12–24 hours after the accident.
   c. Fracture of base of the skull: In this situation, blood appears from the fornix toward the limbus on the nasal side. It usually appears 24 hours after head injury. The posterior limit of the such hemorrhages are pathognomonic of fractures of the base of the skull.
2. Sudden and severe venous congestion: This can lead to rupture of small conjunctival vessels and SCH. This can occur in strangulation, paroxysmal bouts of coughing as in whooping cough, vomiting, epileptic fit, etc. Compression of thorax and abdomen in road traffic accidents can lead to SCH in this fashion.
3. Conjunctival infections: It can occur associated with conjunctivitis due to adenovirus, *Streptococcus pneumoniae, Haemophilus influenzae (H. influenzae)*, etc.
4. Fragility of vessel walls as in old people with atherosclerosis, diabetes and hypertension. Mild exertion in such people can rupture a small conjunctival vessel leading to SCH.
5. Blood dyscrasias like leukemia, hemophilia, idiopathic thrombocytopenic purpura (ITP), etc. can cause SCH.

Treatment

No treatment is required. Blood will absorb by itself. This usually takes a few days to 2–3 weeks depending on the quantity of blood. When SCH occurs without any obvious trauma or conjunctival infections, the patient has to be investigated for the presence of any systemic condition that can lead to SCH.

Chemosis

The chemosis (Fig. 14.5) is an edema of the conjunctiva. In a severe case, the bulbar conjunctiva may protrude as giant folds of the inferior fornix between closed lids (Fig. 14.6).

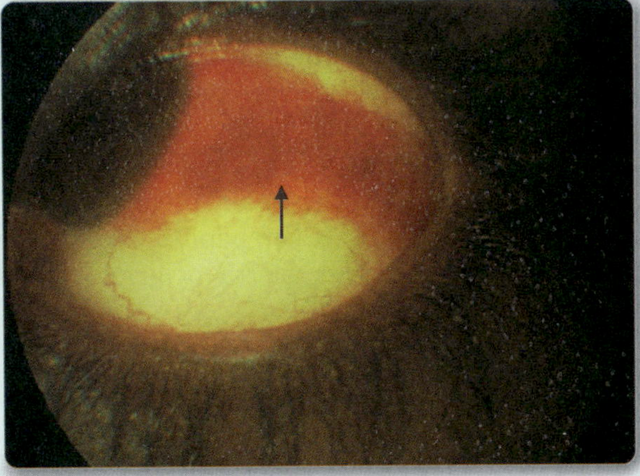

FIGURE 14.4: Subconjunctival hemorrhage

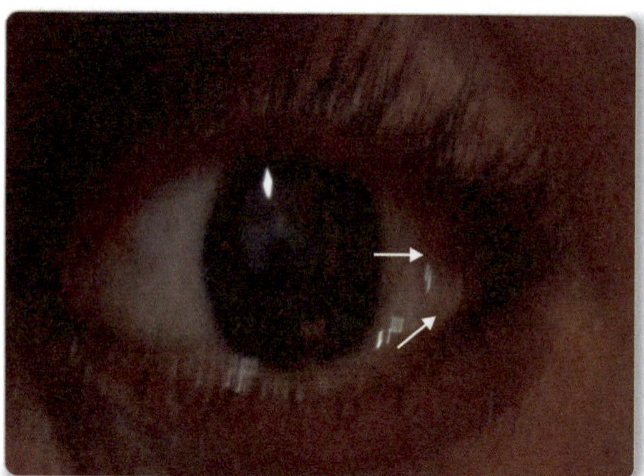

FIGURE 14.5: Chemosis

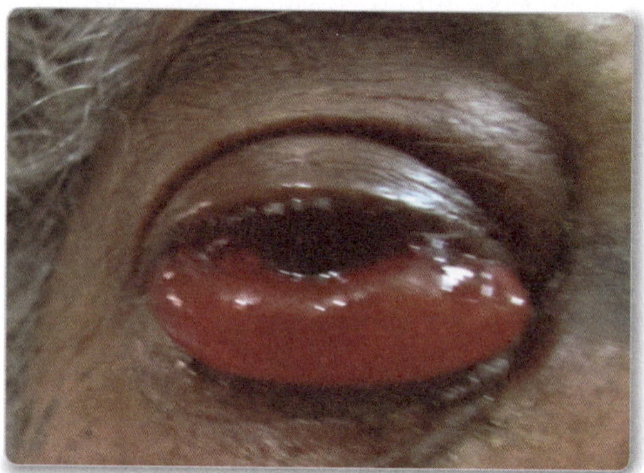

FIGURE 14.6: Severe chemosis

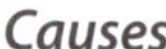

Causes

1. Inflammatory conditions like viral conjunctivitis, any severe inflammation of the anterior segment like severe bacterial conjunctivitis, corneal ulcer or uveitis.
2. Severe infection in surrounding tissues like orbital cellulitis, dacryoadenitis or dacryocystitis can lead to chemosis of conjunctiva.
3. Severe allergic reactions like angioneurotic edema, insect bite, etc.
4. Obstruction to venous circulation at the orbital apex as in tumors and caroticocavernous fistula.
5. Thyrotoxicosis is another cause.

Treatment

Treat the underlying cause.

Papillary Hypertrophy

Papillary hypertrophy is a hypertrophy of the vascular system where a glomerulus-like tuft of new vessels grows into the hypertrophied epithelium. Under the naked eye it is seen as a roughened red conjunctiva, but under the slit lamp the underlying bunch of vessels can be visualized. Papillae are usually seen in any prolonged inflammation of the conjunctiva. Giant papillae are the characteristic feature of spring catarrh or giant papillary conjunctivitis (GPC).

Follicles

Follicles are hyperplasia of the adenoid layer of conjunctiva. It is a tissue reaction to chronic irritation. While papillae are a vascular reaction, follicles are a lymphatic reaction. They appear as multiple discrete pale elevated lesions, often surrounded by a tiny blood vessel. They are more common in the lower fornix except in trachoma where it is more prominent in the upper fornix.

Causes

- Acute viral infection due to adenovirus and herpes simplex
- Chlamydial infection like inclusion conjunctivitis and trachoma
- Allergy to drugs like pilocarpine
- Benign folliculosis in children with adenoids
- Parinaud's oculoglandular syndrome.

Conjunctival Membranes

Pseudomembrane

Pseudomembrane is a translucent pale yellow coagulum of fibrin and leukocytes formed on the palpebral conjunctiva. It can be easily peeled off leaving an intact epithelium.

Causes

Severe infection by adenovirus, gonococci or pneumococci, Stevens-Johnson (SJ) syndrome, etc.

True Membrane

In true membrane, the strands of fibrin firmly permeate among the epithelial cells. Any attempt to peel off the membrane removes the epithelium also, leaving a raw bleeding surface. This feature differentiates it from a pseudomembrane. This can lead to formation of adhesions between the palpebral and bulbar conjunctiva (symblepharon).

Causes

Infection by *Corynebacterium diphtheriae (C. diphtheriae),* ocular pemphigoid and epidermolysis bullosa.

The membranes of lower tarsal conjunctiva and upper tarsal conjunctiva are shown in Figures 14.7A and B.

Cicatrization of the Conjunctiva

Most infections of conjunctiva heal without leaving any cicatrization. The exceptions are trachoma and diphtheritic conjunctivitis. Severe chemical and thermal injuries, epidermolysis bullosa and SJ syndrome are other conditions leading to scarring of conjunctiva.

Symblepharon

Symblepharon is the adhesion between palpebral and bulbar conjunctiva (Fig. 14.8). It is the sequelae when raw surfaces on the palpebral and bulbar conjunctiva remain in contact in the healing stage.

Different Types of Symblepharon

Anterior symblepharon: In this condition the lid margin is adherent to the eyeball. Due to constant movements of the lids and eyeball, these adhesions will become elongated strips of scar tissue between the eyeball and the lid margin.

Posterior symblepharon: Here the adhesion involves the fornices, so that they get obliterated or shallow.

Total symblepharon: Here the two conjunctival surfaces are struck together completely.

Causes

Any severe inflammation leading to cicatrization of the conjunctiva can cause symblepharon formation, e.g. Trachoma, diphtheritic or gonococcal conjunctivitis, Steven-Johnson syndrome, chemical and thermal injuries, and ocular cicatricial pemphigoid.

Complications

Symblepharon can lead to restriction of eye movement and consequently diplopia. Restriction of lid movements can lead to lagophthalmos, exposure keratitis and cicatricial entropion.

Treatment

Prevention of symblepharon formation in situations where it is anticipated, with frequent instillation of lubricating drops and antiseptic ointment. Amniotic membrane transplantation in the 2nd week in severe chemical and thermal injuries, and also in SJ syndrome will decrease symblepharon formation.

Once symblepharon has developed, reconstruction of the ocular surface is done when the inflammation has subsided. Complete excision of all scar tissue is done and the raw surface is covered with a conjunctival autograft, if the other eye is not involved or with amniotic membrane in bilateral cases.

Conjunctival Xerosis

Conjunctival xerosis or xerophthalmia is characterized by dry lusterless condition of the conjunctiva.

Causes

Conjunctival xerosis is due to degenerative changes in the conjunctiva and impaired activity of the mucous glands of the conjunctiva and not due to decreased secretions from the lacrimal glands.

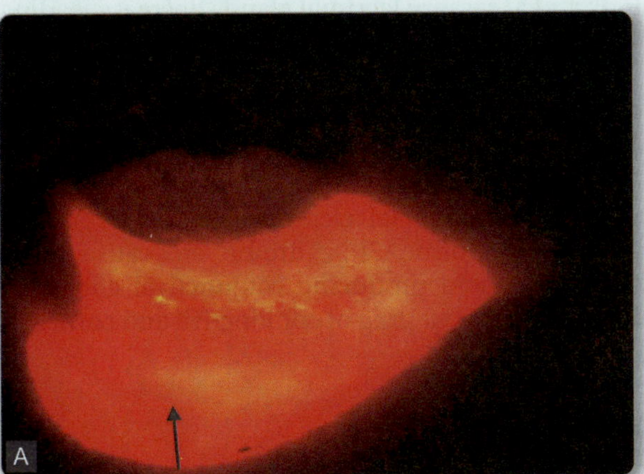

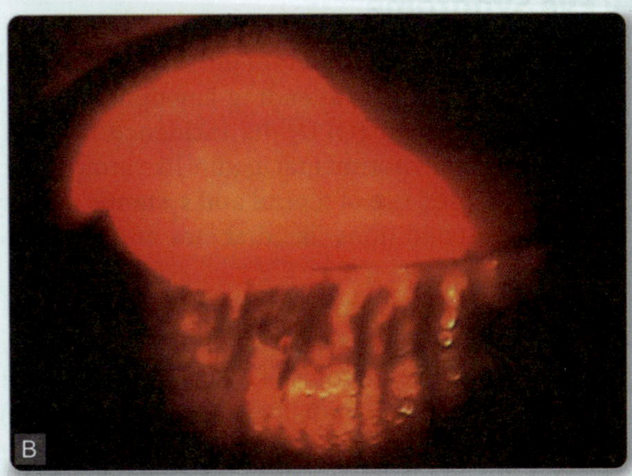

FIGURES 14.7A and B: Conjunctival membranes. **A.** Membrane on lower tarsal conjunctiva; **B.** Membrane on upper tarsal conjunctiva.

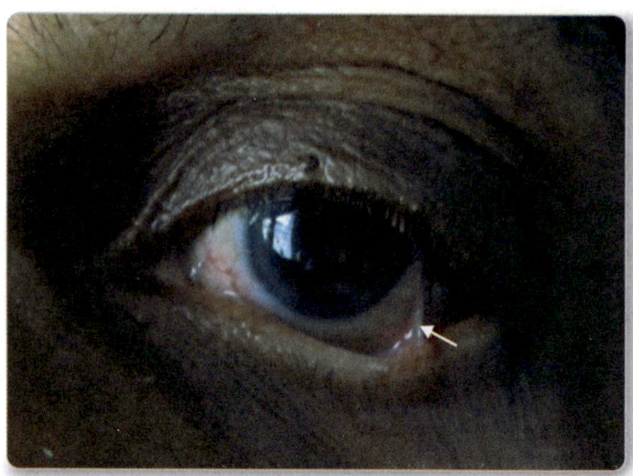

FIGURE 14.8: Symblepharon

Conjunctival xerosis can occur due to local diseases like trachoma, diphtheritic conjunctivitis, chemical and thermal injuries, SJ syndrome, pemphigus, etc. Exposure due to severe ectropion, proptosis or lagophthalmos can lead to xerotic changes on the exposed part of conjunctiva. Vitamin A deficiency is another important cause.

The epithelium becomes epidermoid similar to that of skin. The damaged epithelium gets covered with increased oily secretion from meibomian glands, which further prevents wetting of the epithelium. *C. xerosis* grows profusely within the secretion and hence the name.

Treatment

Treat the underlying cause.

Lubricating eye drops and that containing hydroxypropyl methylcellulose (HPMC), etc. will lessen the symptoms.

Keratoconjunctivitis Sicca/ Dry Eye Syndrome

Keratoconjunctivitis sicca is one of the commonest problems among the patients attending any ophthalmology outpatient department (OPD). Its incidence is slightly increased due to environmental factors like atmospheric pollution, increased use of topical and systemic medications, systemic conditions like diabetes and hypertension, etc.

The term dry eye syndrome has been defined as a multifactorial disease of the tears and the ocular surfaces that results in symptoms of discomfort, visual disturbance and tear film instability with potential damage to the ocular surface. It is accompanied by increased osmolarity of the tear film and inflammation of the ocular surface (DEWS, 2007).

Precorneal Film

Precorneal film plays an important role in maintaining the structural and functional integrity of the ocular surfaces. It consists of three layers:

1. Lipid layer.
2. Aqueous layer.
3. Mucous layer.

Functions of each layer

Lipid layer: It is the outermost layer secreted by the meibomian glands. The functions are:

1. It retards the evaporation of tears.
2. Forms a lubricant for movement of lids over cornea.
3. Also thickens and stabilizes the tear film with the underlying aqueous layers.

Aqueous layer: It is the middle layer secreted by the lacrimal glands. The functions are:

1. The main function is to supply oxygen and other nutrients to the avascular corneal epithelium.
2. Presents smooth optical surface by abolishing any minute irregularities on the corneal surface.
3. Lysozyme and lactoferrin in the tears has some antibacterial action and protect against infections.
4. Helps to wash away epithelial debris, dust, microorganisms, etc. from the conjunctival sac into the lacrimal drainage system.

Mucous layer: It is the inner most layer. It is secreted by the conjunctival goblet cells, the crypts of Henle and glands of Manz.

It forms a loose coating over conjunctival and corneal surfaces rendering their hydrophobic surface wettable by the aqueous layer.

Tear Film Abnormalities

As age advances, the aqueous tear secretion by lacrimal glands and accessory lacrimal glands decrease leading to dry eye.

Patients with Sjögren's syndrome have an autoimmune process leading to lymphocytic infiltration of lacrimal and accessory lacrimal glands resulting in lack of tears.

Diseases that cause chronic inflammation of conjunctiva such as superficial cicatricial ocular pemphigoid, erythema multiforme, SJ syndrome, etc. cause destruction of the mucin producing conjunctival goblet cells. This leads to non-wetting of conjunctiva and cornea, and leads to dry eye.

Mechanism of Dry Eye

Dry eye can be due to:

- Decreased lacrimal secretion

- Increased evaporation
- Meibomian gland dysfunction, which can lead to tear hyperosmolarity.

Dry Eye is a Vicious Cycle

Decreased lacrimal secretion can lead to tear film hyperosmolarity and defective wetting of the ocular surface. This causes damage to surface epithelium. This in turn leads to release of inflammatory mediators, which aggravates the tear film hyperosmolarity by damaging the goblet cells and thus decreasing mucin secretion (Fig. 14.9).

Refractive surgeries, use of contact lenses and topical anesthetics can cause lacrimal hyposecretion by producing neurogenic block.

Types

There are two types of keratoconjunctivitis sicca (KCS):

1. Sjögren:
   a. Primary.
   b. Secondary.
2. Non-Sjögren.

Primary Sjögren's syndrome: This is a dry eye associated with dry mouth (xerostomia), but no other systemic problem will be present.

Secondary Sjögren's syndrome: This is associated with systemic connective tissue disorders like rheumatoid arthritis, systemic lupus erythematosus (SLE), etc.

Non-Sjögren's KCS: This is the more common type, associated with hyposecretion of the lacrimal gland.

Causes

Causes may be:

1. Age related: Tear production decreases with age.
2. The effect of systemic medications.
3. Lacrimal gland obstruction due to conjunctivitis or inflammation.
4. Reflex block from ocular surface as in contact lens wear, refractive surgeries and prolonged use of topical anesthetics.

Evaporative Dry Eye

Evaporative dry eye can be due to intrinsic or extrinsic causes. Intrinsic causes are meibomian gland hyposecretion, low blink rate, etc. which can lead to increased evaporation of tears. Extrinsic causes are vitamin A deficiency, contact lens wear, allergic condition, etc.

Sx Symptoms

Patients rarely complain of dry eye. Usual symptoms are irritation and foreign body sensation caused by the debris in tear film, which accumulate due to slow clearance from the eye. Patients often complain of a pricking sensation caused by the drying of the ocular surface or watering—due to reflex hypersecretion caused by the drying. The symptoms are often worse toward the end of the day when the patient is tired and the blink rate comes down.

Patients with meibomian gland dysfunction complain of heaviness of lids, itching and frequent chalazia.

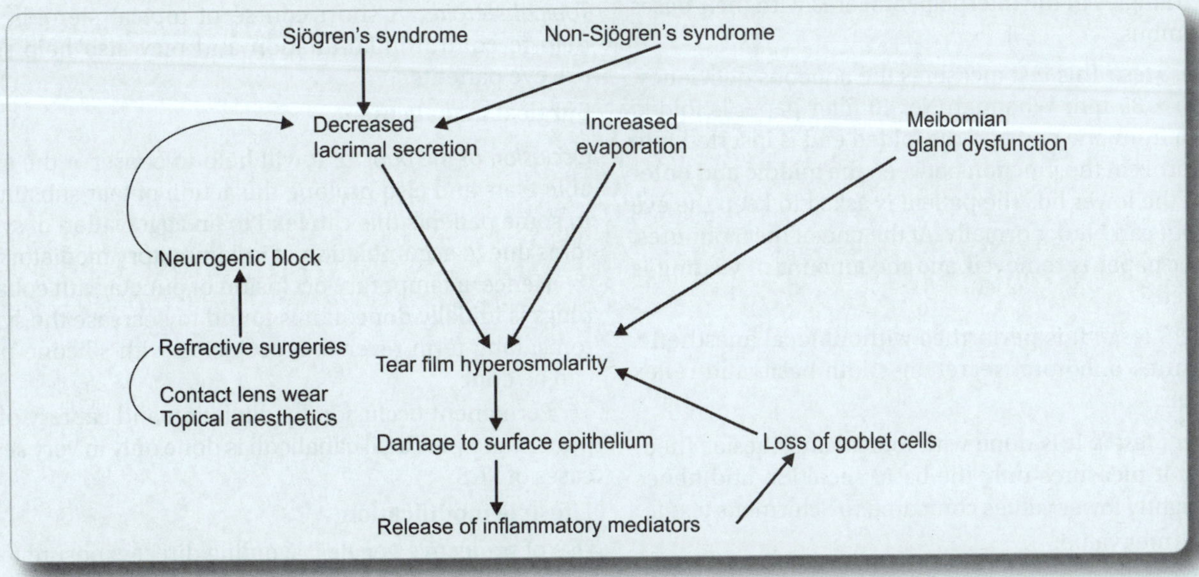

FIGURE 14.9: Vicious cycle of dry eye

Signs

On examination under the slit lamp, the tear film often shows mucous strands and debris caused by mixing of the mucin with lipids due to insufficient aqueous component and decreased clearance from the eye due to decreased tear production.

The normal marginal tear meniscus is smooth and convex, and varies in height from 0.1 to 0.5 mm. In dry eye, it is concave, irregular in height and even absent.

The corneal surface may show punctate epithelial erosion in the lower part of cornea. In severe cases, filaments may be seen on the cornea. The filaments are comma-shaped strands of epithelium and mucin attached at one end to the cornea and the other free end moving with movements of the eye.

Investigations in Dry Eye Conditions

Tear film break-up time (BUT): This is an important index of tear film stability. Fluorescein dye is instilled into the conjunctival sac and the cornea is viewed with the cobalt-blue filter of the slit lamp. The time taken for the first dry spot to appear in the cornea is noted. The test is repeated three times to make sure that the dry spot formation is not due to any local surface problem of the cornea.

Tear break-up time: It is the time interval between the last blink and the appearance of the dry spot. The BUT less than 10 seconds is abnormal.

Rose Bengal staining: Rose Bengal stains the devitalized epithelial cells. When instilled into an eye with dry eye syndrome, the typical staining pattern is the appearance of two triangles in the interpalpebral area with their bases at the limbus.

Schirmer's test: This test measures the aqueous deficiency. A 5 mm × 35 mm Whatman No. 40 filter paper is folded at 5 mm from one end and the folded end is inserted into lower fornix at the junction between the middle and outer third of the lower lid. The patient is asked to keep the eye open, but can blink normally. At the end of the 5 minutes, the filter paper is removed and the amount of wetting is measured.

Schirmer's test I: It is performed without local anesthetic. It measures only total secretion—both basic and reflex secretion.

Schirmer's test II: It is done with topical anesthesia. Theoretically it measures only the basal secretion and hence gives slightly lower values compared to Schirmer's test I.

Schirmer value:

- > 15: No dry eye
- 10–15: Doubtful
- 6–10: Borderline
- < 5: Definite dry eye.

Tear composition assays: Tear film osmolarity, tear lysozyme and lactoferrin assay. These tests are mostly done for research purposes.

Newer imaging techniques: Confocal microscopy can be used to image the tear film, meibomian gland morphology and dry eye-associated corneal neuropathy.

Impression cytology shows decrease in goblet cells in dry eye.

Treatment of Dry Eye

Medical management

Tear substitutes: Eye drops containing hypromellose, hydroxymethyl cellulose, polyvinyl alcohol, sodium hyaluronate, etc. act as tear substitutes and help to lubricate the eye. Short duration of action of eye drops necessitates frequent instillation. Preservatives in tear substitutes can themselves aggravate the dry eye condition. So, preservative-free tear substitutes are better, but they are costlier.

Tear substitute gels: They have more prolonged action and hence, require less frequent instillation, but they can cause transient blurring of vision immediately after instillation. They can be applied at bedtime.

Acetylcysteine: About 5%–10% drops. It is a mucolytic agents useful in filamentary keratopathy.

Cyclosporine: About 0.05%–0.1% eye drops. It helps to control lacrimal gland inflammation and to decrease the frequency of application of tear substitutes.

Topical steroids: A short course of topical steroids may help to control inflammation and may also help some dry eye patients.

Surgical management

Occlusion of the puncta: It will help to conserve the available tears and also prolong the action of tear substitutes. In some patients this can lead to an aggravation of symptoms due to accumulation of inflammatory mediators.

Hence, a temporary occlusion of puncta with collagen plugs is initially done. If it is found to decrease the symptoms, long-term reversible occlusion with silicone plugs can be done.

Permanent occlusion by dilatation and cautery of the puncta and proximal canaliculi is done only in very severe cases of KCS.

Lifestyle modification

Use of protective goggles, avoiding direct exposure to the vent of air conditioners, use of humidifiers, etc. can be done to decrease tear evaporation.

Conjunctival Ulcers

Injuries to conjunctiva usually heal well without any ulceration. An ulcer following injury usually means an impacted foreign body in the wound. Conjunctival ulcers can be produced by specific infections like tuberculosis, primary syphilis or herpes simplex or zoster.

Inflammation of the Conjunctiva

Inflammation of the conjunctiva can be infective or non-infective.

Infective Conjunctivitis

Infective conjunctivitis may be classified depending on the clinical course as (Table 14.2):

- Acute
- Subacute
- Chronic.

TABLE 14.2: Classification of infective conjuctivitis

Acute conjunctivitis	Subacute conjunctivitis	Chronic conjunctivitis
Serous	Simple chronic conjunctivitis	Trachoma
Mucopurulent	Angular conjunctivitis	–
Purulent	Follicular conjunctivitis	–
Membranous	Trachoma	–

Depending on the type of organism it can be:

- Viral
- Bacterial
- Chlamydial
- Parasitic infection.

Depending on the type of exudate or discharge from the eye, it can be classified as:

- Serous (commonly viral, allergic or toxic)
- Catarrhal or mucopurulent (bacterial or chlamydial)
- Purulent (bacterial)
- Pseudomembranous.

Non-infective Types

- Immune mediated
- Hay fever conjunctivitis or perennial allergic conjunctivitis
- Keratoconjunctivitis
- Phlyctenular keratoconjunctivitis
- Atopic keratoconjunctivitis
- Contact lens-induced conjunctivitis
- Immune-mediated disorder of skin and mucous membrane, SJ syndrome, toxic epidermolysis bullosa and pemphigus
- Irritant conjunctivitis caused by smoke, fumes, retained foreign bodies, UV radiation, etc.
- Toxic conjunctivitis (chemicals or drugs induced)
- Dry eye syndrome.

INFECTIVE TYPE OF CONJUNCTIVITIS

VIRAL CONJUNCTIVITIS

Adenovirus Infections

Adenovirus is the common virus that can cause conjunctivitis. It can cause significant morbidity. Spread is via droplets from respiratory tract or ocular infections. An ophthalmology clinic can become the source of infection, if strict aseptic practices like hand asepsis of health personnel, sterilization of tonometers, etc. are not followed.

Clinical Manifestations

They are as follows.

Simple serous conjunctivitis: This is a mild adenoviral infection. There will be some redness and watering, often associated with chemosis of conjunctiva and minimal discharge. Resolves by itself in 7–10 days, unilateral or bilateral.

Pharyngoconjunctival fever: This is caused by adenovirus types 3, 4 and 7 and sometimes type 5. It is often associated with upper respiratory tract infection, fever and preauricular adenopathy. Mild keratitis can also develop and the infection is often self-limiting (Figs 14.10 and 14.11).

Epidemic keratoconjunctivitis (EKC): This is caused by adenovirus types 8 and 19. It runs a prolonged course due to involvement of the cornea, which occurs in 70%–80% of cases. Unlike pharyngoconjunctival fever, it is not associated with any systemic symptoms.

Sx Symptoms

Redness, watering and irritation. Photophobia and blurring of vision occurs when cornea is involved. Often bilateral.

Signs

Conjunctival congestion, SCH and chemosis are seen. Pseudomembrane may form in severe infection.

Corneal Involvement

Appears as punctuate epithelial keratitis. They may resolve within 2 weeks. This may be followed by the appearance

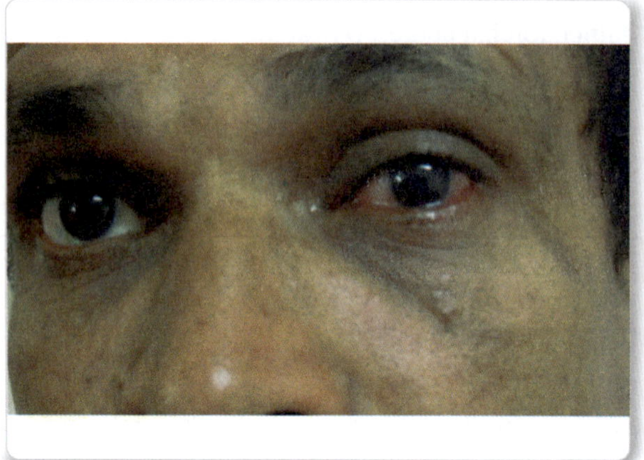

FIGURE 14.10: Pharyngoconjunctival fever

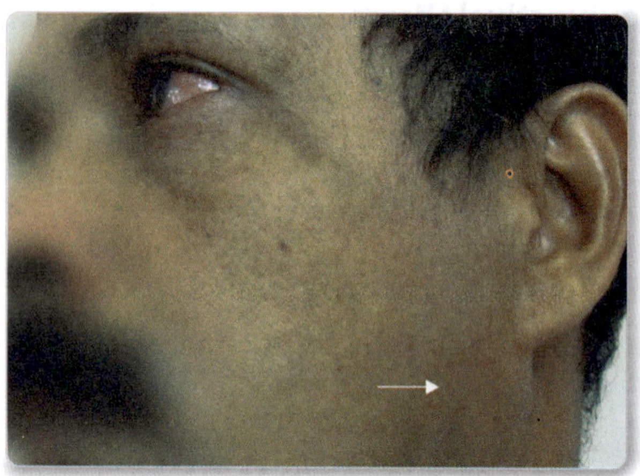

FIGURE 14.11: Preauricular adenopathy in pharyngoconjunctival fever

of subepithelial opacities and stromal infiltrates. They are considered to be immunological reaction to the virus proteins and may take weeks to months to disappear.

Treatment

Mainly supportive treatment with lubricants or anti-inflammatory agents. Antiviral drugs like acyclovir are not effective against adenoviral infection. When subepithelial lesions develop, mild steroid drugs can be given, which has to be tapered off slowly.

Herpes Simplex Virus Infection

Herpes simplex virus (HSV) infection is considered to be a worldwide public health problem. It is estimated that one third of the world population suffers from recurrent infection.

Among the eight types of known herpes virus, ocular lesions are caused by HSV type 1 and 2, varicella-zoster virus (VZV), Epstein-Barr virus (EBV) and cytomegalovirus (CMV). All herpes virus can survive in latent form in the host. HSV type 1 and 2, and VZV establish latent infection in trigeminal ganglion.

Clinical Features

Herpes simplex virus type 1 more commonly causes infection above the waist and HSV type 2 genital infections, but either viruses can cause infection in either location.

Primary HSV infection occur in the skin and mucous membrane innervated by the trigeminal nerve. It can later establish a latent infection in the trigeminal ganglion and reactivation of the virus at a later period can lead to recurrent infections.

Primary HSV infection in the eye often manifests as a unilateral blepharoconjunctivitis and accompanied by preauricular adenopathy. Vesicles on the skin of the lids and eyelid margins are important in making the diagnosis. Epithelial keratitis may develop in primary HSV infection, but subepithelial and stromal lesions are rare.

It is differentiated from adenoviral infection by being often unilateral, by the presence of eyelid vesicles and dendritic epithelial keratitis.

Treatment

Primary ocular HSV is a self-limited infection. Antiviral therapy helps to shorten the natural course of the disease. Acyclovir 3% eye ointment five times daily for 10 days. Other antiviral agents available are vidarabine 2% ointment, trifluridine solution, Ganciclovir 0.15% ophthalmic gel.

Recurrent HSV Infection

The HSV infection can present as:

- Blepharoconjunctivitis
- Epithelial keratitis
- Stromal keratitis
- Iridocyclitis.

The corneal lesions are the most frequent manifestation. Recurrent blepharoconjunctitis infection is indistinguishable from primary blepharoconjunctivitis (refer Chapter 15, 'Cornea').

Herpes Zoster Virus Infection

Primary Infection

Vesicles in the lids and follicular conjunctivitis are the common ocular manifestations in primary infection (Fig. 14.12).

The latent virus in trigeminal ganglion can undergo reactivation and cause condition called herpes zoster ophthalmicus (HZO) due to the involvement of the ophthalmic division. The HZO produces a variety of corneal lesions (refer Chapter 15, 'Cornea').

Molluscum Contagiosum

Spread is by direct contact with infected lesion. A molluscum is a smooth pale umbilicated lesion. When they involve the lid margin, a chronic follicular conjunctivitis, punctate corneal erosions or even corneal pannus may develop. Multiple lesions may develop in immunocompromized persons.

Treatment

Complete excision of the lesions, cryotherapy or incision of the central portion of the lesion and cauterization can cure the condition.

Human Papovavirus Infection

Human papovavirus (HPV) infection can cause papillomatous lesions on the conjunctiva. Lesions at lid margins can lead to chronic follicular conjunctivitis and keratitis.

In any case of chronic intractable conjunctivitis, the lid margins have to be carefully inspected for any molluscum or wart.

BACTERIAL CONJUNCTIVITIS

Different species of bacteria can produce conjunctivitis—mucopurulent, purulent, membranous or pseudomembranous conjunctivitis, depending on the type and virulence of the organism and the immunological status of the host.

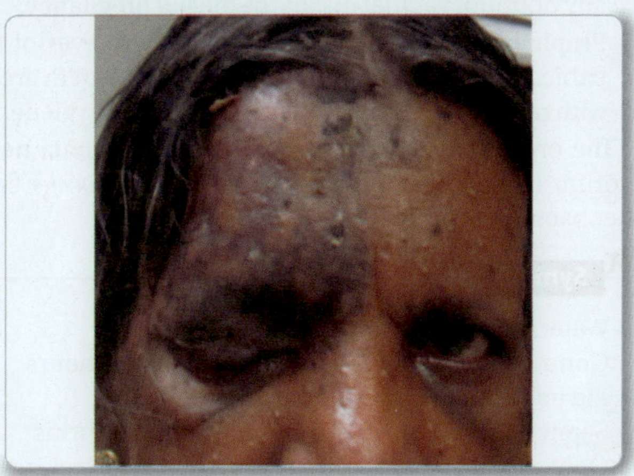

FIGURE 14.12: Herpes zoster ophthalmicus

The mode of spread is by either direct or indirect contact (through contaminated fingers, handkerchiefs, towels, tonometer, etc.) with an infected person's secretions. In unilateral cases, the source of infection may be his/her own lacrimal sac. Nasolacrimal duct obstruction, dacryocystitis and canaliculitis. Must be investigated for any chronic unilateral bacterial conjunctivitis.

Causative Organism

Mild-to-moderate infections are caused by *Staphylococcus aureus, Pseudomonas,* etc. Moderate-to-severe infections are caused by *H. influenzae, Streptococcus pneumoniae (S. pneumoniae)* and *S. aureus.*

The etiological agent of severe purulent conjunctivitis is *Neisseria gonorrhoeae (N. gonorrhoeae)* and *N. meningitidis.* Membraneous conjunctivitis is caused by *C. diphtheriae.*

Types of Bacterial Conjunctivitis

Acute Catarrhal or Mucopurulent Conjunctivitis

Sx Symptoms

Patient usually present with complaints of redness, swelling of the lids and mucoid discharge from the eye. Matting of the lashes with discharge will make opening the eyes difficult on waking up in the morning. Flakes of mucous over the cornea may produce symptoms of colored halos or transient blurring of vision.

Signs

On examination, there will be mild lid edema and matting of the lashes with mucopurulent discharge. The conjunctival vessels will be congested and typically the congestion will be more toward the fornices and relatively less around the cornea in the circumcorneal area.

Treatment

Antibiotic drops at frequent intervals during day time and ointment at bedtime. This has to be given for 5–7 days. Irrigating the conjunctival sac with normal saline will give some comfort to the patient and wash away the discharge and the toxins produced by the organism.

The eyes should not be bandaged, since the condition will be aggravated by the rise of temperature of the conjunctival sac as well as the collection of the secretion within the conjunctival sac by bandaging. Protective dark goggles can be worn.

Culture and sensitivity (C&S) studies of conjunctival swabs are necessary only in patients who are not responding to adequate antibiotic therapy.

Purulent Conjunctivitis

Purulent conjunctivitis is characterized by dramatic onset, copious purulent discharge, severe lid edema and chemosis. Usual causative organism is *N. gonorrhoeae*. It can occur in adults as a sexually transmitted diseases (STD) by direct genital-ocular contact or by genital-hand-ocular contact. It can occur in newborn-ophthalmia neonatorum by spread of infection from mother during vaginal delivery. Infection by *N. gonorrhoeae* has been decreased due to better control of STD and also due to prophylactic treatment in pregnant ladies and newborn. Other organisms like *Haemophilus aegyptius (H. aegyptius)* and *S. aureus* can produce a similar picture, especially in immunocompromised individuals.

Sx **Symptoms**

Purulent conjunctivitis often has a dramatic onset. There will be much lid edema and inability to open the eyes. There will be moderate pain and copious purulent discharge. In adults there may be history of urethritis.

Signs

There will be marked lid edema. The lids will be tense with folds of chemotic conjunctiva hanging out through closed lids. There will be copious purulent discharge. Separation of the lids and examination of the eyeball is often difficult and will require lid retractors. *N. gonorrhoeae* organism can directly invade the intact corneal epithelium. There will be epithelial haziness of the cornea, epithelial defects, marginal infiltrates and peripheral corneal ulcers that can rapidly progress to perforation. Eversion of the lids is difficult and often shows formation of membranes. There will be preauricular adenopathy also.

Complications

1. Corneal ulceration: Perforation and loss of the eye can occur, if prompt treatment is not started.
2. Iridocystitis and its complications can occur.
3. Rarely gonococcal arthritis may develop.
4. Subacute bacterial endocarditis.
5. Septicemia, especially in newborns or immunocompromised persons.

Diagnosis

Diagnosis is confirmed by demonstration of intracellular diplococci in conjunctival scraping.

Treatment

Gonococcal conjunctivitis requires systemic antibiotics in addition to topical medication.

Penicillin was the most effective drug against gonococci in the past, but recently there is increasing prevalence of penicillin-resistant gonococci. It is sensitive to ceftriaxone, a third generation cephalosporin. Ceftriaxone 1 g IV 8 hourly, only for 3 days. A single dose is enough, if there is no corneal involvement. Oral fluoroquinolones can be given to patients with penicillin allergy.

Topical therapy

1. Frequent irrigation of the eye with normal saline.
2. Ciprofloxacin or ofloxacin eye drops, erythromycin eye ointment, etc. can be frequently instilled.
3. Atropine ointment or cyclopentolate drops are also given when there is corneal involvement.
4. Often there is coexisting chlamydial infection also. So, tetracycline or erythromycin ointment is also applied.

Patient may be sent to dermatology department for management of the primary problem. The sex partner of the patient may also be advised to undergo treatment.

Ophthalmia Neonatorum

Ophthalmia neonatorum is any mucoid or mucopurulent or purulent discharge from one or both eyes of an infant in the 1st month of life.

Etiology

The infant gets the infection during its birth from the infected mother.

Neisseria gonorrhoeae was the major etiological agent in the past. But the incidence of gonococcal infection has now come down considerably due to:

1. Better antenatal care to the mother with treatment for any doubtful vaginal discharge during pregnancy.
2. Prophylactic treatment given routinely to eyes of all babies soon after birth. But it is still prevalent in areas with poor public health facilities and poor hygiene.

The organisms now responsible for ophthalmia neonatorum is chlamydia oculogenitalis, *Streptococcus* and other bacteria.

Sx **Symptoms**

- Watering/discharge from the newborn's eye
- Gonococcal infection manifested in first 48 hours
- Lid edema and corneal opacities
- Septicemia, meningitis, pneumonia and arthritis
- Ophthalmia neonatorum by the end of 1st week, etc.

Signs

Any watering or discharge from the newborn's eye should be taken seriously.

Gonococcal infection usually manifests in the first 48 hours. The infant has lid edema and mucopurulent discharge, which soon becomes purulent in nature. It will be difficult to separate the lids and examine the eyes, but utmost care must be taken not to traumatize the corneal epithelium, while retracting the lids with lid retractors. Since, gonococci can invade intact corneal epithelium, any corneal involvement can be considered pathognomonic of gonococcal infection. The typical corneal lesion is a vertically oval ulcer just below the center of the cornea. This is the part of the cornea in contact with the lid margins when the eyes are closed. The ulcer can progress rapidly leading to perforation of the eye and all its complications. Prompt treatment can prevent perforation, but healing of the ulcer can lead to corneal opacities. Corneal opacities in an infant will clear to a large extent compared to that in an adult's eye, but the nebular opacity can interfere with the macular fixation that develop in the first 6 weeks of life. This can cause amblyopia and nystagmus.

Systemic spread of the infection can lead to septicemia, meningitis, pneumonia and arthritis.

Chlamydial infection in a newborn presents as a less severe infection, usually in 5–7 days after birth. Clinical features are watering, mucopurulent discharge and conjunctival congestion. Follicles that we see in an adult chlamydial infection are not seen in an infant, since the infant's conjunctiva develop the adenoid layer only by the 3rd month of life. If the infection is left untreated and progress beyond the 3rd month of life, follicles will appear.

Ophthalmia neonatorum due to other bacteria appear by the end of the 1st week as a non-specific mucopurulent conjunctivitis.

Diagnosis

A presumptive diagnosis is possible in gonococcal ophthalmia neonatorum by the early onset, purulent discharge and corneal involvement. Diagnosis can be confirmed by the presence of gram-negative diplococci in conjunctival scrapings. Scrapings showing plenty of neutrophils, lymphocytes and intracellular inclusion bodies in Giemsa's stain denote a diagnosis of chlamydial infection. Gram stain as well as C&S studies will reveal other bacterial infections.

Treatment

Systemic

In non-disseminated gonococcal infections, a single intramuscular (IM) or intravenous (IV) injection of ceftriaxone at a dose of 100 mg/kg body weight is given. In disseminated infection, the duration of the treatment with ceftriaxone is decided by consultation with infectious diseases specialists.

Topical

Frequent saline irrigation to wash out all discharge, epithelial debri, toxins and organisms.

Fluoroquinolone drops combined with erythromycin or gentamicin eye ointment, if there is corneal involvement.

Cycloplegic drugs like atropine ointment or cyclopentolate drops are also given, if there is corneal involvement.

Systemic treatment is advised for infants born to mothers with active gonococcal infection, even if there is no ocular involvement (American Academy of Pediatrics, 2009. pp. 305-13).

Neonatal Chlamydial Infection

The infection responds well to topical treatment with erythromycin ointment. Since, other chlamydial infections like otitis media can accompany conjunctivitis, systemic erythromycin (12.5 mg/kg oral or IV qid for 14 days) is recommended.

Other bacterial neonatal infection is treated with topical fluoroquinolones or gentamicin ointment. The antibiotic can be modified according to the C&S reports.

Prophylaxis

Crede's method: This is the prophylactic method adopted before the era of antibiotics. One drop of silver nitrate 1% solution is instilled into each eye of the infant soon after the birth in suspected cases of maternal infection. This is no longer in practice now.

Nowadays some antibiotic drops like gentamicin or erythromycin ointment is applied immediately after birth.

Membranous Conjunctivitis

Conjunctival inflammation can be associated with pseudomembrane or true membrane formation. Pseudomembrane formation is often seen in adenoviral infection, SJ syndrome, gonococcal or pneumococcal infections.

True membrane formation is typically seen in diphtheritic infection of conjunctiva. It can also occur in severe bacterial conjunctivitis, usually in immunocompromised or malnourished persons in infections with organisms like β-hemolytic streptococci, *S. pneumoniae, H. aegyptius,* etc.

Diphtheritic infection occurs in non-immunized children, often malnourished or recovering from some systemic infections like measles, whooping cough, etc.

Signs and symptoms

In mild cases, there will be lid edema and mucopurulent or blood stained discharge. The upper and lower palpebral conjunctivita will be covered with a whitish membrane. Peeling off this membrane will leave a raw bleeding surface.

In severe cases, the lids will be indurated and edematous and the discharge from the eye will be minimal. A thick fibrinous exudate will cover the conjunctiva and sometimes extend to the cornea also. This thick membrane covering the conjunctiva can be removed only with difficulty and leave raw bleeding surfaces due to necrosis of the epithelium. This fibrinous membrane is similar to that cover the throat in diphtheria. The preauricular lymph nodes will be enlarged. The diphtheritic organism can invade intact corneal epithelium and corneal ulceration can develop. When the raw conjunctival surfaces heal; symblepharon may develop.

Treatment

Every case of membranous conjunctivitis should be treated as diphtheritic in unimmunized children unless C&S studies prove otherwise.

Diphtheritic antiserum 4,000–10,000 units at 12 hourly intervals combined with systemic injection of crystalline penicillin. Topical crystalline penicillin drops (10,000 units/mL freshly prepared everyday from the pencillin powder available for injection) should be applied at half hourly or hourly interval.

This treatment will be effective against other bacterial infections also.

In non-responsive cases, the topical and systemic antibiotic can be modified based on the C&S studies.

Complications

1. Corneal ulceration—corneal opacity, perforation, blindness.
2. Symblepharon—limitation of ocular movements, diplopia, restriction of lid movements—lagophthalmos.
3. Dry eye.

Angular Conjunctivitis

Etiological agent is *Moraxella lacunata* (gram-negative diplobacilli) or staphylococci. *Moraxella* produces a proteolytic ferment, which will cause destruction of epithelium.

Sx **Symptoms**

The patient will complain of some discomfort and mild discharge.

Signs

There will be conjunctival congestion limited to the intermarginal strip at the outer and inner canthi and congestion of the bulbar conjunctiva in the exposed area between the inflamed lid margins. There will be some excoriation of the neighboring skin also leading to blepharitis-like picture. The rest of the conjunctiva will appear normal, which clinches the diagnosis.

Complication

If left untreated, marginal corneal infiltrates and ulceration can develop.

Treatment

Tetracycline eye ointment is effective against *Moraxella* and has to be applied four times daily for 10–14 days or more till the inflammation subsides.

Zinc can inhibit the proteolytic enzyme. So, proprietary eye lotion containing zinc oxide can be combined with the antibiotic therapy.

CHLAMYDIAL INFECTIONS

Chlamydia trachomatis (C. trachomatis) can cause different types of conjunctival inflammation each associated with different serotypes:

1. Inclusion conjunctivitis: Serotypes DK.
2. Trachoma: Serotype AC.
3. Lymphogranuloma venereum: Serotypes L1, L2 and L3.

Inclusion Conjunctivitis

Inclusion conjunctivitis is a STD seen in young- and middle-aged adults. The affected people has an associated, often asymptomatic genital infection (urethritis in men and cervicitis in women). Often, the mode of spread is by eye contact with contaminated finger or towels. It can spread widely through contaminated water in swimming pools (swimming pool conjunctivitis). The usual incubation period is 1–2 weeks.

Sx **Symptoms**

The disease has an insidious onset unlike adenoviral infection. Patients usually complain of mild discomfort and irritation with minimal discharge.

Signs

There will be moderate conjunctival congestion with follicular hypertrophy, more prominent in the lower palpebral conjunctiva. Occasionally, follicles will appear on the bulbar conjunctiva and semilunar fold. The lesser involvement of upper tarsal conjunctiva and minimal scarring differentiates it from trachoma.

Corneal Involvement

Epithelial keratitis and subepithelial keratitis usually involving the upper part of the cornea can occur. A micropannus not extending more than 3 mm into the cornea may also develop.

Natural Course

The infection has a chronic, but benign course. If left untreated, it will resolve in 6–12 months.

Diagnosis

1. Giemsa stain of conjunctival scraping will show Halberstaedter-Prowazek inclusion bodies. These inclusion bodies are the cluster of elementary bodies of the organism in a carbohydrate matrix.
2. Confirmation of the diagnosis can be made by direct monoclonal antibody immunofluorescent staining of conjunctival smears. This test is very sensitive and give quick results, but not widely available.
3. Enzyme-linked immunosorbent assay (ELISA) test for chlamydial antigen and polymerase chain reaction (PCR) test.
4. Standard single passage McCoy cell culture is used for growing and identifying the organism in laboratory. This test takes 3 days to give a result. Expensive and not required for confirming the diagnosis in view of other quick and sensitive tests available.

All confirmed cases should be sent for investigation for genital infection and also for screening of other STDs.

Treatment

The organism is sensitive to tetracycline, fluoroquinolones, azithromycin and erythromycin. Topical erythromycin, tetracycline or ofloxacin ointment qid is given for 6 weeks:

- Systemic therapy
- Azithromycin 1 g orally as a single dose
- Ofloxacin 300 mg bd orally for 7 days
- Erythromycin 500 mg qid for 14 days
- Doxycycline 100 mg bd for 14 days
- Tetracycline 250 mg qid for 14 days.

Erythromycin, doxycycline and tetracycline are avoided in children below 12 years and in lactating and pregnant mothers.

Trachoma

Trachoma is the leading cause of infectious blindness globally. According to World Health Organization (WHO), trachoma is endemic in over 50 countries in Africa, Middle East, South East Asia and South America. Its prevalence is correlated with poverty, poor sanitation facilities and limited access to healthcare services.

To bring down blindness due to trachoma, trachoma control program was started by Central Government in India in 1963. Later when National Programme for Control of Blindness (NPCB) was started in 1976, the trachoma control program was included in NPCB with the various activities under NPCB; with active preventive measures, the prevalence of trachoma has come down in India. The severity of trachoma and its blinding potential varies in different parts of India. In 2006, rapid assessment of trachoma was conducted in six previously hyperendemic states in India. It was observed that all these states were still having active cases of tractoma, ranging from less than 1% in Gujarat to 15% in Uttarakhand.

Global Elimination of Trachoma (GET) 2020 was launched under WHO in 1997 with the initiative to eliminate trachoma globally as a blinding disease. The control activities are based on SAFE strategy as given below:

- S: Lid surgery
- A: Antibiotics to treat the community pool of infection
- F: Facial cleanliness
- E: Environmental changes.

These activities are given through primary healthcare facilities. The target is global elimination of trachoma by the year 2020.

Clinical Features

Trachoma is an infection caused by serotype A, B, Ba and C of *C. trachomatis.* The disease is prevalent among the poor people living in overcrowded areas with poor conditions of hygiene and limited access to healthcare facilities.

Features of trachomatous follicles:

1. They may assume much larger in size up to 5 mm in diameter, unlike non-trachomatous conditions.
2. More prominent on the upper tarsal conjunctiva, where they may form a prominent row along the upper tarsal border. More in lower tarsal conjunctiva in non-trachomatous causes.
3. They may appear at the limbus, bulbar conjunctiva, caruncle and plica. Rare in other conditions.
4. Soon they become associated with scarring. A horizontal line or a row of stellate scar appears on the upper tarsal conjunctiva—Arlt's line. Scarring is not seen in other conditions (Fig. 14.13).

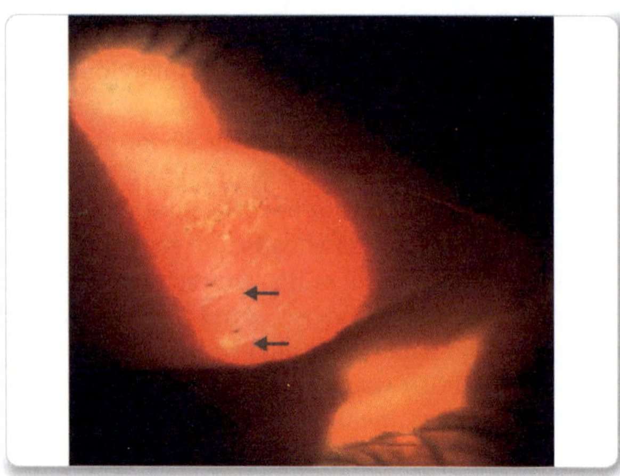

FIGURE 14.13: Scarring

Mode of Spread

The disease is spread by transfer of conjunctival secretions through contaminated fingers, towels, etc. The common fly is an important vector in the spread of the infection.

Sx Symptoms

The disease usually has an insidious onset with some watering, irritation and slight mucopurulent discharge.

The symptoms are so mild and chronic that the patients rarely seek any medical attention. In the later stages, when complications like entropion, trichiasis and corneal ulceration set in, the symptoms are aggravated and the patients seek medical attention for the first time. This is the symptomatically 'pure' trachoma uncomplicated by superadded infection.

But superadded bacterial infections are common, especially in undernourished children living in overcrowded areas and then the symptoms are more aggressive; there will be lid edema and more mucopurulent or purulent discharge.

Trachoma can rarely present as an acute infection—acute trachoma. When there is massive inoculation of the organisms in the eye as in experimental infection or accidental spurting of discharge into the eye of medical personnel during examination of an uncooperative child.

Signs

The disease runs through a prolonged and progressive course.

In the earliest stage, it appears as a mild conjunctivitis with moderate congestion of palpebral conjunctiva and slight mucoid discharge. This is soon followed by the appearance of the papillae, which gives a velvety appearance to the palpebral conjunctiva. Soon the follicles will appear within 2–3 weeks. Initially they may appear in the lower tarsal conjunctiva, but soon becomes more prominent on the upper tarsal conjunctiva and assume the characteristic features of trachomatous follicles, which differentiate them from follicles of other follicular conjunctivitis.

Corneal Changes

The earliest changes are fine epithelial erosion seen only with the slit lamp at the superior limbus. This is followed by a superficial keratitis and later the infiltration will spread into the superficial layers of the stroma also. All these changes are more commonly seen in the superior half of the cornea. Rarely changes may appear all around, but even then, the upper half of the cornea will be affected more.

Trachomatous Pannus

The corneal changes are soon associated with the development of pannus. Pannus is defined as superficial infiltration with vascularization of the cornea. It is most commonly seen in trachoma, but can occur in other conditions also. The pannus seen in trachoma is called trachomatous pannus (Figs 14.14A to C). It can appear in three stages as follows:

1. **Progressive pannus:** The upper part of the cornea close to the limbus becomes cloudy due to lymphoid infiltration. Soon parallel vessels will grow from the marginal loops at the limbus. They are all radially arranged, directed toward the center of the cornea and show little branching. Initially they are situated between the Bowman's membrane (BM) and epithelium.

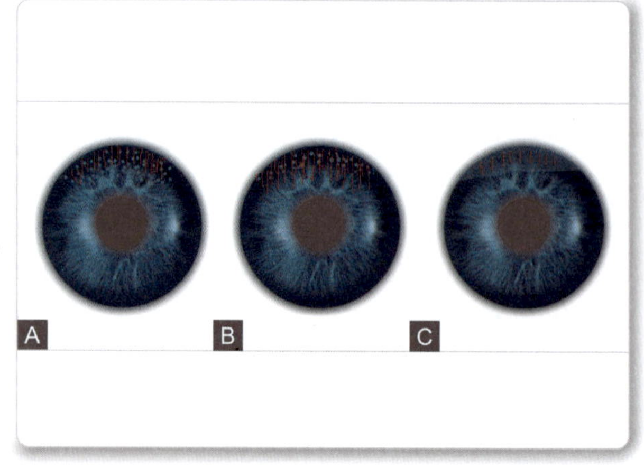

FIGURES 14.14A to C: Types of trachomatous pannus. **A.** Progressive pannus with infiltration beyond the level of blood vessels; **B.** Regressive pannus with blood vessels beyond the level of infiltration; **C.** Healed pannus with ghost vessels.

Later the BM is destroyed and vessels will be seen in the superficial stroma also. The infiltration and cloudiness of the cornea extend beyond the advancing edge of the vessels, which extend up to a horizontal line and it appears as if the vessels are pushing the infiltration forward. This is the typical feature of a progressive pannus.

Rarely vessels will appear and grow all around the limbus.

Follicles may appear at the limbus along with the pannus formation. Later they get absorbed and form depressed scars called Herbert's pits.

2. **Regressive pannus:** Once healing starts, the infiltration tends to recede and the advancing edge of the vessels will appear to be in clear cornea. This appearance is a clear indication of the favorable response to treatment.
3. **Healed pannus:** Even after all the infections have been cured, ghost vessels will be seen at the upper part of cornea appearing as some parallel white lines. If the BM has been destroyed by the pannus, there will also be some scarring in the upper part of the cornea. This arcuate scarring at the upper limbus with a few ghost vessels is evidence of trachoma infection in the past and is called healed pannus (Fig. 14.15).

Lid Changes

The trachomatous infiltration is not confined to the conjunctiva alone. It will invade deep into the tarsal plate causing its thickening and subsequent distortion on healing. The initial changes are thickening of the tarsal plate with drooping of the lids—trachomatous ptosis. There will be scarring and distortion of the lids leading to entropion. The scarring can involve the root of the lashes and cause misdirection of the lashes. This will cause trichiasis. The entropion will aggravate this problem (Fig. 14.16).

The misdirected lashes can rub on the cornea and cause recurrent epithelial erosions, secondary infection and corneal ulcers. This can be a lifelong problem unless the lid abnormalities are surgically corrected.

Corneal Ulceration

Small corneal infiltrates and keratitis are seen at the advancing edge of the pannus. They can get secondarily infected and form large corneal ulcers. They may heal with scarring or progress to perforation and its complications. These ulcerations are the cause of blindness in trachoma.

Sequelae

The corneal opacification and recurrent breakdown and ulceration are the important sequelae. The lid abnormalities—entropion or trichiasis are the other important sequelae, which aggravate the corneal problem (Fig. 14.17).

In addition to this, there will be severe dry eye problem also. The trachomatous infiltration can invade and destroy the lacrimal glands and goblet cells. The scarring can cause occlusion of the ducts of the lacrimal gland. The dry eye problem will aggravate the symptom of irritation and foreign body sensation. Also they facilitate the breakdown of corneal epithelium and subsequent ulceration.

Macallan's Staging of Trachoma

The staging is suggested by Macallan, an English ophthalmologist, who studied trachoma extensively in Egypt.

Stage I: This is the earliest stage before the follicles appear and clinical diagnosis is not possible. There will be conjunctival

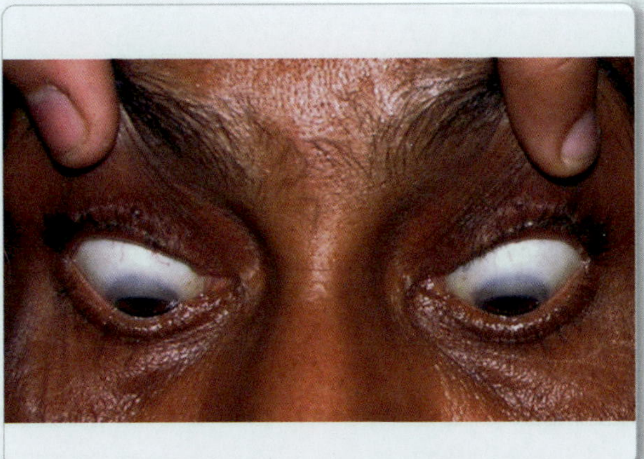

FIGURE 14.15: Healed pannus

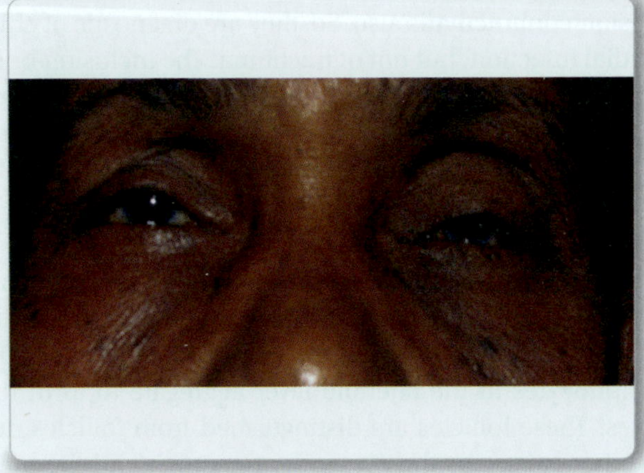

FIGURE 14.16: Ptosis, entropion and trichiasis

congestion and epithelial erosions in the upper part of cornea.

Stage II: This is the stage from the appearance of the follicles up to the appearance of scar tissue. There will be follicles, pannus and epithelial keratitis.

Stage III: Stage of sequelae when scarring has appeared, but infection is still active.

Stage IV: Clinical cure has occurred, but the scarring is giving rise to symptoms and recurrent corneal ulceration.

The WHO grading is a simplified grading system (Table 14.3), which was developed for use by the trained personnel other than ophthalmologists to assess the prevalence in population-based surveys.

TABLE 14.3: WHO classification

Grades	Features
TF	Five or more follicles > 0.5 mm on upper tarsal conjunctiva
TI	Intense trachomatous inflammation—papillary hypertrophy and inflammatory thickening of the upper tarsal conjunctiva
TS	Presence of scarring in upper tarsal conjunctiva
TT	At least one ingrown eyelash touching the globe
CO	Corneal opacity blocking the papillary margin (Fig. 14.17)

Pathology

The *C. trachomatis* is an obligatory intracellular parasite. They are seen as inclusion bodies in the conjunctival epithelial cells called Halberstaedter-Prowazek inclusion bodies—first described by Halberstaedter and Prowazek. Morphologically identical inclusion bodies are seen in inclusion conjunctivitis also. So, they are diagnostic of chlamydial infection, but not of trachoma. The inclusion body initially consists of a number of initial bodies embedded in a carbohydrate matrix. The initial bodies grow and multiply and form a number of elementary bodies. Finally the cell degenerates and the elementary bodies are released, which in turn attack new cells.

There is extensive lymphoid infiltration, which is not confined to the adenoid layer of the conjunctiva. It involves the tarsal plate and the lacrimal glands also. The lymphocytes in the adenoid layer aggregate to form follicles. These follicles are distinguished from follicles due to other causes by the presence of necrosis and the presence of multinucleated giant cells called Leber cells. Later degenerative changes will set in, fibrous tissue will form around the follicles and the tarsal plate will be destroyed and replaced by scar tissue. Contraction of the fibrous tissue will lead to symblepharon formation and distortion of the lids and lashes.

Diagnosis

Diagnosis is mostly based on the following clinical findings:

1. Clinical diagnosis require at least two of the following clinical features:
   a. Follicles on the upper tarsal conjunctiva.
   b. Limbal follicles and their sequelae (Herbert's pits).
   c. Typical tarsal conjunctival scarring.
   d. Pannus most marked on the upper limbus.
   [American Academy for Ophthalmology (AAO) External Disease and Cornea, 2011-2012].
   Giemsa stain will show the inclusion bodies and the Leber cells.
2. Monoclonal antibody immunofluorescent staining of conjunctival smear and PCR are confirmatory tests.
3. Culture of the organism in irradiated McCoy cell culture is expensive.

Treatment

The organism is susceptible to many antibiotics—sulfonamides, tetracycline, erythromycin, azithromycin and rifampicin. The topical antibiotic has to be given for 6-12 weeks or more for complete eradication of the organism. There will be initial dramatic improvement due to eradication of the secondary bacterial infection, which is usually present. The follicle will take few weeks to disappear. The effect of sequelae like trichiasis, dry eye and recurrent corneal surface breakdown will be permanent, even if the infection is completely cured.

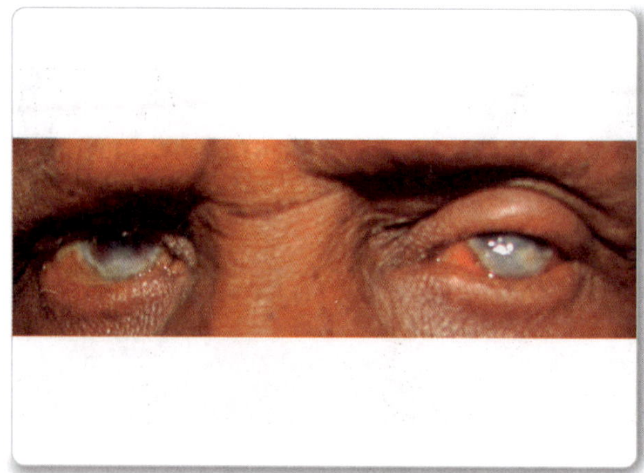

FIGURE 14.17: Bilateral corneal opacity with madarosis, tylosis and upper lid entropion

The WHO recommends community-based management of trachoma by the integrated SAFE strategy. SAFE strategy includes:

1. Surgery to correct advanced stages of the disease like entropion, trichiasis.
2. Antibiotics to treat active infection; using topical tetracycline 1% ointment twice a day for 6 weeks or oral azithromycin as a single dose.
3. Facial cleanliness to reduce disease transmission.
4. Environmental change to increase access to clean water and improved sanitation.

Complications

1. Lid deformation: Entropion, trichiasis and tylosis.
2. Scarring of conjunctiva and cornea: Symblepharon, dry eye and corneal opacities.
3. Blindness: Due to recurrent corneal ulceration.

Granulomatous Conjunctivitis

Granulomatous conjunctivitis is an inflammation of the conjunctiva with granuloma formation. It usually forms part of Parinaud's oculoglandular syndrome. It is a rare disorder with multiple etiology characterized by granulomatous or follicular conjunctivitis associated with preauricular adenopathy.

Causes

Cat-scratch disease (CSD), tularemia, tuberculosis, infectious mononucleosis, lymphogranuloma venereum, fungal infections and syphilis.

The CSD is caused by gram-negative bacillus *Bartonella henselae* transmitted by the scratch or bite of an infected cat. IP 2 weeks.

It usually presents with granulomatous conjunctivitis with preauricular adenopathy.

Diagnosis

It is confirmed by immunofluorescent antibody test and Hanger-Rose cat-scratch skin test.

Treatment

- Oral doxycycline, ciprofloxacin or cotrimoxazole
- Topical treatment with gentamicin, ciprofloxacin or Bacitracin and neomycin combination
- Even without treatment there will be spontaneous resolution in 4–6 weeks.

Lymphogranuloma Venereum

Lymphogranuloma venereum is caused by *C. trachomatis* serotypes L1, L2 and L3. It is a sexually transmitted disease. The vesicles can appear on the lids by contamination. It can burst and form an ulcer with preauricular and submandibular lymphadenopathy.

Treatment

Azithromycin single dose or doxycycline, tetracycline or erythromycin.

PARASITIC INFECTION

Tuberculosis

Usually occurs without any systemic involvement. Appears as conjunctival ulcer, single or multiple with preauricular adenopathy.

Diagnosis

Acid-fast bacilli (AFB) staining of conjunctival scrapings will confirm the etiology.

Treatment

If possible the lesion should be removed completely followed by cauterization. A short course of systemic antituberculosis treatment should also be given.

Syphilis

A primary chancre can appear on the conjunctiva usually associated with oral lesion and preauricular adenopathy.

Diagnosis

It is confirmed by demonstration of spirochaetes by dark ground microscope examination of conjunctival scrapings.

Treatment

Topical tetracycline and systemic penicillin.

Tularemia

Tularemia is an infection caused by *Francisella tularensis*. Infection can be acquired from several animals like cattle sheep, rabbit, deer, etc. by direct skin contact or by bites of an insect vector-like ticks. This disease is widely seen in many countries in America and Asia. In the oculoglandular form, nodules and ulcers appear on the conjunctiva associated with preauricular adenitis. Patient will have constitutional symptoms like fever, myalgia and headache.

Diagnosis

Confirmed by laboratory tests like agglutination test.

Treatment

- Topical gentamicin drops
- Systemic treatment has to be given in consultation with a physician.

Ophthalmia Nodosa

Ophthalmia nodosa is a foreign body reaction caused by caterpillar hair. Follicle-like lesions will appear on the tarsal (usually upper tarsal conjunctiva) with caterpillar hair in the center. Careful slit lamp examination in intractable conjunctivitis will reveal the caterpillar hair. The hair has to be removed or the nodules excised.

Fungal Conjunctivitis

Follicular conjunctivitis with lymphadenopathy can be caused by many fungi like *Aspergillus, Leptothrix, Candida, Nocardia,* etc.

Treatment

Treatment is with topical antifungal agents like miconazole or natamycin.

Rhinosporidiosis

Rhinosporidiosis is a specific type of fungal infection caused by *Rhinosporidium seeberi.* It is widely prevalent in several parts of the world like South India, Srilanka, Central and South America and Africa. It is usually a waterborne infection spread by bathing in contaminated pools or other water source (Fig. 14.18).

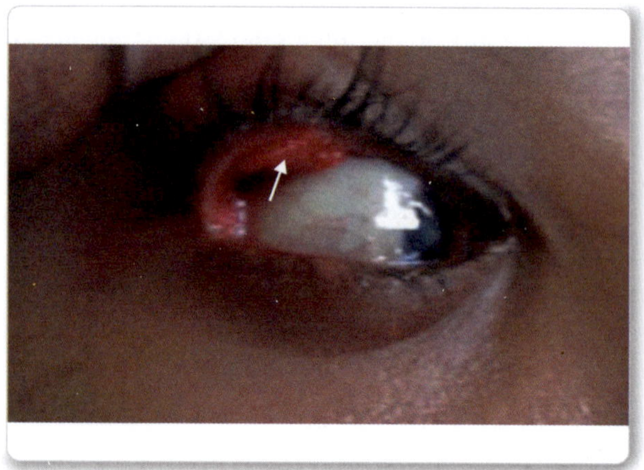

FIGURE 14.18: Rhinosporidiosis

Clinical Features

Rhinosporidiosis usually presents as a sessile or pedunculated fleshy granulomatous growth resembling a strawberry covered with multiple white spots, which are the spores. The granuloma is highly vascular and readily bleeds on touch. The rest of the conjunctiva will be normal. It usually involves the lid margin or fornices. When they appear on the bulbar conjunctiva, the collagenase-like enzymes produced by the organism can cause thinning of the sclera and localized staphyloma formation underneath the granuloma (Figs 14.19A and B).

Rhinosporidiosis can involve the nasolacrimal sac and cause chronic dacryocystitis. It may spread to the nasal cavity and lead to multiple granuloma involving the nasal cavity, sinuses and nasopharynx. Patient usually presents with recurrent epistaxis.

Involvement of all the three areas—conjunctiva, lacrimal sac and nasal cavity is not uncommon.

Diagnosis

It is based on the clinical features and histopathological examination of the excised granuloma.

Treatment

1. Complete excision of the granuloma. Incomplete excision will lead to recurrence.
2. Avoid contaminated swimming pools to avoid reinfection.
3. Scleral staphyloma, if larger, will require reinforcement with lamellar scleral graft using preserved sclera from enucleated eyes.
4. Complete eradication of the organism from other involved sites from lacrimal sac by dacryocystectomy or from nasal cavity by excision of the granulomas is essential to prevent recurrence.

Simple Chronic Conjunctivitis

Causes

Acute bacterial conjunctivitis can go into a chronic stage if:

1. It is not properly treated: The premature stopping of the topical antibiotics, incomplete eradication of organisms due to use of antibiotic steroid combination or use of antibiotic to which the organism was resistant.

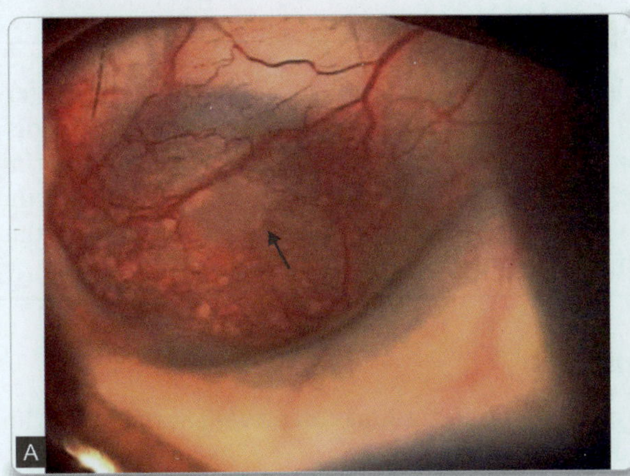

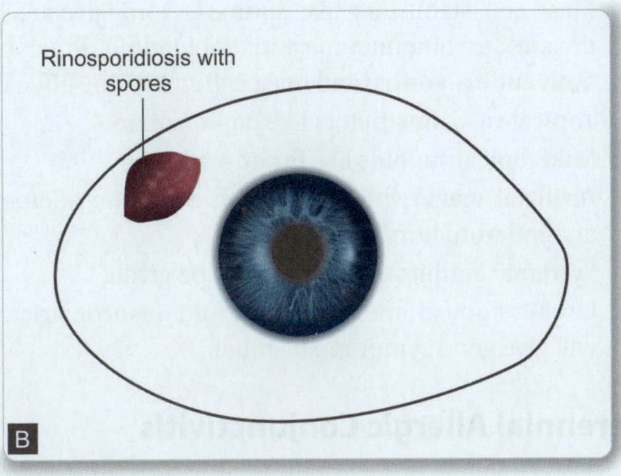

FIGURES 14.19A and B: Rhinosporidiosis. **A.** With staphyloma; **B.** On bulbar conjunctiva (diagrammatic representation).

2. If there is a nearby chronic source of infection like chronic dacryocystitis, blepharitis, molluscum or papillomavirus infection of the lid margins, etc.
3. Chronic irritation: Like retained foreign body in the fornices, inturned lashes, chronic exposure to dust fumes or smoke.
4. Mucus fishing syndrome: Patient keeps on trying to remove the mucus from the eye and traumatizes the conjunctiva and also introduces organisms.

Clinical Features

Patient will complain of grittiness or burning sensation for long duration. There will be minimal discharge during day time, but there will be difficulty in opening the eyes in the morning due to matting of the lashes with discharge.

On examination, the eyes may appear normal, since the bulbar conjunctiva is often not congested except toward the fornices, which is revealed by pulling the lower lid down. The palpebral conjunctiva will be congested and there will be papillary hypertrophy.

Management

Careful examination of the eye and history taking is essential to find out the cause for the chronicity. The nasolacrimal duct should be tested for any evidence of chronic dacryocystitis. Any retained foreign body in the upper fornix should be ruled out. The lid margins should be closely inspected for any small wart or molluscum.

If any specific reason can be found out, it should be eradicated.

A conjunctival swab for C&S studies should be taken and the appropriate antibiotic drops instilled frequently for 7–10 days or till the infection is completely cured. Meanwhile any unhealthy habits of the patients like removing the mucus frequently with fingers or handkerchief should be discouraged.

NON-INFECTIVE TYPE OF CONJUNCTIVITIS

Hay Fever Conjunctivitis or Seasonal Allergic Conjunctivitis

Hay fever conjunctivitis or seasonal allergic conjunctivitis is an IgE-mediated immediate hypersensitivity reaction. The allergen is airborne, typically pollens of some flowering tree or plant and the allergy appear at the time of flowering of plants or trees. When the allergen enters the tear film and comes into contact with the conjunctival mast cells, degranulation of the mast cells and release of histamine and other inflammatory mediators occur.

Clinical Features

On exposure to the allergen, the person will have an attack of intense itching and watering of the eye. The lids will be swollen and the conjunctiva becomes congested and chemotic. This is usually associated with sneezing and rhinitis. Sudden onset and intense itching are the hallmarks of this problem.

Treatment

Avoidance of the allergen is the most effective method, but often not practical. Wearing protective goggles during the flowering season will decrease the intensity of the attack.

1. Cold compresses.
2. Topical antihistamines like chlorpheniramine maleate, azelastine, etc.

3. Mast cell stabilizers like sodium cromoglycate, lodoxamide tromethamine and olopatadine, which has both antihistaminic and mast cell stabilizing effect.
4. Topical vasoconstrictors like naphazoline.
5. Mild topical steroids like fluorometholone.
6. Artificial tears, which will wash away the allergens and inflammatory mediators.
7. Systemic antihistamines can also be given.
8. Usually topical antihistamines and vasoconstrictors will give good symptomatic relief.

Perennial Allergic Conjunctivitis

Perennial allergic conjunctivitis is also an IgE-mediated hypersensitivity reaction. It is less acute, but more persistent than hay fever conjunctivitis and symptoms can occur throughout the year with exacerbations in between. Allergen may be dust mites or fungal allergens.

Clinical Features

Clinical features are recurrent attacks of itching, watering and redness of the eyes associated with sneezing and running nose.

Treatment

Avoidance of allergens as much as possible. Keep the houses as dust free as possible with vacuuming and wet mopping. The pillows and mattresses may be kept mite free by frequent dusting and exposure to sunlight. Long-term use of mast cell stabilizers are very useful in this condition to suppress the mast cell degranulation—sodium cromoglycate and lodoxamide tromethamine.

Topical decongestants and antihistamine will control acute exacerbation. Topical steroids should be used only in severe cases.

Vernal Keratoconjunctivitis (Spring Catarrh)

Vernal keratoconjunctivitis (VKC) is a seasonal bilateral recurring inflammation of the conjunctiva and cornea. Though it is called spring catarrh, acute exacerbation occurs in summer time and in tropical countries the inflammation may be present round the year. Male children are predominantly affected. The disease is often self-limiting and the problem burns out by 25 years of age. The immunopathogenesis appears to involve both type I and IV hypersensitivity reaction.

> *Sx* **Symptoms**
>
> Itching is the main problem associated with watering, redness, photophobia and copious mucoid discharge—often described as 'ropy'. Parents often bring the young children with the main complaint of the child frequently rubbing their eyes. The dictum is that if there is no itching, it cannot be VKC.

Signs

The clinical manifestations can present as palpebral, limbal or both.

Palpebral form: There is a diffuse papillary hypertrophy affecting both upper and lower tarsal conjunctiva, but the upper tarsal conjunctiva is predominantly affected. The palpebral conjunctiva in VKC is described to have a 'cobblestone' appearance (Figs 14.20A to C). The papillae can attain large size, are flat topped and have a pale milky hue due to the hypertrophy of the overlying epithelium and fibrous tissue underneath. But histologically they are hypertrophied papillae.

Limbal form: It occurs predominantly in Asia and Africa. The limbus has a thickened gelatinous appearance. White dots called Horner-Trantas dots may be seen at the limbus. They are aggregates of degenerated eosinophils and epithelial cells and their appearance is an identifying feature of VKC.

Combined form: These patients have both palpebral and limbal involvement.

Corneal Changes

Cornea can be involved in both forms. Punctuate epithelial erosion may appear predominantly in the upper half of the cornea. Pannus may also appear predominantly in the superior limbus, but at times it may involve 360° all around. But the extent of the pannus is limited.

Sometimes non-infectious epithelial ulcers—horizontally oval or shield like in shape may appear in the upper part of the cornea with underlying stromal opacification. They are called shield ulcers. An association between VKC and keratoconus has been reported (Fig. 14.21).

Management

Mild cases may respond to mast cell suppressants like disodium cromoglycate 2% eye drops alone. For acute exacerbations, topical antihistamines or non-steroidal anti-inflammatory drugs (NSAIDs) drops may be effective in mild cases. Moderate-to-severe form will require topical

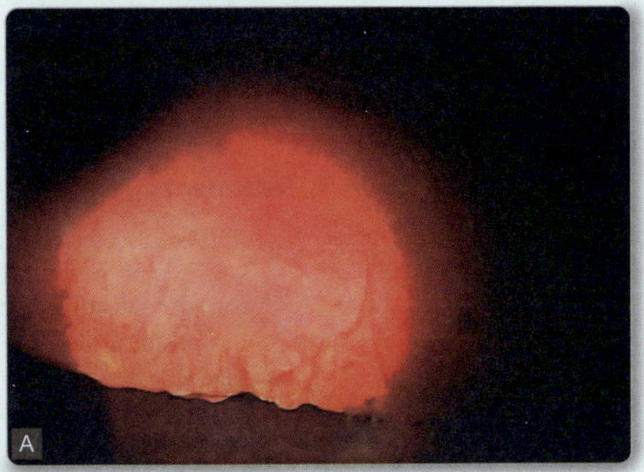

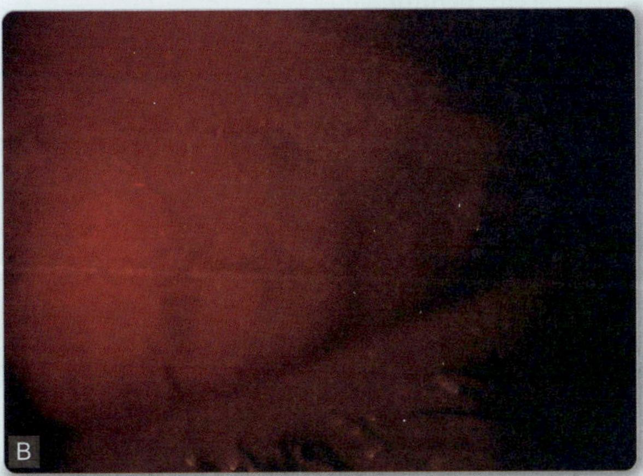

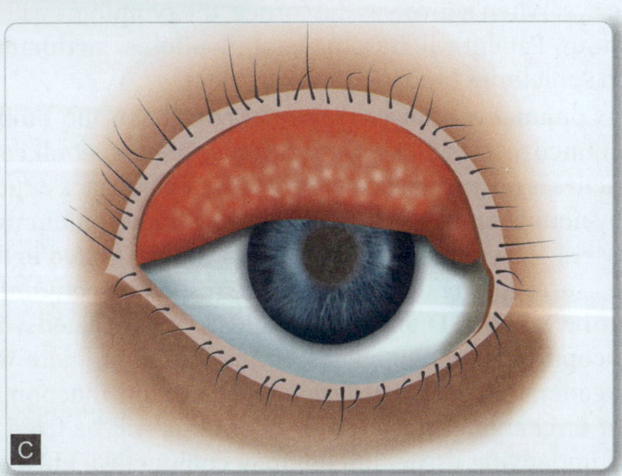

FIGURES 14.20A to C: **A.** Cobblestone appearance of upper tarsal conjunctiva (UTC) in spring catarrh; **B.** Flat-topped papillae on upper tarsal conjunctiva; **C.** Flat-topped papillae in spring catarrh (diagrammatic representation).

steroids, which may be judiciously used and tapered off as soon as the symptoms show some relief. The patient runs the risk of the complications of long-term use of steroids; secondary bacterial infections, glaucoma and cataract, so that misuse of steroids is to be avoided.

Systemic NSAIDs may help to control severe inflammation. In patients with large florid upper papillae, subconjunctival injection of triamcinolone acetonide or dexamethasone 0.5–1 mL into the supratarsal region can be given. The patient has to be closely followed-up for the development of secondary glaucoma.

Topical cyclosporine drops applied 2–4 times daily may be effective in refractory cases of VKC, which do not show significant response to other modalities of treatment.

Phlyctenular Conjunctivitis

Phlyctenular keratoconjunctivitis or phlyctenulosis is a localized corneal and/or conjunctival inflammation that is believed to represent a cell medicated or delayed hypersensitivity response induced by endogenous microbial antigens (AAO External Diseases and Cornea, 2011–2012).

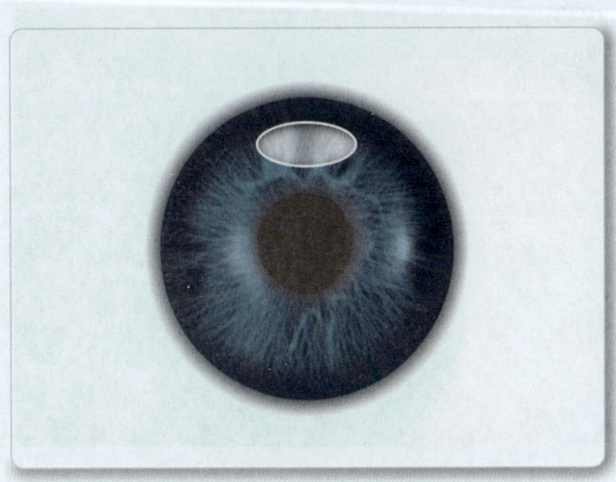

FIGURE 14.21: Shield ulcer

Etiology

In developing countries where malnutrition and tuberculosis are endemic, it is usually an allergic reaction to tuberculous protein. In developed countries, it is frequently associated with *S. aureus* infections as an allergic response to the cell wall component of *Staphylococcus.* Streptococcal infections of tonsil and adenoid may also be other factors. Children are more commonly affected.

Clinical Features

Pure phlyctenular conjunctivitis produces minimal symptoms. There will be mild irritation of the eye. Patients usually approache a doctor with the complaints of redness of the eye. When it involves the cornea, the symptoms will be serious. Patient will have pain, photophobia, lacrimation and sometimes blurring of vision.

Conjunctival phlycten usually appear on the bulbar conjunctiva at or close to the limbus. The palpebral conjunctiva is not involved. A typical phlycten appear as a pale gray nodule or bleb surrounded by engorged conjunctival vessels. The conjunctival congestion will be limited to the area surrounding the phlycten. The rest of the conjuntiva will be normal. Often phlyctenulosis is associated with mucopurulent conjunctivitis. In this situation, there will be generalized conjunctival congestion and mucopurulent discharge. A phlycten at the limbus will be fixed to the underlying tissue. But a purely conjunctival phlycten is not fixed to the underlying episcleral tissue and it can be moved with the conjunctiva by pressure applied by a finger through the lower lid (Figs 14.22A and B).

The phlycten will be initially very small and vesicular and only careful examination of the congested area will reveal it. But they gradually increase in size and reach up to 3–4 mm in diameter. The epithelium over the surface becomes necrotic and it can form a shallow ulcer and heals rapidly without leaving any scar, if it is confined to the conjunctiva.

Treatment

1. Phlyctenular conjunctivitis responds well to topical steroids and when the size of the nodule diminishes, the topical steroids can be tapered off.
2. Systemic or general measures are also important especially in cases with recurring episodes. Children living in areas where tuberculosis is endemic (as in India) have to be investigated for tuberculosis and treated, if it is present. The general health of the child also has to be improved.
3. In cases with no evidence of tuberculosis, child has to be investigated for any source of focal infection in the throat or the lid margin. Swabs may be taken and C&S studies and a course of antibiotics given to eradicate the focal sepsis.

Atopic Keratoconjunctivitis

Atopic keratoconjunctivitis (AKC) is seen in young adults with a history of atopic dermatitis. One third of cases of atopic dermatitis develop this problem, often several years after the onset of the features of this disease.

Clinical Features

The clinical features are similar to VKC, but there are some distinguishing characteristics, as given below:

1. Vernal keratoconjunctivitis affects young children; AKC starts at a higher age usually involving young adults.

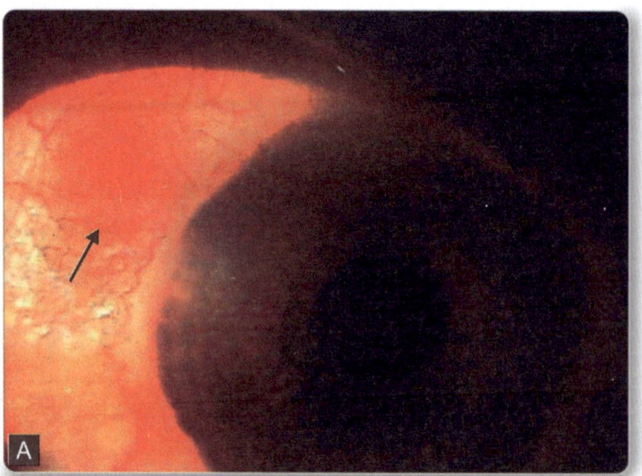

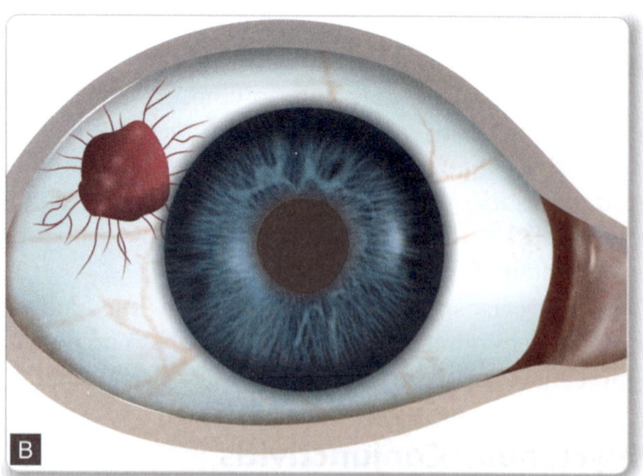

FIGURES 14.22 A and B: Phlycten. **A.** Photograph; **B.** Limbal phlycten with feeder vessels (diagrammatic representation).

2. The AKC does not show seasonal variation like VKC.
3. The VKC usually has a spontaneous resolution after some years. AKC runs a more chronic course. Hence, complications like keratoconus, keratectasia and corneal opacification are more frequent in AKC.
4. The papillae in AKC are much smaller and often the lower lid is more involved than the upper lid.
5. Subconjunctival fibrous tissue will give a pale look to the inferior palpebral conjunctiva and this can lead to symblepharon formation.
6. Cases of AKC are highly susceptible to HSV infection and *Staphylococcus* blepharoconjunctivitis due to altered systemic cell-mediated immunity.

Treatment

Treatment is on the same line as VKC:

1. In patients of severe AKC, topical medications alone may not be sufficient, they may require systemic immunosuppressant agents like cyclosporine (2.0–2.5 mg/kg daily).
2. They have to be closely monitored for any HSV or staphylococcal infections and if present, this will require specific therapy.

Ligneous Conjunctivitis

Ligneous conjunctivitis is a rare chronic disorder characterized by the formation of firm fibrinous pseudomembrane on the conjunctival surface. The cause of ligneous conjunctivitis was unknown till recently. Now it is linked to severe deficiency of type I plasminogen with hypofibrinolysis as the primary defect. The genetic defect in the plasminogen gene is located at chromosome 6q26.

Clinical Features

Often starts in childhood, but can affect all ages. Patients will complain of irritation and foreign body sensation. On eversion of the lids, one or both palpebral surfaces show firm 'woody' pseudomembranes, which recur after peeling off. Similar pseudomembranous lesions are seen in other mucous membrane also as in oral cavity, nasopharynx and vagina, etc.

Management

Bacterial and viral causes for pseudomembranous conjunctivitis should be excluded by culture and conjunctival smear studies.

Medical management includes administration of purified plasminogen, fresh frozen plasma, corticosteroids or azathioprine.

Surgical Management

Excision of the pseudomembrane and cryotherapy or amniotic membrane transplantation:

1. The most suitable treatment for each case has to be decided by trial and error method.
2. Many cases may spontaneously resolve after some months or years.

Contact Lens-associated Allergic Conjunctivitis

Contact lens-associated allergic conjunctivitis has a multifactorial etiology. Similar response has been seen in patients wearing artificial prosthesis or having retained exposed sutures.

Causes

1. It can be due to irritation of the upper tarsal conjunctiva by the edge of an ill-fitting contact lens, roughened surface of a prosthesis or the tip of an exposed suture.
2. It can be an allergy to the contact lens material or a reaction to the protein deposit formed on the lens surface.

Clinical Features

Irritation, watering, itching, redness and mucoid discharge in a patient wearing a contact lens or a prosthesis for variable period of time. On everting the upper tarsal conjunctiva, it will show papillary hypertrophy. The papillae can assume very large size up to 0.3–1 mm in size and then this condition is called GPC. The cornea may show punctate epithelial erosions.

Management

Control the inflammation with topical mast cell stabilizer, antihistamine or steroid drops. Remove the offending contact lens, prosthesis or suture. A new pair of the same type of contact lens or prosthesis can be given. Proper cleaning of the contact lens and the prosthesis should be taught to the patient to avoid deposit formation on them.

If the allergy is to the material of the contact lens or prosthesis, the symptoms will continue. In this situation, replace the soft contact lens with a rigid gas permeable lens or change the prosthesis to one of the different material.

Periodic replacement of the contact lens or prosthesis is essential to prevent recurrence of GPC.

Ocular Cicatricial Pemphigoid

Ocular cicatricial pemphigoid (OCP) is a disease of unknown etiology, which affects people above 50 years of age. It is considered to be a type II hypersensitivity in which cell injury results from antibodies against a cell surface antigen in the basement zone. Antibodies activate complement with a subsequent breakdown of the conjunctival membrane.

Clinical Features

The disease has an insidious onset and both eyes are affected. Patient complains of irritation, watering and photophobia. Subconjunctival vesicles or membranes appear on the conjunctival and subsequent scarring of the conjunctiva leads to shrinkage of the conjunctiva, obliteration of the fornices, symblepharon and ankyloblepharon. Destruction of the glands of the conjunctiva leads to severe dry eye. Cornea involvement includes superficial punctate keratopathy and pannus. The trichiasis, dry eye and corneal exposure due to lid contracture leads to corneal ulceration and loss of vision. There will be similar vesicular lesions on other mucous membranes of the body.

Differential Diagnosis

1. Other vesicular mucocutaneous disorders like epidermolysis bullosa, dermatitis herpetiformis, etc.

   Diagnosis can be confirmed by conjunctival biopsy and immunofluorescent staining.
2. Pseudopemphigoid: It is a similar picture produced by chronic topical drug usage and hypersensitivity reaction to them, e.g. pilocarpine and timolol. The stoppage of the medication will reverse the situation.

Treatment

Topical

- Steroid drops: To control inflammation
- Artificial tears: To control the dry eye
- Antibiotic drops: To control secondary bacterial infection.

Systemic

- Steroids to control acute exacerbation
- Dapsone is sometimes useful in moderate cases
- Cytotoxic agents like methotrexate and cyclophosphamide when steroids fail to control inflammation.

Surgery

- To correct cicatricial entropion and trichiasis
- Punctal occlusion to conserve tears
- Tarsorrhaphy in non-healing corneal epithelial defects
- Keratoprosthesis in end stage disease when everything else fails.

Stevens-Johnson Syndrome

Stevens-Johnson syndrome is an acute severe mucocutaneous vesicular disease. It usually affects young adults. It is a type II hypersensitivity reaction triggered by:

1. Drug allergy (commonly to phenobarbitone, NSAIDs, paracetamol, etc.).
2. Systemic infections (caused by HSV, mycoplasma pneumonia, etc.).
3. Idiopathic.

Clinical Presentation

The syndrome (Figs 14.23A and B) has an acute onset and runs a self-limiting course and can be fatal in some patients. There will be redness, watering and photophobia associated with fever and mucocutaneous eruptions. A history of any drug intake may or may not be present.

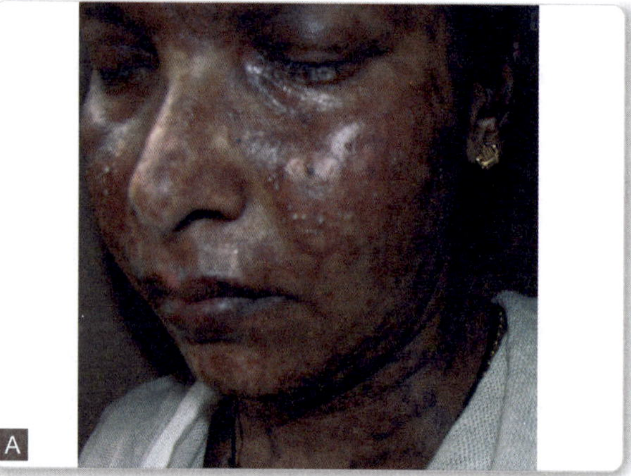

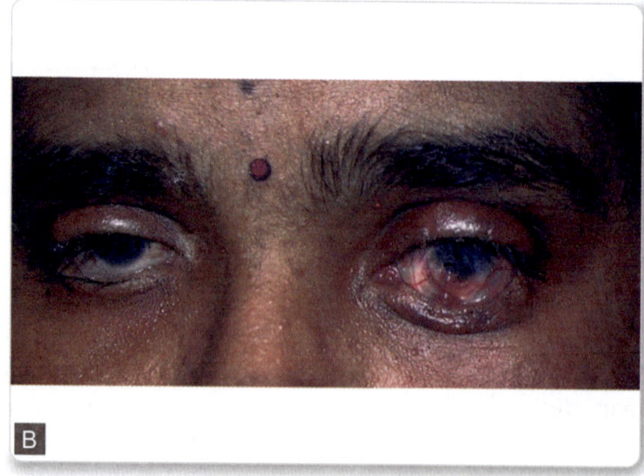

FIGURES 14.23A and B: Stevens-Johnson (SJ) syndrome. **A.** Skin lesions; **B.** Ocular clinical presentation.

There will be intense congestion of conjunctiva with pseudo or true membrane formation. Cornea may be involved with superficial punctate erosion and secondary bacterial infections can set in leading to corneal ulceration. The destruction of the conjunctiva by the inflammation can lead to entropion trichiasis, severe dry eye and symblepharon formation. All these sequelae can cause further damage to the cornea. Recurrent epithelial breakdown, ulceration and corneal opacification can occur.

The cutaneous and other mucous membrane lesions will heal, if the patient survives, but the patient will have lifelong suffering and partial or total visual impairment due to the severe dry eye and corneal problems.

Treatment

In the acute phase, the main aim is to control the inflammation and subsequent permanent damage to the conjunctiva and cornea.

Topical

1. Artificial tears and lubricant gels or antibiotic ointments are applied frequently to keep the raw surfaces from forming adhesions.
2. Topical steroids are applied frequently to control the inflammation.
3. Antibiotics are given topically to prevent or control secondary infection.
4. Amniotic membrane transplantation within the first 2 weeks will help to control the inflammation and its sequelae like symblepharon formation and dry eye.

Systemic

Systemic antibiotics, steroids, IV fluids and electrolytes to control the electrolyte imbalance caused by the generalized vesiculation.

Management of Sequelae

Once the acute phase is over, subsequent management depends on the cicatricial damage that has occurred in the eye.

Patients usually require lifelong artificial tear therapy to control the dry eye.

If symblepharon formation has occurred, adhesion can be mechanically released after all inflammation has subsided and amniotic membrane transplantation can be done.

Corneal opacities will require keratoplasty. But the success rate will be very low due to the dry eye, heavy vascularization of the cornea and the destruction of the limbal stem cells, which are essential for normal epithelialization and maintenance of clarity of the graft. Limbal stem cell from a near relative can be grown on amniotic membrane by tissue culture method and transplanted to the patients' eye. This will increase the chances of success of a subsequent keratoplasty and also decrease the dry eye problem. But the facilities for limbal stem cell transplantation are available only in advanced centers.

DEGENERATIVE CONDITIONS OF CONJUNCTIVA

CONCRETIONS

Concretions are yellowish white spots seen on the palpebral conjunctiva. Histologically they are epithelial cysts filled with epithelial and keratin debris. Usually seen in elderly persons or people who have trachoma or chronic conjunctivitis (Fig. 12.24).

Clinical Features

Usually concretions produce no symptoms. Sometimes they project from the conjunctival surface on the upper tarsal conjunctiva and cause irritation and foreign body sensation.

On examination, they are seen as minute, yellowish, flat or raised lesions on the conjunctiva.

Treatment

If they are producing symptoms, they can be removed with a fine needle after applying topical anesthetic drops in the conjunctival sac.

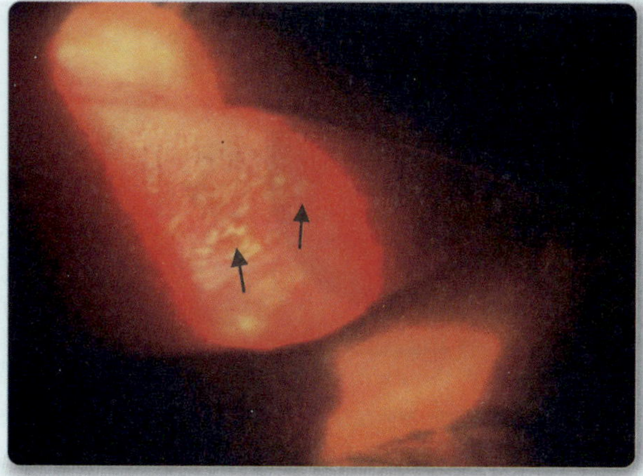

FIGURE 14.24: Concretions

PINGUECULA

Pinguecula is a pale yellowish triangular patch seen in the bulbar conjunctiva close to the limbus within the palpebral aperture. It looks like fat and hence the name (pinguis means fat). But it does not contain fat and it is due to hyaline infiltration and elastotic degeneration of the subepithelial layer of the conjunctiva. It is usually seen in the elderly (Fig. 14.25).

Clinical Features

The disease does not usually produce any symptoms. But it can sometimes get inflamed (pingueculitis) and this can cause pain and watering. It can become very conspicuous when subconjunctival hemorrhage occurs. It can stand out prominently in a background of bright red color of blood.

Treatment

The disease does not require any treatment. If patients feel it is cosmetically ugly, it can be removed surgically. If pingueculitis develops, a short course of topical steroid drop will control the inflammation.

Differential Diagnosis

1. Pterygium: The yellowish color and the apex of the triangle away from the cornea and non-involvement of the limbus differentiate it from a pterygium.
2. Limbal nodules and tumors: The yellowish color and absence of congestion differentiates it from inflammatory and tumor nodules at the limbus.

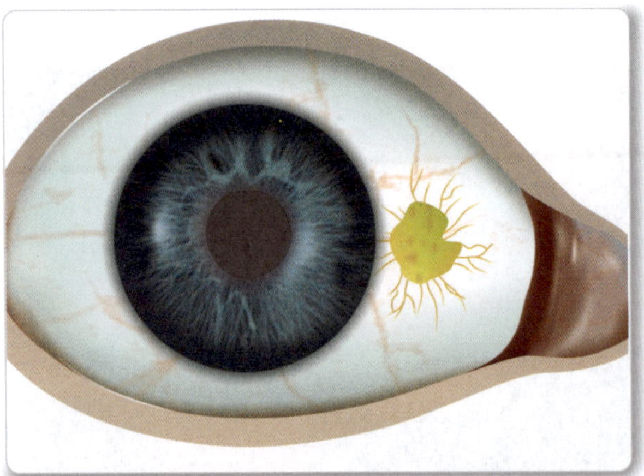

FIGURE 14.25: Pinguecula

PTERYGIUM

Pterygium is a degenerative condition of the subconjunctival tissue, which grows as a fibrovascular triangular tissue covered with conjunctival epithelium onto the cornea, destroying the superficial layers of the stroma and the epithelium (Figs 14.26A to D).

Etiology

It is much more common in the tropical countries. So, UV light plays an important role in its development. Dryness and exposure to irritants like dust, smoke and wind also play a role. Usually seen in the elderly, it can occur in younger people also, who are more exposed to UV light and irritants as an occupational hazard, e.g. fishermen, cooks, people engaged in welding jobs, etc.

Clinical Features

The main complaint of a patient will be the reddish growth in the eye. Pterygium can affect vision, but decrease in vision is rarely one of the presenting complaints.

Signs

A triangular fibrovascular growth is seen at the limbus at the palpebral aperture usually on the nasal side, rarely on the temporal side and sometime on both temporal and nasal side. It can be thin and atrophic, containing only a few vessels and showing minimal growth or thick and fleshy, if it is an actively growing one. A line of pigment may be seen on the cornea anterior to the advancing edge of the pterygium-Stocker's line.

Complications

1. Pterygium can interfere with vision in two ways. It can cause decrease in vision by:
   a. Irregular astigmatism, as it invades the cornea.
   b. As it reaches the pupillary area, it can block the light rays and the vision. This visual problem will persist even after excision of the growth due to the corneal opacity left behind.
2. Recurrent inflammation can occur in a pterygium. This can be controlled with steroid drops.
3. Cystoid degeneration can occur.
4. It can interfere with proper wetting on the cornea leading to 'dellen' formation.

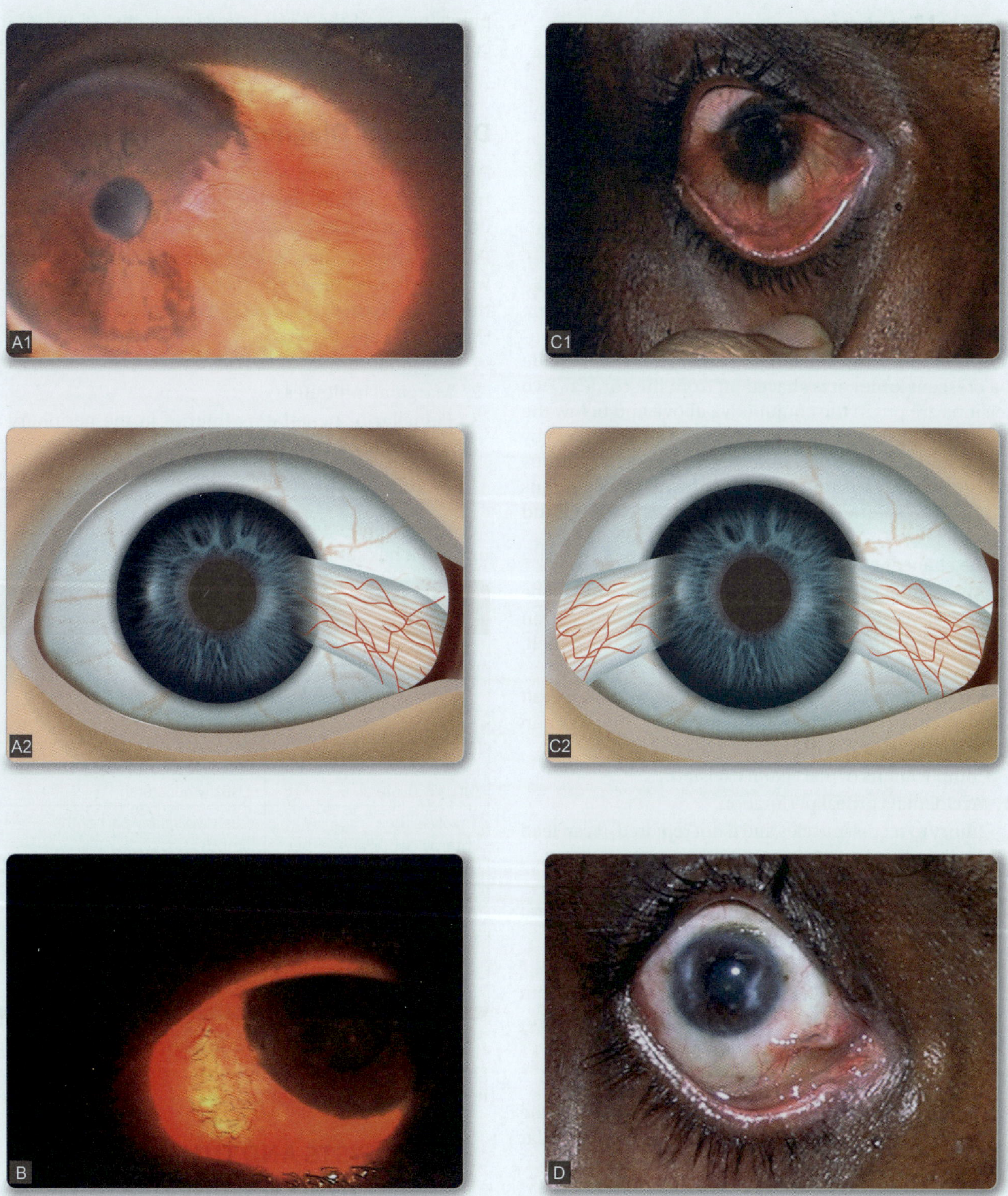

FIGURES 14.26A to D: Excision pterygium. **A1 and A2.** Pterygium; **B.** Appearance after excision; **C1 and C2.** Bilimbal pterygium; **D.** Postoperative picture after excision.

Surgical Treatment

Since there is a high chance of recurrence, surgery is planned only:

1. If it is actively growing and possibility of invading the visual axis is there.
2. If it is cosmetically disfiguring. The surgeries can be any one of the following.

Simple Excision of the Pterygium

Technique: After thorough cleaning and draping of the patient, local anesthetic is injected under the pterygium. With a fixation forceps, the pterygium is held at the limbus and with a sharp knife [Bard Parker (BP) No. 15 blade or a crescent knife], it is shaved off from the cornea. Two incisions are put in the conjunctiva above and below the conjunctival limits of the pterygium and it is removed by cutting off with scissors, midway between the limbus and the canthus without injuring the underlying rectus muscle. The sclera close to the limbus is cleaned and left bare (Figs 14.27A to D).

The chances of recurrences can be minimized by:

1. Application of Mitomycin-C drops (0.4 mg/mL) at the end of surgery to the bare scleral area using cotton tapped applicator (the complications are scleral melt, cataract and iritis).
2. Covering the bare area with a limboconjunctival graft taken from the same eye from the upper limbus or an amniotic membrane graft.

Complications of pterygium excision:

1. Accidental corneal perforation.
2. Injury to rectus muscles and if not repaired, it can lead to diplopia.
3. Bleeding.
4. Scleral necrosis and staphyloma formation, if scleral dissection is deep or mitomycin is used.
5. Recurrence of pterygium.
6. Limbal stem cell deficiency in bilimbal pterygium leading to irritable eye with corneal vascularization.

Lamellar Keratoplasty

Simple dissection of the cornea will leave a scar. So, if the pterygium encroaches onto the pupillary area, a lamellar keratoplasty is needed to obtain a clear visual axis.

McReynold's Operation

The operation is rarely done now. The pterygium is shaved off from cornea and freed from the surrounding conjunctiva by 2 parallel incisions above and below the body of pterygium, and the freed pterygium is buried under the conjunctiva in the inferior fornix and fixed there with sutures. The aim is to prevent recurrence.

Differential Diagnosis

Pinguecula: It is more yellowish in color. The apex of the triangular growth is directed away from the limbus and it does not encroach onto the cornea.

Pseudopterygium: It is a triangular fold of conjunctiva, which gets attached to the periphery of the cornea when there is a persistent raw area in the periphery of the cornea (Figs 14.28A and B) as in:

1. Marginal corneal ulcers.
2. Marginal infiltrates.
3. Lamellar or penetrating injuries in the periphery of the cornea.
4. Such pseudopterygium can occur in chemical injuries, OCP, etc.

A pseudopterygium closely resembles a true pterygium, but it has some differentiating features (Table 14.4).

TABLE 14.4: Differences between pterygium and pseudopterygium

Pterygium	Pseudopterygium
Degenerative process of the conjunctiva	Follows some injury or inflammation in the cornea close to limbus
Seen usually in the elderly	Occur in any age group
Usually bilateral	Usually unilateral
Involves the interpalpebral area either nasal or temporal side	Can involve any part of the limbus
The whole pterygium will be attached to the underlying tissue	Attached to the cornea only at the apex of the conjunctival fold; so a probe can be passed underneath the pseudopterygium

Any other nodule at the limbus like a foreign body granuloma, ophthalmia nodosum, phlycten, papilloma, nevus, malignant melanoma, etc.

CYSTS AND TUMORS OF THE CONJUNCTIVA

The conjunctiva is the common site for the development of benign and malignant tumors. The limbus, which is a transition zone for the surface epithelium, is a common site where these tumors arise. Since, malignant tumors often

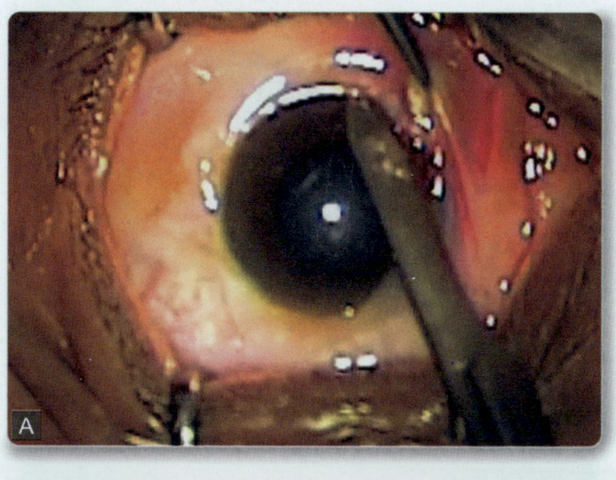

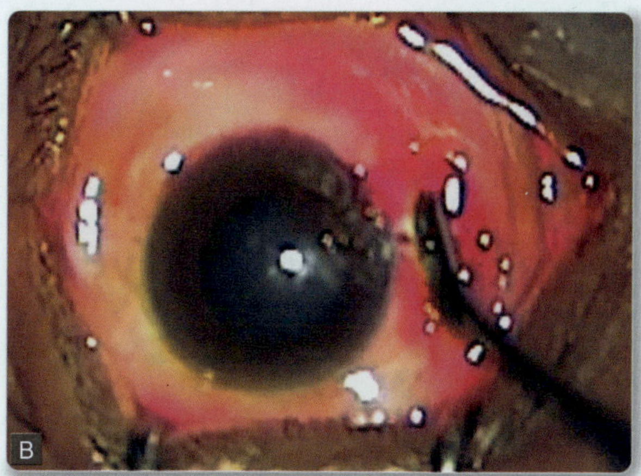

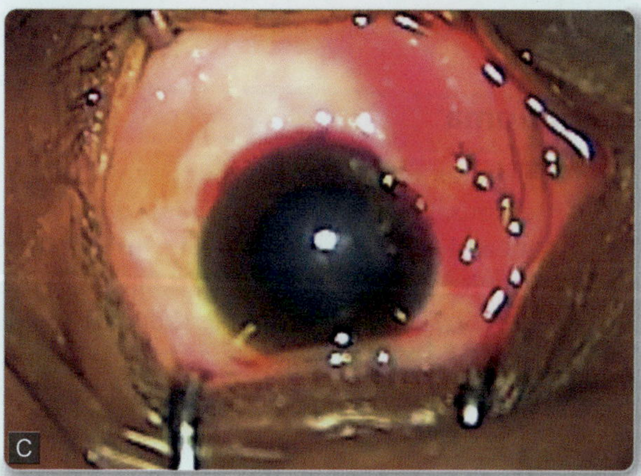

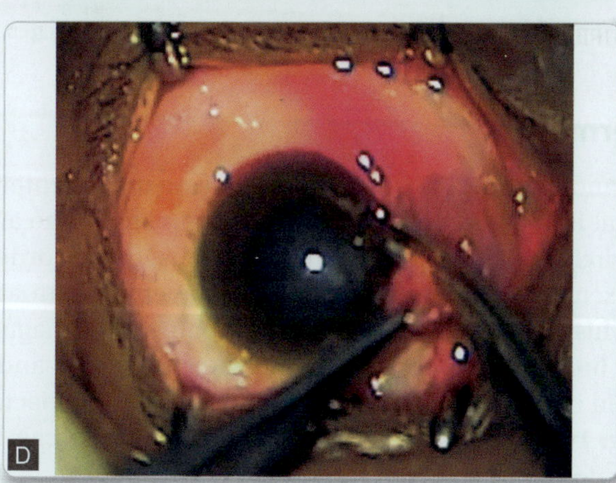

FIGURES 14.27A to D: Excision of the pterygium. **A.** Pterygium is dissected from the cornea; **B.** Cornea is cleaned off all pterygium tissue; **C.** The pterygium is dissected from the sclera; **D.** Pterygium is cut with scissors.

involve the conjunctiva and cornea together, the malignant tumors arising on the ocular surface are often grouped together and termed as ocular surface neoplasia (OSN).

CYSTS OF THE CONJUNCTIVA

1. Thin-walled transparent cysts containing clear fluid can appear on the bulbar conjunctiva or the upper or lower fornices (Fig. 14.29).
2. They are usually due to enlargement of lymphatic vessels due to some obstruction—lymphangiectasia. They can appear as a row of cysts also like a string of beads.
3. They can be retention cysts of the Krause's glands or accessory lacrimal glands when they usually appear on the superior fornix.
4. Epithelial implantation cysts can develop following some injury to the eye. Such cysts are not transparent as the lymphatic cysts.

Cystic degeneration of a long-standing pterygium can occur close to the limbus.

Treatment

1. Small cysts causing no symptoms can be left alone.
2. If cosmetically disfiguring or causing irritation, or foreign body sensation, marsupialization or simple excision of the cysts can be done.
3. Simple puncturing of the cysts with a needle will give only a temporary solution. The cysts will reform soon.

CONGENITAL TUMORS

Congenital tumors are either dermoids or dermolipoma. They are not true neoplasm. They are choristomas—abnormal growth of normal tissue in an abnormal location.

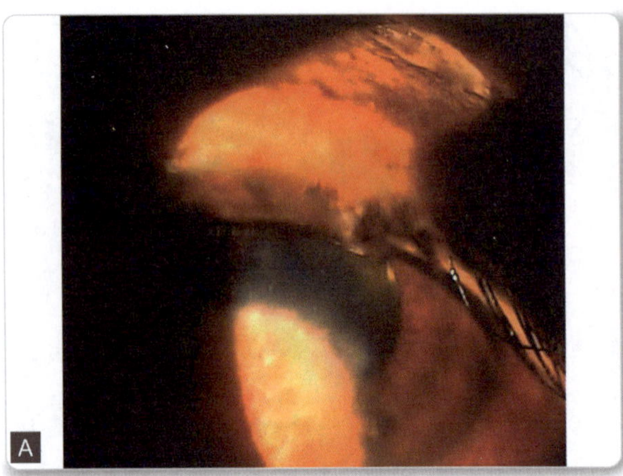

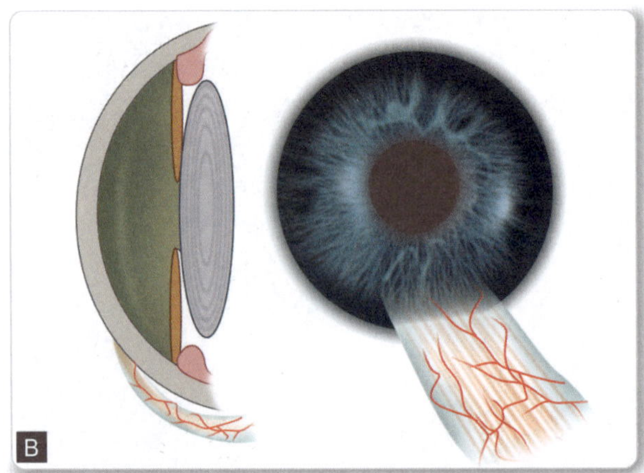

FIGURES 14.28A and B: Pseudopterygium. **A.** Photograph; **B.** Peripheral opacity with pseudopterygium (diagrammatic representation).

Dermoids

Dermoids appear as soft yellow masses at the inferotemporal limbus. Sometimes they can attain larger size and encircle the cornea or rarely include most of the cornea. Presence of hairs, keratinization of the epithelium and the history of presence since birth, confirms the diagnosis. It usually increases in size as the child grows and a rapid increase at the time of puberty has to be expected (Fig. 14.30A). Small cysts causing no symptoms can be left alone.

Treatment

Surgical excision, if it is large and disfiguring. Simple excision will leave a dense scar on the cornea. If the involvement of the cornea is extensive, a lamellar keratoplasty is ideal to avoid the opacity.

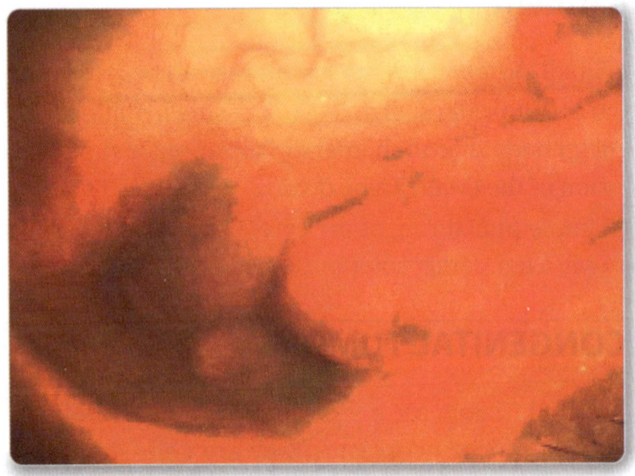

FIGURE 14.29: Conjunctival cysts in lower fornix

Dermolipoma

Usually appears as soft yellow subconjunctival mass at the outer canthus. It is usually continuous with orbital-dermolipoma and so the posterior limit cannot be seen. Though congenital, the mass is detected later in life, often accidentally by everting the upper lid (Fig. 14.30B).

Treatment

Surgical excision should be avoided, since this can damage the nerve supply to lateral rectus and the LPS muscle, and can injure the lacrimal gland or its ducts. This can lead to convergent squint, diplopia, ptosis and dry eye problem. If it is large and disfiguring, careful excision of the anterior portion alone may be done without damaging the nerves, lateral rectus muscle or its nerve supply or lacrimal glands.

Both dermoid and dermolipoma can be associated with other congenital anomalies like accessory auricles, ear deformities, lid coloboma and vertebral anomalies and form Goldenhar's syndrome (Figs 14.31A and B).

ACQUIRED TUMORS

1. Squamous tumors:
   a. Papilloma—sessile or pedunculated.
   b. Pyogenic granuloma.
   c. Intraepithelial neoplasia.
   d. Squamous cell carcinoma (SCC) or ocular surface squamous neoplasia (OSSN).
2. Pigmented tumors:
   a. Pigmented lesions.
   b. Nevus.

c. Junctional nevus.
d. Conjunctival melanoma (Fig. 14.32):
• Pigmented
• Non-pigmented.

3. Miscellaneous tumors:
a. Conjunctival sebaceous gland carcinoma.
b. Conjunctival lymphoma.
c. Kaposi's sarcoma.

Squamous Tumors

Papilloma

Papilloma can be pedunculated or sessile.

Pedunculated papilloma

Pedunculated papilloma is caused by infections by human papilloma virus (HPV). Soft reddish pedunculated masses appear on the palpebral conjunctiva, fornices or caruncle. They often multiple in HIV patients and in children infected by mothers by vaginal passage.

Treatment: The tumor is treated by simple excision or cryotherapy. In recurrent cases, topical Mitomycin-C or subconjunctival interferon α is given.

Sessile papilloma

Sessile papilloma are seen in adults, usually in bulbar conjunctiva close to the limbus and often single. It is not related to papilloma virus infection (Fig. 14.33).

Treatment: It includes excision of the tumor.

Pyogenic Granuloma

Pyogenic granuloma are red fleshy granulation tissue seen in areas where subconjunctival tissue prolapses through surgical or traumatic wounds or bulbar conjunctiva after excision of pterygium and after squint surgery or in an empty socket after removal of the eyeball.

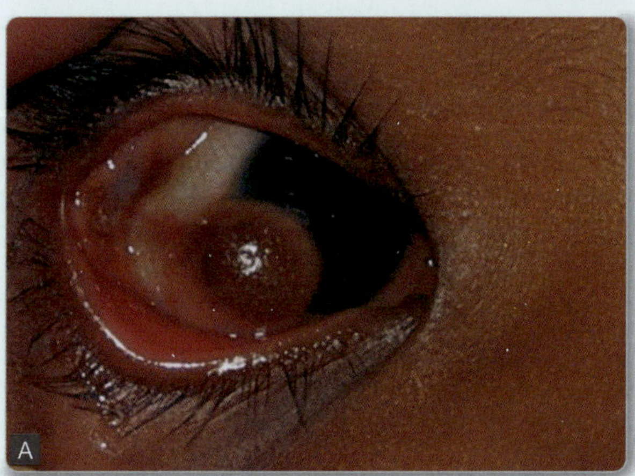
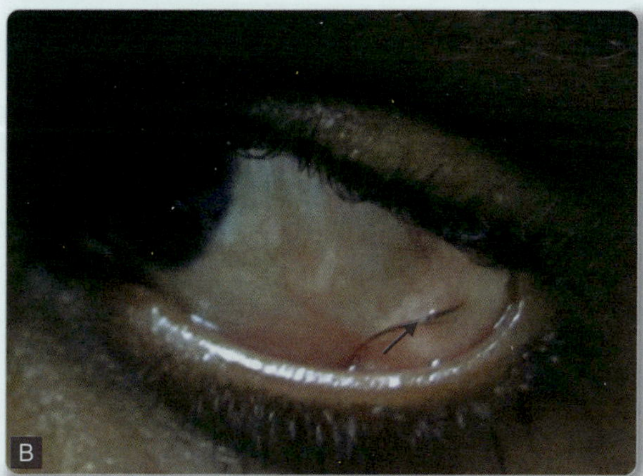

FIGURES 14.30A and B: Dermolipoma. **A.** Limbal dermoid; **B.** Dermolipoma with hair.

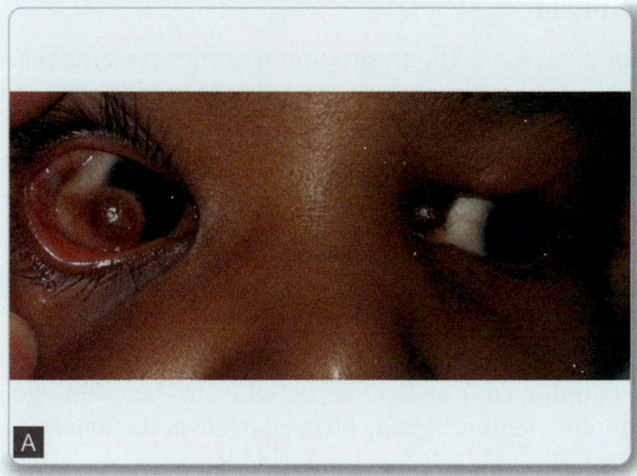
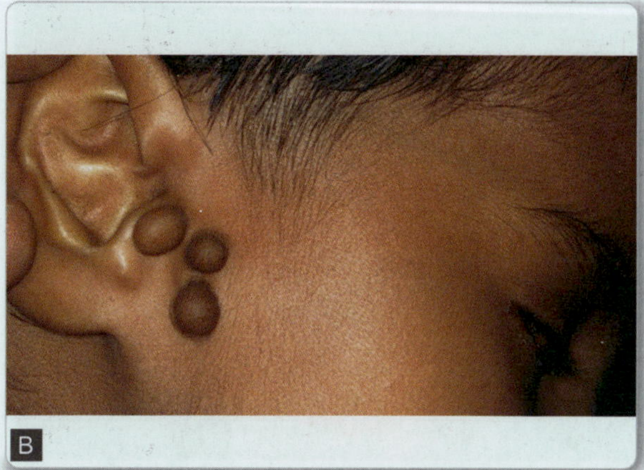

FIGURES 14.31A and B: A. Goldenhar's syndrome; **B.** Goldenhar's syndrome—accessory auricles.

Pyogenic granuloma is a misnomer, since it is neither pyogenic or granulomatous. It is a fibrovascular response to surgical or non-surgical trauma.

Treatment

The granuloma should be excised and the wound in the conjunctiva should be carefully sutured.

Ocular Surface Squamous Neoplasia

Ocular surface squamous neoplasia is the currently used term for precancerous and cancerous epithelial lesions of the conjunctiva and cornea. It includes dysplasia, carcinoma in situ and SCC (Figs 14.34A to C).

Etiology

1. Exposure to UV radiation plays an important role, since higher incidence is seen in people in tropical countries.
2. Human papilloma virus infection: HPV especially type 16 has been demonstrated in the eyes and tissue of OSSN and it may be playing a role in conjunction with other factors in the development of OSSN.
3. Acquired immunodeficiency syndrome (AIDS): Higher incidence of OSSN is reported in patients with AIDS, especially in African countries, and like HPV virus infection, it may be playing a supportive role to other factors like exposure to UV radiation.
4. Stem cell theory: Since OSSN usually arises at the limbus, where the stem cells are located, various risk factors may be acting on these stem cells leading to their abnormal maturation and proliferation leading to formation of OSSN.

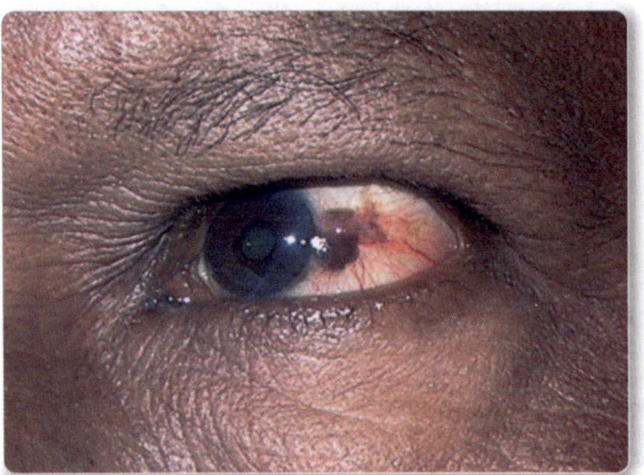

FIGURE 14.32: Conjunctival melanoma

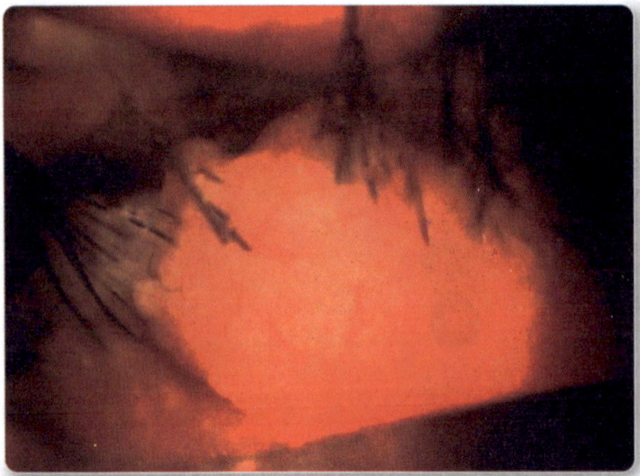

FIGURE 14.33: Sessile papilloma on upper lid margin

Sx Symptoms

Apart from swelling, the patients may complain of some redness and irritation of the eye.

Signs

It is difficult to clinically differentiate between dysplasia, carcinoma in situ and SCC. The usual site of the lesion is the interpalpebral area on the bulbar conjunctiva at or near the limbus. Usually seen as a gelatinous thickening with superficial vessels, which give a papillae-like appearance. It usually spreads over the conjunctiva as well as the nearby cornea. Growth may be rapid or slow, taking months to years. It can appear as nodular lesion when it is usually a SCC or a diffusely spreading growth.

Differential diagnosis

Pinguecula, pterygium, squamous papilloma.

Investigations

Exfoliative cytology with scraping from the conjunctival surface or impression cytology using a filter paper may at times help in identifying the cancer cells, but a negative test does not exclude malignant changes.

Treatment

Surgical excision: The traditional treatment is surgical excision with a surrounding 3–4 mm of normal tissue. This may require superficial sclerectomy or lamellar keratectomy when the lesion is at the limbus. Even when the edges of the excised tissue is free of the neoplasm, the recurrence rate are high up to 15%–50%.

Cryotherapy: To bring down the recurrence rate, surgical excision can be combined with cryotherapy.

Surgical reconstruction: When large areas of ocular surface are bared, a conjunctival autograft from the other eye or amniotic membrane may be used to cover the defect.

Topical chemotherapy: It includes the following:

1. Mitomycin-C: 0.2% four times daily for 2 weeks.

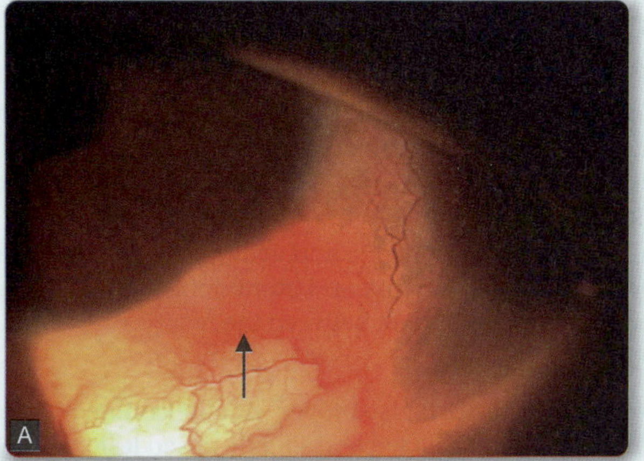

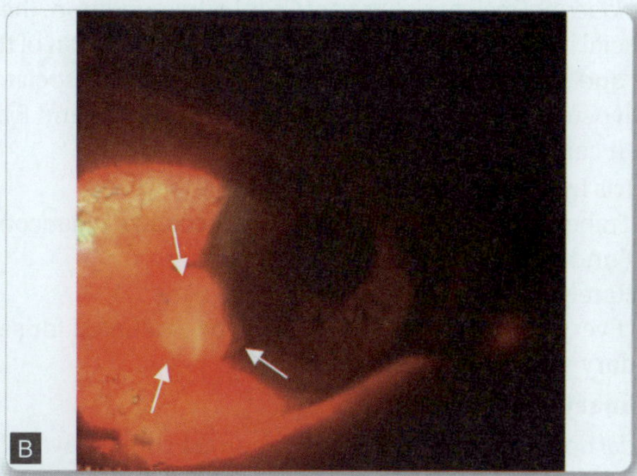

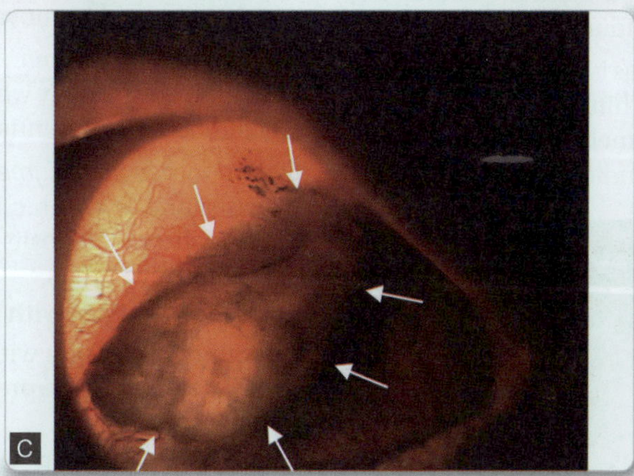

FIGURES 14.34A to C: Ocular surface squamous neoplasia (OSSN). **A.** With feeder vessel at limbus; **B.** OSSN; **C.** An advanced lesion extending up to the pupil.

2. Fluorouracil: 1% drops four times daily for 4 weeks.
3. Interferon-α 2b: As drops or intralesional injection.

These can be used to reduce the recurrence rate.

Conjunctival and Corneal Intraepithelial Neoplasia (CCIN)

Histologically, the dysplastic changes are limited to the deeper layer of the epithelium, but clinically it is difficult to differentiate from SCC when the lesion is flat and slow going. Management is on the same lines as SCC.

Pigmented Tumors

Conjunctival Melanosis

A variety of pigmentation can occur on the conjunctiva. This can be congenital or acquired:

1. Congenital:
   - Ocular melanosis
   - Oculodermal melanosis.
2. Acquired:
   - Racial
   - Primary:
     - With atypia
     - Without atypia.
   - Secondary.

Congenital melanosis: A localized area of pigmentation around an intrascleral nerve or where an anterior ciliary artery enters the globe is common. It is called Axenfeld loop.

Congenital oculodermal melanosis: This appears as multiple areas of episcleral pigmentation. Since the pigmentation is deeper to the conjunctiva, it has a slate-gray color and conjunctiva can be freely moved over it.

Oculodermal melanosis (nevus of Ota): In this condition, there is facial hyperpigmentation in the area of distribution of the 1st and 2nd divisions of the trigeminal nerve associated with ocular melanosis. It is unilateral (Figs 14.35A and B).

It can be associated with:
- Iris hyperpigmentation
- Trabecular hyperpigmentation with secondary glaucoma
- Fundus hyperpigmentation
- Rarely uveal melanoma.

Every case of nevus of Ota has to be evaluated for secondary glaucoma.

Primary acquired type

Racial acquired melanosis: This is a normal conjunctival pigmentation that develops in dark skinned races. It is epithelial pigmentation and usually seen around the limbus and sometimes extends into the surrounding bulbar conjunctiva.

Primary acquired melanosis (PAM): This is an acquired pigmentation developing in the eyes of white races. PAM without atypia is a simple proliferation of melanocytes, while PAM with atypia is a premalignant condition. But the clinical features are the same. And biopsies, often from multiple sites are required to differentiate between the two (Fig. 14.36).

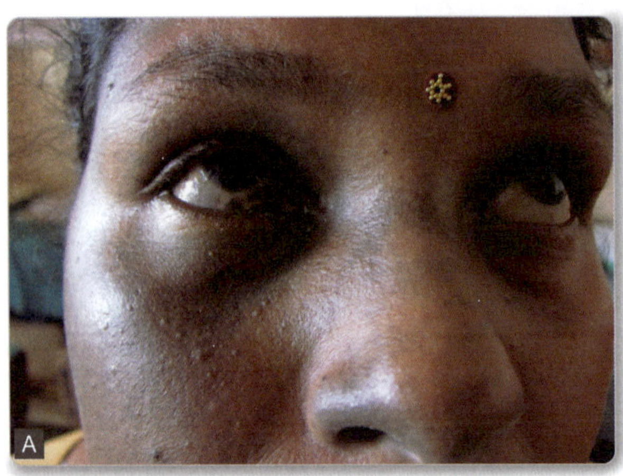

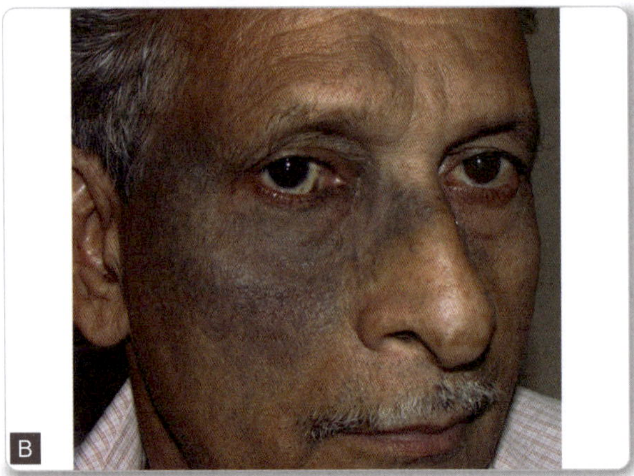

FIGURES 14.35A and B: Oculodermal melanosis. **A.** Nevus of Ota; **B.** Nevus of Ota with iris hyperpigmentation.

Clinical features

Occurs in white people of middle age or above. Multiple flat areas of brown pigmentation appear on any part of the conjunctiva. Since, it involves the epithelium, it moves with the conjunctiva.

Since, PAM with atypia and without atypia is clinically indistinguishable, biopsy and immunohistochemistry are required to differentiate between the two.

Differential diagnosis

Conjunctival nevus: It also moves with the conjunctiva, but it is often more localized and slightly raised lesion.

Episcleral melanosis or oculodermal melanocytosis: It is blue gray in color and immovable.

Conjunctival melanoma: Usually, elevated lesion, but in early stages especially when arising from PAM with atypia, it is difficult to differentiate.

Secondary acquired pigmentation: It can occur in Addison's diseases and is chronic in mascara users. Drug deposits (adrenochrome deposits) can occur in long-term users of adrenaline eye drops.

Treatment in PAM with atypia

1. Surgical excision with cryotherapy or both often cannot eliminate the problem, since it is difficult to cover the entire lesion.
2. Surgical excision with topical mitomycin therapy: This can be used instead of cryosurgery, since it can cover the hidden lesions also and does not produce the complications of cryotherapy.

Prognosis

Recurrence will occur in PAM with atypia after incomplete excision. Progression to malignant melanoma can occur in PAM with atypia.

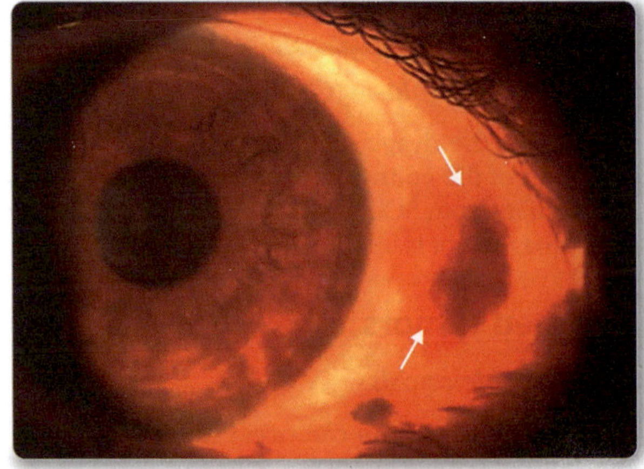

FIGURE 14.36: Primary acquired melanosis

Conjunctival Nevus

Conjunctival nevus is the most common melanocytic tumor of the conjunctiva. It affects all races, but it is more common in white races; it usually appears within the first two decades of life. If they appear later than two decades, it will be a PAM or melanoma.

Site

Commonly near the limbus. It appears on bulbar conjunctiva, plica or caruncle.

Clinical features

A lesion with variable pigmentation that appears within the first two decades, slowly growing in size as the child grows. If it appears in a child, there is some increase in size and pigmentation at the time of puberty and remain stable after puberty.

Signs

A well-circumscribed lesion with variable pigmentation on the bulbar conjunctiva, plica or caruncle, slightly raised or with cystic areas, moves well with the conjunctiva. No feeder vessels.

Treatment

Periodic observation with clinical photographs, if possible. Excision is done for cosmetic reason. Wide excision with cryoapplication to the margin of the conjunctiva around is done to prevent recurrence, if there is a sudden increase in size. If there is a change in pigmentation, increase in size, appearance of feeder vessels or recurrence after a simple excision, all these changes may denote a malignant transformation.

Malignant Melanoma of the Conjunctiva

Malignant melanoma of the conjunctiva is a rare ocular tumor. It accounts for about 2% of all ocular malignancies.

Etiology

No definite etiology is known. Mostly arise from PAM with atypia, pre-existing nevus or as a primary melanoma (least common). There is no association with nevus of Ota or cutaneous malignant melanoma (MM).

Clinical features

Usually seen in the elderly and only one eye is affected. Unlike nevus it can arise from any part of the conjunctiva. Pigmented lesion in the palpebral conjunctiva and fornix should arise high suspicion, since nevus does not develop in these areas. Two types:

1. Arising from PAM with atypia.
2. Arising directly without PAM.

Malignamt melanoma arising from PAM with atypia: Arises as a sudden enlargement or thickening in an otherwise flat lesion. It is usually multifocal and can involve the adjacent skin of the lids.

When arising denovo or from a pre-existing nevus, it is usually solitary, vascularized pigmented or non-pigmented lesion, commonly seen at the limbal area. A limbal lesion can extend into the cornea also, but a primary malignant melanoma (MM) of cornea is very rare.

Differential diagnosis

As follows:

- Conjunctival nevus
- PAM with or without atypia
- Scleral staphyloma
- Squamous papillomas
- Squamous cell carcinoma, which has developed pigmentation.

Points in favor of malignant melanoma

- A pigmented nodule developing after 2nd decade
- Location on the palpebral conjunctiva or fornix
- A sudden increase in size of a nevus
- Prominent feeder vessels
- Recurrence after excision of a nevus or PAM
- A sudden increase in size or thickening in an area of PAM

Confirmation of the diagnosis is by histopathological examination.

Treatment

Wide excision with a margin of 3–5 mm surrounding the lesion.

Adjuvant treatment: They are as follows:

1. Cryotherapy to the surgical margin and/or the surgical bed.
2. Mitomycin-C drops.

Surgical reconstruction of the bare area is often needed with conjunctival autograft or amniotic membrane.

Conjunctival melanoma is not radiosensitive. Spread to regional lymph nodes is treated with excision of lymph nodes and radiotherapy.

Miscellaneous Tumors

Conjunctival Lymphoma

Lymphocytes in the subconjunctival layer can proliferate and undergo malignant transformation. Systemic involvement is seen in 30% of cases (Figs 14.37A and B).

Clinical features

Patients present with complaints of a slow-growing, pinkish swelling in the eye.

Pink salmon or flesh-colored, ill-defined, slightly raised swelling with intrinsic vascularization and feeder vessels are seen often on the bulbar conjunctiva or the inferior

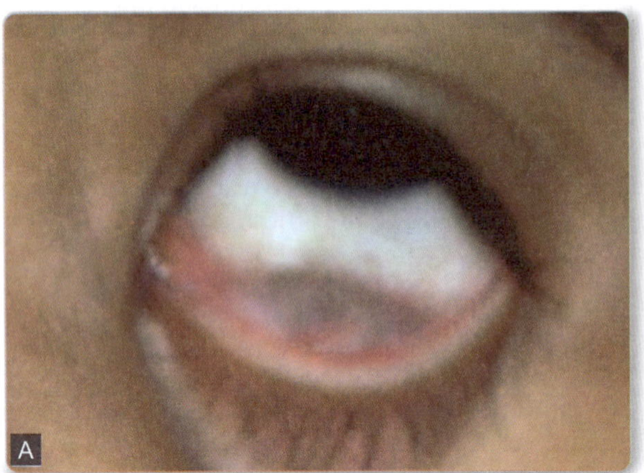

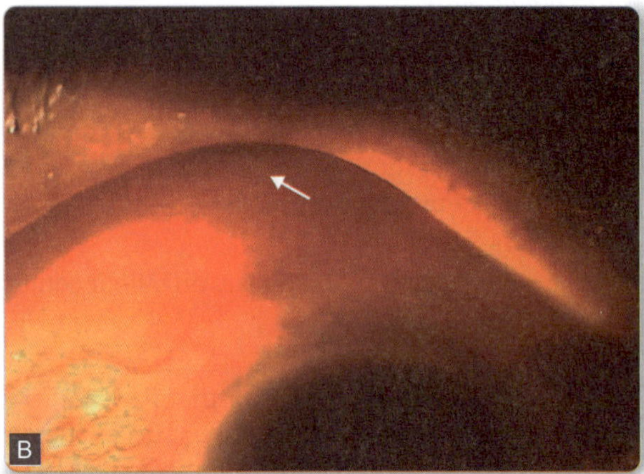

FIGURES 14.37A and B: **A.** Conjunctival lymphoma; **B.** Lymphoma.

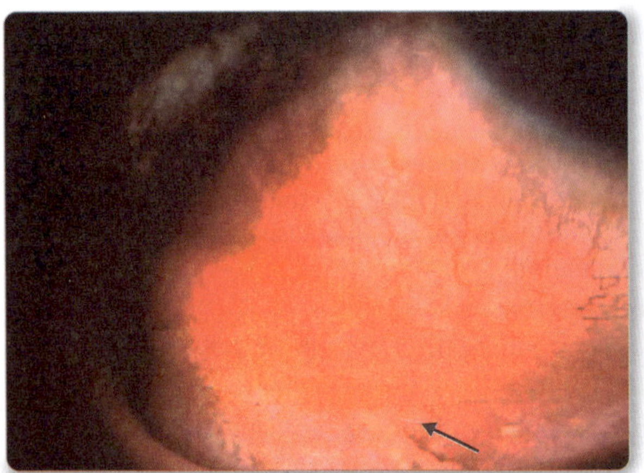

FIGURE 14.38: Sebaceous gland carcinoma in the inferior fornix

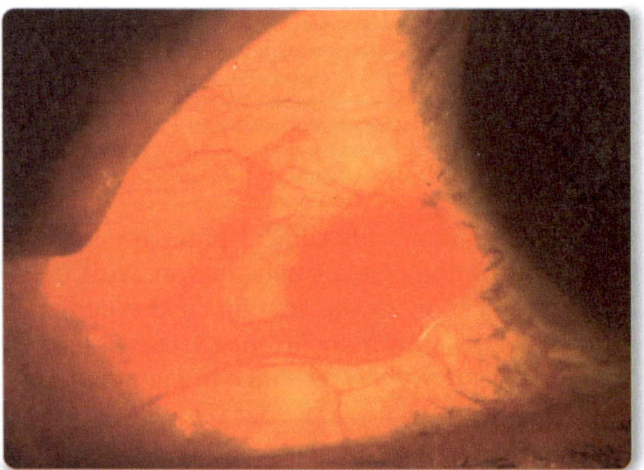

FIGURE 14.39: Conjunctival hemangioma

fornix. They can be bilateral or have posterior extensions into the orbit.

Diagnosis

Diagnosis is confirmed by biopsy.

Treatment

Treatment is wide excision combined with cryotherapy or chemotherapy and local injection of interferon-α 2b.

Kaposi's Sarcoma

Kaposi's sarcoma is seen in patients with AIDS. It is a slow-growing bright red lesion usually seen in the inferior fornix.

Treatment

Excision with cryotherapy or focal radiotherapy.

Sebaceous Gland Carcinoma

Sebaceous gland carcinoma (Fig. 14.38) can rarely develop on the conjunctiva by pagetoid spread from a meibomian gland or Zeis' gland. It often mimics chronic conjunctivitis, but irregular nodular thickening of the palpebral conjunctiva arouses suspicion and diagnosis is confirmed by biopsy.

Treatment

Treatment is by wide excision. Often exenteration will be required to completely eradicate the growth.

Tumors Arising from the Mesenchymal Tissue

Conjunctival hemangioma

Conjunctival hemangioma is extremely rare on the conjunctival surface.

Treatment: Excision can be done after closure of the feeder vessels by application of radiofrequency coagulator or diathermy (Fig. 14.39).

Prognosis of conjunctival tumors on the whole is good, since they are detected early due to the exposed position and most of them show only local spread.

Cornea

15

Girija Devi PS

ANATOMY AND PHYSIOLOGY

Key Features

- Cornea forms the anterior one-fifth transparent wall of the globe of eye
- It forms the major refractive surface of eye (43D–43.5D)
- Cornea with its tear film is a barrier against infection.

Shape/Size

- Cornea is horizontally oval in shape
- Horizontal diameter in adult is 11.5–12 mm
- Vertical diameter is less about 11–11.5 mm.

Development

- Corneal epithelium is derived from the surface ectoderm at 5–6 weeks of gestation
- Corneal stroma, keratocytes and endothelium develop from neural crest in the 7th week of gestation.

Layers of Cornea

Epithelium is stratified squamous and has the following layers (Fig. 15.1):

- Single layer of basal columnar cells lying on basement membrane
- Wing cells of 2–3 rows
- Two layers of squamous surface cells.

Epithelial stem cells are located mainly at the superior and inferior limbus and are indispensable for maintaining healthy corneal epithelium. New epithelial cells are formed from the stem cells and move in a centripetal direction toward the center of the cornea to replace the old cells. Dysfunction of stem cells cause chronic epithelial defect and has to be treated by stem cell transplantation.

Bowman's membrane is the acellular superficial layer of stroma. Stroma constitutes 90% of corneal thickness and consists of regularly oriented collagen fibrils set in a proteoglycan ground substance and interspersed with keratocytes (modified fibroblasts). Descemet's membrane is composed of a fine lattice work of collagen fibrils.

Endothelium consists of a single layer of hexagonal cuboidal cells that cannot regenerate. Endothelium is incapable of multiplication. When the endothelial cell density decreases, the existing cells flatten out to cover the whole of posterior corneal surface. From second to eighth decades of life, the cell density declines from 4,000 to 2,600 cells/mm^2. The endothelium is primarily responsible for maintaining the corneal dehydration and thus corneal transparency. A variation in the endothelial cell size (polymegathism) and variation in cell shape (pleomorphism) correlate with reduced ability of endothelium to maintain corneal transparency.

Cornea with cell count of less than 500 cells/mm^2 are at risk for developing corneal edema.

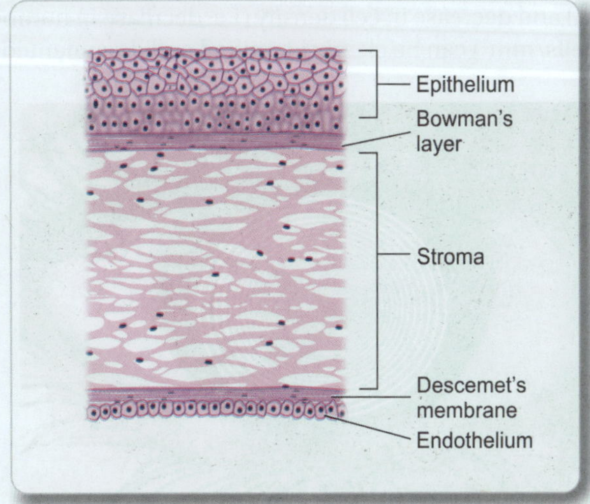

FIGURE 15.1: Anatomy of cornea

Blood Supply of Cornea

Cornea is avascular, which derives nourishment from the superficial episcleral plexus at the limbus and from the aqueous. The oxygen supply comes from the atmosphere through the precorneal tear film.

Nerve Supply of Cornea

Cornea is supplied with ophthalmic division of trigeminal nerve through the long ciliary nerves.

EXAMINATION OF CORNEA

Diagnostic modalities of the corneal pathologies are explained below.

Slit Lamp

Slit lamp is the commonly used equipment in clinical practice to identify corneal lesions, their exact dimensions, depth, edges, the condition of the overlying epithelium, clarity and thickness of the cornea.

Specular Microscopy

Specular microscopy is done by using specular microscope. When the instrument is focused on the posterior corneal surface, an image of the corneal endothelium is seen. This image can be viewed directly and photographed.

The endothelial cells are seen as a mosaic of hexagonal cells of the same size and cell boundaries are clearly defined.

Clinically significant anomalies such as pleomorphism (different abnormal shapes with different number of sides) and polymegathism (variation in individual cell area) and decrease in cell density (i.e. decrease in number of cells/mm^2) can be clearly identified and documented.

Corneal Topography

Computerized corneal topography is an assessment of the anterior surface of cornea and the curvature of the cornea. Normally, the cornea is slightly steeper in the center and flatters toward the periphery.

The different methods of assessment of corneal surface are detailed below.

Window Reflex

The image of a window frame reflected onto the cornea of the patient is assessed for any distortion. Distorted window reflex suggests irregularity of anterior corneal surface.

Placido's Disk

Placido's disk consists of a round disk painted with alternating black and white rings. Disk is held in front of cornea and observer look through the hole (lens) at the center of the disk, at the image of the painted rings, which falls on the cornea. If the image of the rings are distorted the corneal surface is irregular (Figs 15.2A and B).

Keratoscopy

A keratoscope projects an illuminated series of concentric rings onto the anterior corneal surface. A steep cornea will crowd the rings, while a flat cornea will spread them out. Distortion of rings suggest irregular cornea.

Video Keratoscopy

Video keratoscopy is the corneal topography where the image of the Placido's disk on the anterior surface of the cornea is captured by a video cornea and analyzed by computer software and then presented in the form of colored maps.

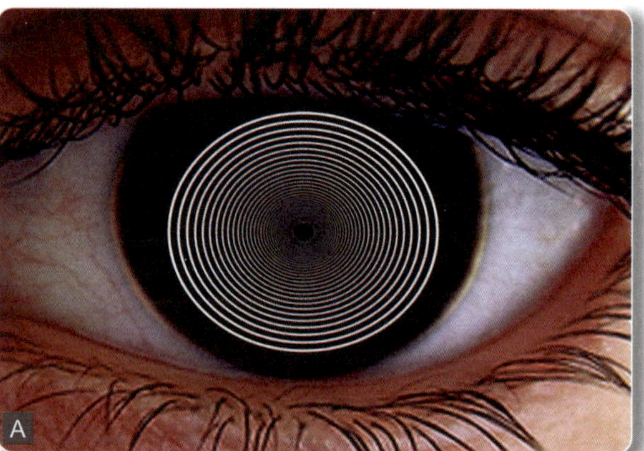

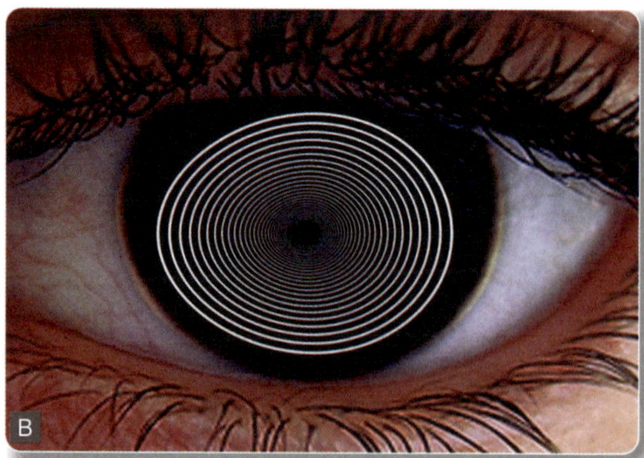

FIGURES 15.2A and B: Corneal reflex with Placido's disk. **A.** Normal; **B.** Astigmatism.

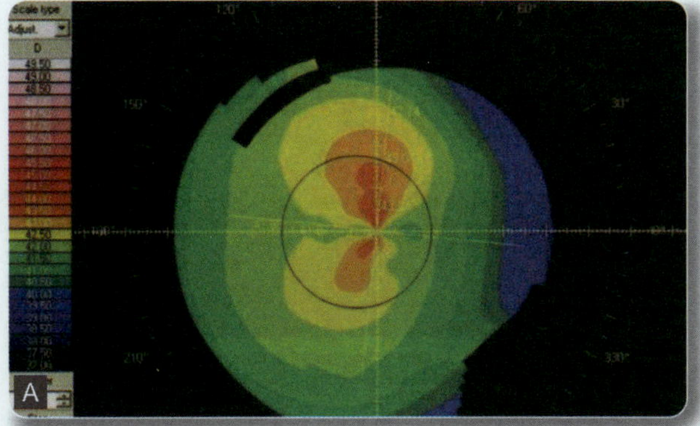

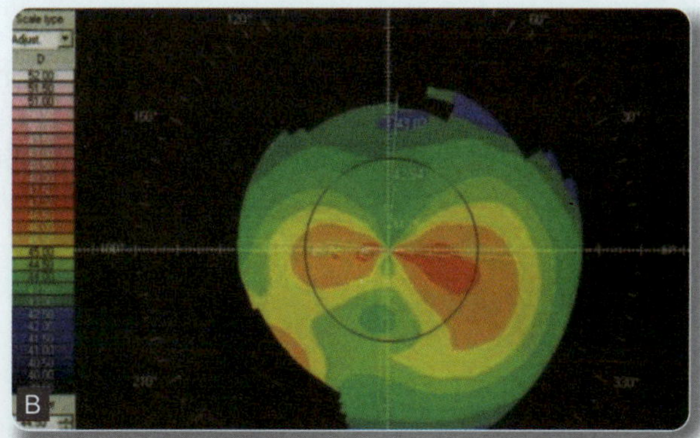

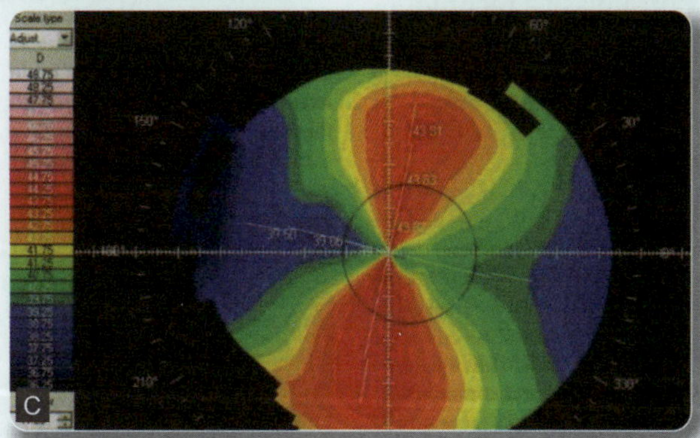

FIGURES 15.3A to C: Corneal topography pictures. **A.** Normal corneal topography; **B.** Against the rule astigmatism; **C.** With the rule astigmatism.

Usual color spectrum for normal corneal powers are green, cool colors such as blue indicates lower than normal corneal powers and warm colors such as red indicates higher than normal powers (Figs 15.3A to C).

Uses: Reinforce the data collected by keratometry and refraction helps early detection of corneal pathologies such as keratoconus and pellucid marginal degeneration and guides the surgeon to plan for refractive surgeries.

Anterior Segment Optical Coherence Tomography

Anterior optical coherence tomography (OCT) is a cross-sectional, three dimensional and high-resolution imaging technology.

Uses: They are as follows:

1. In laser-assisted in situ keratomileusis (LASIK) and other refractive surgeries to directly measure the corneal flap thickness intraoperatively.
2. For accurate anterior chamber depth measurement, which is very essential in assessing the size of phakic intraocular lens.
3. Useful in delineating anterior segment anatomy in case of opaque corneas.

Keratometry

Keratometry is done by using ophthalmometer or keratometer. It is the measurement of the dioptric power of central (3–4 mm) cornea and the radius of curvature of central cornea can be calculated.

Uses: This is needed for calculating intraocular lens power, fitting of contact lenses, etc.

Pachymetry

Pachymeter measures the corneal thickness, which is a sensitive index of endothelial function. The normal average central thickness of cornea is about 540 mm.

Uses: Increase in corneal thickness due to corneal edema occurs in endothelial dysfunction. Pachymeter also helps to diagnose corneal thinning disorder. Central corneal thickness more than 650 mm suggests higher risk for corneal edema after intraocular surgery. It is also of value in refractive surgeries like LASIK, for preoperative measurement of corneal thickness and to plan keratorefractive procedures.

Esthesiometry

Esthesiometry is the measurement of corneal sensation, which is a function of ophthalmic division of trigeminal (V cranial) nerve. Clinically, corneal sensation can be assessed with a wisp of cotton wool and compared with the other eye.

Uses: It is used to quantify the deficit in sensation in unusual cases and for research work.

Confocal Microscopy

Confocal microscopy (CFM) is a non-invasive technique of imaging the corneal layers that provides excellent resolution of each layer of cornea, epithelium, subepithelial nerve plexus, stroma and endothelium.

Uses

In corneal pathologies the uses of CFM are as follows.

Keratoconus: CFM helps in diagnosing very early cases. The morphological changes are mostly confined to corneal apex in early stage.

Corneal dystrophies: CFM clearly defines the changes in the corresponding layer of cornea in dystrophies affecting the different layers of cornea.

In LASIK: CFM is useful for evaluation of the following parameters—corneal flap thickness, interface study, corneal nerve fiber regeneration and residual stromal thickness.

Corneal grafts: To assess the donor cornea and especially to assess the endothelium in the presence of corneal edema CFM is better than specular microscopy. Corneal graft survival is entirely dependent on optimum number of viable endothelial cells. Reinnervation after grafting is also well evaluated with CFM. Graft rejection in epithelial, subepithelial and endothelial grafting can be identified early by CFM.

Intracorneal deposits: As in Wilson's disease, drug toxicity (vortex keratopathy or cornea verticillata), Fabry's disease, hemosiderosis, refractive surgery and long-term use of contact lenses can be studied with CFM.

COMMON CORNEAL LESIONS

Keratitis

Keratitis is an inflammation of the cornea. It can be divided into three types:

1. Superficial keratitis—inflammation involving only epithelium and Bowman's membrane.
2. Deep keratitis—inflammation of stroma.
3. Endothelitis—inflammation of endothelium.

Corneal Ulcer

Corneal ulcer is suppurative inflammation with an epithelial defect. Inflammation can be infective or sterile.

Corneal Infiltrate

When the inflamed cornea has a white or yellowish white patch due to outpouring of leukocytes, it is called corneal infiltrate. The epithelium is usually intact.

Corneal Opacity

Loss of epithelium or any epithelial defect will heal without leaving any opacity. Any injury or inflammation affecting the Bowman's membrane and deeper tissues on healing will interfere with corneal transparency and leave an opacity. A healed corneal lesion, which affects corneal transparency is termed corneal opacity. The five types of corneal opacities are:

1. Nebula.
2. Macula.
3. Leukoma.
4. Adherent leukoma.
5. Anterior staphyloma.

Nebula

Mild opacification of cornea with visible iris details (Fig. 15.4).

Macula

Denser corneal opacification obscuring iris details, but with visible pupillary margins (Fig. 15.5).

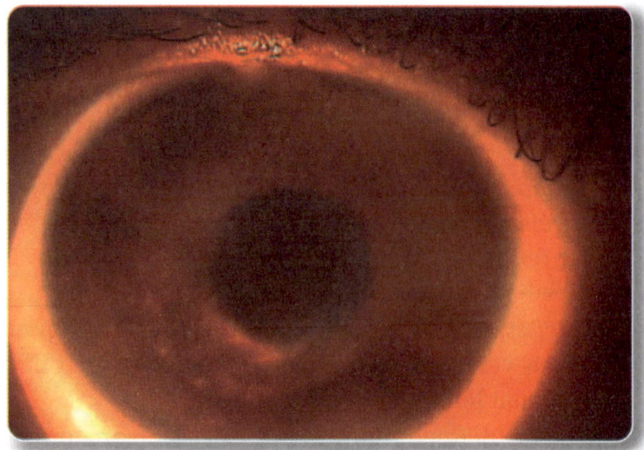

FIGURE 15.4: Nebula

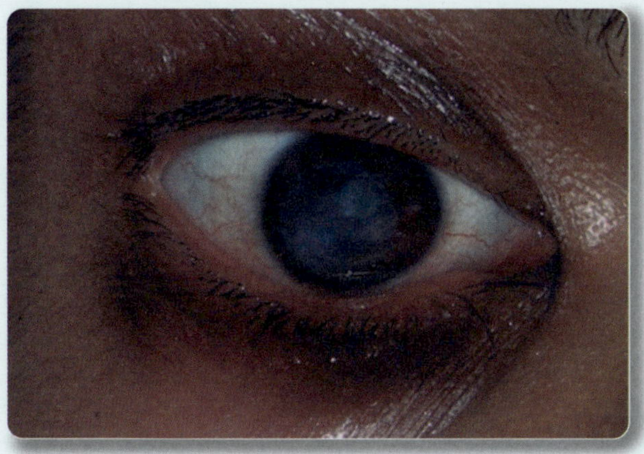

FIGURE 15.5: Macula

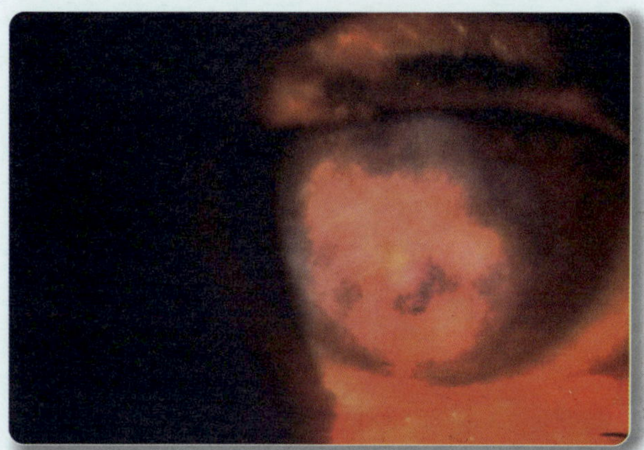

FIGURE 15.6: Leukoma

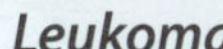

Leukoma

Dense corneal opacity obscuring view of iris and pupil (Fig. 15.6).

Adherent Leukoma

Iris is incorporated in the dense corneal opacity. Attachment of iris can be made out by irregularly shallow anterior chamber, where iris is pulled into the opacity and the iris pigments within the corneal opacity (Figs 15.7A and B). Causes are perforated corneal ulcer, penetrating injury.

Anterior Staphyloma

Anterior staphyloma is an ectatic cicatrix of cornea in which the iris is incarcerated. Raised intraocular pressure (IOP) during healing of a perforated corneal ulcer or penetrating injury leads to the development of an anterior staphyloma (Figs 15.8A and B).

Corneal Edema

Clinically seen as a hazy cornea due to accumulation of fluid between the epithelial cells and also within the stroma between the corneal lamellae. The increase in corneal thickness can be assessed with pachymetry or anterior segment OCT (Fig. 15.9).

Bullous Keratopathy

If the edema persists for a long period, the epithelium is raised into large bullae [bullous keratopathy (BK)]. The bullae rupture exposing the nerve endings causing pain and ocular irritation.

Common causes for BK are:

- Long-standing glaucoma
- Endothelial dystrophies like Fuchs' dystrophy
- Endothelial cell loss during intraocular surgeries.

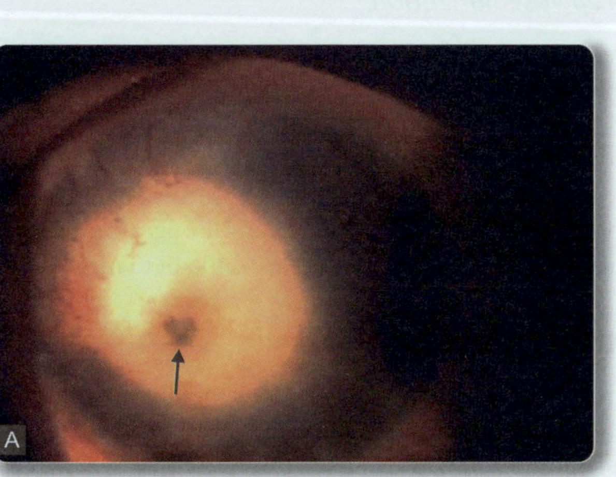

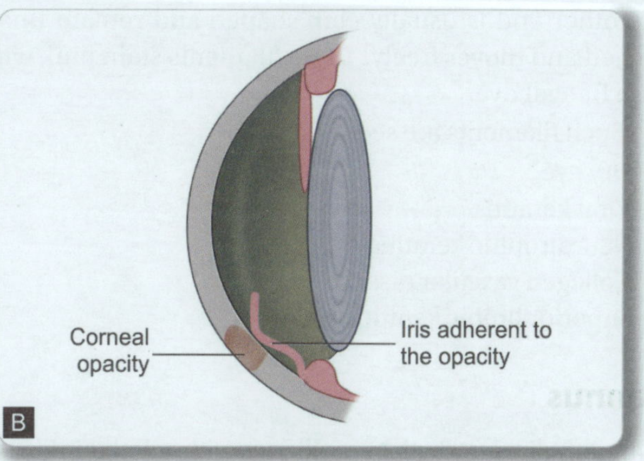

FIGURES 15.7A and B: Adherent leukoma. A. Pigmented spot (black arrow) showing the site of adhesion; B. Diagrammatic representation.

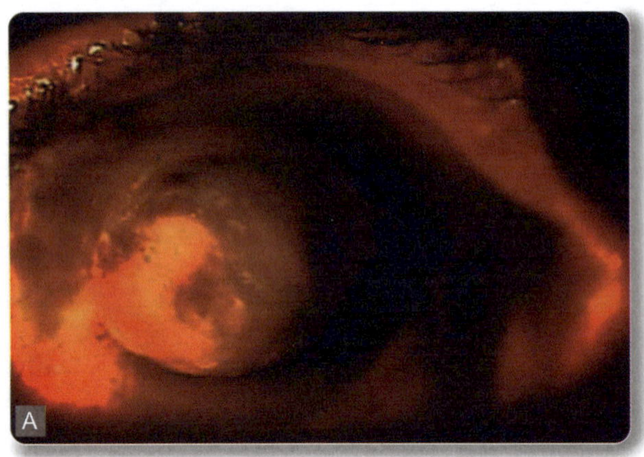

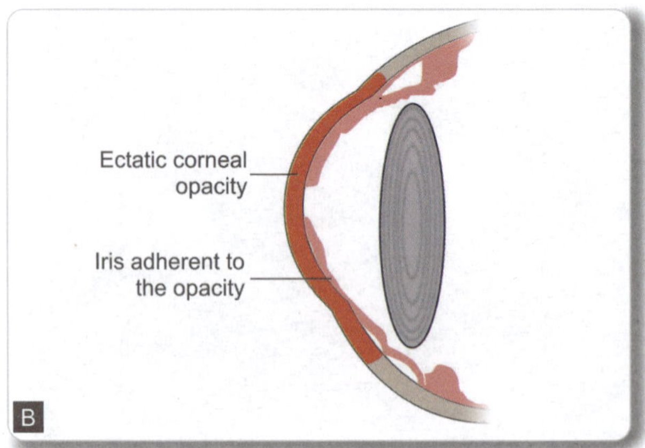

FIGURES 15.8A and B: Anterior staphyloma. **A.** Photograph; **B.** Diagrammatic representation.

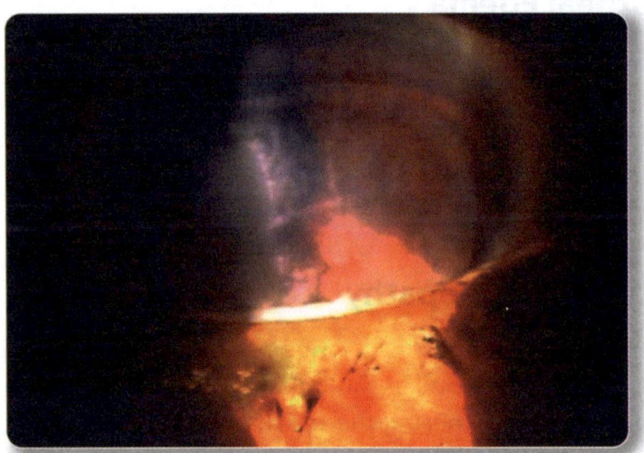

FIGURE 15.9: Corneal edema

Filamentary Keratopathy

Filamentary keratopathy is formation of epithelial threads, which adhere to the cornea by one end, while the other end is usually club shaped and remain unattached and moves freely. These filaments stain pink with rose Bengal dye.

Such filaments are seen in:

- Dry eye
- Viral keratitis
- Neurotrophic keratitis
- Collagen vascular disease
- Superior limbic keratitis, etc.

Pannus

Subepithelial ingrowth of capillaries with cellular infiltrate from the limbus due to inflammatory or rarely degenerative causes (Figs 15.10A and B).

Progressive pannus is characterized by infiltration beyond the vessels and in regressive pannus the vessels extend beyond infiltration.

Cause: Trachoma.

Corneal Vascularization

Corneal vascularization can be superficial or deep.

Superficial Vascularization

Superficial vascularization occurs in superficial infections of cornea, chronic ocular surface irritation as in retained superficial foreign bodies or chronic hypoxia as in chronic contact lens wear. Superficial vascularization is seen as bright red irregularly branching vessels (Figs 15.11 and 15.12A and B).

Deep Vascularization

Deep vascularization occurs in the stroma in chronic deep inflammations of the cornea, e.g. interstitial keratitis (Figs 15.13A and B), deep corneal ulcers, corneal graft rejection, etc. Deep vessels appear parallel since their ingrowth is in between the parallelly arranged corneal lamellae. These appear as bluish area when seen through the overlying stroma and individual vessels are difficult to make out.

Striate Keratopathy

Striate keratopathy are Descemet's membrane folds, may be caused by surgical trauma, ocular hypotony and stromal inflammation. It is seen as an area of corneal haziness with parallel lines. Commonly follows cataract surgery and it is seen in the upper part of cornea near the surgical incision.

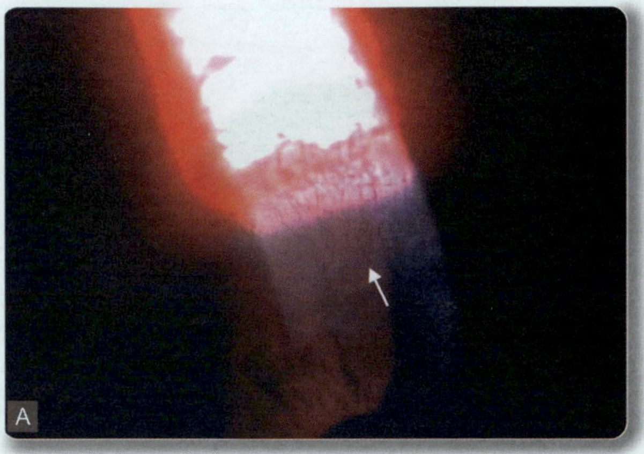

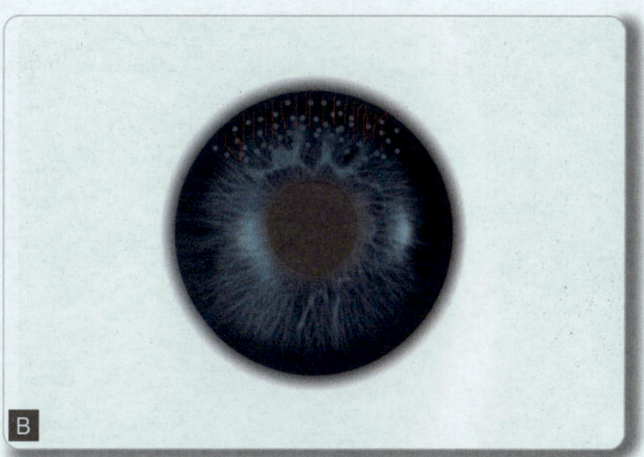

FIGURES 15.10A and B: Pannus. **A.** Photograph; **B.** Diagrammatic representation.

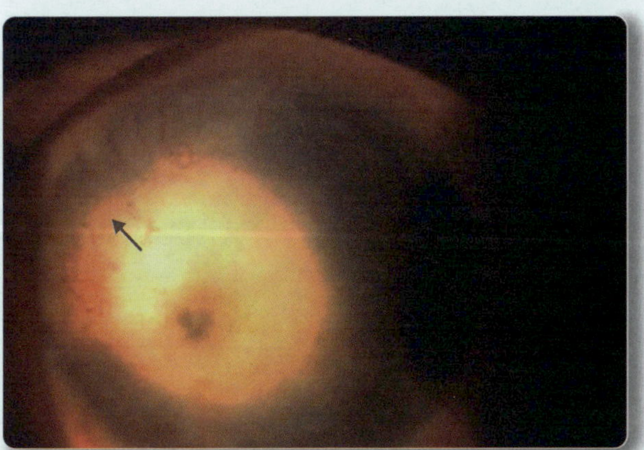

FIGURE 15.11: Superficial vessels in corneal opacity following ulceration

Pigments in Cornea

Iron in siderosis bulbi following retained iron intraocular foreign bodies, Krukenberg's spindle (a vertical area of pigmentation seen on the endothelial surface in pigmentary glaucoma) and copper deposition (chalcosis) in retained copper foreign bodies and Kayser-Fleischer ring in Wilson's disease.

Pseudocornea

Perforations of the cornea get plugged with iris and exudates from the iris vessels will cover the iris and this will form an artificial cornea. This is called pseudocornea (Fig. 15.14). These exudates will get organized by formation of granulation tissue and subsequently by scar tissue to form an adherent leukoma.

INFECTIVE KERATITIS

The etiological agent may be:

- Bacterial
- Fungal

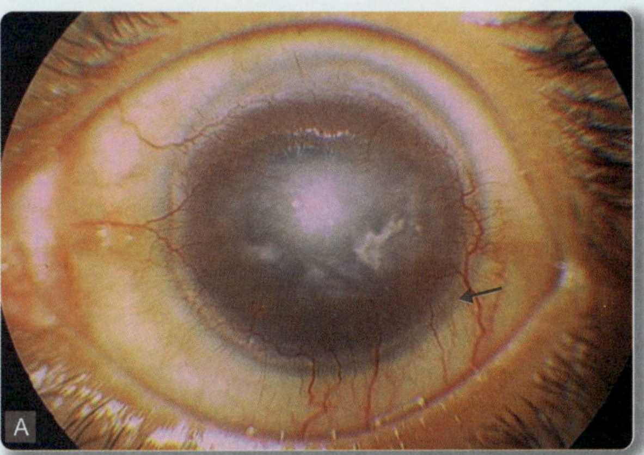

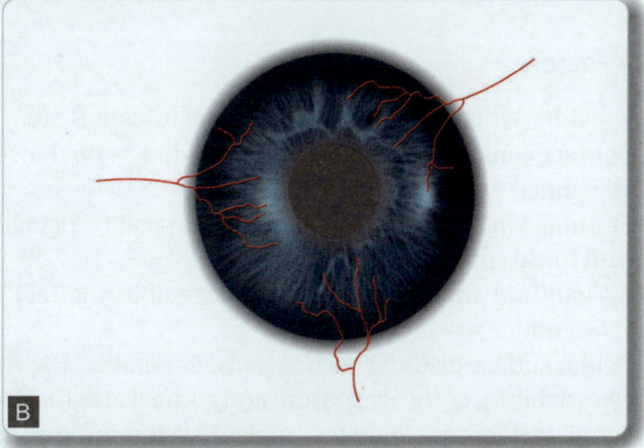

FIGURES 15.12A and B: Superficial vessels in chemical injury. **A.** Photograph; **B.** Diagrammatic representation.

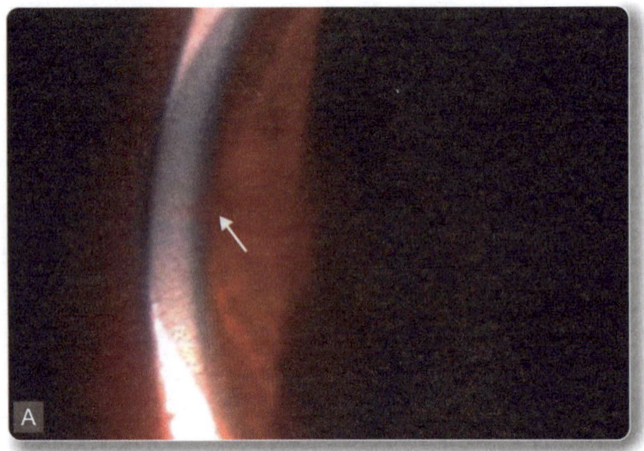

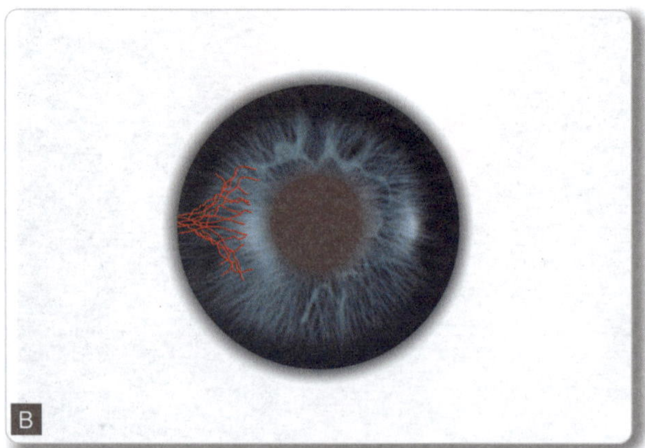

FIGURES 15.13A and B: Deep brush-like vessels. **A.** Photograph; **B.** Diagrammatic representation

- Viral
- Protozoal.

Role of Vital Stains in Infective Keratitis

Fluorescein is the most useful vital dye to delineate areas denuded of epithelium. These areas stain a brilliant yellowish green, when seen through cobalt blue light (Fig. 15.15A) .

Rose Bengal stains diseased and devitalized cells red (Fig. 15.15B). This is of value in the diagnosis of superficial punctate keratitis of viral origin.

Bacterial Keratitis

The common pathogens that cause corneal ulcers are:

- *Pseudomonas aeruginosa* (gram-negative rods)
- *Staphylococcus aureus* (gram- and coagulase-positive cocci)
- *Streptococcus pyogenes* and *Streptococcus viridans*
- Pneumococci.

Risk Factors

Risk factors, which predispose to corneal infection are:

- Contact lens wear—especially extended wear lenses associated with poor lens hygiene
- Trauma, which may be accidental, surgical (especially with loose sutures)
- Agricultural injury (injury with vegetable matter) is also a major risk factor
- Ocular surface disorder such as herpetic keratitis, BK, dry eye, trichiasis, corneal exposure and corneal anesthesia
- Other factors are diabetes, topical/systemic immune suppression.

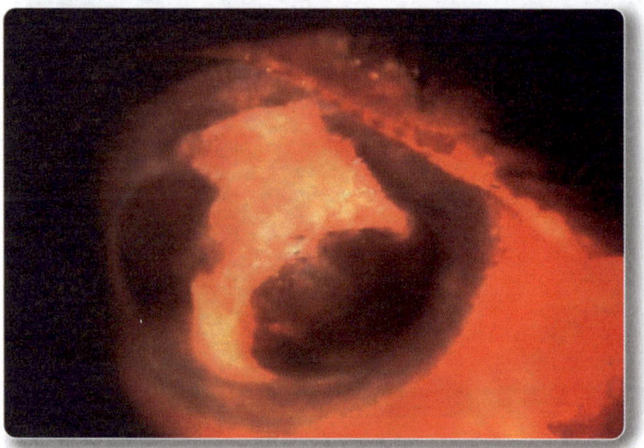

FIGURE 15.14: Pseudocornea

Pathogenesis

Minute corneal abrasions are almost of daily occurrence due to the exposed position of the cornea. But these are not getting infected because:

1. Highly virulent organisms are not normally present in conjunctiva sac.
2. Tear film and the protective mechanisms of the eye are sufficient to overcome infection.

Organisms that can invade intact cornea are *Corynebacterium diphtheriae* and *Neisseria gonorrhoeae*. In most of the corneal infections the pathogenic organisms are carried into the eye by the object causing the injury.

Pathology

Once infection occurs in a corneal abrasion, there is localized necrosis of anterior layers of cornea. The ulcer is saucer shaped and the walls project over the normal surface

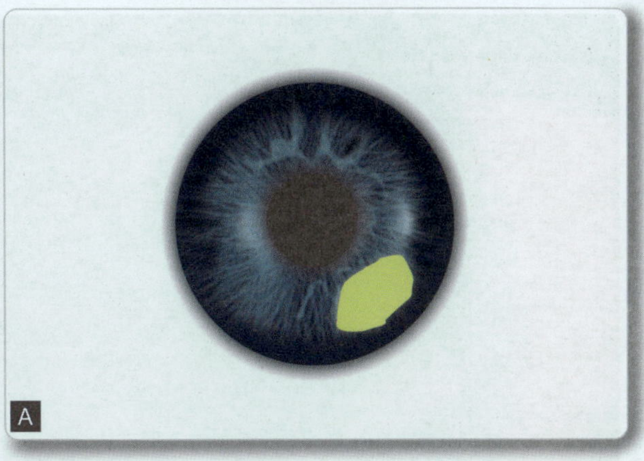

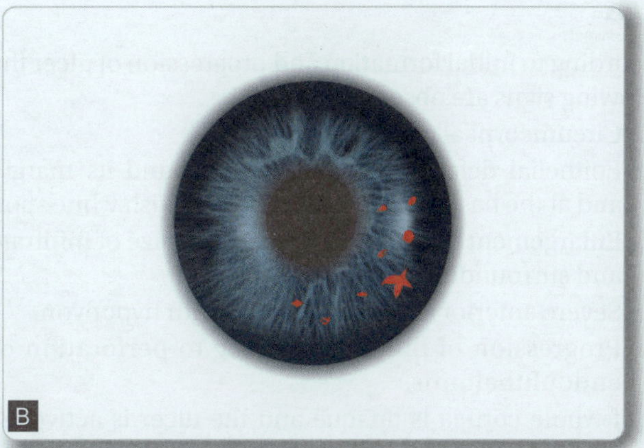

FIGURES 15.15A and B: Epithelial defect taking. **A.** Brilliant yellowish green stain with fluorescein; **B.** Red with rose Bengal stain.

of the cornea due to the surrounding corneal edema. The affected area is packed with leukocytes, which forms an infiltrate. This stage of corneal infiltration with surrounding edema is progressive. Then the sequestrum is cast off the polymorphs, which form a line of defence and dissolve the necrotic materials by phagocytosis. These polymorphs reach the site of infiltration via tears and later from limbal vessels. Corneal vascularization may develop in response to inflammation.

Hypopyon in Corneal Ulcers

If the bacterial colony overcomes the corneal protective mechanism, then the ulcer progresses to hypopyon formation. The toxins produced by the invading organism diffuse into the anterior chamber and produce a sterile inflammation of the anterior uvea and the exudates pouring out will form a hypopyon (Fig. 15.16). This hypopyon in a corneal ulcer is sterile except in fungal infections, where the fungal organisms are seen in the anterior chamber (AC) also. This hypopyon in bacterial ulcers changes position according to position of patient, e.g. hypopyon occurs in temporal limbus when patient lies on his/her side. In fungal ulcers it is more solid in consistency.

If the infection progresses the whole of the stroma can get destroyed. The Descemet's membrane is usually more resistant and it can protrude as a transparent knuckle surrounded by the white infiltrate. This is called descemetocele. The descemetocele can rupture under any sudden rise in IOP or by the invasion of the organisms and lead to perforation of the ulcer. Perforation is associated with some advantages as well as disadvantages. Due to the sudden decrease in IOP and emptying of the anterior chamber the iris-lens diaphragm moves forwards and the iris can plug the defect in the cornea, if it is not central in position. The lowering of the IOP and the contact with the iris will bring more nutrients, cells and factors to fight the infection to the ulcer. This will promote the healing of the ulcer, which was actively progressing till now. But perforation and the sudden lowering of the IOP is associated with some complications also. It can lead to subluxation or even extrusion of the lens or massive bleeding from the choroidal blood vessels.

If the infection is brought under control, the infiltrate will decrease in size and epithelium will grew over the ulcer and healing by scarring will occur. Any injury or infection, which destroys the Bowman's membrane and involves underlying stroma results in scarring.

Sx Symptoms

Early stages—foreign body sensation, mild pain, photophobia, blurring of vision and watering of eyes.

Later pain becomes severe, discharge and lid edema occurs and there will be considerable drop in vision.

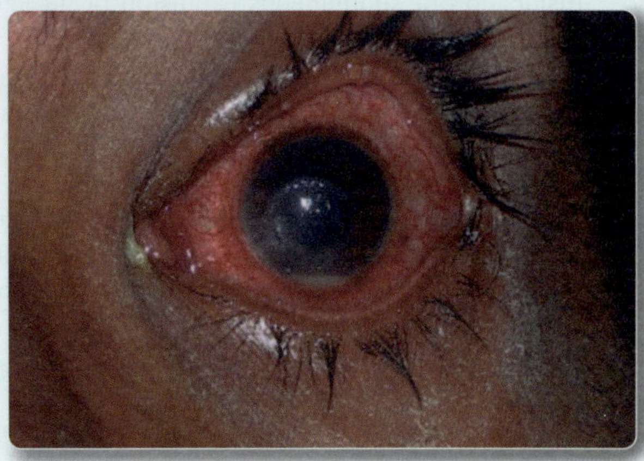

FIGURE 15.16: Hypopyon in bacterial ulcer

Signs

According to initial formation and progression of ulcer the following signs are observed:

1. Circumcorneal congestion.
2. Epithelial defect with infiltration around its margin and at the base, which appears as a grayish white spot.
3. Enlargement of ulcer with increase in size of infiltrate and surrounding corneal edema.
4. Severe anterior chamber reaction with hypopyon.
5. Progression of the ulcer leading to perforation or endophthalmitis.

If whole cornea is opaque and the ulcer is active, B-scan should be performed to rule out endophthalmitis.

Differential Diagnosis

- Fungal keratitis
- Sterile infiltrates in contact lens wearers
- Marginal keratitis.

Complications of Corneal Ulcers

1. Secondary glaucoma occurs due to the proteinaceous exudates in the anterior chamber. This exudation occurs because of the iritis set up by the toxins liberated by the organisms causing the corneal ulcer.
2. Descemetocele (keratocele) occurs when ulcers extend in depth destroying the whole thickness of cornea except Descemet's membrane (Figs 15.17A to C).
3. Perforation of corneal ulcer occurs when the weak floor of the ulcer gives way. This can give rise to some major complications. These include:
   a. Rupture of major choroidal vessels leading to expulsive hemorrhage.
   b. If perforation occurs, suddenly the suspensory ligament ruptures causing subluxation or anterior dislocation or spontaneous expulsion of the lens and vitreous through the perforation.
   c. If perforation is opposite, in some part of iris, iris prolapse occurs and it seals the opening as aqueous escapes (Fig. 15.18).
4. The prolapsed iris will get covered with exudates to form a 'pseudocornea' (Figs 15.19A and B). Scarring occurs over the iris and anterior synechia results. Anterior synechia is adhesion of iris to posterior corneal surface. These include:
   a. If perforation occurs opposite pupil, corneal fistula results (Figs 15.20A and B).
   b. The absent AC following perforation leads to closure of the angle with peripheral anterior synechia and secondary glaucoma.

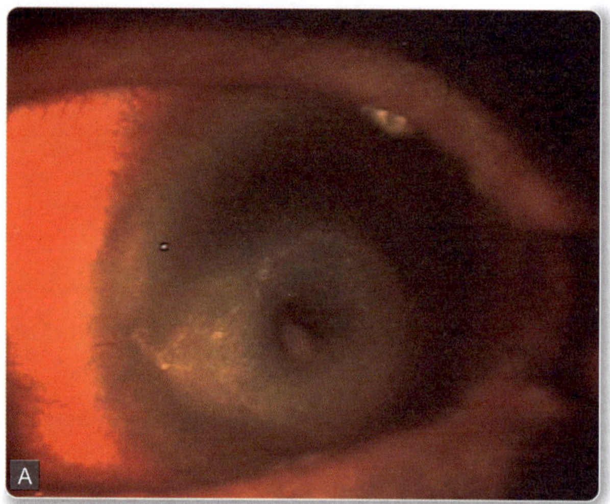

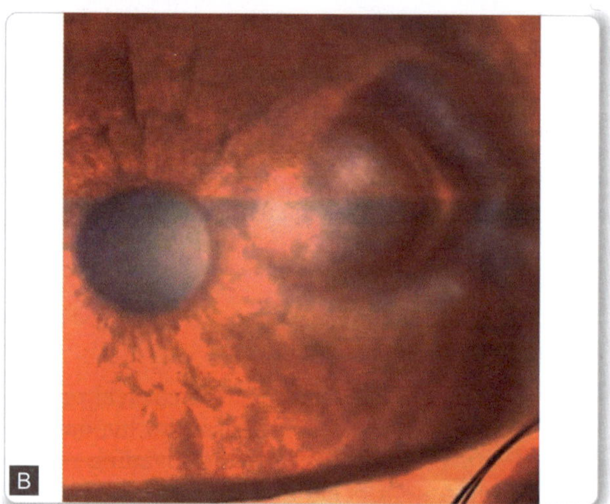

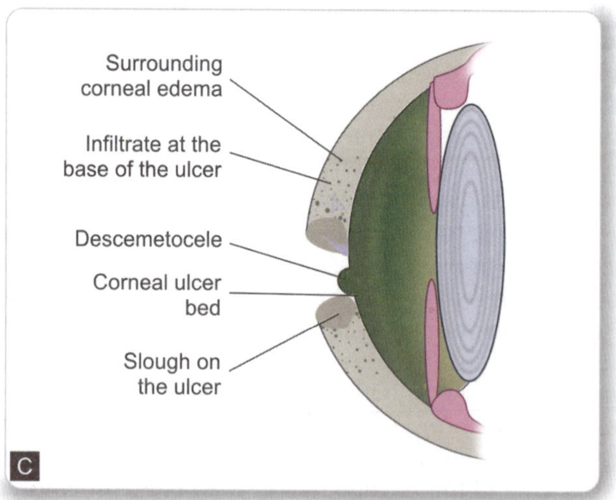

FIGURES 15.17A to C: Descemetocele. **A.** In an ulcer; **B.** In corneal melting in rheumatoid arthritis; **C.** In a corneal ulcer—diagrammatic representation.

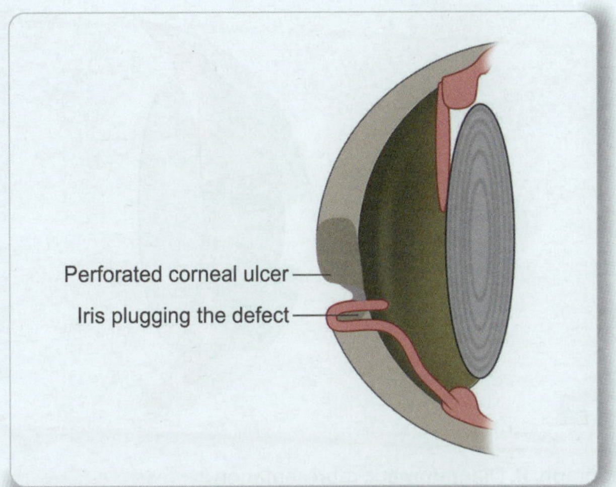

FIGURE 15.18: Diagrammatic representation of iris prolapse in a perforated ulcer

c. This secondary glaucoma leads to ecstatic scar tissue—anterior staphyloma develops.
d. Spread of infection inside the eye can lead to panophthalmitis.

5. Corneal opacity occurs as a result of healing of corneal ulcer by scarring. These opacities interfere with vision, if it occurs in the pupillary region.
6. Complicated cataract can occur due to the effect of toxins diffusing into the anterior chamber.

Management of Bacterial Ulcer

Management of bacterial ulcer includes:

1. Control of risk factors.
2. Control of infection.
3. Management of the complications and sequel (after healing).

Control of Risk Factors

Control can be done by:

1. Any retained foreign bodies in the ulcer or in the upper fornix should be removed.
2. Remove any inturned lashes rubbing the cornea.
3. Risk factors like dacryocystitis should be treated with dacryocystectomy.
4. If any steroid drugs are used, these are stopped and contact lenses discontinued.
5. If it is a case of exposure keratitis due to lagophthalmos, a lateral tarsorrhaphy is required.
6. If diabetic, strict control should be achieved and maintained.
7. If there is any evidence of malnutrition or vitamin A deficiency especially in a child, it should be corrected.

Control of infection: This process includes identification of the organisms and application of the appropriate antibiotic at optimum dose.

As soon as diagnosis of corneal ulcer is made, scrapings are taken from ulcer for Gram/Giemsa stain culture and sensitivity studies for bacterial agents, and KOH mount for identifying the causative organism if it is fungal. This should be done before starting any antibiotics, since it will be difficult to identify the organism after starting antibiotics.

If the patient is already on antibiotics, but the response is poor and/or the microbiological investigations fail to identify the organism, stop all topical antibiotics for 12-24 hours and then take scrapings. But in case of

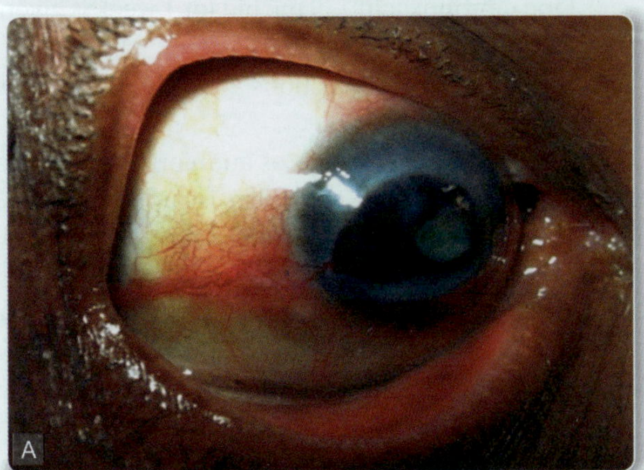

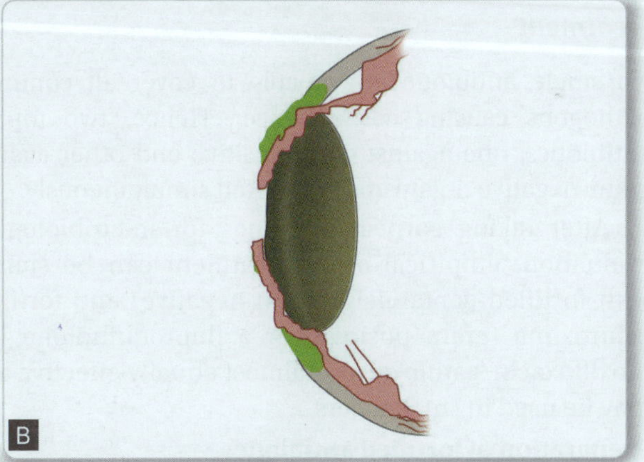

FIGURES 15.19A and B: Perforated ulcer with iris and cataractous lens plugging the defect. **A.** Photograph; **B.** Diagrammatic representation.

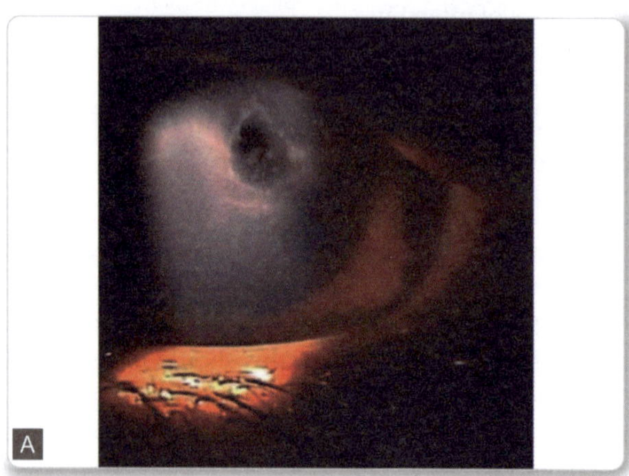

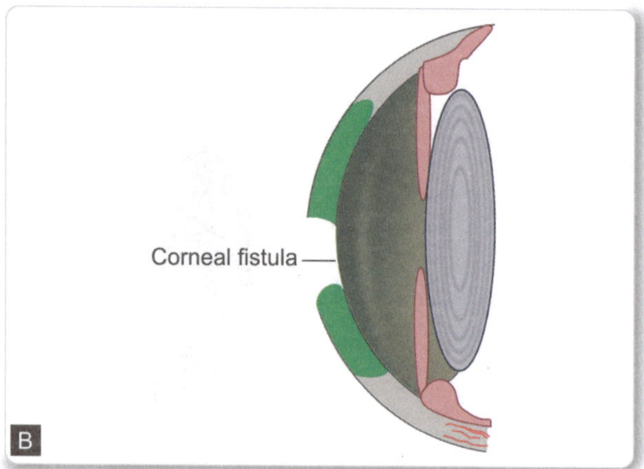

FIGURES 15.20A and B: Corneal fistula. **A.** Photograph; **B.** Diagrammatic representation

severe infection, and rapidly progressing ulcer topical antibiotics cannot be stopped.

Method of Taking Scraping

Put preservative-free local anesthetic drops. Scrape the base and margins directly, where multiplying organisms are found and after removing all sloughs covering the ulcer. Corneal spatula or the tip of needle is used. Scrapings are transferred to slide for staining or a slide with KOH to identify fungi and also to inoculate into culture media for culture and sensitivity studies. The culture media used are blood agar, chocolate agar (for bacteria) (Fig. 15.21A) and Sabouraud's dextrose agar (for fungi) (Fig. 15.21B). In addition to corneal scrapings, contact lenses and swab from inflamed lids may also be cultured that helps to identify, which the source in difficult cases.

Treatment

No single antibiotic is available to cover all common pathogens causing corneal ulcer. Hence, two topical antibiotics, one against gram positive and other against gram-negative organisms are started simultaneously.

After taking corneal scrapings for microbiological evaluation, empirical-based treatment can be started with fortified gentamicin (gram negative) and fortified cefuroxime (gram positive) or a fluoroquinolone like moxifloxacin/gatifloxacin is almost equally effective and may be used in small ulcers.

Preparation of fortified antibiotics

1. Gentamicin—15 mg/mL (1.5%): 2 mL of gentamicin injection (40 mg/mL) is added to 4 mL of the gentamicin eye drop preparation.
2. Cefuroxime, cefazolin, ceftazidime eye drops 50 mg/mL (5%). Parenteral antibiotic of 500 mg is diluated with 2.5 mL of sterile water and added to 7.5 mL preservative-free artificial tears. Stable for 24 hours in room temperature or 96 hours in refrigerator. The problem with topical fortified preparation is the short shelf-life and decreased sterility.

Therapeutic regimen

1. Topical antibiotics are initially used at hourly intervals for 48–72 hours (day and night). The aim is to destroy the invading organisms as quickly as possible before much damage occurs to the cornea. Frequency can be reduced to 2 hourly in waking hours for further 48 hours and then four times daily for 1 week depending on the response to treatment. Treatment is continued till epithelium heals.

   Oral ciprofloxacin 750 mg bid for 1 week is given in cases of peripheral ulcers.

   Subconjunctival injections are given only in cases of poor compliance.

   Indications for change of antibiotic, if a resistant pathogen is isolated and ulcer is progressing. Even if a resistant pathogen is isolated there is no need to change the antibiotics, if the ulcer is healing.
2. Mydriatics—atropine 1% or cyclopentolate 1% are used to prevent iritis and its complications.
3. Topical steroids are contraindicated in fungal and keratitis. Can be used in bacterial keratitis to reduce inflammation once the infection is brought under control. But is of no value as the final visual outcome is not affected though it suppresses inflammation and gives temporary comfort.

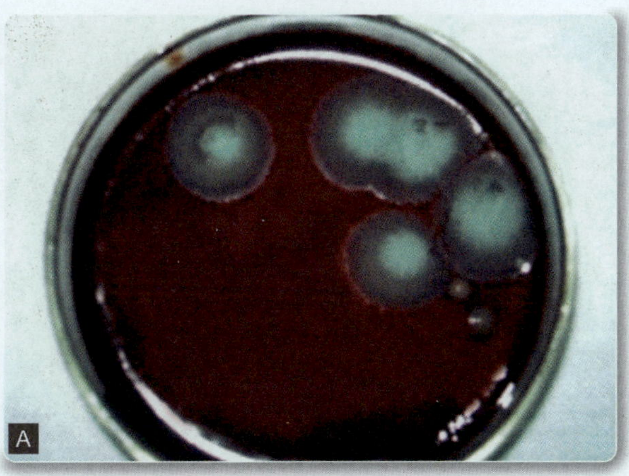

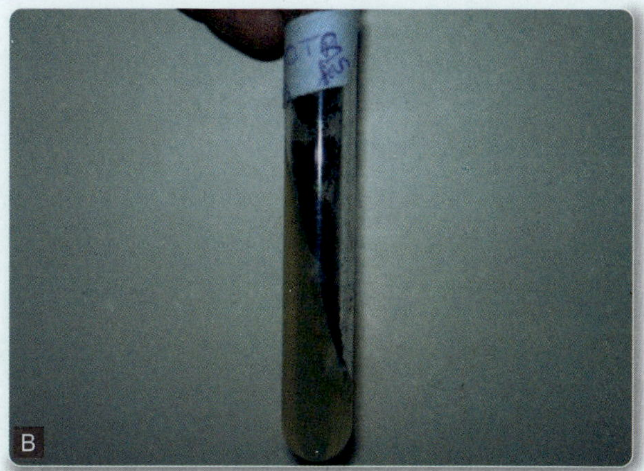

FIGURES 15.21A and B: Culture media used for bacterial and fungal growth. **A.** Bacterial growth on blood agar plate; **B.** Fungal growth on Sabouraud's medium.

Fortified eye drops (Table 15.1) are prepared from the injectable preparation of the antibiotic, diluted with sterile water or commercially available eye drops.

TABLE 15.1: Organisms and the effective antibiotics

Organism	Antibiotic eye drops
Gram-positive cocci	Fortified cefazolin, moxifloxacin or gatifloxacin
Gram-negative cocci	Fortified ceftriaxone, fortified ceftazidime, moxifloxacin or gatifloxacin
Gram-negative rods	Tobramycin, fortified tobramycin or fluoroquinolones (ciprofloxacin, ofloxacin, moxifloxacin or gatifloxacin)
Mixed infection	Fortified cefazolin with fortified tobramycin or fluoroquinolones

Assessment of healing and progressing ulcers is shown in Figures 15.22A to C and diagrammatically in Figures 15.23A and B.

Visual rehabilitation is needed when vision is affected by scarring. Irregular astigmatism by scarring outside pupillary region may be corrected by rigid gas permeable (RPG) lenses, but only 3 months after epithelization of ulcer.

Lamellar keratoplasty or penetrating keratoplasty (PKP) may be needed to improve vision in cases of corneal opacities involving pupillary region.

Factors promoting healing

1. Lubrication with preservative-free artificial tears (expensive and not absolutely essential).
2. Closure of eyelids by taping lids closed and by lateral tarsorrhaphy (especially, if there is lagophthalmos or neurotrophic factors).
3. Bandage contact lenses to provide the regenerating corneal epithelium from damage by constant lid rubbing (only after the infection has been brought under control).
4. Amniotic membrane graft may be needed when there is failure of epithelialization of ulcer.
5. Limbal stem cell transplantation when there is stem cell deficiency or in chemical injuries, cicatricial conjunctivitis (as in cicatricial pemphigoid).
6. Botulism toxin injection into upper eyelid paralyses levator palpebrae superioris (LPS) and induces ptosis and provides healing.
7. Autologous serum drops promote healing of non-healing or sterile ulcers and punctate epithelial erosion and success rate of 51%–86% (Table 15.2).

TABLE 15.2: Healing vs progressing ulcer

Features	Healing ulcers	Progressing ulcers
Size of ulcer	Ulcer becomes smaller and size of epithelial defect decreases	Ulcer becomes larger and epithelial defect increases
Surrounding cornea	Cornea surrounding ulcer clears as corneal edema subsides	Surrounding cornea become hazy due to corneal edema
Infiltrate	Infiltrate decreases in size and cornea starts healing	Corneal infiltrate increases and spreads to deeper layers
Anterior chamber reaction	Anterior chamber reaction decreases and hypopyon disappears	Hypopyon increases

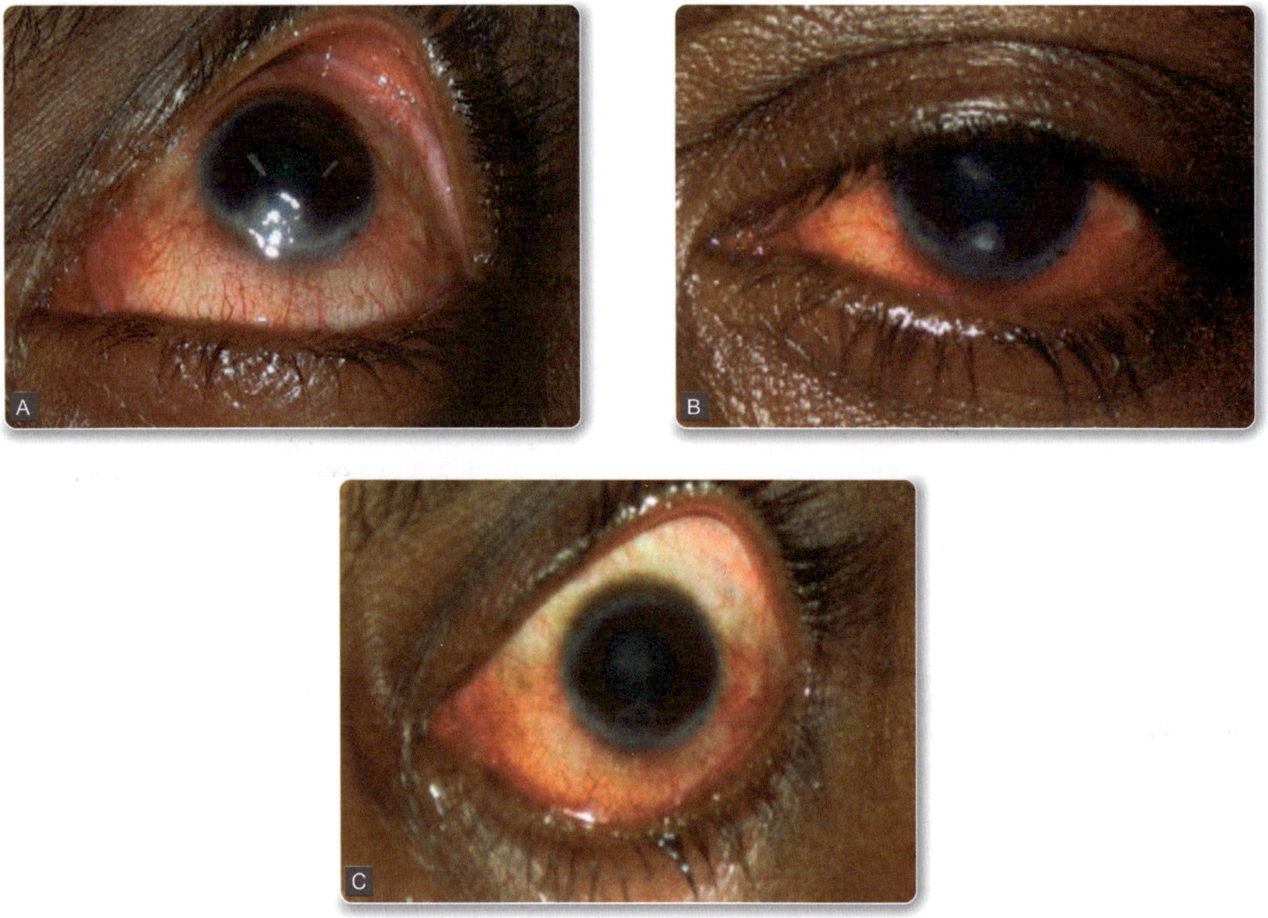

FIGURES 15.22A to C: Corneal ulcer. **A.** Active ulcer; **B.** Healing ulcer with opacity; **C.** Healed ulcer with opacity.

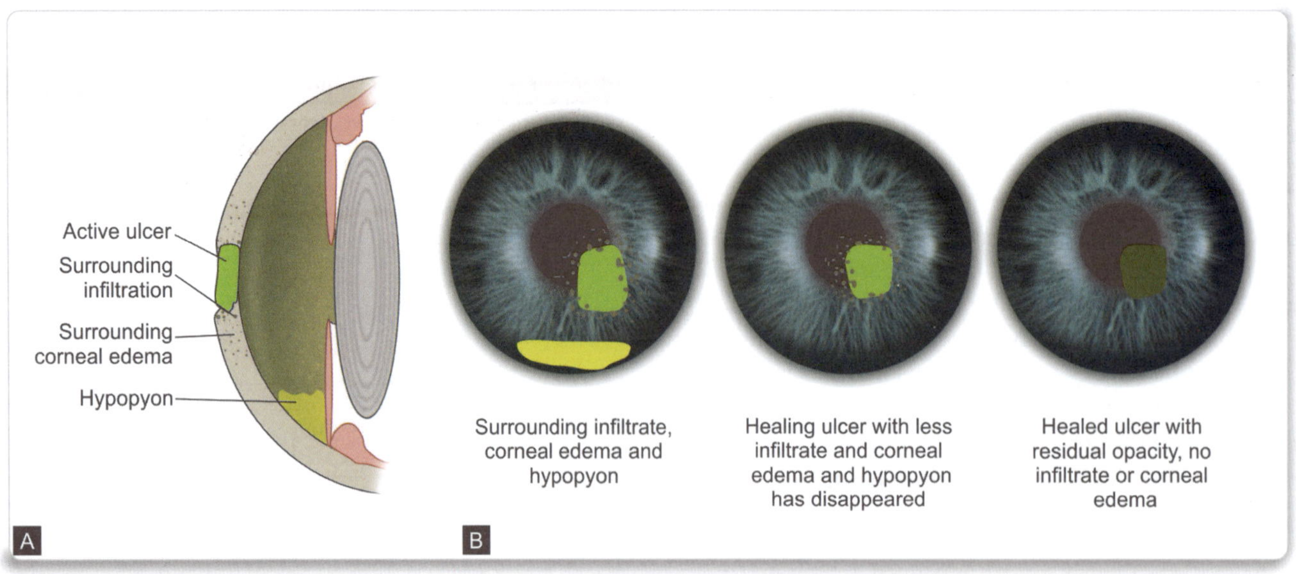

FIGURES 15.23A and B: Corneal ulcer. **A.** Active hypopyon corneal ulcer (diagrammatic); **B.** Stages of a healing corneal ulcer.

Management

Management of non-healing ulcer

If cornea fails to heal despite proper antibiotic and suppuration progresses, look for specific reasons like:

1. Deep impacted foreign body in cornea.
2. Impaired corneal sensation to rule out neuroparalytic keratitis (needs tarsorrhaphy for faster healing).
3. Local causes like dacryocystitis.

Emergency dacryocystectomy is needed in chronic dacryocystitis (need to take away the source of infecting organism):

1. Failure to isolate the correct organism. Repeat culture using same media as well as specific media for *Mycobacterium, Acanthamoeba,* etc. Change to the sensitive specific antibiotic.
2. Mechanical debridement, which can be done by careful scraping with the BP knife to remove necrotic material from ulcer and allow antibiotic to act.
3. Finally corneal biopsy may be needed to isolate the causative organism.
4. Systemic conditions like diabetic mellitus and immunocompromised situations hinder healing and must be ruled out.

Management of impending perforation

Case of impending perforations are those with deep ulcers and corneal thinning with descemetocele. Care should be taken to prevent sudden perforation as sudden perforation causes sudden decrease in IOP from the baseline, subluxation and dislocation of lens, vitreous hemorrhage, etc. Perforation can also cause shallow anterior chamber leading to peripheral anterior synechiae (PAS) and secondary glaucoma:

1. Avoid coughing and straining or those actions that cause increase in IOP leading to perforation.
2. Pressure bandage to give external pressure.
3. A 250 mg of acetazolamide four times daily or oral glycerine daily may be given to reduce IOP. Timolol 0.5% bid topically can also be used.
4. Controlled paracentesis to get the advantages of perforation (promotion of healing) and at the same time avoid the complications of sudden lowering of IOP.

Fungal Keratitis

Organisms

Majority of the cases of fungal infection of cornea are caused by a small number of filamentous fungi and yeasts.

Filamentous fungi: Fusarium, Aspergillus.

Yeasts: Candida species.

Risk Factors

- Corneal trauma with vegetative matter
- Contact lens wear
- Use of topical steroid drops and systemic steroids
- Dry eye and neurotrophic cornea.

Clinical Features

Clinical features of filamentous fungal infection: They are:

1. Insidious onset and gradually progressive ulcer.
2. Dry ulcer with feathery margin.
3. Satellite lesions surrounding stroma may show hyphae under high magnification.
4. Immune ring may develop around the ulcer, which may be partial or complete.
5. Hypopyon develops when ulcer progresses (Figs 15.24A and B). Fungal filaments may be seen, though not always inside the anterior chamber.

Yeast infections: Most common yeast causing corneal infections is *Candida albicans.* Usually seen in immunologically weak people, neurotrophic corneas, severe dry eye, etc. Yeasts give rise to superficial ulcers, deep ones are rare.

Treatment

Principles

1. Avoid specific treatment prior to definite diagnosis (demonstration of fungi by KOH mount or fungal culture) or start treatment only if the clinical signs of fungal ulcer are present and the ulcer fail to respond to antibiotics.
2. Topical treatment is best.
3. Supplementation with systemic antifungals is helpful where healing is delayed.
4. Avoid topical and systemic steroids.
5. Therapeutic keratoplasty is the last resort.
6. Duration of treatment is 4–6 weeks or more, if the ulcer is large.

Antifungal agents

Polyenes: Natamycin and amphotericin B.

Imidazoles: Miconazole, clotrimazole and ketoconazole.

Azoles: Fluconazole and itraconazole.

These are administered as topical drops or ointment.

Treatment of fungal ulcers

1. Debridement epithelium over the ulcers helps in better penetration of antifungal agents.
2. Natamycin is treatment of choice in filamentous fungal infection. A 5% suspension of natamycin is used hourly for first 48 hours and then tapered. Frequent

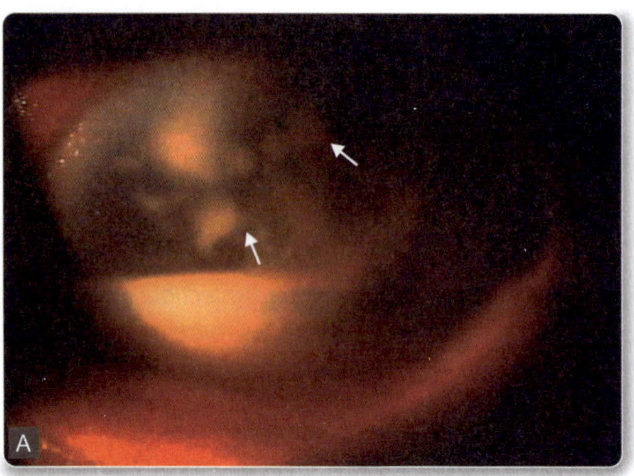

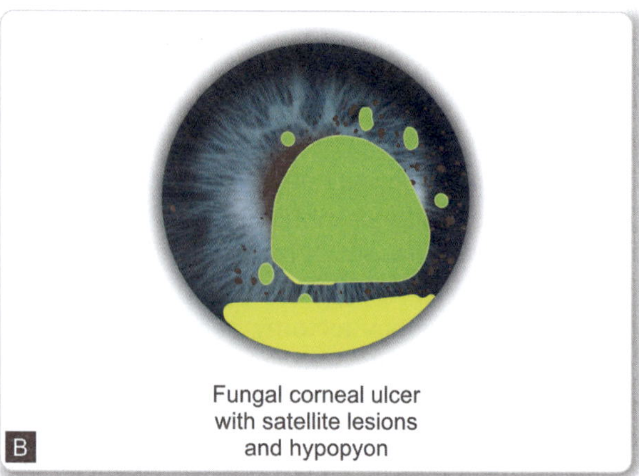

FIGURES 15.24A and B: Fungal corneal ulcer. **A.** Fungal corneal ulcer with hypopyon and satellite lesions; **B.** Diagrammatic representation.

debridement is necessary since natamycin has poor penetration.

3. *Candida* ulcers are best treated by amphotericin B. Eye drops, which are constituted from systemic preparations (injection vial 0.15% solution) is effective and well tolerated. It is a fungicidal drug and it is used hourly for the first 24 hours and then tapered.
4. Amphotericin B can also be used as injections systemically as an additive to topical treatment, but not preferred as there are many side effects.
5. Systemic antifungals are fluconazole (200–400 mg/day) effective mainly against yeasts and ketoconazole (200–600 mg/day) effective mainly against filamentous fungi.
6. Duration of treatment is at least 4–6 weeks or longer and fungal infection regress slowly.
7. Voriconazole drops and intrastromal injection (0.5 mg in 1 mL around the ulcer at multiple sites in deep stromal fungal ulcers) are the latest in the armamentarium in the fight against fungal ulcers.

Viral Keratitis

Organisms

- Herpes simplex virus
- Herpes zoster virus
- Adenovirus.

Adenovirus produces mainly conjunctival infection. Corneal involvement occurs in epidemic keratoconjunctivitis. Subepithelial nummular lesions can develop as a result of antigen-antibody reaction (refer Chapter 14 'Conjunctiva').

Herpetic keratitis leading to corneal opacity is an important cause of unilateral blindness in developing countries.

Herpes simplex is caused by DNA virus. Herpes simplex virus has two subtypes—HSV-1 and HSV-2 according to clinical and immunological properties. HSV-1 cause infection above waist, affecting the lips and eyes and HSV-2 below waist (herpes genitalis).

Primary HSV-1 infection occurs even in skin and mucosal surfaces innervated by V cranial nerve. Latent infection of trigeminal ganglia can occur even in the absence of recognized primary infection. Reactivation of virus may follow in any of the three branches of V cranial nerve.

Primary Infection

Occurs uncommonly in children below 6 months of age due to protection conferred by maternal antibodies.

Clinical Features

Clinical features are fever and mild blepharoconjunctivitis.

Vesicles on eyelid margins and skin are important diagnostic features. Follicular conjunctivitis and blepharitis are common, while corneal involvement is rare and occurs as superficial punctate keratitis.

Recurrent infection due to reactivation of virus lying latent in trigeminal ganglia.

Clinical Manifestation

- Epithelial keratitis—punctate epithelial keratitis, dendritic keratitis, geographic ulcers

- Stromal keratitis
- Metaherpetic keratitis.

Epithelial keratitis

Starts as punctate epithelial keratitis (Figs 15.25A and B). Lesions coalesce to form linear dendritic ulcers (Figs 15.26A and B). The ends of the dendrites have characteristic terminal buds. Corneal sensation is diminished. The dendritic ulcer develops into geographic ulcer.

The branches or dendrites broaden and coalesce to form irregular-shaped ulcers. These lesions stain with rose Bengal and fluorescein.

Differential diagnosis: Includes the diagnoses of:

- Herpes zoster keratitis
- Healing corneal abrasions
- Toxic keratopathy.

Treatment: As follows:

1. Topical antiviral drugs: Acyclovir is the most frequently used drug as it is effective and relatively non-toxic. A 3% eye ointment is applied five times daily and should be given till lesions heal. It acts preferentially on virus laden cells only. It penetrates the corneal epithelium and stroma and reaches therapeutic concentrations in aqueous also. Hence, the drug is useful in stromal keratitis also. About 99% of epithelial lesions heal in 2 weeks.
2. Trifluorothymidine 1% eye drops are applied 2 hourly and then tapered.
3. Vidarabine and ganciclovir are other antivirals that can be used (Table 15.3).
4. Debridement with sponge may be used in dendritic keratitis, which helps by removing the virus laden cells.

Disciform keratitis (stromal)

Etiology: Exact etiology is not known. It may be HSV infection of keratocytes in stroma and endothelium or a hypersensitivity reaction to viral antigen in cornea. It is primarily an endotheliitis. There may be associated iridocyclitis.

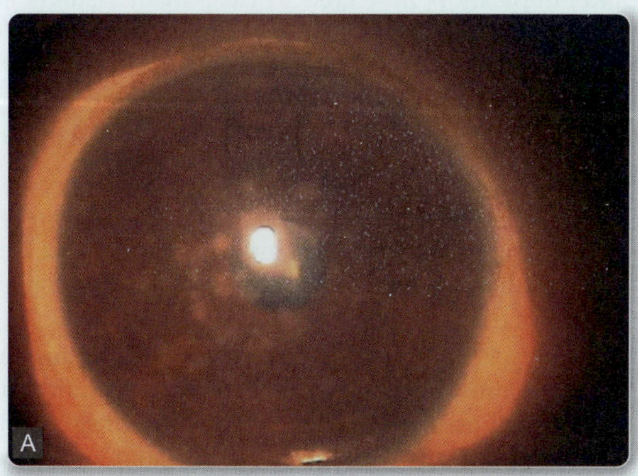

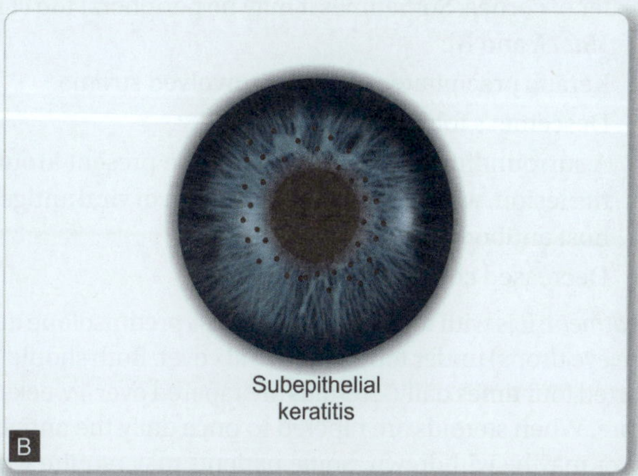

FIGURES 15.25A and B: Epithelial keratitis **A.** Photograph; **B.** Diagrammatic representation.

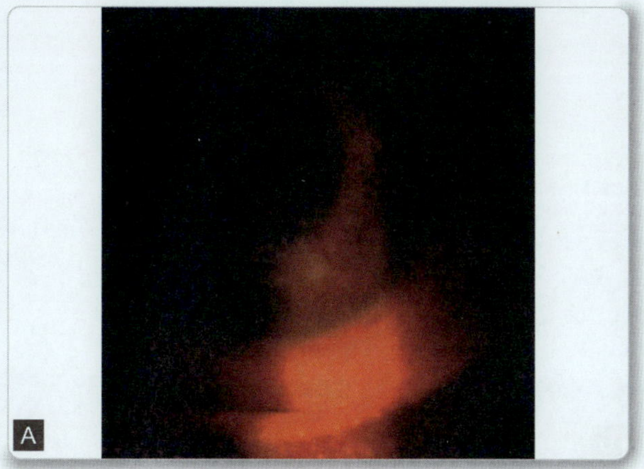

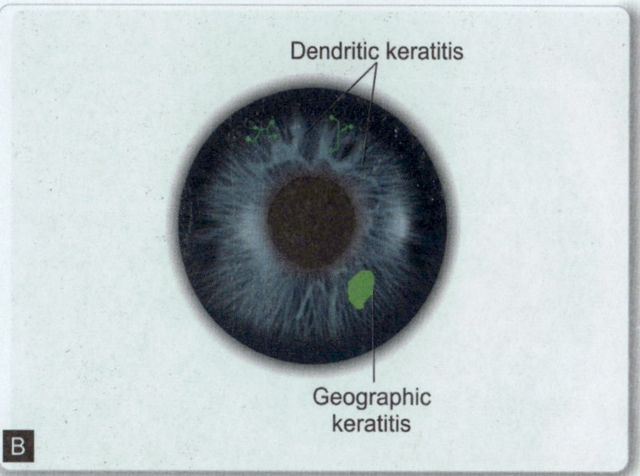

FIGURES 15.26A and B: Dendritic keratitis. **A.** Photograph; **B.** Diagrammatic representation.

TABLE 15.3: Antiviral agents		
Vidarabine	3% ophthalmic ointment	5 times/day × 10 day
Acyclovir	3% ophthalmic ointment	5 times/day × 10 day
Trifluridine	1% ophthalmic solution	8 times/day × 10 day
Ganciclovir	0.15% gel	5 times/day till epithelium heals then 3 times/day × 7 day

Sx **Symptoms**

Patient usually presents with decreased vision, which may be associated with halos as central portion of cornea is commonly involved.

Signs: Includes the following.

1. Disk-shaped stromal corneal edema usually in the center of cornea. Sometimes it may be peripheral too (Figs 15.27A and B).
2. Keratic precipitates under the involved stroma.
3. Descemet's folds may be present.
4. A surrounding immune thing may be present around the lesion, which indicates deposition of viral antigen-host antibody complexes.
5. Decreased corneal sensation.

Treatment: It is with topical steroids (0.5% prednisolone acetate eye drops) under topical antiviral cover. Both should be started four times daily. Steroids are tapered over 4 weeks or more. When steroids are tapered to once daily the antiviral cover may be withdrawn. Some patients may require weak steroid like fluorometholone for several months.

Stromal necrotic keratitis

Stromal necrotic keratitis is a suppurative stromal inflammation, which may be severe and may progress rapidly (Fig. 15.28). It may be clinically indistinguishable from bacterial and fungal keratitis.

Treatment: Oral antiviral drugs preferred as topical drugs can cause toxicity. Necrotizing herpetic keratitis is very sensitive to topical steroids and twice a day dose will control the inflammation. Frequent use of unpreserved corneal tear substitutes to promote epithelial healing.

Metaherpetic ulcers (neurotrophickeratopathy)

Develops in patients with reduced corneal sensation due to postherpetic infection. It is not an active viral disease.

Treatment: Consider the following:

1. Lubricants to promote healing, punctal cautery and bandage contact lens.
2. Tarsorrhaphy indicated in cases that fail to respond to conservative treatment.
3. Keratoplasty is indicated in cases with visually significant stromal scarring. But should be deferred till the eye has been quiet for several months because of chance of recurrence of viral keratitis in new graft.
4. Amniotic membrane transplantation may be done in persistent epithelial defects.

Herpetic eye disease study (HEDS) result

1. Topical corticosteroids are indicated in stromal keratitis as these significantly decrease inflammation and shorten duration of keratitis.
2. Oral acyclovir is not beneficial in non-necrotizing stromal keratitis. But in necrotizing stromal keratitis, it is beneficial as this helps to reduce local drug toxicity. Oral antivirals do not prevent the development of stromal keratitis or iritis in cases of epithelial keratitis.

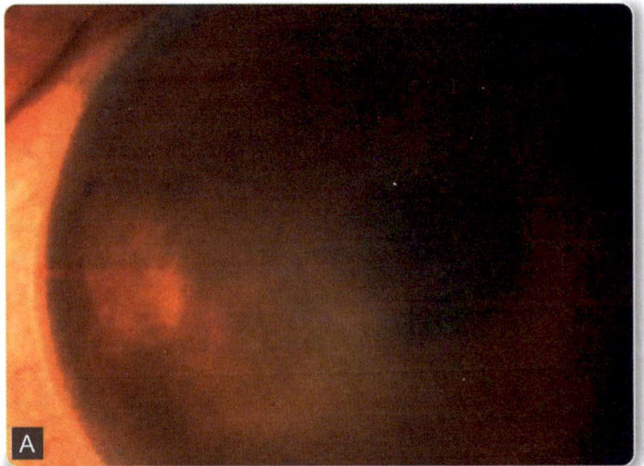

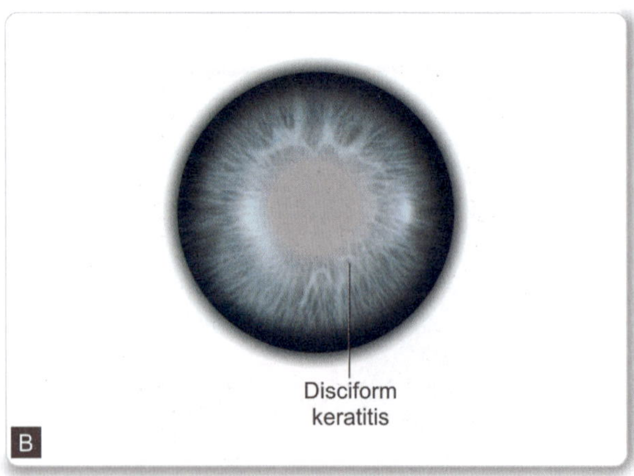

FIGURES 15.27A and B: Disciform keratitis. **A.** Photograph; **B.** Diagrammatic representation.

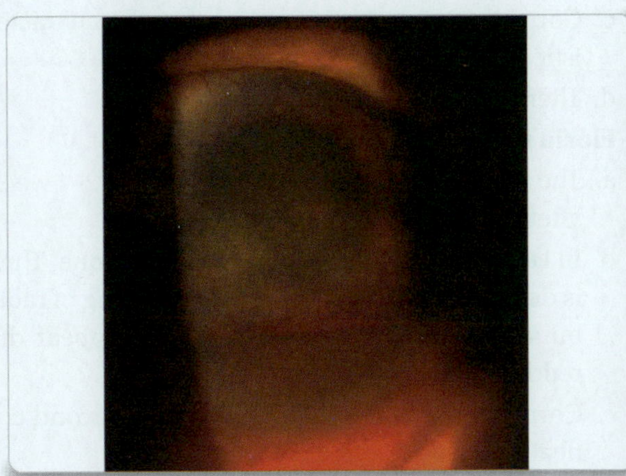

FIGURE 15.28: Necrotizing stromal keratitis

3. These reduce the recurrence rate in cases of recurrent HSV stromal keratitis. Hence, long-term prophylaxis is recommended for recurrent HSV stromal keratitis (oral acyclovir 400 mg bid for 12 months).

Herpes simplex virus vaccine

A lot of work is being done, but still no active or passive vaccine is available.

Herpes Zoster Ophthalmicus

Herpes zoster ophthalmicus (HZO) is caused by varicella zoster virus (VZV) that causes chickenpox.

Mechanism: Varicella zoster virus and herpes zoster virus (HZV) are morphologically identical, but antigenically different. After an attack of chickenpox, the virus travels in a retrograde manner and lodges in cranial nerve sensory ganglia or dorsal root ganglia, where it remains dormant for decades. These viruses get activated especially when cellular immunity has faded. In most patients with zoster ophthalmicus, the focus of infection is the gasserian ganglion. The disease occurs in old people from sixth to ninth decades and in those who are on systemic immunosuppressants, those with malignancies, HIV infection and other debilitating diseases.

Clinical features: Presents as a painful vesicular dermatitis typically localized to a dermatome on thorax or face. The vesicular lesions never cross the midline. In HZO the ophthalmic division of trigeminal nerve is affected:

1. Prodromal phase: Characterized by fever, malaise and headache 3–5 days before onset of skin eruptions.
2. Skin lesions: Appears as painful maculopapular rashes along the distribution of ophthalmic division of trigeminal nerve. Lesions do not cross the midline:
   a. Within 24 hours vesicles appear.
   b. Vesicles pass through the pustular stage, crust and dry after 2–3 weeks.
   c. Residual skin destruction and scarring occurs (Fig. 15.29). Disease does not spread once crusting is complete.
3. Ocular manifestation of HZO: Ocular involvement may be due to:
   a. Direct viral invasion.
   b. Antigen-antibody reaction.
   c. Corneal anesthesia—neurotrophic keratitis.
4. Hutchinson's sign: Involvement of the external nasal nerve, which supplies the side of—tip of nose and root of nose correlates significantly with corneal involvement.
5. Epithelial keratitis: It develops in 50% of patients within 2 days of onset of disease. Fine dendritic lesions develop without terminal bulbs. Can be treated with topical antivirals.
6. Nummular keratitis: Usually develops about 10 days after onset of rashes. Characterized by subepithelial deposits with stromal haze. Treated by topical steroids, which is slowly tapered.
7. Stromal keratitis: It develops 3 weeks after onset of disease and responds to topical steroids.
8. Disciform keratitis: It is less common with HZO, but may lead to corneal decompensation. It is also treated with topical steroids.
9. Neurotrophic keratitis with reduced sensation occurs in about 50%. Treatment is by promotion of epithelial healing by tarsorrhaphy.
10. Secondary bacterial infection may occur.
11. Postherpetic neuralgia (pain) persists after the rash has healed. It occurs in 75% of patients over 70 years of age. The pain may be constant or intermittent worse at night and may be severe causing depression.

Treatment of systemic disease: Oral acyclovir 800 mg five times for 3-7 days. The drug should be started within

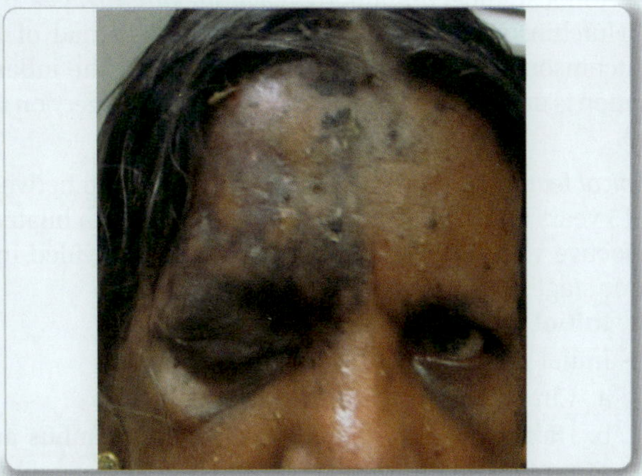

FIGURE 15.29: Herpes zoster ophthalmicus

72 hours of onset of signs to reduce the severity of the attack and the risk of postherpetic neuralgia. Systemic treatment also reduces the risk of ophthalmic complication by 50%.

Other oral antivirals: It include the following:

1. Valaciclovir 1 g 8th hourly, famciclovir 750 mg daily and zidovudine 125 mg daily are equally effective, but expensive.
2. Systemic steroids—prednisolone 40–60 mg daily should be used only in conjunction with systemic antivirals.

Treatment of postherpetic neuralgia: As follows:

- Topical—local anesthetic creams may be beneficial
- Systemic—simple analgesics such as paracetamol up to 4 g daily
- Non-steroidal anti-inflammatory drugs (NSAIDS) are ineffective. Carbamazepine 400 mg daily can be given for severe pain.

Interstitial Keratitis

Interstitial keratitis is an inflammation of corneal stroma without primary involvement of epithelium or endothelium. It may be infective or allergic in origin.

Etiology: Interstitial keratitis (IK) occurs in:

- Congenital syphilis (usually bilateral)
- Tuberculosis
- Leprosy
- Sarcoidosis
- Cogan's syndrome (IK with deafness tinnitus and vertigo).

Syphilitic Interstitial Keratitis

Etiology: Occurs in cases where the infection is passed on to the child from mother in the primary, secondary or early latent phase of disease (within first 2 years of infection).

Interstitial keratitis is allergic manifestation to *Treponema pallidum* and the stromal inflammation occurs due to local antigen-antibody reaction. Often IK is a part of Hutchinson's triad of congenital syphilis (triad of IK, Hutchinson's teeth and vestibular deafness). The inflammation is usually triggered off by an injury or surgery on the eye.

Clinical features: Manifestations in child develop between 5–15 years of life. The child usually presents with bilateral defective vision. The clinical picture can be divided into three stages.

1. **Initial progressive stage**
   Initial progressive stage is characterized by:
   a. Circumcorneal congestion.
   b. Hazy patches in cornea starting near limbus and progressing toward center due to cellular infiltration and edema.
   c. Corneal vascularization, which has the characteristic salmon patch appearance.
   d. There is associated anterior uveitis.
2. **Florid stage**
   a. The whole cornea becomes hazy within 2–4 weeks after the onset of inflammation.
   b. In severe cases, the cornea appears opaque. There is deep corneal vascularization consisting of radial bundles of brush-like vessels, which appear dull reddish-pink (salmon patches).
   c. Corneal haze and infiltration extends beyond corneal vessels.
   d. There may be profound uveitis.
3. **Stage of regression**
   a. Cornea starts clearing from periphery to center.
   b. As cloudiness disappear, vessels become obliterated and appear as fine opaque lines (ghost vessels).
   c. Cornea takes weeks or months to clear, but little improvement occurs after till 18 months.

Diagnosis: It is confirmed by other systemic features also.

Parasitic Keratitis

Protozoal keratitis are:

- Acanthamoeba
- Microsporidia.

Acanthamoeba Keratitis

Acanthamoeba are free-lying ameba found in soil, freshwater, well water, swimming pools, etc. The cystic form is lightly resilient and under favorable conditions cysts turn into trophozoites, which produce a wide variety of enzymes, which enables tissue penetration and destruction.

The organism can contaminate contact lenses and their cleaning solutions. Once they adhere to hydrogel lenses, infection is certain as they can penetrate intact corneal epithelium. Acanthamoeba keratitis (Figs 15.30A to C), which is a blinding disease is a threat to contact lens wearers. It can occur in non-contact lens users also due to contact of the eye with contaminated water or injury with contaminated vegetable matter.

Clinical features: These includes:

1. History of contact lens wear.
2. Trauma with vegetable matter and exposure to contaminants in water.

Sx Symptoms

Pain, which is very severe and disproportionate to the signs is usually the presenting symptom. It is due to perineuritis. Other symptoms are blurred vision, photophobia, blepharospasm, watering.

Signs: The earliest signs are similar to viral epithelial keratitis and advanced lesions may look like fungal ulcers (refer Figs 15.30B and C).

1. The characteristic feature of *Acanthamoeba* infection of the cornea is necrotizing stromal keratitis.
2. Focal anterior stromal infiltrates and perineural infiltrates are seen.
3. Limbitis and scleritis may develop.
4. Coalescence and enlargement of infiltrates leads to ring abscess (refer Fig. 15.30A).
5. Corneal opacification occurs and also corneal melting can occur at any stage.
6. Vascularization is very uncommon.

Investigations: They are as follows.

Staining: Using periodic acid-Schiff or calcofluor white, which are fluorescent dyes with an affinity for amebic agents and fungi. Culture of scraping and inoculating in non-nutrient agar seeded with dead *E. coli.*

Polymerase chain reaction (PCR): Positive PCR can diagnosis *Acanthamoeba.* The CFM can demonstrate cysts at early stage.

Treatment: There are as follows:

1. Debridement to remove infected epithelium.
2. Dual therapy with amebicides is effective only against trophozoites:
   a. Propamidine isethionate 0.1% and polyhexamethylene biguanide (PHMB) 0.02%.
   b. Hexamidine and chlorhexidine 0.02%.
   c. Neomycin—polymyxin antibiotic drops or ointment has some action against *Acanthamoeba.*

   Antibiotic-like ciprofloxacin to cover coexistent gram-negative infection.

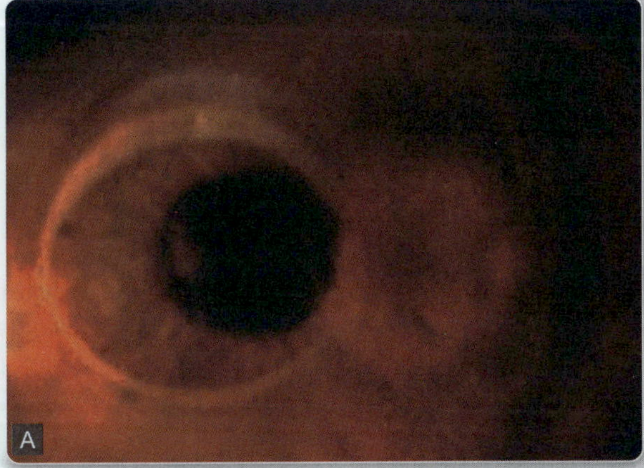

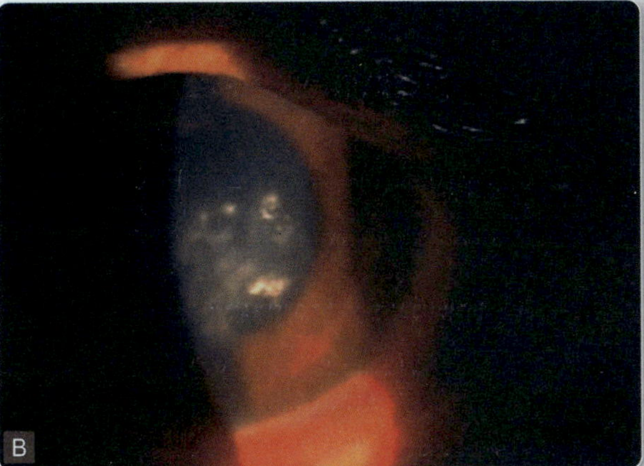

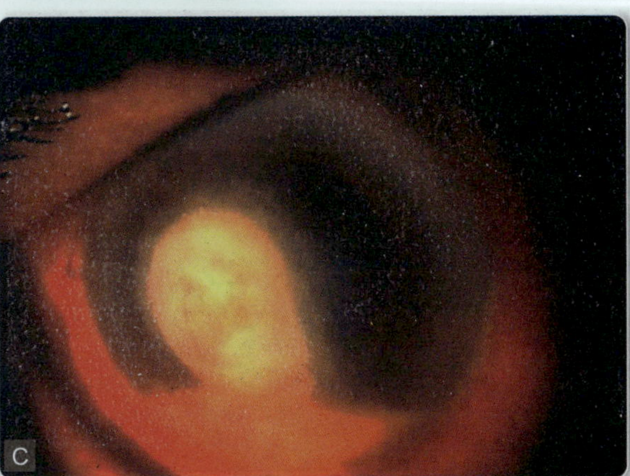

FIGURES 15.30A to C: Acanthamoeba keratitis. **A.** Ring infiltrates in the acanthamoeba keratitis; **B.** Early stage; **C.** Advanced stages.

3. Topical steroids are avoided as these contribute to prolonged viability of cysts.
4. Pain is controlled with systemic NSAID like ibuprofen.
5. Keratoplasty can be done for residual scarring. But it should be done only after infection is controlled. Otherwise recurrence in graft can occur.

Microsporidial Keratitis

Microsporidia are intracellular spore-forming protozoa causing opportunistic infections in individuals with acquired immunodeficiency syndrome (AIDS). Human infection with *Microsporidia* was rare before AIDS became prevalent.

Clinical features: These includes the following:

- Bilateral epithelial keratitis
- Stromal keratitis
- Scleritis and endophthalmitis
- Corneal biopsy shows spores and characteristic intracellular parasites.

Treatment: Fumagillin suspension (10 mg/mL) is applied as drops into the eye hourly for 24 hours and then tapered.

Antiretroviral treatment together with this can restore immunity and help healing. If refractory to topical therapy, albendazole 400 mg daily is given for 2 weeks and then repeated 2 weeks later with a second course. If albendazole fails oral itraconazole can be given.

BACTERIAL HYPERSENSITIVITY-MEDIATED CORNEAL DISEASE

Marginal Keratitis

Marginal keratitis are small superficial ulcer situated near the limbus. Ulcers are usually less than 1 mm in size, with or without epithelial defect. Associated uveitis is rare. These ulcers develop as a reaction to staphylococcal exotoxins (*Staphylococcus aureus*). The culture of corneal lesions are negative for *S. aureus,* but the organism can be isolated from lid margins.

Signs and Symptoms

Mild irritation, watering, photophobia, associated *Staphylococcus* blepharitis or conjunctival congestion may be seen.

Lesions of 1 mm occur inside the limbus discrete opacities with clear areas (Figs 15.31A and B).

Treatment

Topical fluoroquinolone eye drops 4 times for 1 week. Systemic tetracyclines may be needed in recurrent cases. Once the infection is controlled, the mild topical steroid drops are given.

Phlyctenular Keratoconjunctivitis

Phlyctenular keratoconjunctivitis is primarily a conjunctival disease, which may affect the cornea also. It is a presumed, delayed hypersensitivity reaction to staphylococcal cell wall antigen or tuberculoprotein or associated with helminthic infection.

Clinical Features

Usually children or young adults are affected and presents with pain, photophobia, watering and blepharospasm. Corneal phlycten starts as a gray nodule near the limbus. Nodule may break up into an ulcer. Limbal phlycten extends progressively onto cornea leading to fascicular ulcer,

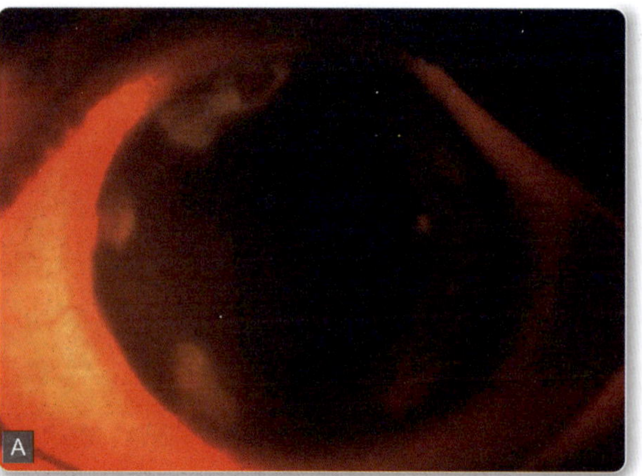

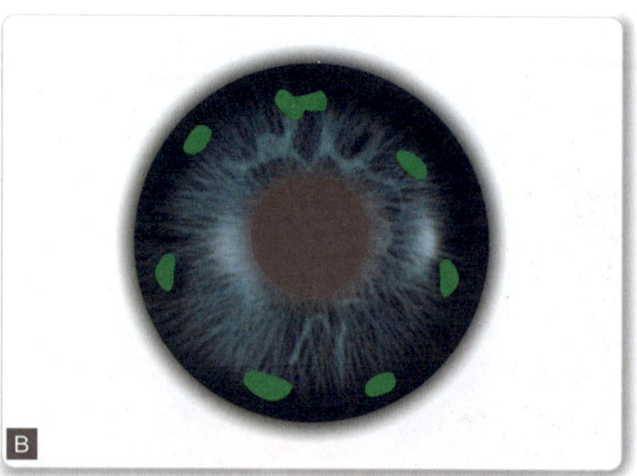

FIGURES 15.31A and B: Marginal keratitis. **A.** Photograph; **B.** Diagrammatic representation.

which is a vascularized corneal ulcer. The characteristic feature of a fascicular ulcer is severe blepharospasm and heavy vascularization, which is out of proportion to the size of the ulcer (Figs 15.32A and B). Sometimes corneal thinning and even perforation can occur.

Treatment

Treatment is by using topical steroids, which suppresses the hypersensitivity reaction and promote healing. It is also important to treat the staphylococcal infection, tuberculous infection and helminths to eradicate the source of antigen.

Focus of staphyloccocal infection should be identified and X-ray of chest and Mantoux test done to rule out tuberculosis.

Differential Diagnosis

- Peripheral corneal ulceration
- Mooren's ulcer (Figs 15.33A to C)
- Peripheral ulcerative keratitis.

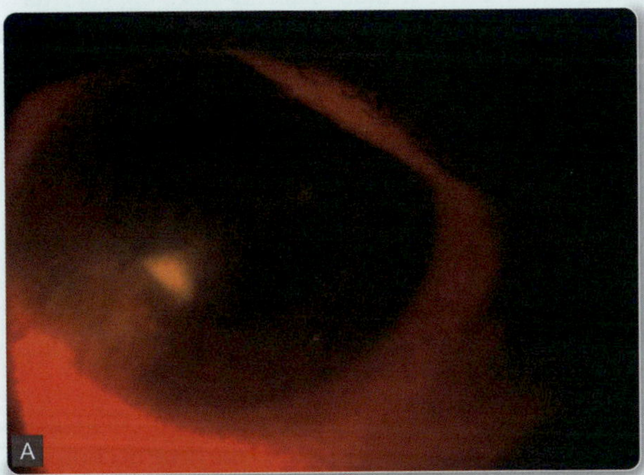

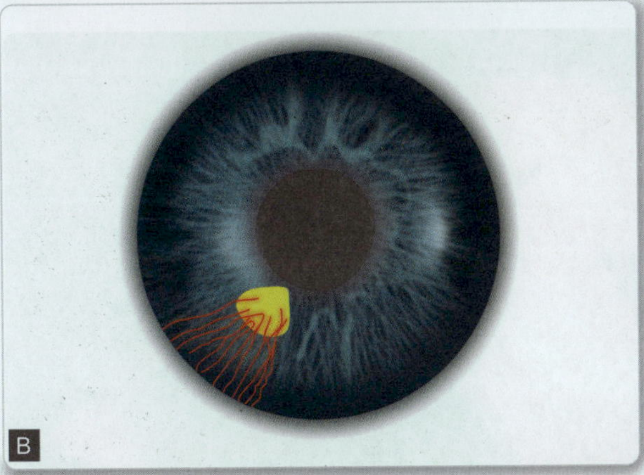

FIGURES 15.32A and B: Fascicular ulcer. **A.** Photograph; **B.** Diagrammatic representation.

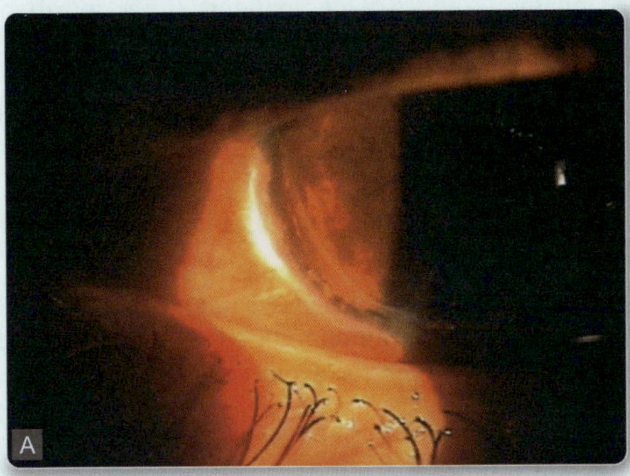

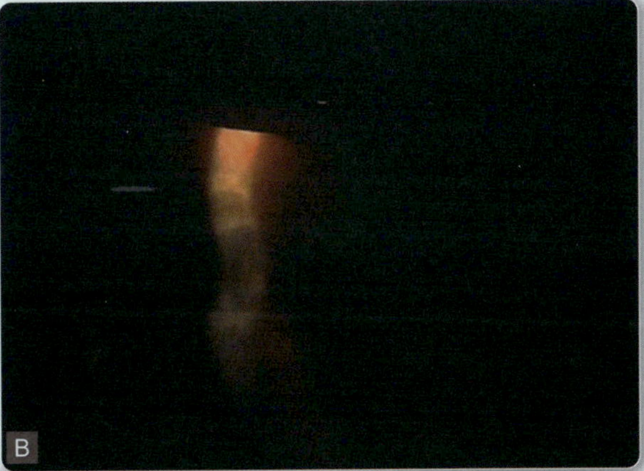

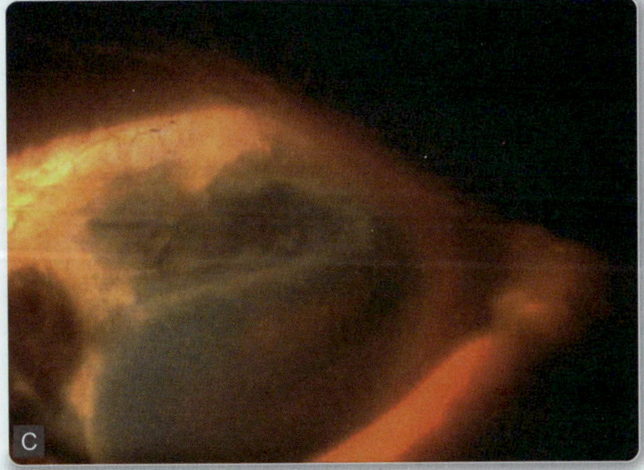

FIGURES 15.33A to C: Mooren's ulcer. **A.** Early stage; **B.** Peripheral corneal thinning; **C.** Perforated Mooren's ulcer.

Mooren's ulcer

Mooren's ulcer is an uncommon painful severe form of peripheral ulceration of cornea characterized by progression along the corneal periphery and later central spread. The ulceration mainly affects stroma. Two clinical types of Mooren's ulcer has been identified.

1. Unilateral—affects older patients (after fourth decade) and is more responsive to medical and surgical treatment.
2. Bilateral—occurs in younger age groups and is the more severe form, which is more painful and resistant to treatment.

Mooren's ulcer is more common in males than in females and rare in children.

Pathogenesis: Exact pathogenesis is unknown, but the disease appears to be an autoimmune reaction to a specific corneal antigen, which results in collagenolytic destruction of cornea.

Sx **Symptoms**

Symptoms include severe pain (more in bilateral type) photophobia, lacrimation and defective vision.

Signs: Peripheral ulcer, which undermines the epithelium and superficial stroma and has characteristic overhanging edges. The typical progression in a radial fashion along the limbus with overhanging edges at the advancing end with or without healing at the other end is the typical picture. Some slow progression toward the center of the cornea also occurs, especially in a rapidly progressing type.

Ulcer rarely perforates. The sclera is not involved unlike other peripheral ulcerative keratitis (PUK). Healing is characterized by corneal thinning vascularization and scarring.

Complication: These include the following:

1. It can cause severe irregular corneal astigmatism.
2. Secondary bacterial infection is common.
3. Perforation may occur.
4. Cataract and glaucoma may be seen.

Treatment: These are as follows:

1. Aggressive treatment with topical corticosteroids may help in some cases (less severe and unilateral cases).
2. Wide conjunctival resection to have bare sclera extending 2'O clock on either side of ulcer and 4 mm posteriorly.
3. Following limbal conjunctival resection, tissue adhesive can be applied to lesion with bandage contact lenses over the glue.
4. Topical cyclosporine drugs may be used in unilateral cases.
5. Systemic cytotoxic chemotherapy may be needed to arrest progressive corneal destruction especially in bilateral cases methotrexate, azathioprine or cyclophosphamide can be given. This is highly successful. The drugs are continued for 6 months and then tapered if possible.
6. Corneal surgeries keratoplasty or even section for cataract surgery can trigger an activity even in burnt out cases of Mooren's. Hence, patients with Mooren's should be immune suppressed before surgery. Graft can be lysed by reactivation of disease.

Peripheral ulcerative keratitis

In PUK there is severe peripheral corneal infiltration and ulceration with corneal thinning, and progresses along corneal periphery and also centrally, and is unresponsive to topical form of therapy. It is usually seen in systemic collagen vascular diseases and it may precede or follow the onset of systemic illness.

Pathogenesis: The PUK generally occurs in patients with autoimmune disease due to deposition of antigen-antibody complexes in peripheral cornea associated with limbal vasculitis (Fig. 15.34). There is inflammatory cell infiltration and release of enzymes leading to peripheral ulceration and thinning of cornea.

Clinical features: The PUK is crescent-shaped peripheral corneal ulcers. Associated scleritis and episcleritis are usually present and ulcer spreads along the corneal periphery with thinning. The corneal ulceration may extend into sclera too unlike Mooren's.

Associated systemic diseases may be:

1. Rheumatoid arthritis: 30% of rheumatoid arthritis patients have bilateral PUK as shown in Figure 15.35.
2. Wegener's granulomatosis is the second most common association of PUK.

Treatment: High dose of systemic steroids have to be used to control acute disease.

Cytotoxic therapy is required for long-term management of the disease. Cyclophosphamide is the drug of choice. Other options are methotrexate, azathioprine and cyclosporine.

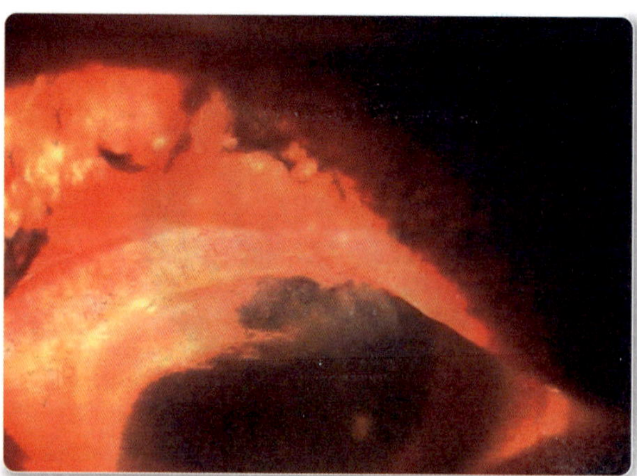

FIGURE 15.34: Peripheral ulcerative keratitis

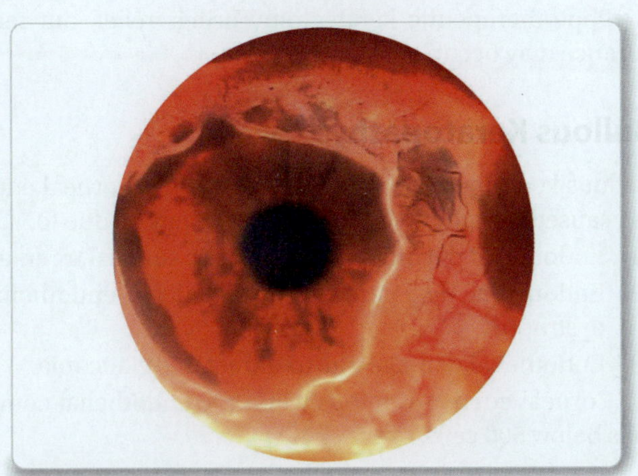

FIGURE 15.35: Contact lens cornea in rheumatoid arthritis

Neurotrophic Keratitis

Neurotrophic keratitis (NTK) is due to paralysis of sensory supply to cornea, i.e. paralysis of ophthalmic division of trigeminal nerve. Disruption of the sensory pathways lead to reduced reflex tearing and decreased cell division (mitosis inhibition). This effect on mitosis and reflex tearing interferes with normal healing after trauma and microtrauma to cornea and desiccation leading to ulceration.

Causes

Causes of NTK are as follows:

1. Varicella-zoster keratitis and HSV keratitis are the most common causes of NTK.
2. Trauma to ophthalmic division of trigeminal nerve by injuries or surgeries.
3. Stroke, irradiation to regions near orbit for malignancies, multiple sclerosis, etc.
4. Decreased sensation occurs in diabetic, herpes, hereditary sensory neuropathy like familial dysautonomia (Riley-Day syndrome).

Clinical Features

1. Neurotrophic keratopathy occurs in central or inferior paracentral cornea.
2. Ulcers are usually oval in shape.
3. Progression of the ulcer may be virtually asymptomatic because of corneal anesthesia.
4. Progression occurs from punctate keratopathy to persistent epithelial defects, which enlarges and then stromal edema and infiltration occur. Then stromal breakdown occur leading to non-healing neurotrophic ulcer.

Treatment

1. For mild punctate keratitis preservative-free lubricant drops can be used.
2. Avoid all potentially toxic topical medications.
3. For persistent epithelial defects and stromal lysis, patching and bandage contact lens may be tried.
4. Topical autologous serum has been demonstrated to promote healing.
5. Tarsorrhaphy, either temporary or permanent has the best healing response.
6. Botulinum toxin injection to induce protective ptosis.
7. Amniotic membrane grafts and conjunctival flaps over the ulcer may be required for severe cases.
8. Lid diseases including blepharitis, entropion, ectropion, facial palsy, etc. must be aggressively treated.

Lagophthalmos and Exposure Keratitis

Lagophthalmos is defective lid closure can occur due to an abnormality of the lids or an abnormal position of the eyeball.

Exposure of eye can occur in these clinical situations leading to drying of cornea in spite of normal tear production and normal cornea. Drying leads to desiccation and epithelial loss. These epithelial defects become infected to form corneal ulcers.

Causes of Corneal Exposure

Paralysis of facial nerve may be idiopathic (Bell's palsy) result of surgery for acoustic neuroma or parotid gland tumors.

Mechanical exposure as in cicatricial pemphigoid, burns of face (Fig. 15.36), trauma causing contracture of eyelids.

Contraction of skin of face as in xeroderma pigmentosa, ichthyosis, etc. Symblepharon and severe ectropion can cause exposure.

Abnormal globe positions, such as proptosis or exophthalmos. Deep coma may also cause globe exposure.

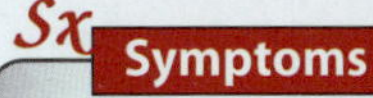

Symptoms

Symptoms are those of dry eye.

Signs

1. Lesions usually appear in inferior third of cornea.
2. There is drying and desiccation of epithelium which breaks down.
3. Stromal edema and breakdown also occurs.

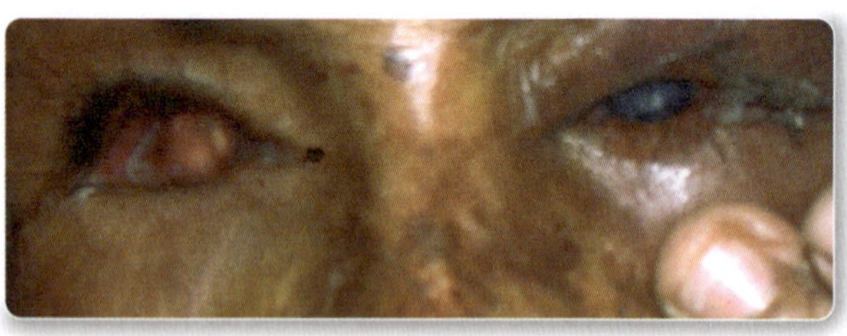

FIGURE 15.36: Severe facial burns with cicatricial contracture of lids of both eyes and tarsorrhaphy done in left eye to protect the already damaged cornea. Right eye lost due to burns and exposure keratitis.

4. There may be super added secondary bacterial infection which may be viral/bacterial.
5. Finally perforation or healing without perforation takes place.

Treatment

If the exposure is reversible as in Bell's palsy, artificial tears (without preservative) is used during day and ointments used at night.

Taping of lids at night and bandage contact lenses is useful. Temporary tarsorrhaphy can be done, which is released when cause of exposure is cured. Lateral or medial or central tarsorrhaphy is done in proptosis. Severe proptosis can be managed by orbital decompression.

OTHER TYPES OF KERATITIS

Infectious Crystalline Keratitis

Infectious crystalline keratitis is a rare type of infective keratitis caused by *Streptococcus viridans* and occurs in case of long-term topical steroid therapy as in the postoperative period of PKP. Slowly progressing gray-white branching opacities are seen in anterior and mid-stroma.
Treatment: Topical antibiotics for a long period.

Thygeson's Superficial Punctate Keratitis

Thygeson's superficial punctate keratitis is also uncommon, idiopathic keratitis, which is often bilateral and affects young adults . It presents with elevated epithelial lesions with subepithelial haze. The common differential diagnoses are viral keratitis, staphylococal hypersensitivity and punctate epitheliopathy.
Treatment: With lubricants and low dose of topical steroids, which needs to be tapered off. Cyclosporine eye drops may also be used.

Phototherapeutic keratectomy brings relief, but reccurence may occur.

Bullous Keratopathy

Bullous keratopathy (Fig. 15.37) is a chronic corneal edema caused by endothelial damage and may be due to:
1. Endothelial decompensation due to surgical trauma.
2. Endothelial degeneration as in Fuchs' endothelial dystrophy.
3. Endothelial damage due to intractable glaucoma.

Corneal edema develops when the endothelial count falls below 500 cells/mm^2.

Signs and Symptoms

Symptoms are pain, irritation, foreign body sensation and decrease in vision. Decrease in vision occurs due to loss of corneal transparency. Ocular pain, irritation and foreign body sensation are due to rupture of epithelial bullae and exposure of nerve endings. Stromal edema and epithelial edema leading to increase in corneal thickness and epithelial bullae can be visualized. Microbial infection of cornea may occur as complication.

Treatment

1. Hypertonic saline for local application to decrease edema.
2. Topical application of carboxymethyl cellulose to decrease pain and foreign body sensation.
3. Penetrating keratoplasty is treatment of choice for patients with visual potential.
4. Those with poor visual prognosis can be treated by any one of the following:
   a. Anterior stromal puncture.

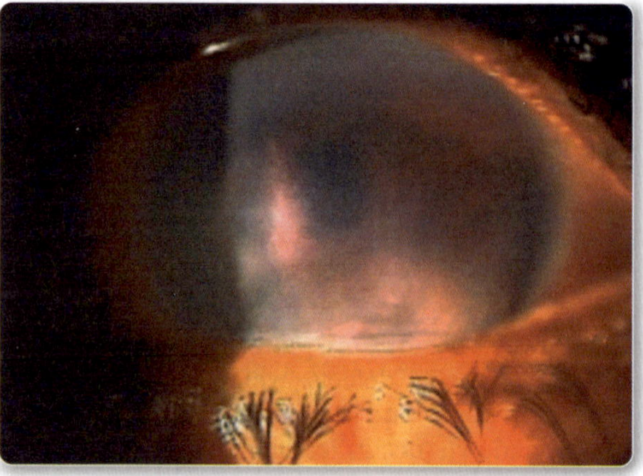

FIGURE 15.37: Bullous keratopathy

b. Excimer laser photoablation.
c. Conjunctival flap to cover the cornea after epithelial debridement (Gundersen's flap).
d. Amniotic membrane transplantation after epithelial debridement.

Photophthalmia

Photophthalmia is a corneal manifestation caused by exposure of cornea to ultraviolet rays (311–290 nm wavelength). Ultraviolet rays cause desquamation of corneal epithelial cells leading to multiple corneal erosions.

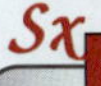

Symptoms

The symptoms develop 4–6 hours after exposure to ultraviolet rays. Symptoms are severe pain, photophobia, blepharospasm, edema of conjunctiva, etc.

Causes

1. Exposure to bright flash of short circuit.
2. Exposure to industrial welding.
3. Snow blindness (ultraviolet rays are reflected from snow).

Treatment

1. Prophylaxis by wearing glasses, that cut off ultraviolet rays, e.g. Crookes glass.
2. Lubricant eye drops.
3. Bandage eyes for 24 hours, which allow epithelium to regenerate.

Filamentary Keratitis

Filamentary keratitis is a condition characterized by formation of epithelial filaments, which adhere to cornea at one end and the other end moves freely. These are deposition of mucus and cellular debris on epithelial strands. These filaments cause considerable irritation and foreign body sensation.

Causes

1. Keratoconjunctivitis sicca is the most common cause.
2. Ptosis/occlusion of eye.
3. Neurotrophic keratitis.
4. Superior limbic keratoconjunctivitis.
5. Recurrent corneal erosions, after corneal graft or refractive surgery and drug toxicity.

Clinical Features

1. Foreign body sensation and irritation in eye.
2. Filaments of epithelial cells and mucus are seen on the cornea that move with blink. Epithelial defect is seen at the base of the filament.
3. Filaments stain with rose Bengal.

Treatment

1. The underlying cause (e.g. dry eye) should be treated.
2. All unnecessary drugs should be stopped (to prevent toxicity) short-term topical steroids help healing.
3. Mechanical removal of filaments relieves irritation.
4. Mucolytic agents like acetylcysteine 10% and bandage contact lenses are useful.

Recurrent Epithelial Erosions

Epithelial defects of cornea usually heal quickly and permanently, but sometimes there is recurrent breakdown of epithelium for several years after the initial episode. This is because there is an abnormally weak attachment between the epithelium and basement membrane. Minor injuries such as opening eyes after sleep causes tearing of epithelium.

Causes

Trauma usually with finger nail of child and can lead to recurrent corneal erosions.

1. Erosions associated with corneal dystrophy.
2. Erosions associated with diabetes mellitus.

Sx **Symptoms**

1. Typically pain on waking up in the morning.
2. Prior history of trauma.
3. Epithelial defect usually in interpalpebral region.

Signs

Signs of epithelial dystrophy (fingerprint lines, intraepithelial microcysts, filamentary keratitis, bullae, etc.). Loose sheet of epithelium hanging on corneal surface may be seen.

Treatment

1. Lubricants as preservative-free drops during day time and lubricant ointment at night for 1–3 weeks.
2. Hypertonic saline drops during day and ointment at night.

3. Bandage contact lens.
4. Phototherapeutic keratectomy, i.e. excimer laser ablation after epithelial debridement (superficial keratectomy) to remove the abnormal epithelium and basement membrane.
5. Anterior stromal punctures for localized areas not involving visual axis.

First three procedures promote healing and last two remove abnormal epithelium and basement membrane.

Superior Limbic Keratoconjunctivitis

Superior limbic keratoconjunctivitis usually affects middle-aged women. About 20%–50% of patients has associated thyroid dysfunction and hence should be investigated for thyroid disease and 25% are associated with keratoconjunctivitis sicca.

Clinical Features

Bilateral chronic inflammation of the superior tarsal and bulbar conjunctiva.

1. Papillary hypertrophy and hyperemia of superior tarsal conjunctiva.
2. Hyperemia of superior bulbar conjunctiva.
3. Punctate epithelial erosions and corneal filaments in superior cornea are common.

Treatment

1. Liberal use of topical lubricants.
2. Mucolytic agents like 10% acetylcysteine.
3. Occlusion of puncta.
4. Soft contact lenses.
5. Resection of superior limbic conjunctiva may help in resistant cases.

Xerophthalmia

Xerophthalmia is a spectrum of ocular diseases caused by vitamin A deficiency (Box 15.1). Vitamin A is essential for synthesis of retinal pigments and conjunctival glycoproteins. Deficiency occurs due to dietary deficiency of the vitamin or defective absorption. Vitamin A deficiency is responsible for 1 lakh new cases of blindness, worldwide, every year.

Sx **Symptoms**

The main symptom of the patient is night blindness (nyctalopia).

BOX 15.1: WHO grading of xerophthalmia
XN: Night blindness
X1: Conjunctival xerosis and Bitot's spots
X2: Corneal xerosis
X3: Corneal ulceration X3a: Corneal ulceration or keratomalacia affecting less than one-third cornea X3b: Corneal ulceration or keratomalacia affecting more than one-third cornea
XS: Corneal scar
XF: Xerophthalmic fundus

Signs

1. Conjunctival signs:
   a. Dryness of conjunctiva in the interpalpebral zone with keratinization.
   b. Bitot's spots: These are triangular patches of keratinized epithelium in interpalpebral zone on the temporal aspect of bulbar conjunctiva (Fig. 15.38).
2. Corneal signs:
   a. Dry luster less cornea due to xerosis of cornea.
   b. Keratinization of cornea.
   c. Keratomalacia, which is sterile corneal melting by necrosis and liquefaction of cornea. Keratomalacia can lead to perforation or whole cornea may necrose off.
3. Retinal signs:
   a. Retinopathy with yellow peripheral dots.
   b. Electroretinography (ERG) shows decreased amplitude in advanced cases.

Treatment

1. Keratomalacia is treated as a medical emergency often with hospitalization.
2. Oil-based vitamin A preparations are given orally and aqueous based preparation is given parenterally.
3. Vitamin A is administered in 3 doses. First dose is to be given at diagnosis, the second after 24 hours and third after 2 weeks. Oral oil-based preparations are preferred, but water soluble preparations of vitamin A in half the dose are given as injections if the child is having profuse diarrhea or vomiting.
4. Oral preparations of vitamin A (injections in half the dose):
   a. Children less than 6 months—retinyl palmitate 50,000 IU.
   b. Children 6–12 months or weight less than 8 kg—retinyl palmitate 10,000 IU.

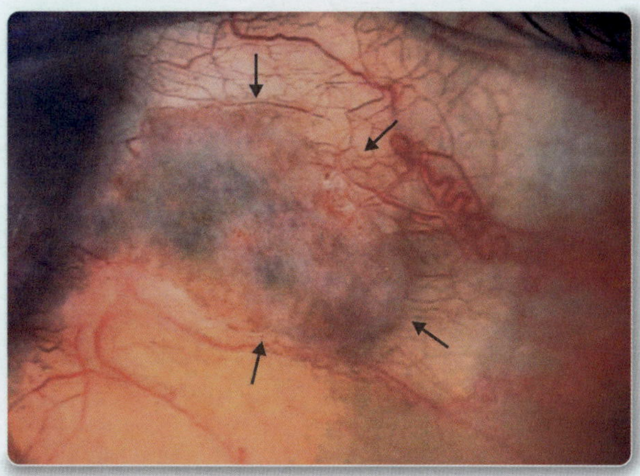

FIGURE 15.38: Bitot's spots

c. Child more than 12 months and weight less than 8 kg—retinyl palmitate 200,000 IU.

CORNEAL DYSTROPHIES

Dystrophies are usually hereditary progressive bilateral non-inflammatory diseases of cornea. These manifest as bilateral, usually central, corneal opacities that are non-vascularized (Table 15.4).

Corneal dystrophies can be classified into:

1. Epithelial dystrophies.
2. Dystrophies of Bowman's layer.
3. Stromal dystrophies.
4. Granular dystrophies.
5. Endothelial dystrophies.

TABLE 15.4: Characteristics of corneal dystrophy

Dystrophy	Deposited material	Staining
Lattice	Amyloid	Congo red
Granular	Hyaline	Masson's trichrome
Macular	Mucopolysaccharide (glycosaminoglycans)	Alcian blue (Prussian blue)

Epithelial Dystrophies

Common epithelial dystrophies are the following.

Cogan's Epithelial Basement Membrane Dystrophy

Cogan's epithelial basement membrane dystrophy is usually sporadic and rarely autosomal dominant with incomplete prevalence. History shows thickening of basement membrane.

Clinical manifestations: These are as follows:

1. About 10% of patients develop recurrent corneal erosions by third decade and the remaining 90% are asymptomatic throughout life.
2. On slit-lamp biomicroscopic examination, the following lesions may be visible; dot-like opacities, epithelial microcysts, subepithelial map-like pattern and fingerprint-like lines.

Treatment: For recurrent corneal erosions.

Meesmann Epithelial Dystrophy

Meesmann epithelial dystrophy is a rare type of epithelial dystrophy, which is AD. It is characterized by tiny intraepithelial cysts, which are maximum centrally. Corneal sensation may be reduced.

Treatment: Only lubricants are usually required.

Other Epithelial Dystrophies

The other epithelial dystrophies are:

1. Lisch epithelial dystrophy.
2. Gelatinous drop-like corneal dystrophy.

Bowman's Layer Corneal Dystrophy

Bowman's layer corneal dystrophy also know as Reis-Bucklers corneal dystrophy. It is inherited as an AD trait, shows replacement of Bowman's membrane by fibrous tissue, which can interfere with vision and presents with subepithelial opacities similar to granular dystrophy.

Treatment

Initially treatment of recurrent erosion, later excimer laser keratectomy, phototherapeutic keratectomy, lamellar keratoplasty or even PKP may be needed.

Other dystrophies affecting the Bowman's membrane is Behnke dystrophy (honeycomb-shaped corneal dystrophy).

Stromal Dystrophies

Lattice Dystrophy Type 1

1. Autosomal dominant inheritance with locus at *5q31* gene (Figs 15.39A and B).
2. Characterized by amyloid deposition in corneal stroma that stains with congo red.
3. Onset at the end of first decade with recurrent corneal erosions.
4. Refractive lines in the anterior corneal stroma, subepithelial white dots and diffuse stromal haze appear in central cornea, while periphery remains clear.

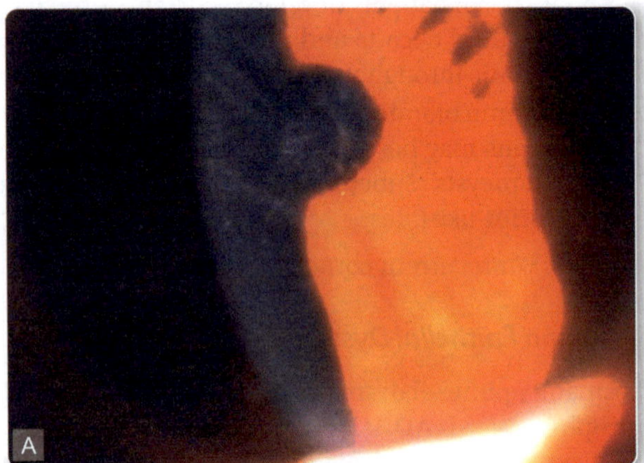

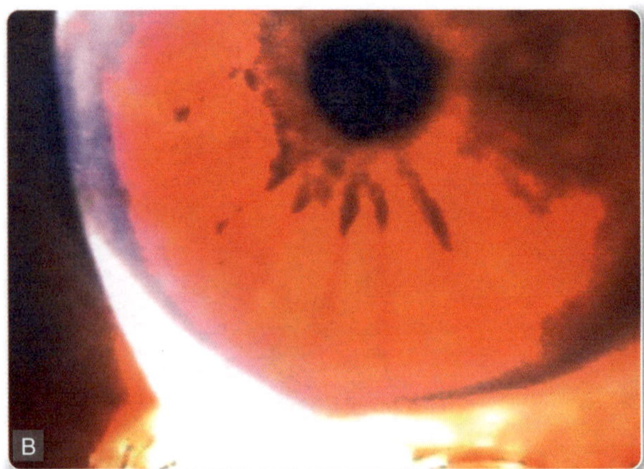

FIGURES 15.39A and B: Lattice dystrophy

5. Corneal sensation is reduced and vision drops.

Treatment: By deep anterior lamellar keratoplasty (DALK), but recurrence in graft may occur.

Lattice Corneal Dystrophy Type II

1. Also AD inheritance gene locus at *9q34*.
2. Has systemic amyloidosis-like 'mask-like' facial expression, protruding lips, progressive cranial and peripheral neutropathy, dry and lax skin, etc. Amyloidosis may also affect heart and kidney.

Granular Dystrophies

Granular Dystrophy Type I (Groenouw Type I)

1. Inheritance is AD with gene locus at *5q31*.
2. Characterized by hyaline deposition in corneal stroma, which stain bright red with Masson's trichrome.
3. Small, white, sharply demarcated opacities in corneal stroma with clear stroma in between opacities.
4. Gradual confluence of opacities occur and stroma becomes hazy leading to drop in vision.
5. Periphery is usually spared.

Treatment: It is by DALK or PKP.

Granular Dystrophy Type II (Avellino Corneal Dystrophy, Combined Granular-lattice Dystrophy)

1. Inheritance is AD and both hyaline and amyloid deposition occurs in stroma.
2. Superficial opacities similar to type I granular dystrophy is seen along deep linear lattice opacities.

Treatment: Not usually required.

Macular Dystrophy (Groenouw Type II)

Macular dystrophy (Fig. 15.40) is the least common type of corneal stromal dystrophy and is due to an inborn error in keratin sulfate metabolism:

1. Inheritance is autosomal recessive with gene locus at *16q22*.
2. Characterized by deposition of glycosaminoglycans in corneal stroma that stains with Prussian blue.
3. There is stromal haze and gray-white deposits in central cornea leading to drop in vision.

Treatment: By PKP, but late recurrence in graft may occur.

Endothelial Dystrophies

Fuchs' Endothelial Dystrophy

1. Fuchs' dystrophy (Fig. 15.41) is more common in females and associated with increased prevalence of open angle glaucoma.

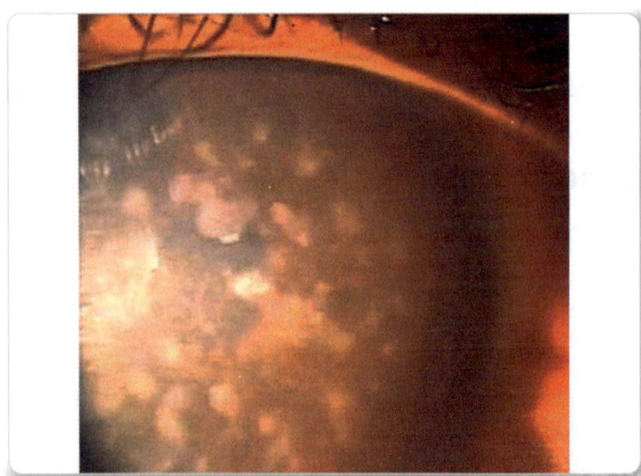

FIGURE 15.40: Macular dystrophy

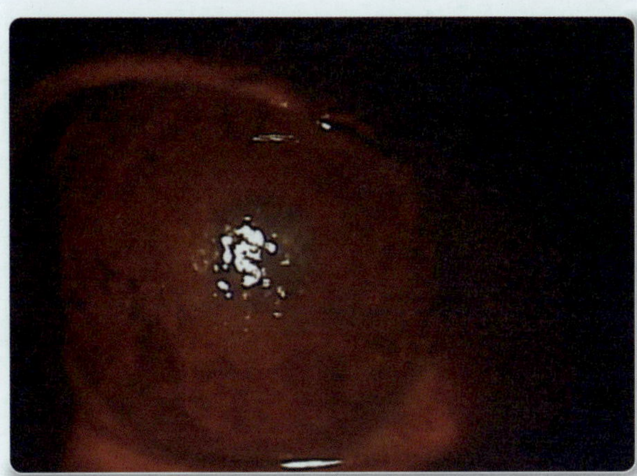

FIGURE 15.41: Fuchs' dystrophy

2. Characterized by bilateral accelerated endothelial cell loss.
3. Cornea guttata are the first changes seen.
4. As endothelial cell count decreases, corneal edema develops leading to drop in vision.
5. Later subepithelial fibrosis develops.

Treatment: They are as follows:

1. Conservative treatment in the form of sodium chloride 5% drops or ointment (to reduce corneal edema) reduction of IOP and using hair drier to speed up corneal dehydration.
2. Bandage contact lenses provide comfort by protecting the exposed nerve endings.
3. Penetrating keratoplasty is the standard procedure, but recently this has been replaced by endothelial keratoplasty.

Posterior Polymorphous Dystrophy

Posterior polymorphous dystrophy is a rare and usually asymptomatic condition, which does not require any treatment.

Congenital Hereditary Endothelial Dystrophy

Corneal edema is present at birth. Visual impairment if severe can lead to amblyopia and hence early surgery is preferred.

CORNEAL DEGENERATIONS

1. Age-related degenerations (Table 15.5):
   a. Arcus senilis.
   b. Vogt limbal.
   c. Cornea farinata.
   d. Crocodile shagreen.

TABLE 15.5: Difference between corneal degenerations and dystrophy

Degeneration	Dystrophy
Opacity is often peripherally located	Often centrally located
May be asymmetric in two eyes	Bilateral and symmetric
Presents later in life, associated with aging	Presents early in life, hereditary
Progression can be slow or rapid	Progression is usually slow

2. Epithelial and subepithelial degenerations:
   a. Spheroidal degeneration.
   b. Coats white ring.
3. Peripheral corneal degenerations:
   a. Terrien's marginal degeneration.
   b. Pellucid marginal degeneration.
4. Postinflammatory degenerative changes:
   a. Salzmann's nodular degeneration.
   b. Lipid keratopathy.
   c. Band keratopathy.
5. Endothelial degenerations:
   a. Peripheral corneal guttae.
   b. Melanin pigmentation of endothelium.

Arcus Senilis

Arcus senilis is the most common peripheral opacity and usually occurs without any predisposing cause. Sometimes this may be associated with familial or non-familial dyslipoproteinemias:

1. Stromal lipid deposition starts in superior or inferior cornea. Spreads circumferentially to form a band, which is about 1 mm broad.
2. Central border of band is diffuse, but peripheral border is sharp and separated from limbus by a clear zone, which differentiates it from other peripheral opacities.
3. This lucid interval occasionally undergo mild thinning (senile furrow).

Treatment

No treatment is needed.

Lipid Keratopathy

The common type of lipid keratopathy is associated with previous ocular injury or disease that has resulted in corneal vascularization like herpes simplex or herpes zoster disciform keratitis. Primary lipid keratopathy is very rare.

Treatment

1. Argon laser photocoagulation of arterial feeder vessels.
2. Needle point cautery of the feeder vessels.
3. Penetrating keratoplasty may be required, but the visual outcome is poor because of corneal vascularization, thinning and decreased corneal sensation.

Band Keratopathy

Bend keratopathy is characterized by deposition of calcium in the Bowman's layer, epithelial basement membrane and anterior stroma. Usually occurs in diseased and degenerating eye (Fig. 15.42).

Causes are chronic anterior uveitis (especially in children), severe keratitis, chronic corneal edema or abnormalities of calcium metabolism. Hereditary causes include familial cases and ichthyosis:

1. Peripheral calcification starts in interpalpebral area with a clear area between the limbus and the peripheral margin of the band.
2. Gradual central spread of band with small holes and clefts in the opaque band.
3. Advanced lesions may become nodular due to calcium deposition and cause.
4. Diagnosed by the site; the interpalpebral area at the level of Bowman's membrane, clear area at the limbus, presence of holes and clefts and the usual tendency to start from the limbus on either side and slowly advance toward the center.

Treatment

1. Chelation with ethylenediaminetetraacetic acid (EDTA) is simple and effective for mild cases. First the epithelium and larger chips of calcium are scraped off with No. 15 BP blade, cornea is then treated with a cotton-tipped applicator dipped in 1.5%–3% EDTA.
2. The cornea is rubbed with a cotton-tipped applicator dipped in a solution of EDTA (1.5%–3%) until all calcium has been removed and also allow adequate time for chelation to occur (15–20 minutes).
3. Re-epithelialization can take many days and recurrences can occur.
4. Other modalities of treatment include excimer laser keratectomy and lamellar keratoplasty.

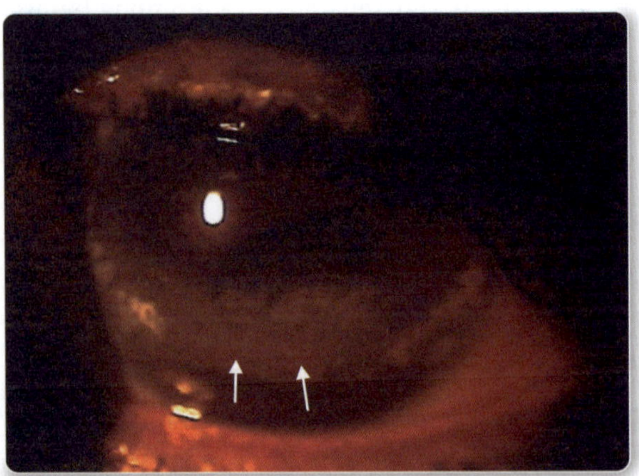

FIGURE 15.42: Band keratophathy

Spheroidal Degenerations

Spheroidal degeneration is a degenerative condition seen in men, who work outdoors, as the main risk factor is exposure to ultraviolet rays. Visual impairment may occur only rarely. This is a fairly common degeneration.

Clinical Sign

Amber-colored granules in superficial stroma of interpalpebral fissure.

Treatment

1. Sunglasses for protection from ultraviolet rays.
2. Excimer laser keratectomy, superficial keratectomy or lamellar keratoplasty.

Salzmann's Nodular Degeneration

1. Occurs usually in case of long-standing keratitis.
2. Common causes are trachoma, IK and phlyctenulosis.
3. Corneal lesions appear as gray white or nodular opacities in superficial stroma, usually in the periphery.
4. Treatment is by lubricant drops and superficial keratectomy.

Endothelial Degenerations

Peripheral corneal guttae or Hassall-Henle bodies, which are wart-like excrescences that appear in peripheral part of Descemet's membrane.

Peripheral Degenerations

Peripheral degenerations are:

1. Terrien's marginal degeneration may be unilateral or bilateral:
   a. Begins superiorly and spreads peripherally, rarely involves.

b. Characterized by stromal thinning and vascularization. But spontaneous perforation is rare.
2. Pellucid marginal degeneration.

CORNEAL ECTASIAS

Corneal ectasias are of three types:
1. Keratoconus.
2. Pellucid marginal degeneration.
3. Keratoglobus.

Keratoconus

Keratoconus is a common progressive disorder (prevalence of about 50 per 1 lakh population) in which the central or paracentral cornea undergo progressive stromal thinning and protrusion (Fig. 15.43). Both eyes are usually affected, sometimes only one eye has typical keratoconus, but the other eye shows steepening and protrusion on topography with myopic astigmatism. The role of heredity has not been defined, but most cases do not have positive family history (Table 15.6).

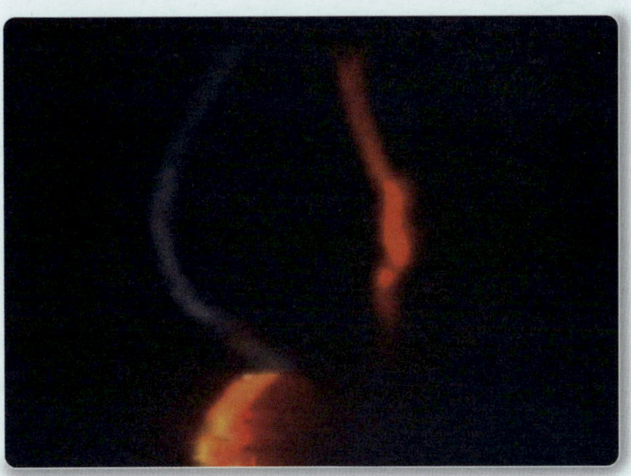

FIGURE 15.43: Conical cornea in keratoconus

Clinical Features

1. Patient presents with unilateral defective vision due to progressive myopia and astigmatism. Approximately 50% of patients progress to keratoconus in the normal fellow eye within next 15–16 years.
2. Corneal stromal thinning is seen in central or paracentral region of cornea with apical protrusion of cornea (Figs 15.44 and 15.45).
3. Retinoscopy shows scissor reflex.
4. Distant direct ophthalmoscopy shows oil droplet appearance.
5. Vogt's striae are seen; these are vertical lines in deep stroma.
6. Fleischer ring is seen at the base of protrusion due to iron deposition in the epithelium.
7. Myopia and astigmatism cause by corneal protrusion.
8. Rizzuti sign—conical reflex on nasal cornea when pen light is shone from temporal side.
9. Munson's sign—protrusion of lower lid on looking down (Fig. 15.46).

Diagnosis

1. Placido's disk examination shows irregularity of circles due to alteration in corneal curvature.
2. Keratometry shows malalignment of mires.
3. Corneal topography (Fig. 15.47) is the most sensitive method for detecting early keratoconus and for monitoring its progression.
4. Pachymetry mapping and ultrasonic pachymetry shows thin zone of cornea to be present.
5. Computerized videokeratography is another recent investigation to detect keratoconus suspects and diagnose keratoconus.

Grading of Keratoconus

Keratoconus can be graded by keratometry values and by size of cone.

TABLE 15.6: Differences between keratoconus, pellucid marginal degeneration and keratoglobus

Features	Keratoconus	Pellucid marginal degeneration	Keratoglobus
Incidence	Most common	Less common	Rare
Laterality	Bilateral (may be unilateral)	Bilateral	Bilateral
Age of onset	Puberty	20–40 year	At birth
Sites of thinning	Central or inferior para central	Inferior	Greatest in periphery
Scarring	Common	Not usual	Mild

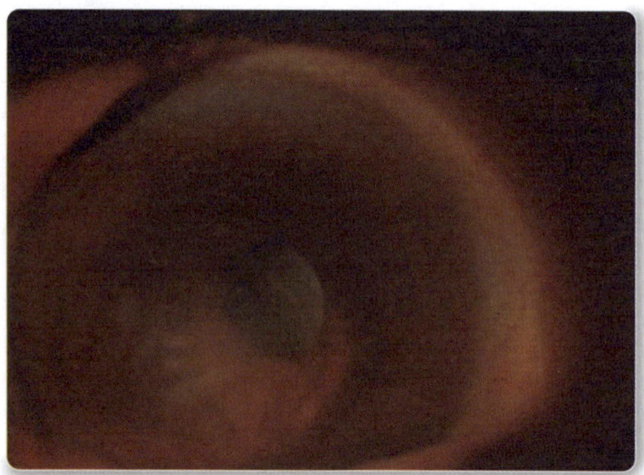

FIGURE 15.44: Inferior paracentral cone

FIGURE 15.45: Corneal thinning in keratoconus

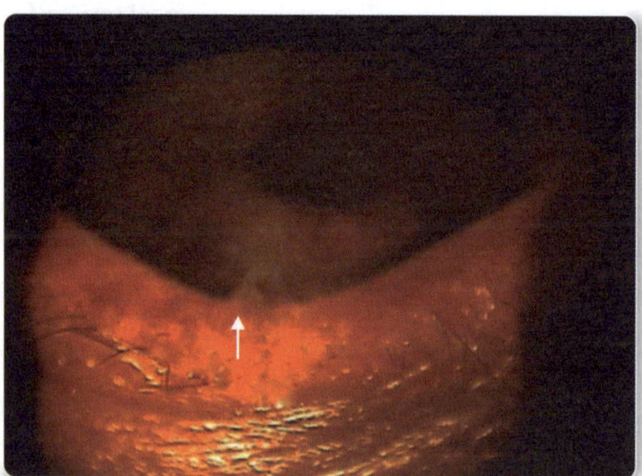

FIGURE 15.46: Munson's sign in keratoconus

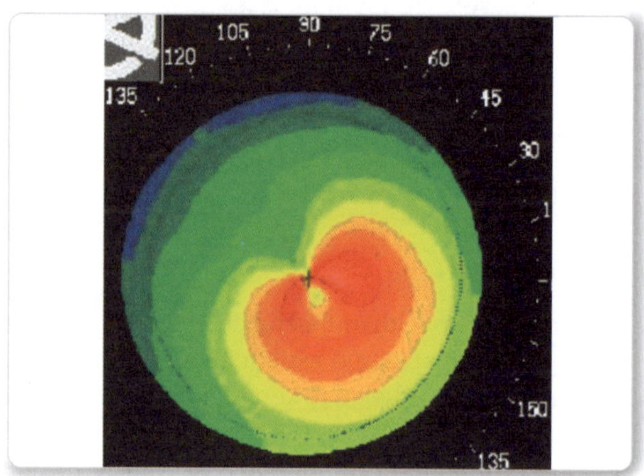

FIGURE 15.47: Corneal topography in keratoconus

1. It can be graded by keratometry:
   - Mild (< 48D)
   - Moderate (48D–54D)
   - Severe (> 54D).
2. It can be graded by size of cone:
   - Nipple cone (< 5 mm)
   - Oval cone (5–6 mm)
   - Globus cone (> 6 mm in size).

Complications

Acute hydrops: It is a sudden corneal edema developing as a result of breaks in Descemet's membrane and influx of aqueous humor into the cornea. This causes a sudden fall in vision and clouding of the cornea. Healing occurs spontaneously within 6–12 weeks resulting in corneal scarring. Then visions depends on the site and extend of scarring.

Associations

1. Ocular associations are vernal keratoconjunctivitis, aniridia, ectopia lentis, retinitis pigmentosa and persistent rubbing.
2. Systemic associations are Down syndrome, Marfan syndrome and osteogenesis imperfecta.

Treatment

1. Spectacle correction and soft contact lenses are given in early stages.
2. Rigid contact lenses are required for higher degrees of astigmatism.
3. Toric contact lenses are the special lenses designed for keratoconus.
4. Keratoplasty is indicated when the vision cannot be corrected even with rigid contact lenses. The PKP has

good visual prognosis. The DALK can be done successfully before an attack of acute hydrops occurs.

5. Intrastromal corneal segment (INTACS) implantation provides moderate visual improvement.
6. Collagen crosslinking is a newer method of treatment, which can be combined with INTACS. Cornea is treated with UV light, after sensitizing the cornea by treating it with riboflavin drops. This is considered to be effective in slowing down or arresting the progression of protrusion of the cornea.
7. Hydrops is treated conservatively with topical hypertonic agents, patching or soft contact lenses. Cycloplegics are given for ciliary pain. Keratoplasty is not done in case of acute hydrops till it has healed by scarring.

Pellucid Marginal Degeneration

Pellucid marginal degeneration is a bilateral uncommon condition characterized by thinning of the inferior peripheral cornea in the absence of inflammation and vascularization. Etiology is not known. There is also protrusion of cornea above the thinned region leading to myopia and astigmatism. This presents around 40–50 years of age. Corneal topography shows a butterfly pattern.

Treatment

1. Spectacles.
2. Contact lenses—soft toric contact lenses are enough in early stages.
3. Surgery options are eccentric PKPs, crescentic lamellar keratoplasty and intracorneal ring implantation.

Keratoglobus

Keratoglobus is a rare congenital condition typically present from birth, but is not hereditary. It is strongly associated with blue sclera and Ehlers-Danlos syndrome and may be due to a defect in collagen synthesis. Both cornea are globular in shape and entire cornea is thinned. The corneal curvature is 50D–60D and anterior chamber is deep. Corneal diameter may be slightly increased.

Differential Diagnosis

1. Congenital glaucoma (IOP is raised).
2. Megalocornea (no thinning of cornea).

Treatment

Treatment is with contact lenses. Results with surgery are poor.

CONGENITAL ANOMALIES OF CORNEA

Microcornea

Microcornea is not very common:

1. May be unilateral or bilateral.
2. Adult horizontal cornea diameter is 10 mm for lens.
3. Cornea is clear.
4. There may be associated hypermetropia or shallow anterior chamber, but other dimension are normal.
5. Ocular associates are glaucoma (open or closed angle), congenital cataract and leukoma (Fig. 15.48).
6. Syndromes associated with microcornea are Ehlers-Danlos, Weill-Marchesani, Waardenburg, etc.

Megalocornea

1. Bilateral non-progressive corneal enlargement of cornea due to defective growth of optic cup (Fig. 15.49).
2. Histologically the cornea is normal, but the corneal diameter is 13–16.5 mm.
3. High myopia and astigmatism may be present.
4. Pigment dispersion with trabecular dysgenesis may be present.
5. Lens subluxation may be present.
6. Systemic associations are Alport's syndrome, Marfan syndrome, Ehlers-Danlos syndrome, Down syndrome, osteogenesis imperfecta (common with systemic disorders of collagen synthesis), etc.

Differential Diagnosis

1. Buphthalmos, but IOP is normal and cornea clear.

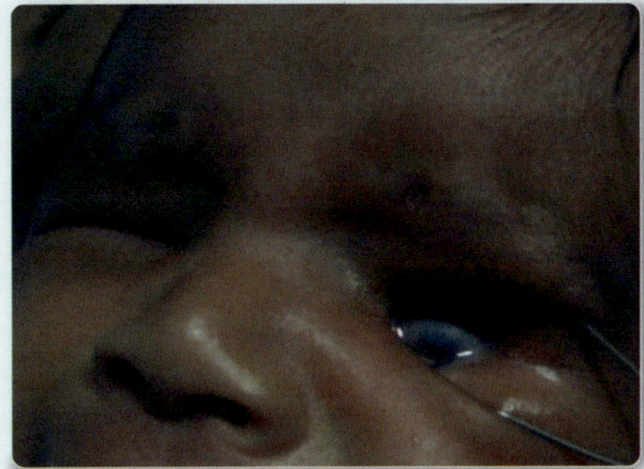

FIGURE 15.48: Microphthalmos with microcornea

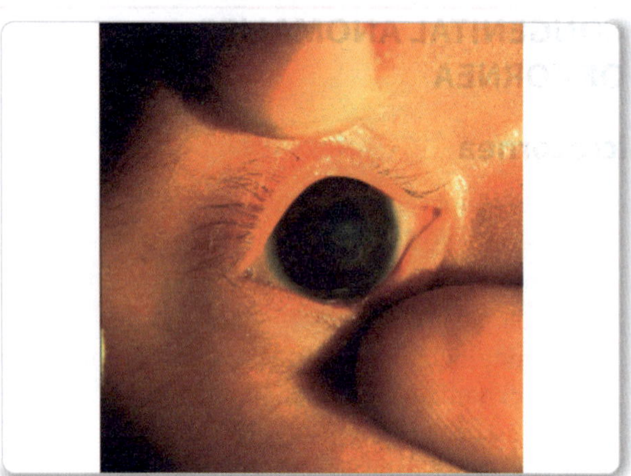

FIGURE 15.49: Megalocornea

Sclerocornea

1. Sclerocornea is a non-inflammatory non-progressive scleralization of peripheral cornea that makes the cornea appear small, occasionally entire cornea is involved (Fig. 15.50).
2. Usually sporadic, but AD and autosomal recessive (AR) cases have been reported.
3. Usually bilateral.

Cornea Plana

1. Rare bilateral condition.
2. Cornea is flat with radius of curvature less than 43D and readings of 30D–35D are common.
3. Sclerocornea is also flat cornea, but is distinguished by loss of transparency.
4. Usually causes hypermetropia, but any type of refractive error may be caused by variation in size of globe.

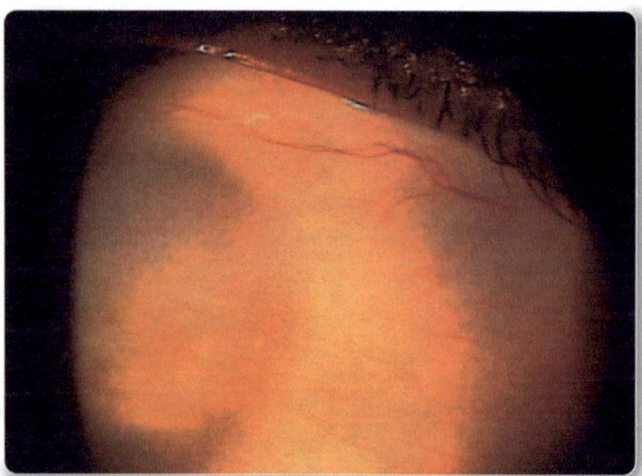

FIGURE 15.50: Sclerocornea

5. Treatment includes correction of hypermetropia and detection and management of associated glaucoma.

Posterior Keratoconus

1. Presence of localized indentation on posterior central or paracentral cornea.
2. Anterior corneal surface is normal.
3. Unilateral and non-progressive.

CONTACT LENSES

Types

Contact lenses are of two main types:

1. Rigid gas permeable lenses.
2. Soft contact lens.

Special Type of Lenses

Toric soft contact lenses: For correction of astigmatism more than 1.5D.

Bifocal soft contact lenses: For correction of presbyopia.

Cosmetic contact lens: Colored contact lenses used for changing the color of the eyes.

Bandage contact lenses: To promote healing of corneal lesions.

Use

Optical

Indications are to improve visual acuity, which cannot be achieved by spectacles:

1. Irregular astigmatism associated with keratoconus can be corrected with rigid lenses (when spectacles have failed).
2. Superficial corneal irregularities—visual acuity can be improved as the rigid surface of contact lens provide a smooth refracting surface, thus visual acuity can be improved.
3. Anisometropia, where binocular vision cannot be achieved with spectacles as in cases of unilateral aphakia.

Cosmetic

1. To avoid spectacles and improve appearance.
2. Soft contact lenses with painted iris and clear pupil to change color of eyes.
3. Soft contact lenses with painted iris and pupil painted black to improve appearance in cases with disfiguring corneal opacities without vision.

Promotion of Healing

1. Bandage contact lenses to promote healing in cases of persistent epithelial defects and recurrent corneal erosion.

Pain Relief

1. Bandage contact lenses are used in cases of BK, filamentary keratitis, etc. The exposed corneal nerve endings are covered and protected from irritation by lid movements.

Complications

Hypoxic Keratitis

Hypoxic keratitis occur due to insufficient oxygen transmission through the contact lens. This manifests as punctate keratitis. Chronic hypoxia causes corneal vascularization.

Infective Keratitis

Contact lens wearers are prone to microbial keratitis because the resistance of cornea is lowered in long-term lens wear. If the cleaning of the lenses is not proper, organisms will colonize in the lens leading to keratitis. Contact lens wearers are at risk of acanthamoeba keratitis also.

Allergic Manifestation

Giant papillary conjunctivitis and superficial punctate keratitis are the common manifestations.

Treatment of Complications of Contact Lens Wear

1. Discontinue lens wear, this will relieve hypoxic and allergic manifestations. Topical steroids may be helpful.
2. Treatment of infection when present.

Sclera

16

Girija Devi PS, Lekshmi H

ANATOMY AND PHYSIOLOGY

The sclera is the tough, white, opaque, outer covering of the posterior four fifth of the eyeball and is composed of collagen and elastin.

It is 1 mm thick posteriorly, 0.66 mm at the insertion of the rectus muscle, 0.33 mm beneath the rectus muscles and is thinnest just behind the muscle insertions. Sclera consists of three ill-defined layers as follows:

1. Sclera proper.
2. Outer episclera.
3. Inner lamina fusca that blends with the suprachoroidal and supraciliary lamellae of the uveal tract.

The three vascular layers that cover the anterior sclera are given below:

1. The conjunctival vessels: Most superficial.
2. The superficial episcleral plexus: Vessels show a radial configuration.
3. The deep vascular plexus: Lies adjacent to the sclera and show maximal congestion in sclcritis.

External examination in daylight is extremely important in localizing the level of maximal congestion. The sclera is pierced by anterior ciliary arteries and episcleral veins anteriorly and the vortex veins, posterior ciliary nerves and vessels, and optic nerve posteriorly. The optic nerve axons leave the eyeball through the lamina cribrosa of the sclera.

Pathophysiology

The sclera consists of only one type of tissue; fibrous tissue and it is relatively avascular. So, the reaction to trauma or infection is minimal, slow to appear and also slow to respond to treatment. The inflammation of sclera is often allergic, either to external allergens or autoimmune in nature.

INFLAMMATION OF SCLERA

Scleral inflammation is of two types:

1. Superficial/Episcleritis.
2. Deep/Scleritis.

Episcleritis/Superficial

Episcleritis (Fig. 16.1) is a common, recurrent, usually benign and frequently bilateral condition.

Pathology

Anatomically, dense lymphocytic infiltration of the subconjunctival and episcleral tissues is seen in episcleritis. It is often regarded as an allergic response to an endogenous toxin. An underlying cause is found only in a minority of patients. In case of multiple recurrences, a work up for underlying causes should be done.

Causes

Causes of recurrent episcleritis:

- Autoimmune connective tissue disorders
- Sjögren's syndrome
- Rheumatoid arthritis
- Gout
- Herpes zoster
- Syphilis
- Tuberculosis (TB)
- Rosaceae.

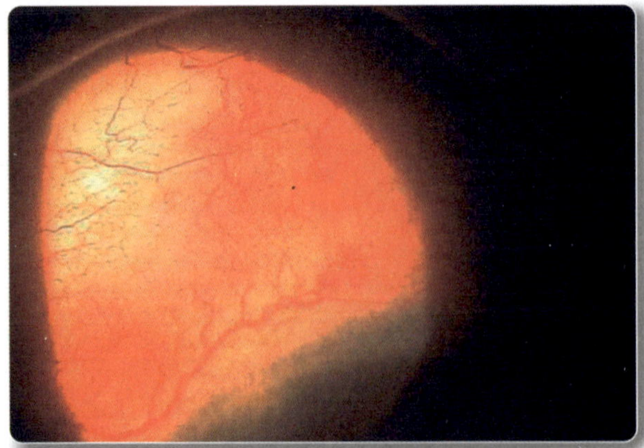

FIGURE 16.1: Episcleritis

Clinical Presentation

Clinically episcleritis occurs in two forms:

1. Simple or diffuse episcleritis: This condition accounts for majority of cases and predominantly affects young adults commonly females. It has a tendency to recur in the same eye or in both eyes together.

   Presentation is with redness and mild discomfort. The redness may be sectoral or diffuse usually in the interpalpebral area. The large episcleral vessels are engorged and run in a radial direction beneath the conjunctiva. Mild tenderness may be present.
2. Nodular episcleritis: This is characterized by the formation of one or more tender nodules in the interpalpebral area with associated episcleral congestion. It is usually self-limiting, but may last longer than a simple episcleritis.

Episcleritis is diagnosed clinically by localizing the site of inflammation to the episclera. The episcleral inflammation is superficial with a bright red or salmon pink color in natural light unlike the violaceous hue in cases of scleritis. In addition, the redness in episcleritis unlike that associated with scleritis, will blanch with the application of 2.5% topical phenylephrine.

Differential diagnosis: Local cause like foreign body (FB) or granuloma in case of an episcleral nodule, pinguecula, etc.

Management

If mild cases, the disease can be treated with a weak topical steroid like fluorometholone prescribed four times a day and this relieves the discomfort and inflammation. Rarely in moderate to severe inflammation, more frequent and potent steroids are required. Once the inflammation starts subsiding, steroids can be tapered off. Patients on topical steroids must be reviewed weekly to evaluate the clinical response and to look for steroid-induced complications, especially any rise in intraocular pressure (IOP).

Along with topical steroids, oral non-steroidal anti-inflammatory drugs (NSAIDs) may be helpful; indomethacin, ibuprofen, etc.

Scleritis/Deep

Scleritis is a granulomatous inflammation of the sclera. Scleritis is a much more severe ocular inflammatory condition than episcleritis.

Etiology

Scleritis is caused by an immune mediated, typically immune-complex vasculitis that frequently leads to destruction of the sclera. It is less common than episcleritis. It occurs most often in 4th to 6th decades of life and is more common in women. About one half of scleritis cases are bilateral at some time in their course.

Clinical Presentation

The onset of scleritis is usually gradual extending over several days. Most patients with scleritis develop severe aching or piercing ocular pain, which may worsen at night and occasionally awaken them from sleep. It may be referred to other regions of head or face on the involved side. The globe is often tender to touch. The inflamed sclera has a violaceous hue best seen in natural sunlight due to the engorgement of deep vessels. Scleral edema often with the overlying episcleral edema is noted by slit lamp examination.

Associated Systemic Diseases

About 45% of patients with scleritis particularly of the necrotizing type have one of the following systemic diseases:

1. Rheumatoid arthritis: By far the most frequent association and 1:200 patients with this disease develop scleritis.
2. Connective time disorders including Wegener's granulomatosis, polyarteritis nodosa and systemic lupus erythematosus (SLE).
3. Miscellaneous conditions: Relapsing polychondritis, herpes zoster and surgically induced necrotizing scleritis (SINS).

Classification

The classification of scleritis is given below:

1. Anterior scleritis are of two types:
   a. Non-necrotizing: Diffuse or nodular.
   b. Necrotizing: With or without inflammation.
2. Posterior scleritis.

Anterior scleritis

Diffuse versus nodular anterior scleritis

Diffuse anterior scleritis is characterized by a zone of scleral edema and redness (Fig. 16.2). A portion of the anterior sclera (< 50%) is involved in 60% cases and the entire anterior segment is involved in 40% of cases. In nodular anterior scleritis the scleral nodule is deep red or purple in color, immobile and separated from the overlying episcleral tissue, which is elevated by the nodule (Figs 16.3 and 16.4). It may be single or multiple and usually seen 3–4 mm from limbus. Nodular non-necrotizing anterior scleritis often occurs with herpes zoster ophthalmicus (HZO).

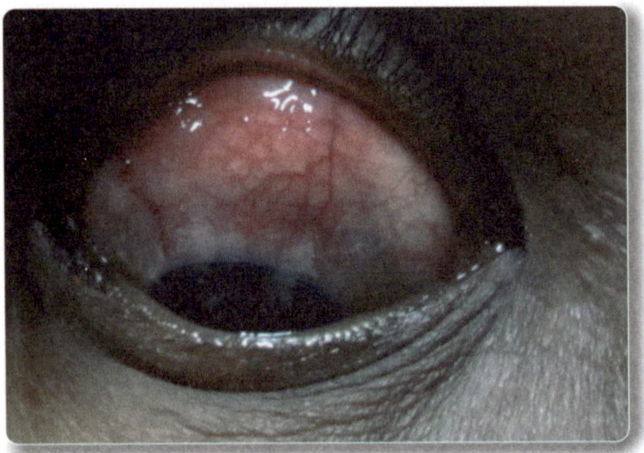

FIGURE 16.2: Diffuse scleritis

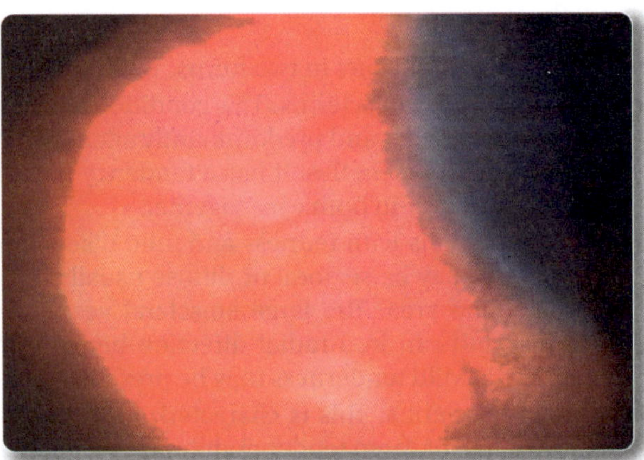

FIGURE 16.3: Nodular scleritis

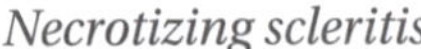

Necrotizing scleritis

Necrotizing scleritis is the most destructive form of scleritis.

Necrotizing scleritis with inflammation

Here, the patient presents with severe pain. On examination, a localized area of inflammation (Fig. 16.5) is noted initially with the edges of the lesion more inflamed than the center. In more advanced disease, an avascular edematous area of sclera is seen. Untreated, necrotizing scleritis may spread posteriorly to the equator and circumferentially until the entire anterior globe is involved. The sclera may develop a blue-gray appearance due to thinning, which allows visibility of the underlying choroid.

Necrotizing scleritis without inflammation

Necrotizing scleritis without inflammation is also known as scleromalacia perforans. This clinical presentation is distinct from the other forms of anterior scleritis, because symptoms like redness, edema and pain are absent in this condition.

Scleromalacia perforans typically occurs in patients with long standing rheumatoid arthritis. This type of scleritis is generally painless. As the disease progresses, the sclera thins and the underlying dark uveal tissue becomes visible. In many cases, the uvea is covered only with a thin connective tissue and conjunctiva.

Complications of anterior scleritis

- Acute infiltrative stromal keratitis
- Sclerosing keratitis (Figs 16.6 and 16.7)
- Peripheral ulcerative keratitis (Fig. 16.8)
- Uveitis (refer Fig. 16.6)
- Glaucoma
- Hypotony and choroidal detachment
- Scleral perforation
- Staphyloma (Fig. 16.9).

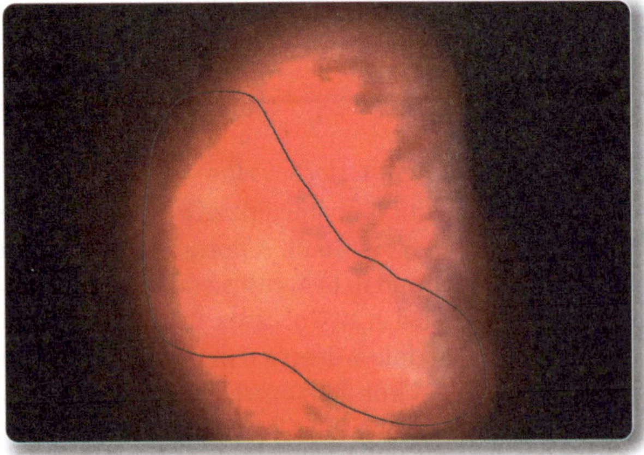

FIGURE 16.4: Nodules in scleritis

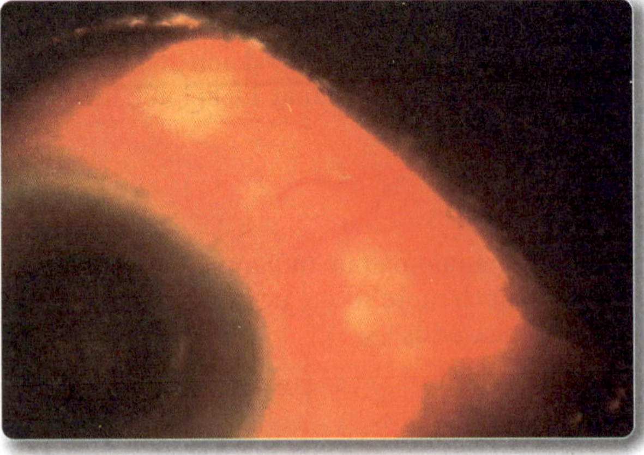

FIGURE 16.5: Advanced stage of necrotizing scleritis with inflammation

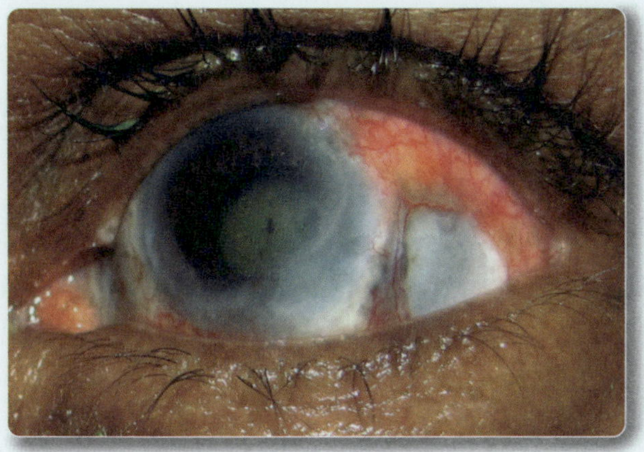

FIGURE 16.6: Sclerokeratouveitis with scleral thinning

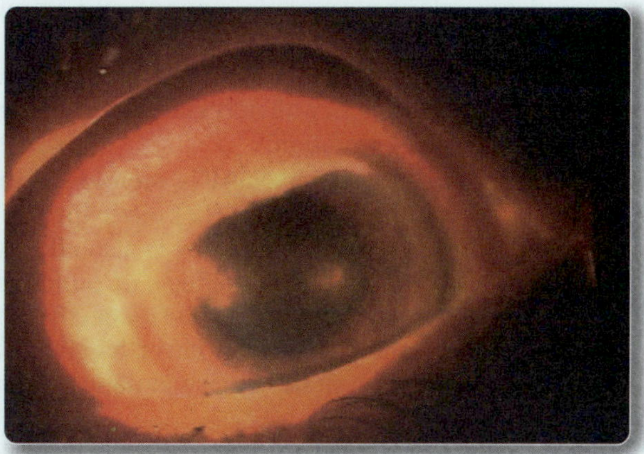

FIGURE 16.7: Sclerosing keratitis

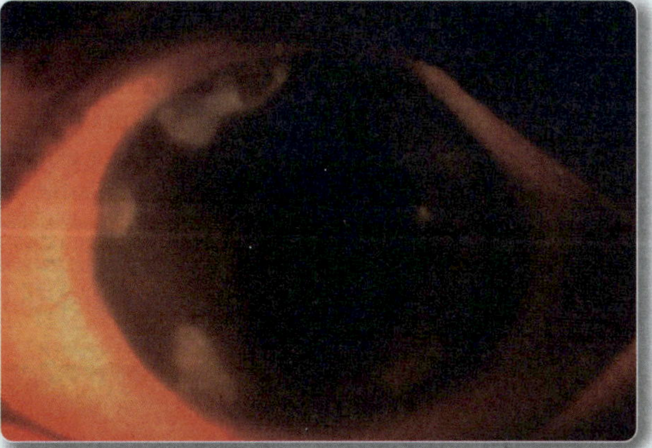

FIGURE 16.8: Peripheral ulcerative keratitis

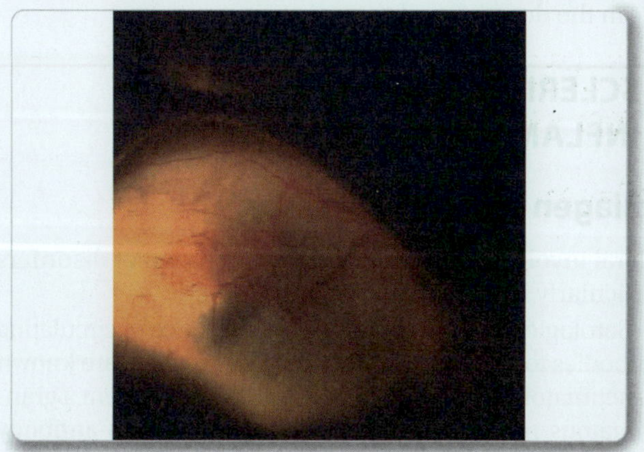

FIGURE 16.9: Staphyloma

Posterior scleritis

Clinical features

Posterior scleritis presents with pain, proptosis, visual loss and occasionally, restriction of eye movements. Choroidal folds, exudative retinal detachment (RD), papilledema and angle-closure glaucoma secondary to choroidal thickening may develop and helps in a clinical diagnosis. The pain may be referred to other parts of the head.

Diagnosis is by B-scan ultrasound, which shows the typical T sign due to thickened posterior sclera and fluid in the sub-Tenon's space. Computed tomography (CT) scan or magnetic resonance imaging (MRI) may be helpful in establishing the diagnosis.

Investigations in Scleritis

- Complete blood count
- Rheumatoid factor
- Mantoux test
- Antinuclear antibodies (ANAs), Venereal Disease Research Laboratory (VDRL) test, lupus erythematosus (LE) cell
- X-ray of chest and sacroiliac joints.

Treatment

In patients with diffuse or nodular scleritis, one or more of the following drugs are recommended:

1. Oral NSAIDs.
2. Oral prednisolone 1 mg/kg as a single dose in the morning for 1 week, when can be tapered to 20 mg/day over the subsequent 2–3 weeks.
3. Oral immunosuppressants such as cyclophosphamide, methotrexate, cyclosporin or azathioprine in cases resistant to steroids or when steroids are not tolerated.

Immunosuppressive therapy is best given in conjunction with a rheumatologist.

4. Necrotizing scleritis: Systemic steroids and immunosuppressants are recommended. Abundant lubricants are important in scleromalacia perforans. Scleral patch grafting may be necessary if there is any significant risk of perforation.
5. Posterior scleritis: Systemic NSAIDs, steroids or immunosuppressants. Intravenous (IV) methylprednisolone administered as pulse therapy is also effective and helps in reducing the side effects of prolonged oral steroids. Local steroids tend to be ineffective and subconjunctival injection should never be given for fear of perforation of globe. Biopsy is dangerous as well as uninformative.
6. Infectious scleritis, if identified, is treated with appropriate topical and systemic antimicrobial agents. Panophthalmitis, if severe, will warrant IV antibiotics in the doses given for meningitis.

SCLERITIS IN SPECIFIC INFLAMMATORY DISEASES

Collagen Vascular Diseases

Scleral involvement is common in this group of disorders particularly in rheumatoid arthritis (RA).

Serological features of RA are the presence of circulating antibodies to immunoglobulin molecules, which are known as rheumatoid factor. Scleral nodules in RA represent a granulomatous response to focal deposits of antigen-antibody complexes. The primary event of RA is possibly a cryptogenic bacterial or viral infection in susceptible individuals, provoking an inappropriate immunological response.

Histologically, the typical scleral lesion assumes the characteristic combination of a proliferative infiltration by chronic inflammatory cells surrounding a central area of fibrinoid necrosis.

Clinical Manifestation

Episcleral rheumatoid nodules: May appear and disappear.

Necrotizing nodular scleritis: A violent and painful anterior scleritis often circumferential in its extent, characterized by extensive swelling and the appearance of one or more yellow nodules usually proceeds to necrosis leading eventually to necrosis of sclera and exposure of the underlying uvea.

Scleromalacia perforans: Similar necrosis of the sclera occurs with exposure of the uvea, but without painful symptoms.

Massive granulomas of the sclera: Proliferative changes are predominant.

Brawny scleritis: Sclera becomes so thickened as to simulate an intraocular or orbital tumor.

Infective Causes

Suppurative bacterial infection: Virulent organism such as *Pseudomonas* causing an endophthalmitis may spread to infect the sclera and episcleral tissue leading to panophthalmitis.

Treatment

High doses of IV broad-spectrum antibiotics and careful watch for further spread into the orbit and subsequent cavernous sinus thrombosis. Surgical measures:

1. Intravitreal injection of antibiotics.
2. Vitrectomy.
3. Evisceration of the globe if the eye has no PL and all measures to contain the infection fail.

Gumma: Seen in tertiary syphilis but now uncommon.

Tuberculosis: Form of scleritis may be secondary, due to an extension from the conjunctiva, iris, ciliary body or choroid. It may also be primary, forming a localized nodule, which caseates and ulcerates. Nodule should be excised or scraped and the tissue examined for the organisms.

Treatment consists of systemic antituberculosis treatment (ATT) with local lubricating drops. The comparison of phlycten, episcleritis and scleritis is given in Table 16.1.

TABLE 16.1: Comparison of phlycten, episcleritis and scleritis

Phlycten	Episcleritis	Scleritis
Mild symptoms: Irritation, mild discomfort	Moderate pain	Severe pain
No tenderness	Mild tenderness	Severe tenderness
Conjunctival nodule, moves with conjunctiva on finger pressure	Superficial scleral nodule fixed to underlying tissues	Deep nodule fixed to deeper tissues
Localized congestion of conjunctival vessels only	Localized or diffuse congestion of episcleral vessels	Congestion of deeper vessels with a purplish hue
No complications	Complications are rare	Uveitis, keratitis and secondary glaucoma are common complications
Resolves leaving no scar	Scleral thinning can occur	Scleral thinning or staphyloma can occur

Staphyloma

Staphyloma is an ectasia of the outer coats (cornea, sclera or both) of the eye with incarceration of uveal tissue. It results from a weakening of the eye wall caused by a variety of inflammatory and degenerative diseases of these structures. The raised IOP associated with these conditions also contributes to the formation of staphyloma. It usually occurs at sites where sclera is weakened by passage of blood vessels.

Classification

Depending on the site affected, staphylomas are classified as (Fig. 16.10):

- Anterior
- Intercalary
- Ciliary
- Equatorial
- Posterior.

Anterior staphyloma: This commonly occurs following a sloughing corneal ulcer, which perforates and heals with the formation of a pseudocornea by the organization of exudates and lying down of fibrous tissue. The anterior chamber is flat and secondary glaucoma supervenes leading to outward protrusion of the weak anterior surface of the eye resulting in an anterior staphyloma. It can be total or partial depending on whether the whole or part of the cornea is involved (Fig. 16.11).

Intercalary staphyloma: It is seen in the part of sclera up to 2 mm from the limbus (Fig. 16.12). It is lined by the root of iris and most anterior part of ciliary body. At this region, the sclera is weakened by the presence of anterior ciliary veins and canal of Schlemm. The common predisposing lesions are penetrating injuries in limbal region, marginal corneal ulcer, anterior scleritis, scleromalacia perforans, scleral thinning after cataract surgery and secondary glaucoma.

Ciliary staphyloma: This affects the ciliary region that includes the zone up to 8 mm behind the limbus (Fig. 16.13).

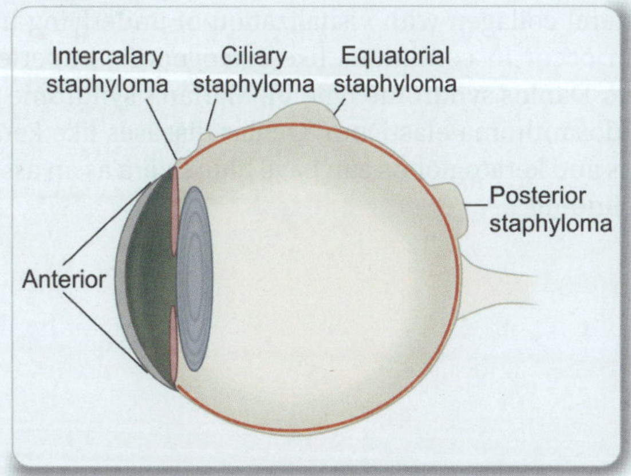

FIGURE 16.10: Types of scleral staphyloma

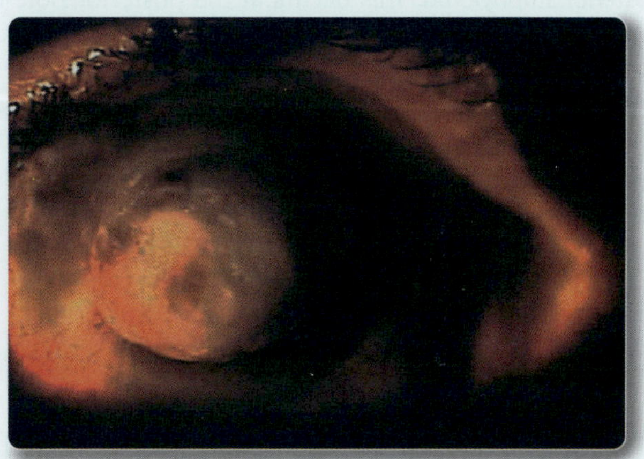

FIGURE 16.11: Anterior staphyloma

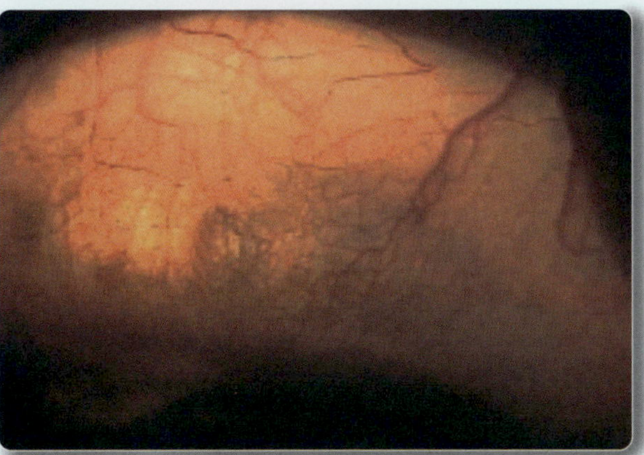

FIGURE 16.12: Intercalary staphyloma

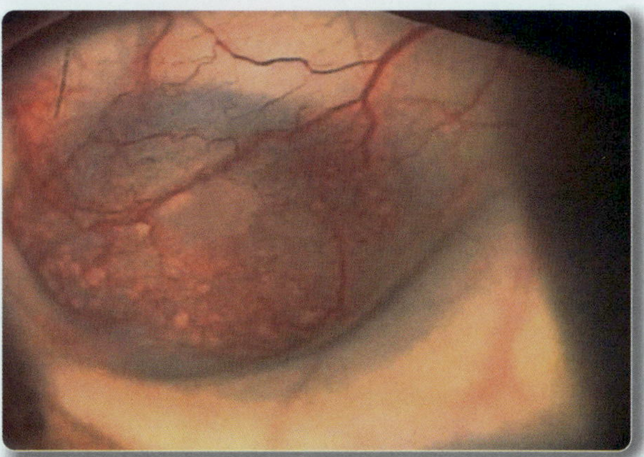

FIGURE 16.13: Rhinosporidiosis with ciliary staphyloma

The ectatic area is lined by the ciliary body and has a bluish color with a lobulated appearance. Here the sclera is weakened by the passage of anterior ciliary arteries. It is differentiated from an intercalary staphyloma by the location of the anterior ciliary arteries, which are seen to emerge at the anterior border of the bulge in case of a ciliary staphyloma. Developmental glaucoma, end-stage glaucomas, scleritis and trauma to the ciliary region are a few conditions that can predispose to a ciliary staphyloma. Rhinosporidiosis of the bulbar conjunctiva is often associated with thinning and staphyloma formation of the underlying sclera, probably by collagenase-like enzymes produced by the invading organism.

Equatorial staphyloma: This occurs at the equatorial region of the eyeball about 14 mm from the limbus and is lined by choroid. Here the sclera is inherently weak due to the passage of vortex veins. Scleritis, degenerative myopia and chronic glaucoma are the predisposing factors leading to equatorial staphyloma.

Posterior staphyloma: This occurs at the posterior pole of the eye and is lined by the choroid. Degenerative high axial myopia is the most common cause. It is seen in indirect ophthalmoscopy as a crescentic shadow in the macular region with the retinal vessels seen dipping down into the region. A posterior outward curvature of the globe can be seen in B-scan ultrasound.

Treatment

Inflammatory diseases like scleritis, corneal ulcer, keratomalacia due to vitamin A deficiency should be promptly treated to prevent formation of staphylomas.

Scleroplasty: Local excision of the staphyloma with placement of a scleral patch graft can be done in some cases.

Scleral resection: Here, the entire staphyloma is excised, especially in equatorial staphylomas. The peripheral edges of the protruding area may be drawn together with mattress sutures and the staphyloma is excised or buckled inwards (Young's operation).

Large unsightly eyes can be treated with staphylectomy and keratoplasty or enucleation with placement of an implant.

Congenital Abnormalities of Sclera

Blue Sclera

Bluish discoloration is caused by thinning or transparency of scleral collagen with visualization of underlying uvea. It can occur in conditions like osteogenesis imperfecta, Ehlers-Danlos syndrome type VI, Marfan's syndrome and pseudoxanthoma elasticum. Ocular diseases like keratoconus and keratoglobus can have blue sclera as an associated finding.

Uvea

17

Girija Devi PS, Kanchana

ANATOMY AND PHYSIOLOGY

Uvea is the middle vascular coat of the eye, which has got three parts:

1. Iris.
2. Ciliary body.
3. Choroid.

Choroid

Choroid is the posterior most part of the uveal tract and its inner surface is in contact with retina. The choroid consists of mainly blood vessels with a non-vascular limiting layer on either side. The choroid is firmly attached to the edge of the optic disk and to the sclera more firmly, where vessels perforate the eye.

Microscopic structure of choroid, from outside towards inside is following.

Suprachoroidal Lamina

Suprachoroidal lamina consists of flattened laminae consisting of collagen fibers. The laminae join each other at acute angles and contain potential spaces in between which can get distended with fluid in choroidal effusions. The suprachoroidal lamina contains some fibroblasts and melanocytes also.

Stroma of Choroid

Stroma of choroid is the layer of blood vessels. The larger vessels are seen on the outer aspect and the smaller vessels on the inner aspect of the stroma. It contains loose collagenous tissue and plenty of melanocytes, which give choroid its characteristic color. The size of the vessels decrease from outside toward inside and the innermost layer close to the retina called choriocapillaris contains only capillaries.

Choriocapillaris

Choriocapillaris is the layer of capillaries, which give nourishment to the outer layers of the retina. The capillaries of choriocapillaris have wide bore and have fenestrations through which fluid and nutrients can easily diffuse out. The choriocapillaris stops at the ora serrata.

Basal Lamina of Choroid/Bruch's Membrane

Basal lamina of connective tissue is 2 microns in thickness. The stromal fibers are firmly attached to its outer aspect, while the inner aspect is firmly adherent to the pigment layer of the retina.

Ciliary Body

Ciliary body is the forward continuation of choroid. The whole ciliary body forms a ring behind the limbus, but on sagittal section it is triangular in shape and has got two parts such as a posterior smooth part called pars plana and an anterior part with ciliary process called pars plicata.

Microscopically it contains the following layers from outside toward inside:

1. Supraciliary lamina: It resembles that of choroid and it is its forward continuation.
2. Stroma: Ciliary body stroma contains non-striated muscles arranged in three bundles are:
   a. Longitudinal/Meridional.
   b. Circular fibers.
   c. Radial fibers.
3. Layer of pigmented epithelium: This is the forward continuation of the pigment layer of the retina.
4. Layer of non-pigmented epithelium: It is the forward continuation of the inner layers of the retina in a modified fashion and this is the innermost layer.
5. Internal limiting membrane.

6. Ciliary processes: These are finger-like projections form pars plicata, about 70–80 in number and are the site of aqueous production. It consists of blood vessels alone and it is the most vascular region of the eye.

Iris

Iris is the anterior most part of uveal tract attached circumferentially to the anterior surface of ciliary body. At its central part there is a 3–4 mm aperture called pupil.

Anterior surface is divided into ciliary zone and pupillary zone by a zigzag line called collarette (Fig. 17.1). Posterior surface is brown or black in color.

Layers of Iris from Anterior to Posterior

1. Anterior limiting layer: This is a surface condensation of the stroma of the iris. It consists of star-shaped connective tissue cells and pigment cells. The color of the iris depends on the amount of pigment cells in this layer.
2. Iris stroma: This layer contains muscles and vessels. The sphincter papillae is a circular band of plain muscle fibers, 1 mm broad, placed close to the pupillary margin. The stroma consists of collagenous fibers in a mucopolysaccharide ground substance. The main bulk of it is the radially arranged blood vessels, which follow a sinus course to accommodate the changes in the pupillary size.
3. Anterior epithelial layer: The forward continuation of the pigmentary layer and the pigmented layer of the ciliary epithelium.
4. Posterior pigmented epithelial layer: The forward continuation of the sensory retina and the non-pigmented epithelial layer of the ciliary body.

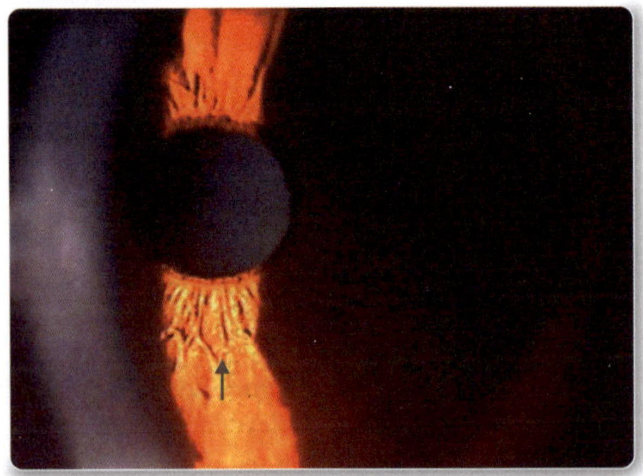

FIGURE 17.1: Normal anatomy of iris. The arrow shows the collarette. The part behind it is the ciliary zone and the part beyond it is the pupillary zone.

Both layers are pigmented and become continuous with each other at the pupillary margin. The anterior epithelium, derived from the outer layer of the optic cup, gets modified to form the dilator papillae muscle situated mainly in the peripheral portion of the iris. The posterior epithelium formed from the internal layer of the optic cup is heavily pigmented. The blue color of the eyes of the lightly pigmented people is due to this dark pigment in the posterior epithelium seen through the translucent stroma.

Blood Supply of Uveal Tract

Uveal tract is highly vascular and is supplied by three groups of arteries, which are given below:

1. Short posterior ciliary arteries: This arise from the ophthalmic artery as two main trunks and then divides into 10–20 branches, which pierce sclera around optic nerve and supply the choroid.
2. Long posterior ciliary arteries: These are two in number; one nasal and one temporal. The long posterior ciliary arteries run in the suprachoroidal space to reach the ciliary body anteriorly where it anastomose with each other and also with anterior ciliary arteries to form major arterial circle, which supply ciliary body.
3. Anterior ciliary arteries: These are branches from muscular branches of the ophthalmic artery—two each from superior rectus (SR), inferior (IR), medical rectus (MR) and one from later rectus (LR) muscles. These pierce the sclera near limbus to enter the ciliary body and anastomose with long posterior ciliary artery to form circulus arteriosus iridis major near root of iris, branches from which go radially in the iris towards the pupil. Just outside the pupillary border these anastomose and form circulus arteriosus iridis minor.

CONGENITAL ANOMALIES OF UVEAL TRACT

Congenital Aniridia

Congenital aniridia (Figs 17.2A and B) is the congenital absence of iris. It is a very rare condition with genetic predisposition. Associated anomalies—glaucoma, Wilms' tumor, mental retardation and genitourinary anomalies.

Polycoria

Very rare condition in which more than one pupil are present (Fig. 17.3).

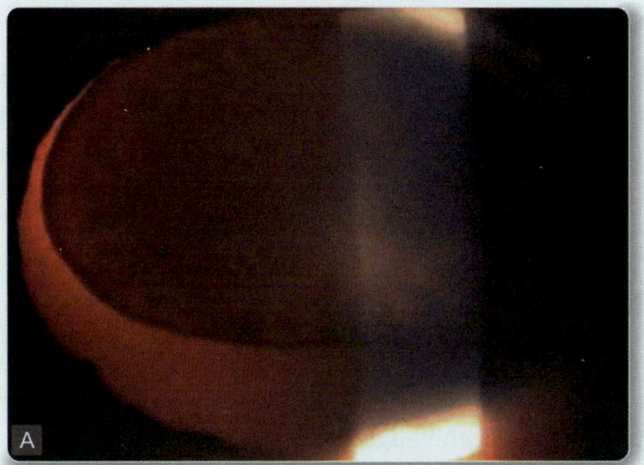

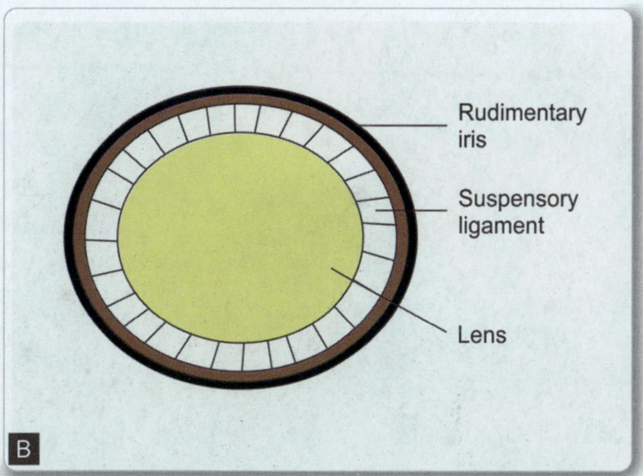

FIGURES 17.2A and B: Aniridia. **A.** Photography; **B.** Diagrammatic representation.

Corectopia

Corectopia refers to a condition where the pupil is eccentrically placed (Fig. 17.4).

Heterochromia of Iris

Heterochromia of iris refers to the variation in the iris color. A difference in the color between two eyes is called heterochromia iridum (Fig. 17.5) and when one sector of iris differs in color from another in the same eye it is called heterochromia iridis (Fig. 17.6).

Persistent Pupillary Membrane

Persistent pupillary membrane is due to the continued existence of part of the anterior vascular sheath of the lens; a fetal structure, which normally disappears shortly before birth. Fine threads stretchy across the pupil or may be anchored down to the lens capsule (Fig. 17.7). These can be distinguished from postinflammatory synechiae as there always come from the anterior surface of the iris just outside the pupillary margin from the position of the circulus arteriosus iridis minor.

Coloboma

Coloboma occurs due to defective closure of embryonic fissure. Colobomas can occur in the iris, ciliary body, lens, choroid and optic disk. Typical iris coloboma occurs in the inferonasal quadrant since this is the site of embryonic fissure (Figs 17.8A and B).

Chorioretinal Coloboma

A coloboma of the fundus appears as an oval or comet-shaped defect with the rounded apex toward the disk with

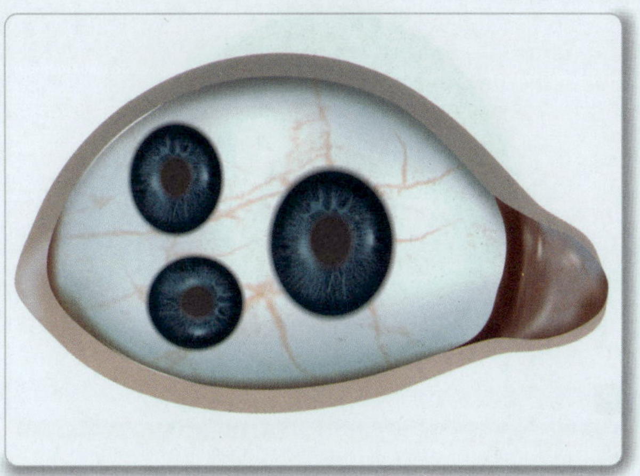

FIGURE 17.3: Polycoria

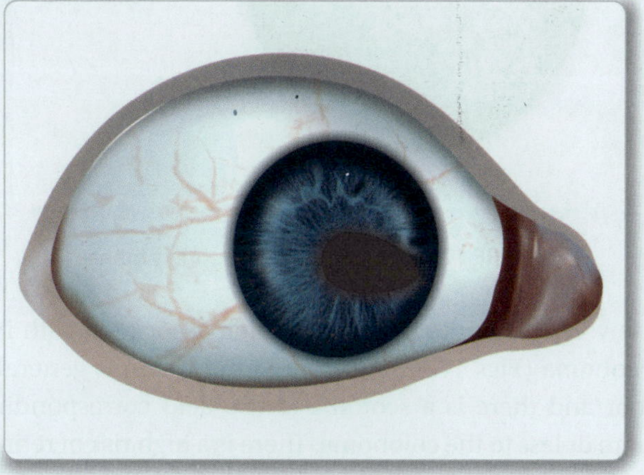

FIGURE 17.4: Corectopia

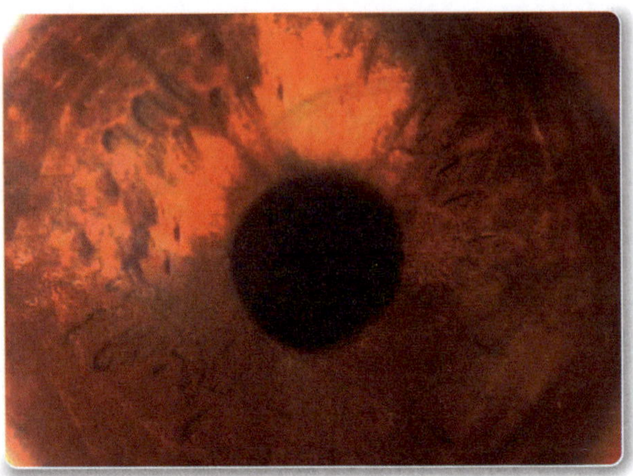

FIGURE 17.5: Heterochromia iridis

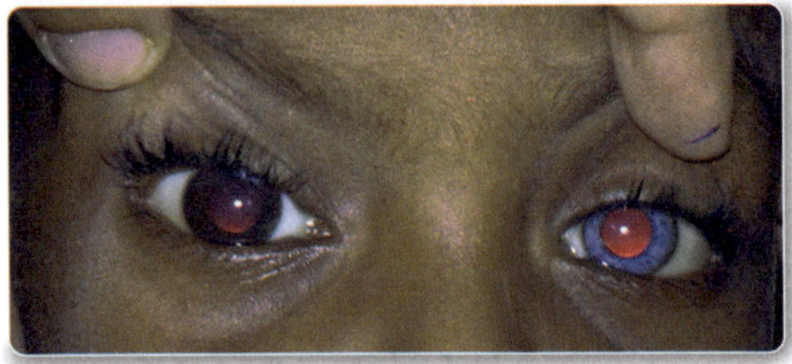

FIGURE 17.6: Heterochromia iridum and ocular albinism in Waardenburg syndrome

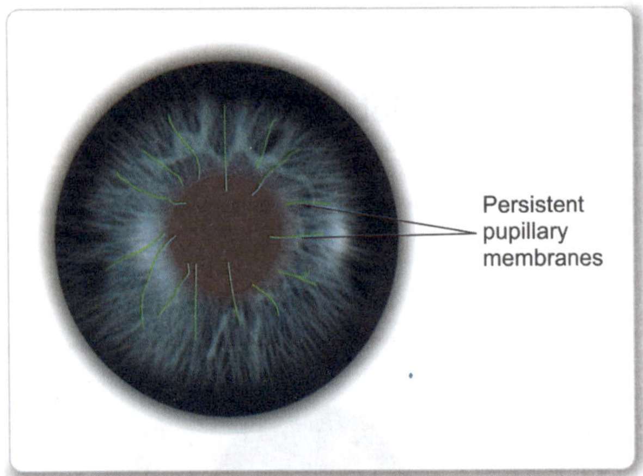

FIGURE 17.7: Persistent pupillary membrane

Coloboma

Coloboma occurs due to defective closure of embryonic fissure. Colobomas can occur in the iris, ciliary body, lens, choroid and optic disk. Typical iris coloboma occurs in the inferonasal quadrant since this is the site of embryonic fissure (refer Figs 17.8A and B).

Chorioretinal Coloboma

A coloboma of the fundus appears as an oval or comet-shaped defect with the rounded apex toward the disk with a few vessels at the edges. It is often associated with iris coloboma (Figs 17.9A and B). Central vision is generally poor and there is a scotoma in the field corresponding more or less to the coloboma. There is a high risk of retinal detachment and prophylactic laser delimitation along the edges of the coloboma is sometimes advocated.

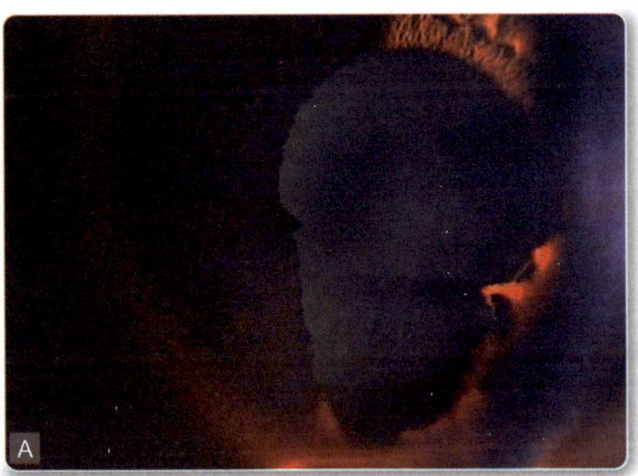

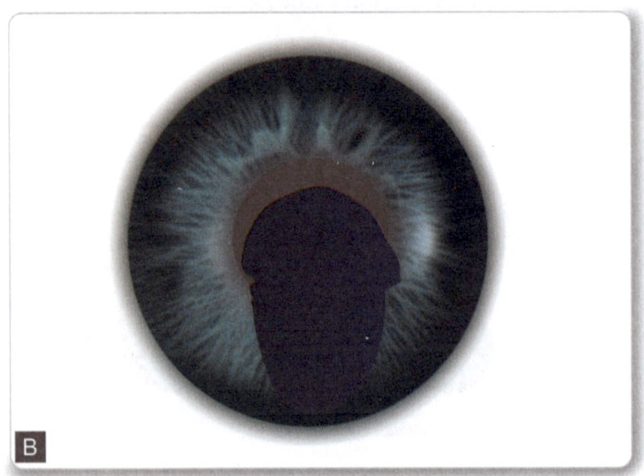

FIGURES 17.8A and B: Iris coloboma. **A.** Coloboma of choroid; **B.** Diagrammatic representation.

a few vessels at the edges. It is often associated with iris coloboma (Figs 17.9A and B). Central vision is generally poor and there is a scotoma in the field corresponding more or less to the coloboma. There is a high risk of retinal detachment and prophylactic laser delimitation along the edges of the coloboma is sometimes advocated.

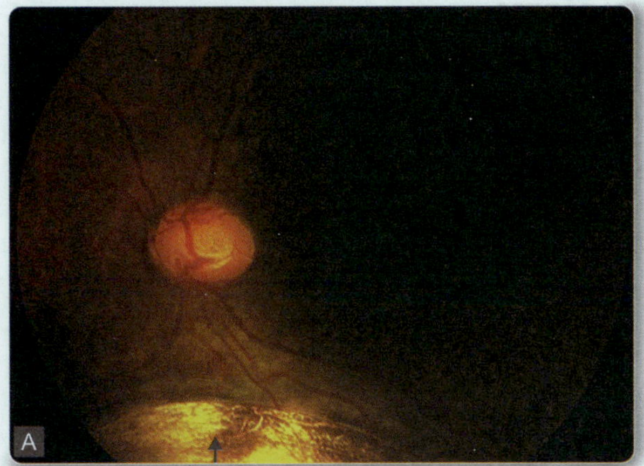

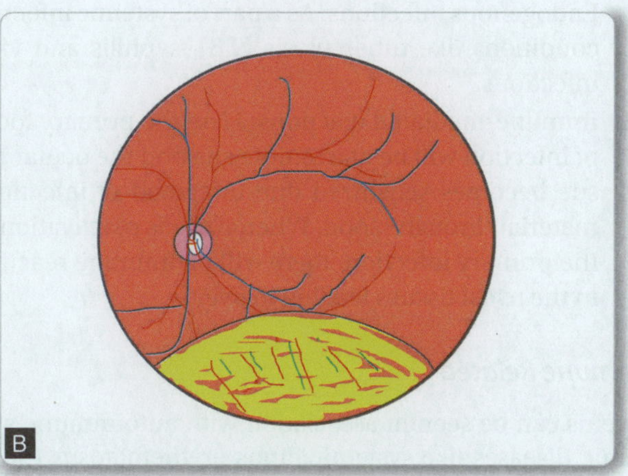

FIGURES 17.9A and B: Coloboma of the choroid. **A.** Photograph; **B.** Diagrammatic representation.

UVEITIS

Uveitis is the inflammation of uveal tissue. According to the anatomical site involved, it can be iritis, cyclitis or choroiditis. Inflammation of one part of uvea will usually lead to contiguous inflammation of the other parts of uveal tissue as well. This is due to the anatomical continuity as well as the common blood supply, but the inflammation can be predominant in one particular part of choroid and hence named accordingly.

Classification

Different types of classifications exists for uveitis according to anatomical site, etiology and pathology.

The International Uveitis Study Group (IUSG) recommended a classification according to the anatomical location.

According to anatomical site, uveitis can be classified as the following:

1. Anterior uveitis:
   - Iritis
   - Anterior cyclitis
   - Iridocyclitis.
2. Intermediate uveitis:
   - Posterior cyclitis
   - Pars planitis
   - Hyalitis
   - Basal retinochoroiditis.
3. Posterior uveitis:
   - Choroiditis (focal/multifocal/diffuse)
   - Chorioretinitis
   - Retinochoroiditis
   - Neurouveitis.
4. Panuveitis:
   - Inflammation of all the layers of uvea.

According to etiology, uveitis can be classified as the following:

- Idiopathic
- Infective
- Immune related
- Neoplastic
- Traumatic
- Toxic.

According to pathology, two types of uveitis are recognized:

- Granulomatous
- Nongranulomatous.

Etiopathogenesis of Uveitis

Idiopathic

Despite various types of modern investigation modalities, determining the exact cause of uveitis is difficult. A definite etiology can be identified only in a few cases. Those cases with no definite cause identified are called idiopathic.

Infective

Most of the time the uveal inflammation is due to an immunological reaction and not due to direct infections. The infective agent acts as a foreign antigen and uveitis sets in only in late stages, when hypersensitivity is established:

1. Exogenous infections: These usually follow a penetrating trauma or a perforated corneal ulcer and are commonly suppurative in nature.
2. Secondary infections: From adjacent ocular structures (like cornea, sclera, etc.).

3. Endogenous infections: As a part of systemic infective conditions like tuberculosis (TB), syphilis and viral infections.
4. Immune-mediated reactions: Here the primary focus of infection will be at a remote site and the ocular tissue becomes sensitized due to spread of infectious material through blood. When there is reactivation of the primary infection, there will be immune reaction in the uveal tissues leading to uveitis.

Immune Related

Uveitis can be seen in association with autoimmune systemic diseases like systemic lupus erythematosus (SLE), sarcoidosis, Wegener's granulomatosis, ankylosing spondylitis, rheumatoid arthritis, etc.

Many of the uveitis are much more common in people with certain human leukocyte antigen (HLA):
- HLA-B27: Ankylosing spondylitis; Reiter's syndrome
- HLA-B5: Behçet's disease
- HLA-A29: Birdshot chorioretinopathy.

Traumatic

Uveitis can follow an accidental injury or following an operative injury. It can occur due to direct mechanical injury with microbial invasion or foreign bodies inside the eye initiating an immunological reaction.

Toxic

Toxins can be either endogenous or exogenous. Endogenous toxins can be either autotoxins or microbial toxins. Exogenous toxins mainly include organic and inorganic chemicals, especially drugs (cytotoxic drugs, miotics).

Neoplastic

Some systemic or intraocular tumors can present with features similar to uveitis and these are called masquerade syndromes.

Intraocular tumors: Retinoblastoma, iris melanoma, reticulum cell carcinoma.

Systemic malignancies: Leukemia, lymphomas, histiocytic sarcomas.

ACUTE ANTERIOR UVEITIS

Acute anterior uveitis is usually iridocyclitis, but sometimes iritis can be the predominant inflammation or sometimes it can be cyclitis alone.

Symptoms

The earliest symptoms are slight blurring of vision, mild pain, redness, photophobia and lacrimation. If left untreated symptoms can aggravate and marked drop in vision can occur.

The absence of any mucopurulent discharge and the pain usually in the area of distribution of the trigeminal nerve and the blurring of vision should arouse suspicion.

Pain

Pain is the predominant symptom in acute anterior uveitis. It will be mild to dull aching pain in chronic uveitis.

Redness

Toxins produce hyperemia of anterior ciliary vessels leading to circumcorneal congestion. This is one of the earliest signs. In any red eye, if there is circumcorneal congestion, more careful evaluation by slit lamp examination is warranted to confirm or rule out anterior uveitis.

Photophobia

Photophobia is also a warning sign that the condition is not simple conjunctivitis.

Defective Vision

In early phases there will be only mild blurring of vision, but later stages there is marked deterioration.

Causes of defective vision in uveitis: These are following:
1. Cornea: Corneal edema, keratic precipitates (KPs) on endothelium.
2. Anterior chamber (AC) reaction: Cells and flare and hypopyon if present.
3. Pupil: Miosis, pupillary exudates, occlusio pupillae.
4. Complicated cataract, cyclitic membrane: In late stages of improperly treated cases.
5. Associated complications like macular edema, papillitis, secondary glaucoma.

Signs

Signs of acute anterior uveitis are:
1. Visual acuity.
2. Circumcorneal congestion.
3. Changes in pupil.
4. Iris changes.
5. Changes in cornea.

6. Anterior chambers signs.
7. Lens changes.

The earliest signs are circumcorneal congestion and a small, sluggishly reacting pupil.

Visual Acuity

Visual acuity will be slightly reduced in mild cases, but can be profoundly decreased in chronic and severe cases.

Circumcorneal Congestion

Circumcorneal congestion is one of the earliest signs, which should raise the suspicion of uveitis and differentiates it from conjunctivitis.

Changes in Pupil

1. The pupil (Fig. 17.10) will be small and sluggishly reacting. This is easier to make out in unilateral cases by comparing with the uninvolved normal eye. The reasons for the small sluggish pupil include:
   a. The water logging of the loose stroma with massive exudation from the blood vessels.
   b. Engorgement of the radially arranged vessels.
   c. The toxins liberated will irritate both sphincter and dilator papillae, but the action of the more powerful sphincter muscle overcomes that of the dilator and the pupil constricts.
2. If treatment is not promptly given adhesions will develop between the pupillary margin and the lens surface, [posterior synechiae (PS)] (Fig. 17.11) and this will make the pupil irregular in shape.

Iris Changes

Change in normal iris color and pattern: In acute stages iris will be muddy in color with loss of iris pattern.

Posterior synechiae: It is the adhesion between the posterior surface of iris and the lens capsule.

Causes of PS formation: As follows:

1. Normally the posterior surface of the iris is slightly in contact with the anterior lens surface. In acute iritis with the accompanying pupillary constriction more of the posterior surface comes into contact with the anterior lens surface.
2. The exudation of fluid from the blood vessels of iris will be pouring out from both anterior as well as posterior surface of the iris and this will cause adhesion of the iris to the lens surface.
3. The sluggish pupillary reaction promotes this adhesion.

If strong mydriatics like atropine is applied before the adhesions between the iris and the lens get organized these adhesions can be broken, and the pupil will get dilated. But pigments from the pigment cells on the posterior surface of the iris will be left on the anterior lens capsule as a permanent evidence of iridocyclitis. These pigments form a ring on the lens (Figs 17.12 and 17.13).

If application of mydriatics is delayed and the adhesions get organized by formation of granulation tissue, the pupil will dilate only in areas where no permanent adhesions have formed, and this will result in irregular festooned pupil (Fig. 17.14).

Posterior synechiae can be initially segmental, but if the pupil is not promptly dilated with strong mydriatics the adhesions can extend all around the pupil and result

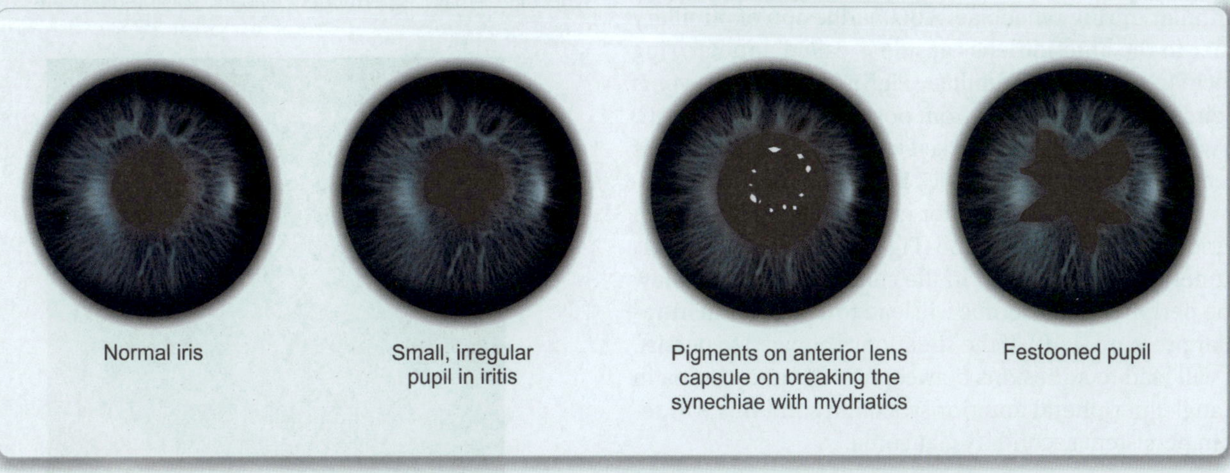

FIGURE 17.10: Changes in pupil in iritis

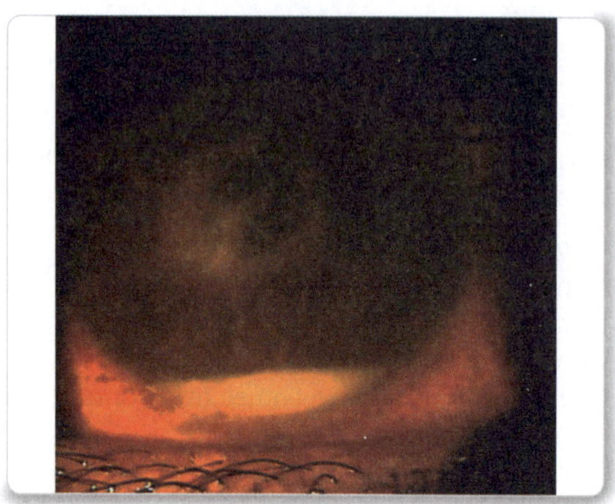

FIGURE 17.11: Hypopyon and exudates covering the pupil in severe anterior uveitis

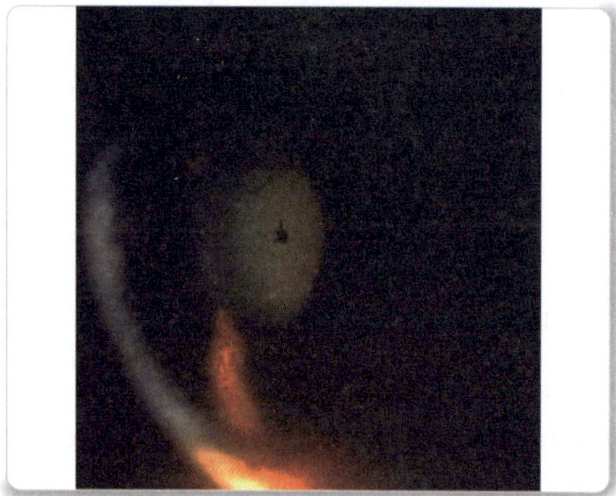

FIGURE 17.12: Acute anterior uveitis with keratic precipitates (KPs) posterior synechiae and pigments on anterior lens capsule where synechiae have broken.

in annular or ring synechiae. A 360° adhesion of pupillary border to the anterior lens capsule is called annular/ring synechiae or seclusio pupillae (Fig. 17.15). This prevents the circulation of aqueous from posterior chamber to AC. The whole pupil can get blocked with exudates and this is called occlusio pupillae (Figs 17.16A and B). Hence, aqueous will collect in the posterior chamber pushing the iris anteriorly forming iris bombe (Figs 17.17A and B). This is a funnel-shaped AC, deep in the center and very shallow in the periphery. Iris bombe will lead to acute rise in intraocular pressure (IOP). If the situation is allowed to persist, this will lead to adhesions between the iris and cornea in the angle, peripheral anterior synechiae, and this will result in persistent secondary glaucoma.

Iris nodules: Iris nodules can be seen in granulomatous uveitis (Fig. 17.18).

Koeppe's nodules are seen at the pupillary borders and these initiate synechiae formation. Busacca nodules are seen nearer the collarette in the iris stroma and are seen in granulomatous uveitis (Fig. 17.19).

When the whole of the posterior surface of iris is plastered onto the lens capsule, it is called total PS. Posterior synechiae can occur in acute or chronic uveitis, but more in chronic cases.

Iris neovascularization: There are seen in chronic cases only.

Changes in Cornea (Visualized with a Slit Lamp)

Keratic precipitates: These are cellular deposits on the corneal endothelium. The cells in the exudates pouring into the AC from the iris will stick to endothelial cells damaged by the toxins in the inflammatory exudates. Along with

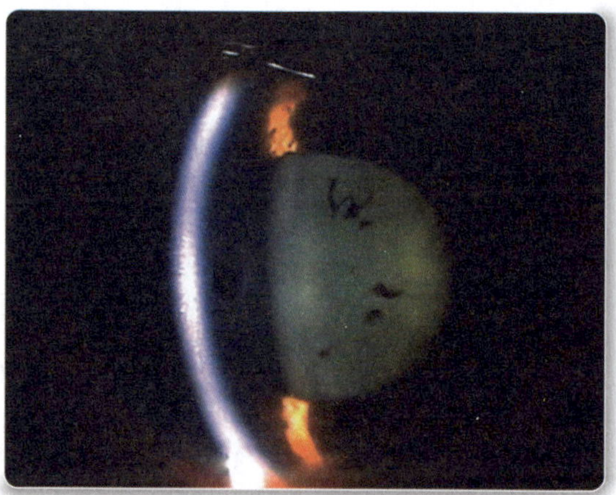

FIGURE 17.13: With treatment keratic precipitates (KPs) have decreased, pupil has become more dilated and the synechiae have all broken pigments on anterior lens capsule from broken posterior synechiae remain as permanent evidence of anterior uveitis.

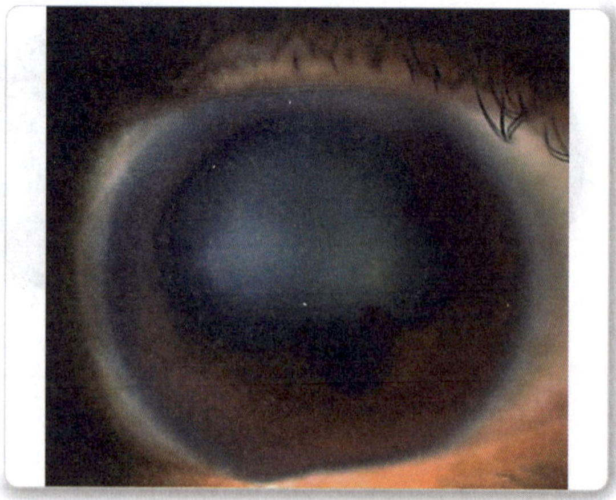

FIGURE 17.14: Festooned pupil

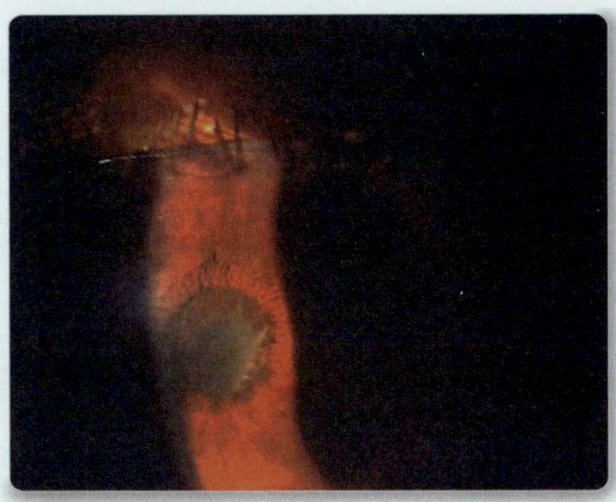

FIGURE 17.15: Seclusio pupillae

the altered endothelium, the centrifugal forces of the convention currents in the AC lead to these cells coming in contact with the damaged endothelium and these get stuck on the endothelium. These KPs are visualized with the help of a slit lamp. The KPs are usually concentrated in a triangular zone with the base inferiorly on the lower part of the cornea. This is called Arlt's triangle.

The morphology of the KPs varies according to the clinical condition, viewed with the help of a slit lamp:

1. Small and medium sized KPs: Non-granulomatous uveitis.
2. Mutton fat (large KPs): Seen in granulomatous uveitis. These are large, greasy KPs, which are deposits of white blood cells mainly lymphocytes (refer Figs 17.19 and 17.20).
3. Fresh KPs: In acute uveitis, usually white, round with a hydrated appearance (Fig. 17.21A).
4. Old KPs: In chronic uveitis or resolved cases. Here the KPs will be crenated, flat and pigmented (Fig. 17.21B).
5. Stellate KPs: In Fuchs' heterochromic iridocyclitis and herpetic uveitis.

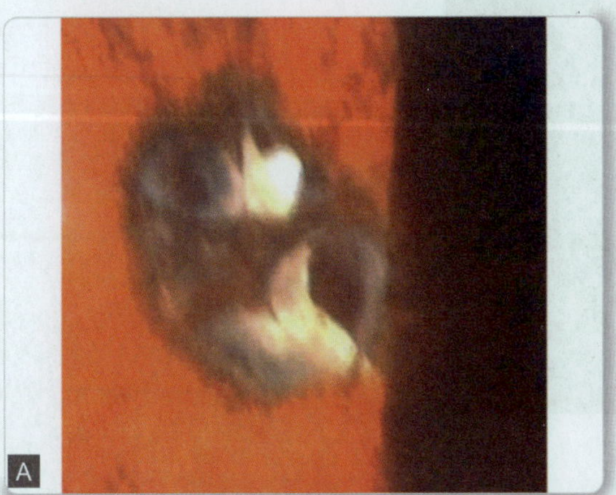

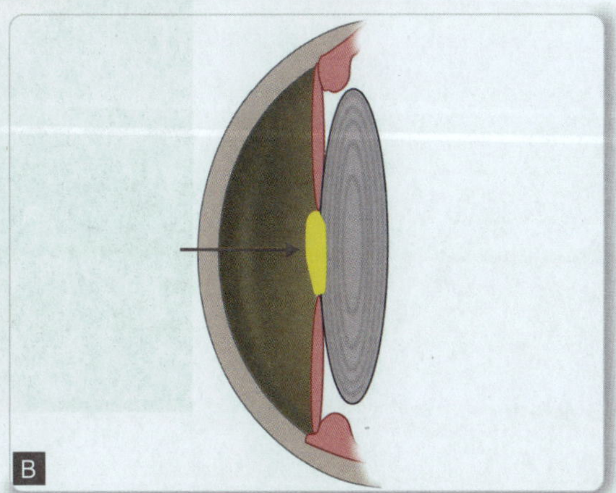

FIGURES 17.16A and B: Occlusio pupillae. A. Photograph; B. Diagrammatic representation.

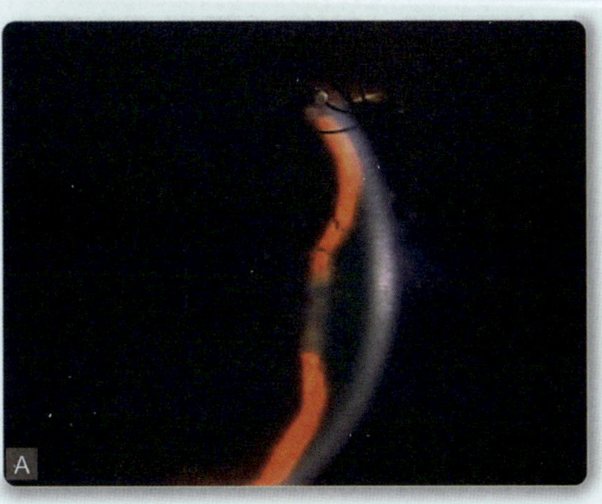

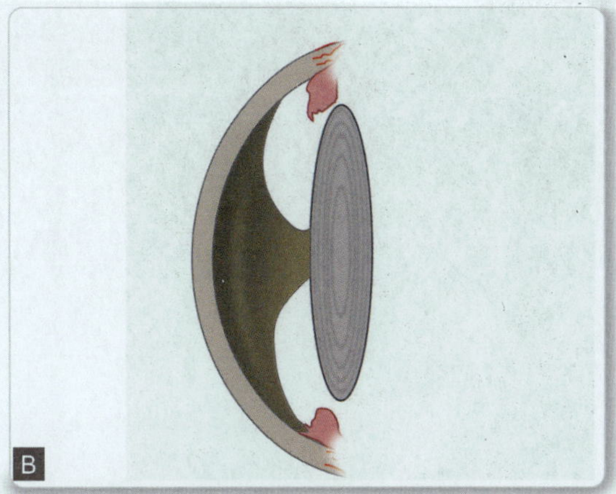

FIGURES 17.17A and B: Iris bombe. A. Photograph; B. Ring synechiae with iris bombe.

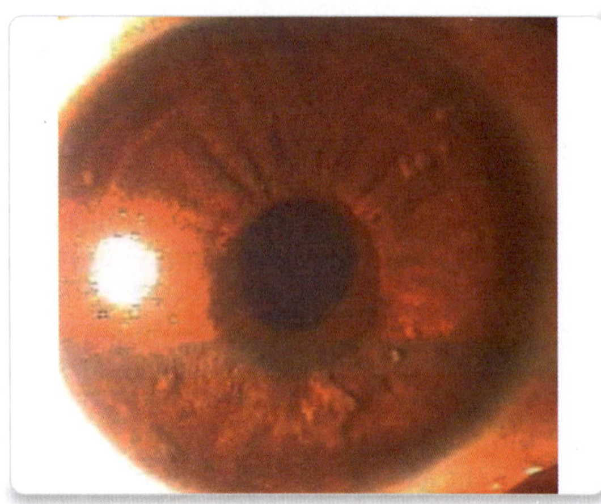

FIGURE 17.18: Iris nodules with ectropion uvea

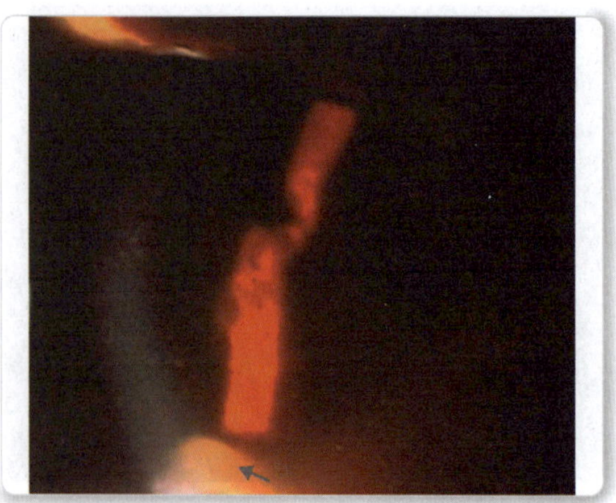

FIGURE 17.19: Granulomatous uveitis with mutton-fat keratic precipitates and granuloma at angle (black arrow)

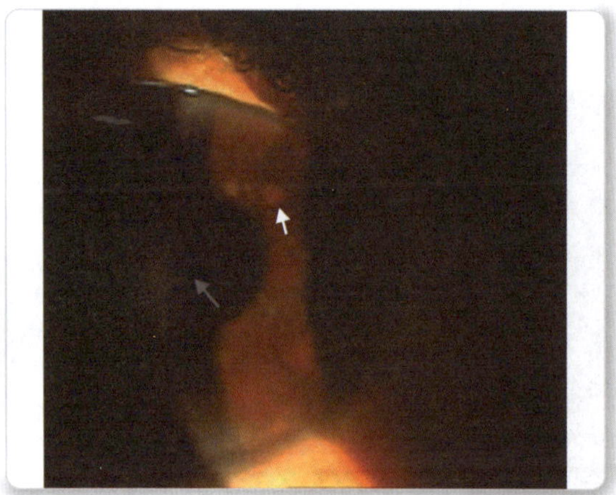

FIGURE 17.20: Granulomatous uveitis with mutton-fat keratic precipitates (black arrow) and iris nodules (white arrow)

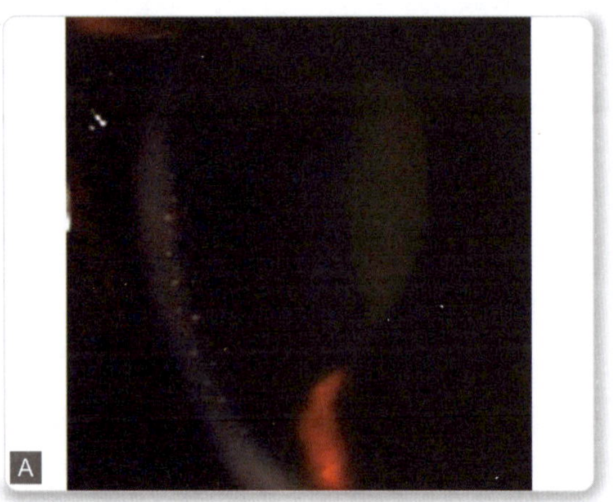

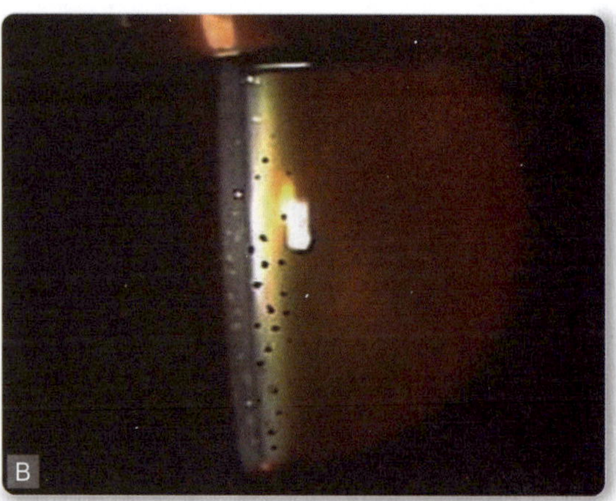

FIGURES 17.21A and B: Slit lamp section showing keratic precipitates (KPs). **A.** Fresh KPs; **B.** Pigmented KPs.

Corneal edema: It can occur due to endothelial damage by toxins or when there is secondary rise in IOP.

Anterior Chamber Signs

Aqueous cells: Cells in the AC can be detected by slit lamp examination (Table 17.1). It indicates activity and severity of the disease.

TABLE 17.1: Cell grading by slit lamp examination

Grading of cells	Number of cells seen with 2 × 1 mm slit
0	No cells
1+	5–10 cells/field
2+	10–20 cells/field
3+	20–50 cells/field
4+	Greater than 50

Anterior chamber flare: Due to inflammation there will be breakdown in the blood aqueous barrier and proteins leak into the AC. These proteins in the AC produce flare.

This is the Tyndall effect produced by the cells and proteins in the aqueous, when a beam of light passes through it (similar to what happens when a beam of sunlight passes into a darkened room) (Fig. 17.22). The grading of flare detailed in Table 17.2.

TABLE 17.2: Grading of flare

Grading of flare	Characteristic
0	Nil
1+	Faint
2+	Moderate (iris and lens details clear)
3+	Marked (iris and lens can be seen, but details hazy)
4+	Intense (fibrinous exudates)

Hypopyon: This is pus in the AC. This pus is sterile since it is a collection of the cellular components of the inflammatory exudates. Presence of hypopyon denotes a severe inflammatory reaction.

Characteristically seen in Behçet's disease and any severe uveitis. It may be present in fungal endophthalmitis and postoperative endophthalmitis also.

Hyphema: Seen in herpetic uveitis.

Changes in the angle: There will be deposition of cellular exudates in the angle and later, there will be synechial closure of angle, both of these can lead to increased IOP.

Lens Changes

When PS have formed and these are broken by applying strong mydriatics like atropine, this will leave behind pigments from the posterior epithelium on the anterior lens capsule (Fig. 17.23). These are much larger and irregularly distributed compared to a Vossius ring left on the anterior lens surface by blunt trauma. These pigments will remain as permanent sequel of an attack of uveitis (refer Figure 17.10). Once PS has organized these are not broken by even atropine and the PS will remain permanently.

In course of time, localized lenticular opacities develop on the anterior lens capsule below the PS.

The toxins and the inflammatory exudates in the aqueous will interfere with metabolism of the lens leading to the development of complicated cataract in the posterior cortex (Figs 17.24A to C).

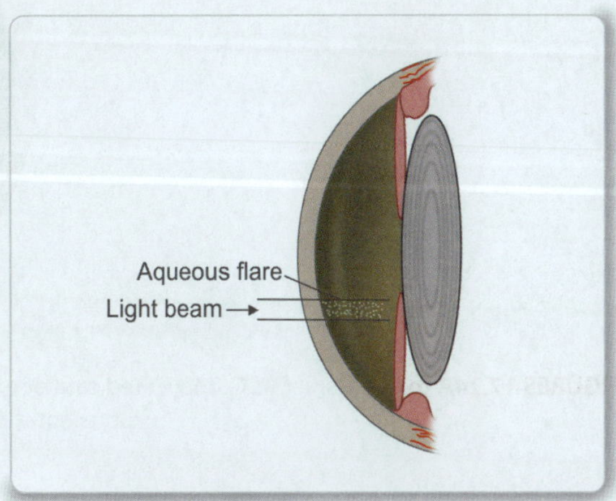

FIGURE 17.22: Aqueous flare

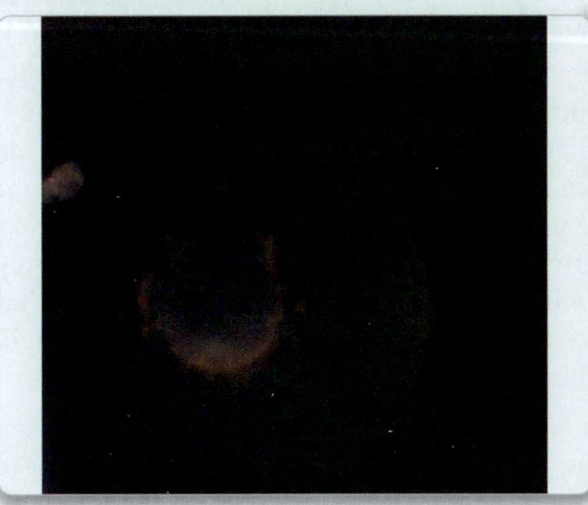

FIGURE 17.23: Pigments and exudates on lens surface after the posterior synechiae have broken

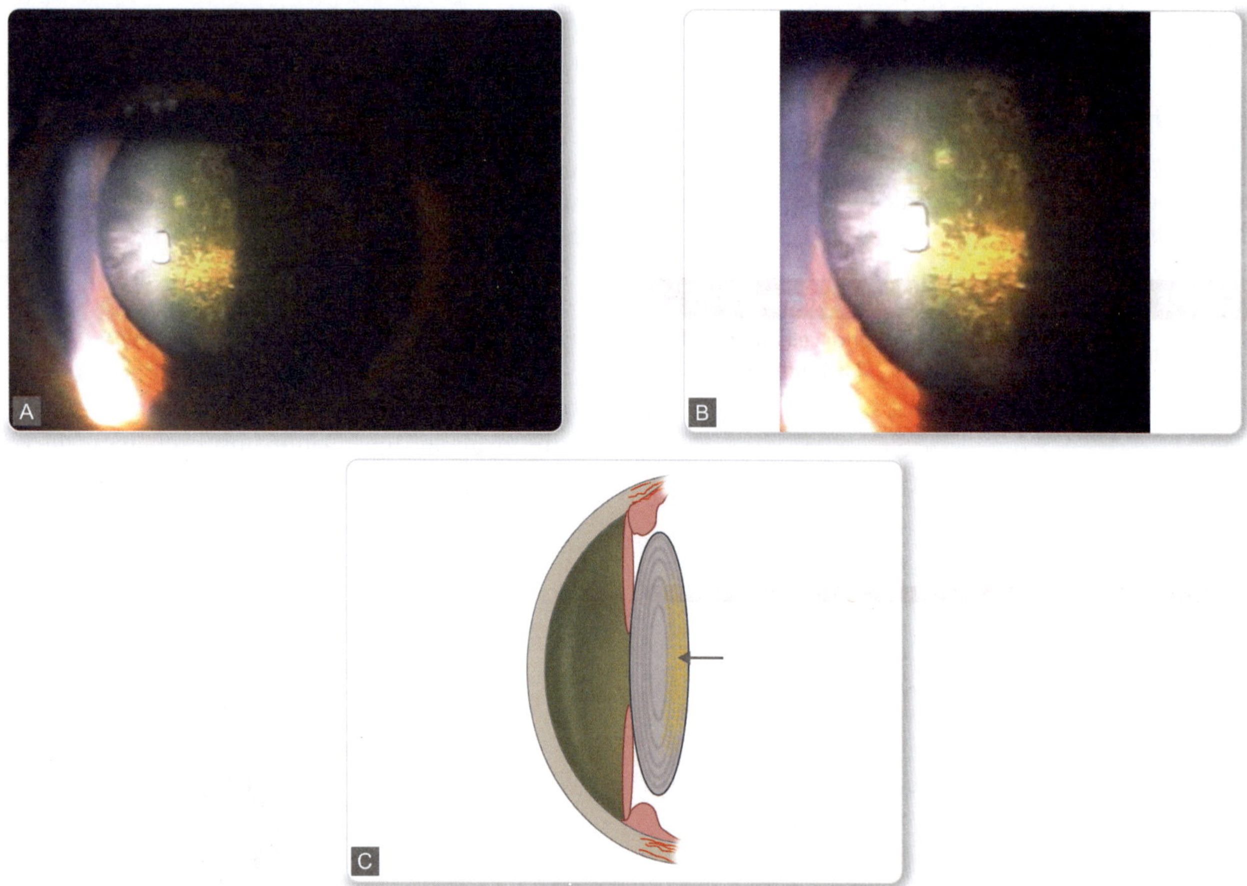

FIGURES 17.24A to C: Cataract. **A.** Complicated cataract; **B.** S/I photograph showing bread crumb appearance; **C.** Diagrammatic representation of complicated cataract.

Complications of Anterior Uveitis

Secondary Glaucoma

Glaucoma or rise in IOP can occur early in the disease or late.

Hypertensive uveitis: In early cases there is no anatomical obstruction to the circulation of aqueous at the pupil or the angle, but the trabecular meshwork can get clogged with inflammatory cells and exudates. An inflammation of the trabecular meshwork (trabeculitis) can also cause an early rise in IOP. This rise in IOP can be controlled by controlling the inflammation with intensive use of anti-inflammatory agents (both topical and systemic) and topical antiglaucoma drugs.

Secondary angle-closure glaucoma: In the late stages angle-closure glaucoma can occur. Because of iris bombe formation the peripheral iris is pushed anteriorly and there is closure of angle due to peripheral anterior synechiae (adhesions between the iris and the cornea).

Steroid-induced glaucoma: It can also occur in chronic cases due to prolonged use of steroids.

Complicated cataract: Most commonly it is a posterior subcapsular cataract. It can occur due to the actual disease process or due to chronic steroid usage.

Plastic Iridocyclitis

Cyclitic membrane may form behind the lens (called plastic iridocyclitis). Exudates poured into the posterior chamber can get organized behind the lens to form a cyclitic membrane. Organization and contraction of these fibrous bands will pull on the ciliary body leading to its detachment, and finally degeneration and atrophy of the ciliary processes resulting in hypotony and phthisis bulbi.

Adjacent Choroiditis

Inflammation can spread to the adjacent choroid by contiguity.

Cystoid Macular Edema, Macular Degeneration, Papillitis

Cystoid macular edema (CME), macular degeneration, papillitis complications are caused by the prostaglandins and other immunomodulators liberated into the eye by the uveal inflammation and reaching the posterior segment.

Band Keratopathy

Band keratopathy occurs in long-standing chronic uveitis, when there is calcium deposition in Bowman's layer of the cornea (Figs 17.25A to C).

Phthisis Bulbi

Phthisis bulbi is the end stage condition. Due to chronic inflammation, there is degeneration of the ciliary body with loss of aqueous production, chronic hypotony, which eventually leads to a shrunken eyeball; phthisis bulbi (Fig. 17.26).

CHRONIC ANTERIOR UVEITIS

If an acute inflammation of uvea lasts longer than 4–6 weeks, it can be considered to be a chronic uveitis. In chronic anterior uveitis, the symptoms are comparatively less, and usually present with mild pain, minimal congestion and mainly defective vision. Examination of the eye will show evidence of prolonged inflammation like multiple dense PS leading to a festooned pupil.

In chronic uveitis iris atrophy and localized areas of iris hyperpigmentation and hypopigmentation may be seen. Complications like complicated cataract, secondary glaucoma, cystoid macular edema and band keratopathy may be present.

Granulomatous and Non-granulomatous Uveitis

Two types of uveitis were first described by Alan Churchill Woods based on the clinical features. The granulomatous inflammations are presumed to be associated with specific infections like TB, sarcoidosis, etc. and non-granulomatous uveitis to be immune mediated. Many a time such a watertight distinction into one or other type is often not possible. The differences between the two clinical types are given in Table 17.3.

Hypertensive Iridocyclitis of Posner and Schlossman

Hypertensive iridocyclitis clinical syndrome is often mistaken for an acute congestive attack. The patient presents with recurrent attacks of mild pain, colored halos and some drop in vision. There will be some corneal edema and the IOP will be high. The AC will be of normal depth and careful examination will reveal a few KPs, which will

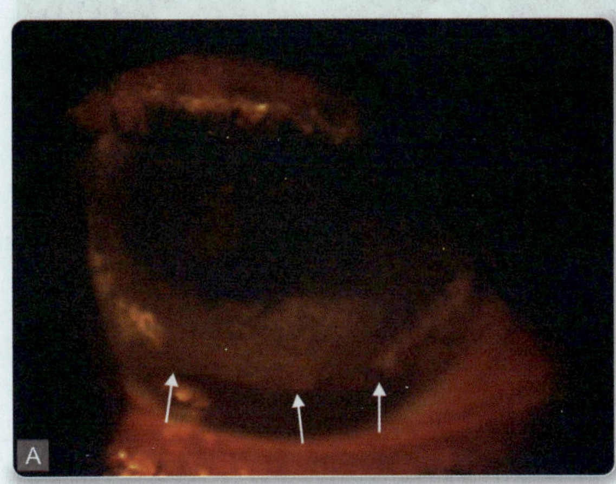

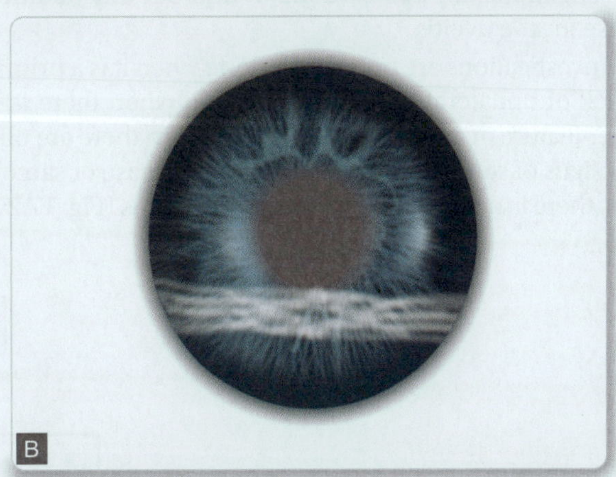

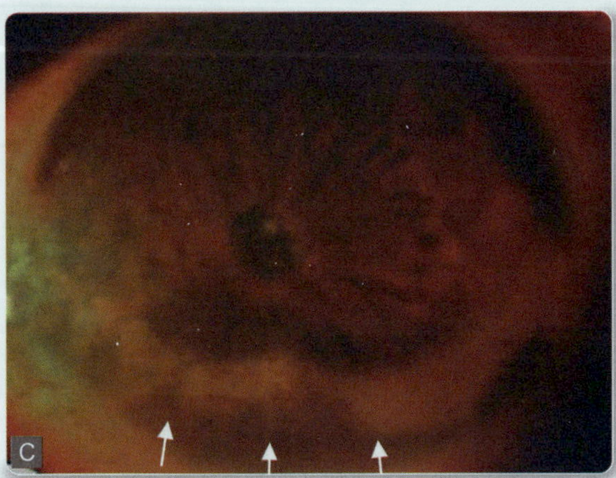

FIGURES 17.25A to C: Band keratopathy. A. Photograph; B. Diagrammatic representation; C. Band keratopathy with occlusio pupillae

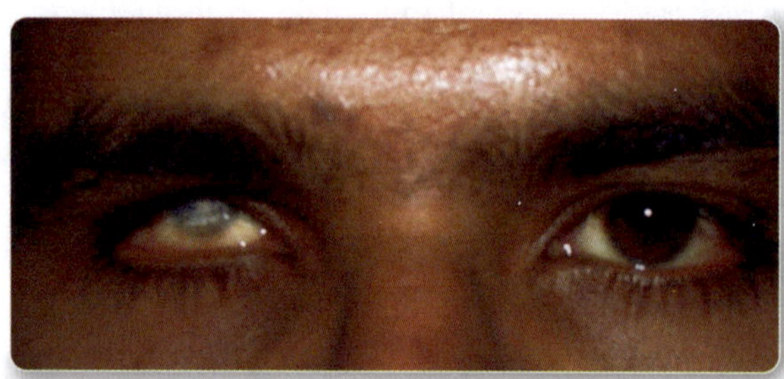

FIGURE 17.26: Phthisis bulbi

clinch the diagnosis. The cause of this condition is considered to be trabeculitis.

Treatment with topical steroids will control the inflammation and the glaucoma. Topical antiglaucoma drugs may also be given to tide over the acute rise in IOP.

INVESTIGATIONS IN UVEITIS

Investigations are mainly done to find out any definitive cause for the uveitis.

Investigations are not usually done when it is a primary attack of unilateral anterior uveitis and when there is no other feature of any systemic disease. When there are obvious signs of some diseases like Behçet's disease or sarcoidosis, there is no need for further investigations (Fig. 17.27).

Indications for Investigations

1. Recurrent non-granulomatous uveitis.
2. Granulomatous uveitis.
3. Bilateral uveitis.
4. Some systemic clues are there, but no definite diagnosis could be made out from clinical appearance.
5. To confirm any HLA association.

Common Investigations

1. Complete blood counts.
2. Skin tests: Mantoux test for TB, pathergy test for Behçet's disease.
3. Serological tests:
   a. For syphilis:
      i. Venereal Disease Research Laboratory (VDRL), rapid plasma reagin (RPR), fluorescent treponemal antibody-absorption (FTA-ABS) test.
      ii. Microhemagluttination *Treponema pallidum* (MHA-TP) test.
   b. For toxoplasmosis: Immunofluorescent antibody test, enzyme-linked immunosorbent assay (ELISA).
   c. Antinuclear antibody (ANA): For juvenile rheumatoid arthritis.

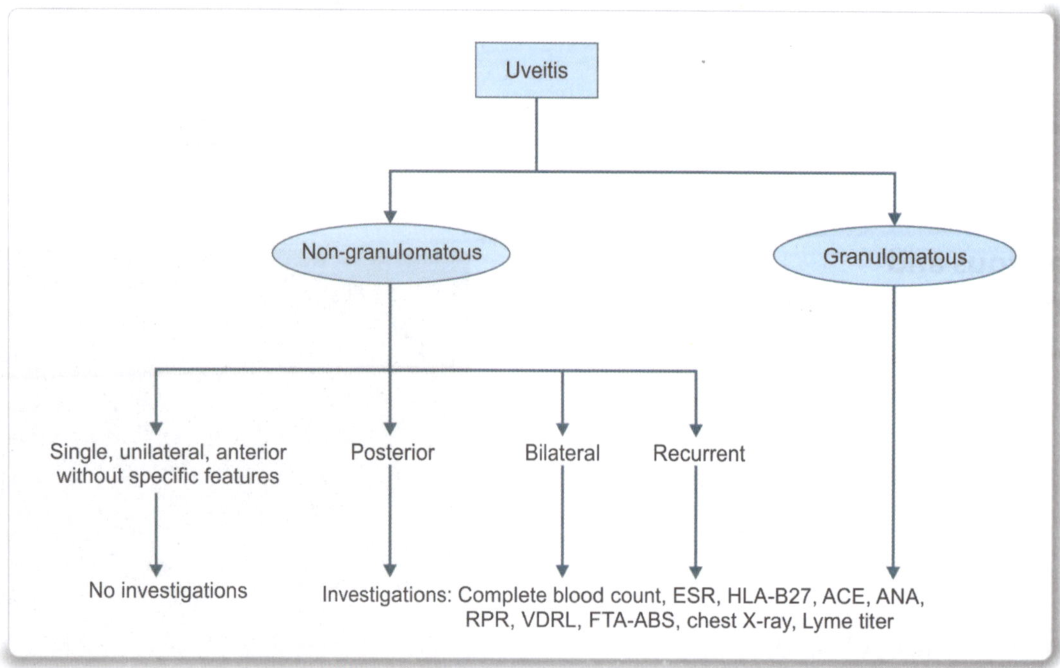

FIGURE 17.27: Investigations in uveitis. ACE, angiotensin-converting enzyme; ANAs, antinuclear antibodies; ESR, erythrocyte sedimentation rate; FTA-ABS, fluorescent treponemal antibody-absorption; RPR, rapid plasma reagin; VDRL, Venereal Disease Research Laboratory.

TABLE 17.3: Differences between granulomatous and non-granulomatous uveitis

Granulomatous uveitis	Non-granulomatous uveitis
Onset is usually insidious	Acute onset
Minimal symptoms	Severe inflammatory symptoms seen
Mutton-fat KPs are seen	Fine KPs seen
Iris nodules and granulomas may be present	Iris nodules not seen
Broad based and thick synechiae are seen	Synechiae are fine and filamentous

   d. Enzyme assay:
      i. Angiotensin-converting enzyme and serum lysozyme—usually used for sarcoidosis.
      ii. Antineutrophil cytoplasmic antibody (ANCA)—Wegener's granulomatosis and polyarteritis nodosa (PAN).
4. HLA typing:
   a. B27—ankylosing spondylitis and Reiter's syndrome.
   b. A29—birdshot chorioretinopathy.
   c. B51—Behçet's disease.
5. Urine examination: To rule out urinary infections.
6. Stool examination: Cysts and ova in stools to be checked to rule out parasitic infestations.
7. Radiological examinations: X-ray may help in reaching at differential diagnosis:
   a. X-ray chest is useful in TB, sarcoidosis (hilar lymphadenopathy).
   b. X-ray spine and sacroiliac joint is helpful in spondyloarthropathies, e.g. bamboo spine in ankylosing spondylitis.
   c. X-ray paranasal sinuses help to rule out any foci of infections.

TREATMENT

Treatment of uveitis involves mainly anti-inflammatory and immunosuppressive drugs. If any specific etiology like infection is found out, it should be treated with appropriate drugs concurrently. Treatment can be topical, periocular or systemic.

Topical Mydriatic Cycloplegic

Topical mydriatic cycloplegic prevent formation of PS and break any PS already formed.

These are very useful in the acute phase of the disease as it promotes comfort by relieving the ciliary spasm, and prevent many complications like occlusio and seclusio pupillae, iris bombe and secondary glaucoma.

Commonly used drugs include long-acting drugs (atropine 1%) and short-acting drugs (homatropine 2% and cyclopentolate in mild cases).

Preventing PS and breaking any already formed is important in preventing complications like iris bombe and secondary glaucoma. Due to the long duration of action of atropine, it can cause PS in dilated pupil. So, atropine is indicated if the synechiae has already formed since stronger mydriatics like atropine is needed to break them. Once the acute phase is over, to prevent the further formation of synechiae short-acting mydriatics can be used.

Subconjunctival mydricaine: If atropine fails to break the already formed dense synechiae, subconjunctival mydricaine (0.3 mL) can be given. Mydricaine contains atropine, adrenaline and procaine.

Topical Steroids

Topical steroids are very effective in anterior uveitis as anti-inflammatory agents. The frequency of instillation depends on the severity of inflammation. Commonly used ones are topical prednisolone, dexamethasone, betamethasone, etc. Severe inflammations like a hypopyon uveitis require prednisolone acetate drops to be applied every hourly to control the inflammation. Milder cases require less frequent instillations. The topical steroids are tapered off as the inflammation comes down. This is judged by the level of aqueous flare and cells. Presence of cells in aqueous means the inflammation is still active. Tapering dose of steroids has to be continued for 2 weeks after all inflammation has subsided as shown by the absence of cells in aqueous. Chronic inflammation can cause a permanent breakdown of the blood-aqueous barrier and the proteins coming to the aqueous due to this, can produce aqueous flare even when the inflammation has subsided. So, the presence of flare alone without cells shows the chronic nature of the condition, not activity and does not require any treatment.

Periocular Steroids

Periocular steroids are commonly used for intermediate or posterior uveitis. But if the anterior uveitis is very severe and systemic steroids are contraindicated, periocular steroids can be given. 0.5 cc of triamcinolone acetonide is given as a subtenon injection. This is useful in non-compliant patients with severe inflammation.

Systemic Steroids

Systemic steroids are used in intermediate and posterior uveitis. In severe anterior uveitis not responding to topical or repository steroids or in non-complaint patients, systemic steroids are given.

Treatment should be started with a large dose and then tapered slowly according to response. Prednisolone 1 mg/kg/day is a common starting dose. Side effects mainly depend on the dosage and duration of the treatment. These include dyspepsia, gastritis, peptic ulcers, hypertension, obesity, hyperglycemia, aseptic necrosis of femur, cataract, glaucoma, flaring up of systemic infections, growth retardation in children, etc.

Systemic Antimetabolites and Immune Modulators

Systemic antimetabolites and immune modulators are usually used as steroid sparing agents in very severe cases. When patient develops severe complications due to steroids or intolerance or non-responsiveness to steroids, immunosuppressants are given, e.g. azathioprine, methotrexate, cyclosporin, etc.

These are very useful in sarcoidosis, Behçet's disease, Vogt-Koyanagi-Harada (VKH) syndrome and sympathetic ophthalmia (SO).

Non-steroidal Anti-inflammatory Drugs

Non-steroidal anti-inflammatory drugs (NSAIDs) are rarely used to decrease inflammation and pain when steroids are contraindicated.

Biological Blockers

Biological blockers include:

1. Anti-TNF-α therapy—infliximab, adalimumab.
2. Interleukin-2 (IL-2) 2 receptor antagonist—daclizumab.

INTERMEDIATE UVEITIS

Intermediate uveitis is also known as chronic posterior cyclitis or pars planitis, and effects pars plana of the ciliary body and periphery of the choroid.

Pars planitis is a subset of idiopathic uveitis, where there is snow banking or snowball formation of exudates over the pars plana and peripheral retina near the ora serrata. The diagnosis is mainly clinical, but investigations are necessary to rule out systemic associations.

Intermediate uveitis can be idiopathic or associated with systemic conditions.

Clinical Features

Due to its insidious onset, a long period elapses before it becomes symptomatic. Hence, any systemic causes are difficult to determine.

Symptom is mainly blurring of vision associated with vitreous floaters. There will not be any pain or redness of the eyes. Even though, initially symptoms are unilateral, condition is typically bilateral and often asymmetrical.

Clinical signs include minimal aqueous cells and flare, few KPs, anterior vitritis, snowball-like exudates in the periphery of vitreous, snow banking, where fibrovascular plaques are seen in the pars plana region. Peripheral retina may show periphlebitis patches. The cells and flare are usually the spread of inflammatory exudates into the AC and this is called 'spillover uveitis'.

Later in the course of disease, papillitis, CME, epiretinal membrane, cataract, glaucoma, cyclitic membrane, retinal detachment, etc. can occur, which can lead to severe diminution of vision.

Complications

- Cystoid macular edema, epiretinal membrane formation
- Peripheral periphlebitis, exudative or tractional retinal detachment (RD)
- Vitreous hemorrhage
- Cataract
- Glaucoma.

Management

Investigations

Investigations should be done to rule out sarcoidosis, syphilis, multiple sclerosis, toxocariasis and Lyme disease.

Treatment

Majority of the cases has minimal problems and resolve spontaneously and do not need any treatment. Treatment is indicated when there are vision-threatening problems like intense vitritis, macular edema, etc.

Main line of management is steroids (posterior subtenon injection or systemic steroids) or immunosuppressants, when steroids have already been used and failed.

Vitrectomy is indicated in cases with intractable macular edema, epiretinal membrane formation, persistent vitreous hemorrhage or tractional RD.

POSTERIOR UVEITIS

The inflammation of the choroid (choroiditis) is the characteristic feature of posterior uveitis and since the retinal layers are in close proximity to choroid, these are often involved together, and hence the general terminology for the lesion is chorioretinitis.

Classification

Posterior uveitis is classified according to the number and location of the areas involved:

1. Based on the type of lesion:
   a. Diffuse/Disseminated choroiditis is seen as multiple small scattered areas of inflammation in the posterior pole (due to syphilis/TB). Later it forms atrophic patches. Complicated cataract due to impaired lens nutrition occurs (Fig. 17.28).

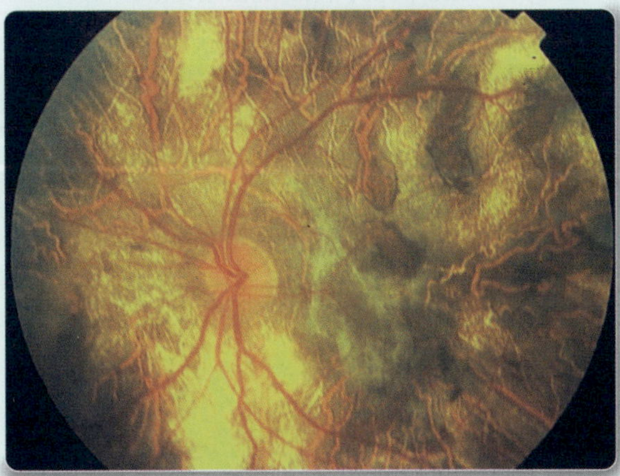

FIGURE 17.28: Disseminated choroiditis

   b. Multifocal choroiditis: In this condition, the lesions are fewer, and more discrete, mainly seen in the periphery and also called anterior choroiditis (Fig. 17.29).
2. Based on location of lesion (circumscribed/localized/focal choroiditis) (Fig. 17.30):
   a. Central choroiditis: Affects the posterior pole or macular region.
   b. Juxtacecal or juxtapapillary choroiditis (Jensen): Usually occurs in young persons as an oval, exudation of about the size of the disk occurring close to the disk (Figs 17.31A and B).

Symptoms

1. Floaters with or without diminution of vision.
2. Usually painless condition since choroid does not have pain nerve endings.
3. Metamorphopsia: Due to raised lesions, (macropsia/micropsia) retinal contour altered and distortion of image occur.
4. Photopsia: Due to retinal irritability.
5. Black spot (positive scotoma): A black spot in front of the eye.
6. Negative scotoma: A defect in the field of vision (in later stages).
7. No symptoms of pain or redness unless the anterior uvea is also involved.

Signs

In the initial stages, the lesion can be identified by fundus examination.

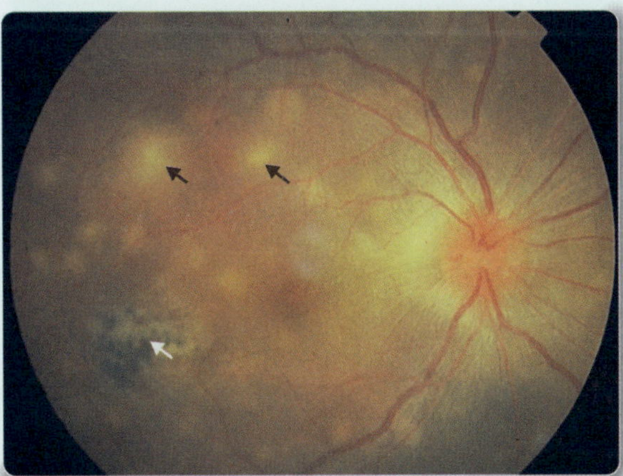

FIGURE 17.29: Multifocal choroiditis showing healed lesion (white arrow) and active lesions (black arrows)

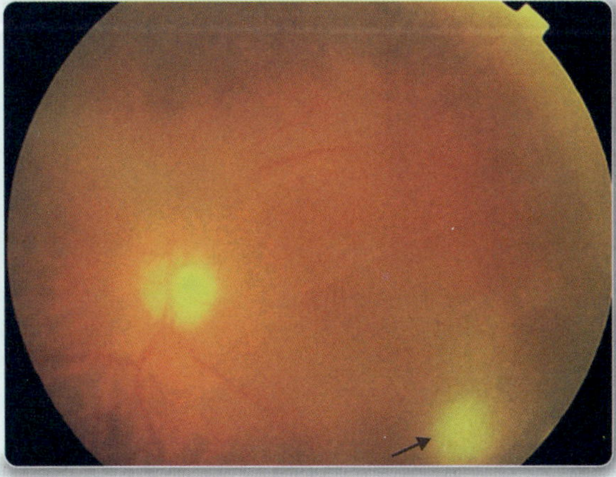

FIGURE 17.30: Focal choroiditis with vitritis (black arrow)

Active Stage

A choroiditis lesion is seen as an yellowish raised lesion with retinal vessels passing above it and overlying retinal edema. Opacities in vitreous and vitreous haze may be present (Fig. 17.32A).

Healed Stage

Atrophic choroiditis patch is white in color with pigmentation of borders (Fig. 17.32B).

Complications

- Panuveitis
- Complicated cataract
- Vitreous degeneration
- Retinal detachment
- Retinal and choroidal neovascularization (CNV).

Treatment

- Nonspecific: Systemic and topical corticosteroids
- Specific: It is given after identifying the underlying cause.

INFECTIOUS UVEITIS

Infectious uveitis includes bacterial, spirochetal, viral, protozoal and fungal disease.

Classification

1. Anterior uveitis:
   - Granulomatous: Leprosy, tuberculosis
   - Non-granulomatous: Syphilis, viral
   - Intermediate uveitis: Lyme disease, toxocariasis.
2. Posterior uveitis:
   - Choroiditis and retinitis: Toxoplasmosis, TB, cytomegalovirus (CMV), herpetic uveitis

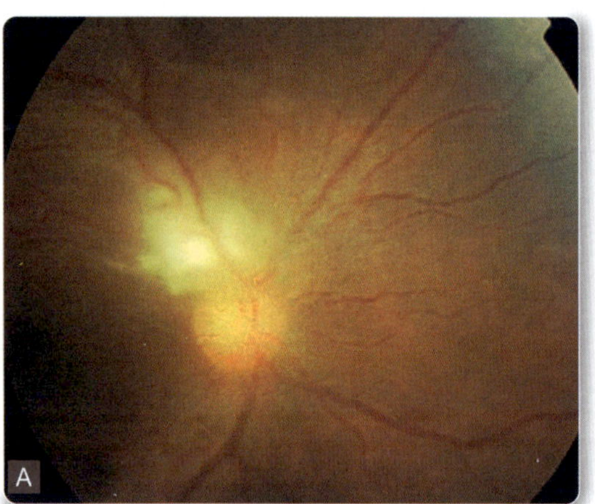

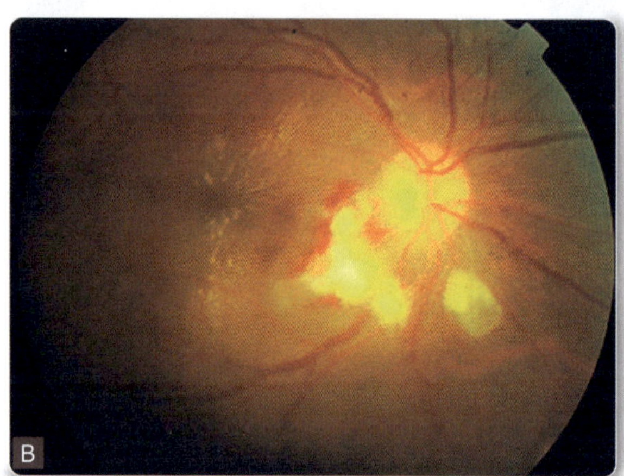

FIGURES 17.31A and B: Juxtapapillary choroiditis

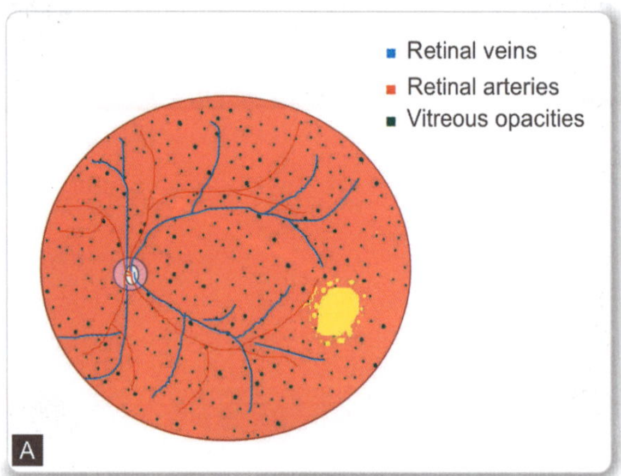

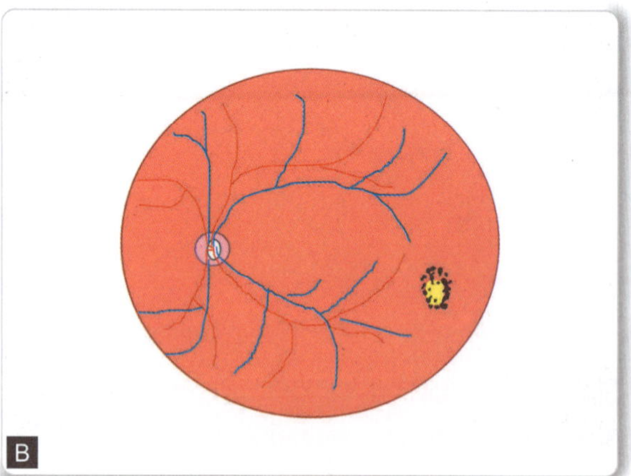

FIGURES 17.32A and B: Choroiditis. **A.** Active choroiditis; **B.** Healed choroiditis with surrounding pigmentation and clear media.

- Neuroretinitis: Syphilis, cat scratch disease, Lyme disease
- Panuveitis: TB, syphilis, Lyme, herpetic
- Vasculitis: TB, syphilis, toxoplasmosis, CMV.

Tuberculosis

Tuberculosis can produce varied and widespread inflammatory damage to the eye and can mimic various disease entities.

Pathogenesis

1. It can occur as a direct ocular infection from an exogenous source and can involve ocular adnexa, conjunctiva, sclera or cornea. It is relatively rare.
2. It may also result from a hypersensitivity reaction to distant foci of infection. For example, episcleritis, phlyctenulosis and Eales' disease. This is probably the commonest mode of involvement.
3. Hematogenous spread from pulmonary or extrapulmonary sites can also occur.

Clinical Presentation

Conjunctival granulomas, keratitis, scleritis, anterior uveitis, intermediate uveitis, diffuse uveitis, solitary and multiple choroidal granulomas, subretinal abscesses and optic neuritis, optic disk edema, optic atrophy and choroidal granulomas may also occur along with TB meningitis.

Tuberculous iritis: It can be granulomatous (military or solitary) or non-granulomatous.

Tuberculous choroiditis: It can occur as choroidal tubercles or as solitary large tuberculomas or as multifocal choroiditis due to hypersensitivity reaction to tuberculoprotein.

Investigations

Investigations methods are complete blood count, ESR, Mantoux, chest X-ray.

Newer methods: PCR [aqueous or vitreous or fine needle aspiration cytology (FNAC) sample] and QuantiFERON-TB gold test.

Treatment

Antituberculosis treatment: Four drugs given for 6–12 months [isoniazid (INH), rifampicin, pyrazinamide and ethambutol]. Topical and systemic steroids with cycloplegics are also required.

Leprosy

Uveal involvement is seen commonly in the lepromatous form and involves the anterior part, iris and ciliary body, and rarely a peripheral choroiditis can occur.

Uveal involvement can occur as:

1. Initial bacteremia, which seeds bacilli in ciliary body, iris, autonomic nerve fibers, etc. followed by hypotony, atrophy of iris stroma and dilator muscles and low-grade uveitis leading to cataract and secondary glaucoma.
2. Acute granulomatous type of uveitis, postsynechiae, hypopyon and glaucoma.
3. Lepra pearls or iris pearls, which contains clumps of both dead and live lepra bacilli on the iris surface or in the aqueous.

Treatment

Antileprotic drugs: Dapsone 50–100 mg is the drug of choice. Rifampicin, ofloxacin, clofazimine and minocycline are used in various regimens in combination with dapsone.

Spirochetal Uveitis

Syphilis caused by *Treponema pallidum.*

Clinical Features

Transmitted transplacentally or by sexual contact. Among the three stages of syphilis, panuveitis occur more commonly in secondary and tertiary stages and in congenital syphilis.

Ocular Manifestations

1. Primary syphilis:
   - Chancres of eyelid and conjunctiva.
2. Secondary syphilis:
   - Blepharitis and madarosis
   - Conjunctivitis
   - Keratitis
   - Iris roseola, iridocyclitis
   - Episcleritis and scleritis
   - Chorioretinitis (Fig. 17.33)
   - Vitritis
   - Exudative RD
   - Perivasculitis.
3. Tertiary syphilis:
   - Gummas of eyelids
   - Unilateral interstitial keratitis
   - Punctate stromal keratitis
   - Bilateral periostitis of orbital bones

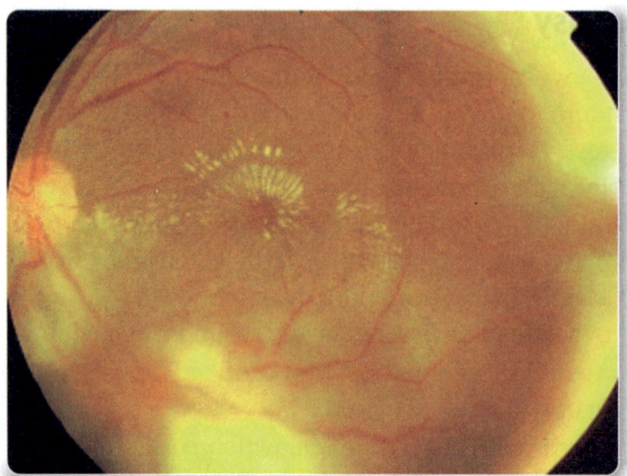

FIGURE 17.33: Chorioretinitis with perivasculitis in syphilis

- Episcleritis and scleritis
- Anterior and posterior uveitis
- Venous and arterial occlusive disease
- Exudative RD
- Pseudoretinitis pigmentosa
- Choroidal neovascular membrane (CRNVM)
- Argyll Robertson pupil (ARP), oculomotor palsies.

4. Congenital syphilis:
   - Bilateral interstitial keratitis
   - Pigmentary retinitis
   - Glaucoma, keratouveitis.

The typical manifestation in congenital syphilis is bilateral interstitial keratitis, which is rarely seen now due to investigation and treatment of mothers in antenatal period.

Investigations

Commonly used screening tests are VDRL and RPR. FTA-ABS is more sensitive.

Treatment

1. Penicillin IV or IM.
2. Ocular syphilis is treated like neurosyphilis.
3. Intravenous (IV) penicillin G 18–24 million units for 10–14 days followed by IM penicillin 2.4 million units for 3 weeks.
4. Tetracycline 500 mg or doxycycline 100 mg bid × 14 days given in patients with penicillin allergy.

Lyme Disease

Uveitis may take in the form of granulomatous iridocyclitis, intermediate uveitis, retinal vasculitis and rarely neuroretinitis.

Leptospirosis

Most important ocular manifestation of leptospirosis is uveitis. It exist as two clinical subtypes such as anterior or diffuse. Posterior uveitis is seen as vitritis, choroiditis, vasculitis, papillitis and panuveitis.

Investigations

1. Isolation of organism: ELISA.
2. Isolation of DNA: Microscopic agglutination test (MAT), polymerase chain reaction (PCR).

Treatment

Doxycycline 100 mg bid × 14 days.

Protozoal Uveitis

Protozoal uveitis is ocular toxoplasmosis definitive hosts are cats. Intermediate hosts are man and other animals like cattles, pigs, etc. Spread of infection:

1. Ingestion of undercooked meat (bradyzoites).
2. Food contaminated by feline excreta (oocysts).
3. Transplacental spread.

Congenital toxoplasmosis is more common than the acquired form.

Clinical Presentation

Focal necrotizing retinitis: Congenital infections will be detected later as bilateral or unilateral chorioretinal scars. Macula is preferentially involved resulting in punched out, heavily pigmented scars at the macula (Fig. 17.34). In acquired infections, the most common presentation is a reactivation of a healed lesion

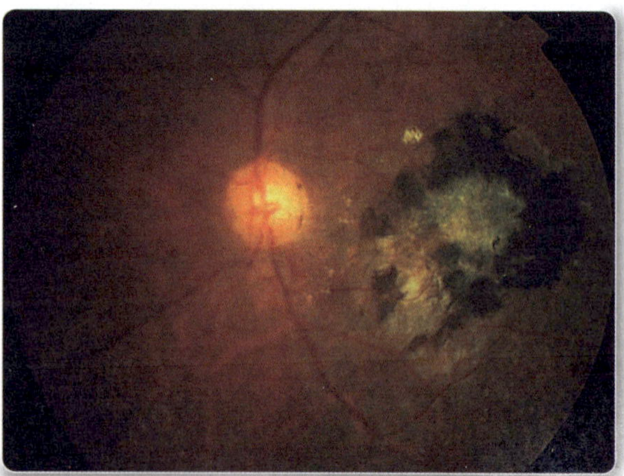

FIGURE 17.34: Healed toxoplasma chorioretinal scar at macula

(active lesion adjacent to an old pigmented scar) with intense vitritis giving rise to 'headlight in fog' appearance (Fig. 17.35).

This reactivation of a healed lesion is a characteristic feature of toxoplasmosis. The parasite goes into spore form when it comes into contact with the antitoxoplasma drugs and remain in a dormant form within a healed lesion for years. When conditions become favorable these organisms may start a new lesion adjacent to the healed scar.

Investigations

1. Serology for toxoplasma antibodies: ELISA test for IgG and IgM levels. A positive IgM is an indicator of recent infection.
2. In aqueous tumor PCR can be done.
3. The fundus fluorescein angiography (FFA), indocyanine green angiography (ICG) confirms activity of the lesion and can detect complications.
4. Optical coherence tomography (OCT) can detect complications like epiretinal membrane, vitreomacular traction, CME and choroidal neovascular membranes (CNVMs) underneath a healed lesion.

Treatment

Indications of treatment: Macula, optic nerve or papillomacular bundle involvement, severe vitritis causing visual impairment, immunosuppression, etc.

Use a combination of drugs for 3–4 weeks minimum. Antitoxoplasma agents commonly in use are given in Table 17.4.

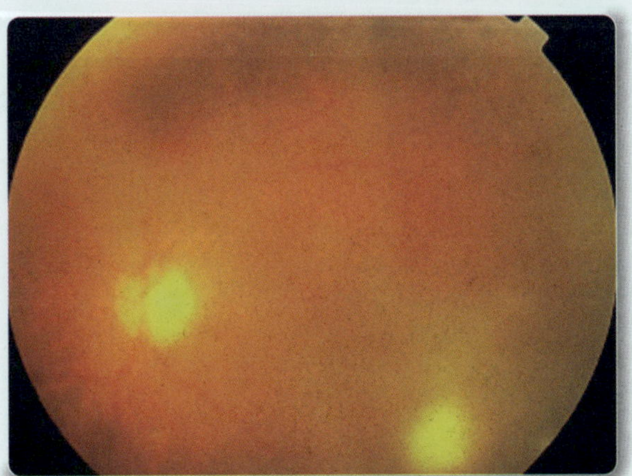

FIGURE 17.35: Active toxoplasmosis; headlight in fog appearance

Toxocariasis

Toxocariasis infestation occur by larval forms of dog roundworm *(Toxocara canis)* or cat *(Toxocara cati)* results in toxocariasis.

TABLE 17.4: Drugs for toxoplasmosis

Drugs	Dosage
Pyrimethamine	75 mg/day loading dose 25 mg/day maintenance × 4 week
Sulfadiazine	2 g loading dose 1 g qid × 4 week
Clindamycin	300 mg qid × 4–6 week
Azithromycin	500 mg bid × 4–6 week
Atovaquone	750 mg qid orally
Cotrimoxazole	960 mg bid

Ocular Toxocariasis

Ocular toxocariasis is caused by infestation with roundworms of dogs *T. canis.* Man gets the infestation by accidental ingestion of the ova shed in dog's feces through contaminated food or water. Children playing with pet dogs are at risk of getting this disease. It takes three forms:

1. Peripheral granuloma lies at or anterior to equator. It is usually asymptomatic, but tractional bands may extend from the granuloma to the posterior pole and this may cause macular heterotopia, tractional and rhegmatogenous RD (Fig. 17.36).
2. Posterior pole granuloma lie in macular area and seen in children between 6 and 14 years of age.

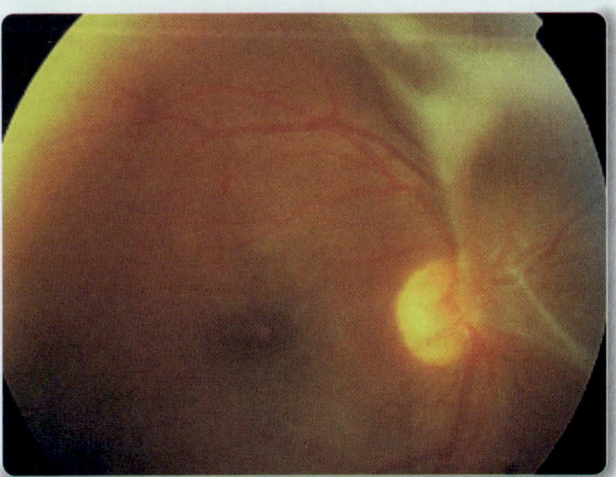

FIGURE 17.36: Peripheral granuloma with traction bands extending to optic disk

3. Chronic endophthalmitis present as leukocoria in children between 2 and 9 years of age. It can lead to formation of cyclitic membrane and RD.

Investigations

- Blood counts: Eosinophilia.
- ELISA: To detect antibodies.

Treatment

Systemic and periocular steroids to suppress inflammation.Anthelmintics such as thiabendazole and diethylcarbamazine have a limited role.

Cysticercosis

Cysticercosis is the infestation with cysticercus cellulosae larval form of the tapeworm *Taenia solium*. Common sites are vitreous cavity and subretinal space.

The larvae in the subretinal space or vitreous cavity can release toxins, which produce an intense inflammatory reaction causing intense vitritis, panuveitis and exudative RD and can end in blindness.

Cysts can appear under the conjunctiva, orbit or lids, or rarely appear as free floating cysts in the AC. Cysts clinically appear as translucent mass with a dense white spot at one region.

Treatment

Systemic steroids to control the inflammation and surgical removal of cysts or larvae from the eye. Computed tomography scan of head should be done to rule out neurocysticercosis.

Viral Uveitis

Viruses belonging to the herpesviridae family [HSV-I and II, herpes zoster virus (HZV), CMV and Epstein-Barr virus (EBV)] produce uveal inflammation. Manifestations may be nonspecific or distinct clinical syndromes.

Herpetic Uveitis

1. Anterior uveitis presents with fine small (stellate) KPs scattered all over the endothelium with mild AC reaction. Characteristic features are sectorial iris atrophy, hyphema and secondary glaucoma. It may occur with or without corneal involvement.
2. Acute retinal necrosis (ARN) is a panuveitis, which is caused by HSV and varicella zoster. It appears as multifocal yellow-white retinal infiltrates, which spread and coalesce, and the posterior pole is affected last. When the lesions heal, it leaves behind extensive areas of white necrotic retina with pigmented borders. It will be accompanied by granulomatous anterior uveitis.

Treatment: Intravenous acyclovir for 14 days. A 750 mg loading dose followed by 500 mg 8th hourly. This is followed by oral acyclovir 800 mg five times daily for 3–6 months.

Prognosis: It is poor.

HIV-related Uveitis

1. Retinal microangiopathy: Non-infectious retinal microangiopathy develops in 60% of the patients with acquired immunodeficiency syndrome (AIDS). It is characterized by cotton-wool spots, which may be associated with retinal hemorrhages and microaneurysms.
2. Cytomegalovirus retinitis: The CMV retinitis eventually affects 40% of patients with AIDS and its appearance usually signifies severe systemic involvement. It occurs in two forms:
   a. Indolent CMV retinitis.
   b. Fulminating retinitis.
3. Pneumocystis carinii choroiditis: The presence of choroidal involvement can be an important sign of extrapulmonary systemic dissemination.
4. Other fundus lesions: Progressive outer retinal necrosis (PORN) (Fig. 17.37) is caused by varicella-zoster virus. It is a rapidly progressive necrotizing retinitis, which responds poorly to antiviral therapy and most patients become blind in both eyes within a few weeks. PORN is distinguished from acute retinal necrosis

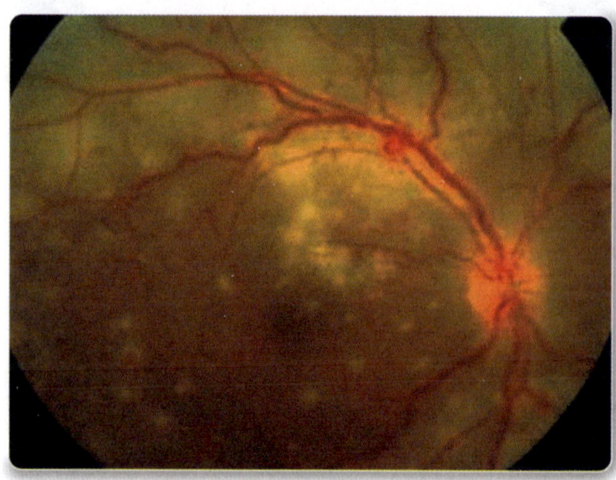

FIGURE 17.37: Progressive outer retinal necrosis

by the absence of inflammation and early involvement of the posterior pole.

Treatment: Ganciclovir is initially given IV (induction) every 12 hours for 2–3 weeks and then every 24 hours.

Intravitreal ganciclovir, in the form of either injection or slow-release devices, appears to be as effective as IV therapy IV cidofovir may also be used.

Fungal Uveitis

Presumed ocular histoplasmosis syndrome caused by *Histoplasma capsulatum* that is endemic in certain regions of the world (like Mississippi valley).

Candidiasis: Candida species are commensal yeasts of low virulence for healthy persons. These may be cause serious disease with altered host defense like patients on long term immunosuppressants.

Clinical Presentation

Multifocal discrete yellow-white lesions, which coalesce, invade retina and vitreous. It form cotton-ball colonies or string of pearls.

Treatment

Intravitreal amphotericin B plus systemic antifungals like flucytosine, ketoconazole, etc.

PURULENT UVEITIS, ENDOPHTHALMITIS AND PANOPHTHALMITIS

Purulent exogenous uveitis is caused by infected wounds, whether accidental or following surgeries or corneal ulcer.

Endophthalmitis

Endophthalmitis is an intraocular inflammation affecting the inner coats of the eye with exudation into the vitreous. When the whole of the eye including the sclera is involved, it results in panophthalmitis. It can be of two types:

1. Acute postoperative occurs one to several days after surgery. Chief organisms are staphylococci *(Staphylococcus epidermidis* and *Staphylococcus aureus),* streptococci, gram-negative bacteria *(Pseudomonas, Proteus)* and anaerobes.
2. Delayed onset postoperative occurs a week to a month or more after surgery. Causes may be *Propionibacterium acnes,* fungi, etc.

Post-traumatic common causes are *Staphylococcus epidermidis,* fungi, etc. (Fig. 17.38).

Endogenous Endophthalmitis

Endogenous endophthalmitis (Fig. 17.39) is usually metastatic in origin. Usually seen in septicemia, immunosuppressed persons or in HIV infection. *Bacillus, Streptococcus, Staphylococcus, Mucor, Candida,* etc. are implicated.

Clinical Features

Symptoms: Severe pain, lid edema and decreased vision.

Signs: Lid edema, discharge, chemosis, infiltrate at the wound, wound abscess, hypopyon, pupillary exudates, poor red reflex and reduced visual acuity.

Proptosis and painful limitation of extraocular movements indicate panophthalmitis.

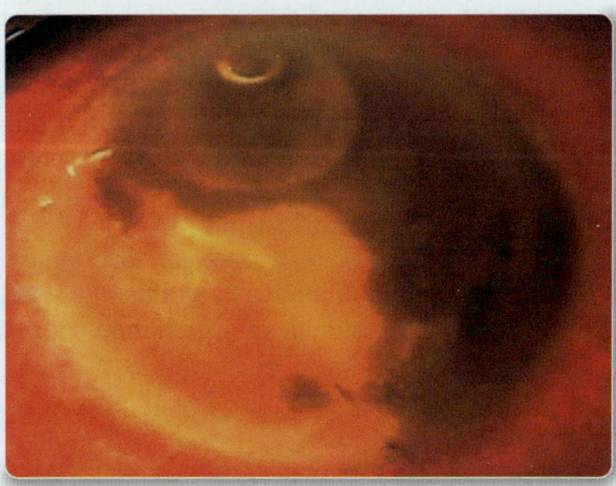

FIGURE 17.38: Post-traumatic endophthalmitis

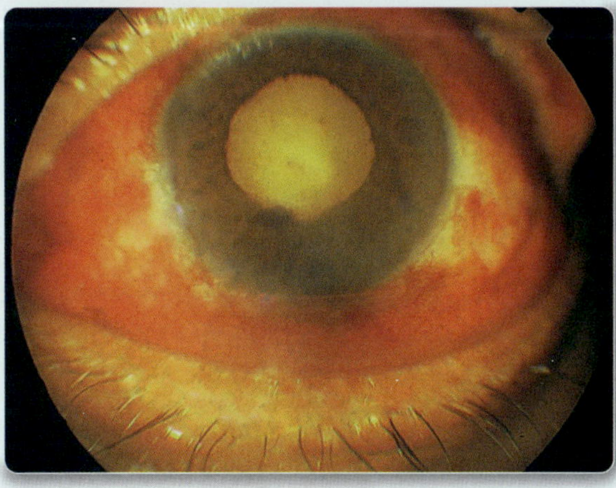

FIGURE 17.39: Endogenous endophthalmitis with yellow reflex at pupil

Investigation

Vitreous tap or biopsy or AC tap to isolate the organism.

Treatment

Intravitreal broad-spectrum antibiotics; vancomycin and ceftazidime or amikacin:

1. If fungal: Amphotericin B.
2. Pars plana vitrectomy is done if visual acuity on presentation is light perception or worse or if patient does not respond to intravitreal antibiotics within 48 hours.
3. Evisceration: If the eye has no perception of light and develops signs suggestive of panophthalmitis.

NON-INFECTIOUS UVEITIS

Ankylosing Spondylitis

Ankylosing spondylitis is a chronic progressive disease affecting the joints of spine and adjacent soft tissue of young men starting in 3rd decade (Fig. 17.40). Sacroiliac joint is the commonly involved joint. Majority are HLA-B27 positive.

It can present as acute anterior uveitis with fibrinous exudates in the AC.

Behçet's Disease

Behçet's disease is an obliterative vasculitis of a possible immune etiology with a significant association with HLA-B5 antigen.

Clinical Features

1. Systemic:
    - Oral ulcers
    - Genital ulcers
    - Skin lesions; erythema nodosum
    - Arthralgia/Arthritis
    - Thrombophlebitis
    - Gastrointestinal dysfunction
    - Meningoencephalitis.
2. Ocular:
    - Recurrent acute iritis with mobile transient hypopyon (Fig. 17.41)
    - Chronic iridocyclitis
    - Keratoconjunctivitis
    - Episcleritis
    - Diffuse vascular leakage (retinal/macular edema/disk edema)
    - Retinitis/Periphlebitis/Infraction/Necrosis/Vascular obliteration
    - Vitritis
    - Optic atrophy.

Reiter's Disease

Reiter's disease usually affects young males with HLA-B27 positivity. Non-specific urethritis, pauciarticular, large joint arthritis and conjunctivitis are the chief manifestations. Recurrent acute iridocyclitis can occur, which usually responds to conventional therapy.

Sarcoidosis

Sarcoidosis is a multisystem granulomatous inflammatory disorder characterized by localized granuloma formation involving the lungs, lymph nodes, skin, central nervous system (CNS) and eye.

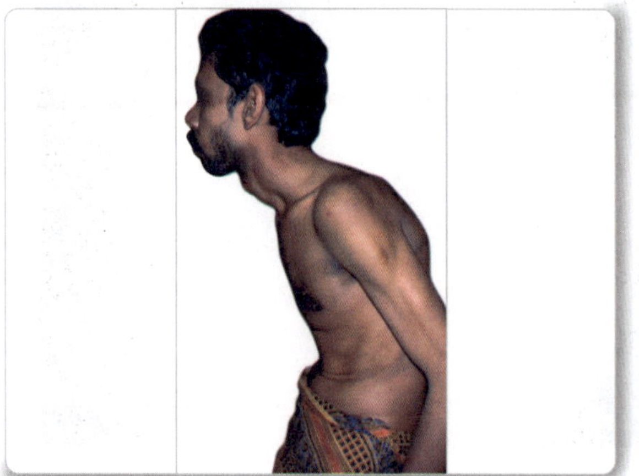

FIGURE 17.40: Person with ankylosing spondylitis

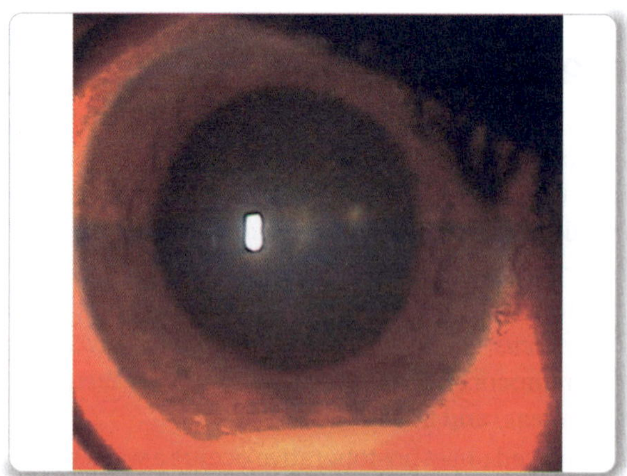

FIGURE 17.41: Hypopyon uveitis

Clinical Features

1. Anterior uveitis is the most common presentation; unilateral at onset, bilateral involvement is typical.
2. Granulomatous uveitis with medium to large mutton-fat KPs.
3. Iris—Koeppe and Busacca nodules.
4. Anterior and PS common.
5. Recurrent exacerbation can lead to complication like secondary glaucoma, cataract and CME.
6. Posterior uveitis: Presents with periphlebitis of mid-peripheral or peripheral venules with perivascular cuffing with or without focal narrowing, perivascular exudation; candle wax dripping.
7. Retinal neovascularization.
8. Preretinal and vitreous involvement: Snowball opacity in inferior vitreous.
9. Retinitis is rare, but has grave prognosis because of association with CNS sarcoidosis.
10. Choroidal lesion: Choroidal granuloma may be seen.
11. Optic nerve involvement may be seen as edema, infiltration, swelling associated with adjacent retinitis or progressive atrophy.
12. Dacryoadenitis can cause pain, proptosis and exposure keratopathy if severe infiltration of lacrimal gland; keratoconjunctivitis sicca (KCS).
13. Rarely isolated orbital or extraocular muscle (EOM) granulomas occur.

Lens-related Uveitis

Phacoanaphylactic Uveitis

Phacoanaphylactic uveitis follows a traumatic or operative perforation of lens after a latent period of 1–2 weeks. It may present as a severe acute granulomatous uveitis with PS, mutton-fat KPs, etc.

Phacotoxic Uveitis

Phacotoxic uveitis occurs as a toxic reaction to lens protein liberated from a surgical or traumatic break of lens capsule, or from leaking of hypermature lens matter through lens capsule.

Sympathetic Ophthalmia

Sympathetic ophthalmia is a bilateral granulomatous inflammation of entire uveal tract of unknown etiology, clinically characterized by an insidious onset, and a progressive course with exacerbations and almost invariably follows a penetrating wound involving uveal tissues of one eye.

Pathogenesis

Believed to be an autoimmune response to a retinal, retinal pigment epithelium (RPE) or choroidal antigen that involves a cell-mediated immune response.

Clinical Features

The eye, which has suffered the injury is called the exciting eye and the other eye, which is subsequently inflamed is called the sympathizing eye. May appear as anterior uveitis or choroiditis to a severe panuveitis with mutton-fat KPs. Focal elevated choroidal infiltrates are common in midperiphery; Dalen-Fuchs spots:

1. Papillitis and exudative RD may occur in severe cases.
2. Chorioretinal scarring frequently seen when inflammation subsides ('sunset glow' fundus).

Diagnosis

Usually occurs within 3 months of injury to exciting eye earliest within 9–10 days of injury. History of a penetrating wound and a bilateral panuveitis serves as basis for diagnosis.

Fundus fluorescein angiography: Multiple persistent foci of leakage from which dye may spread coalescent pools of dye are seen in areas of exudative RD.

Ultrasonography: Shows choroidal thickening.

Differential Diagnosis

- Harada's syndrome
- Bilateral phacoanaphylactic endophthalmitis.

Treatment

Prophylaxes are the following:

1. May be prevented by enucleating the injured eye within 2 weeks of injury. Enucleation after that time is not preventive.
2. Prophylactic corticosteroids do not prevent development of SO.
3. Anti-inflammatory therapy helps to suppress the inflammation as soon as possible and helps to continue treatment for an extended period. Topical steroids may control very mild cases, but usually needs large doses (1–1.5 mg/kg) prednisolone initially. Later on dosage may be tapered and maintenance therapy given till 3–6 months.
4. Immunosuppressant may be given in cases where steroids either do not control inflammation or produce unacceptable side effects.

Complication

Complications are band keratopathy, cataract, glaucoma, macular edema and scarring, RD, phthisis bulbi.

Vogt-Koyanagi-Harada Disease

Idiopathic bilateral (B/L) chronic granulomatous uveitis involving the eye with associated extraocular involvement including pleocytosis in cerebrospinal fluid (CSF), dysgeusia, alopecia, poliosis and vitiligo.

Entities

Vogt-Koyanagi syndrome: Characterized by chronic anterior uveitis associated with alopecia, vitiligo and dysacusis.

Harada's disease: Characterized by bilateral exudative uveitis primarily in posterior segment of the eye accompanied by CSF pleocytosis.

Pathogenesis

1. Mainly 40–50 age group.
2. Due to autoimmune reaction to melanocytes.

Clinical Features

Four stages of clinical features are the following.

Prodromal: Flu-like symptoms such as fever, headache, etc. and within 1–2 days patients complain of blurring of vision, photophobia, and injection of bulbar conjunctiva, ocular pain and metamorphopsia.

Uveitic: Cells in both AC and B/L exudative RD in typical cases.

Chronic phase: Elevation of neural retina, which gradually disappears with absorption of subretinal fluid. Depigmentation occurs in fundus, which give rise to sunset glow appearance, following degeneration of RPE.

Sugiura's sign—depigmentation of corneal limbus noticed in the chronic phase.

Recurrent: The anterior uveitis is more predominant than posterior. Retinal vasculitis and CNVM can develop as secondary reaction to the long-standing choroidal inflammation.

Diagnosis

Fundus fluorescein angiography: Early stage subretinal exudation seen as multiple pinpoint hyperfluorescent spots at the level of RPE, which gradually enlarge. Dye leaks through RPE and accumulates in subretinal space.

Indocyanine green: Hypofluorescence due to choroidal nonperfusion. CNV may also be visualized.

Ultrasonography: Diffuse thickening of posterior choroid, serous detachment of retina, etc.

CSF analysis: Pleocytosis is seen in 80% patients within 1 week.

Differential Diagnosis

Sympathetic ophthalmia, central serous retinopathy, posterior scleritis, acute posterior multifocal placoid pigment epitheliopathy (APMPPE).

Treatment

Early active cases:

1. High doses of steroids should be given. IV methylprednisolone followed by oral steroids for 2–3 months with gradual tapering.
2. Topical steroids and cycloplegics.
3. Immunosuppressant like azathioprine, cyclophosphamide and cyclosporine can be used when there is intolerance to steroids.

Complications

- Posterior subcapsular cataract
- Secondary angle-closure glaucoma
- Choroidal neovascular membrane.

UVEITIS OF UNKNOWN CAUSES

- Fuchs' heterochromic iridocyclitis
- Posner-Schlossman syndrome
- Drug induced
- Schwartz syndrome
- White dot syndrome
- Serpiginous choroidopathy.

Fuchs' Heterochromic Iridocyclitis

- Fuchs' heterochromic iridocyclitis is a low-grade idiopathic chronic cyclitis
- Mainly in 35–40 years
- Unilateral (U/L) involvement typically
- Patients have a quiet appearing eye with decreased vision due to development of cataract
- S/L examination shows fine, stellate KPs, which cover the entire corneal endothelium
- Mild AC reaction with minimal flare, no synechiae, iris heterochromia (involved iris to appear light colored)
- Gonio: Fine, friable vessels are seen crossing the trab meshwork in 20%–30% cases

- A surgical intervention into the AC produces filiform hemorrhage from these vessels termed as Amsler sign
- Complications: Cataract, glaucoma.

Posner-Schlossman Syndrome

- Present as acute unilateral elevation of IOP
- More in 30–60 years male
- Patient complains of blurring of vision and periorbital discomfort
- On examination (O/E): Non-injected eye with paucity of anterior chamber cells with occasional small non-pigmented KPs
- IOP elevated despite open angle
- Rx: lowering IOP during the period of glaucomatocyclitic crises
- Due to inflammatory components, therapy with topical steroids may shorten duration of IOP rise.

Drug-induced Anterior Uveitis

- Rifabutin is used in Rx or prophylaxis of *Mycobacterium avium,* complex infection in AIDS
- Cidofovir: Typically U/L anterior uveitis with mild cellular reaction and fibrinoid response.

Schwartz Syndrome

- Described as increased IOP with open angle, anterior uveitis and rhegmatogenous RD
- Management: Surgical Rx of RD, topical IOP lowering agents.

White Dot Syndrome

Inflammatory disorders of unknown cause involving outer retina, RPE or choroid or a combination:

- Unilateral (U/L) or bilateral (B/L)
- 2nd to 6th decade
- Variable inflammatory cells in AC and vitreous humor depending on disease
- Serological evaluation is negative
- Usually self-limiting, but variable prognosis depending on the disease
- Include APMPPE, multiple evanescent white dot syndrome (MEWDS), birdshot chorioretinopathy, punctate inner choroidopathy (PIC).

Serpiginous Choroidopathy

Serpiginous choroidopathy (Fig. 17.42) is an uncommon, idiopathic, chronic progressive bilateral disease usually occurs between 4th and 6th decades.

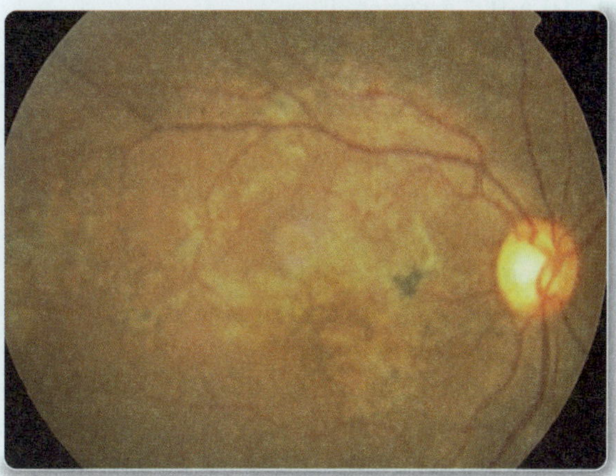

FIGURE 17.42: Serpiginous choroidopathy

Clinically, active lesions consist of deep, cream-colored lesions with hazy borders usually starts around optic disk and spreads outward in all directions. Successive attacks result in extension of lesion from the peripapillary area in an irregular, snake-like manner and hence the name. Inactive lesions consist of residual, scalloped, atrophic punched out areas.

Complication

Choroidal neovascular membrane can occur occasionally.

Treatment

Systemic steroids and/or immunosuppressants.

UVEITIS IN CHILDREN

Uveitis is a potentially vision threatening condition in the pediatric population.

Anterior Uveitis in Children

In children the major causes of anterior uveitis are listed below:

1. Idiopathic.
2. Infectious:
   a. Bacterial.
   b. Viral.
   c. Parasitic.
   d. Fungal.
3. Noninfectious:
   a. Traumatic:
      i. Due to blunt injury; intraocular foreign body (IOFB) has to be ruled out.

b. HLA-B27 associated:
   i. Ankylosing spondylitis.
   ii. Reiter's syndrome.
   iii. Psoriatic arthritis.
   iv. Inflammatory bowel disease (Crohn's disease and ulcerative colitis).

c. Sarcoid-associated uveitis.

d. Juvenile rheumatoid arthritis (JRA) associated:
   i. Most common cause of uveitis in children (20%).
   ii. More common in girls.
   iii. Uveitis tends to develop after arthritis.

Main causes to be ruled out are TB, syphilis, leprosy, herpes, varicella and HIV. Three major groups are of anterior uveitis in children are given below:

1. Systemic: Usually seen in children less than 5 years. Clinical features include fever, lymph node enlargement, hepatosplenomegaly, rashes, pericarditis, etc. Ocular involvement is uncommon.
2. Polyarticular: Here five or more joints are involved. About 7%–14% cases have uveitis. Constitute about 40% of JRA.
3. Pauciarticular: Constitute about 40% of JRA, four or less joints are involved. About 78%–91% have uveitis.

Girls of pauciarticular group with antinuclear antibody (ANA) positivity and negative RA factor has got the highest risk of developing uveitis.

Intermediate Uveitis

Intermediate uveitis accounts for 25% of all pediatric uveitis. Common causes of visual loss are due to cataract, CME, band keratopathy, glaucoma, retinal detachment, vitreous hemorrhage and optic disk edema.

Posterior Uveitis

Common causes are:

- Toxoplasmosis
- Toxocariasis
- Postviral
- Sarcoidosis
- Masquerade syndrome.

These are primary neoplasms or secondary deposits in the eye, which simulate uveitis or produce uveal inflammation and may be mistaken as uveitis. Conditions are given below:

- Retinoblastoma
- Leukemia
- Juvenile xanthogranuloma
- Retinitis pigmentosa
- Intraocular foreign body
- Peripheral retinal detachment.

Toxoplasmosis

Congenital systemic toxoplasmosis can occur in three forms:

1. Inactive at birth.
2. Active at birth with 3 'Cs' (convulsions, intracranial calcifications, chorioretinitis).
3. Recurrent (just like acquired).

Bilateral macular scar represents congenital variety. Active white retinitis in the absence of a scar represents acquired disease. An active patch of retinitis adjacent to older scar represents either congenital or acquired disease.

Toxocariasis

Toxocariasis is caused by *Toxocara canis.* It is usually unilateral. Three forms of presentations occur in children:

1. Chronic endophthalmitis:
   a. Younger age group; 2–9 years.
   b. Severe visual loss due to vitritis and leukocoria.
   c. Signs of anterior uveitis will be present.
2. Posterior pole granuloma:
   a. Occurs in children between 6 and 14 years.
   b. Leukocoria and strabismus will be there.
   c. Solitary white elevated mass in the macula with overlying vitritis will be seen.
3. Peripheral granuloma:
   a. Seen in older children; it presents with poor vision and strabismus.
   b. Spherical whitish lesion in the retinal periphery associated with tractional bands causing macular heterotopia.

Syphilis-associated Uveitis

Ocular involvement can be seen either acquired or congenital form.

Acquired form: Vitritis chorioretinitis, vasculitis, optic neuritis and optic atrophy are the features.

Congenital form: Salt and pepper fundus with optic atrophy may be seen.

Iritis and interstitial keratitis are the other ocular findings.

Rubella-associated Uveitis

Ocular involvement occurs both in congenital and acquired forms.

Congenital rubella: Salt and pepper fundus with pale optic nerve. Cataract, glaucoma are other ocular associations.

Acquired form: Conjunctivitis, iritis, bilateral retinitis, cataract and glaucoma.

Masquerade Syndromes

Masquerade syndromes are a group of disorders that occur with intraocular inflammation and often misdiagnosed as chronic idiopathic uveitis. Many are malignant disorders; early diagnosis and prompt treatment critical.

Malignant

- Intraocular lymphoma
- Non-Hodgkin's lymphoma of CNS:
  - Systemic non-Hodgkin's lymphoma metastatic to eye
  - Hodgkin's lymphoma.
- Carcinoma metastasis to eye: Renal, lungs, breast
- Uveal melanoma
- Diffuse hyperplasia of uvea
- Childhood malignancies: Retinoblastoma, leukemia, medulloepithelioma, juvenile xanthogranuloma, etc.
- Paraneoplastic conditions: Carcinoma-associated retinopathy.

Non-malignant Disorders

- Intraocular foreign body
- Retinal detachment
- Retinal degenerations
- Pigment dispersion syndrome
- Myopic degeneration
- Postoperative infections: Fungal, *Propionibacterium acnes*
- Drug induced: Rifabutin, didanosine, cidofovir.

Careful evaluation of the case history and examination of the eye are essential to differentiate the condition from a true uveitis. The management will depend on the underlying cause.

Neovascularization of the Iris (Rubeosis Iridis)

Neovascularization of the iris (NVI) or rubeosis iridis occurs commonly in eyes having proliferative diabetic retinopathy or central retinal vein obstruction (Fig. 17.43).

It is characterized by the development of new, branching and enlarged vessels in the iris. It usually starts at pupillary border and can occur in the angle of the AC. NVI may be associated with signs of iritis.

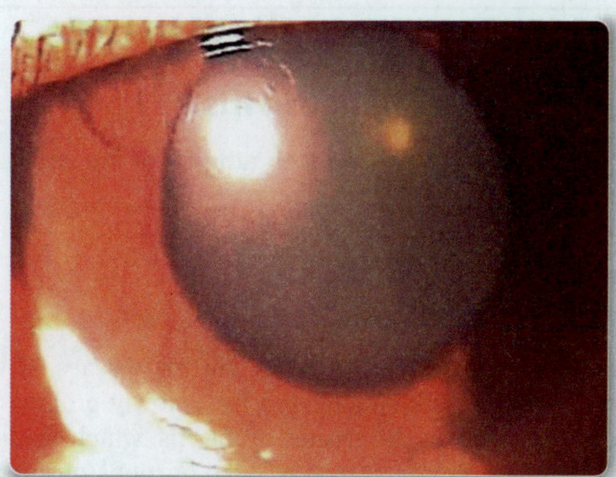

FIGURE 17.43: Neovascularization of iris

Complication

1. Secondary glaucoma: A rise in IOP occurs, initially with an open AC angle and later results in an intractable secondary angle-closure glaucoma (neovascular glaucoma).
2. Recurrent hyphema due to bleeding from the new vessels, which will aggravate the secondary glaucoma.

Treatment

1. Panretinal photocoagulation of an ischemic retina prevents the development of neovascular glaucoma.
2. If the ocular media are hazy, anterior retinal cryopexy would be as effective.
3. A trabeculectomy with adjuvant administration of mitomycin C or a drainage implant is used to control the raised IOP. The visual prognosis is poor.
4. If the eye is blind and painful, enucleation can be done.

Uveal Effusion Syndrome

A diagnosis of idiopathic uveal effusion syndrome is made after excluding all other inflammatory and hydrostatic causes of uveal effusion. The basic pathogenesis is a transudation of fluid from the vascular uvea with extravasation from the choriocapillaris into the suprachoroidal space and within the uveal tissues. The result is bilateral choroidal and ciliochoroidal effusion and subsequent detachment.

Iris Nevus

Iris nevus is usually benign and is due to congenital aggregation of pigment cells (Fig. 17.44).

DEGENERATIVE CHANGES IN UVEA

Degenerative Change in Iris

Depigmentation of the iris with atrophy of the stroma is seen in old people.

Essential (Progressive) Atrophy of the Iris

Essential atrophy (Fig. 17.45) of the iris disease of unknown etiology is characterized by a slowly progressive atrophic change in the tissues of the iris, which leads to the complete disappearance of large portions of this tissue. It forms part of the iridocorneal endothelial (ICE) syndromes (Fig. 17.46).

Synechiae, corectopia, iris atrophy from ischemia, ectropion uveae, dyscoria (abnormal shape of the pupil), polycoria (more than one pupil due to secondary holes in the iris) and nodules in the iris, glaucoma, etc. may be present.

Iridoschisis

Iridoschisis usually occurs as a degenerative senile phenomenon. A high incidence of glaucoma (almost 50%) is reported and is usually of the angle-closure type.

Iris Cysts

Iris cysts are uncommon, unilateral lesions, which may be primary or secondary.

Primary iris cysts: These may arise from either the iris pigment epithelium or rarely, the stroma. These may be epithelial cysts or stromal cysts.

Secondary iris cysts: Develop following intraocular surgery (Fig. 17.47), ocular trauma or prolonged use of long-acting miotics like pilocarpine.

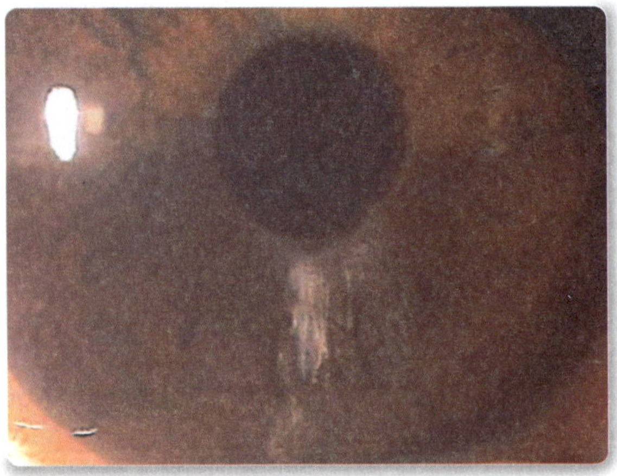

FIGURE 17.44: Iris nevus

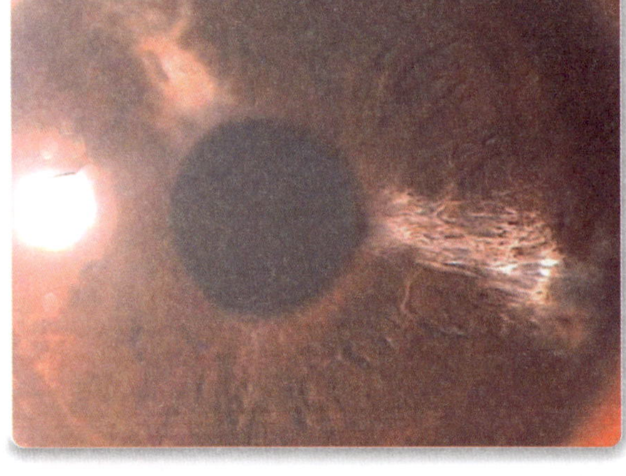

FIGURE 17.45: Essential (progressive) atrophy of the iris

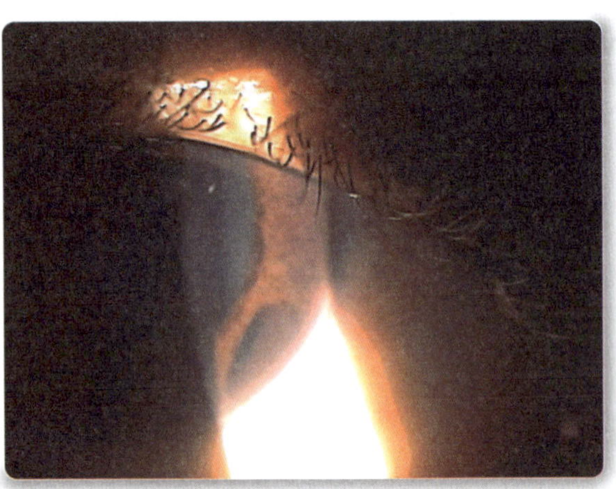

FIGURE 17.46: Iridocorneal endothelial syndrome

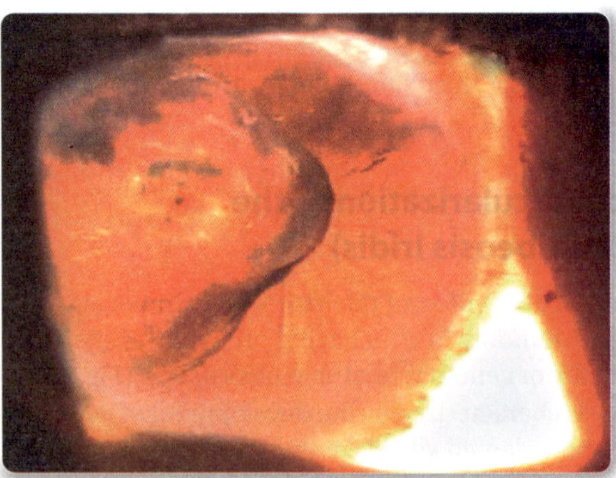

FIGURE 17.47: Iris cyst

Pigment Dispersion Syndrome

Pigment dispersion syndrome is associated with dispersion of iris pigment in the anterior segment of the eye because of mechanical rubbing of the posterior surface of the iris against the zonules of the lens. Melanin from the iris neuroepithelium is phagocytosed by the corneal endothelial cells, seen on slit lamp examination as a vertical spindle (Krukenberg's spindle). There is deposition of melanin pigment in the trabecular meshwork (Sampaolesi's line) and glaucoma.

Degenerative Changes in the Choroid

Secondary Degenerations

Secondary degenerations following inflammatory lesion culminating in localized spots of complete atrophy.

Primary Choroidal Degenerations

Central choroidal atrophy is most commonly the result of myopia or obliterative vasosclerosis due to aging. Degenerative changes are common in pathological axial myopia; these are particularly marked around the optic disk and in the central area of the fundus involving the choroid and retina (Fig. 17.48).

In the majority of cases of moderate myopia, there is a myopic crescent (refer Fig. 17.48). This is a white crescent at the temporal border of the disk or it may form an annular crescent all around the disk. There is a gradual disappearance of the small vessels of the choroid with the development of lacunae forming irregular areas of atrophy.

Small hemorrhages and occasionally choroidal thromboses are not uncommon in the macular area. Choroidal thromboses may give rise to the sudden formation of a circular claret colored or black spot at the fovea, which may persist (Foster Fuchs' spots). Linear breaks in Bruch's membrane (called 'lacquer cracks') may be seen as fine lines.

Degenerative changes, typically those of cystoid and lattice degeneration are also common at the periphery of the retina. These may lead to the formation of retinal holes resulting in a retinal detachment.

Essential (Gyrate) Atrophy of the Choroid

Essential atrophy condition is due to defective activity of the enzyme ornithine ketoacid aminotransferase and is an inborn error of amino acid metabolism. Usually starts as areas of irregular chorioretinal atrophy in early adult life, which finally coalesces so that practically the entire fundus disappears, with preservation of only the macula.

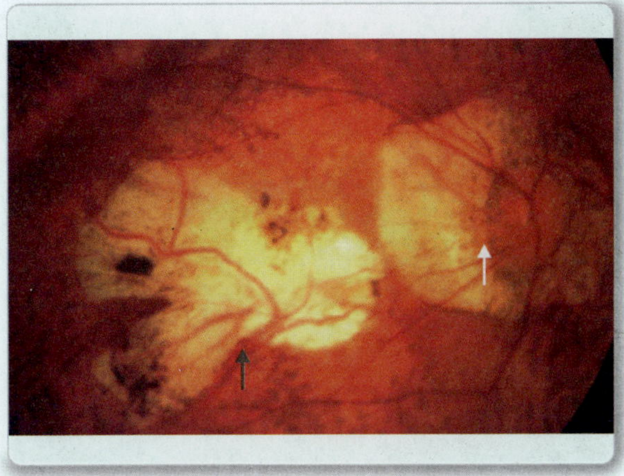

FIGURE 17.48: Myopic chorioretinal degeneration (black arrow) with myopic crescent (white arrow)

Choroideremia

Choroideremia is a hereditary degeneration and the most prominent symptoms are night blindness; and extreme concentric contraction of the visual fields.

Albinism

Albinism is a genetically determined, heterogeneous group of disorders of melanin synthesis in which either the eyes alone (ocular albinism) or the eyes, skin and hair (oculocutaneous albinism) may be affected. The latter may be either tyrosinase positive or tyrosinase negative.

Signs: As follows:

1. Visual acuity is usually less than 6/60 due to foveal hypoplasia.
2. Nystagmus is usually pendular and horizontal. It usually increases in bright illumination and tends to lessen in severity with age.
3. The iris is diaphanous and translucent giving rise to a pink-eyed appearance (Fig. 17.49).
4. The fundus lacks pigment and shows conspicuously large choroidal vessels. There is also foveal hypoplasia with absence of the foveal pit and lack of vessels forming the perimacular arcades. Associated optic nerve hypoplasia is uncommon (Fig. 17.50).
5. The optic chiasma has fewer uncrossed nerve fibers than normal so that the majority from each eye crosses to the contralateral hemisphere. This can be demonstrated by visual evoked potential.
6. Other features commonly seen include high refractive errors of various types, positive angle kappa, squint and absence of stereopsis.

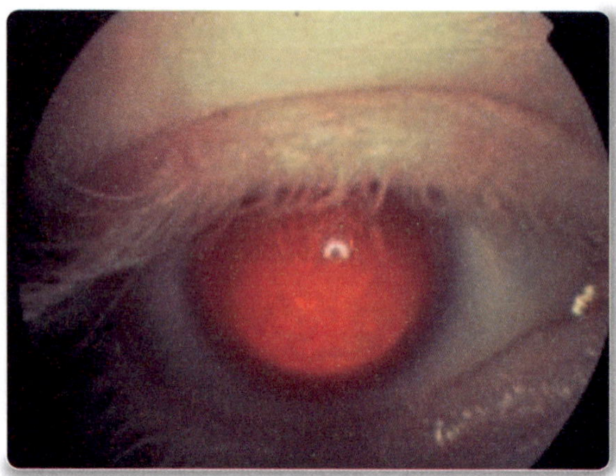

FIGURE 17.49: Ocular albinism

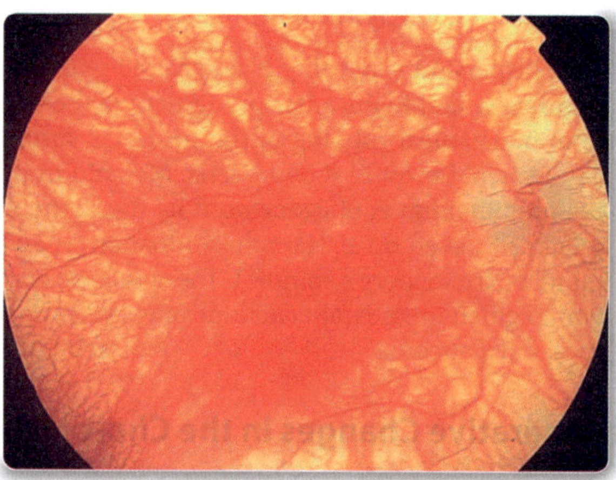

FIGURE 17.50: Fundus in albinism with visible choroidal vessels due to lack of pigment in retinal pigment epithelium layer

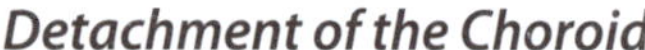

Detachment of the Choroid

Detachment of the choroid is a condition in which severe exudation or bleeding occurs into the suprachoroidal space, which results in globular elevation of the choroid, which will be seen as dark globular lesions through the pupil. It includes the following.

Causes: Severe choroidal inflammations like SO, VKH, postoperative inflammation or expulsive hemorrhage.

Choroidal detachment is often present in eyes, which have been lost by plastic iridocyclitis or glaucoma and this may also result from severe hemorrhage or a neoplasm. This condition also commonly occurs soon after intraocular operations such as trabeculectomy with excessive filtration.

The AC is shallow and on ophthalmoscopic examination the detached choroid is seen through the pupil as a dark mass. It may also be visible as a dark-brown mass by oblique illumination, the IOP of the eye remains low.

Diagnosis: Confirmed by ultrasound scan.

Treatment: Treat the underlying cause. Control the inflammation with systemic steroids. If there is any wound leak or overfiltration after trabeculectomy that has to be corrected. Sclerotomy and drainage of the suprachoroidal fluid or blood may be required if other measures fail.

Lens

18

Girija Devi PS

APPLIED ANATOMY

The lens is a unique structure in the body. It consists of only one type of cell—epithelium enclosed in a capsule, which is the basement membrane of the epithelial cells. It is biconvex in shape. The circumference of the lens is called the equator. The centers of the anterior and posterior capsules are called the anterior and posterior poles respectively. The lens capsule is elastic and it molds the lens substance during accommodation. The anterior capsule is thicker than the posterior capsule and it is thinnest at the posterior pole. Consequently, the change in curvature during accommodation takes place more on the posterior surface.

All epithelial layers in the body grow and multiply, and the oldest cells get thrown off. Similarly, the lens epitheliums also grow and multiply, but these cannot get discarded since it is completely enclosed by the capsule.

The epithelial cells on the anterior capsule and the equatorial region show the maximum mitotic activity. The newly formed cells elongate, lose their organelle and form lens fibers. As new and new lens fibers are formed, the older ones get buried and compacted. It loses their organelle including the nucleus, mitochondria, etc. and the protein content increases. The oldest fibers occupy the most central part of the lens and the newest fibers occupy the most superficial part. The innermost fibers form the embryonic nucleus and the next layer is the fetal nucleus, which corresponds to the lens fibers formed by the time the child is born; next is the infantile nucleus corresponding to the lens at puberty and finally the adult nucleus corresponding the lens in early adult life. The most superficial soft lens fibers form the cortex (Fig. 18.1).

For practical purposes, from the surgeon's point of view, the innermost hard biconvex mass is the nucleus, the not so hard layer covering this nucleus is the epinucleus and the soft superficial layers, which can be easily removed by irrigation and aspiration is the cortex.

The lens does not have blood supply or nerve supply. Since it contains only epithelium, it cannot undergo any inflammatory process. As it does not contain nerve fibers, any injury or diseases of the lens cannot produce pain.

BIOCHEMISTRY

The lens is mostly composed of water (66%) and 33% of its weight is proteins. The protein content is twice in that of most tissues. Lens proteins, depending on their water solubility, are divided into two groups—water-soluble protein (called crystallins) and water-insoluble proteins. In a young lens, 80% of the protein is water-soluble type. As age increases, lens proteins aggregate to form larger particles, which are water-insoluble. So, as age advances, the water-soluble proteins decrease and the concentration of water-insoluble proteins increase. The increase in water-insoluble proteins does not affect its transparency. But its concentration is much more in cataractous lenses (Fig. 18.2) compared to clear lenses of the same age and the concentration correlates with the degree of opacification.

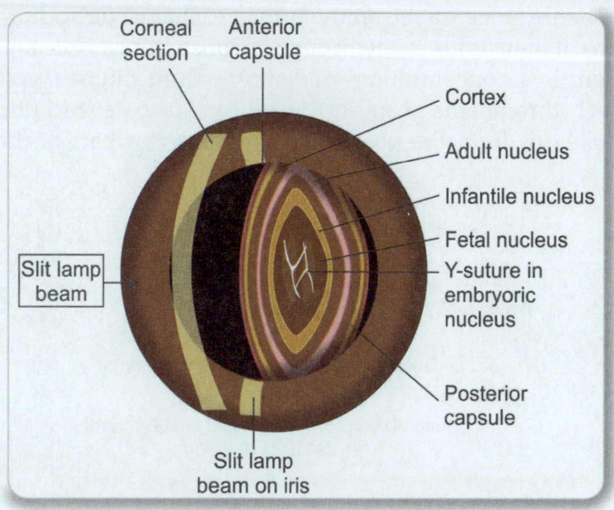

FIGURE 18.1: Layers of the lens as seen with a slit lamp

In addition, in cataracts, proteins are highly cross-linked by non-disulfide bonds also. In nuclear cataracts, the insoluble proteins contain yellow to brown pigments, which give them their characteristic color.

Metabolism

Maintenance of transparency of the lens depends on its metabolism. Lens depends on glucose for its energy requirements. Glucose enters the lens from the aqueous by passive diffusion and by a metabolic transfer process. The O_2 concentration in the lens is low. So, the metabolism is mainly by anaerobic glycolysis. The metabolic waste products diffuse into the aqueous.

When the blood sugar level rises (in uncontrolled diabetes), excess glucose will reach the lens via aqueous. In this situation, the sorbitol pathway will be activated. Since the enzyme polyol dehydrogenase, which converts sorbitol to fructose is not very efficient within the lens and the lens capsule is poorly permeable to sorbitol, retention of sorbitol occurs in the lens. This increases the osmotic pressure within the lens drawing in water and leading to swelling and opacification of the lens (Fig. 18.3).

A similar process occurs when galactose reaches the lens in excess in disorders of galactose metabolism.

Maintenance of Lens Water and Cation Balance

Proper maintenance of water and electrolyte balance is important for maintaining lens transparency. Lens has higher level of potassium ions and amino acids than the surrounding aqueous, but lower levels of sodium and chloride ions, and water. Potassium, amino acids and other molecules are actively transported into the anterior lens substance via the epithelium in exchange for sodium ions. It then diffuses out through the posterior capsule and there is a concentration gradient. Sodium diffuses passively through the posterior capsule and its concentration decreases from the posterior to the anterior part of the lens where it is exchanged for potassium by the epithelial cells. The lens contains higher concentration of calcium. The high concentration of calcium in the lens epithelial cells and lens fibers are maintained by the calcium pump (Ca^{2+}-ATPase). Low- or high-levels of calcium can interfere with lens metabolism. The amino acid transport takes place on the anterior surface by the lens epithelium based on sodium pump. The waste products of metabolism leave the lens by simple diffusion.

PATHOLOGY

Being comprised of only epithelium and its basement membrane (capsule) the pathological changes the lens can undergo are mainly degenerative either due to age or various toxic, metabolic or traumatic insults—resulting in loss of transparency.

Changes with Increasing Age

As the age increases, and more and more new lens fibers are added, the lens increases in weight and thickness. The soluble protein fraction aggregate and undergo chemical modification to form insoluble proteins. These protein aggregates increase the refractive index of lens and increases the scattering of light making the lens appear gray in diffuse illumination, without affecting the transparency of the lens or vision. The glutathione and potassium concentration decreases with age and the sodium and calcium concentration increases.

Pathology of Age-related Cataract

Genetic and multifactorial factors play a role in the pathogenesis of cataract. The etiopathogenesis of cataract is still not completely understood.

Three types of age-related cataract can occur:

1. Nuclear.
2. Cortical.
3. Posterior subcapsular.

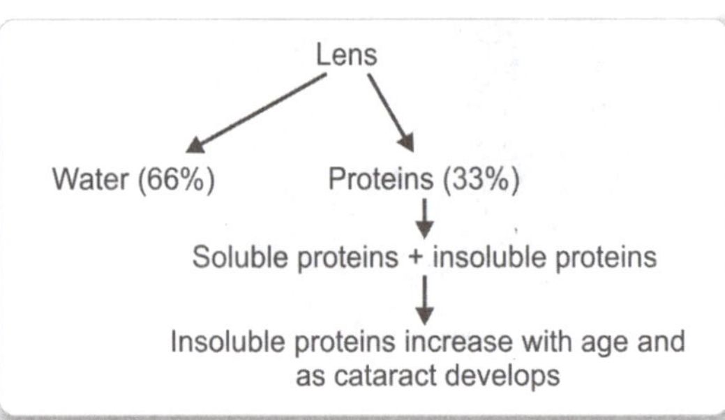

FIGURE 18.2: Biochemistry of lens

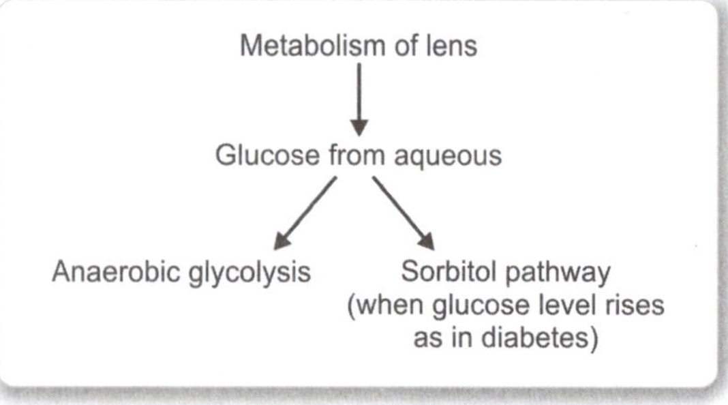

FIGURE 18.3: Metabolism of lens

Most people show changes suggestive of more than one type.

Nuclear Cataract

Histopathologically, the nuclear cataract shows an exaggeration of the normal age-related changes. The insoluble protein aggregates show many pigmented components, which give the nuclear cataract its color that ranges from yellow, amber, brown and finally black as the cataractous changes progress. Histopathologically, the only distinguishing feature from normal age changes is an increased number of lamellar membrane whorls in nuclear cataracts under the electron microscope.

Cortical Cataract

In cortical cataract, there is disruption of the structure of the mature lenses fibers. There is loss of permeability of the cell membrane leading to loss of metabolites from the affected lens fibers. This leads to protein oxidation and precipitation. Vacuoles and fluid clefts appear between cortical lamellae leading to **lamellar separation**. Wedge-shaped opacities appear near the periphery of the lens with the pointed ends of the wedge toward the center of the lens. Initially this involves the middle portion of the lens fibers with the anterior and posterior ends remaining clear. Later the anterior and posterior areas are also involved and the opacities extend up to the center of the lens interfering with vision. The adjacent fibers are also subsequently affected thus increasing the width of the wedges. Finally, the whole of the lens will be involved resulting in mature cataract. Meanwhile, the nucleus will undergo progressive sclerosis.

If the condition is allowed to progress, it reaches the stage of hypermature cataract. There will be progressive liquefaction of the cortex and escape of fluid through the capsule. The capsule becomes wrinkled and shrunken with sometimes calcareous deposits and cholesterol crystals over it. Thus, capsule encloses the sclerotic nucleus in **hypermature sclerotic cataract.** Sometimes, the capsule remains impermeable to the liquefied cortex and the brown or black nucleus remains within the fluid cortex sinking to the lowest part of the lens, which depends on the position of the head. This is called **morgagnian cataract.**

Posterior Subcapsular Cataract

Posterior subcapsular (PSC) cataract is located in the posterior cortex usually in the central position. It is usually seen in younger population compared to the people affected with nuclear or cortical cataract. Similar PSC cataract can occur due to various other causes like trauma, ocular inflammation, use of steroids, etc.

Histopathologically, there is a posterior migration of lens epithelial cells to the central part of the posterior capsule, which undergo enlargement and degeneration. These swollen cells are called Wedl cells or bladder cells.

CONGENITAL ANOMALIES

Congenital Aphakia

Congenital aphakia is a rare anomaly often associated with other congenital anomalies of the eye. Either the lens fails to develop from the surface ectoderm (primary aphakia) or lens gets absorbed during the stage of development (secondary aphakia).

Lenticonus

Lenticonus is a localized conical protrusion of the anterior or posterior surface of the lens (Fig. 18.4). The anterior lenticonus may be associated with Alport's syndrome. The posterior lenticonus is more common and often bilateral.

Lentiglobus

In lentiglobus condition, there is a localized globular protrusion of the anterior or posterior surface of the lens (Fig. 18.5). The posterior lentiglobus is more common and is often associated with localized posterior polar cataract.

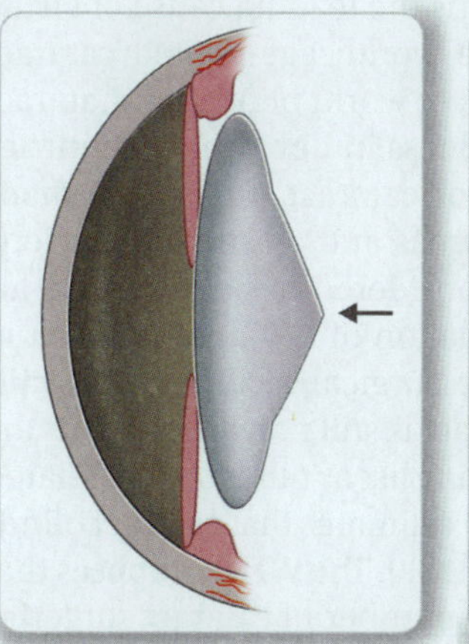

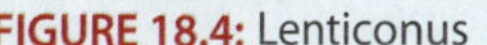

FIGURE 18.4: Lenticonus

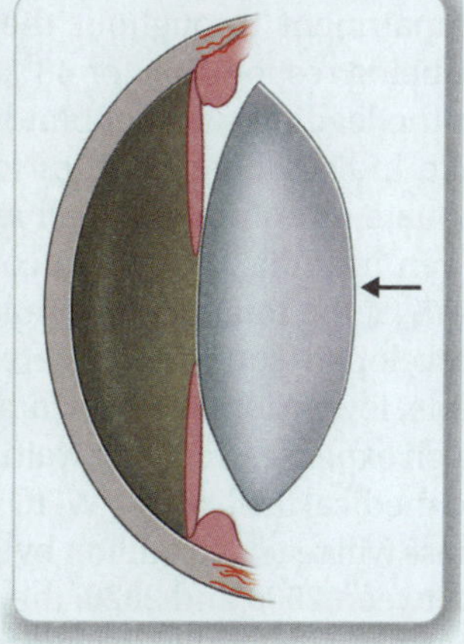

FIGURES 18.5: Lentiglobus

Lens Coloboma

Lens coloboma is a localized indentation of the equator of the lens (Fig. 18.6). The zonules in the region of the coloboma are weak or absent. This is often situated inferiorly and associated with coloboma of the uveal tract. It is due to defective closure of fetal fissure. Often there are localized cortical opacities near the coloboma.

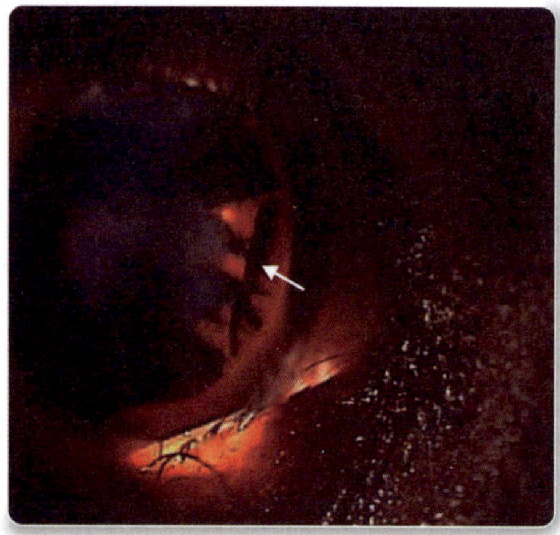

FIGURE 18.6: Lens coloboma with hypertrophied ciliary processes

Peters Anomaly or Anterior Segment Dysgenesis Syndrome

Peters anomaly is due to defective or incomplete separation of the lens vesicle from the surface ectoderm during development. There will be localized corneal opacities with adhesion between the lens and the cornea. Other lens anomalies that can occur with Peters anomaly are anterior polar cataract and microspherophakia.

Microspherophakia

In microspherophakia, the lens is smaller in shape and more spherical. The edge of the lens can be seen on dilatation of the pupil (Fig. 18.7). The spherical lens can block the pupil and can cause secondary angle-closure glaucoma.

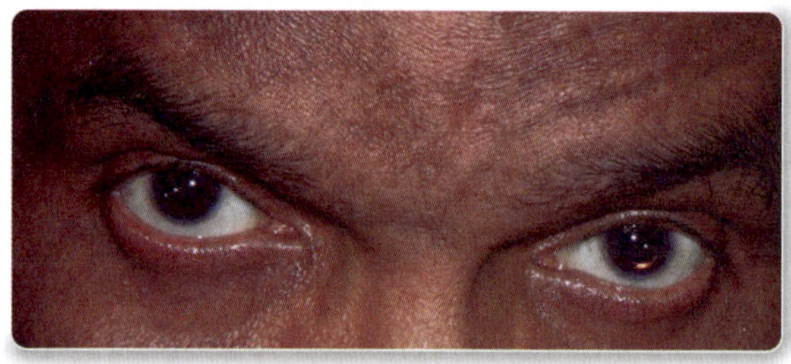

FIGURE 18.7: Microspherophakia

CATARACT

Cataract is defined as a congenital or acquired opacification of the lens or its capsule.

The word cataract is derived from the Latin word 'cataracta', means 'a cascade' or 'waterfall'. In ancient times it was believed that cataract is due to some 'bad humor' flowing in front of the lens and blocking vision.

Epidemiology

According to WHO, cataract is the leading cause of visual impairment throughout the world; age-related cataract is being responsible for 48% of world blindness. Cataract is the leading cause of blindness in developing countries like India, where facilities for cataract surgery are inadequate or do not reach all areas and all strata of society. Even in India, cataract is considered to be the cause for 50% of the total blind population of 150 million. Even in developed countries, where surgical facilities are available, low vision due to cataract is still prevalent due to the high expenses and long waiting list or other factors related to medical facility. The WHO estimates that cataract blindness will reach 40 million by 2020. The WHO proposes that between 2000 and 2020, the number of cataract surgeries performed worldwide have to be tripled to keep pace with the needs of the population.

Classification of Cataract

There is no internationally accepted uniform classification for cataract. It can be classified as given in Table 18.1.

Congenital

Congenital cataract is a lenticular opacity, which is present at birth.

Infantile Cataract

Infantile cataract is a lenticular opacity, which develops during the first year of life. Since most congenital cataracts are not noticed at the time of birth and are detected later, usually within the first year of life, both terms are often used synonymously.

Clinical features

Congenital cataract:

1. Can be unilateral or bilateral.
2. Can occur alone or associated with other congenital or inherited abnormalities.
3. Occurs in various morphological patterns and are named accordingly.

TABLE 18.1: Classification of cataract	
Congenital	**Acquired**
Zonular cataract	**Age-related cataract** Cortical cataract Nuclear cataract PSC cataract
Anterior polar cataract	**Metabolic cataract** Diabetes mellitus Galactosemia Wilson's disease Myotonic dystrophy
Posterior polar cataract	**Drug-induced cataract** Corticosteroids Phenothiazines Miotics Amiodarone Statins
Blue dot cataract	**Traumatic cataract** Contusion injury Penetrating injury Chemical injury Radiation injury Electrical injury
Nuclear cataract	**Complicated cataract** Chronic Uveitis Retinitis pigmentosa Long-standing retinal detachment High myopia Absolute glaucoma
Membranous cataract	
Sutural cataract	

4. The damage is usually limited to a particular area of the lens and does not progress or progresses very slowly.

Etiology

1. One-third cases form part of a syndrome or a disease:
   a. Genetic and metabolic diseases:
      - Down syndrome
      - Marfan syndrome
      - Lowe syndrome
      - Galactosemia
      - Alport's syndrome
      - Myotonic dystrophy
      - Fabry's disease.

   b. Maternal infections:
      - Rubella
      - Cytomegalovirus
      - Chickenpox
      - Syphilis
      - Toxoplasmosis.

   c. The ocular anomalies:
      - Aniridia
      - Peters anomaly.
2. One-third cases occur as an isolated inherited condition.
3. One-third cases are due to undetermined causes.

Lamellar or Zonular Cataract

Lamellar cataracts are the most common congenital cataract.

Causes

1. Usually inherited as an autosomal dominant trait.
2. These may also occur due to a period of maternal malnutrition.
3. Lack of vitamin D can interfere with the development of structures of epithelial origin. The enamel of the permanent teeth is also formed at this time and along with a lamellar cataract, these children usually have transverse lines across the permanent incisors and canines.

Influenced by genetic factors or toxic insult, the lens fibers formed at a particular period during the fetal stage or early infancy is affected. A sharply demarcated zone of opacity is formed. The earlier in life is the insult, the smaller and deeply buried will be the opacity and lesser the interference with vision. The lens fibers within and outside this zone of opacification will be clear.

Clinical features

In diffuse illumination a sharply demarcated disk-shaped opacity will be seen with clear lens matter in front of it. In cross sectional view with the slit lamp, the opacity will have a clear center and surrounded by clear lens outside (Figs 18.8A and B).

In some cases, there will be linear opacities surrounding the disk of opacity like the spokes of a wheel. These are called riders.

The extent to which these interfere with vision depends on the size and situation of the lamellar opacity. Small and deeply buried lamellar cataracts rarely interfere with vision and need no treatment. If these are larger, it can interfere with vision and need surgery. Lamellar cataracts rarely progress.

Anterior Capsular (Polar) Cataract

Causes

1. The cataract is frequently inherited as autosomal dominant condition or occurs due to a delayed formation of the anterior chamber (AC) during intrauterine life.

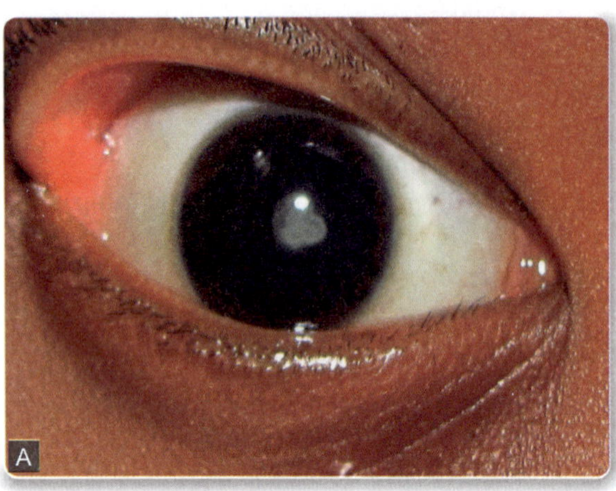

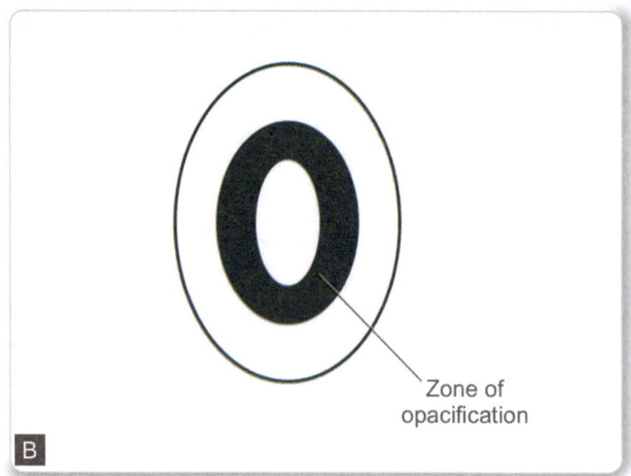

FIGURES 18.8A and B: Zonular cataract. **A.** Photograph; **B.** Diagrammatic representation of opacification zone.

2. Sometimes it can follow an intrauterine sepsis with corneal ulceration or following ophthalmia neonatorum. The corneal ulcer perforates and temporarily comes into contact with the anterior lens capsule leading to its opacification.

Clinical features

Anterior polar cataract (Fig. 18.9A) is usually small, bilateral and involves the capsule and the subcapsular cortex at the anterior pole. Sometimes a white plaque forms on the capsule, which projects into the AC in a pyramidal fashion and it is called **anterior pyramidal cataract** (Fig. 18.9B). When it involves the anterior subcapsular cortex, as the child grows and more and more lens fibers are formed, the anterior subcapsular cataract (Fig. 18.10) gets separated from the capsular opacity by the newly formed lens fibers and gets buried into the deeper layers of the cortex.

Anterior polar cataract is usually non-progressive and does not interfere with vision and hence require no treatment.

Posterior Polar Cataract

Causes

Posterior polar cataract may be inherited as an autosomal dominant trait or occurs associated with other congenital abnormalities like posterior lenticonus or persistence of the posterior part of the vascular sheath of the lens.

Clinical features

Posterior polar cataracts (Fig. 18.11) are much larger than the anterior polar variety. Since situated closer to the nodal point of the eye, these interfere with vision and often require surgical management.

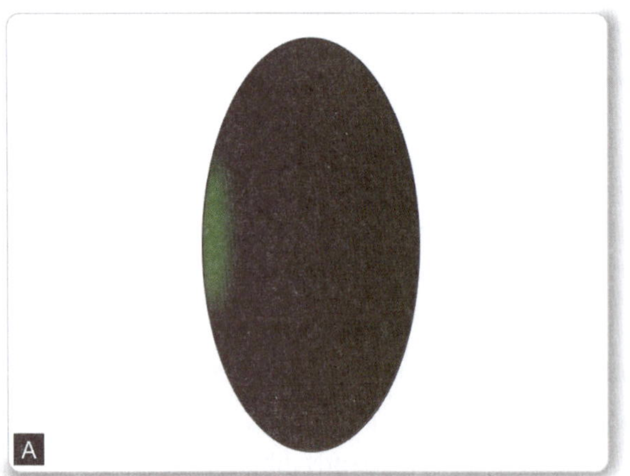

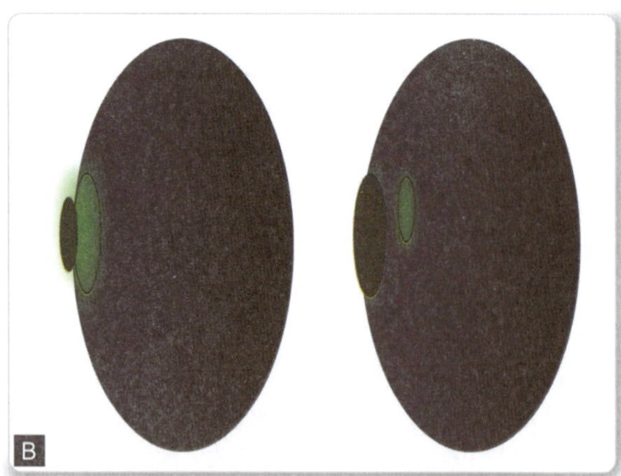

FIGURES 18.9A and B: **A.** Anterior polar cataract; **B.** Anterior pyramidal cataract (early and late forms).

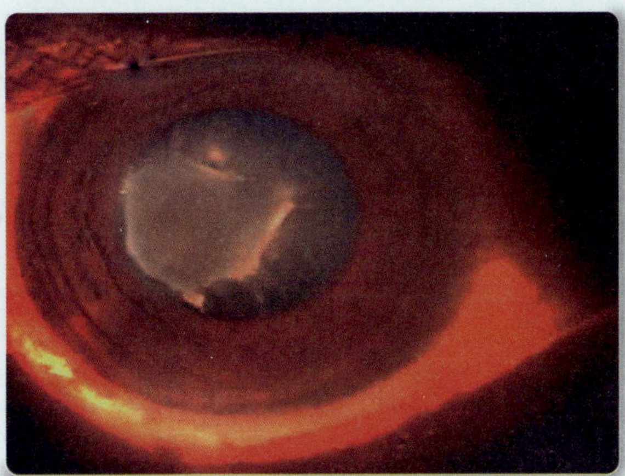

FIGURE 18.10: Anterior capsular cataract

Sutural Cataract

Sutural cataract is usually inherited as an autosomal dominant trait. These are opacification seen in a Y-shaped or stellate pattern seen along the sutural lines of the lens (Fig. 18.12). These are usually bilateral and symmetrical, and do not interfere with vision.

Coronary Cataract

Coronary cataract consists of a corona of club-shaped opacities situated in the cortex. These are situated in the periphery of the lens and can be seen only if the pupil is dilate. These do not interfere with vision and are non-progressive. These are often accidently detected when the eyes of a child or a young adult are dilated for checking refraction or for fundus evaluation (Fig. 18.13). The condition is also inherited as an autosomal dominant trait.

Cerulean or Blue Dot Cataract

Cerulean cataract consists of multiple small bluish opacities scattered all over the lens (Fig. 18.14). These do not interfere with vision.

Congenital Nuclear Cataract

In the congenital nuclear cataract, there is opacification of the embryonic nucleus alone or of both embryonic and fetal nuclei (Figs 18.15A to C). It is often associated with other congenital anomalies like microphthalmos (Figs 18.16A and B).

Progressive Type of Congenital Nuclear Cataract

Progressive type of congenital nuclear cataract can occur in association with maternal rubella infection in the first trimester of pregnancy.

At the time of birth, only the nucleus will be opaque or at times the whole lens will be pearly white in color. The nuclear cataract will subsequently progress to total opacification of the lens. Since rubella cataract grossly interferes with vision, surgery has to be done at the earliest depending on the extent of opacification of the lens. Congenital rubella cataract is often associated with other ocular abnormalities like congenital glaucoma, microphthalmos and pigmentary retinopathy. Systemic manifestations are deafness, mental retardation and cardiac abnormalities.

The systemic problems increase the risk for life during surgery. Live virus particles will be present in the lens up to the age of 3 years and the release of these virus particles will lead to severe postoperative inflammation.

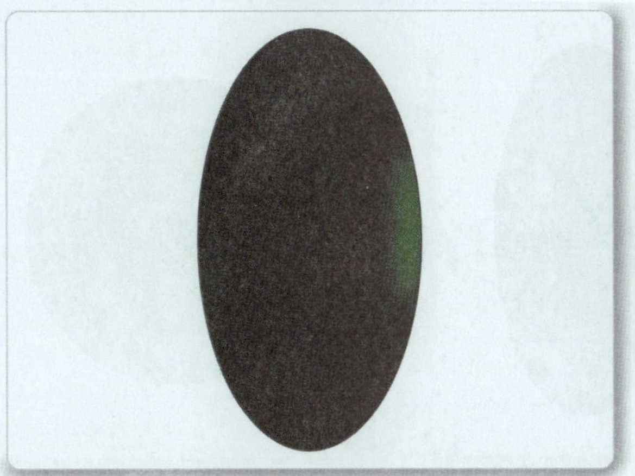

FIGURE 18.11: Posterior polar cataract

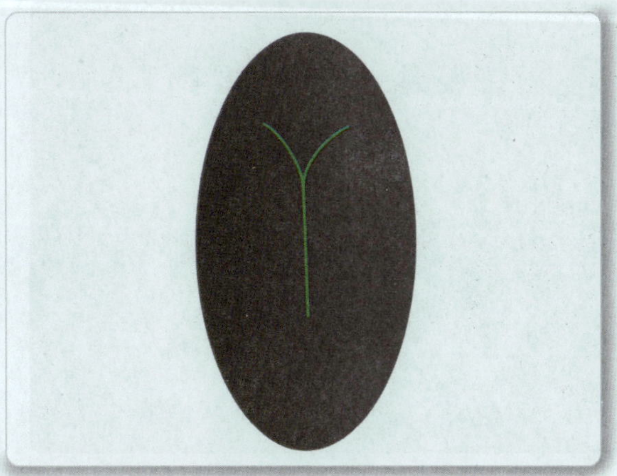

FIGURE 18.12: Sutural cataract

FIGURE 18.13: Coronary cataract

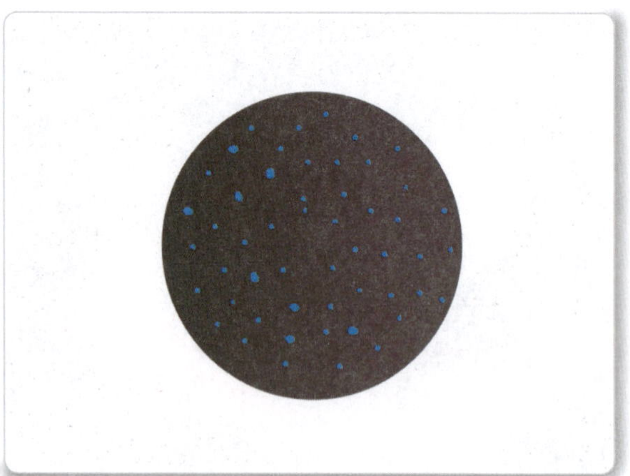

FIGURE 18.14: Blue dot cataract

Membranous Cataract

Membranous cataract (Fig. 18.17) results from absorption of the lens material in intrauterine life, leaving the opacified anterior and posterior capsules that fuse together to form a dense, white membranous cataract. These cause significant visual impairment and require surgery.

Acquired Cataract

Age-related Cataract

Age-related cataract was formerly called 'senile cataract'. The new term is age-related cataract, since it can occur in middle-aged people also and age is one of the important factors in its etiology. Etiology of it is multifactorial and not completely known.

Heredity: It is seen to run in families and affect the family members around the same age. Studies of identical twins and familial association have shown that genetic factors play a role in the development. The gene responsible has not yet been identified.

The depletion of the ozone layer and UV light are also considered to be important risk factors.

Clinical features

Three types of age-related cataract can occur:

1. Cortical.
2. Nuclear.
3. Posterior subcapsular.

Most people show changes suggestive of more than one type, but only one type of opacification will be predominant in them.

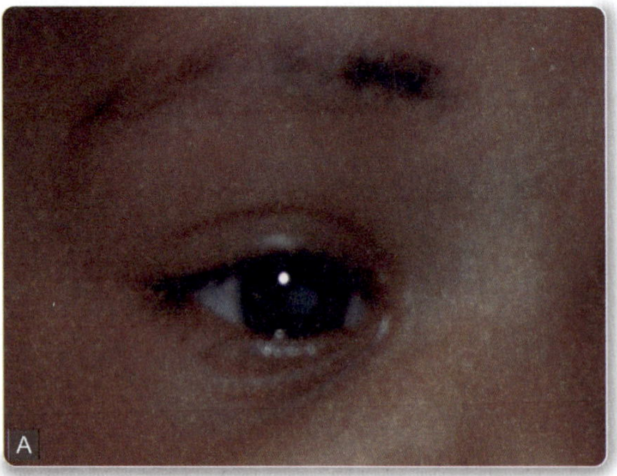

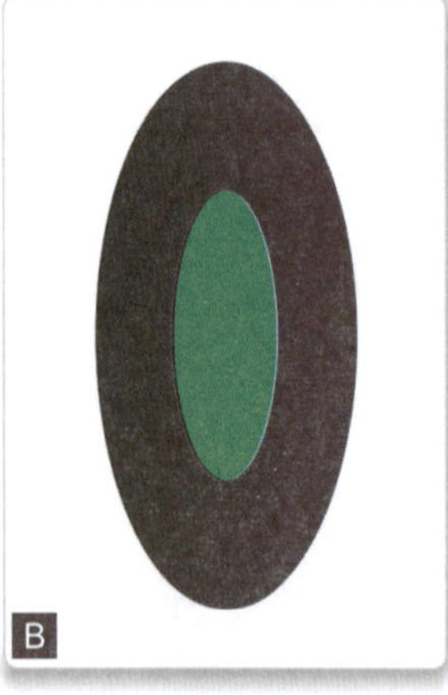

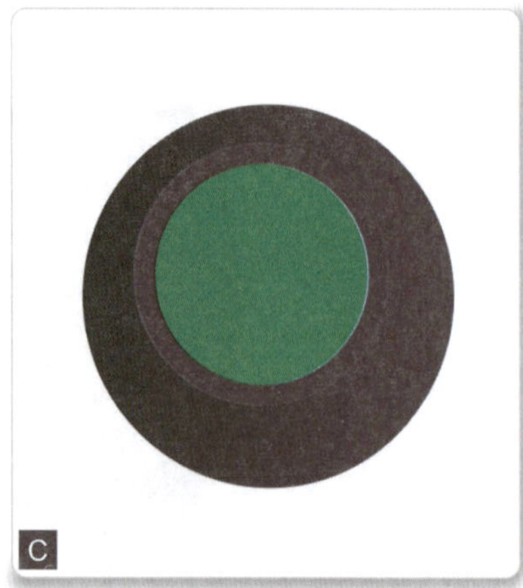

FIGURES 18.15A to C: Congenital nuclear cataract. **A.** Photograph; **B and C.** Diagrammatic representation.

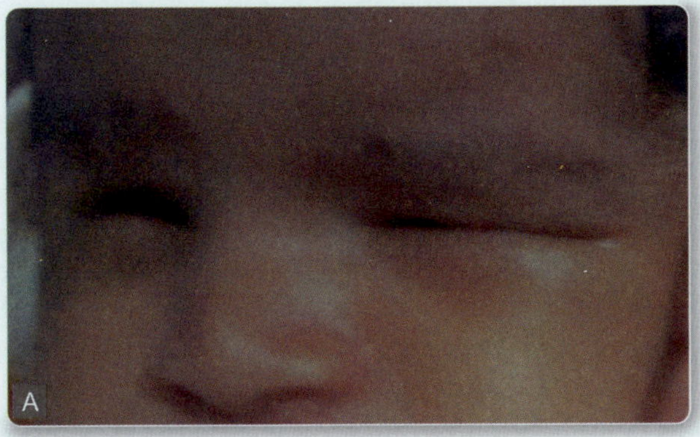

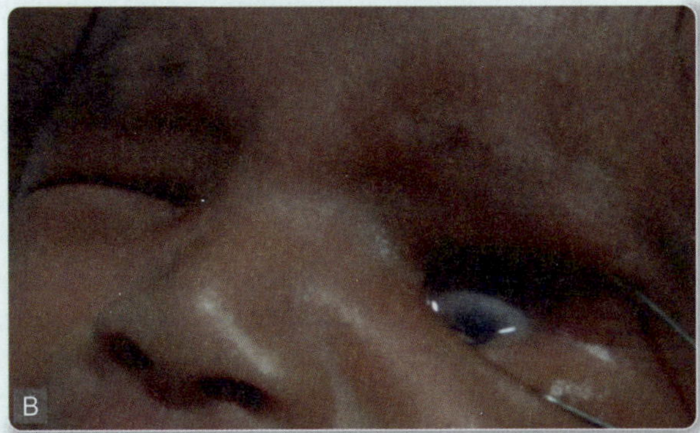

FIGURES 18.16A and B: Microphthalmos with corneal and lenticular opacities

Cortical Cataract

Normally a cortical cataract progresses in five stages and the symptoms also vary depending on the stage of the cortical cataract (Fig. 18.18):

1. Stage of lamellar separation: Under the slit lamp water clefts and vacuoles are seen in the anterior and posterior cortex.
2. Incipient cataract: Wedge-shaped opacities start appearing in the peripheral cortex with their pointed ends toward the center of the lens.
3. Intumescent cataract: The disintegration of lens fibers with loss of intracellular contents leads to imbibition of water into the lens. This leads to increase in the thickness of the lens and it becomes more spherical. This can lead to shallowing of the AC and lens-induced secondary glaucoma. This is called phacomorphic glaucoma. The stage of intumescence can follow the stage of lamellar separation, but in slowly progressing cataract intumescence usually occur as the lens opacity matures.
4. Mature cataract: Here the whole of the lens become opaque.
5. Hypermature cataract: If no surgery is undertaken even at the stage of mature cataract and the condition is allowed to progress, the cataract will go into the stage of hypermaturity. The whole cortex becomes liquefied and the fluid can leak through the capsule, leaving behind a thickened shrunken capsule forming a loose bag containing the nucleus—**hypermature sclerotic cataract.** If the capsule remains impermeable to the liquefied material, the lens becomes a pearly white fluid-filled bag with a brown or black nucleus sinking to its bottom. This is called **morgagnian cataract.**

Stage of lamellar separation: In the early stages of lamellar separation patient usually complains of colored halos around bright light and also glare, while driving at night. This is due to the scattering of the light by the fluid vacuoles in the lens. These colored halos can be differentiated from the halos seen in narrow angle glaucoma by the Fincham's test.

Fincham's stenopaic test: A stenopaic slit is passed before the eye across the visual pathway. As it passes the halos

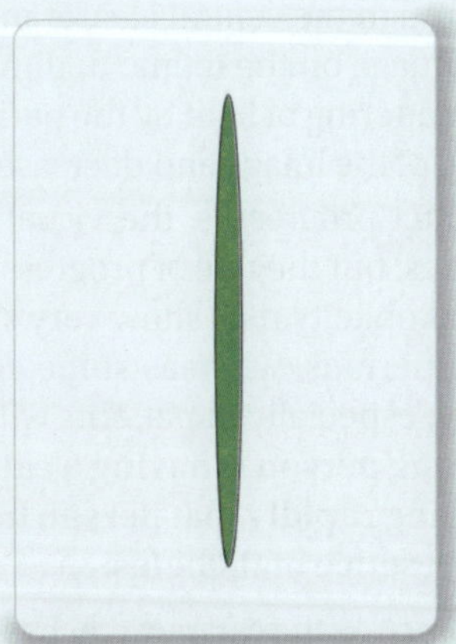

FIGURE 18.17: Membranous cataract

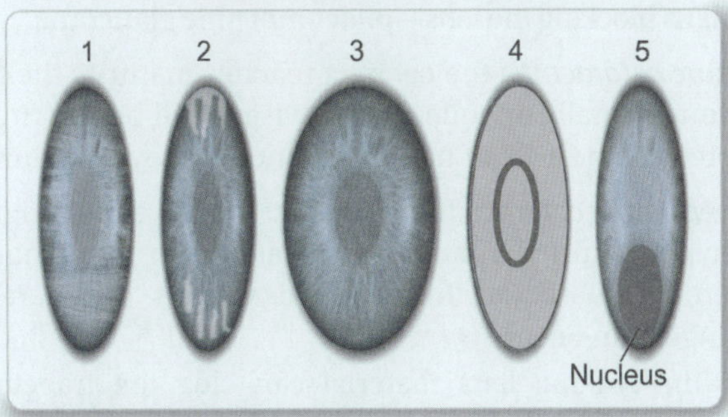

FIGURE 18.18: Stages of senile cortical cataract. **1.** Stage of lamellar separation; **2.** Stage of incipient cataract; **3.** Intumescent cataract; **4.** Mature cataract; **5.** Hypermature cataract.

due to a lenticular opacity is broken into segments, which rotate as the slit is passed. If the halos are due to narrow angle glaucoma, it remains unaffected by the slit, only its intensity may be somewhat decreased as the slit passes before the eye (Fig. 18.19).

Changes in the refractive index in different parts of the lens can lead to monocular diplopia or polyopia. There will be some decrease in the visual acuity and this can be corrected to some extent with spectacles in the early stages of cataract. But, as the lenticular opacity progresses, the refractive index of the lens keep changing and the patient will need frequent change of glasses.

Sx Symptoms

The symptoms are solely visual and depend on location of the opacification and stage of the disease.

Stage of incipient cataract: Since the wedge-shaped opacities are mainly in the periphery of the lens, the patient will have better vision in bright light. This is due to the contraction of the pupil in bright light, which diminishes the scattering of light by the peripheral wedge-shaped opacities and the light passing through the central clearer pupillary area will form a sharper image on the retina. In dim light, as the pupil dilates, the scattering of light by the peripheral opacities leads to blurring of the image and decrease in vision.

As the cataract progresses, the visual acuity progressively deteriorates, but the rate of progression varies greatly. Some cortical opacity may show very slow progression over prolonged periods, whereas some cortical cataracts progress rapidly, especially in patients with diabetes mellitus. So, **if a young person is having a cataract or if cataract is progressing rapidly that person has to be investigated for the presence of diabetes.**

Intumescent cataract: As the cataract reaches the intumescent stage, the patient can present with symptoms of pain and redness due to secondary glaucoma produced by the swollen lens blocking the lens—**phacomorphic glaucoma**.

Mature cataract: As the cataract reaches maturity the lens becomes totally opaque and the vision will be very much decreased to CFCF or hand movements or even PL only.

Hypermature cataract: If the cataract is allowed to progress to hypermaturity, a morgagnian cataract or hypermature sclerotic cataract is formed and various degenerative changes can occur:

1. The leaking lens material can clog the trabecular meshwork and can cause lens particle glaucoma or phacotoxic glaucoma.
2. The lens material can produce hypersensitivity reaction and inflammation of the uvea. Lens-induced uveitis and this inflammation can in turn lead to secondary glaucoma called phacolytic or phacoanaphylactic glaucoma.

The suspensory ligaments also degenerate as the cataract reaches the hypermature stage leading to subluxation or dislocation of the hypermature cataractous lens. This displaced lens can block the pupil and cause secondary glaucoma. Thus, a hypermature cataract can cause secondary glaucoma by several mechanisms.

Signs

In the stage of lamellar separation, the fluid vacuoles and clefts can be visualized under the slit lamp. The wedge-shaped cortical opacities are better visualized after dilation of the pupil.

As the wedges increase in size and fuse together, a diffuse cortical opacification will be seen usually with the more superficial cortex remaining transparent. In this stage the immature cataract will act like a mirror—the clear superficial cortex acting as the glass of a mirror and the white opacity underneath as the silvering behind the mirror. When torchlight is thrown into the eye from one side with the patient looking straight, the iris will throw a semilunar shadow on the white opacity within the pupillary area. This will be seen on the same side as the light and its position changes when the direction of the beam of light is changed (Fig. 18.20). The demonstration of the iris shadow is a clear indication that the cataract is still immature. When the lens is totally opaque, no iris shadow is seen. This test was important in the age of intracapsular cataract extraction, when the time of surgery is decided by the maturity of the cataract.

When the opacity reaches the hypermature stage and a morgagnian cataract is formed it will have a milky-white hue and the brown nucleus will be seen through the milky cortex in the lower part of the lens (Fig. 18.21A).

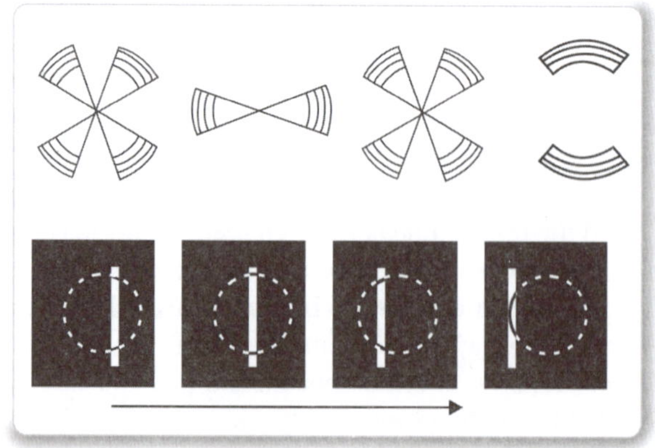

FIGURE 18.19: Fincham's test. In cataract the halos break into segments when the stenopaic slit is passed, but not in narrow angle glaucoma.

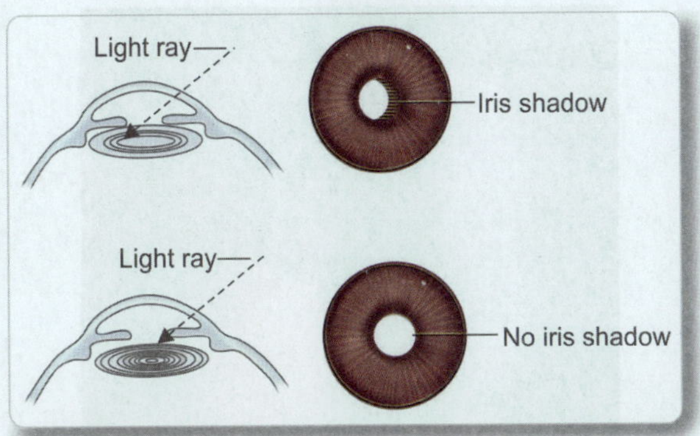

FIGURE 18.20: Iris shadow and stage of cataract. In immature cataract iris shadow is seen, but not in mature cataract

In a sclerotic hypermature cataract when the fluid lens material has gone out of the capsule, the capsule will be wrinkled and shrunken, and often show calcareous or shining cholesterol crystal deposits on it (Fig. 18.21B). The brown nucleus will be showing some movements in the loose capsular bag devoid of all cortical maternal.

If the leaking lens material accumulates in the AC it can simulate a hypopyon. Since it is composed of lens particles and macrophages that have engulfed the lens particles, it is a pseudohypopyon. These lens particles can causes secondary glaucoma with pain, redness and rise in intraocular pressure (IOP) or it can cause a hypersensitivity reaction showing all the features of iritis and secondary glaucoma. The presence of a hypermature cataract will point to the cause of the inflammation (Figs 18.22A and B) and rise in IOP. When the suspensory ligaments degenerate and there is subluxation of the hypermature cataract, the AC will be deep and there will be tremulousness of the iris (Figs 18.23A and B). The hypermature cataract can get dislocated into the AC or the vitreous cavity, often following some trivial trauma. If it is posteriorly dislocated the eye will appear aphakic, but there will be no history of any surgery. After dilatation of the pupil, examination of the fundus will reveal the opaque lens in the lower part of the vitreous cavity. A posteriorly dislocated lens is better tolerated by the eye, but if it is dislocated anteriorly into the AC, it can block the pupil leading to acute use in IOP and secondary glaucoma.

Nuclear Cataract

A nuclear cataract is often bilateral and symmetrical, and tends to progress slowly.

Signs

Since the opacification involves the nucleus, which occupies the center of the lens, the opacity will look denser in the center. The characteristic change of color of the nuclear cataract from yellow to amber, brown and finally up to black helps to distinguish it from other types of cataract and also help to assess the density of the opacity (Fig. 18.24). When it reaches the brown or black color (cataracta brunescens or cataract nigra) a casual examination of the eye will fail to reveal the cataract, due to the dark color of the pupil. On dilation of the pupil and examination under the slit lamp the brown or black cataract will be revealed (Fig. 18.25).

Here also, when the color of the cataract is yellow or amber (Fig. 18.26), iris shadow can be demonstrated.

Posterior Subcapsular Cataract

Posterior subcapsular cataract was earlier called the cupuliform cataract. The posterior subcapsular cataract forms a central opacity in the posterior cortex (Figs 18.27A and B). Since it is situated closer to the nodal point, the degree of loss of vision will be out of proportion to the size of the cataract.

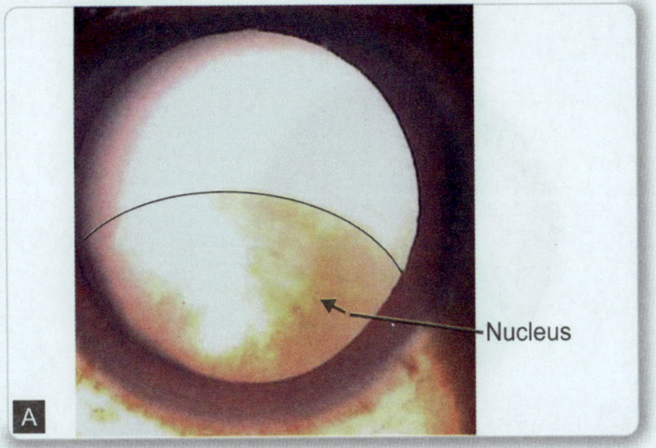

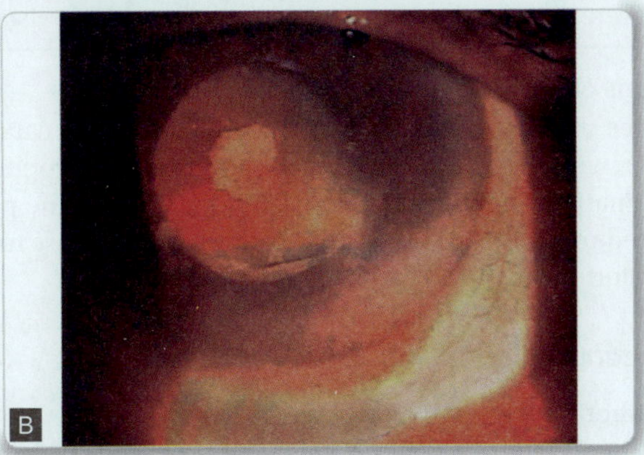

FIGURES 18.21A and B: Hypermature cataract. **A.** Hypermature morgagnian cataract with brown nucleus sinking to lower part of lens; **B.** Hypermature sclerotic cataract.

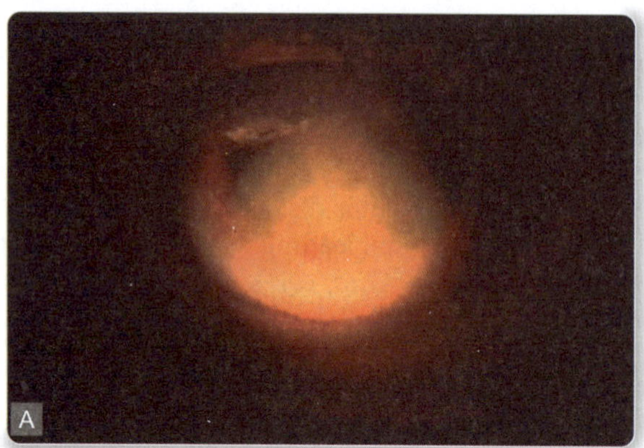

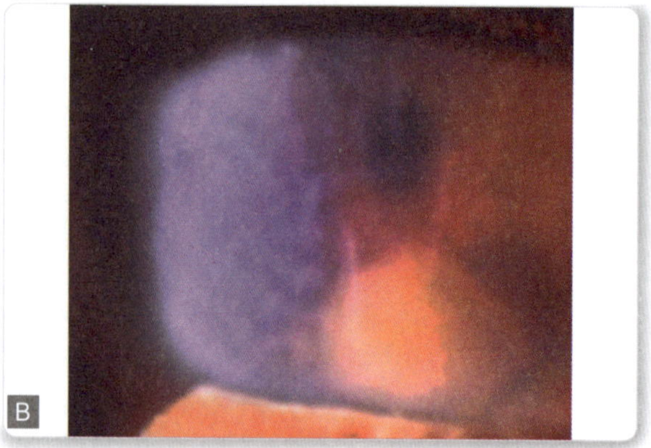

FIGURES 18.22A and B: Hypermature cataract with nucleus in anterior chamber. **A.** Clear cornea; **B.** Cornea decompensated with corneal edema.

Sx Symptoms of nuclear cataract

The symptoms are visual and the distant vision is affected more than the near vision. The vision in bright light is very poor. As the pupil constricts it cuts off the light rays more and the visual acuity decreases. In dim light the pupil dilates and the light rays entering through the clearer periphery of the lens enable the person to see better. The increase in refractive index of the nucleus produces a 'myopic shift' to the refraction of the eye. This 'index myopia' will compensate for the presbyopia and a person who needed glasses for reading finds that he can read without glasses. This improvement in near vision due to early nuclear cataract is called **second sight**. Occasionally, the marked difference in the refractive index between the nucleus and the cortex can produce monocular diplopia. The progressive color change of the nucleus from yellow to brown affects the color discrimination, the blue end of the spectrum is affected more.

As the cataract progresses, the temporary improvement in near vision will be gone and the patient will have severe decrease in acuity for near as well as distant vision.

Signs of posterior subcapsular cataract

Since the drop in vision is considerable and the cataract seen with a torchlight examination is minimal, proper examination under the slit lamp after dilatation of the pupil is required. This will reveal the central opacity close to the posterior capsule to confirm the diagnosis.

Metabolic Cataract

Diabetic cataract

Diabetes can affect the refractive index (refer Refractive Error) as well as the transparency of the lens. The typical diabetic cataract is called the snowflake cataract.

Snowflake cataract

Mechanism: As the blood glucose level rises, aqueous concentration of glucose also rises and glucose reaches the lens in excess via passive diffusion. Some of the excess glucose is converted into sorbitol. Further metabolism of sorbitol is slow in the lens and sorbitol accumulates in the lens.

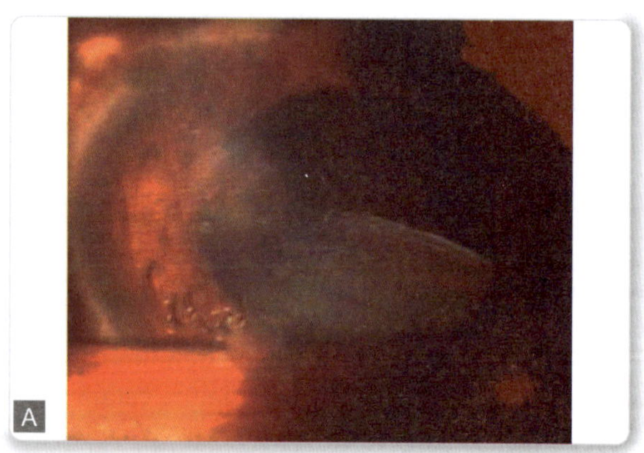

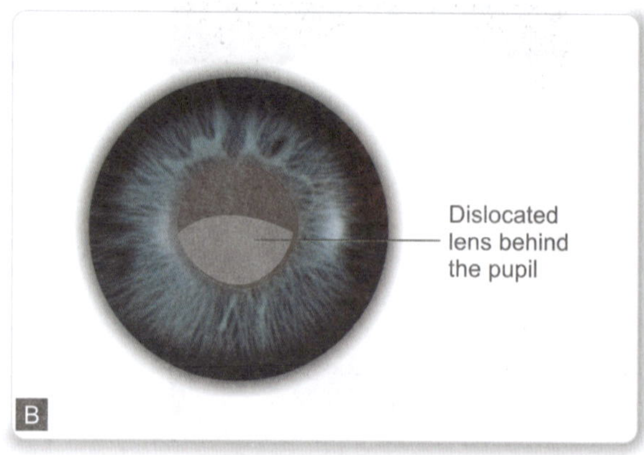

FIGURES 18.23A and B: Subluxation of hypermature cataract. **A.** Photograph; **B.** Diagrammatic representation.

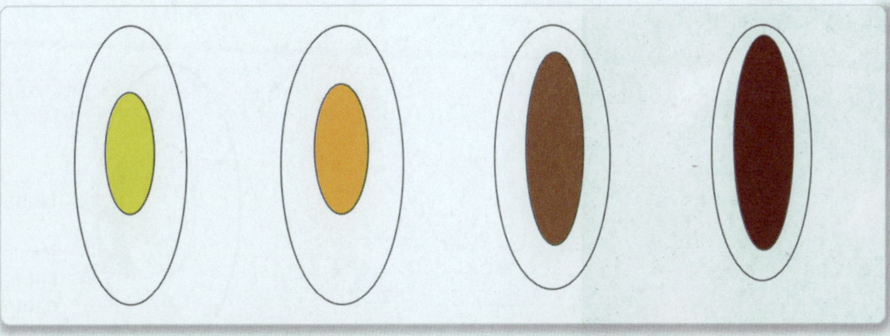

FIGURE 18.24: Stages of nuclear cataract

Sx Symptoms

The early symptoms are glare and poor vision in bright light. The near vision will be much more affected than the distant vision.

This increases the osmotic pressure within the lens, and hydration and swelling of the lens. This can increase the refractive index of the lens and induce myopia. If the diabetic state remains uncontrolled, as in an undetected or poorly controlled juvenile diabetic, bilateral subcapsular opacities can appear in both anterior and posterior cortex due to disintegration of the lens fibers. These opacities resemble snowflakes and hence named snowflake cataract. The opacity rapidly progresses through intumescence to total opacification of the lens. Such typical snowflake cataract is nowadays rarely seen.

Age-related cataract in diabetes

Age-related cataract in diabetes is indistinguishable from age-related cataract in non-diabetic persons by clinical appearance. But it tends to occur at a younger age and progress more rapidly in diabetic persons than non-diabetic people.

So, if a young person has cataract or if the cataract is progressing rapidly, that person has to be investigated for the presence of diabetes.

Galactosemia

Galactosemia is characterized by an inborn error of metabolism of galactose. The child is unable to convert galactose to glucose and galactose accumulates in the body. This galactose reaches in excess into the lens also where it is converted to dulcitol. The excess galactose and dulcitol increase the osmotic pressure in the lens and cause hydration and subsequent opacification of the lens.

Galactosemia is an inherited autosomal disease. Galactosemia can result from deficiency of one of the three enzymes involved in the metabolism of galactose.

The more severe form called the classic galactosemia is caused by a defect in the enzyme galactose-1-phosphate uridyl transferase. The child shows malnutrition, hepatosplenomegaly, jaundice, mental retardation and cataract within the first few weeks of life itself. The diagnosis is confirmed by the demonstration of galactose in urine.

Galactokinase or epimerase deficiency is a milder form with galactosemia and cataract without the other systemic features and appear later in life.

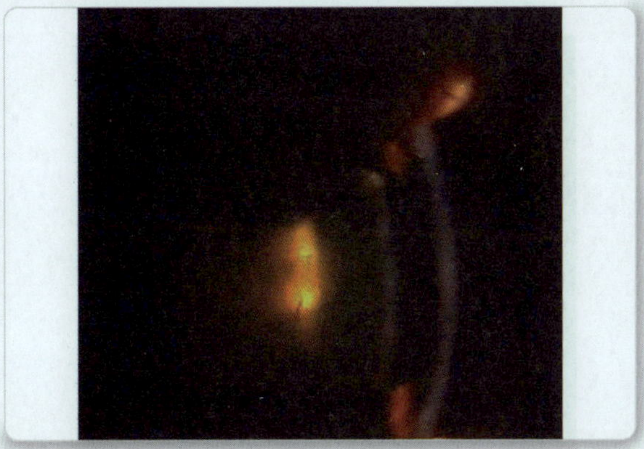

FIGURE 18.25: Nuclear cataract (brown nucleus)

FIGURE 18.26: Nuclear cataract (amber colored)

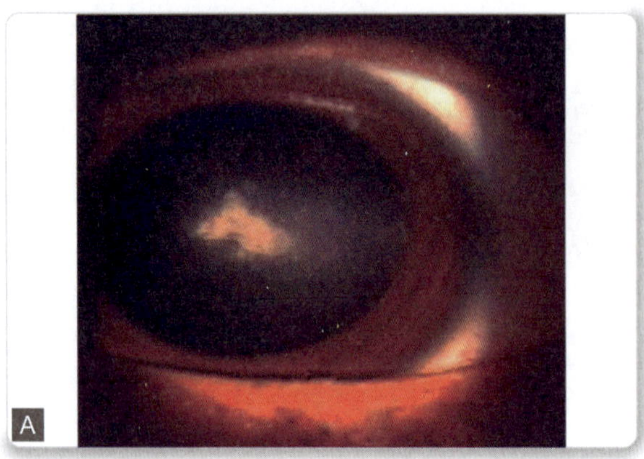

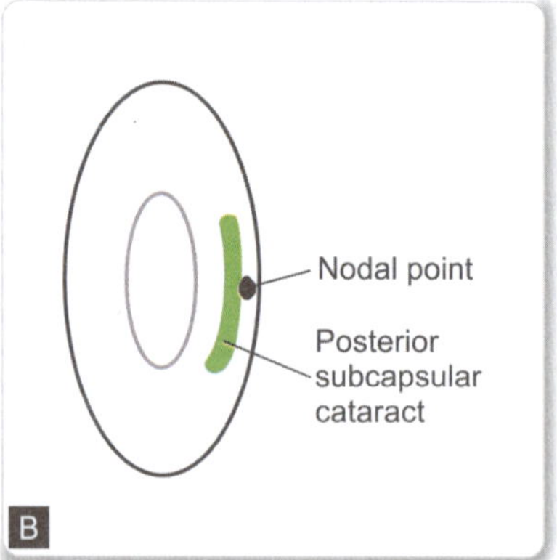

FIGURES 18.27A and B: Posterior subcapsular cataract. **A.** Photograph; **B.** Diagrammatic representation.

Clinical features: Patients with the classic galactosemia develop bilateral cataract within the first few weeks of life. The nucleus and the deep cortex are opacified to appear as an 'oil droplet' appearance. It will progress to total opacification of the lens if left untreated. If classic galactosemia is detected early in life, and milk and milk products are avoided from the diet, the cataract may get arrested or may ever reverse. If detected later, but the patient survives, surgery can be done after improvement of the general condition.

Hypocalcemia

Hypocalcemia usually develops due to destruction of the parathyroid glands during thyroid surgery, as part of parathyroid tetany. It can occur as an idiopathic condition also. Cataract formation can be prevented by supplementation of calcium and parathyroid hormone.

Clinical features: It appears as iridescent opacities in both anterior and posterior cortex, usually separated from the capsule by a clear zone. If left untreated it can progress to total opacification of the lens. The cataract can be surgically treated with good visual prognosis.

Myotonic dystrophy

The patients with myotonic dystrophy develop a characteristic cataract called Christmas tree cataract (Fig. 18.28) with tiny iridescent crystal-like opacities appearing in both anterior and posterior cortex. These crystals are composed of whorls of plasmalemma from the lens fibers. These shiny crystals have given it its name. The opacities may remain stationary or progress to PSC cataract and subsequent complete opacification. Prognosis for surgery is good.

Wilson's disease

In addition to the characteristic Kayser-Fleischer ring these patients can develop a characteristic sunflower cataract. Cuprous oxide, which is a reddish brown pigment, is deposited in the anterior capsule and subcapsular cortex in a stellate pattern. In most cases, this cataract does not seriously affect vision.

Down syndrome

Punctate subcapsular cataract can occur in children with Down syndrome. Sometimes it can progress to the total opacification.

Atopic cataract

Patients suffering from severe dermatological problems like atopic dermatitis, scleroderma, keratosis follicularis, etc. can develop cataract, as part of the systemic diseases or as complication of long-term steroid therapy.

Drug-induced Cataract

Corticosteroids

Long-term use of corticosteroids—both topical and systemic, can induce cataract. It is related to the dose as well as duration of therapy unlike glaucoma induced by steroids. Often long-term treatment lasting for one or more

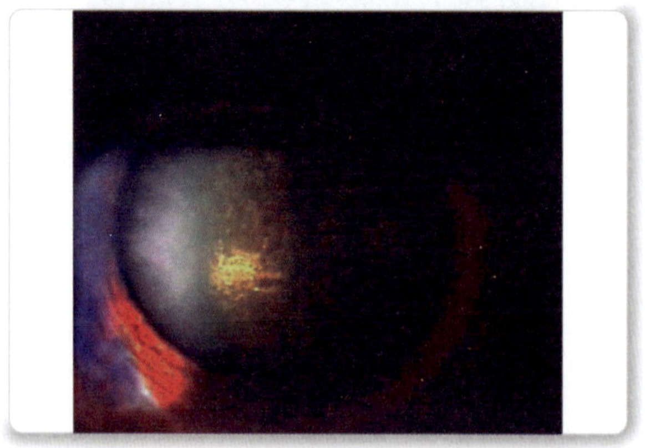

FIGURE 18.28: Christmas tree cataract

years is required for the development of cataract. The exact relationship between total dose, duration of treatment—daily, alternate day or weekly therapy and the development of cataract is still unclear. The cataract is initially posterior subcapsular. It can progress to involve the anterior capsular and the whole of the lens to produce total cataract. Cessation of therapy can arrest the progress of cataract or sometimes its regression, especially in children.

All people on long-term steroid therapy, whether topical or systemic, should undergo periodic ocular examination for development of cataract and glaucoma.

Phenothiazines

Phenothiazines, especially chlorpromazine, on long-term use lead to pigment deposits on the anterior lens capsule centrally. These deposits appear to be related to the dose and duration of treatment. These deposits rarely affect vision.

Amiodarone

On long-term use, this drug can cause stellate pigment deposition on the anterior capsular along with deposits on the cornea. Rarely affect vision.

Miotics

Long-term use of anticholinesterase drugs, especially echothiophate or pilocarpine, can induce cataract formation involving the posterior capsule.

Statins

Studies in dogs have shown that statins are cataractogenic in high doses. Long-term use in humans has not shown increased risk for development of cataract. Simultaneous use of simvastatin and erythromycin or grapes or grape products, which increases the statin level in blood, may be associated with increased risk for developing cataract.

Other drugs, which are cataractogenic, are busulfan and allopurinol.

Traumatic Cataract

Traumatic cataract can be due to direct injury to the lens or by physical forces like radiation, electric current and chemicals, etc.

Concussion cataract

Vossius ring: A sudden blunt force over the eye can cause anteroposterior flattening of the eye and the iris will be pressed against the lens. This will leave a ring of pigment corresponding to the pupillary margin of a contracted pupil on the anterior lens capsule. This is called Vossius ring. This is only a pigment deposition and not a lenticular opacity. It does not interfere with vision, but is a permanent sign that the eye has undergone a concussion injury.

A concussion cataract can take various forms depending on the damage produced by the mechanical force.

Causes: As follows:

1. Mechanical damage to the lens fibers.
2. Alteration in the semipermeability of the capsule.
3. Actual rupture of the capsule can also occur if the force is considerable. A tear in the capsule can lead to a localized or generalized opacification of the lens depending on the size of the tear.

Most common manifestation of a concussion cataract is a rosette cataract.

It usually appears in the posterior cortex a variable period after the injury. Sometimes it can occur in the anterior cortex also or both anterior and posterior cortex will be involved.

There is a star-shaped opacification due to accumulation of fluid at the sutural lines and sometimes opacities will be seen radiating from these sutural opacities.

An early rosette cataract appears within a few days after the injury and a late rosette cataract appears a few months to 1–2 years after the injury. In early rosette cataract, the opacities are seen radiating from the sutural lines, while in late rosette cataract the opacities are radiating from spaces in between the lines (Fig. 18.29). It is usually more compact than the early rosette cataract.

The rosette cataract may remain stationary or progress and can cause significant drop in vision. If vision is significantly affected, surgery can be done. Before undertaking surgery, a detailed evaluation is essential to rule out the effects of injury on other parts of the eye and to decide whether the decrease in vision is due to cataract or some other effect of concussion.

Cataract due to penetrating injuries

If the tear in the capsule (Fig. 18.30) is large, aqueous entering the lens will cause total opacification of the lens

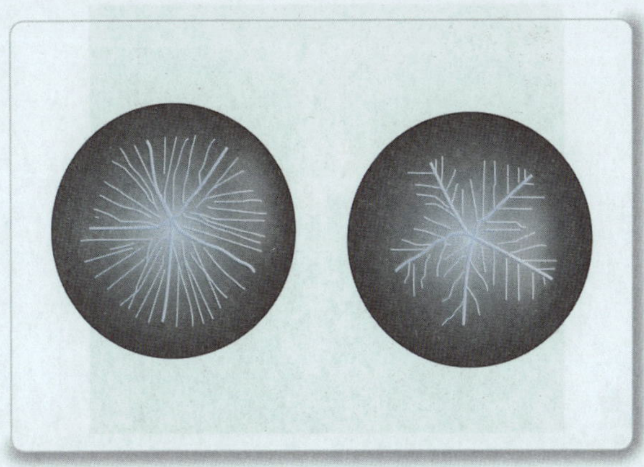

FIGURE 18.29: Rosette cataract (late and early types)

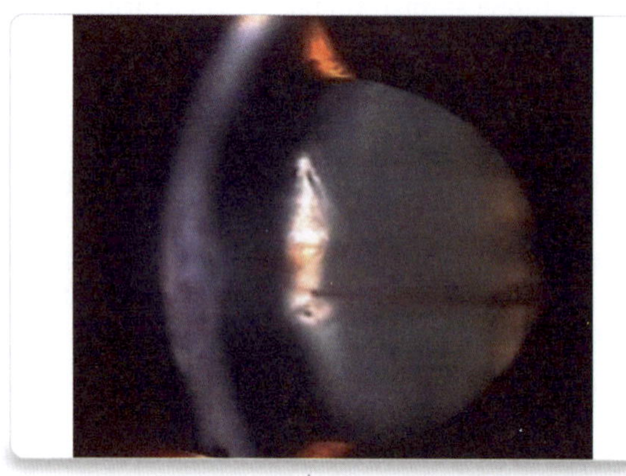

FIGURE 18.30: Linear tear in the capsule due to trauma with opacification of the lens

within a few hours (Figs 18.31A and B). The lens will be swollen up causing shallowing of the AC and secondary glaucoma. The lens material will be liberated into the aqueous, which can aggravate the glaucoma by blocking the trabecular meshwork. The lens material can irritate the iris and produce uveal inflammation, which in turn can add onto the secondary glaucoma.

If the wound in the capsule is smaller, a gradual opacification of the lens will occur taking a few days to weeks.

The patient has to be closely followed up for development of any secondary glaucoma due to shallowing of the AC. Time of cataract surgery is decided by the healing of the penetrating corneoscleral injury as well as the presence or absence of any sequelae like glaucoma or uveitis. If glaucoma cannot be medically controlled, cataract surgery has to be done at an early date without waiting for the healing of the wound and the inflammation to come down. If there is no secondary glaucoma, cataract surgery can be done as an elective procedure after all inflammation has subsided.

If the wound in the capsule is very small as in a needle prick injury, the cataract will be localized to the area of the injury and progress very slowly or remain stationary. Surgery is decided by the effect of the cataract on vision.

Infrared or heat cataract

Infrared or heat cataract occurs as an occupational hazard in people engaged in glass manufacturing or iron works—people who have to work close to furnaces and thus to high temperatures. The heat will be absorbed by the pigment on the iris and ciliary body, and the lens is affected indirectly by the heat from the iris and ciliary body. It is impossible to produce infrared cataract in albino animals in experimental conditions or people with lightly pigmented eyes.

The infrared cataract appears as a small compact disk of opacity in the posterior cortex. Its smaller size and more compact appearance differentiate it from a complicated cataract. It may slowly progress to involve the whole of the cortex. In addition to the opacification, there will be true exfoliation of the capsule, i.e. splitting of the capsule into sheets, which curl up into large whorls in the pupillary area.

Irradiation cataract

Irradiation cataract develops in people treated with X-rays, gamma rays or neutrons for malignancies in or the surrounding areas of the eye, e.g. malignant melanoma of the choroid or carcinoma of the maxillary sinus. Survivors of atomic explosion or technicians not properly protected can also be affected. The radiation affects the multiplying lens epithelium at the equator. The damaged lens fibers will appear as opacities close to the posterior pole.

It appears as a disk of opacity similar to infrared cataract, but it can progress rapidly to total involvement of the lens. The prognosis for cataract surgery is often very good.

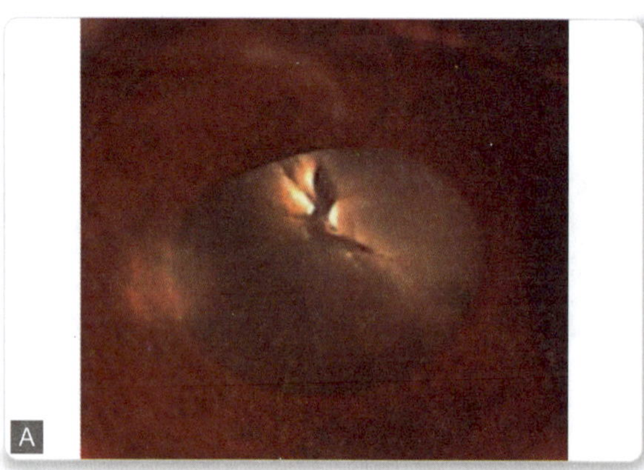

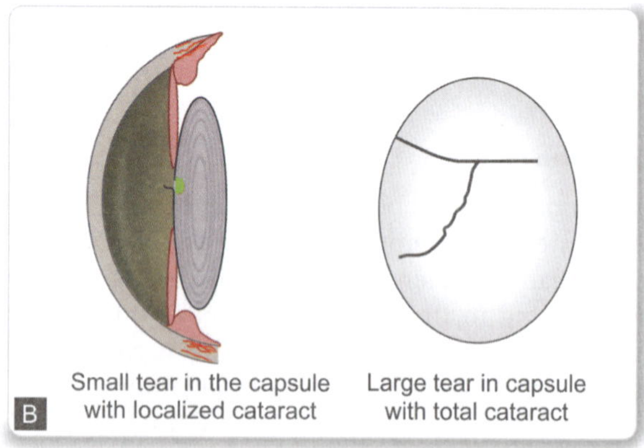

FIGURES 18.31A and B: Traumatic cataract. **A.** Photograph; **B.** Diagrammatic representation.

Electric cataract

Electric cataract develops in people struck by lightning or electric shock if the current passes through the eye. The cataract starts as subcapsular opacities, which can progress rapidly. The prognosis after surgery depends on whether the retina and choroid are damaged by the passage of the electric current.

Complicated cataract (secondary cataract)

Secondary cataract is a cataract which develops as a complication of some other ocular pathology. **It has to be suspected in any unilateral cataract or cataract in a young person**. But the complicated cataract can be bilateral also, if the ocular pathology is bilateral as retinitis pigmentosa or high myopia.

The most common cause for complicated cataract is chronic anterior uveitis. The other causes are:

1. Acute angle-closure glaucoma (where the opacities appear as punctate anterior subcapsular opacities called glaukomflecken).
2. Degenerative myopia.
3. Degenerative conditions of the posterior segment like retinitis pigmentosa, Leber congenital amaurosis and gyrate atrophy.

Clinical features: The typical complicated cataract appears in the posterior cortex, with ill-defined edges and extending peripherally as well as anteroposteriorly. Under the slit lamp it has a breadcrumb appearance and show a display of multiple colors—polychromatic luster (Fig. 18.32). Since the opacity is situated close to the nodal point of the eye, vision will be seriously impaired at an early stage.

The prognosis for vision depends on the underlying cause for the complicated cataract. If it is due to uveitis, surgery is undertaken only after the inflammation has completely subsided. The surgical trauma can cause a flare up of the uveal inflammation. So surgery is done under systemic steroid cover only.

Management of cataract: The management of cataract is surgical. There is no scientifically proven medical treatment that can reverse the opacification of the lens. Lot of research is going on in this field. Aldose reductase inhibitors, which block the conversion of glucose to sorbitol, were found to prevent cataract in experimental animals, but their use in human being is yet to be evaluated.

Non-surgical techniques: Many non-surgical techniques can be tried in people with cataract to improve their vision:

1. Spectacles: Careful refraction and spectacle correction can improve vision in many patients with early lenticular opacity. But there will be fluctuations in the refractive index and consequently in the refractive power of the lens with progression of the cataract. So, frequent change of spectacles is required in patients with cataract.
2. Pupillary dilatation: In people with small central lenticular opacity, pupillary dilatation with mydriatics or laser pupilloplasty will improve the vision. This is especially useful in children with congenital nuclear or lamellar cataract, in whom the opacity is often stationary. In children, mydriatics with minimal cycloplegic action like tropicamide should be used since cycloplegia will interfere with near vision.
3. Low vision aids: The patients in whom surgery is delayed or not possible due to some medical reasons, various low vision aids like magnifying glasses or close circuit television can be used to improve near vision and facilitate reading.

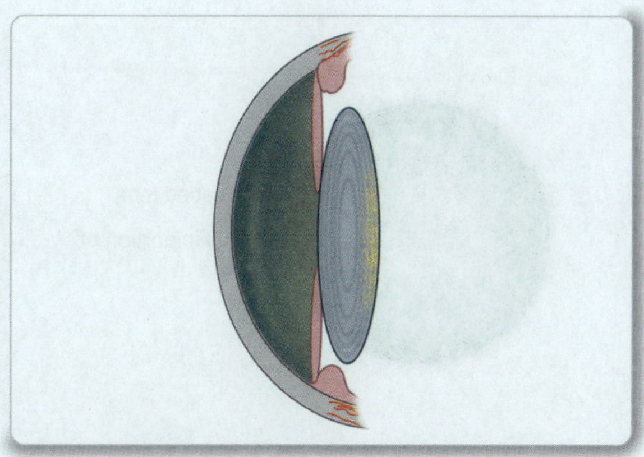

FIGURE 18.32: Complicated cataract with breadcrumb-like appearance and polychromatic luster

The treatment of cataract is primarily surgery and this is discussed in Chapter 28, Surgery for Cataract.

DISPLACEMENT OF THE LENS OR ECTOPIA LENTIS

Ectopia lentis is a displacement of the lens from its natural position. This can be:

1. Subluxation.
2. Dislocation.

It is called subluxation when the displacement of the lens is partial and part of the lens is in the pupillary area. Part of the zonules obviously must be intact (Fig. 18.33).

In dislocation the lens is completely displaced from its natural position. Here the zonules are completely torn. If the lens is dislocated into the AC, it is called anterior dislocation and if it is displaced into the vitreous cavity, it is called posterior dislocation.

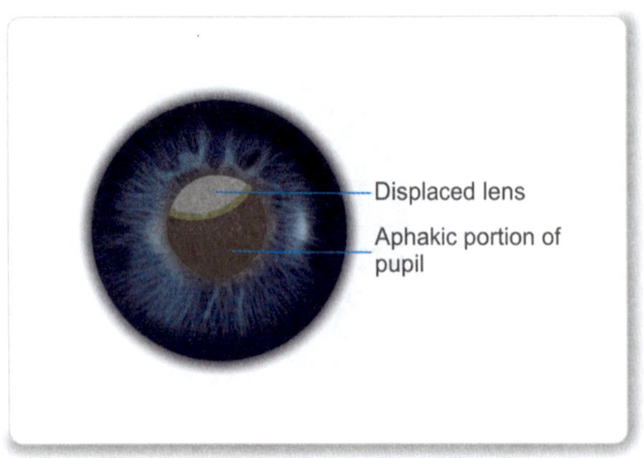

FIGURE 18.33: Subluxation of lens

Ectopia lentis may be hereditary or acquired:

- Hereditary ectopia lentis:
  - May be isolated
  - Have systemic association
  - Associated with an ocular abnormality also.
- Hereditary ectopia lentis with systemic association seen in:
  - Marfan syndrome
  - Homocystinuria
  - Weill-Marchesani syndrome
  - Sulfite oxidase deficiency
  - Hyperlysinemia
  - Ehlers-Danlos syndrome.
- Hereditary ectopia lentis without systemic association:
  - Hereditary ectopia lentis
  - Ectopia lentis et pupillae
  - Aniridia
  - Iris coloboma
  - Congenital glaucoma.
- Acquired displacement of the lens:
  - Trauma
  - Anterior uveal tumors
  - Hypermature cataract.

Hereditary Ectopia Lentis with Systemic Association

Marfan Syndrome

Marfan syndrome is an autosomal disorder of connective tissue. It is an abnormality of fibrillin, a connective tissue component. This leads to ocular, cardiac and skeletal abnormalities. Affected persons are very tall with long limbs and fingers (arachnodactyly), loose flexible joints and high-arched palate and foot. The cardiac abnormalities are enlargement of the aortic root, dilatation of descending aorta and mitral valve prolapse. The cardiac abnormalities lead to shortened life expectancy.

Ocular abnormalities: Bilateral and symmetrical displacement of the lens is seen in 80% of cases. The lens is displaced **upwards and temporally.** The lens may be microspherophakic and this can lead to pupillary block. The zonules are intact, but stretched unlike the broken zonules seen in homocystinuria. The pupil is small and shows poor dilatation.

The patients are usually myopic. The connective tissue abnormality leads to retinal and vitreous degeneration resulting in retinal detachment in the 2nd and 3rd decade, of life.

Homocystinuria

Homocystinuria is an autosomal recessive disorder caused by an abnormality in the enzyme cystathionine β-synthase. Homocysteine accumulates in the plasma and gets excreted in the urine.

The clinical manifestations involve the skeletal system, central nervous system (CNS), vascular system and the eyes. The affected individuals are tall with skeletal abnormalities like scoliosis chest deformities and osteoporosis. The CNS abnormalities are mental retardation and seizures. The affected individuals are prone to thromboembolic diseases involving various organs, cardiomegaly and hypertension.

Ocular abnormalities: The main ocular change is a displacement of the lens usually downwards and it may get displaced into the AC.

The abnormalities develop after birth and get worse with age.

Management: If detected early and the biochemical abnormality is corrected by dietary management (low methionine and high cysteine diet) and supplementation of coenzymes like pyridoxine and cyanocobalamin, the systemic problems can be controlled. If this is done early in life, ectopia lentis can be prevented.

Diagnosis is confirmed by detecting homocysteine in urine. There is a high-risk for surgery under general anesthesia due to risk of thromboembolic episodes. So, surgery for the management of the ectopia lentis is risky.

Weill-Marchesani Syndrome

The people affected by Weill-Marchesani syndrome are physically opposite to Marfan syndrome—short stature with short limbs and fingers. They have stiff joints and are usually mentally subnormal.

The ectopia lentis is usually displaced downwards and bilateral, and occurs in the 2nd decade. The lens is usually microspherophakic and the displacement can lead to pupillary block and secondary angle-closure glaucoma.

Hyperlysinemia

Hyperlysinemia is rare inborn error of metabolism caused by a deficiency in lysine-ketoglutarate reductase. The ectopia lentis is associated with hypotonic muscles, lax joints, seizures and mental retardation.

Sulfate Oxidase Deficiency

Sulfate oxidase deficiency is a rare autosomal recessive disorder of sulfur metabolism. In addition to ectopia lentis the other manifestations are seizures and mental retardation. It is usually fatal by the age of 5 years.

Ehlers-Danlos Syndrome

Ehlers-Danlos syndrome is occasionally associated with ectopia lentis.

Hereditary Ectopia Lentis Without Systemic Associations

Hereditary Ectopia Lentis

Hereditary ectopia lentis is a condition with autosomal dominant inheritance. The lens is displaced upward and temporarily, and it is usually bilaterally symmetrical. It may be present at birth or develop later. Late-onset hereditary ectopia lentis is often associated with glaucoma.

Ectopia Lentis et Pupillae

Ectopia lentis et pupillae is a rare autosomal recessive condition. There is a bilateral displacement of the pupil, usually inferotemporally with lens displaced in the opposite direction, i.e. superonasally. The pupils are often slit like and small and they show poor dilatation with mydriatics and the lens is often microspherophakic.

Aniridia and Iris Coloboma

Aniridia and iris coloboma are congenital anomalies, which are sometimes associated with lens displacement.

Congenital Glaucoma

In congenital glaucoma there is enlargement of the eyeball and consequent stretching, and sometimes rupture of the zonules leading to displacement of the lens.

Acquired Displacement of the Lens

Trauma

Trauma is a common cause for displacement of the lens. It can be a closed globe- or open-globe injury. A trauma that can produce a displacement of lens has to be with considerable force and there will be associated damage to other parts of the globe and the visual prognosis is often poor.

Anterior Uveal Tumors

Tumors of the ciliary body can cause mechanical displacement of the lens.

Hypermature Cataract

The zonules also show degenerative changes once the cataract reaches the hypermature state. At this stage, trivial trauma can cause a displacement of the lens anteriorly or posteriorly.

Clinical Features of Displacement

Once the lens is displaced from its position, the peripheral portion of the lens may be occupying the visual axis. The vision will be variably decreased due to the irregular astigmatism of the peripheral portion of the lens or the pupil may be partly phakic and partly aphakic with the edge of the lens bisecting the pupil. The aphakic portion can be corrected with strong convex glasses and some patients will get reasonably good vision. The phakic portion will have marked irregular astigmatism and the vision cannot usually be improved with glasses. Sometimes patients will experience uniocular diplopia. If the lens is microspherophakic, it may remain mobile, i.e. sometimes it may be in the AC and sometimes in the posterior chamber. If it is displaced anteriorly, it can cause pupillary block and there will be severe pain and redness due to the sudden elevation of IOP. If the lens is displaced posteriorly into the vitreous, apart from the visual problems there will be minimal symptoms. If it is displaced into the AC (Figs 18.34A and B), the corneal endothelium can get damaged by the contact with the lens and corneal edema can develop.

Signs of Displacement

The AC is deep or irregular in depth. The iris will show tremulousness (iridodonesis). If the edge of the lens is

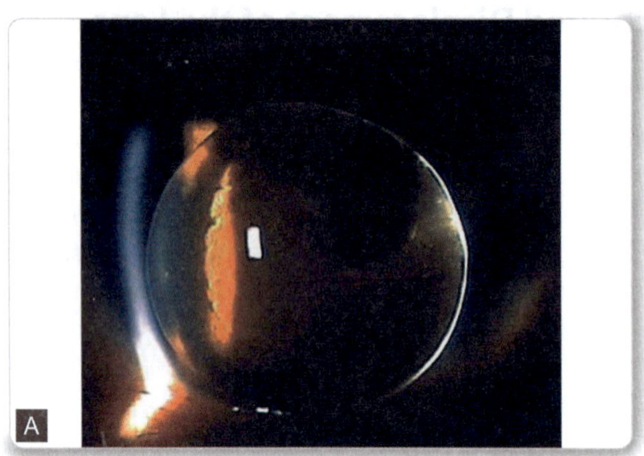

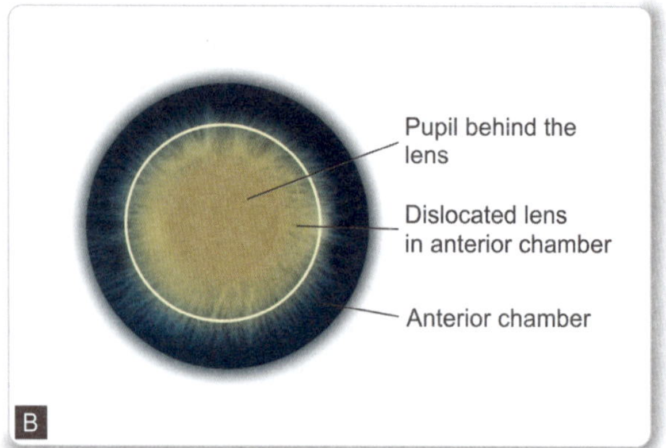

FIGURES 18.34A and B: Microspherophakia with lens dislocated into anterior chamber. **A.** Photograph; **B.** Diagrammatic representation.

seen in the pupillary area, part of the pupil will be aphakic. Even if the lens is covering the pupil in normal condition, dilating the pupil will reveal the displacement of the lens.

Management of Displacement

Management depends on the effect on vision and the presence or absence of secondary glaucoma.

Spectacle Correction

If spectacles correct the astigmatism, it can be prescribed. Often the accommodation is defective and the patient will require near vision correction, irrespective of the age.

Surgical Removal of the Lens

Surgical removal of the lens has to be done if the visual improvement with spectacles is unsatisfactory or the patient develops secondary angle-closure glaucoma due to pupillary block or displacement of the lens into the AC.

Surgery will be invariably associated with vitreous loss and consequently, there is a high-risk of postoperative retinal detachment.

So, phacoemulsification or lensectomy with automated anterior vitrectomy is the ideal surgical option.

Visual rehabilitation is with spectacles or contact lenses. Posterior intraocular lens (IOL) is not possible and sutured scleral fixated IOL or AC IOL is not suitable for patients with metabolic abnormalities.

Vitreous

19

Girija Devi PS

ANATOMY

Vitreous is a clear gel with a slightly denser consistency compared to egg-white, filling the posterior segment of the eye. It is composed mostly of water (99%). It also contains collagen and hyaluronic acid and it is mostly acellular. Its total volume is 4 mL and it is the largest single structure of the eye. It is almost spherical except at its anterior surface (Fig. 19.1). The anterior surface is concave to accommodate the crystalline lens. It is firmly attached to the vitreous base. The vitreous base is a circular band of 4 mm broad, extending 2 mm to the pars plana and 3 mm posterior to the ora serrata. The collagen fibrils are densely packed at the vitreous base, which gives a firm anchorage to the vitreous at this area. Even in conditions with total posterior vitreous detachment or massive vitreous loss during surgery, the attachment to the vitreous base will be retained. The vitreous is also attached to the edge of the optic disk, along the major blood vessels and in the area surrounding the foveola at a diameter of 500 microns. The attachments at these sites are not as firm as at the vitreous base; and separation from these attachments can occur in old age, trauma, etc.

The main function of vitreous is to provide structural support to the retina and acts as a shock absorber on rapid ocular movements and deformation of the eye as in a blunt trauma, but this mechanical support does not have much practical importance. An eye in which vitreous has been removed by vitrectomy, can still have normal retinal function and the retina will remain attached.

NORMAL AGE CHANGES

A disintegration of the gel structure otherwise called liquefaction can occur mostly in the central part of the vitreous cavity where the density of the collagen fibrils are the least. These areas will be seen as optically empty spaces under slit lamp.

The aging process at the vitreoretinal interface will lead to separation of the vitreous from the internal limiting membrane of the retina. This is called posterior vitreous detachment. This is mainly due to collapse of the gel structure in the center of the vitreous cavity due to liquefaction (Fig. 19.2).

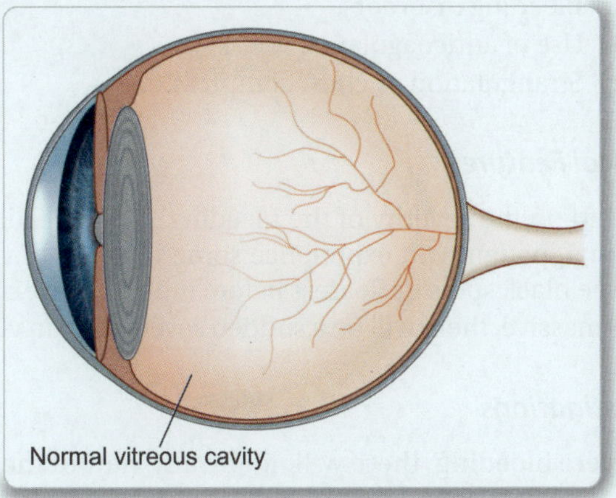

FIGURE 19.1: Normal vitreous cavity

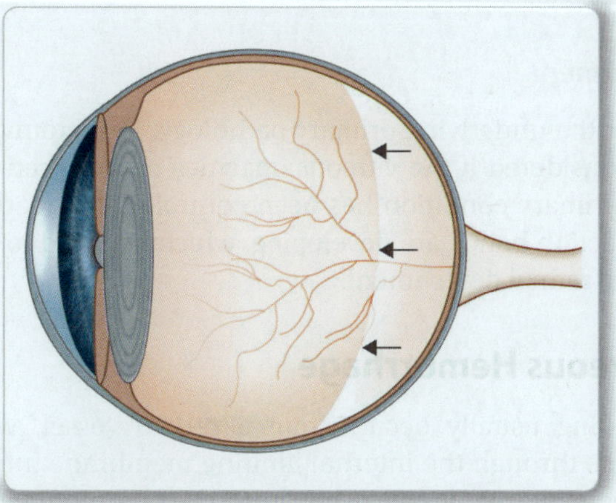

FIGURE 19.2: Posterior vitreous detachment

PATHOLOGICAL CHANGES

Vitreous opacities—various types of opacities can accumulate in the vitreous in many pathological conditions.

Muscae Volitantes

Muscae volitantes are fine spots, sometimes shaped like a fly or a worm seen in bright light against a pale background. These appear to move when the eye is moved and remain stationary when the eye is not moving. These are microscopic opacities in the vitreous—caused by posterior vitreous detachment or vitreous liquefaction as in myopia or old age. These are very common in myopic eyes.

Management

A detailed fundus examination after dilatation is essential to rule out any pathological conditions causing floaters like vasculitis or retinal tear causing avulsion of a blood vessel in the periphery.

Once any ocular abnormalities are ruled out, patient should be reassured that this is only a normal physiological phenomenon. Patient should be asked to simply ignore these spots.

Vitritis

Vitritis is an inflammatory reaction of the vitreous. The vitreous per se cannot get inflamed due to its physiological structure. The inflammatory reaction is a spread of inflammatory cells and exudation from nearby structures—ciliary body, choroid or retina.

Clinically it appears as a dense vitreous haze, which can obscure the fundus view.

Treatment

Treat the underlying primary pathology. Vitrectomy may be considered if the vitreous opacities persist even after the primary condition has been controlled by treatment or traction bands are developing, which can lead to tractional retinal detachment.

Vitreous Hemorrhage

Bleeding usually occurs from a retinal vessel, which breaks through the internal limiting membrane into the vitreous. Rarely it can occur from the choroidal vessels as in expulsive hemorrhage or from the ciliary body as in cases of severe trauma (Fig. 19.3).

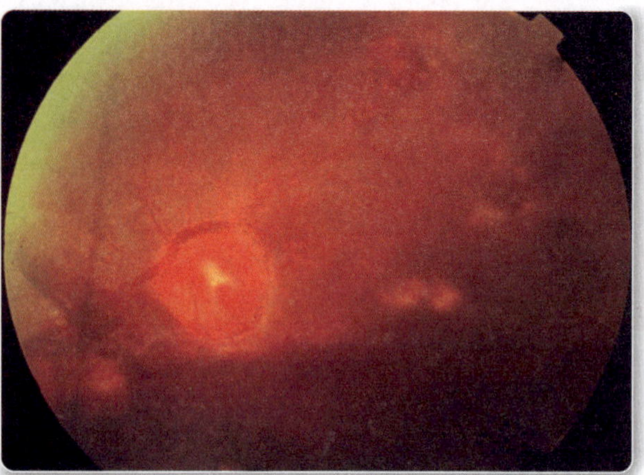

FIGURE 19.3: Disk showing new vessels with vitreous hemorrhage in lower part of vitreous cavity

Causes

1. Proliferative retinopathies:
   a. Diabetic retinopathy.
   b. Neovascularization of disk (NVD) or neovascularization elsewhere (NVE) following retinal vein occlusion.
   c. Eales' disease.
   d. Vasculitis.
   e. Sickle-cell disease.
2. Miscellaneous retinal conditions:
   a. Wet, age-related macular degeneration (ARMD).
   b. Retinal macroaneurysms or telangiectasias.
   c. Retinal tear causing avulsion of a retinal vessel.
   d. Expulsive hemorrhage.
3. Trauma:
   a. Contusion or penetrating injuries.
   b. Iatrogenic—intra- or post-operatively.
4. Systemic conditions:
   a. Bleeding disorders.
   b. Use of anticoagulants.
   c. Strangulation or chest compression.

Clinical Features

Depend on the severity of the bleeding. If the bleeding is minimal, patient will experience some blurring of vision and see black spots or floaters before the eye. If the bleeding is massive, there will be a sudden severe drop in vision.

Investigations

In severe bleeding, there will not be any view of the fundus. B-scan ultrasonography will help to confirm the diagnosis and also reveal any associated problems like retinal detachment.

Treatment

Treatment depends on the primary pathology. Any primary cause like bleeding disorders or use of anticoagulants, if present has to be dealt with.

The blood in the vitreous cavity will get absorbed spontaneously in most of the cases within 2–3 months. Meanwhile patient is instructed to avoid further bleeding—avoid straining, coughing or stooping. While sleeping, patient is asked to keep the head elevated on two pillows.

If the blood is not getting absorbed or the bleeding is so massive that reabsorption is difficult, pars plana vitrectomy is done to remove the blood.

Asteroid Hyalosis (Benson's Disease)

Asteroid hyalosis is a degenerative condition where tiny white globules of calcium phosphorylate accumulate in the vitreous. These are seen as tiny white globules in the vitreous on fundus examination. These move when the eye is moved and do not settle to the bottom of the eye on resting. It is unilateral in majority of patients. It is seen in people of advanced age and men are more affected. The exact cause is not known. These rarely affect vision and require no treatment.

Synchysis Scintillans

Synchysis scintillans is a condition in which a shower of bright shining cholesterol crystals are seen in the vitreous cavity on fundus examination.

Causes

Synchysis scintillans may follow an old vitreous hemorrhage and the shiny crystals are degradation products of erythrocytes. Sometimes these may occur without any apparent reason and also in blind eyes.

Clinical Features

Synchysis scintillans is seen as shower of shiny-golden crystals on fundus examination.

The crystals move when the eye is moved, but unlike asteroid hyalosis, these settle down inferiorly when the eye is at rest.

Treatment

Synchysis scintillans rarely affect vision and require no treatment. But these can interfere with proper visualization of the fundus in case of diabetic retinopathy. Also, rarely these can affect vision. In these situations, vitrectomy is indicated.

Amyloidosis

Vitreous opacities can develop in patients with familial amyloidosis. These can be unilateral or bilateral. These opacities are initially perivascular, but later it appears in the vitreous as 'glass wool-like' opacities, which can show attachment to the posterior lens capsule.

If these are sufficiently dense as to interfere with vision, these can be removed by vitrectomy.

Retina

20

Biju John, Girija Devi PS, Mahadevan, Pappa P

ANATOMY

The retina is the innermost layer of the eye and is derived from neuroectoderm. It is composed of two layers namely the outer retinal pigment epithelium (RPE) and the inner neural retina, with a potential space between the two layers.

Embryology

The retina develops from a diverticulum of the forebrain (prosencephalon). Optic vesicle develops from the forebrain, which then invaginates to form a double-walled bowl, the optic cup. The outer wall becomes the pigment epithelium and the inner wall later differentiates into the nine layers of the retina.

Histology

The retina consists of 10 layers. The individual layers of the retina are as follows (Fig. 20.1):

1. **Retinal pigment epithelium**: A single cubic layer of heavily pigmented epithelial cells. It is more firmly attached to the choroid than the layer of the rods and cones. The pigment cells are taller at the macula and give a darker hue to this area.
2. **Layers of rods and cones:** It contains the actual photoreceptors, rods and cones.
3. **Outer limiting membrane:** Sieve-like plate of processes of glial cells through which rods and cones project. It appears as a fenestrated membrane.
4. **Outer nuclear layer:** This layer contains the nuclei of the rods and cones, first order neuron. The axons of these neurons extend into the outer plexiform layer.
5. **Outer plexiform layer:** It contains synapses between the axons of the first neuron and dendrites of the second neuron.
6. **Inner nuclear layer:** It contains the cell nuclei of the bipolar nerve cells, the second order neuron, also horizontal cells and amacrine cells.
7. **Inner plexiform layer:** It consists of synapses between the axons of the second order neuron and dendrites of the third order neuron.
8. **Layer of ganglion cells:** It contains the cell nuclei of the multipolar ganglion cells, the third order neuron (data acquisition system).
9. **Layer of optic nerve fibers:** It is formed by the axons of the third neuron.
10. **Inner limiting membrane:** It is formed by glial cell fibers separating the retina from the vitreous body.

In retinal detachment the pigment epithelium remains with the choroid when the retina proper separates, opening up the potential space of the optic vesicle.

The photoreceptors are close to the choroid, its source of nutrition and light rays have to travel through all the other layers of the retina to reach the photoreceptors.

Different Zones of Retina

Macula Lutea

Macula lutea is functionally the most important part of the retina. The macula lutea is a flattened oval area approximately 5.5 mm in diameter, in the center of the retina, enclosed by the superior and inferior temporal vessels.

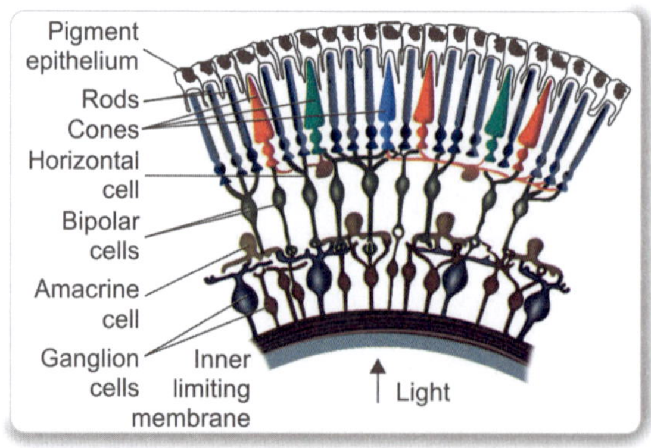

FIGURE 20.1: Layers of the retina

Fovea Centralis

The central 1.5 mm of the macula is called fovea centralis and is situated 2 disk diameters (DD) temporal to the optic disk (1 DD = 1.5 mm).

A depressed area, which is 0.35 mm in diameter in the center of the fovea is called foveola. The foveola contains only cones and is the area with maximum visual acuity.

The central 0.8 mm of the fovea centralis, which includes the foveola is also completely avascular and is referred to as the foveal avascular zone.

Optic Disk

The optic disk is placed 3–4 mm to the nasal side of the fovea. It is a vertical oval, with average dimensions of 1.76 mm horizontally and 1.92 mm vertically. There is a central depression of variable size called optic cup. The optic disk represents the beginning of optic nerve and is the point where the axons of retinal ganglion cells come together. The optic disk is also the entry point for the major blood vessels that supply the retina.

Vascular Supply to the Retina

The inner layers of the retina (the inner limiting membrane up to the inner nuclear layer) are supplied by the central artery of the retina. This originates at the ophthalmic artery, enters the eye within the optic nerve and branches on the inner surface of the retina. The central artery is a genuine artery with a diameter of 0.1 mm. It is a terminal artery without anastomoses and divides into four main branches.

The outer layers (outer plexiform layer to the pigment epithelium) contain no capillaries. These are nourished by diffusion, primarily from the richly supplied capillary layer of the choroid.

The retinal arteries are normally bright red and have bright red reflex strips that become paler with advancing age, and do not show a pulse.

The retinal veins are dark red with a narrow reflex strip and may show spontaneous pulsation on the optic disk. Pulsation in the retinal veins is seen normally in 80%–90% of people. But pulsation in the retinal arteries is abnormal.

The walls of the vessels are transparent, so that only the blood will be visible on ophthalmoscopy. In terms of their structure and size, the retinal vessels are arterioles and venules, although these are referred to as arteries and veins.

Venous diameter is normally 1.5 times greater than arterial diameter. Capillaries are not visible.

Nerve Supply to the Retina

The neurosensory retina has no sensory supply. Disorders of the retina are painless because of the absence of sensory supply.

PHYSIOLOGY

The neuronal component of the retina consists of rods and cones that transduce light signals into electric impulses, which are amplified and integrated through circuitry involving bipolar, horizontal, amacrine and ganglion cells, and transmitted through the nerve fiber layer to the optic nerve.

EXAMINATION OF THE FUNDUS

Examination of the posterior segment of eye (vitreous, optic nerve head or disk, vessels, retina, choroid) is performed with the aid of an ophthalmoscope (Figs 20.2A and B). A satisfactory examination of the posterior pole can usually be made through an undilated pupil, provided that the media (aqueous, lens and vitreous) are clear. However, a greater extent of the peripheral posterior segment can be examined through a dilated pupil. Ophthalmoscopy is best done in a darkened room. Abnormalities in fundus examination are shown in Figures 20.3A to D.

For optimum dilated fundus examination, mydriatic agents commonly used are cyclopentolate 0.5% or tropicamide 1% with phenylephrine 2.5%; the latter should be used with caution in any patient with a history of significant cardiovascular disease. No mydriatic agent should be instilled in an eye in which a shallow anterior chamber is suspected. An estimate of the anterior chamber depth can be made by illuminating it from the side with a penlight.

If the iris seems abnormally close to the cornea, dilation is contraindicated because of the risk of inducing acute angle-closure glaucoma.

Ophthalmoscopes

There are many forms of ophthalmoscopes, the most commonly used being handheld direct ophthalmoscopes designed to provide a direct magnified view (14X). The source of illumination is projected by means of a mirror or prism coinciding with the observer's line of vision through the aperture.

Technique of Direct Ophthalmoscopy

The ophthalmoscope is held close to the observer's eye and approximately 15 cm from the patient's eye in the observer's right hand to examine the patient's right eye and in the observer's left hand to examine the patient's left eye. The observer uses right eye for the patient's right eye and left eye for the patient's left eye. The patient should have no glasses on, have chin straight and be fixating on a distant target with the eye as steady as possible. From time

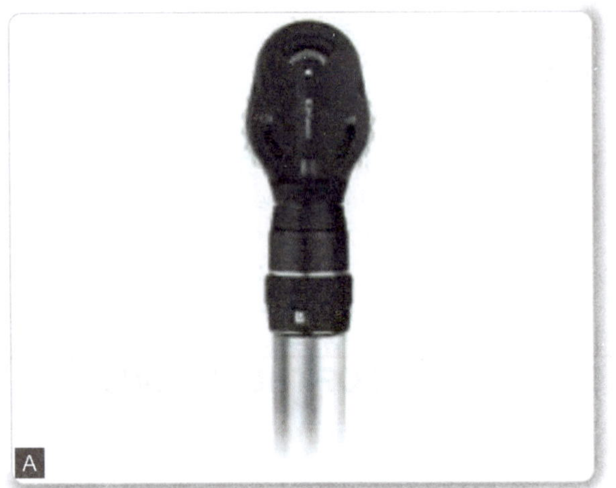

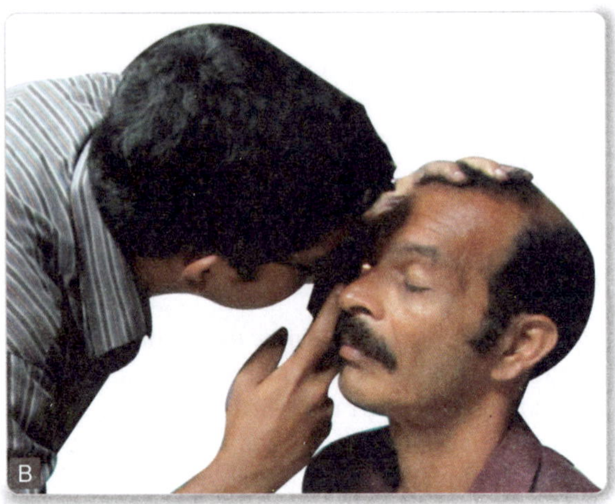

FIGURES 20.2A and B: Direct ophthalmoscopy. **A.** Ophthalmoscope; **B.** Method of examination.

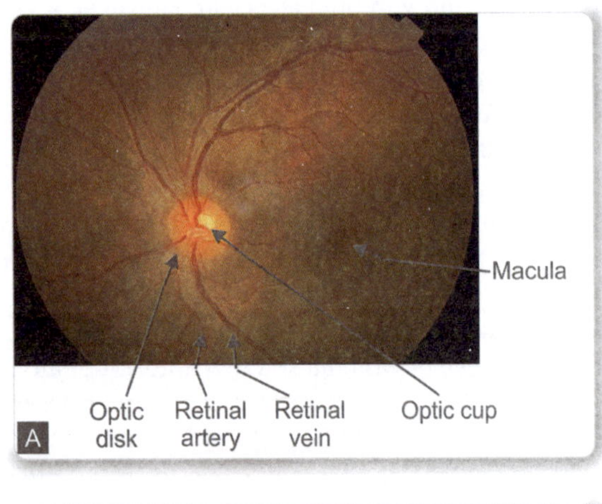

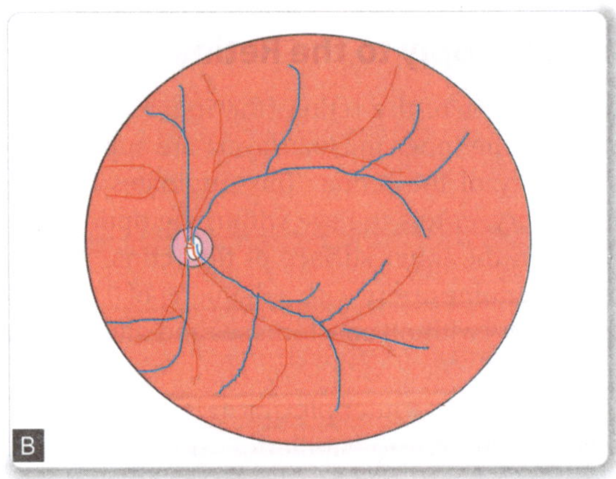

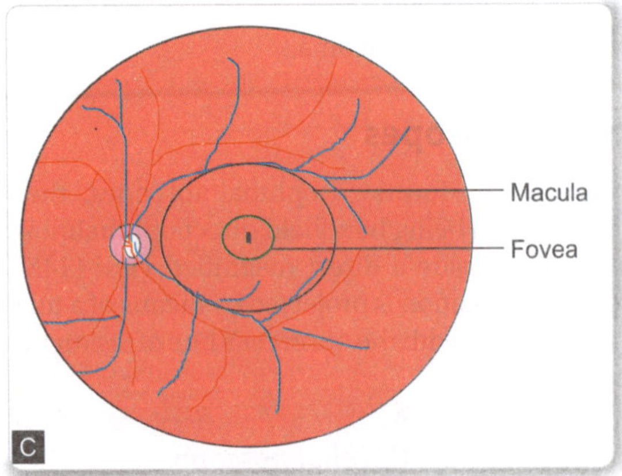

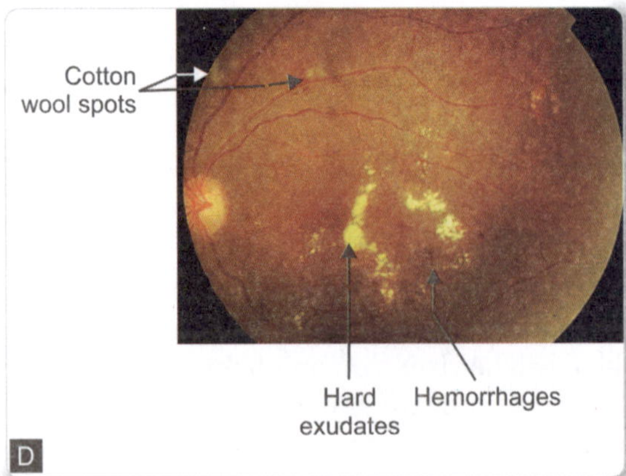

FIGURES 20.3A to D: Retina. **A.** Normal retina; **B.** Diagrammatic representation; **C.** Anatomical landmarks; **D.** Abnormalities seen on fundus examination.

to time the patient may have to be reminded to refixate on a distant target to avoid accommodation from interfering with the observer's level of focus within the eye. The physician may have to adjust the ophthalmoscope power setting to accommodate for the patient's or his/her own refractive error—red-numbered minus lenses are used for myopic errors and black-numbered plus lenses are used for hypermetropic errors. Eyes that have undergone cataract removal, but no lens implantation (aphakia) should be examined with a +8 to +12 lens to obtain a view of the fundus. If both patient and examiner have normal eyes and the lens is set at 0, a red reflex will be seen and is considered normal. Moving the ophthalmoscope as close to the patient's eye as possible, the observer uses black or positive lenses.

Lens settings of +4 to +8 will focus the ophthalmoscope on the anterior segment to reveal corneal opacities or changes in the iris and lens. The retina in a normal eye will focus at 0, provided that no refractive error is present. By decreasing the power of the lens from positive toward negative, the depth of focus will become greater so that the examiner may move from the anterior segment progressively through structures until the vitreous and retina are reached.

Vitreous opacities such as hemorrhages and floaters should be localized and noted, and changes in the posterior segment structures focused and studied.

The optic nerve head should be brought into focus and examined. This structure is generally circular to oval with vertical orientation and pink in color. The temporal side is usually lighter pink than the nasal side. The center of the disk may have some depression, which is referred to as the physiologic cup, the bottom of which may be fibrous in appearance and represents the fibers of the lamina cribrosa of the sclera. Normal cupping is round and may vary from absence to 80% involvement of the nerve head. In the presence of extensive, vertically elongated or asymmetric cupping, glaucoma should be suspected. In optic atrophy the entire nerve head will be pale; in papilledema or papillitis it will be swollen and congested.

The size of the normal nerve head may vary with the refractive error of the patient, being small in hypermetropic patients and large in myopic patients.

Retinal arteries and veins (AV): The arteries are red and smaller than the slightly darker veins in about a 2:3 ratio. Because of a thicker wall, the arteries have a shiny central reflex stripe. It is not the vessels, but the column of blood traversing these vessels that is seen through the transparent walls.

Hemorrhages: These appear bright red in color and take various shapes. Round hemorrhages may occur in patients with diabetes mellitus and are located deep in the retina, usually the outer plexiform layer and flame-shaped hemorrhages are commonly found in patients with high blood pressure and blood dyscrasias. The flame-shaped hemorrhages are located in the nerve fiber layer.

Exudates: These are of two types; hard exudates and soft exudates. They are seen in the posterior pole. The hard exudates are clumps of lipids and lipoproteins and appear as discrete yellowish areas arranged in a circinate fashion, as clumps or as plaques. Soft exudates appear as white fluffy areas with feathery margins and these are nerve fiber layer infarcts.

The macular area located temporal to about 2 DD to the optic nerve head, which is darker than the surrounding retina and have a lustrous central area called fovea centralis. This appears as a small area of dark red with a tiny yellow light reflex at the center of the fovea called foveal reflex. The foveal reflex dulls with age or certain drug-induced retinal toxicities.

The periphery of the fundus can be examined by the movement of the ophthalmoscope in various directions as well as by having the patient move the eye in various quadrants horizontally and vertically. The periphery is better visualized with the indirect ophthalmoscope (Fig. 20.4).

Indirect Ophthalmoscopy

Indirect ophthalmoscopy is a technique generally used by specialists and involves the use of a head mounted, prism-directed light source coupled with use of double aspheric (+14, +20 or +28) diopter condensing lenses to see the retinal image (Fig. 20.5).

The image covers approximately 10 times the area usually seen in the field of the direct ophthalmoscope, but is smaller than a direct ophthalmoscope (3X), although the larger field of view gives great perspective to the entire

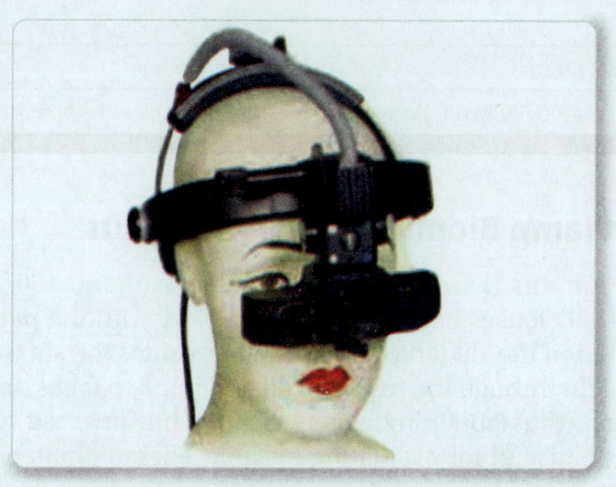

FIGURE 20.4: Indirect ophthalmoscope

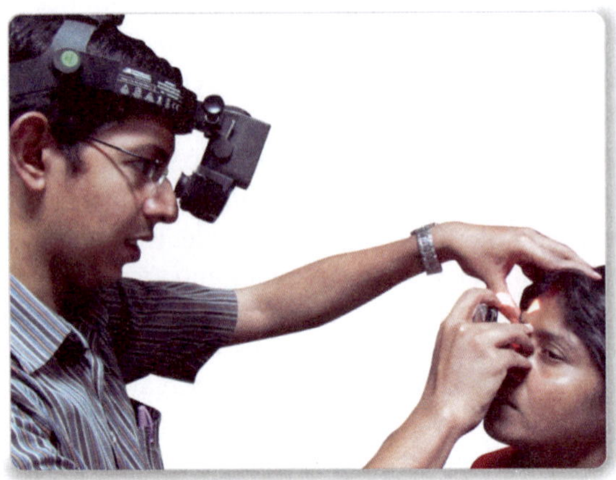

FIGURE 20.5: Examination with indirect ophthalmoscope

fundus and is helpful in locating multiple lesions or in evaluating retinal detachment. Since the fundus is viewed with both eyes a stereoscopic view is obtained, elevation or depressions of various lesions are better visualized. Another advantage is stronger illumination, which allows light to pass through opacities of the vitreous and the fundus, which are poorly visualized with the direct ophthalmoscope due to opacities of the media are better visualized with indirect ophthalmoscope (Table 20.1). Since the image seen through an indirect ophthalmoscope is inverted and right side is seen on the left side, there is a learning curve in proper visualization with this equipment.

TABLE 20.1: Direct vs indirect ophthalmoscopy

Direct ophthalmoscopy	Indirect ophthalmoscopy
More magnified image	Lesser magnification
Area visualized is less	Panoramic view
Area up to the equator visualized	Up to the retinal periphery visualized
Viewed with one eye alone	Viewed with both eyes and hence stereoscopic vision
Straight image	Inverted image
Poor visibility in hazy media	Better visibility in hazy media

Slit lamp Biomicroscopy of Fundus

The fundus is seen by use of double aspheric +60, +78 or +90D lenses handheld before the eye with the patient seated in the slit lamp. The examiner shines the slit beam straight through the (usually) dilated pupil to focus on the retina, thus obtaining a stereoscopic, but inverted view. This is useful for evaluating macular edema, optic nerve lesions or other posterior pole lesions. It is less useful for the peripheral retina beyond the equator.

COMMON INVESTIGATIONS

Common investigations used for diagnosis of vitreoretinal diseases are detailed below.

Fluorescein Angiography

Fluorescein angiography (Fig. 20.6) is the study of retinal and choroidal vasculature using fluorescein sodium, which is a fluorescent vital dye.

Principle

Fluorescence is a physical property of certain substances that on exposure to light of short wavelength, absorbs the shorter wavelength light and emits light of longer wavelength in a characteristic spectral range. Sodium fluorescein, a yellow-red substance, absorbs light between 485 and 500 nm in aqueous solution and exhibits a maximum emission between 525 and 530 nm.

The value of fluorescein angiography is based on the fact that fluorescein dye does not penetrate healthy RPE and normal retinal capillaries, because of the tight endothelial junction present in the latter. Fluorescein does leak freely from the normal choriocapillaris, but it cannot reach the retina due to the impermeability of the RPE. Under optimum conditions, the smallest retinal capillaries (5–10 μm in diameter) can be seen with this technique, a feat impossible by ophthalmoscopy or by color photography.

Technique

A 5 mL bolus of 20% sodium fluorescein is rapidly injected via the antecubital vein and rapid retinal photographs are taken with a fundus camera. This special camera contains an excitatory filter in the course of the beam of light with maximum transmission between 485 and 500 nm that

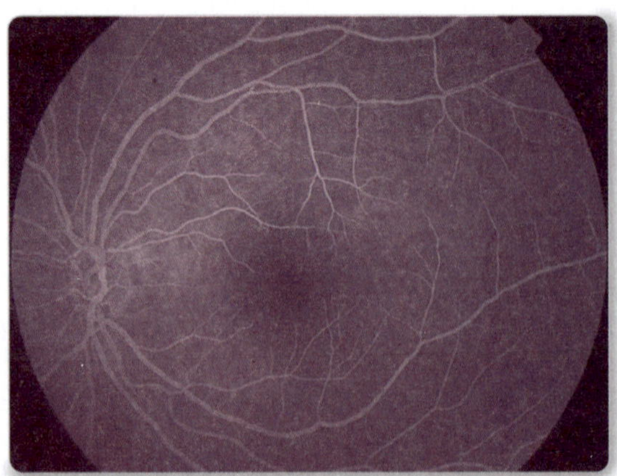

FIGURE 20.6: Normal fundus fluorescein angiography

allows the passage of only the required wavelength of light to stimulate the fluorescein dye and a barrier filter peaking close to the maximum of the fluorescein emission curve (between 525 and 530 nm) that allows only the light rays emitted by the dye to reach the observer's eye.

Use in Retinal and Choroidal Disease

Fluorescein angiography is of particular value in elucidating small vessel disease such as diabetic retinopathy, outlining clearly such changes as microaneurysms (Fig. 20.7), shunt vessels and sites of capillary occlusion and early neovascularization. Vascular abnormalities within the retina commonly leak fluorescein because of damage to the endothelium. New vessels, both those anterior to the retina and those arising from the choroid under the retina, characteristically leak fluorescein because of the absence of tight endothelial junctions. Angiography provides a valuable means of identifying such vessels in macular degeneration, diabetes, sickle cell disease and retinal vein obstruction. It also provides a means of assessing the efficacy of treatment, particularly photocoagulation, in eliminating these vessels and in sealing leaks from vascular abnormalities within the retina, as in clinically significant diabetic macular edema.

Electrophysiology

There are three major electrophysiologic tests used in the investigation of the visual system.

Electrooculography

Electrooculography (EOG) measures slow changes in the standing potential of the retina caused by the interaction of the RPE with the photoreceptors.

Technique: Electrodes are attached to the skin over the orbital margin opposite the medial and lateral canthi and the potential difference between the electrodes is amplified and recorded, as the patient is asked to look back and forth at targets to the right and left. Recordings are done after both light and dark adaptation. The maximum height of the potential in light divided by the minimum height of the potential in dark gives the Arden ratio, which is normally 1.85 or greater. Its principal diagnostic usefulness is in distinguishing best vitelliform degeneration (in which the ratio is abnormal, but the electroretinography is normal) from other macular diseases such as Stargardt's disease or pattern dystrophies.

Electroretinogram

Electroretinogram (ERG) reflects the chain of graded electric responses from each layer of the retina. The human response, for clinically useful purposes, is a biphasic wave, an early negative A wave, generated by the rods and cones, followed by a larger positive B wave, generated in the Müller and the bipolar cell layer (Fig. 20.8). The recording is done with a corneal contact lens electrode and a reference electrode on the forehead. Cone responses predominate

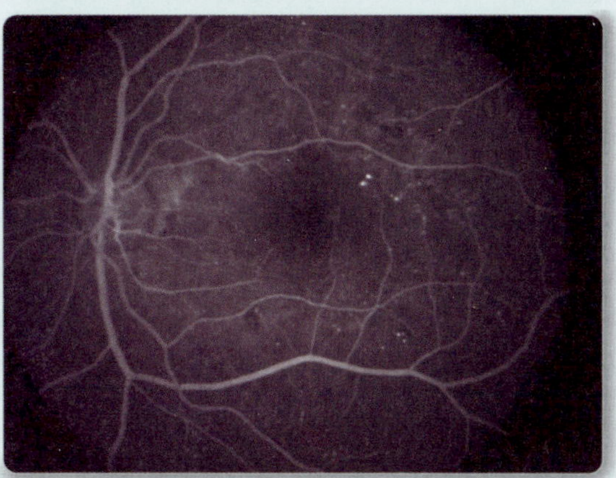

FIGURE 20.7: Fundus fluorescein angiography showing microaneurysms

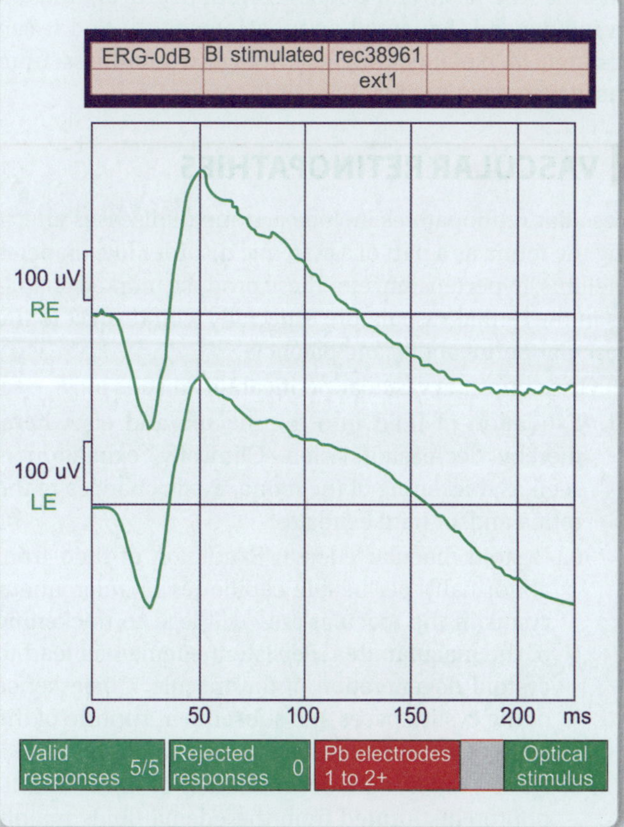

FIGURE 20.8: Electroretinogram

under photopic testing conditions, when a bright flash stimulates the retina. Rod responses predominate in a scotopic environment when a dim flash is used. A bright flash under scotopic conditions elicits a combined response. In addition, the ERG can distinguish the differences in response between the rods and cones to flickering flash; only the cones respond at 30 Hz, because these have a much higher temporal resolution than the rods. The ERG is very useful in evaluating early retinal function loss before ophthalmoscopic changes are evident. The ERG is normal in diseases involving only the ganglion cells and the higher visual pathway, such as optic atrophy.

Visual Evoked Response

Visual evoked response (VER) is the response of the electroencephalogram recorded at the occipital pole and is a macula-dominated response, due to the disproportionately large projection of the macular retina in the occipital cortex. The VER can be recorded using an intense flash stimulation or pattern stimulation. The VER is the only clinically objective technique available to assess the functional state of the visual system beyond the retinal ganglion cells. The flash VER can assess retinocortical function in infants and demented or aphasic patients, and it can distinguish patients with psychological blindness from those who have an organic basis for poor vision.

VASCULAR RETINOPATHIES

Vascular retinopathies include a group of diseases affecting the retina as a part of a systemic disorder like diabetes mellitus, hypertension, etc. These produce marked changes in the retinal vasculature especially with respect to the vascular permeability and patency.

The abnormal vascular permeability results in:

1. Exudation of fluid into the macula and elsewhere, thereby decreasing vision. Clinically, exudation is seen as thickening of the retina, cystic changes in the retina and/or hard exudates:
   a. Cystoid macular edema: Exudation of fluid from abnormally permeable capillaries or microaneurysms in the macular area will lead to thickening of the macular area. Persistent edema will lead to cystoid degeneration of the macula. Coalescence of the cystic spaces and subsequent rupture of the walls of the cysts can lead to macular hole.
   b. Hard exudates are accumulation of lipids and lipoproteins formed from the edema fluids mainly in the outer plexiform layer. These have a pale yellow color and can take various arrangements and shapes like a circinate pattern in diabetic retinopathy or a fan or star-like arrangement at macula in hypertensive retinopathy. These hard exudates may get slowly absorbed, but take several months to 1–2 years to disappear. On fluorescein angiography, the leakage can be diffuse in new vessel formation or specific, such as that coming from a microaneurysm.
2. Retinal ischemia: This is seen as capillary dropout on fluorescein angiography. Capillary dropout may correlate with soft exudates or cotton-wool spots (CWSs). These are white fluffy areas of a disk diameter in size with feathery or ill-defined edges, hence the name 'soft exudates'. This feature plus their bright white appearance has also earned them the eponym CWSs. A CWS results when there is interruption of axoplasmic flow in the nerve fiber layer secondary to closure of a precapillary arteriole. CWSs are seen in diabetic retinopathy, hypertension, anemia, leukemia, collagen vascular diseases, dysproteinemias, endocarditis, preretinal macular fibrosis and acquired immunodeficiency syndrome (AIDS). The CWSs disappear in 4–6 weeks. Retinal ischemia may also correlate with widespread retinal whitening as seen in acute central retinal artery occlusion. More commonly, however, there is no retinal whitening in areas of capillary dropout, which can only be detected on fluorescein angiography.
3. Ischemia can cause visual loss in the following ways:
   a. Ischemia can lead to breakdown of inner blood-retinal barrier (the tight junctions between the endothelium of the retinal capillaries) and retinal edema especially at the macula.
   b. Vascular endothelial growth factor (VEGF) released by partially ischemic tissue may induce the proliferation of new vessels on the disk or surface of the retina. These new vessels become tightly bound to the posterior vitreous. These leak fluid into it. This fluid induces contraction of the vitreous gel resulting in traction on the new vessels, which can then bleed into the vitreous cavity. Depending on the size of the hemorrhage, only a few floaters might be seen or there can be a sudden and severe decrease in vision.
   c. The blood components can cause further contraction of the vitreous and further bleeding, setting up a vicious cycle of recurrent hemorrhaging and the traction can lead to pulling and detachment of the retina under and around the new vessels (traction retinal detachment). If the fovea is involved, vision will decrease.

d. Rubeosis iridis: VEGF can induce new vessel formation on the iris and trabecular meshwork blocking Schlemm's canal, leading to severe pressure elevations (neovascular glaucoma).

In diabetic retinopathy, posterior proliferative changes predominate with vitreous hemorrhages and traction retinal detachments, whereas in central retinal vein occlusion, neovascular glaucoma is more common. In artery occlusions, total ischemia with destruction of the perifoveal capillary network is the mechanism of visual loss. New vessel formation either anteriorly or posteriorly is rare, presumably because little VEGF is produced by totally ischemic tissue.

Management

Management of the vascular retinopathies consists of treatment of the underlying medical condition:

1. **Laser photocoagulation:** Depending on the underlying cause, laser photocoagulation has been shown in controlled clinical trials to be of visual benefit:
   a. By decreasing the exudation of fluid into the macula by closing the leaking microaneurysms and by increasing the reabsorption of fluid.
   b. Lessen the retinal complications of new vessel growth. This is done by converting portions of hypoxic retina to ischemic retina by the laser burns and thus decreasing the liberation of VEGFs. This will lead to regression of new vessel growth.
2. **Pars plana vitrectomy:** It is useful in managing vitreous hemorrhages and traction retinal detachments.

Diabetic Retinopathy and Hypertensive Retinopathy

Diabetic retinopathy is an ocular microangiopathy. Diabetic retinopathy is one of the main causes of acquired blindness in the industrialized countries. Approximately 90% of all diabetic patients have retinopathy after 20 years.

Diabetic retinopathy and hypertensive retinopathy are described in detail in the Section 10 'Systemic Diseases and the Eye'.

Retinal Vein Occlusion

Retinal vein occlusion (RVO) occurs as a result of circulatory dysfunction in the central vein or one of its branches.

It can manifest itself as:

1. Central retinal vein occlusion (CRVO): It is a type of occlusion in which the occlusion of the central retinal vein occurs at or behind the cribriform plate.
2. Branch retinal vein occlusion (BRVO): Here the occlusion occurs is at one of the branches of the retinal vein at an AV crossing.

Epidemiology

Retinal vein occlusion ranks as the second most frequent retinal disorder after diabetic retinopathy.

Associations

Systemic disorders associated with retinal vein occlusion include atherosclerosis, arterial hypertension and diabetes mellitus.

Frequent underlying ocular disorders include glaucoma and retinal vasculitis.

Risk Factors

1. Age: More than 50% of cases occur above 65 years.
2. Hypertension: Especially if the BP is not adequately controlled.
3. Hypercholesterolemia: It can lead to sluggishness of circulation and lead to venous occlusion.
4. Diabetes mellitus.
5. Oral contraceptive pills: This is the most common risk factor in younger females.
6. Raised intraocular pressure (IOP): It leads to stagnation of circulation in the eye and kinking of vein at the edge of the cup. Every case of CRVO has to be carefully evaluated to rule out glaucoma.
7. Smoking: It can add onto the risk for vein occlusion.
8. Atherosclerosis: It is the most important risk factor for BRVO. The artery and vein share a common adventitious sheath at the A-V crossing. The sclerotic artery compresses the vein leading to endothelial damage in the vein and thrombus formation. It plays a risk factor in CRVO also since retinal artery and vein shares a common sheath behind the cribriform plate.

Rare Causes

Hyperviscosity syndromes like polycythemia, myeloma, leukemia, homocystenemia, etc. Thus, both arterial and venous changes contribute to venous occlusion.

Etiopathogenesis

Occlusion of the central vein of the retina or its branches is frequently due to local thrombosis at sites, where sclerotic arteries compress the veins. In central retinal vein occlusion, the thrombus lies at the level of the lamina cribrosa;

in branch retinal vein occlusion, it is frequently at an arteriovenous crossing. Other mechanisms implicated are venous stasis and inflammation (vasculitis).

Whatever be the mechanism of the occlusion, it leads to backup of blood in the retinal vascular system and increased resistance to venous blood flow. This increased resistance causes stagnation of blood and ischemia of inner retinal layers in the affected areas. Increased blood pressure in the venous system causes breakdown of inner retinal barrier at the retinal capillary endothelium, leading to bleeding as well as abnormal leakage of fluid in the retinal layers causing macular edema. In addition to the ischemic damage to the retina, ischemia is supposed to give rise to release of angiogenic factors, which stimulates abnormal vascularization of the posterior and anterior segment.

Classification

1. Branch retina vein occlusion.
2. Central retinal vein occlusion:
   a. Non-ischemic (Fig. 20.9).
   b. Ischemic (Fig. 20.10).
3. Hemiretinal vein occlusion.

Ischemic and non-ischemic CRVO: One differentiates non-ischemic and ischemic CRVO depending on the extent of capillary occlusion demonstrated with the aid of fluorescein angiography.

Clinical Features

Clinically, patients with CRVO typically present with sudden loss of central vision. Transient obscurations of vision can also occur, but are less common. Vision loss at presentation is related to the extent of macular damage from intraretinal edema (most common), hemorrhage or capillary non-perfusion. Vision loss is more in the ischemic type than in the non-ischemic type (Table 20.2).

TABLE 20.2: Ischemic CRVO* vs non-ischemic CRVO

Ischemic CRVO	Non-ischemic CRVO
More ischemic damage to retina as shown by more areas of capillary dropout on FFA†	Less ischemic damage
Vision less than 6/60	Vision 6/60 or better
RAPD‡ present	RAPD absent
Venous tortuosity and hemorrhages are more	Venous tortuosity and hemorrhages are less
Visual prognosis poor	Visual prognosis better
Risk of complications like neovascularization and glaucoma are more	Less chance for complications

*CRVO, central retinal vein occlusion; †FFA, fundus fluorescein angiography; ‡RAPD, relative afferent pupillary defect.

In BRVO, vision loss at presentation is related to the extent of macular damage and can range from severe blurring in temporal BRVO to completely asymptomatic as in nasal branch vein occlusions. In nasal BRVO the symptom is usually a field defect. Since the macula is spared, this will cause minimal symptoms and may go undetected.

In the acute phase in CRVO, all four quadrants show venous dilation and tortuosity, superficial and deep intraretinal hemorrhages and/or CWSs. There is usually disk edema and there may be macular edema. The characteristic fluorescein angiographic findings in CRVO include delayed venous filling and capillary non-perfusion, which may be obscured by the retinal hemorrhages.

In BRVO similar fundus findings are seen except that these are confined to a portion of the retina in the area of vascular occlusion. Also disk edema will not be there (Fig. 20.11).

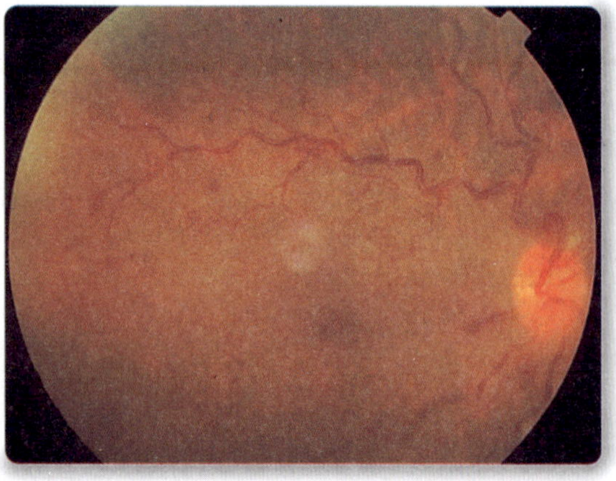

FIGURE 20.9: Non-ischemic central retinal vein occlusion

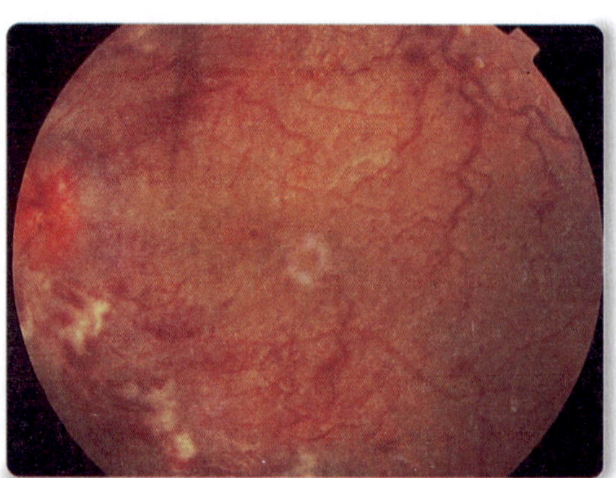

FIGURE 20.10: Ischemic central retinal vein occlusion

Differential Diagnosis

Other forms of vascular retinal disease must be excluded, especially diabetic retinopathy.

Clinical Course and Prognosis

Visual acuity improves in approximately one third of all patients, remains unchanged in one third and worsens in one third despite therapy.

Complications

Complications are retinal neovascularization, vitreous hemorrhage, tractional retinal detachment and rubeosis iridis with neovascular glaucoma.

Management

1. Evaluation for any risk factors: An internist should be consulted to verify or exclude the possible presence of an underlying disorder as mentioned in the risk factors. Such risk factors when identified should be managed properly, so as to prevent further vascular occlusions in other major organs as well as to prevent recurrence of venous occlusion particularly in the fellow eye.
2. Evaluation for primary open-angle glaucoma (POAG): Since POAG is an important risk factor, all cases of venous occlusions should be checked for the presence of it, especially the normal other eye has to be carefully evaluated.
3. Investigation: Fundus fluorescein angiogram (FFA) in the acute phase will not give much information, since the profuse hemorrhages will mask the areas of capillary dropout and the new vessels will take around 3 months to appear. The neovascular glaucoma following CRVO is called 100th day glaucoma.

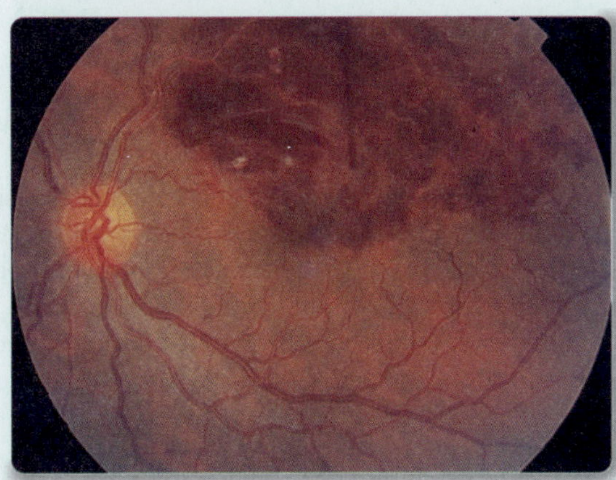

FIGURE 20.11: Acute superotemporal branch vein occlusion

Treatment

1. No specific treatment is available to prevent or reverse ischemic damage. Close follow-up is required to detect and manage complications.
2. In the acute stage of vein occlusion, medical therapies like antiplatelet drugs and anticoagulants have been used with very limited benefits to improve retinal venous flow. The main line of management is control of risk factors, if any.
3. Close follow-up of patient for the development of complications like neovascularization of the retina and/or angle and the development of glaucoma, and also persistent macular edema.
4. Treatment of neovascularization is panretinal photocoagulation.

The neovascularization is mostly preretinal or on the optic disk in branch retinal vein occlusion, whereas in CRVO it will be more in the anterior segment in the form of rubeosis iridis and neovascularization of the angle.

For BRVO, it is recommended that sector laser photocoagulation is applied once retinal or optic disk neovascularization occur. Photocoagulation is applied to the sector of retinal capillary closure. The 500 micron burns at the retina are used and are applied in a scatter pattern to the affected sector. A quadrant usually requires 400–500 burns.

In CRVO, which has resulted in rubeosis iridis or neovascularization of the angle or neovascular glaucoma, the same type of laser photocoagulation has to be done, so as to cover most of the area of the retina outside the posterior pole. This is referred to as panretinal photocoagulation. About 1,500–2,000 burns each sized 500 microns are required.

Management of Macular Edema in RVOs

Grid Laser photocoagulation: In BRVO, grid laser photocoagulation to the edematous area is beneficial. Here gentle burns of 100–200 microns are given in a grid pattern to the areas of vascular leakage, but avoiding the foveal avascular zone.

However, grid photocoagulation is not effective in the treatment of macular edema due to CRVO. In fact the options are quite limited here.

Intravitreal injections: Anti-VEGF agents like ranibizumab and bevacizumab, and long-acting depot steroids like triamcinolone are being increasingly used as intravitreal injections nowadays to treat macular edema in BRVO and CRVO.

Prophylaxis

Early diagnosis and prompt treatment of underlying systemic and ocular disorders is important.

Prognosis

The prognosis for vision in BRVO depends on the involvement of macula and the amount of capillary occlusion.

In BRVO involving the upper and lower nasal branches prognosis for vision is good, since the macula is not affected.

In temporal BRVOs, visual prognosis depends on the damage to the macula. If the capillary non-perfusion is so severe as to produce neovascularization of the fundus or the anterior segment, vision can be severely affected due to vitreous hemorrhage or neovascular glaucoma. In ischemic type, whatever be the treatment given not only that the visual prognosis is poor but the patient also carries risk for ending up with a painful blind eye due to neovascular glaucoma (Figs 20.12 and 20.13).

In non-ischemic type of CRVO the visual prognosis is fairly good.

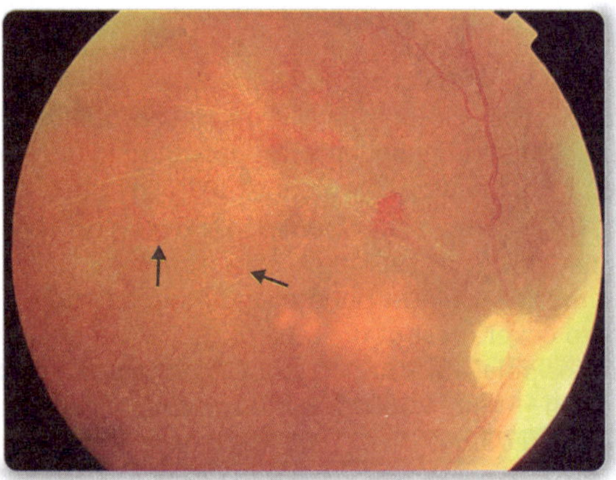

FIGURE 20.12: Old upper temporal BRVO with neovascularization (black arrows) (BRVO, branch retinal artery occlusion)

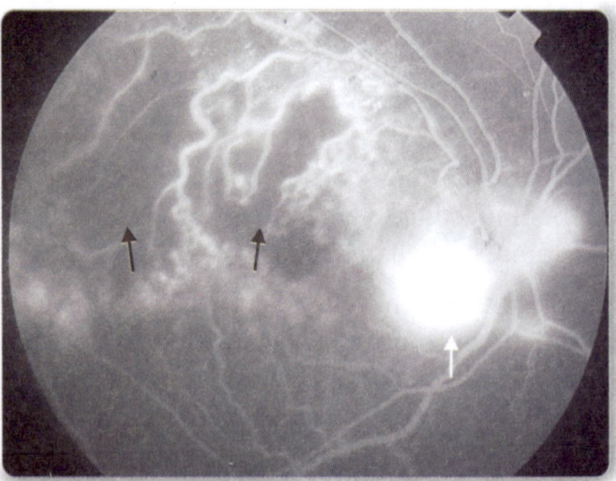

FIGURE 20.13: Branch retinal artery occlusion. Disk new vessels (white arrow) and areas of capillary dropout (black arrows) in old BRVO-FFA (FFA, fundus fluorescein angiogram).

Retinal Arterial Occlusion

Definition

Occlusion of the central retinal artery or one of its branches can lead to infarction of the area of the retina supplied by it often resulting in severe functional impairment of the involved area. This is referred to as central retinal artery occlusion and branch retinal artery occlusion, respectively.

Epidemiology

Retinal artery occlusions occur significantly less often than vein occlusions.

Etiology

1. The most common cause of retinal arterial occlusion is embolization of the retinal vascular tree due to emboli arising from the major arteries supplying the head or from the left side of the heart. The emboli may be:
   a. Fatty material from atheromas.
   b. Calcium deposits from diseased heart valves.
   c. Septic and non-septic fibrin.
   d. Platelet thrombi.
2. In the absence of visible emboli, other causes to be considered are:
   a. Giant-cell (temporal) arteritis.
   b. Collagen vascular diseases.
   c. Oral contraceptives.
   d. Increased orbital pressure in conditions such as retrobulbar hemorrhage and endocrine exophthalmos.
   e. Rare causes include sickle cell disease and syphilis.

Sx **Symptoms**

In CRAO, the patient generally complains of sudden, painless unilateral blindness.

In BRAO, the patient will notice a blurring of vision or visual field defects corresponding to the area of supply of the branch artery. If one of the temporal branches is involved, macula will be affected (since macula receives almost equal amount of blood supply from both superior and inferior temporal branches) and this can cause marked drop in vision.

Sometimes, there will be history of transient obscurations of vision preceding the sudden occlusion.

Signs

Anterior segment may be unremarkable except for a relative afferent pupillary defect (RAPD), which may be present in case of a CRAO. The diagnosis is typically made by ophthalmoscopy.

Fundus changes: In the acute stage of CRAO, the retina appears grayish white due to edema of the layer of optic nerve fibers and is no longer transparent. Only the fovea centralis, which contains no nerve fibers, remains visible as a 'cherry-red spot' because the red color of the choroid shows through at this site in sharp contrast to surrounding white retina (Fig. 20.14). The arteries will be narrow and the smaller branches will be invisible. The column of blood will be seen to be interrupted. This is called 'cattle-truck appearance'. Rarely one will observe an embolus.

Some patients will have a cilioretinal artery (artery originating from the ciliary arteries instead of the central retinal artery supplying the macular area to a variable extent). Patients with a well-developed cilioretinal artery will exhibit normal perfusion in the area of vascular supply at the macula and their loss of visual acuity will be less. Rarely a cilioretinal artery alone may be affected and a cilioretinal artery occlusion will lead to loss of central vision alone (Fig. 20.15).

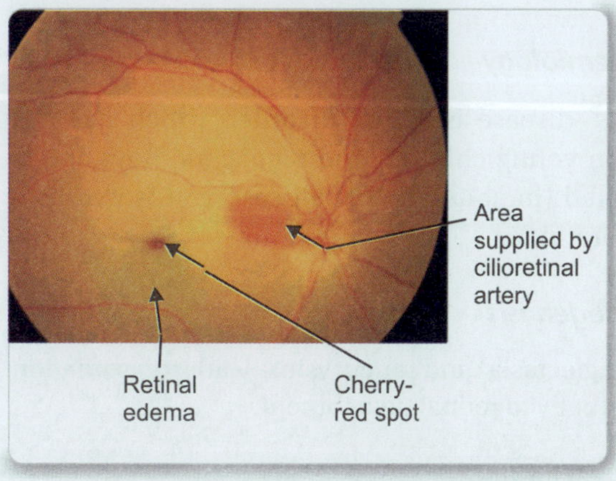

FIGURE 20.14: Central retinal artery occlusion

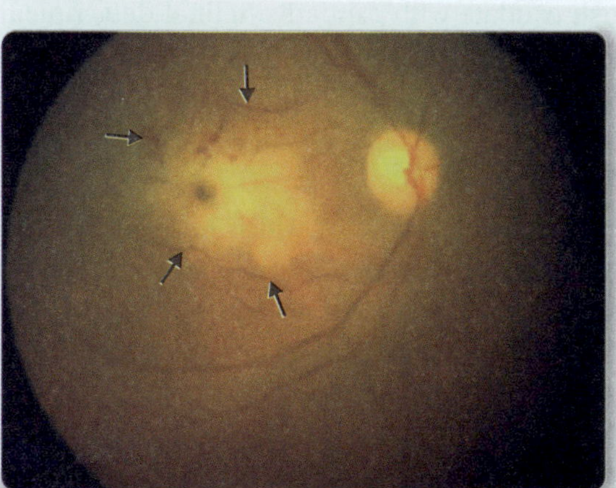

FIGURE 20.15: Cilioretinal artery occlusion (area within the black arrows shows whitening of retina and cherry-red spot)

Late picture: The cherry-red spot and the retinal edema will disappear in a few weeks. The retina will show a diffuse atrophy and the artery and its branches will remain narrow and sometimes show sheathing especially, near the disk. The optic disk will become pale—consecutive optic atrophy.

In branch retinal artery occlusion, a retinal edema will be found in the area of vascular supply of the involved branch (Fig. 20.16). A sectoral area of retinal whitening will be seen corresponding to the area of supply of the involved branch. If a temporal branch is involved a cherry-red spot will be seen.

Visual Field Testing

Visual field testing will reveal a total visual field defect in central retinal artery occlusion and a sectoral defect in branch occlusion.

Differential Diagnosis

1. Other causes of cherry-red spot: It can be seen in lipid-storage diseases such as Tay-Sachs disease, Niemann-Pick disease or Gaucher's disease.
2. Central retinal vein occlusion—in this condition the visual loss is not as sudden or severe as in CRAO and the fundus picture is different.

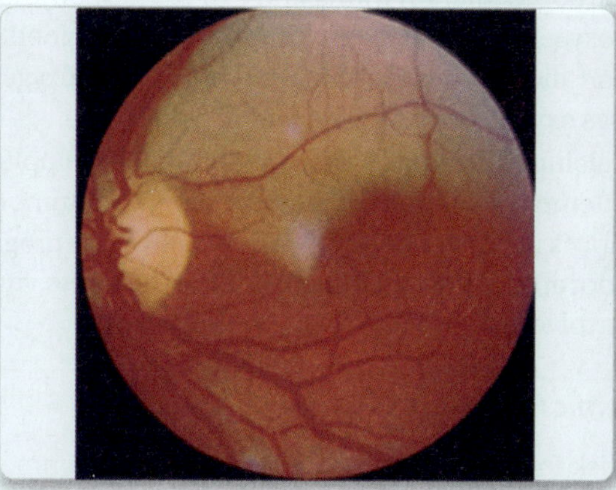

FIGURE 20.16: Branch retinal artery occlusion

Management

Investigations: Obtain a complete blood count to evaluate anemia, polycythemia and platelet disorders.

Sickle cell disease may case retinal artery occlusion (RAO) in black patients and may warrant additional studies. Evaluate the erythrocyte sedimentation rate (ESR) for excluding giant cell arteritis and other systemic vasculitis.

Measure fibrinogen level, antiphospholipid antibodies, prothrombin time (PT), activated partial thromboplastin time (aPTT) and serum protein to evaluate for coagulopathies.

Obtain cholesterol, triglycerides and lipid profile panel to evaluate for atherosclerotic disease. Evaluate blood cultures for bacterial endocarditis and septic emboli.

Consultation

Should be seen by a physician or cardiologist to exclude the various systemic problems outlined already many of which have significant mortality rate.

Treatment

Emergency treatment can be given to drive the embolus to a peripheral smaller vessel and thus restore circulation, if the patient is seen within a couple of hours after the incident.

Ocular massage, medications that reduce intraocular pressure or paracentesis are applied in an attempt to decrease the intraocular pressure and thus open up the vessel. It is often unsuccessful even when initiated immediately. The retina will suffer irreparable damage, if the blood supply is cut off for more than 1 hour.

Carbogen therapy (inhalation of 5% carbon dioxide, 95% oxygen) can be used to improve retinal blood flow. Carbon dioxide dilates retinal arterioles and oxygen increases oxygen delivery to ischemic tissues.

Calcium antagonists or hemodilution are applied in an attempt to improve vascular supply. Thrombolysis therapy is no longer performed due to the poor prognosis (it is not able to prevent blindness) and the risk to vital tissue involved.

Systemic Prophylaxis

The risk for developing a stroke is high in the immediate period after a CRAO. A thorough systemic evaluation for any general risk factors and their management is essential for reducing the risk for life.

Antiplatelet therapy or oral anticoagulants may be indicated in patients with cardiac problems. Smoking should be strongly discouraged.

Clinical Course and Prognosis

The prognosis is poor because irreparable damage to the inner layers of the retina occurs within 1 hour. Blindness usually cannot be prevented in CRAO. The prognosis is better where only a branch of the artery is occluded unless a macular branch is affected.

Coats' Disease

Definition

Congenital retinal telangiectasia with vascular anomalies that nearly always presents unilaterally and can lead to exudation and eventually to exudative retinal detachment.

Epidemiology

Coats' disease is a rare disorder, which manifests itself in young children and teenagers. Boys are usually affected (in about 90% of all cases). It is nearly always unilateral.

Pathogenesis

Telangiectasia and aneurysms lead to exudation and eventually to retinal detachment.

Clinical Findings

Ophthalmoscopy will reveal telangiectasia, subretinal whitish exudate with exudative retinal detachment and hemorrhages involving the macula and surrounding area.

Differential Diagnosis

All causes of leukocoria of which retinoblastoma is the most important condition, but retinoblastoma rarely affects children above 2 years of age.

Other causes include retinopathy of prematurity, toxocariasis, persistent hyperplastic primary vitreous.

Treatment

The treatment of choice is laser photocoagulation or cryotherapy to destroy anomalous vasculature.

Prognosis

If left untreated, the disease will eventually cause blindness due to total retinal detachment. Treatment is effective in preventing blindness in about 50% of all patients.

Eales' Disease

Eales' disease is an idiopathic, bilateral occlusive inflammation of the peripheral retinal veins (periphlebitis) leading to capillary occlusion and neovascularization (Figs 20.17A and B). More common in Asian countries and rare among the white races, males are more commonly affected. A relationship to hypersensitivity to tuberculoproteins is considered to be an etiological factor.

The disease proceeds in three steps:

1. Recurrent episodes of periphlebitis.
2. Capillary occlusion and retinal ischemia.
3. Neovascularization and its sequel like recurrent vitreous hemorrhage, tractional RD, rubeosis iridis and neovascular glaucoma.

Clinical Features

Patients usually comes with a history of seeing floaters with some blurring of vision caused by a small vitreous bleed. If the vitreous hemorrhage is massive, there will be a sudden black out. Repeated similar episodes can occur and the vision usually improves after the initial attacks spontaneously.

Sx Symptoms

The patient, usually a teenage male presents with profound loss of vision in one eye. Rarely presents as leukocoria (white pupil) or unilateral strabismus.

Signs

Depends on the stage of the disease. Initially, the areas of periphlebitis appear as sheathing along an area of the veins with some retinal hemorrhages near it. This may progress to a picture of branch vein occlusion. As the retinal hemorrhages clear the involved veins show sheathing and appear like white threads and there will be extensive areas of capillary drop out as revealed by a fluorescein angiogram (refer Fig. 20.17B). This is followed by the development of new vessels at the junction between the perfused and non-perfused retina. This will result in recurrent vitreous hemorrhages and its complications.

Investigations

Patient has to be evaluated for any inflammatory vascular diseases like collagen vascular disorders. Only when all causes for vasculitis are ruled out, a diagnosis of Eales' disease can be made. Any active TB infection or hypersensitivity to tuberculoproteins also has to be evaluated.

Treatment

In the stage of active periphlebitis, a course of systemic steroids will control the inflammation and reduce the damage to the retina.

Once extensive capillary dropout and subsequent vitreous hemorrhage has started, laser photocoagulation to all the areas of capillary dropout is required to decrease the release of VEGF, thus leading to the regression of new vessels. Vitrectomy will be required in cases with persistent vitreous hemorrhages and tractional RD. Intravitreal injections of anti-VEGF factors are another option.

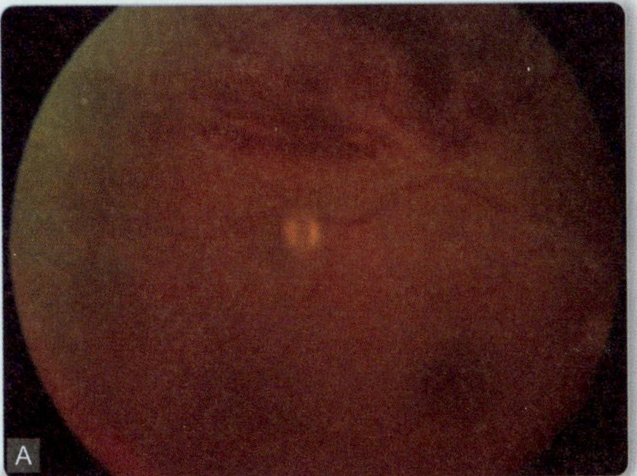

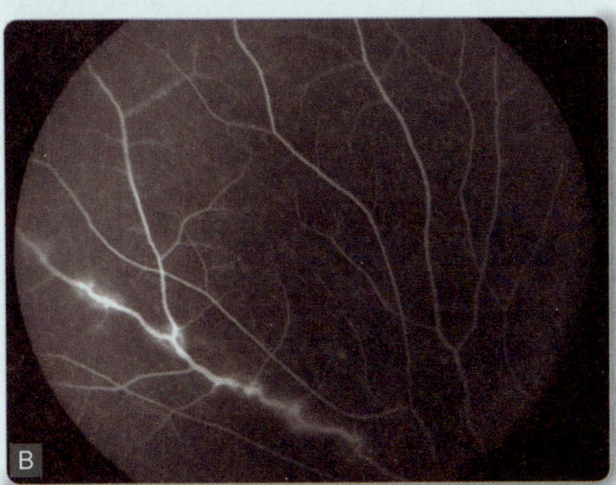

FIGURES 20.17A and B: Eales' disease. **A.** Fundus picture; **B.** Fundus fluorescein angiography.

Complications

Complications are tractional RD, neovascular glaucoma and complicated cataract.

Retinopathy of Prematurity

Definition

Retinopathy of prematurity (ROP) is a disease that affects immature vasculature in the eyes of premature babies.

Epidemiology

The disorder is rare. Infants with birth weight below 1,500 g are at increased risk of developing the disorder. The danger of ROP increases with short gestational age and low birth weight. Most of these babies might have been given oxygen, which aggravates the risk for developing ROP. Retinopathy of prematurity is not always preventable despite optimum care and strict monitoring of partial pressure of oxygen.

Etiopathogenesis

Normal retina is gradually vascularized from the optic disk to the periphery during the final half of gestation, the temporal periphery finally becoming vascularized shortly after term. The earlier in the gestational period an infant is born, the less the vessels have grown out. Preterm birth and exposure to oxygen disturbs the normal development of the retinal vessels. The developing vessels may be arrested in their growth by excessive oxygen in the developing peripheral retina, which obliterates the newly forming vessels. When normal blood vessel growth is interrupted in this way, the vanguard of mesenchymal tissue builds up and forms a ridge that may be interrupted or continuous, peripheral to the retinal vasculature. The peripheral avascular retina becomes hypoxic and releases humoral agents, including vascular endothelial cell growth factor, which stimulate blood vessel growth. In severe cases, extraretinal neovascular proliferation on the surface of the retina and in the vitreous may occur. This results in vitreous hemorrhage, retinal detachment and in the late scarring stage, retrolenticular fibroplasia as vessels and connective tissue fuse with the detached retina (Fig. 20.18).

Findings

The typical fundus findings form the basis of diagnosis of ROP is explained further.

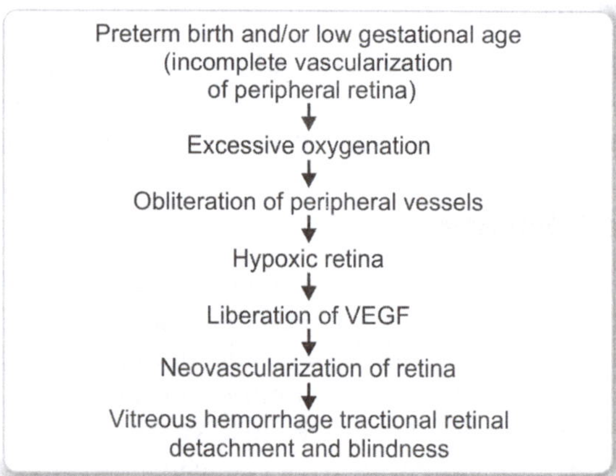

FIGURE 20.18: Showing the course of ROP (ROP, retinopathy of prematurity; VEGF, vascular endothelial growth factor)

Sx Symptoms

After an initially asymptomatic clinical course, the baby will show poor development of vision. The child may not fix or follow a light. In severely affected children, vitreous hemorrhage or retinal detachment will be accompanied by secondary strabismus. Leukocoria can occur in the retrolenticular fibroplasia stage.

Stages

A generally accepted international classification of ROP has been developed to standardize communication and criteria for evaluating treatment.

Stage 1: It is the appearance of a distinct demarcation line separating the peripheral avascular retina from vascularized posterior retina.

Stage 2: It involves the formation of a ridge that is elevated and has width.

Stage 3: It includes extraretinal fibrovascular proliferative tissue growing off the posterior edge of the ridge into the vitreous or onto the surface of the retina.

Stage 4: It exhibits a subtotal retinal detachment without involving the fovea (4A) and a retinal attachment involving the fovea (4B).

Stage 5: It is a total retinal detachment.

Any of the stages of ROP may exhibit dilatation and tortuosity of the posterior retinal blood vessels in which case a '+' is added to the number of the stage and is termed as 'plus' disease.

The location and extent of ROP are described by dividing each retina into three zones with the disk, where the retinal blood vessels begin at the center of concentric circles, which are as given below.

Zone 1: It has a radius that extends from the disk about twice as far as from the disk to the macula.

Zone 2: It extends all the way to the ora serrata on the nasal side and a little bit anterior to the equator on the temporal side.

Zone 3: It is a crescent that involves the remaining superior, inferior and temporal retina. The retina is also divided into clock hours (Fig. 20.19).

Differential Diagnosis

Other causes of leukocoria such as retinoblastoma or cataract should be considered.

Examination and Treatment

Premature infants who are born with a birth weight of less than 1,250–1,500 g or a gestational age less than 32 weeks should be examined beginning around 4 weeks of age and every 2–3 weeks thereafter until the vessels have reached the ora serrata. If ROP is discovered, the patient should be followed more closely, depending on the activity and severity of the abnormalities. If stage 3+ ROP is reached (Fig. 20.20), involving 5 hours or more of the circumference of the retina continuously or 8 hours intermittently, one should consider treating with confluent cryotherapy or indirect diode laser therapy to the entire avascular retina.

Prophylaxis

Partial pressure of oxygen should be kept as low as possible and ophthalmologic screening examinations should be performed.

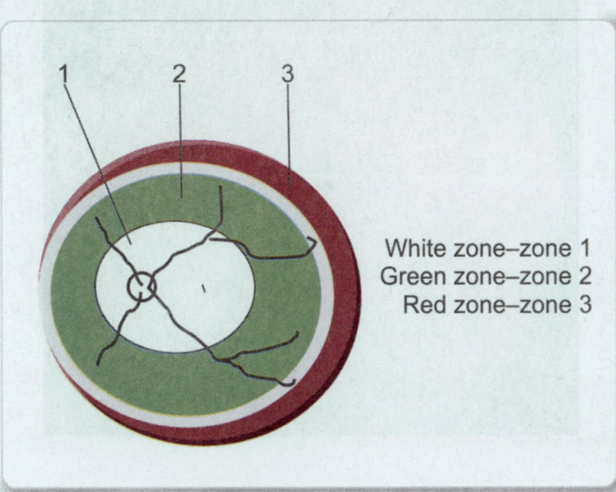

FIGURE 20.19: Zones of retina

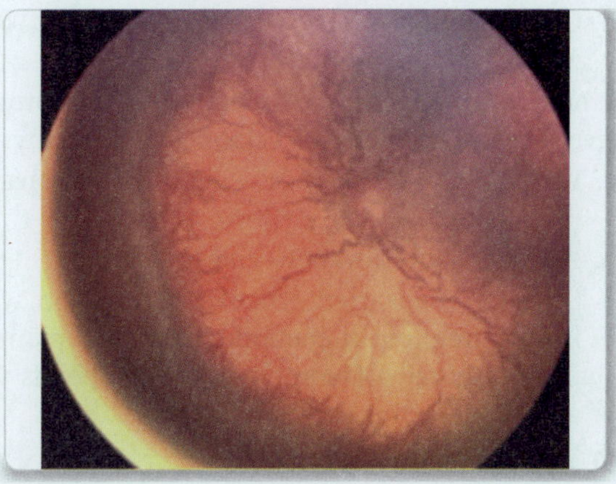

FIGURE 20.20: Stage 3, zone 2+ retinopathy of prematurity

Early detection of retinopathy of prematurity is particularly important.

Clinical Course and Prognosis

Stage 1 and 2 retinopathy resolves spontaneously in 85% of all affected children.

Sickle Cell Retinopathy

Sickle cell retinopathy is a retinopathy associated with sickle cell disease. The causative factor is the occlusion of the small peripheral vessels due the blood abnormalities and consequent retinal hypoxia.

Sickle Cell Disease

The mutant hemoglobins S and C are alleles of hemoglobin and cause sickle trait (HbAS), sickle cell disease (HbSS) and hemoglobin SC disease.

The initial event in the retinopathy associated with this condition is intravascular sickling, hemostasis and thrombosis. Any hemoglobinopathy may cause non-proliferative or proliferative retinopathy, but severe proliferative disease is more common in HbSC and S-Thal than HbSS, which causes more systemic complications. The incidence of significant visual loss is about 4%.

Fundus findings can be classified as follows:

1. Non-proliferative sickle retinopathy is characterized by:
   a. Salmon patch hemorrhages occurring after peripheral retinal arteriolar occlusion.
   b. Refractile spots, which are reabsorbed hemorrhages leaving hemosiderin deposition.
   c. Black sunburst lesions, which are areas of RPE hypertrophy and hyperplasia with posthemorrhagic hemosiderin.

   d. Central retinal artery occlusion may also occur with or without retinopathy.
2. Proliferative sickle cell retinopathy: The five progressive stages of proliferative sickle cell retinopathy are:
   a. Peripheral arteriolar occlusion due to intravascular sickling.
   b. Peripheral arteriovenous anastomosis.
   c. Sea fan (retinal arterial) neovascularization, which is most frequent at about the equatorial plane superotemporally. Fluorescein angiography is valuable for detecting early sea fans.
   d. Vitreous hemorrhage.
   e. Retinal detachment, which usually begins in areas affected by fibrovascular proliferation and local vitreous traction.

Treatment

Application of low-energy scatter argon laser photocoagulation to the involved ischemic areas induces regression in neovascular fronds. Pars plana vitrectomy is useful in treating patients with vitreous hemorrhage.

Prophylaxis

All diagnosed cases of sickle cell disease should undergo periodic fundus evaluation for early detection of proliferative changes and prompt laser treatment to prevent blindness.

ACQUIRED MACULAR DISORDERS

Age-related Macular Degeneration

Age-related macular degeneration (ARMD) is a degenerative condition affecting the macula resulting in significant ocular morbidity. It is a leading cause of irreversible blindness in developed countries. With increase in the life expectancy of people of our country, the incidence of ARMD is increasing here also.

It is characterized by the presence of drusen and retinal pigment epithelial changes in the macula with some degree of vision loss or subretinal neovascularization with marked loss of vision. It is usually seen in patients over 50 years and the prevalence increases as the age increases.

Risk Factors

Age-related macular degeneration has a multifactorial etiology both genetic and environmental factors play a role:

1. Age: Increasing age is an important risk factor.
2. Race: More common in white races. Melanin pigment plays some protective role.
3. Heredity: Risk is more, if a family member has ARMD.
4. Smoking: Increases the risk of developing ARMD.
5. Other factors: High dietary intake of saturated fats and cholesterol, hypertension, oxidative stress and drug intake like chlorpromazine, chloroquine, etc.

Classification

Two major types are:
1. Dry or non-exudative ARMD.
2. Wet or exudative ARMD.

Dry ARMD (non-exudative)

Dry ARMD is characterized by drusen and geographical atrophy of RPE (Fig. 20.21). It is the major form (around 90%). Drusen are extracellular deposits located between RPE and the Bruch's membrane. These consist of metabolic waste products from RPE and immune complexes. These are common in old people, but large soft or confluent drusen associated with hyperpigmentation of RPE are associated with increased risk for visual loss.

Clinical features

There is only mild-to-moderate gradual impairment of vision in these patients. The near vision is more affected and people may experience some difficulty in reading small print even with proper glass correction.

Fundus findings

The macula shows varying amount of hard and soft drusen. Hard drusen are smaller well-defined yellow excrescences where as soft drusen are larger and paler lesions with ill-defined borders. RPE shows varying amounts of hyper and hypopigmentation. The foveal reflex is

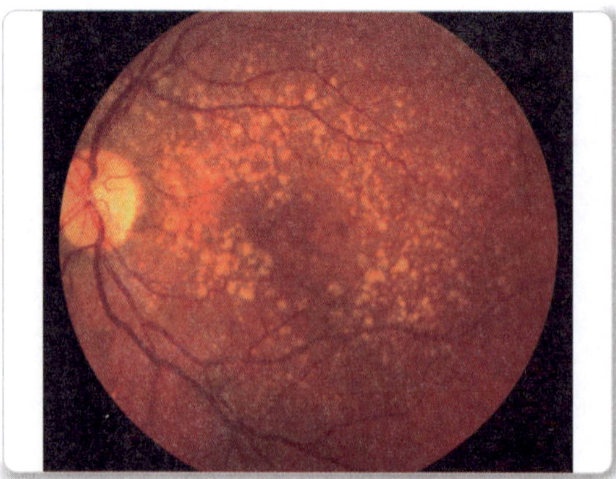

FIGURE 20.21: Dry age-related macular degeneration with drusen at the macula

often absent. Presence of large confluent soft drusen increases the risk of progression to wet type of ARMD.

Treatment

There is no effective treatment.

Observation

Since patients with soft drusen are at the risk for developing choroidal neovascular membranes and exudative ARMD, they should be instructed to report immediately, if they experience any sudden blurring of vision or distortion of images.

The age-related eye diseases study (AREDS) has shown some beneficial effect for high doses of antioxidant vitamins (C, E and β carotene) in reducing the risk for progression of visual loss.

Wet ARMD (exudative)

Wet ARMD is the less common variety of ARMD. In dry ARMD, vision loss is gradual; whereas in wet ARMD, there is loss of central vision within a few days. Two important features of this disease are retinal pigment epithelial detachment and choroidal neovascularization (Fig. 20.22). Choroidal neovascularization consists of proliferation of fibrovascular tissue from choriocapillaris into the subretinal space. Choroidal neovascularization may precede or follow the development of retinal pigment epithelial detachment. Fundus fluorescein angiogram is used to identify the membrane (Fig. 20.23). Subsequently, the membrane may cause leakage of fluid resulting in sensory retinal detachment and subretinal hemorrhage, which can breakthrough to form a vitreous hemorrhage and finally disciform scarring. Disciform scar is the end stage and appears as a subretinal fibrovascular scar with areas of hyperpigmentation (Figs 20.24A and B).

Clinical features

Patient usually presents with a sudden drop in vision. They may experience a black central field defect and metamorphopsia (distortion of images) due to the distortion of fovea because of subretinal fluid. They may experience

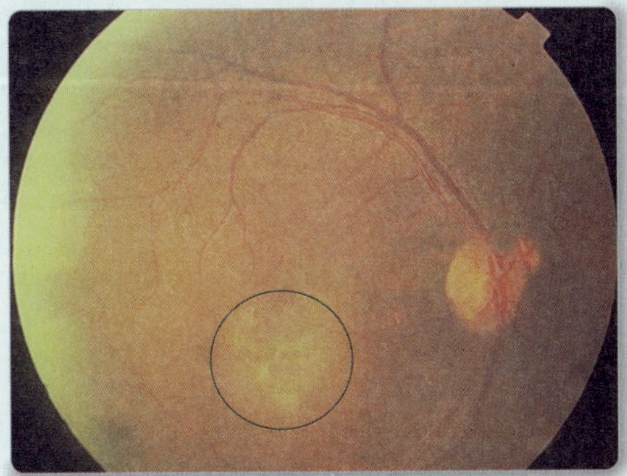

FIGURE 20.22: Wet age-related macular degeneration with exudation at macula

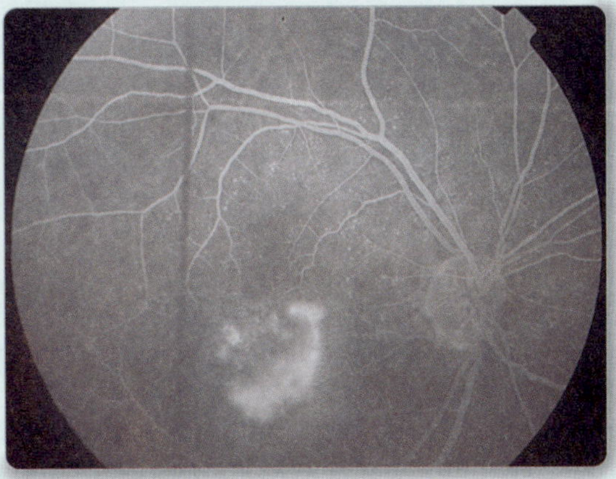

FIGURE 20.23: Fundus fluorescein angiogram of wet age-related macular degeneration showing choroidal neovascular membrane

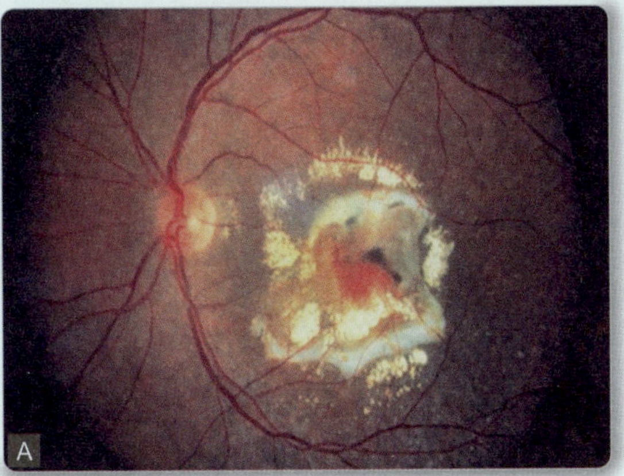

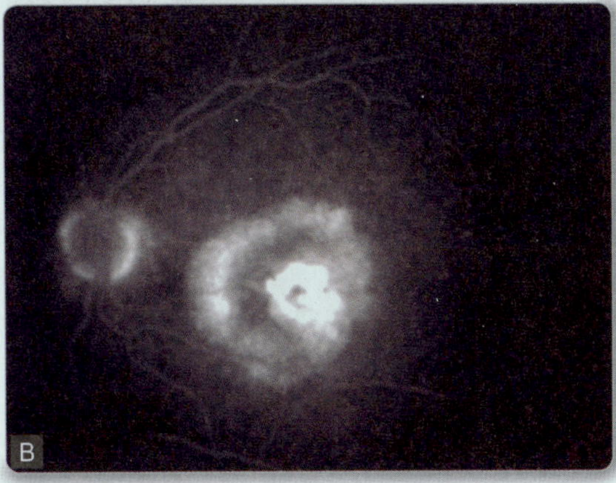

FIGURES 20.24A and B: Wet age-related macular degeneration. **A.** With disciform scar; **B.** Fundus fluorescein angiogram.

some difficulty in color discrimination and slow recovery of visual function after exposure to bright light.

Careful biomicroscopic examination of the macula is essential to detect the early changes. There will be areas of hemorrhages, subretinal fluid and pigment epithelial detachments (Figs 20.25A and B).

Investigations

1. Fundus fluorescein angiography will reveal the site, size and extent of CNVMs and pigment epithelial detachment.
2. Indocyanine green angiogram: This is indicated where the CNVMs are masked by hemorrhage. This angiogram is done with the dye namely indocyanine green using infrared light. This angiogram helps to reveal CNVMs, which are masked by overlying blood and fluid, and not properly visualized with FFA.
3. Optical coherence tomography (OCT) gives a cross-sectional picture of the architecture of retina and reveal the CNVMs and pigment epithelial detachments (PEDs).

Treatment

Wet ARMD treatment includes:

1. Laser photocoagulation is effective for well-defined extrafoveal membranes, but not for membranes close to fovea.
2. Photodynamic therapy—here a photosensitive dye is injected intravenously and the application of a continuous nonthermal laser is done on the CNVM. This photosensitive (verteporfin) accumulates in the CNVM, which absorbs the laser energy that is not intense enough to cause damage to normal tissue.
3. Anti-vascular endothelial growth factor (anti-VEGF) is the main stay of treatment. The agents used are bevacizumab, ranibizumab, pegaptanib sodium given as intravitreal injections. These can cause regression of the CNVMs and stabilize or slightly improve vision. The injections are expensive and have to be repeated.

Central Serous Retinopathy

Central serous retinopathy (CSR) is a self-limiting disease in the young adults, more commonly in males, characterized by localized detachment of sensory retina at the macula (Fig. 20.26) because of fluid collection under the sensory retina due to a presumed dysfunction of a focal area of RPE and the etiology is unknown.

Risk Factors

The risk factors are psychological stress, type A personality, pregnancy, some hormonal or metabolic dysfunction.

Clinical Features

Patient presents usually with complaints of a black area in front of the eye (large central scotoma) or distortion of images (metamorphopsia). Visual acuity is usually reduced to 6/36–6/9, but usually correctable to 6/6 with plus glasses. Fundus examination will show a retinal elevation at the macula surrounded by a ring reflex. In some patients, small subretinal precipitates will be present, suggestive of longstanding CSR. Spontaneous resolution occurs in 2–3 months, but it can recur.

Fundus fluorescein angiogram is useful in making a definite diagnosis.

Two types of fluorescein angiographic patterns (Figs 20.27A and B) are seen. They are:

1. Ink blot: Common, a hyperfluorescent spot that slowly increases in size.
2. Smoke stalk: Less common, a hyperfluorescent spot that increases in a vertical fashion.

ILM
IS/OS
RPE
BM
Caliper
64
A

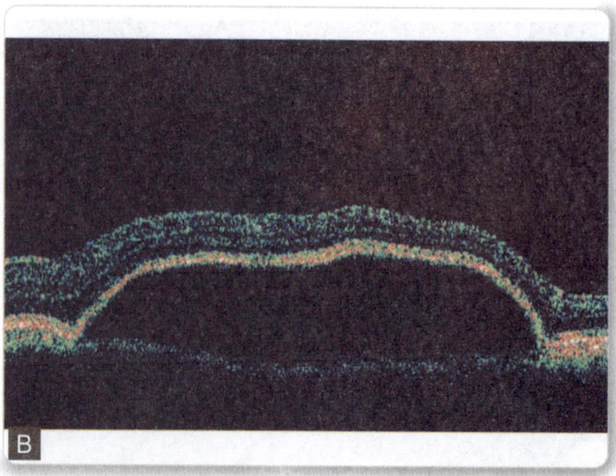

FIGURES 20.25A and B: Optical coherence tomography. **A.** Normal; **B.** Picture showing pigment epithelial detachment.

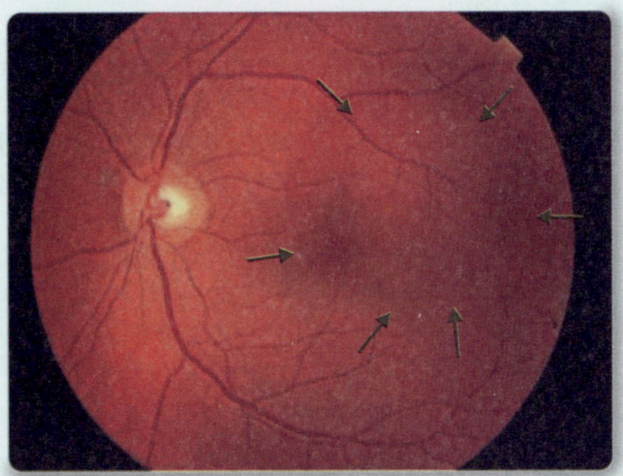

FIGURE 20.26: Central serous retinopathy

Treatment

About 80% of the CSR spontaneously resolves within 2–3 months in the first attack.

Laser photocoagulation is necessary in recurrent CSR or if the first attack does not resolve in 4 months. If the patient is a professional, laser photocoagulation may be done even in the first attack to shorter the episode. Laser is not possible, if the leak is within the foveal avascular zone (Fig. 20.28). Laser done here will cause permanent visual damage. Recurrence is common with this disease.

Macular Hole

Macular hole is a partial or full thickness defect in the retina at macula.

Etiology

Idiopathic macular hole (Fig. 20.29) is thought to be caused by the perifoveal vitreous contraction, which elevates the retina in the foveal region.

Other causes of macular hole are high myopia, blunt trauma and solar retinopathy.

Stages

- Stage 1a: Impending hole
- Stage 1b: Occult hole
- Stage 2: Full thickness hole with pseudo-operculum
- Stage 3: Full thickness hole with partial posterior vitreous detachment (PVD)
- Stage 4: Full thickness hole with total PVD.

Investigation

Optical coherence tomography will reveal the stages of a macular hole formation (Fig. 20.30).

Clinical Features

Visual acuity is reduced to 6/60 or less. Unilateral macular hole is noticed by chance by the patient when the fellow eye is closed. On fundus examination a round punched out area with a surrounding cuff of retinal detachment is usually seen. When a narrow slit beam is centered over the hole, patient will report that the beam is interrupted in full thickness macular hole (Watzke-Allen test).

Treatment

Indication for treatment are full thickness macular holes associated with a visual acuity worse than 6/18 and a duration less than 1 year. Vitrectomy with peeling of internal limiting membrane to relieve traction at the macula is the treatment for macular hole.

Photoretinitis

Photoretinitis is otherwise called 'eclipse blindness' is caused by watching a solar eclipse with naked eyes or by exposure to the flash of the short-circuiting of a strong

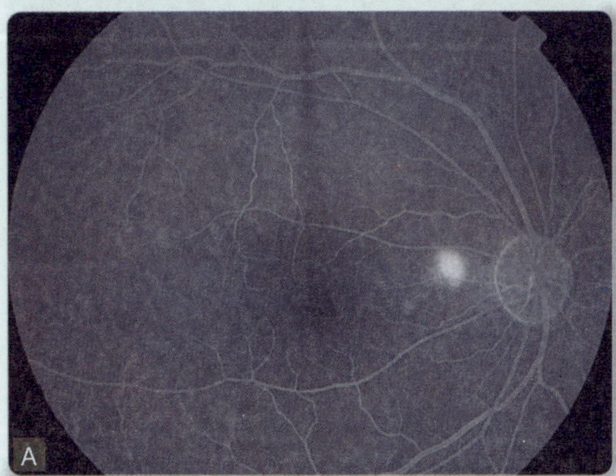

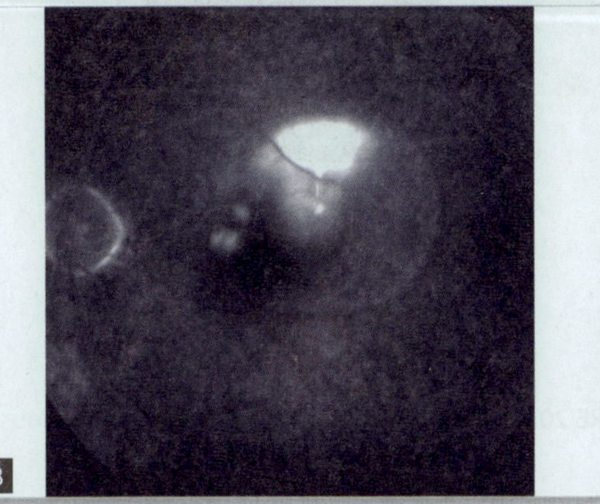

FIGURES 20.27A and B: FFA in central serous. A. Ink-blot pattern of hyperfluorescence; B. Late picture with dye spreading to reveal the subretinal fluid collection.

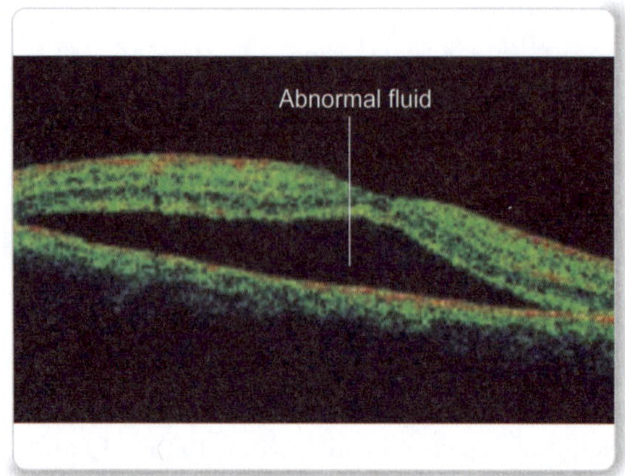

FIGURE 20.28: Optical coherence tomography showing fluid between the pigment epithelium and the sensory retina

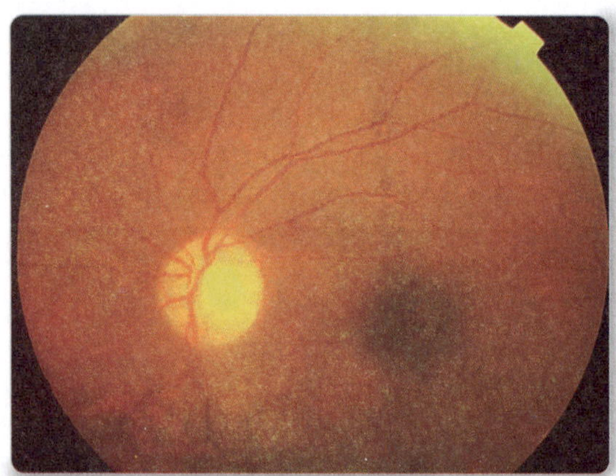

FIGURE 20.29: Macular hole

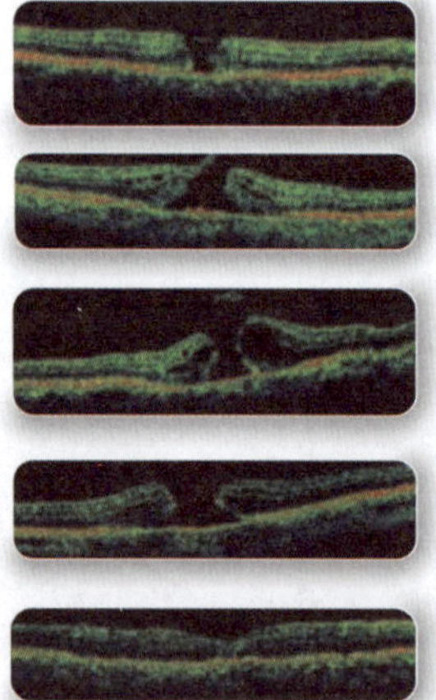

FIGURE 20.30: Optical coherence tomography of various stages of a macular hole

current. This is due to a thermal burn produced at the fovea by the large amount of UV and infrared rays that reach the retina and get focused on the fovea.

Clinical Features

There will be a persistence of the after image of the bright scene immediately following the exposure. This is followed by a positive scotoma (a black area) in front of the eye. A negative scotoma and a permanent decrease in vision is the end result.

Initially the retina appears normal, but soon a pale area surrounded by a reddish ring appears at the macula. Soon an atrophic scar develops at the macula with some pigmentation. Later a macular hole can develop. These changes are permanent.

Treatment

No treatment is effective. So, prevention is important. Never watch a solar eclipse with naked eyes, only through special protective goggles that give protection from short-wavelength rays.

Commotio Retinae

Commotio retinae are macular clouding caused by a contusion injury to the eye.

Clinically, there is some blurring of vision and the macular area will show a 'cherry-red spot.' In mild cases the clouding will disappear with full recovery of vision. More severe damage can lead to some pigmentary degeneration and even macular hole formation. In severe cases, choroidal rupture with retinal hemorrhages can occur with permanent decrease in vision.

Treatment

No effective treatment. A course of systemic steroids can be tried.

RETINAL DETACHMENT

Retinal detachment (RD) is a separation of the retina proper from the pigment epithelium.

The pigment epithelial layer remains attached to the choroid and the potential space of the optic vesicle is opened up in RD.

Classification of RD is as follows:

1. Rhegmatogenous or primary detachments.
2. Non-rhegmatogenous or secondary detachments: It can again be divided as:
   a. Tractional.
   b. Exudative detachment.

The comparison of primary and secondary RD is given in Table 20.3.

TABLE 20.3: Comparison of primary and secondary retinal detachment (RD)

Features	Rhegmatogenous	Tractional	Exudative RD
History	Aphakia, myopia, blunt trauma	DM*, ROP†, penetrating trauma	Malignant HT‡, renal failure, eclampsia
Retinal break	Present	Absent	Absent
Extent	May extend to ora, convex and surface corrugated	Localized and concave	Central or peripheral, convex and smooth surface
Subretinal fluid	Clear	Clear	Turbid with shifting fluid
Intraocular pressure	Low	Normal	Variable
Transillumination	Normal	Normal	Blocked

*DM, diabetes mellitus; †ROP, retinopathy of prematurity; ‡HT, hypertension.

Rhegmatogenous Retinal Detachment

Rhegmatogenous retinal detachment affects 1 in 10,000 of population and the second eye can also be eventually affected in 10% of cases. Myopia is the commonest condition associated with RD.

Etiopathogenesis

Certain changes in the retina and vitreous are essential for a RD to occur:

1. The word rhegma means 'break', as the name indicates rhegmatogenous retinal detachments are usually caused by a break or full thickness defect is the inner sensory layer of the retina. But, a break alone in not enough to cause separation of the two layers of the retina. Two more conditions should exist to cause the mechanical separation of the two layers:
   a. Dynamic vitreous traction: Vitreous traction can be dynamic (occurring during ocular movements) or static (persistent traction unrelated to ocular movements) rhegmatogenous detachment is associated with dynamic vitreous traction. When there is total or partial posterior vitreous detachment with vitreous liquefaction and abnormal adhesions of vitreous to retina, ocular movements will lead to increased pull on the retina at the areas of adhesion and this will lead to mechanical separation of the two layers of the retina.
   b. Liquefaction of the vitreous, which will lead to entry of fluid from the vitreous through the hole to the subretinal space.

If the vitreous is not liquefied and there is no dynamic traction on the retina, RD will not occur even in the presence of a retinal hole.

Breaks are usually caused by retinal degeneration which are commonly seen in the periphery of the retina in:

1. Myopic eyes.
2. Ocular trauma and vitreoretinal traction.

Types of retinal breaks include:

1. Holes or circular defects.
2. Flap or horseshoe tears.
3. Giant retinal tears (tears involving more than one quadrant).
4. Dialysis (disinsertion of the retina at ora serrata).

The upper temporal segment is the commonest site of a retinal tear (60%).

Degenerations, which predispose to retinal detachment include lattice degeneration, white without pressure, diffuse chorioretinal degeneration, vitreoretinal tufts, meridional folds and enclosed oral bays.

Lattice degeneration: This is a common degenerative change seen in 8% of population. This is the commonest peripheral degeneration leading to RD and it is commonly seen in myopic eyes. It is seen in the periphery characterized by arborizing lines arranged in a lattice pattern with associated retinal thinning and vitreous liquefaction (Fig. 20.31). Most common site is the upper temporal quadrant and it is seen parallel to the ora.

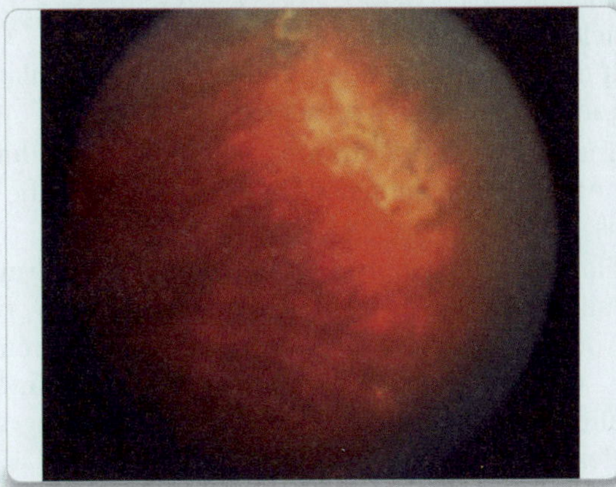

FIGURE 20.31: Lattice degeneration

The progressive thinning in the area of lattice degeneration leads to the formation of retinal breaks at the posterior border or atrophic holes within the lattice itself. Vitreous traction is usually present along the posterior border of the lattice and this pull will lead to retinal detachment. Not all cases of lattice degeneration lead to detachment and hence needs only regular follow-up. Prophylactic treatment with laser is indicated in lattice degeneration with flap or horseshoe tears in high myopia, if there is RD in the follow eye or the affected eye is aphakic.

White without pressure: Discrete well-defined areas of retinal whitening are seen in the retinal periphery usually indicating vitreous traction. Similar picture can sometimes be seen on indentation of the retinal periphery during examination with indirect ophthalmoscope and hence the name for this degeneration. It is commonly associated with giant retinal tears and retinal detachment.

Diffuse chorioretinal degeneration: Commonly seen in myopic eyes, it can follow chorioretinal inflammations (like acute retinal necrosis) also. Thinning of the retina in these areas leads to hole formation and if it is associated with partial posterior vitreous detachment, vitreous traction can lead to RD.

Meridional fold: It is a small radial fold of thickened retina usually seen in the upper nasal quadrant. It often shows a small hole at its apex.

Degeneration not predisposing to retinal detachment: Paving stone/cobblestone degeneration, RPE hypertrophy and hyperplasia and peripheral cystoid degeneration.

Sx **Symptoms**

The symptoms are visual:
- Flashes of light (photopsia)
- Floaters
- Field defect and failing visual acuity.

If the detachment does not involve the macula, visual acuity may be well preserved.

The earliest symptoms are flashes of light produced by the irritation of the sensory epithelium due to the vitreous traction.

Floaters are produced by the vitreous detachment and slight bleeding into the vitreous produced by rupture of small blood vessels at the edge of the retinal tears. Sometimes larger vessels may be torn in this manner producing significant vitreous bleeding and sudden drop in vision. The RD will be detected when the vitreous hemorrhage clears.

As the retina separates a field effect will be experienced by the patient corresponding to the detached retina. If the separation is sudden and massive, the patient will feel like a curtain falling before the eye. If the macula is not involved, good visual acuity will be retained, but the RD can progress and can also involve the macula in course of time.

Signs

Anterior segment
- Pupil may show RAPD
- The intraocular pressure is often low compared to the other eye
- Chronic retinal detachment may show anterior uveitis.

Posterior segment

The detached retina will lose its pink color and appear pale blue in color and convex in contour and show waves or undulations (Fig. 20.32). The retinal vessels in the detached area will appear darker in hue and they lose their reflex streak. If there is a large volume of subretinal fluid, the retina will be much elevated from its bed—this is called bullous RD (Fig. 20.33).

Extend of detachment depends on the position of the hole or tear according to the Lincoff rule. Tobacco dusting of the vitreous may be seen due to pigment deposition.

Long-standing retinal detachment may show thinning and cyst formation, pigmented lines, proliferative vitreoretinopathy (PVR) changes and funnel-shaped RD.

Proliferative vitreoretinopathy is subretinal or epiretinal membrane formation seen in long-standing RDs and RDs following trauma. PVR gives rigidity to the detached retina and fixed retinal folds. PVD is an important cause for failure of retinal detachment surgery.

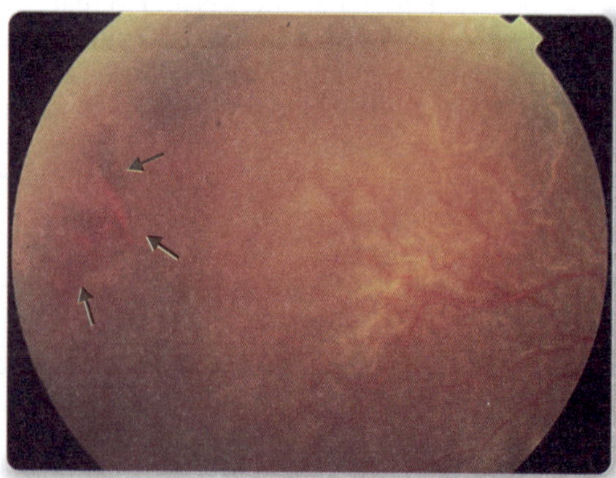

FIGURE 20.32: Retinal tear in retinal detachment (black arrows)

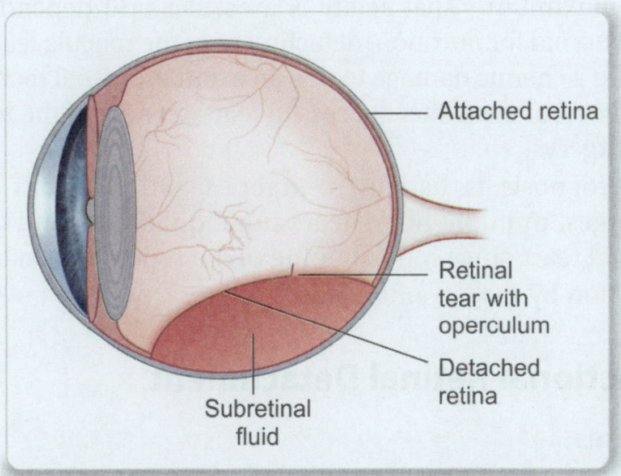

FIGURE 20.33: Retinal detachment with subretinal fluid

Management

Principle: A RD may be associated with more than one retinal break and it is essential that all breaks are identified and localized accurately. All these holes have to be sealed to stop fluid traffic through these holes.

Investigations

Retinal examination with indirect ophthalmoscope is a must to know the:

1. Extent of detachment.
2. Position of all holes/tear.
3. Presence of vitreoretinal traction.
4. Presence of shifting fluid.

Goldmann three-mirror lens also can be used for retinal evaluation.

Examination with indirect ophthalmoscope: With the pupil well-dilated with mydriatics, a thorough examination of the retina is done up to the ora serrata with the help of scleral indentation. All breaks should be detected and their exact locations identified by their distance from anatomical landmarks like optic disk, major vessels and ora serrata, and also by the meridian of their location according to the clock hours. All these details are marked on a detailed fundus drawing.

B-scan ultrasonography: This is used in diagnosing RD in eyes with opaque media due to cataract or vitreous hemorrhage.

Differential Diagnosis

1. Tractional and exudative RD: Differentiated by the characteristic clinical appearance.
2. Degenerative retinoschisis: This condition is characterized by a split in the sensory retina into two layers at the level of the outer plexiform layer. It appears as a smooth immobile elevation of the retina usually anterior to the equator and the surface may show snowflake-like lesions (Figs 20.34A and B). The inner layer may show breaks, but rarely both layers can develop holes and this can lead to rhegmatogenous RD.

The common differences between retinal detachment and retinoschisis are given in Table 20.4.

TABLE 20.4: Retinal detachment (RD) vs retinoschisis

Features	RD	Retinoschisis
Surface	Corrugated	Smooth and glistening
Scotoma	Relative	Absolute
Pigment in vitreous	Present	Absent
Reaction to photocoagulation	Absent	Present

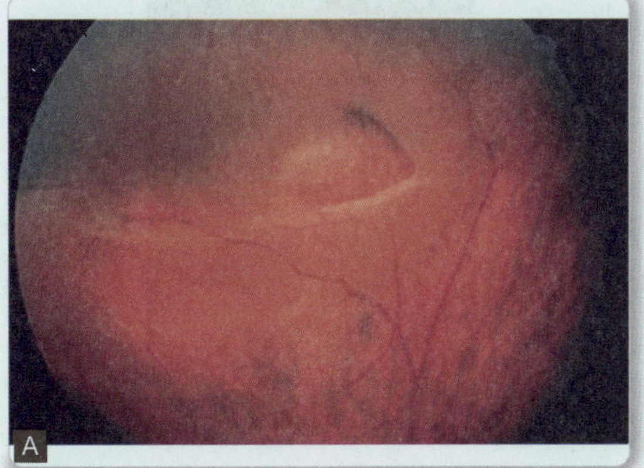

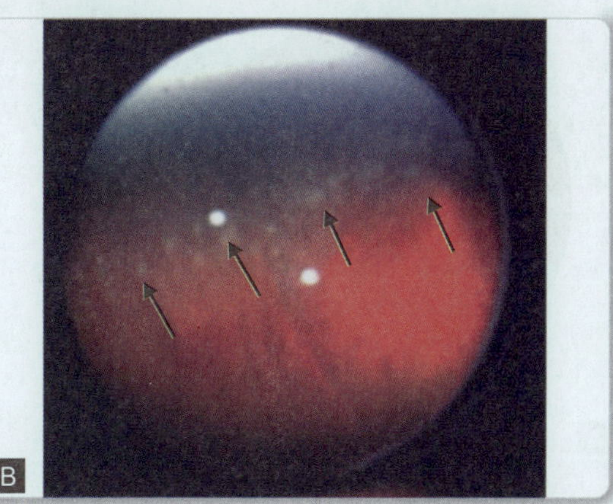

FIGURES 20.34A and B: Snowflake degeneration

Steps in RD Surgery

1. Sealing of all retinal holes: This will stop all fluid traffic into the subretinal space and the remaining fluid in the subretinal space will get spontaneously reabsorbed bringing the detached retina to its normal anatomical position. This sealing is done by inducing an aseptic inflammation around the retinal break by cryotherapy, laser photocoagulation or diathermy.
2. Bringing the retina and choroid in contact: The detached retina and the choroid have to be brought in apposition at the site of the retinal break to create a firm adhesion. This is done by external tamponade by indenting the sclera with silicon bands sutured into place at the site of the retinal breaks or this scleral band can be an encirclage band, which will also decrease the vitreous traction. If there is severe vitreous traction at the breaks, the external tamponade has to be supplemented with internal tamponade by injecting gases or silicon oil after doing a vitrectomy.
3. Drainage of subretinal fluid: In bullous RDs there is a large volume of subretinal fluid (Figs 30.35A and B), drainage of this subretinal fluid is also done through a small opening made into the subretinal space through the sclera and choroid.
4. Pars plana vitrectomy: In case of old RD with PVR changes like funnel RD (Fig. 20.36), pars plana vitrectomy is done to peel the membranes, relieve the fraction and then internal tamponade is done.

Prognosis

Prognosis is good, if it is a fresh retinal detachment with a single break without PVR changes. Prognosis is less, if the macula is detached. Since the center of the fovea with the maximum visual acuity is avascular and depends on the choroid for nutrition, detachment of the macula leads to severe ischemic damage to this area and the visual recovery will be poor even after successful reattachment of the retina by surgery.

Prognosis is bad in resurgeries, old RD with PVR changes, multiple holes/tears in all quadrants and giant retinal tears since repositioning of the retina to its natural position by surgery often fails.

Tractional Retinal Detachment

Causes

- Diabetes
- ROP
- Penetrating injury and venous occlusion.

Etiopathogenesis

In tractional retinal detachment (TRD) situation there is persistent traction on some portion of the retina due to contraction of fibrovascular proliferations in the vitreous. This persistent pull elevates the retina at the site of pull on the retina (Figs 20.37A and B). The RD in TRD is concave in configuration, localized and the effect on vision depends on the site involved. This traction can lead to retinal tears also leading to rhegmatogenous RD, and both TRD and rhegmatogenous RD can exist together.

Clinical Features

Since, TRD is associated with extensive damage to retina and vitreous symptoms due to the RD per se is insignificant. There will be a long history of poor visual acuity depending on the extent of damage to the macula and the vitreous

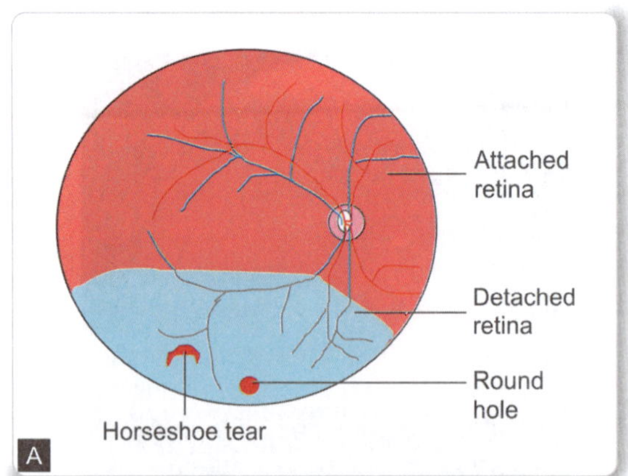

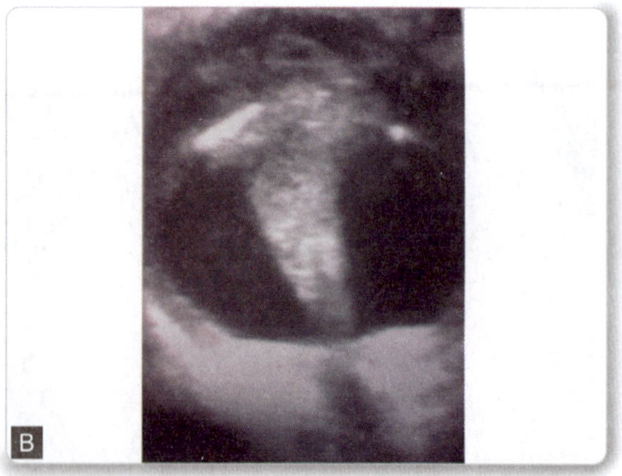

FIGURES 20.35A and B: Retinal detachment. **A.** Rhegmatogenous retinal detachment with retinal break; **B.** Ultrasound showing funnel RD.

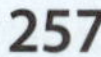

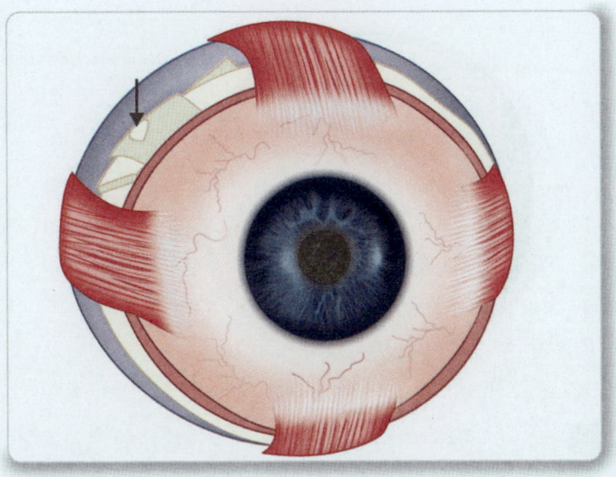

FIGURE 20.36: Eye with encirclage band after retinal detachment surgery

hemorrhage or proliferation. The tractional RD is often detected on routine examination of the fundus. The involved retina is usually a small area and the RD is concave in configuration and shows no undulations. The tractional RD is often stationary and not progressive.

Management

Proper evaluation is done by indirect ophthalmoscopy and B-scan ultrasonography.

Simple TRD can be relieved by vitrectomy and release of traction. External tamponade with scleral encirclage with silicone bands and internal tamponade with intravitreal gases or silicon oil may be required depending on the extent of vitreous traction.

Traction with a retinal break and secondary rhegmatogenous RD needs combined pars plana vitrectomy with scleral buckling procedures.

Exudative Retinal Detachment

Causes

Exudative retinal detachment seen in retinal or choroidal disease like choroidal melanoma, systemic hypertension, eclampsia, renal failure, etc. Here the detachment is due to the exudate collected in the potential space between retina proper and RPE.

Clinical Features

The collection of exudation under the retina leads to a smooth globular elevation of the retina (Figs 20.38A and B). The fluid is often turbid and assumes a dependent position 'shifting subretinal fluid'.

Treatment

Treatment is non-surgical since it is caused by systemic diseases, neoplasia and inflammatory condition. Treatment of the primary cause can correct the detachment.

HEREDITARY RETINAL AND CHOROIDAL DYSTROPHIES

Hereditary retinal and choroidal dystrophies are usually bilateral diseases with symmetric involvement. These dystrophies can be classified in various ways, which are as given below:

1. Anatomical level of involvement.
2. Hereditary pattern.
3. Clinical features and electrophysiological studies. Electroretinography (ERG) and kinetic visual field examination are the most useful tests to diagnose this retinal degeneration.

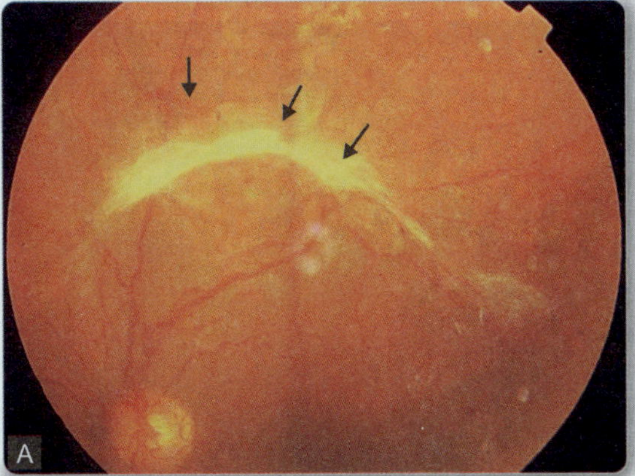

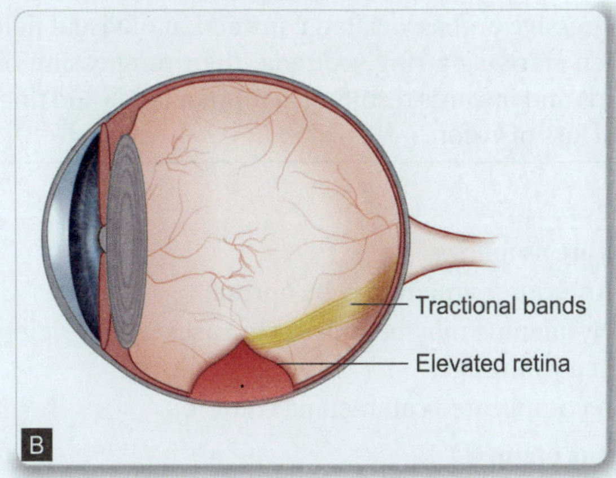

FIGURES 20.37A and B: Tractional retinal detachment **A.** Photograph; **B.** Diagrammatic representation.

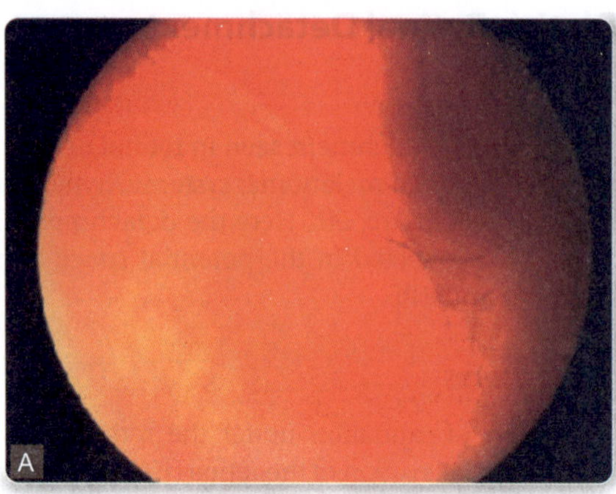

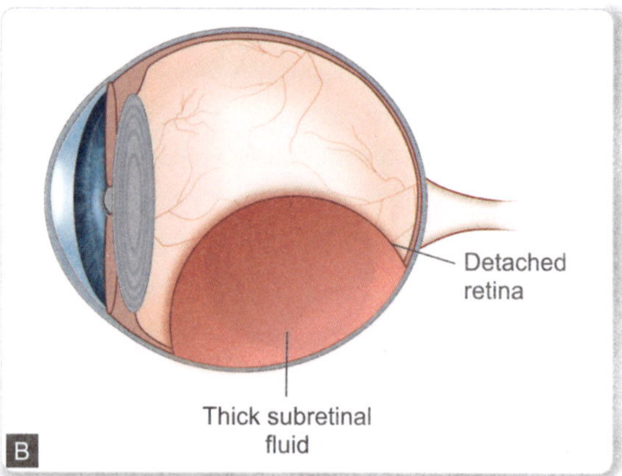

FIGURES 20.38A and B: Exudative retinal detachment. **A.** Photograph; **B.** Diagrammatic representation.

Diffuse Photoreceptor Dystrophies

The commonest type is retinitis pigmentosa (RP).

Retinitis Pigmentosa

Retinitis pigmentosa is a slow degenerative disease of the retina, which affects the photoreceptors primarily the rods, occurring in both eyes beginning in childhood and resulting blindness in middle or advanced age.

Types

Retinitis pigmentosa can be of two types:

1. Primary.
2. Secondary.

Secondary RP can occur when associated with systemic anomalies like Usher's syndrome (associated deafness), Laurence-Moon-Biedl syndrome (hypogonadism, polydactyly, mental retardation, obesity).

Sx **Symptoms**

Defective vision in the dark (night blindness), which is progressive and associated contraction of visual fields, which starts as a ring scotoma, then progressing outwards and inwards resulting in tubular fields and finally total loss of vision.

Signs

Signs are as follows:

1. Anterior segment may be normal.
2. Nystagmus may be present in cases who develop RP at a young age.
3. A complicated cataract may develop.

Fundus picture

The optic disk will show a waxy pallor. The retinal vessels will be attenuated and thread like. Bone corpuscle-shaped pigments will be seen along the vessels, starting at the equatorial area and slowly progressing toward the center as well as the periphery (Fig. 20.39).

Macula may show cystoids changes, cellophane maculopathy or atrophic changes.

Investigations

Electroretinogram: It is diagnostic even in early stage and helps to diagnose or exclude the condition in family members of RP cases. ERG is markedly subnormal or completely extinguished.

Visual fields: It show a ring scotoma in the early stages, which slowly expands toward the center as well as the periphery till a tubular field remains. This tubular field may also get extinguished with time resulting in total blindness.

Complications

Include complicated cataract, cystoid macular edema, cellophane maculopathy and vitreous floaters, which may present as a masquerade syndrome.

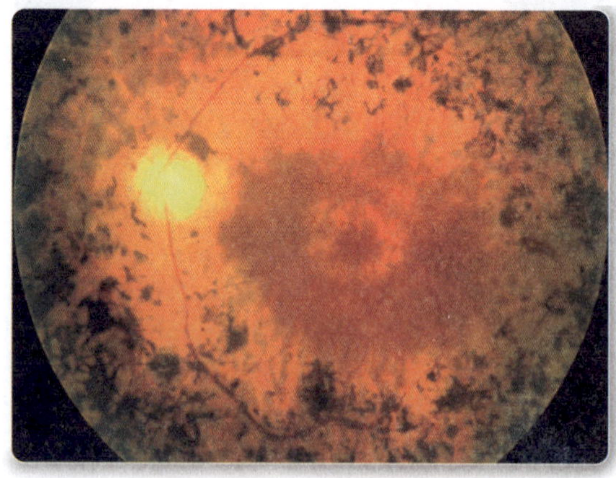

FIGURE 20.39: Retinitis pigmentosa

Variants of RP

Various types of RP are as follows.

Sectoral RP: When only 1 or 2 sectors of the fundus are involved and acquired damage should be ruled out (Fig. 20.40).

Central/pericentral/inverse RP: When the macula is involved first by the disease or the central 20° or 30° of retina is affected.

Unilateral RP: when only one eye is involved, acquired causes like trauma, vascular occlusion, syphilis, drug toxicity, etc. should be ruled out. ERG is not much affected as in a case of true RP.

Retinitis pigmentosa sine pigmento: It is a type of RP with same symptom, but without visible pigmentation of the retina.

Retinitis punctata albescens: It is a type with same symptom, but retina shows small white dots distributed uniformly over the fundus instead of the bone spicule pigmentation.

Genetic inheritance

The different inheritance pattern includes:

- Autosomal dominant RP—rare, but severe form
- Autosomal recessive type—most common
- X-linked RP
- Sporadic type.

Management

Measures include:

1. Regular ophthalmic evaluation at the intervals of 1–2 years.
2. Genetic counseling of affected parents.
3. Posterior subcapsular (PSC) cataract is a complication and cataract extraction may improve vision.
4. Cystoid macular edema, if present, can be treated with oral acetazolamide or intravitreal injection of steroids.

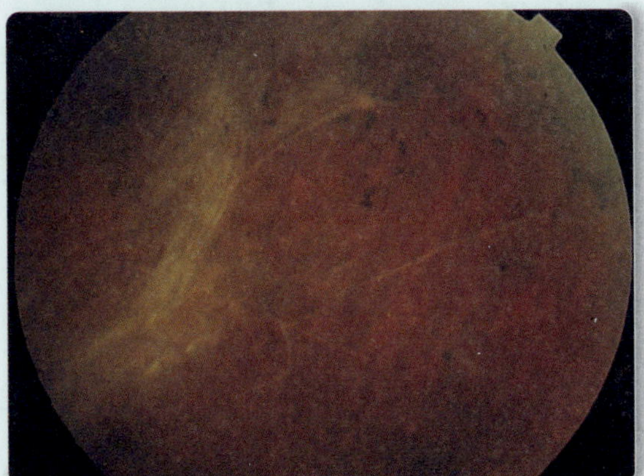

FIGURE 20.40: Sectoral RP like picture produced by vascular occlusion

5. Nutritional supplementation with vitamin A, vitamin E and omega-3 fatty acids may help to slower the progression of visual loss.
6. Low vision aids.
7. Ultraviolet light absorbing sunglasses to prevent photopic damage.
8. Transplantation of retinal cells and genetic modification are under trial.

Macular Dystrophies

Macular dystrophies are a group of inherited macular conditions, which affect the central vision. Usually cause legal blindness at a younger age. Low vision aids are beneficial to these patients.

Stargardt's Disease

Stargardt's disease is the commonest juvenile macular dystrophy. Inheritance is autosomal recessive and is closely related to fundus flavimaculatus.

The classic Stargardt's disease starts between 8 and 14 years of age characterized by discrete yellowish round or pisiform flecks at the level of RPE. If the flecks are widely scattered throughout the fundus, the condition is called fundus flavimaculatus. Macula shows a beaten-bronze appearance (Fig. 20.41).

Fundus fluorescein angiography shows dark choroid due to accumulation of lipofuscin-like pigment in the RPE. EOG is affected and ERG can be affected in later stages.

Differential diagnosis of Stargardt's disease include condition, which cause bull's eye maculopathy like cone rod dystrophy, chloroquine retinal toxicity, ARMD, chronic macular hole and central areolar choroidal dystrophy.

Vitelliform Degeneration

Best Disease or Best Vitelliform Dystrophy

Autosomal dominant maculopathy characterized by lipofuscin accumulation in the macula.

Fundus examination shows a yellow yolk-like (vitelliform) macular lesion in childhood and which breaks down to leave a scrambled egg appearance. About 20% of patients may develop choroidal neovascular membrane with 6/60 vision.

Electroretinography is normal, but the EOG is abnormal and Arden' ratio is less than 1.5. EOG abnormality is always the marker for the disease even in patients in early stage with normal fundus.

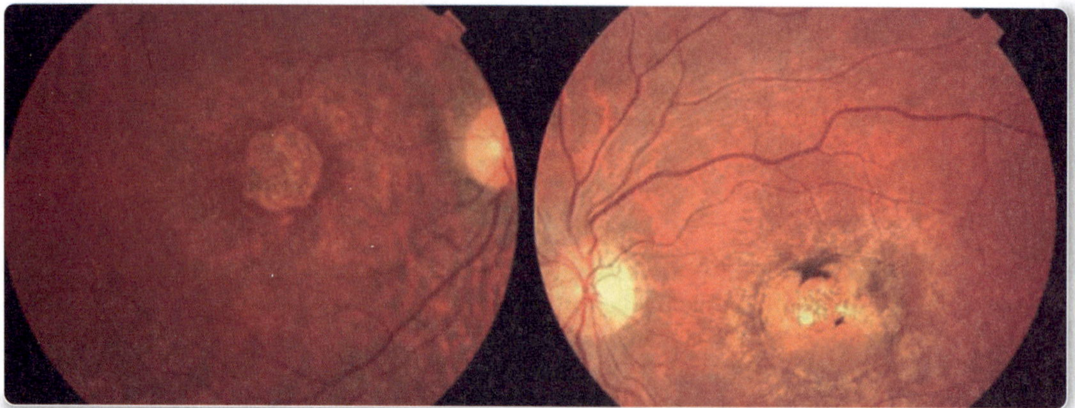

FIGURE 20.41: Stargardt's disease—early and late stage

Adult Onset Vitelliform Lesions

Usually seen in 4th to 6th decade with bilateral round or oval yellowish subfoveal lesions, one-third disk diameter in size with mild blurring and metamorphopsia. EOG is normal or minimally subnormal and the differential diagnosis include drusenoid RPE detachment and basal laminar drusen with exudation.

Familial (Dominant) Drusen

Usually develops at younger age than ARMD. Autosomal dominant inheritance with numerous drusen typically extending beyond the arcades and nasal to optic disk. ERG and EOG are normal and visual acuity is good since the drusen are extrafoveal. These patients have higher risk for developing ARMD.

Choroidal Dystrophies

Choroidal dystrophies include a number of condition in which a primary retinal or RPE disease result in atrophy of the choriocapillaris.

Diffuse Degenerations

Choroideremia

X-linked recessive disease characterized by pigmentary changes in the fundus, night blindness and field constriction (Fig. 20.42).

The features that are different from RP include marked atrophy of choroids and RPE, normal retinal vessels and absence of optic atrophy. The disease primarily affects the RPE and choriocapillaris.

Gyrate atrophy

Autosomal recessive dystrophy caused by mutations in the gene for ornithine aminotransferase. Plasma ornithine levels are high, which is toxic to RPE and choroids.

Clinically, retinal examination show geographical peripheral paving stone-like atrophy of RPE and choriocapillaris, which progress to scalloped border at junction of normal and abnormal RPE (Fig. 20.43).

The common symptoms include night blindness, visual field loss and decrease in visual acuity.

Treatment include dietary restriction of arginine and vitamin B_6 treatment.

Regional and Central Choroidal Dystrophies

Autosomal dominant condition, which affects macular area causing atrophy of RPE and choriocapillaris in macula. Differential diagnosis includes toxoplasmosis, ARMD and bull's eye maculopathies. The two main types are:

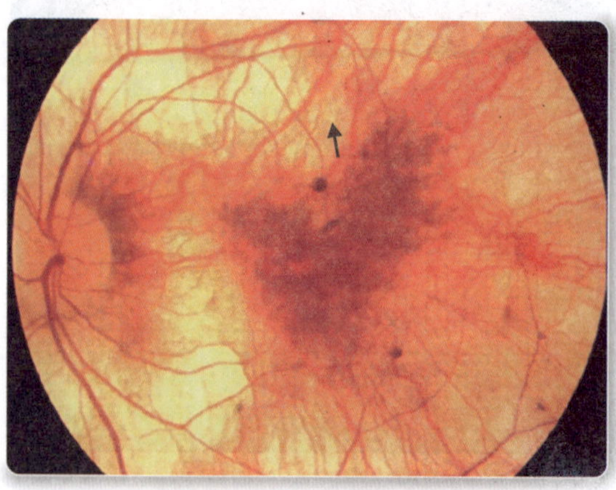

FIGURE 20.42: Choroideremia

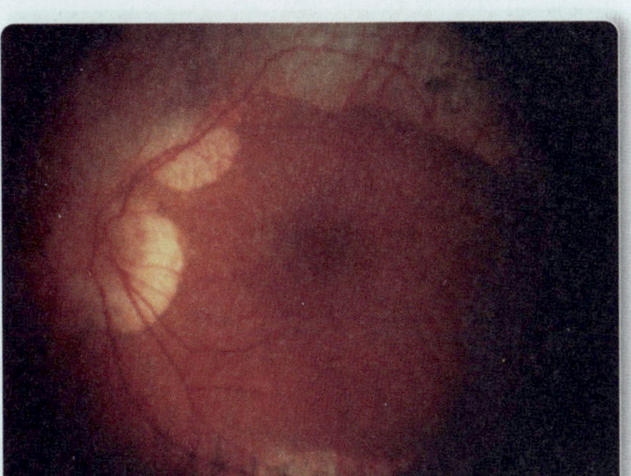

FIGURE 20.43: Gyrate atrophy

1. Central areolar choroidal dystrophy: Characterized by depigmentation of macula, which progress to round or oval area of sharply demarcated geographic atrophy (Fig. 20.44). Visual acuity is usually 20/200.
2. North Carolina macular dystrophy: Begins in infancy with a cluster of yellowish white lesions at macular area, which progresses to excavated or staphylomatous lesion. Visual acuity ranges from 20/20 to 20/200.

Inner Retinal and Vitreoretinal Dystrophies

X-linked Retinoschisis

Retinoschisis refers to a splitting of the neurosensory retina usually in the outer plexiform layer resulting in a loss of field of vision corresponding to the area of retinoschisis. It can be:

1. Degenerative peripheral retinoschisis.
2. Congenital X-linked recessive retinoschisis.
3. Secondary due to vitreoretinal fraction, myopia and vein occlusion.

Congenital X-linked retinoschisis is characterized by foveal schisis, which appears as small, cystoid spaces and fine radial striae in the central macula. No leakage of fluorescein is seen and visual acuity is usually 20/200. ERG shows a negative wave form with absence of b wave.

The retina is vulnerable to mechanical injury and treatment includes refractive correction and correction of strabismus and genetic counseling.

Goldmann-Favre Syndrome

Autosomal recessive disorder characterized by night blindness, increased sensitivity to blue light, retinal pigmentary changes, optically empty vitreous, unusual ERG abnormalities and macular schisis.

Retinal Degeneration Associated with Systemic Disease

Metabolic Diseases

Albinism: Clinically characterized by diminished visual acuity (5/60–6/60), nystagmus, photophobia, iris transillumination defects, hypopigmented fundus and foveal hypoplasia (Fig. 20.45). Two types are there:

1. Ocular albinism: X-linked recessive disorder affecting the eye alone.
2. Oculocutaneous albinism: Autosomal recessive type with tyrosinase negative or positive forms. As the name suggests it involves the eye as well as the skin.

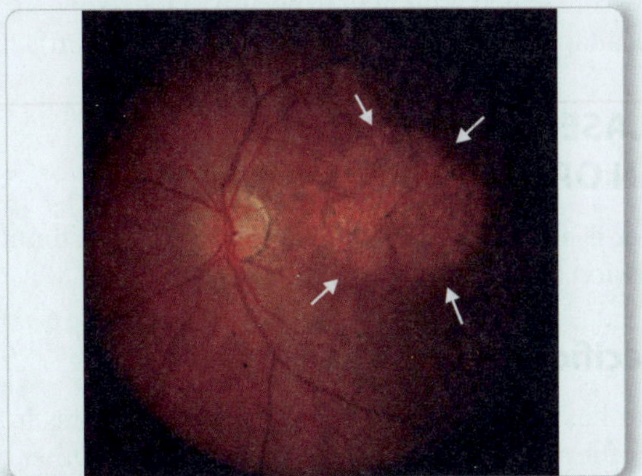

FIGURE 20.44: Central areolar choroidal dystrophy

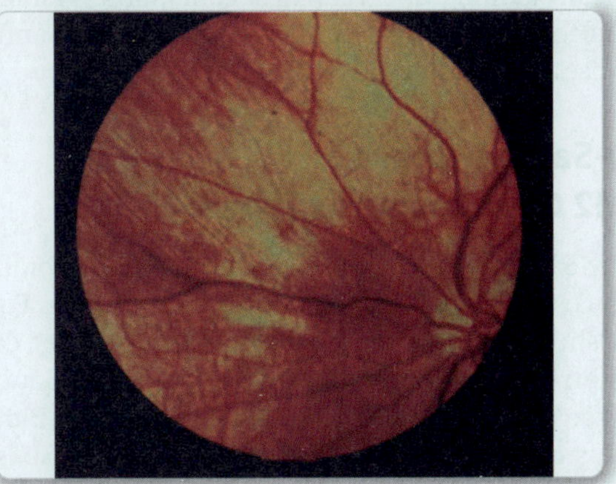

FIGURE 20.45: Fundus in albinism

Central Nervous System Metabolic Abnormalities

Batten Disease

Batten disease caused by accumulation of waxy lipopigments within the lysosomes of neurons and other cells. Characteristic features are progressive dementia, seizures and visual loss with pigmentary retinopathy. Infantile and juvenile types are associated with pigmentary retinopathies. Infantile type is similar to Leber's congenital amaurosis, while juvenile form shows bull's eye maculopathy with retinitis pigmentosa-like picture.

Abetalipoproteinemia

Abetalipoproteinemia is a autosomal recessive disorder leading to fat-soluble vitamin deficiency with acanthocytosis. Retinal changes are similar to retinitis punctata albescens and are a reversible condition with vitamin A therapy.

Refsum's Disease

Refsum's disease characterized by pigmentary retinopathy with reduced ERG, ataxia, polyneuropathy, anosmia, hearing loss and cardiomyopathy. Diagnosis is by elevated plasma levels of phytanic acid.

Mucopolysaccharidosis

Mucopolysaccharidosis occurs due to deficiency of lysosomal enzymes resulting in accumulation of incompletely metabolized mucopolysaccharides within lysosomes.

All have autosomal recessive trait except type II (Hunter), which is X-linked recessive. Hurler-Scheie syndrome are characterized by coarse facies, mental retardation, corneal clouding and retinal degeneration. Hunter has retinal change, but no corneal clouding and Sanfilippo show severe pigmentary retinopathy.

Tay-Sachs Disease (GM2 Gangliosidosis Type I)

In Tay-Sachs disease glycolipid accumulation in brain and retina causes mental retardation and blindness. Fundus may show a cherry-red spot (Fig. 20.46). Other causes of cherry-red spot include Sandhoff disease, Gaucher's disease and Niemann-Pick disease. Niemann-Pick disease is caused by absence of sphingomyelinase isoenzyme and type A is more associated with cherry-red macula.

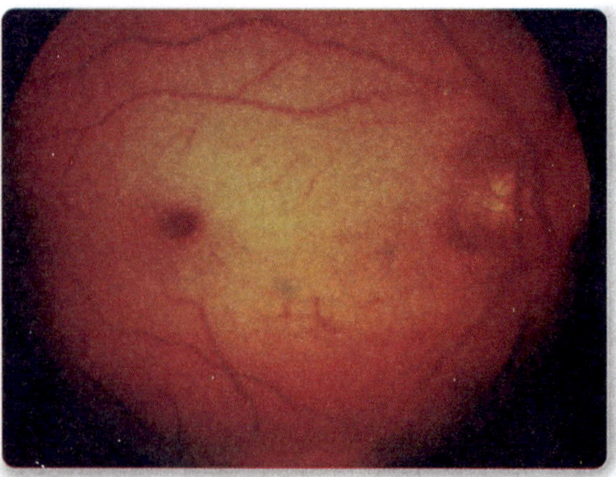

FIGURE 20.46: Cherry-red spot in Tay-Sachs disease

Night Vision Abnormalities

Congenital Stationary Night Blindness

Congenital stationary night blindness (CSNB) genetic types are X linked, AR and AD types. Visual acuity is from normal to 20/200 and the fundus appearance is normal. ERG shows a negative wave form.

Fundus Albipunctatus

Affected people show night blindness, normal visual acuity and color vision.

Fundus show a striking array of yellowish white dots in posterior pole and ERG is normal. Differential diagnosis is retinitis punctata albescens, which also show reduced ERG and attenuated blood vessels and is a variety of RP.

Oguchi's Disease

Oguchi's disease is a retinal circulation defect rather than visual pigments. The fundus shows a peculiar yellowish iridescent sheen after light exposure that disappears after dark adaptation (Mizuo-Nakamura phenomenon).

LASERS AND CRYOTHERAPY IN OPHTHALMOLOGY

Laser is an acronym for light amplification by stimulated emission of radiation.

Specific Features of a Laser Beam

Laser has unique properties, which differentiates it from any other source of light—natural or artificial. Other types of light consist of different wavelengths and these are emitted in all directions and tend to diverge as it travel through any medium. So, it is difficult to converge it to a single point to give a pinpoint powerful beam. Laser is emitted by certain atoms, which can exist in different energy levels. The lowest energy level is 'the ground state', which is the stable one. When stimulated by a radiational field of appropriate wavelength, the atom goes to the higher energy level called 'excited state'. This state is unstable and it gives out a photon of light of a particular wavelength and comes back to the ground state. The emitted photon in turn stimulates another atom to emit a photon of the same wavelength. So, in a short time a high-intensity beam of a specific wavelength is produced—a laser beam. The properties of laser are monochromaticity, coherence and collimation with limited divergence, thus delivering large amount of energy to a small area.

Laser Tissue Interaction

Different lasers produce different types of reactions on tissues.

Photocoagulation

The temperature of the tissues rises to 35°C–50°C causing denaturation of proteins and coagulation of tissues, e.g. argon laser, neodymium-doped yttrium aluminum garnet (Nd:YAG) laser.

Photovaporization

The tissue temperature rises above 100°C resulting in tissue vaporization, e.g. CO_2 laser.

Photodisruption

Very high temperatures up to 1,500°C are produced at microscopic level resulting in tissue disruption or tearing by the hydrodynamic and acoustic shock waves and mechanical stress factors, e.g. pulsed Nd:YAG laser doing posterior capsulotomy, ruby laser, etc.

Photoablation

In photoablation, there is no rise in tissue temperature, but the intermolecular bonds are disrupted resulting in tissue loss at microscopic level with no damage to nearby tissue, e.g. excimer laser used in LASIK.

Photodynamic Reaction

Certain photosensitives like porphyrins, chlorophyll and certain dyes, which accumulate in a particular tissue like malignant cells or CNVMs in ARMD are used to absorb and concentrate the action of the laser at the targeted cells. When exposed to the laser light of specific wavelength these photosensitives absorb the light energy to release singlet oxygen or free radicals, which destroy the targeted cells (e.g. malignant cells or the CNVMs in ARMD).

Types of Lasers

Several types of lasers for ophthalmic use are given in Table 20.5.

Mode of delivery of lasers to eye can be through slit lamp, indirect ophthalmoscope or endophotocoagulation via fiber optic probe (used during vitrectomy to seal retinal tears directly).

Laser Effects and Uses

Photocoagulation

Argon, krypton, diode and frequency-doubled Nd:YAG (Fig. 20.47) are based on this effect. The absorbed light depends on pigments in tissue and has thermal effect coagulating and denaturing cellular elements. Photocoagulation

TABLE 20.5: Lasers commonly used in ophthalmology

Name	Type	Wavelength	Effects produced
Argon	Gas	488–515	Photocoagulation
Krypton	Gas	647	Photocoagulation
Diode	Semiconductor	780–850	Photocoagulation, photodynamic therapy
Nd:YAG	Solid state	1,062	Photodisruption
Frequency-doubled Nd:YAG	Solid state	532	Photocoagulation
Excimer	Gas	193	Photoablation
Femtosecond	Solid state	1,053	Photodisruption
Carbon dioxide	Gas	10,600	Photovaporization

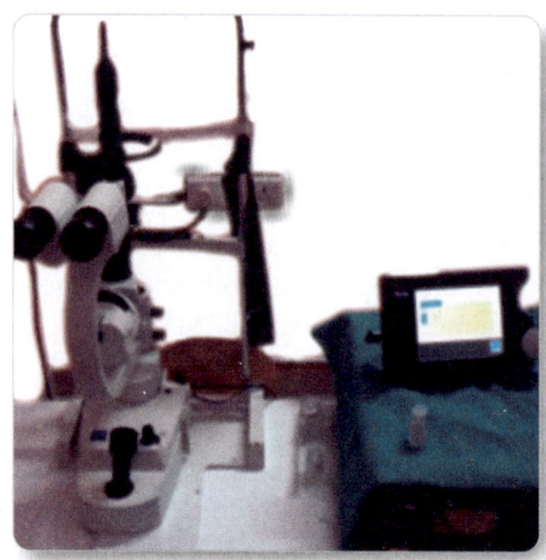

FIGURE 20.47: Frequency-doubled Nd:YAG laser with slit lamp delivery system

depends on pigments in tissue and has thermal effect coagulating and denaturing cellular elements. Photocoagulation is used for destroying new vessels, producing chorioretinal adhesions in the sealing of retinal breaks in retinal detachment and for destruction of RPE.

Indications: Photocoagulation is indicated in:

1. Retina and choroid:
   a. Panretinal photocoagulation for proliferative diabetic retinopathy and focal or grid laser for diabetic macular edema (Figs 20.48 and 20.49).
   b. Venous occlusions.
   c. Peripheral retinal vascular diseases like retinopathy of prematurity, Eales' disease, Coats' disease.
   d. Age-related macular degeneration, central serous retinopathy.
   e. Small intraocular tumors.
2. Glaucoma—to reduce the intraocular pressure by performing:
   a. Laser peripheral iridotomy in narrow angle glaucoma.
   b. Argon laser trabeculoplasty, selective laser trabeculoplasty for POAG.
   c. Cyclophotocoagulation in absolute glaucoma.
   d. Argon laser suture lysis after trabeculectomy.
3. Iris and pupil:
   a. Photomydriasis for dilation of pupil in patients with undulating pupil.
   b. Coreoplasty for up drawn pupil.
   c. Laser sphincterotomy.

Complications: These are foveal burns, macular edema, macular pucker, decreased field of vision, contraction of fibrous tissue, choroidal hemorrhage, etc.

Photodisruption

Neodymium-doped yttrium aluminum garnet laser is based on this mechanism (Fig. 20.50). The laser beam ionizes the electrons from molecules of the target tissue producing the physical state of plasma and the resultant shock waves have an incising or cutting effect on tissues.

Indications: Photocoagulation is indicated in:

1. Nd:YAG laser capsulotomy for posterior capsular opacification.
2. Peripheral iridotomy in narrow angle glaucoma.
3. YAG laser vitreolysis in aphakic/pseudophakic malignant glaucoma.
4. Phacolysis for doing laser-assisted cataract surgery by way of photodisruption.
5. Q switched frequency-doubled Nd:YAG laser used for selective laser trabeculoplasty by photothermolysis of peripheral trabecular meshwork in POAG.

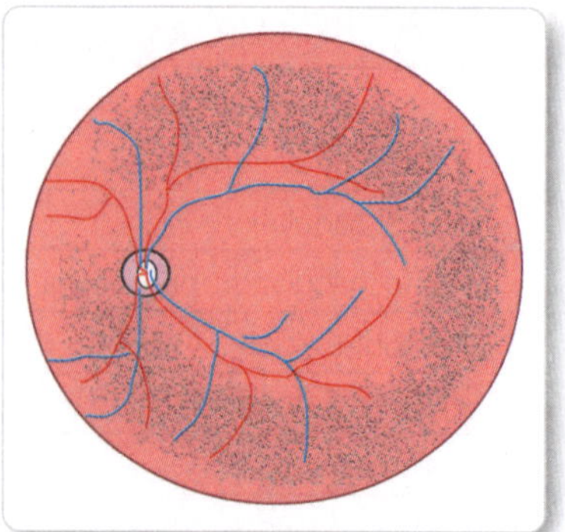

FIGURE 20.48: Retinal burns in panretinal photocoagulation

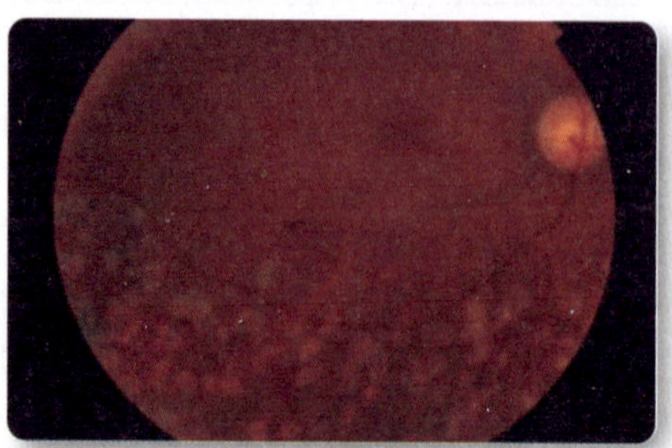

FIGURE 20.49: Sector panretinal photocoagulation for BRVO

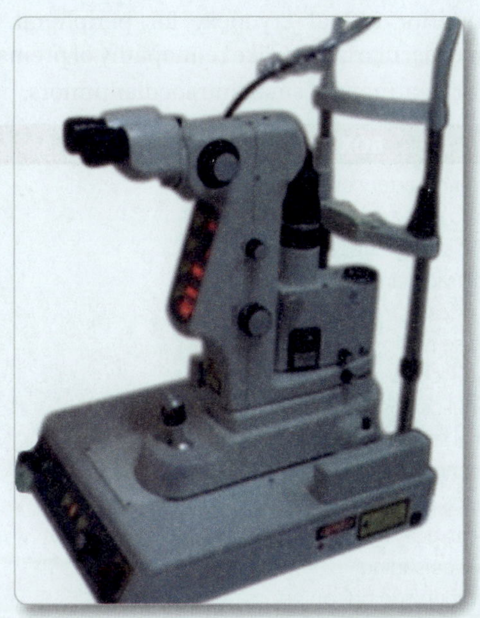

FIGURE 20.50: Nd:YAG laser capsulotomy machine

Photoablation

The excimer laser or excited dimer laser is a combination of a rare gas and a halide. It has wavelength in the ultraviolet range of which the most commonly used is 193 nm argon fluoride. These are used in corneal tissue remodeling in refractive surgeries. These act by ablative photodecomposition, which breaks intramolecular chemical bonds of corneal tissue and ejects the molecular fragments out.

Indications: Photoablation is indicated in:

1. Photorefractive keratectomy (PRK) used to correct low myopia up to 4D. The corneal epithelium is removed and anterior stroma is ablated.
2. Laser-assisted in situ keratomileusis (LASIK) used to correct myopia ranging from 1 to 15D. It involves ablation of the mid stromal tissue after raising a corneal flap and then repositioning the flap.
3. Phototherapeutic keratectomy (PTK) for corneal dystrophies, degenerations and scars.
4. Femto-LASIK is new generation lasers called femtosecond titanium sapphire lasers with intralasik software. It creates a precise corneal flap by photodisruption under lower IOP than needed for conventional LASIK, followed by excimer laser ablation. It is a long wavelength laser of 1,053 nm with laser pulse in femtosecond range (one quadrillionth of a second).

Photodynamic Therapy

A photosensitive dye is injected intravenously (verteporfin) followed by diode laser (690 nm) irradiance corresponding to the absorption peak of dye. The resultant photochemical action is used for treating subretinal neovascular membranes as in age-related macular degeneration, high myopia, etc.

Cryotherapy

Cryotherapy or cryopexy involves use of intense cold in the management of certain ocular conditions. The temperature within the cryoprobe from a cryounit (Fig. 20.51) ranges from –40°C to –100°C. The various gases used are nitrous oxide, freon or compressed carbon dioxide. It is based on the principle of Joule-Thomson effect. The size of cryotip (Table 20.6), gas and duration of freezing influences the temperature produced inside the tissues.

TABLE 20.6: Size of cryotips

Vitreous	1 mm
Cataract extraction	1.5 mm
Retina	2.5 mm
Cyclocryotherapy	4 mm

BOX 20.1: Causes of night blindness

Retinitis pigmentosa
Vitamin A deficiency
Fundus albipunctatus
Congenital stationary night blindness
Oguchi's disease
Pathological myopia
Peripheral cortical cataract
Certain medicines like phenothiazines
Refractive surgeries
Panretinal photocoagulation

Mechanism of Action and Uses

Extracellular and intracellular ice crystal formation occurs by rapid freezing, which destroys cell membranes, producing ischemic necrosis. Vascular occlusion and tissue adhesion are also produced by rapid freezing and slow thawing:

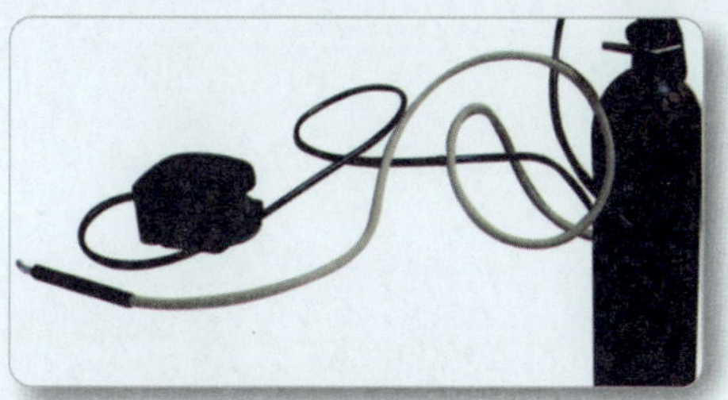

FIGURE 20.51: Cryotherapy unit

BOX 20.2: Tubular visual fields

Advanced glaucoma
Retinitis pigmentosa
Central retinal artery occlusion with spared cilioretinal artery
Aura of migraine
Severe peripheral cortical cataract
Altitude sickness
Hallucinogenic drugs
Hypoxia
Mercury poisoning
Use of optical equipments like telescope, binoculars, microscopes, diving masks, etc.

1. Lids: Trichiasis, lid warts, molluscum, tumors. It can cause lash destruction and melanocyte depigmentation.
2. Conjunctiva: For destruction of papillae in spring catarrh.
3. Lens: Used for ICCE by adherence of the cryoprobe to the lens by ice ball formation.
4. Ciliary body: Cyclocryotherapy for absolute glaucoma and neovascular glaucoma by producing aseptic tissue necrosis at the tips of the ciliary processes and thus decreasing aqueous production.
5. Retina:
   a. For closing retinal breaks by producing adhesions between retina and RPE.
   b. Anterior retinal cryopexy for peripheral retinal neovascularization like retinopathy of prematurity.
   c. For treatment of small intraocular tumors.

BOX 20.3: Cherry-red spot

Central retinal artery occlusion
Commotio retinae
Metabolic storage diseases
Mucopolysaccharidosis
Hurler's disease
Hunter disease
Niemann-Picks disease
GM1 gangliosidoses
Lysosomal storage disorders
Leber's congenital amaurosis
Quinine toxicity
Dapsone toxicity
Methanol poisoning
Carbon monoxide poisoning

Complications

Complications are pain, transient rise in intraocular pressure, uveitis, hyphema, hypotony, anterior segment ischemia, etc. The causes of night blindness, tubular visual fields and cherry-red spots are give in Box 20.1 to 20.3 respectively.

Glaucoma

21

Girija Devi PS, Susan Philip, Thomas George T

The word 'glaucoma' comes from the Greek word 'glaucosis' described by Hippocrates in 400 BC, which means clouded or bluish-green hue. It may be due to corneal edema because of raised intraocular tension or rapid evolution of cataract (cataract and glaucoma were not distinguished until 1705).

Glaucoma is currently defined as a family of ocular diseases characterized by progressive optic neuropathy with associated visual function loss. It is often, but not always, associated with increased IOP.

Glaucoma is the second most common cause of irreversible blindness in the world.

World Health Organization (WHO) survey in 1995 has shown that 5.1 million people are bilaterally blind from glaucoma, 20% more have tubular fields. Prevalence of glaucoma in India is 2.5% in people above 40 years (recent population-based surveys).

Glaucoma has been nicknamed as the 'silent thief of sight' because the loss of vision normally occurs gradually over a long period of time and is often only recognized when the disease is quite advanced. Once lost, this damaged visual field cannot be recovered. Worldwide, it is the second leading cause of blindness after cataracts.

With appropriate screening, usually glaucoma can be identified early and its progress can be arrested with appropriate treatment before significant visual loss occurs.

CLASSIFICATION

1. Primary glaucoma without other known ocular or systemic disorders:
   a. Open-angle glaucoma:
      - Chronic open-angle glaucoma
      - Normal tension glaucoma.
   b. Angle-closure glaucoma.
   c. Combined mechanism glaucoma.
2. Developmental glaucoma:
   a. Primary congenital glaucoma.
   b. Primary infantile glaucoma.
   c. Primary juvenile glaucoma.
   d. Axenfeld-Rieger syndrome.
   e. Peters' anomaly.
   f. Aniridia.
   g. Other developmental anomalies.
3. Secondary glaucoma associated with other ocular and systemic disorders:
   a. Glaucoma associated with disorders of corneal endothelium:
      - Iridocorneal endothelial (ICE) syndrome
      - Fuchs' endothelial dystrophy
      - Posterior polymorphous dystrophy.
   b. Glaucoma associated with disorders of the iris and ciliary body:
      - Pigmentary glaucoma
      - Iridoschisis
      - Plateau iris
      - Iris and ciliary body cysts.
   c. Glaucoma associated with disorders of the lens:
      - Pseudoexfoliation syndrome
      - Glaucoma associated with cataracts
      - Glaucoma associated with lens dislocation.
   d. Glaucoma associated with disorders of the retina, choroid and vitreous:
      - Neovascular glaucoma (NVG)
      - Glaucoma associated with retinal detachment and vitreoretinal diseases.
   e. Glaucoma associated with intraocular tumors:
      - Malignant melanoma
      - Retinoblastoma
      - Metastatic carcinoma
      - Benign tumors.
   f. Glaucoma associated with inflammations such as uveitis, keratitis, episcleritis and scleritis.
   g. Steroid-induced glaucoma.

h. Glaucoma associated with ocular trauma.
i. Glaucoma associated with hemorrhage.
j. Glaucoma following intraocular surgery:
   - Malignant glaucoma
   - Glaucoma in pseudophakia and aphakia
   - Epithelial, fibrous and endothelial proliferation
   - Glaucoma associated with corneal surgery
   - Glaucoma associated with vitreoretinal surgery.
k. Glaucoma associated with elevated episcleral venous pressure.

PRIMARY OPEN-ANGLE GLAUCOMA

Definition

Primary open-angle glaucoma (POAG) can be defined as a multifactorial progressive optic neuropathy with a characteristic acquired loss of optic nerve fibers in a person with open anterior chamber angles. It results in:

1. Characteristic visual field abnormalities due to cupping and atrophy of the optic disk following retinal ganglion cell death.
2. Optic disk cupping.
3. Increased IOP. It is the risk factor associated with the development of the disease and is not the disease itself. Patients can develop optic neuropathy of glaucoma in the absence of documented elevated IOP. This condition has been termed 'normal- or low-tension glaucoma'.

Glaucoma Suspects

Glaucoma suspects are people who are likely to be having POAG or at a high risk for developing POAG (e.g. family members of patients with POAG). These include:

1. Some people can have elevated pressure in the absence of nerve damage or visual field loss. This condition has been termed 'ocular hypertension'. They are at more risk to develop glaucoma and are considered to be glaucoma suspects.
2. Patients with typical glaucomatous optic nerve head (ONH) changes, but with normal IOP and visual field, are also termed as glaucoma suspects.

Pathophysiology

The exact cause of glaucomatous optic neuropathy is not known. A combination of risk factors affecting axonal health has been identified. These include elevated IOP, family history, race, age older than 40 years and myopia.

The three major theories concerning how IOP can initiate glaucomatous damage in a patient include:

1. Vascular theory, which states that optic neuropathy is due to ischemia of the optic nerve.
2. Mechanical theory, which states that optic neuropathy is due to compression of the axons at cribriform plate.
3. The current observation is that the pathogenesis of glaucomatous optic neuropathy is due to obstruction to axoplasmic flow. It can be due to vascular or mechanical causes or both. It may be that the vascular ischemia plays a major role in the optic nerve damage in those with lower IOP and direct mechanical compression in those with higher IOP.

Intraocular pressure is the only clinical risk factor, which is treatable. Several studies have shown that the visual field loss increases rapidly as IOP rises above 21 mm Hg and more, and if pressures are higher than 26–30 mm Hg.

Central corneal thickness (CCT) and diurnal variation should be taken into account when determining the IOP. If CCT is less, the IOP will be recorded as lower than the actual value (more chance of developing POAG, if CCT is < 555 micron). A diurnal variation of more than 8 mm Hg can be seen in POAG cases. The normal diurnal variation in IOP is 5 mm Hg or less. The IOP recorded in routine OP checkup may be normal, but at the peak of the diurnal variation, the IOP may be elevated.

When POAG is associated with increased IOP, the cause for elevated IOP is the increased resistance to aqueous outflow through the trabecular meshwork.

Various theories suggested the reason for increase in resistance to outflow, which include:

1. Loss of trabecular endothelial cells.
2. Loss of giant vacuoles in the inner wall endothelium of the Schlemm's canal.
3. Loss of normal phagocytic activity.

Disk cupping and nerve fiber layer loss of up to 40% can occur before actual visual field loss is detected.

Risk Factors

1. Elevated IOP: It is the most important of these risk factors because it is the main clinically treatable risk factor for glaucoma. According to Ocular Hypertension Treatment Study (OHTS), in patients with IOPs ranging from 24 to 31 mm Hg, but with no clinical signs of glaucoma, the average risk of developing glaucoma over 5 years is 10%. That risk is reduced by 50%, if patients are preemptively started on IOP-lowering therapy.

In some patients, the first sign of elevated IOP can be presentation with sudden loss of vision due to a central retinal vein occlusion (CRVO).

2. Race: Prevalence of POAG is 3–4 times higher in Blacks than in Caucasians.
3. Family history: The prevalence in first-degree relatives of patients with POAG is 7–10 times higher than in general population. The inheritance is multifactorial and polygenic. Mutation of myocilin gene in GLCIA locus is seen in juvenile open-angle glaucoma and GLCIE locus is associated with normal tension glaucoma.
4. Age: People older than 40 years are at risk factor for the development of POAG, with up to 15% of people affected by the seventh decade of life.
5. Other risk factors include:
   a. Myopia more than 4D.
   b. Thin corneas: CCT is less than 555 microns.
   c. Diabetes mellitus.
   d. Vasospasms, e.g. migraine.
   e. Hypertension: Prevalence of glaucoma is higher if diastolic perfusion pressure (sitting diastolic pressure) is less than 55 mm Hg.
   f. Cerebral and cardiovascular diseases.

Screening

Ideally, everyone over the age of 40 years should be screened for POAG due to its chronic insidious nature and also due to the fact that once optic nerve damage has occurred it is irreversible. First-degree relatives of the patients, diabetics and myopes over 40 years should be regularly examined to detect early glaucoma.

Clinical Features

People in the high-risk group should be carefully evaluated periodically for any features of POAG.

Sx Symptoms

Patients will not usually present with any symptoms or visual complaints until late in the disease course in POAG because of the silent nature of glaucoma.

In some patients, a positive history of chronic headache, frequent change of presbyopic glasses and delayed dark adaptation can be elicited. But primarily it is the ophthalmologist's duty to diagnose POAG, especially when a person comes for presbyopic correction by evaluation of the optic disk, by proper fundus examination, and by IOP recording and field testing, if needed.

Diagnosis

To diagnose a patient with POAG, two of the following clinical features should be present with an open-angle recorded by gonioscopy:

1. Elevated IOP.
2. Glaucomatous changes at the optic disk.
3. Typical glaucomatous field changes.

Intraocular Pressure Measurement

There are several methods for measuring IOP:

1. Applanation tonometry (using Goldmann applanation tonometer).
2. Non-contact tonometry.
3. Indentation tonometry (using Schiötz tonometer).

Applanation Tonometry

Applanation tonometry is the most accurate method. In applanation tonometry, the IOP is inferred from the force required to flatten (applanate) a constant area of the cornea (3.06 mm). Goldmann tonometry is considered to be the gold standard test and is the most widely accepted method.

Method: The patient sits at the slit lamp with applanation tonometer attachment. Fluorescein is instilled into the conjunctival sac. A special disinfected prism is mounted on the tonometer head attachment of the slit lamp and then placed against the cornea. Two green semicircles are visualized by looking through the slit lamp using a cobalt blue filter. The force applied to the tonometer head is then adjusted using a dial connected to a variable tension spring until the inner edges of the green semicircles in the viewfinder meet (Figs 21.1A and B). At this point the reading on the dial gives the IOP.

Central corneal thickness must be determined to know the accuracy of IOP measured by applanation tonometry.

The Perkins tonometer is a type of portable applanation tonometer useful in children, patients unable to cooperate with a sitting slit lamp examination or in anesthetized patients, who need to lie flat.

Non-contact Tonometry (Air-puff Tonometry)

Non-contact tonometer uses a rapid air pulse to applanate (flatten) the cornea. Corneal applanation is detected via an electro-optical system. Estimation of IOP is done by detecting the force of the air jet at the instance of applanation. This method is useful in mass screening of a large number of persons and can be done by a trained non-medical personnel also.

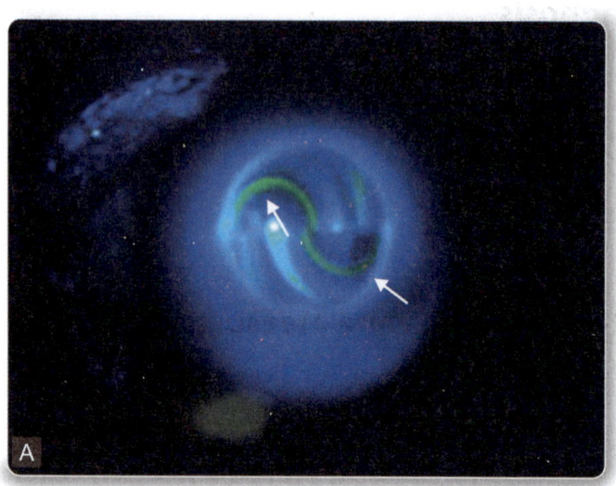

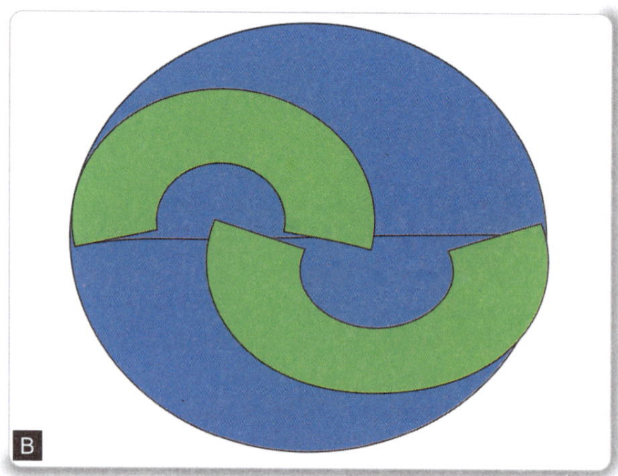

FIGURES 21.1A and B: Green semicircles seen with the inner edges in contact. **A.** Photograph; **B.** Diagrammatic representation.

Indentation Tonometry

Principle

Indentation tonometry measures the depth of corneal indentation made by a small plunger carrying a known weight. The higher the IOP, the harder it is to push against and indent the cornea. The weight of the plunger is 5 mg, but for very high levels of IOP, extra weights, i.e. 7.5 or 10 mg can be used to make the plunger push harder. The movement of the plunger is measured using a calibrated scale. The Schiötz tonometer is the most common device to use this principle. Corneoscleral rigidity will affect the accuracy of measurement of IOP. If the ocular rigidity is high, falsely high values will be obtained and if it is low, falsely low IOP reading is obtained.

Glaucoma should be suspected if:

1. If IOP of more than 21 mm Hg and is measured by applanation tonometry.
2. Diurnal variation of more than 8 mm Hg is recorded.
3. An asymmetry in IOP of more than 5 mm Hg between the two eyes is noted.
4. Normal tension glaucoma, if IOP is less than 21 mm Hg, but other features like optic disk cupping and field changes are present.
5. Glaucomatous changes in the fundus involve:
    a. Optic nerve head.
    b. Peripapillary area.
    c. Nerve fiber layer.

Optic nerve head changes: Proper evaluation of the ONH is important. In the examination of the optic nerve, the things to be evaluated are the neuroretinal rim and the optic cup.

Neuroretinal rim (NRR): This is the nerve fiber layer seen on the optic disk between the disk margin and the optic cup edge (Figs 21.2A and B). Normal NRR has a uniform pink color (slightly paler on the temporal side) and a characteristic configuration—broadest inferiorly followed by the superior, nasal and temporal parts. Changes in configuration are smooth without any sudden distortion or notching.

Cup-disk ratio (CDR): It is the diameter of the cup as a fraction of the disk measured in the vertical meridian. Optic disk can be examined with the direct ophthalmoscope, but the ideal method is to stereoscopically examine for evidence of glaucomatous damage with slit lamp biomicroscopy using a 90D lens. Optic disk changes over the years should be recorded with stereophotographs or objective topographic examination with scanning laser ophthalmoscope. If these are not available, serial drawing over the years should be made to assess any progress while on treatment.

Typical glaucomatous ONH changes include the following:

1. The CDR, especially in vertical meridian of more than 0.5 (Fig. 21.3).
2. An asymmetry of more than 0.2 between the two ONHs (Fig. 21.4).

Contour of NRR changes can be:

1. Progressive enlargement of the cup (Figs 21.5A and B).
2. Notching or thinning of disk rim particularly at superior and inferior poles (because nerve fibers at the superior and inferior poles of the disk can often be affected first) (Figs 21.6A and B).
3. Optic disk hemorrhages (Fig. 21.7): It may precede other signs of glaucoma. It is a sign of uncontrolled glaucoma and a significant risk factor for future progressive ONH damage. It can lead to localized damage of retinal nerve fiber layer (RNFL). It is more commonly seen in normal tension glaucoma.

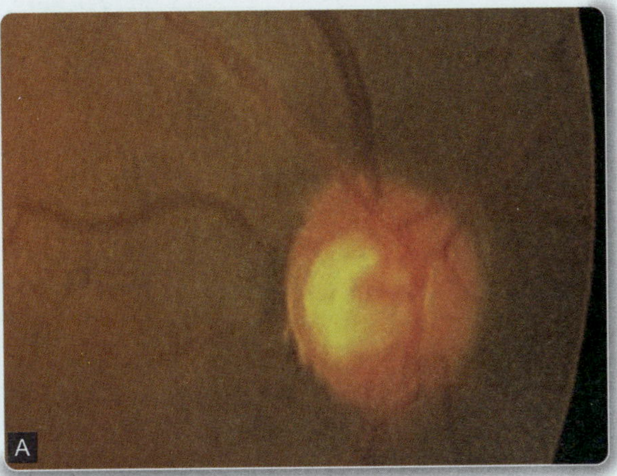

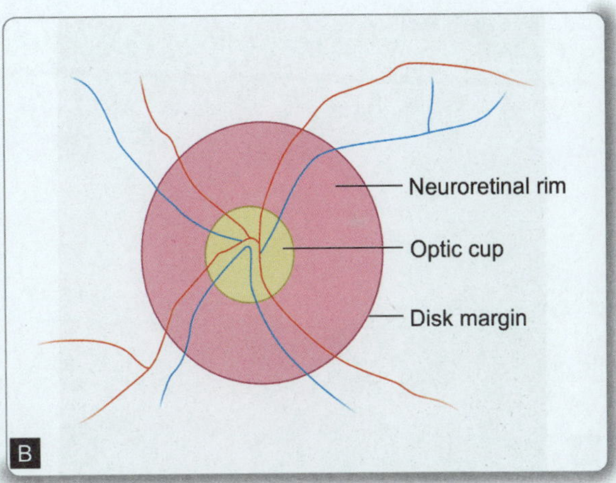

FIGURES 21.2A and B: Optic disk. **A.** Photograph; **B.** Diagrammatic representation.

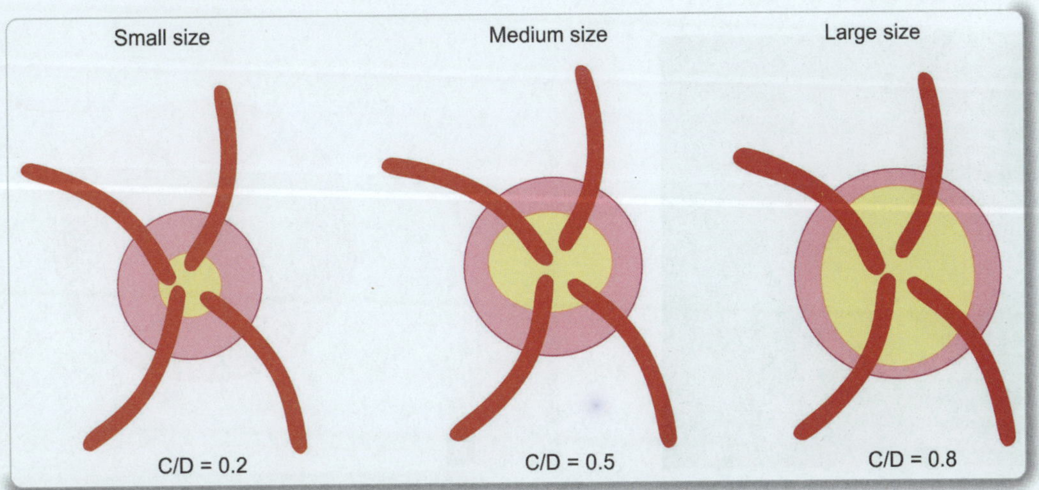

FIGURE 21.3: Difference in the size of the cup depending on the size of the disk

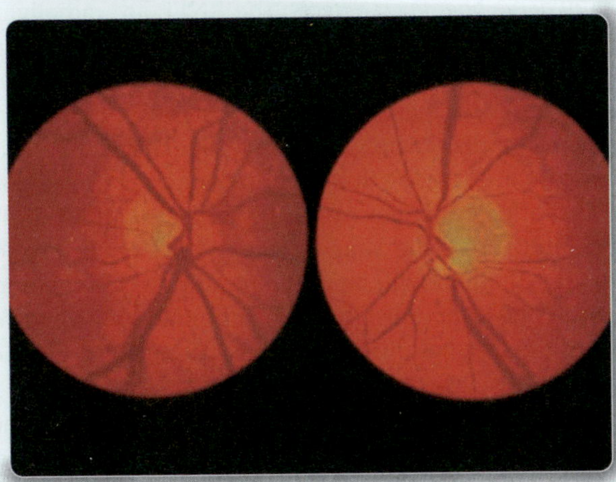

FIGURE 21.4: Asymmetric cupping

Peripapillary changes: The following are the peripapillary changes (Fig. 21.8).

Zone beta: Chorioretinal atrophy with baring of sclera and large choroidal vessels surrounding the disk. It is usually seen more in POAG patients. In asymmetric glaucoma, it is more in worse affected eye.

Zone alpha: Irregular hyper- and hypo-pigmentation of retinal pigment epithelium surrounding zone beta. Though it can be larger in glaucomatous eyes, it is not as specific as zone beta in glaucoma.

Baring of circumlinear vessel: Circumlinear vessel is a small arteriole or vein lying superficially on NRR at its inner edge going toward macula. On NRR loss, this vessel is isolated. It may be seen in other optic nerve diseases and in large physiologic cups (Fig. 21.9).

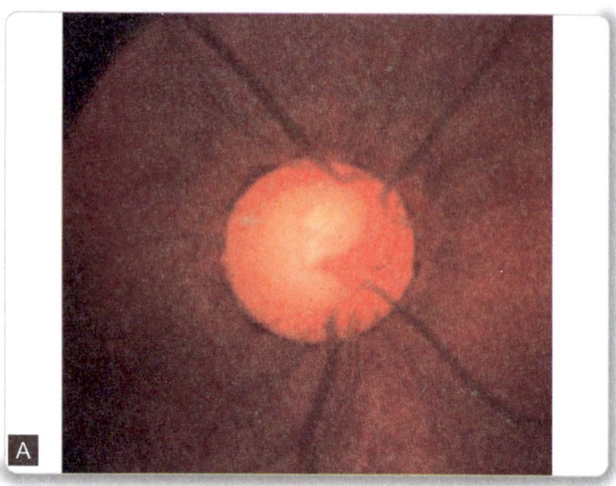

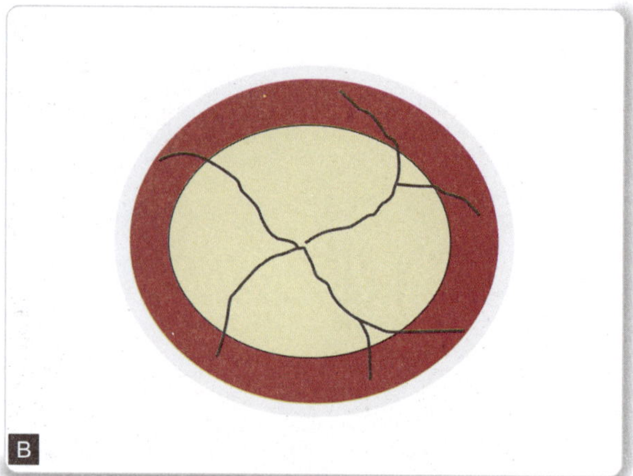

FIGURES 21.5A and B: Generalized enlargement of the cup. **A.** Photograph; **B.** Diagrammatic representation.

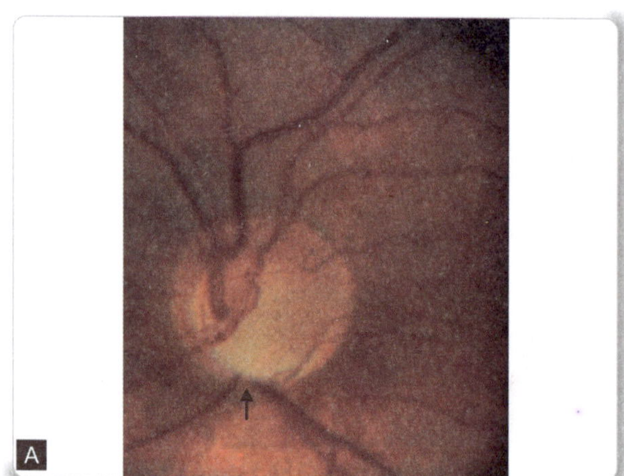

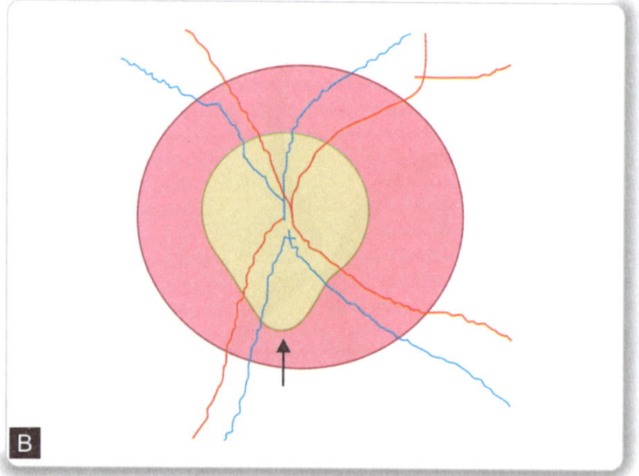

FIGURES 21.6A and B: Notching at inferior pole (black arrow). **A.** Photograph; **B.** Diagrammatic representation.

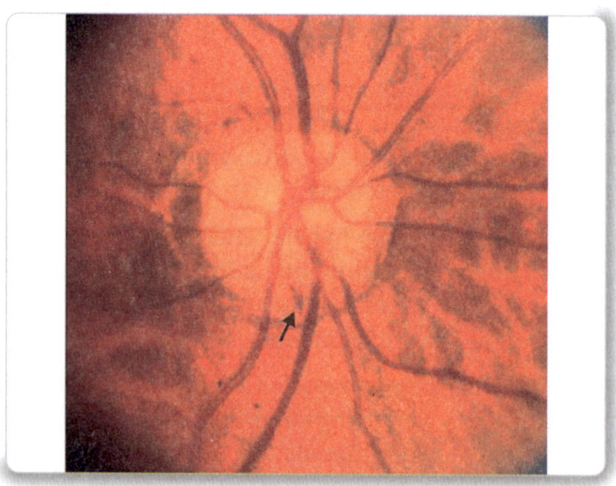

FIGURE 21.7: Optic nerve head hemorrhage

Retinal nerve fiber layer defects: The RNFL are radially oriented striations extending from the disk produced by the nerve fibers converging to the optic disk (Fig. 21.10A). These are more clearly visualized at superior and inferior poles of the disk, where the nerve fiber layer is thickest and these are curving in an arc-like manner. These fibers are first affected in glaucoma. The defects can be slit like (Fig. 21.10B), wedge shaped (Fig. 21.11) or diffuse loss (Fig. 21.12). There will be corresponding visual field loss also. It is best seen on fundus examination with red-free light and dilated pupil. The defects are seen as areas lacking striations.

Scanning laser ophthalmoscopy and optical coherence tomography (OCT) are the newer imaging techniques to detect early ONH, retinal nerve fiber and peripapillary defects.

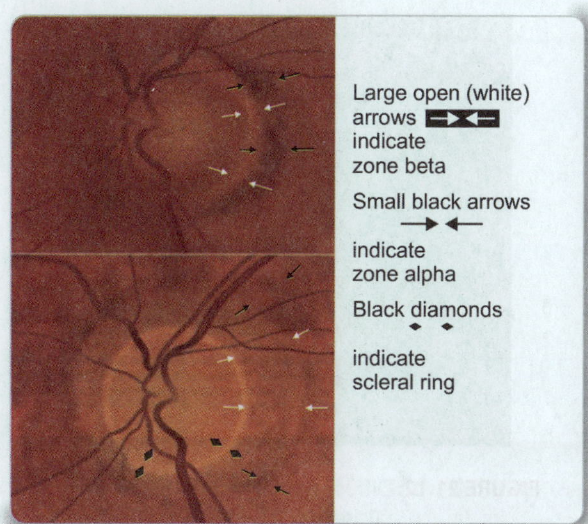

FIGURE 21.8: Peripapillary changes in glaucoma

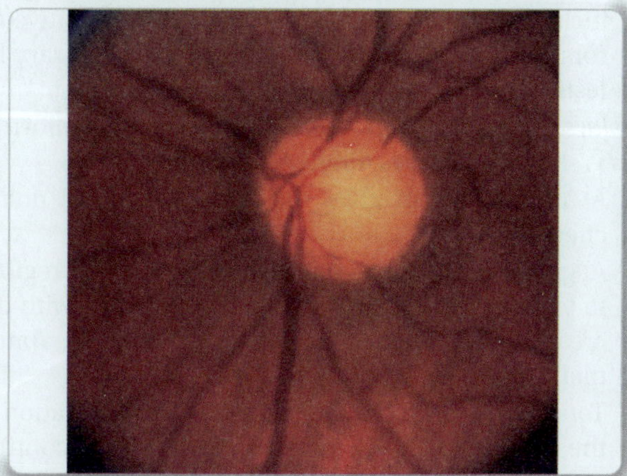

FIGURE 21.9: Glaucomatous cupping with baring of circumlinear vessel

Visual Field Examination

Normal Visual Field

Visual field is described by Traquair as the island hill of vision surrounded by the sea of darkness. The field of vision is often depicted as a three-dimensional hill, with the peak sensitivity to stimuli occurring at the point of fixation under photopic conditions, decreasing rapidly in the 10° around fixation and then decreasing very gradually for locations further in the periphery. The normal visual field extends from the point of fixation, 60° superiorly, 70° inferiorly, 60° nasally and 90° temporally (Fig. 21.13).

Perimetry

Perimetry refers to the clinical assessment of visual field. There are two types of perimetry:

1. Automated static perimetry: In static perimetry, nonmoving stimuli of varying luminance is presented to each position of a number of predetermined locations; so as to get the threshold luminance value in each position. It is compared with age matched normal. Over the last two decades automated perimetry has become the gold standard for assessing visual function in a glaucoma patient, e.g. Humphrey perimeter, Octopus perimeter.
2. Manual kinetic perimetry: In kinetic perimetry, a moving stimulus of fixed size and intensity is moved from non-seeing area in the periphery to seeing area in different meridians and a chart is plotted along the

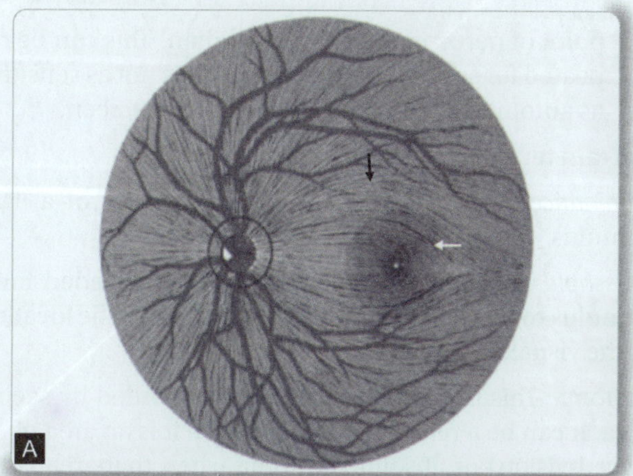

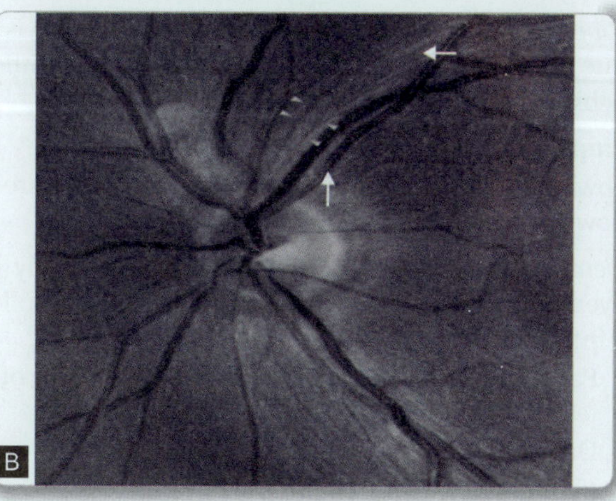

FIGURES 21.10A and B: Retinal nerve fiber layer (RNFL). **A.** Normal arrangement of RNFL arcuate fibers (black arrow), papillomacular bundle (white arrow); **B.** Slit like defects in RNFL.

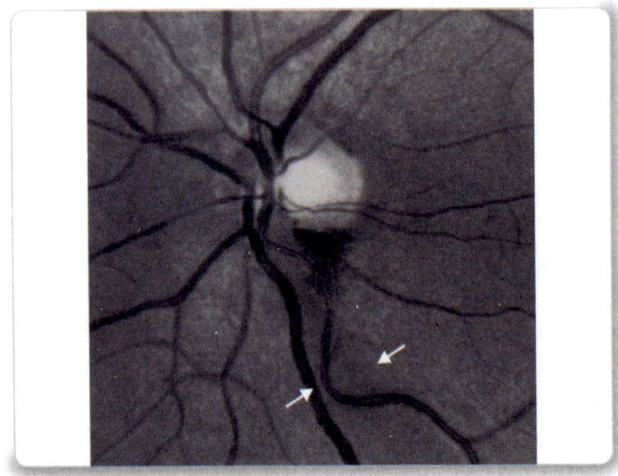

FIGURE 21.11: Wedge-shaped defects in retinal nerve fiber layer

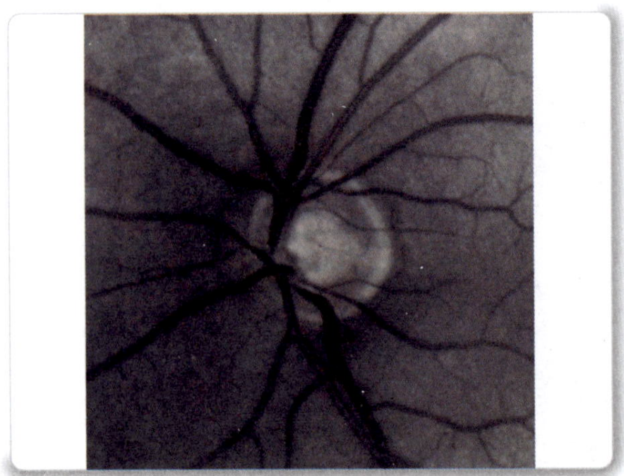

FIGURE 21.12: Diffuse retinal nerve fiber layer loss (loss of striations)

point of perception in each meridian. This can be repeated for stimuli of different size. It is not as sensitive as automated perimetry, e.g. Bjerrum's screen.

Certain terms used in perimetry

Luminance: This is the intensity or brightness of a light stimulus.

Threshold: This is the degree of brightness needed for a stimulus to be detected by the person at a specific location of the visual field.

Scotoma: This is a non-seeing area surrounded by seeing area. It can be a relative scotoma (when it is an area of reduced vision) or absolute scotoma when that area is totally blind.

Decibel: It represents the intensity of luminance and is not a true unit of luminance and may vary between perimetry machines.

Humphrey visual field

Stepwise interpretations of Humphrey visual field are the following.

Patient and test details: The test details are typically displayed on the top of the printout and include the following information:

1. Patient's name, date of birth and age at the time of the test.
2. Date and time of the test.
3. Refractive error correction used during test.
4. Type of test performed including the type of stimulus used, the background light level and the testing strategy employed.
5. Details on the method of fixation monitoring.
6. Information to help in judging the reliability of the test including the rate of fixation losses, false positive errors, false negative errors and the time necessary for testing.

Displays the sensitivities across the visual field: This information is shown in several different ways:

1. A numerical plot gives the threshold for all points checked.
2. A gray-scale plot graphically demonstrates regions to visual field loss by displaying the regions with decreased sensitivity in darker tones. Areas of abnormally high sensitivity are shown as white.
3. Total deviation plot: This plot shows the deviation of the patient's result from that of age-matched controls at each test location. Each test location is graded as normal or abnormal at a defined level (p value) compared to a normative population. The lower the p value, the greater its clinical significance and the lesser likelihood of the defect having occurred 'by chance'.
4. Pattern deviation plot: This plot is similar to total deviation plot except that it is adjusted for any generalized depression, such as that caused by a cataract or miosis. Each test location is graded as normal or abnormal at a defined level (p value) compared to a normative population. The lower the p value, the greater its clinical significance and the lesser likelihood of the defect having occurred 'by chance'. Pattern deviation plot should be carefully inspected for early detection or progression of glaucomatous visual field loss.

Summary measures of visual field performance: Several measures are provided as a summary of the visual field and they are:

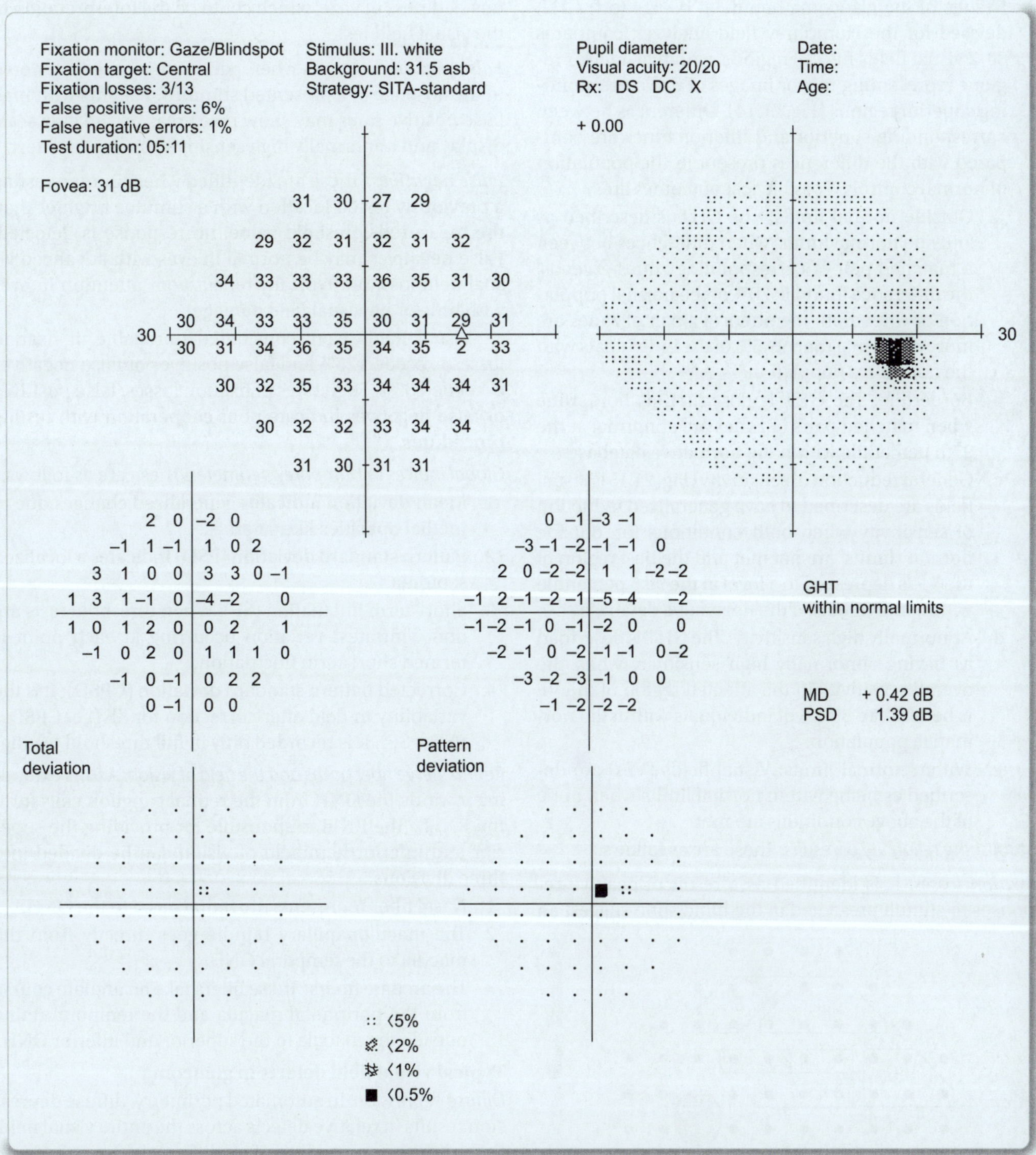

FIGURE 21.13: Normal visual field (asb, apostilbs; GHT, glaucoma hemifield test; MD, mean deviation; PSD, pattern standard deviation; SITA, Swedish interactive threshold algorithm). *Note:* Refer same abbreviations for Figures 21.15, 21.17 to 21.19.

1. Results of the glaucoma hemifield (GHT) test: GHT, devised for the Humphrey field analyzer, compares 30-2 visual fields into 10 regions, with five inferior regions representing mirror images of five corresponding superior regions (Fig. 21.14). Differences between corresponding superior and inferior zones are compared with the differences present in the population of normal controls. Possible test outcomes are:
   a. Outside normal limits: The GHT is described as 'outside normal limits' when differences between a matched pair of corresponding zones exceeds, the difference found in 99% of the normal population or when both members of a pair of zones are more abnormal than 99.5% of the individuals with the normative population.
   b. Borderline: The GHT is described as borderline when matched pairs of zones are abnormal at the 97th percentile within the normative database.
   c. General reduction of sensitivity (Fig. 21.15): Visual fields are described to have generalized reduction of sensitivity when both conditions for 'outside normal limits' are not met and the best region of the VF is depressed to a level at the 99.5 percentile within individuals of the normative database.
   d. Abnormally high sensitivity: The GHT is described as having abnormally high sensitivity when the overall sensitivity in the affected region of the VF is better than 99.5% of individuals within the normative population.
   e. Within normal limits: Visual fields (VFs) are described as being within normal limits when none of the above conditions are met.

Establishing reliability of results: These are as follows.

Fixation losses: It is identified as a result of positive responses to stimuli presented in the blind spot, suggest an unsteadiness of gaze, which could be the interpretation of the visual field test.

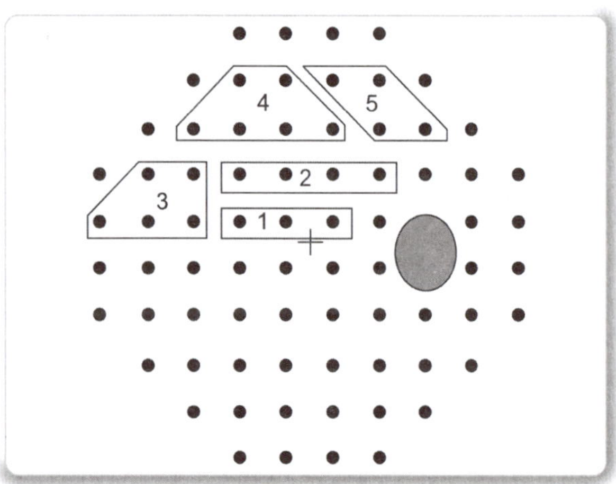

FIGURE 21.14: Glaucoma hemifield

False positives: Occurs when patient responses are noted in the absence of a presented stimulus. Patients with high false positive rates may show pale areas on the gray scale display and abnormally high sensitivity on the GHF test.

False negatives: These are identified when, upon retesting a previously tested location with a stimulus brighter than the measured threshold value, no response is detected. False negatives may be normal in eyes with advanced visual field loss, but typically reflect poor attention in eyes with little or no visual field damage.

Visual fields were considered unreliable, if fixation losses exceeded 25% and false positives or false negatives exceeded 33%. High rates of fixation losses, false positives or false negatives indicate poor cooperation with testing procedures.

Global indices in Humphrey perimeter: These are as follows:

1. Mean deviation indicates generalized changes due to medial opacities like cataract.
2. Pattern standard deviation (PSD) indicates a localized scotoma.
3. Short-term fluctuation (SF): When threshold tests are done, intratest variation occurring at each point is termed short-term fluctuation.
4. Corrected pattern standard deviation (CPSD): It is the variability in field after correction for SF (i.e. CPSD = PSD – SF). It is recorded only in full threshold testing.

Retinal nerve fiber paths and the field of vision: Axons extending towards the ONH from the retinal ganglion cells form the RNFL. The RNFL responsible for providing the superior and inferior hemifield of vision can be divided into three divisions:

1. Nasal fiber represents the retina nasal to the ONH.
2. The maculopapillary bundle goes directly from the macula to the temporal ONH.
3. The arcuate fibers: These fibers take an arcuate course from the peripheral macula and the temporal retina outside the macula to the superior and inferior ONH.

Typical visual field defects in glaucoma

Diffuse depression: In automated perimetry, diffuse depression results in relative defects across the entire visual field. Early diffuse depression is often difficult to detect because thresholds may remain within the normal range, but these may be depressed from previous examinations or the baseline status.

Paracentral defects: Circumscribed paracentral defects are early sign of localized glaucomatous damage. It is found along the course of the nerve fiber bundle. These are most

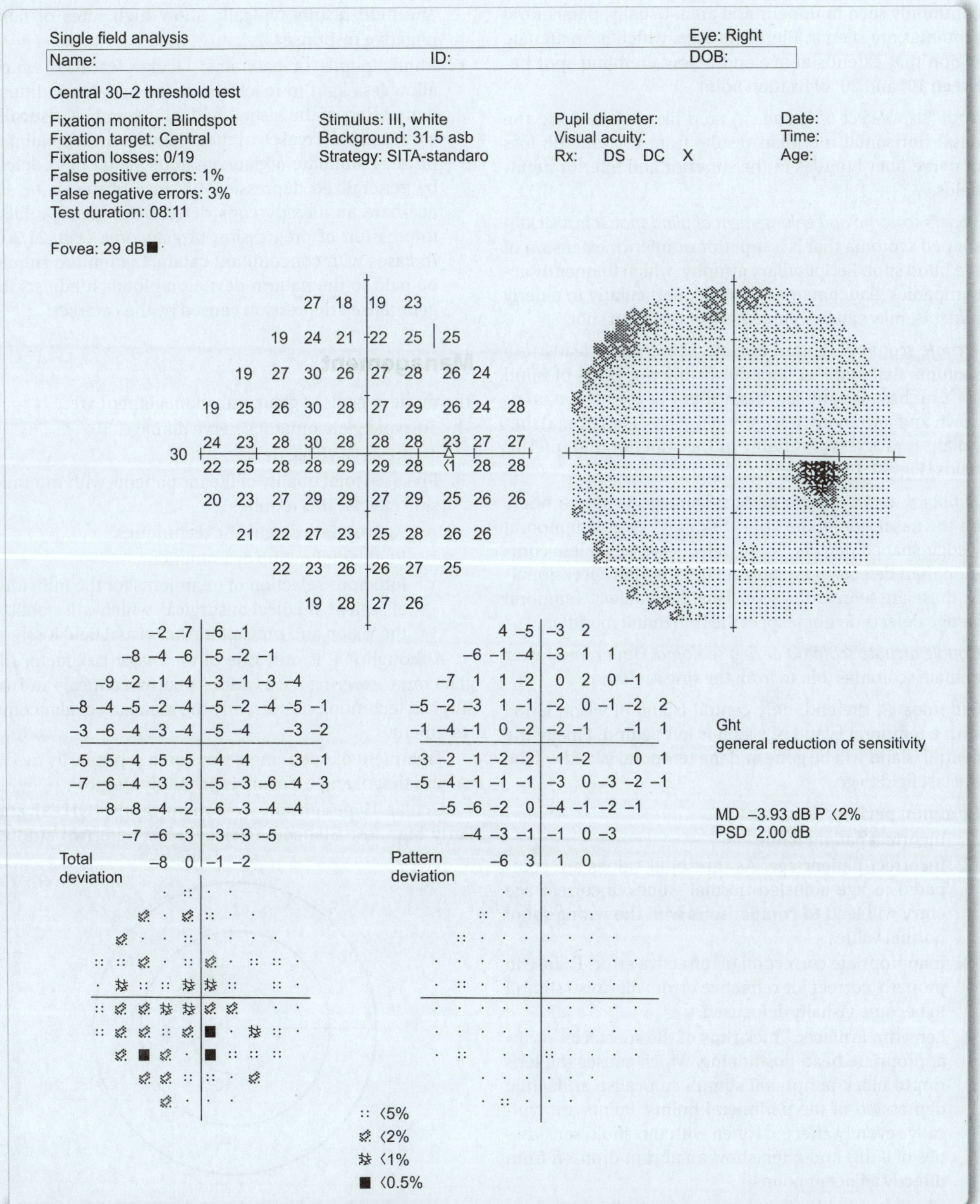

Single field analysis Eye: Right

Name: ID: DOB:

Central 30–2 threshold test

Fixation monitor: Blindspot
Fixation target: Central
Fixation losses: 0/19
False positive errors: 1%
False negative errors: 3%
Test duration: 08:11

Stimulus: III, white
Background: 31.5 asb
Strategy: SITA-standard

Pupil diameter:
Visual acuity:
Rx: DS DC X

Date:
Time:
Age:

Fovea: 29 dB ■

27 18 | 19 23
19 24 21 | 22 25 | 25
19 27 30 26 | 27 28 26 24
19 25 26 30 28 | 27 29 26 24 28
24 23 28 30 28 | 28 28 23 27 27
30
22 25 28 28 29 | 29 28 ‹1 28 28
20 23 27 29 29 | 27 29 25 26 26
21 22 27 23 | 25 28 26 26
22 23 26 | 26 27 25
19 28 | 27 26

-2 -7 | -6 -1
-8 -4 -6 | -5 -2 -1
-9 -2 -1 -4 | -3 -1 -3 -4
-8 -4 -5 -2 -4 | -5 -2 -4 -5 -1
-3 -6 -4 -3 -4 | -5 -4 -3 -2
-5 -5 -4 -5 -5 | -4 -4 -3 -1
-7 -6 -4 -3 -3 | -5 -3 -6 -4 -3
-8 -8 -4 -2 | -6 -3 -4 -4
-7 -6 -3 | -3 -3 -5
-8 0 | -1 -2

Total deviation

4 -5 | -3 2
-6 -1 -4 | -3 1 1
-7 1 1 -2 | 0 2 0 -1
-5 -2 -3 1 -1 | -2 0 -1 -2 2
-1 -4 -1 0 -2 | -2 -1 -1 1
-3 -2 -1 -2 -2 | -1 -2 0 1
-5 -4 -1 -1 -1 | -3 0 -3 -2 -1
-5 -6 -2 0 | -4 -1 -2 -1
-4 -3 -1 | -1 0 -3
-6 3 | 1 0

Pattern deviation

Ght
general reduction of sensitivity

MD −3.93 dB P ‹2%
PSD 2.00 dB

:: ‹5%
‹2%
‹1%
■ ‹0.5%

FIGURE 21.15: General reduction of sensitivity

commonly seen in upper nasal area. Usually, paracentral scotomas are seen in Bjerrum's area, which is an arcuate region that extends above and below the blind spot between 10° and 20° of fixation point.

Nasal step defect of Roenne: A step-like defect along the nasal horizontal meridian results from asymmetric loss of nerve fiber bundles in the superior and inferior hemifields.

Seidel's scotoma and enlargement of blind spot: It is a sickle-shaped scotoma that is a superior or inferior extension of the blind spot. Peripapillary atrophy, which frequently accompanies glaucomatous damage, particularly in elderly patients, may cause enlargement of the blind spot.

Arcuate scotoma: Loss of arcuate nerve fibers leads to a scotoma that starts at superior or inferior poles of blind spot, arches over the macula, widens as they curve up or down and terminates abruptly at the nasal horizontal meridian. It progresses variably in the superior and inferior fields (Figs 21.16 to 21.19).

Temporal wedge-shaped defects: Damage to nerve fibers on the nasal side of the optic disk may result in temporal wedge-shaped defects. These defects are much less common than defects in the arcuate distribution. Occasionally, these are seen as the sole visual field defect. Temporal wedge defects do not respect the horizontal meridian.

Double arcuate scotoma or ring scotoma: Upper and lower arcuate scotomas join to form the ring scotoma.

End stage: At the end, only central island of vision along with a temporal island of vision is left behind. Finally the central island will be gone and the temporal island will be the last field to go.

Common perimetric errors

1. Incorrect patient name.
2. Incorrect patient age: As threshold values are compared to age-adjusted normal values, incorrect age entry will lead to comparisons with the wrong set of normal values.
3. Inappropriate correction of refractive error: Failure to properly correct for refractive error will cause stimuli to become visually defocused.
4. Lens rim artifacts: Thick rims of the spectacles or inappropriate head positioning, which causes the lens rim to block peripheral stimuli can cause artifactual depression of the peripheral points. Points are typically severely affected (often with threshold sensitivities of 0 dB) and often show an abrupt drop-off from directly adjacent points.
5. Cloverleaf fields: This pattern of visual field defects reflects poor visual attention and/or malingering. The field results typically show high rates of false negative responses.
6. Miotic pupils or cataracts: Ocular features, which allow less light to reach the retina can cause diffuse depression of the visual field, along with statistically significant decreases in mean deviation. A small pupil may simulate a glaucomatous visual field defect by generalized depression because of miosis or exacerbate an already constricted field, giving a false impression of progression of glaucoma (Fig. 21.20). In cases with concomitant cataract, attention should be paid to the pattern deviation plot as it adjusts for generalized depression caused by the cataract.

Management

The modern goals of glaucoma management are:

1. To avoid glaucomatous nerve damage.
2. To preserve visual field.
3. Preserve total quality of life for patients with minimal side effects. This requires:
   a. Appropriate diagnostic techniques.
   b. Regular follow-up examinations.
   c. Judicious selection of treatments for the individual patient, medical or surgical, which will stabilize the vision and prevent further visual field loss.

Although IOP is only one of the major risk factor for glaucoma, lowering it via various pharmaceuticals and/or surgical techniques is currently the mainstay of glaucoma treatment.

Treatment of open-angle glaucoma is primarily medical and that of angle closure is primarily surgical.

Ocular Hypertension Treatment Study (OHTS) and Early Manifest Glaucoma Trial (EMGT) are two studies

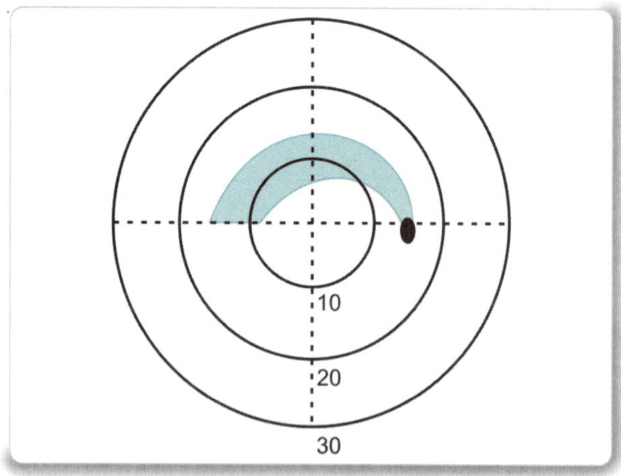

FIGURE 21.16: Arcuate scotoma

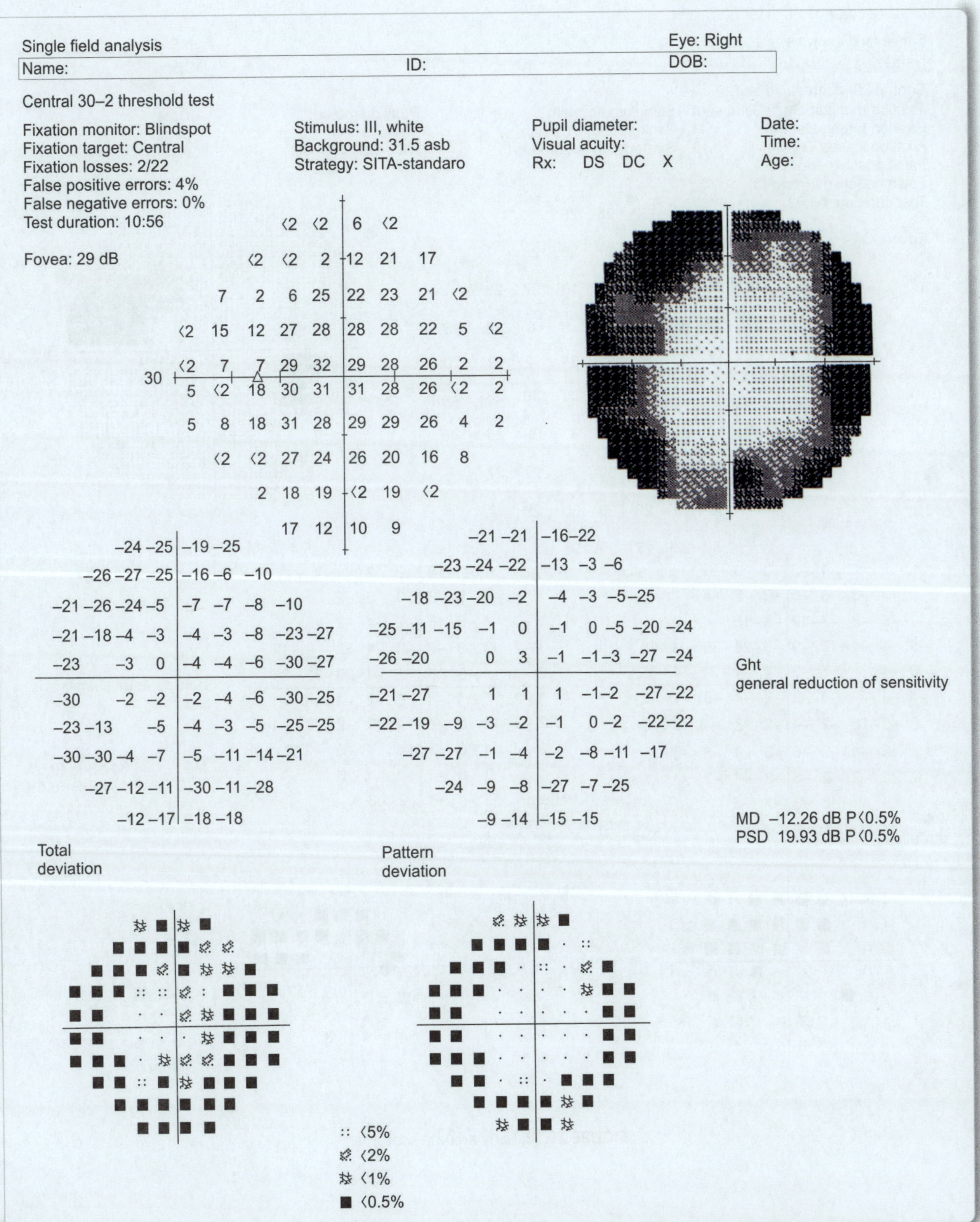

FIGURE 21.17: Double arcuate scotoma

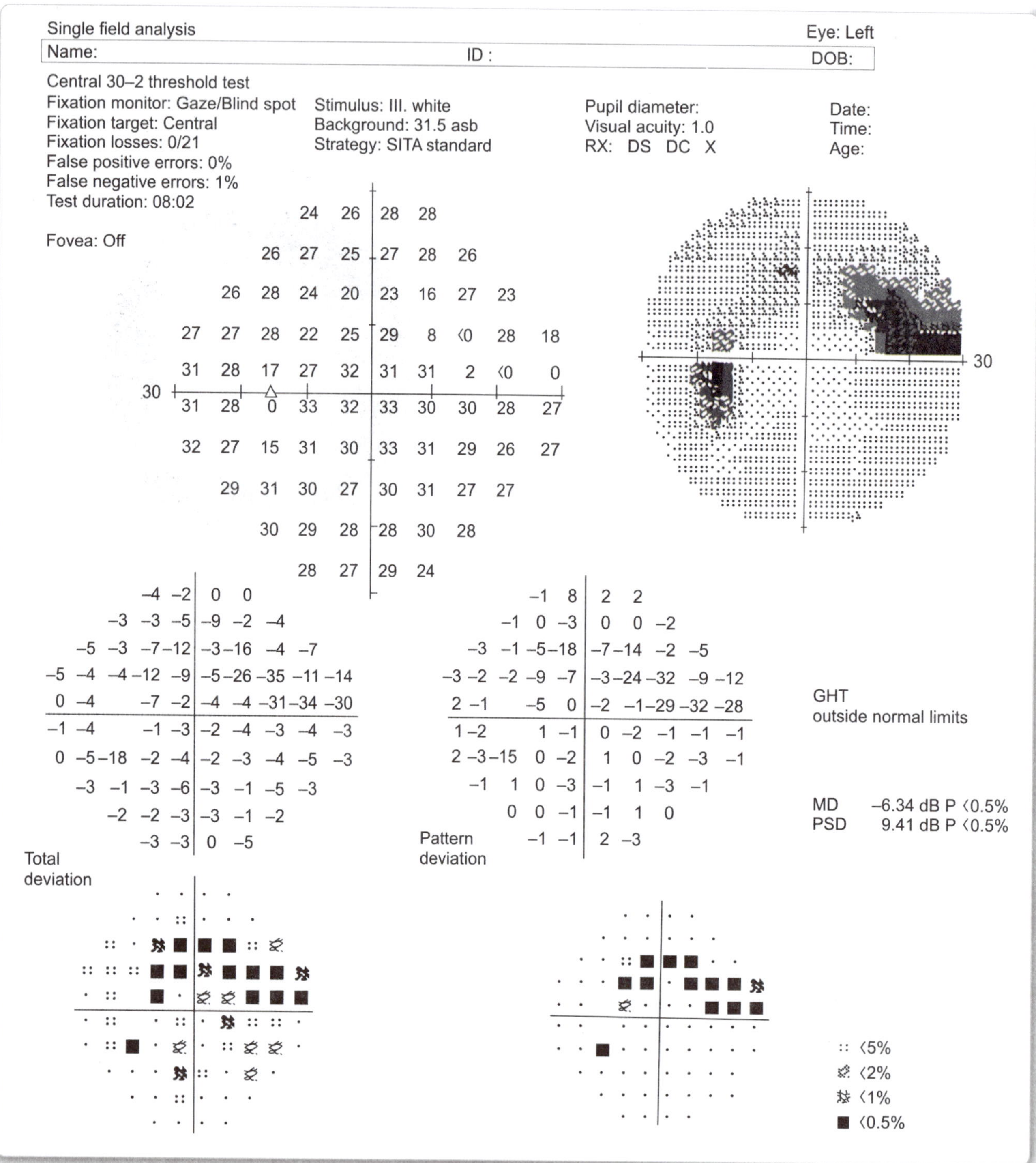

FIGURE 21.18: Early arcuate scotoma

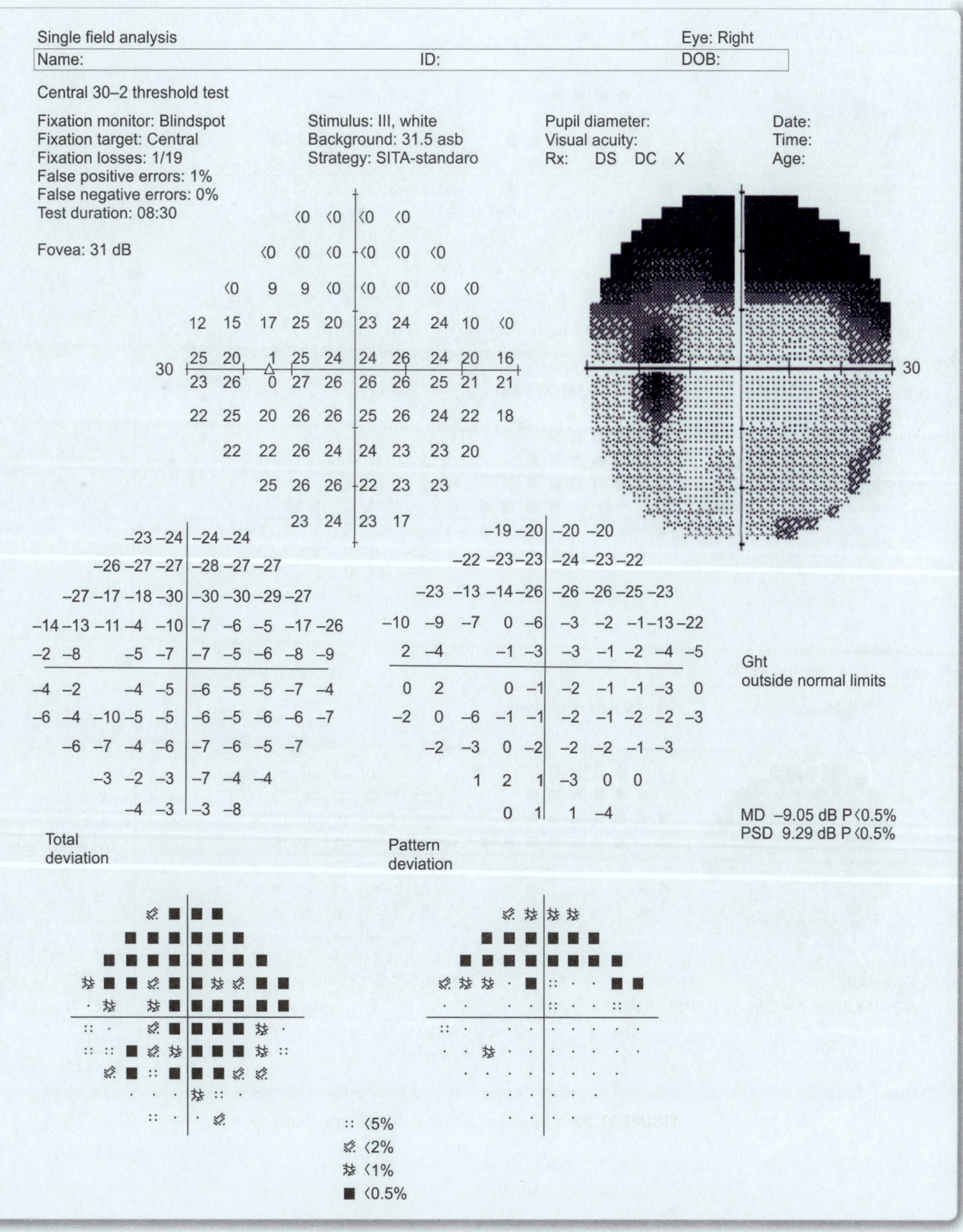

FIGURE 21.19: Advanced superior arcuate scotoma

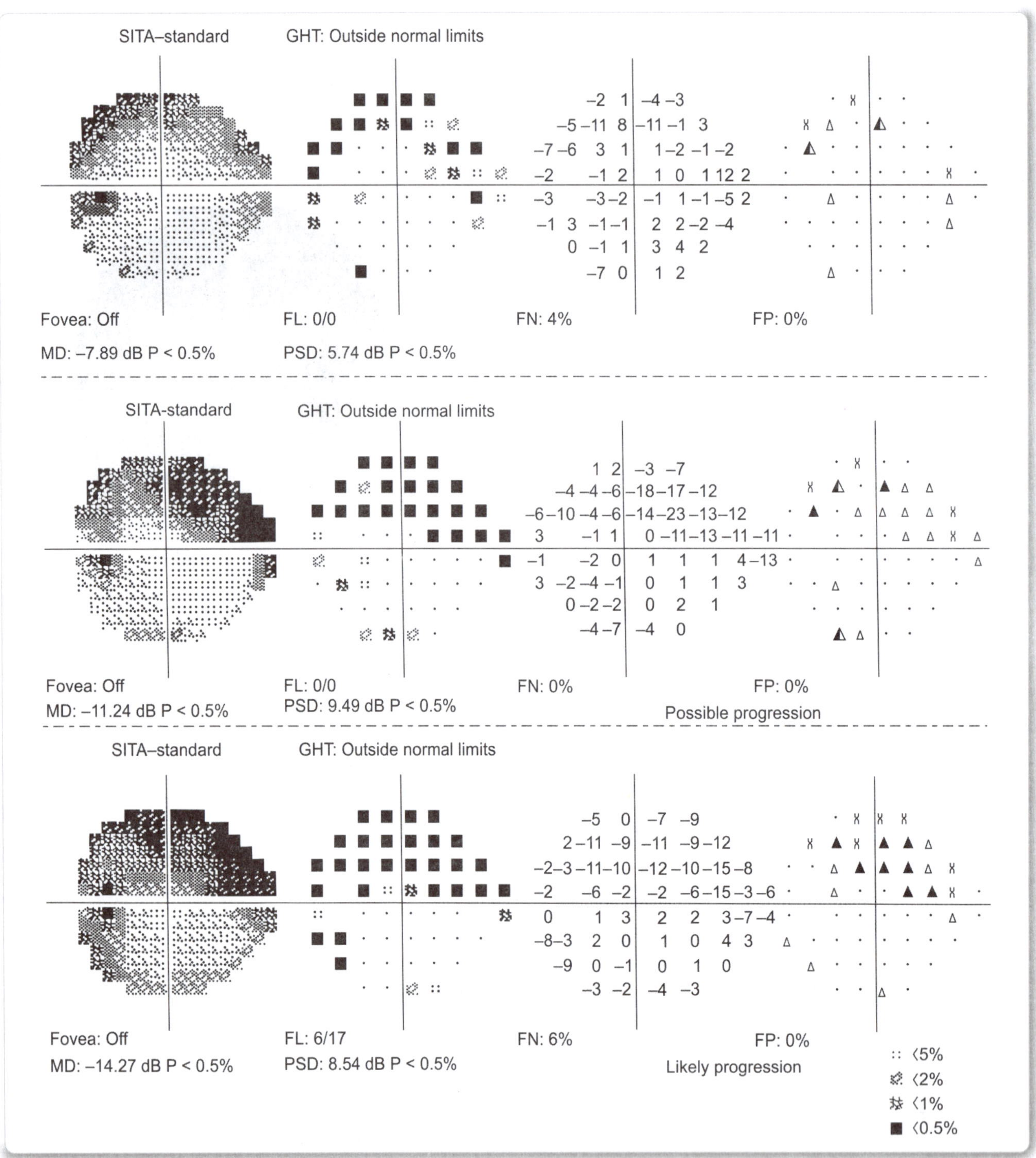

FIGURE 21.20: Progression of field defects in glaucoma

done, which help in decision making of when to start treatment, especially in a patient with early glaucoma.

Ocular Hypertension

Ocular hypertension (OHT) can be defined as elevated IOP in the absence of identifiable optic nerve damage or visual field loss.

Ocular Hypertension Treatment Study

The OHTS trial is a multicenter randomized controlled clinical trial comparing observation with medical therapy for OHT. Result is topical ocular hypotensive medication was effective in delaying or preventing the onset of POAG. 1 out of 22 OHT went on to develop early field loss in 5 years without treatment.

Early Manifest Glaucoma Trial

Multicenter randomized controlled clinical trial comparing observation with betaxolol and laser trabeculoplasty for early open-angle glaucoma. Early glaucoma can be defined as raised IOP with disk changes and early 24-2 field loss. One out of seven patients with early glaucoma progressed in 5 years without treatment.

Conclusion

If the follow-up is done properly, then there is no need to treat all preperimetric (before development of field defects) glaucoma. Before starting treatment, consider side effects of drugs, cost of treatment and labeling of the patient as a glaucoma patient:

- OHT with IOP < 26 mm Hg ⟶ follow-up with fields
- OHT with IOP > 26 mm Hg ⟶ initiate treatment
- OHT with field changes ⟶ initiate treatment.

End Point for Treatment

Target IOP: Aim for a target IOP of 20%–30% reduction in IOP from baseline. If the pretreatment IOP is 30 mm Hg try to bring it down to 22–20 mm Hg, then follow-up the patient. If there is progression in field defects, reset the target IOP by 20%–30% from the 'new baseline' IOP, i.e. try to bring it down from 22 to 15 mm Hg.

Medical Management

Beta blockers

Method of action: By decreasing aqueous inflow, about 20%–30% reduction in IOP occurs, e.g. timolol, betaxolol, levobunolol, metipranolol, carteolol.

Side effects: Hypotension, bradycardia, heart blocks, reduce response to exertion, bronchospasm, mask hypoglycemia, depression, loss of libido, etc.

Parasympathomimetics

Method of action: It is by increasing outflow via trabecular meshwork, e.g. pilocarpine, carbachol, echothiophate, phospholine. These are rarely used now.

Side effects: Loss of accommodation, compensated by increased depth of focus, retinal detachment, iris cyst, etc.

Alpha-agonists

Method of action: It is by decreasing aqueous production and increasing aqueous outflow. About 20%–30% reduction in IOP occurs, e.g. apraclonidine, brimonidine.

Side effects: Burning sensation, follicular conjunctivitis, allergies, headache, drowsiness, dry mouth and nose.

Prostaglandin analogs

Method of action: It is by increasing uveoscleral outflow. About 20%–35% reduction in IOP occurs, e.g. latanoprost, bimatoprost, travoprost and unoprostone.

Side effects: Redness, foreign body sensation, iris and skin pigmentation, increase in number and length of eyelashes.

Topical carbonic anhydrase inhibitors

Method of action: It is by decreasing aqueous production. About 20%–30% reduction in IOP occurs, e.g. dorzolamide and brinzolamide.

Side effects: Metallic taste, hypersensitivity and rarely corneal edema.

Combining drugs

By combining two drugs, though we get 20%–30% reduction individually, together these give only 20%–30% reduction plus an addition of 5%–10% reduction. 1 + 1 = 2 as far as adverse effects goes, e.g. we have combinations of brimonidine with timolol, dorzolamide with timolol and prostaglandins with timolol.

Add/Switch

When the first drug fails to achieve target IOP, it is preferable to switch to another group than add on as:

1. The side effects add up.
2. Long-term allergy/sensitization can occur.

Still we often need multiple drugs. In that case try combination as separate first and if it is effective, combine.

Reduction of side effects

Reduction of side effects can be achieved by applying one drop in cul-de-sac, by closing the eye gently, by wiping excess of drug, by punctal occlusion and by asking the patient not to squeeze the eyelids (to prevent lacrimal pump mechanism).

Compliance issues

Treatment is susceptible to non-compliance as the treatment is lifelong and expensive, and no obvious benefit like improvement in vision occurs. Compliance improves with patient education, improved accessibility to health care and rapport between clinician and patient.

Follow-up

In general, if IOP is stable on treatment, do twice monthly IOP checkup and disk assessment, and field testing every 6–12 months. Complete evaluation including systemic diseases review, gonioscopy, and field and disk assessment is done yearly.

Role of Surgery

Indications for filtration surgery:

1. If target IOP is not achieved medically.
2. If patient cannot afford the medicines.
3. Regular follow-up is not possible due to lack of access to ophthalmologist.
4. Patient shows non-compliance to medical treatment.
5. When glaucomatous optic neuropathy worsens or is expected to worsen at any given level of IOP and the patient is on maximum tolerated medical therapy (MTMT).

Argon laser trabeculoplasty

Argon laser trabeculoplasty (ALT) uses a laser beam focused through a goniolens to treat at the border between anterior and posterior trabecular meshwork. A full treatment consists of 100 spots placed over the entire 360° of the trabecular meshwork. This may be divided between two sessions consisting of 50 spots over 180°. Aqueous outflow improves after the procedure. The IOP reduction obtained is usually in the 7–10 mm Hg range and it may last up to 3–5 years following ALT. Unfortunately, the decrease in IOP is not usually permanent. Approximately, 10% of treated patients will return to pretreatment IOP for each year following treatment.

Complications: A brief, but potentially significant increase in IOP after the procedure (therefore, alpha-agonists are often used either preoperatively or postoperatively for prophylaxis of this occurrence); transient iritis or corneal opacities; peripheral anterior synechiae and hyphema.

Trabeculectomy

An alternate outflow pathway is created to increase passage of aqueous from the anterior chamber to the subconjunctival space, creating a filtering bleb and thereby, lowering IOP (refer Chapter 29 'Glaucoma Surgery').

Ciliary body ablation

Indications: This is a destructive procedure. This procedure is indicated as a last resort for patients who have failed medical management and other surgeries or for those patients who have limited visual potential (often 6/60 or less) or reached the absolute glaucoma stage.

Principle: By destroying a portion of the non-pigmented ciliary epithelium, aqueous humor production is decreased. This will bring down the IOP.

Methods: The ciliary body epithelium can be destroyed by cyclocryotherapy, diathermy, ultrasound, transscleral Nd:YAG or diode laser (known as cyclophotocoagulation) or a newer endoscopic laser.

Public Education

Glaucoma, especially POAG being a silent thief of sight, it is necessary to diagnose POAG early by improving public awareness. Manage and follow-up each patient systematically. Also there is no need to treat all preperimetric glaucoma, if these can be followed up.

All patients and their relatives should be made aware that glaucoma is not curable, but can be medically or surgically controlled, damage to vision is not reversible and glaucoma requires lifelong treatment and follow-up.

PRIMARY ANGLE-CLOSURE GLAUCOMA

Primary angle-closure glaucoma (PACG) is the type of glaucoma occurring due to closure of the trabecular meshwork by the root of the iris, occurring as an anatomical variation.

Epidemiology

Incidence Data

The incidence of PACG varies among different ethnic populations.

Primary angle-closure glaucoma is estimated to be one tenth the number of cases as POAG among White Caucasian population. Mongoloid races have a much higher rate of prevalence for PACG.

Descending order of prevalence (roughly) can be: Inuit (Eskimos), East Asian (Chinese, Filipino, Vietnamese), Indian subcontinent and those of European origin.

Factors

Demographic Factors

Age: The risk of PACG goes up with age. Most often occurs in the sixth or seventh decade, though commonly it can present by the fourth decade.

Gender: Women are more commonly affected with a relative risk of 2–3 times compared to men. This probably reflects the fact that women have approximately 10% less ocular volume and have narrower angles.

Heredity: Most cases are sporadic in nature. Some studies do show some familial influence. The configuration of the anterior chamber is considered to have a polygenic inheritance and that probably is the reason for lack of family history in most patients.

Refractive error: Prevalence of PACG is higher in hypermetropic individuals.

Miscellaneous: Finding that acute PACG occurs more in winter months has been made in the past.

Predisposing Factors

Primary angle-closure glaucoma essentially occurs in a small crowded eye (Figs 21.21A and B). In eyes, predisposed to angle-closure glaucoma, the average corneal diameter, anterior chamber depth and axial length are less, but the lens size and volume do not come down proportionally and this leads to a crowded anterior chamber, especially in the periphery at the angle of the anterior chamber.

Another mechanism, plateau iris, involves the peripheral iris root being inserted at an angle to the ciliary body. This will lead to angle closure by the root of the iris on dilatation of the pupil even though the anterior chamber will be of normal depth.

Mechanisms

Angle closure occurs often as a combination of the following mechanisms elaborated below. In a given case, one mechanism would prevail more than others.

Relative Pupillary Block

The most important mechanism is the relative pupillary block. In a normal eye, the iris is slightly in contact with the lens at the pupillary margin (Fig. 21.22A). In a crowded anterior chamber the crystalline lens is pushing the iris forward and is partially jutting out (Fig. 21.22B). In this state, the iris exerts a posterior pressure on the lens causing resistance to flow of aqueous. This is maximal in the mid-dilated position.

On the constricted state, the pupil is positioned tangential to the lens and is not able to effectively grip the lens. In the mid-dilated position, the sphincter muscle of the iris exerts a centripetal or inward force on the part of lens jutting anterior to it (refer Fig. 21.22B). The centrifugal action of the dilator pupillae muscle (Fig. 21.22C) also is slanted backward and a small part of the vector is hence pressing on the anterior capsule of the lens. This gives maximal resistance to aqueous flow through the pupil into the anterior chamber from its source, ciliary body that secretes it into the posterior chamber. The relaxed peripheral portion of the iris in the mid-dilated position is pushed forward by the increased IOP in the posterior

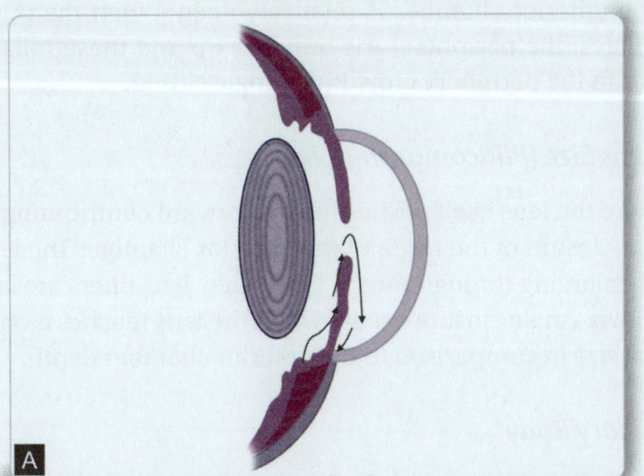

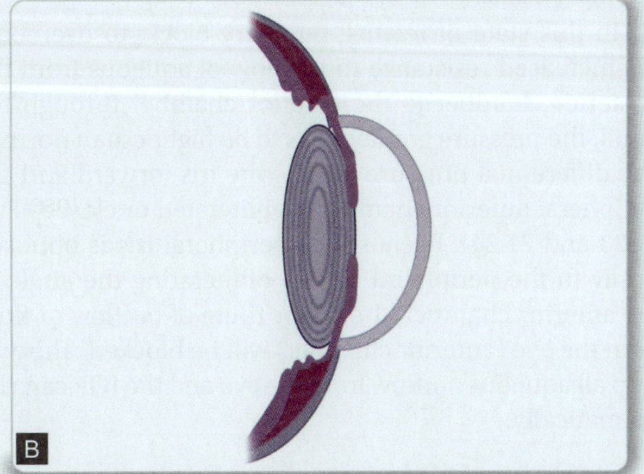

FIGURES 21.21A and B: Predisposing factor. **A.** Normal eye with flow of aqueous shown by arrows. Aqueous is secreted by the ciliary body into the posterior chamber and flows through the pupil into the anterior chamber to the angle of the anterior chamber, where it traverses the trabecular meshwork to the canal of Schlemm and from these to episcleral veins; **B.** In an eye predisposed to angle closure, the anterior chamber is shallow and a relatively normal sized lens juts into the same predisposing to a pupillary block.

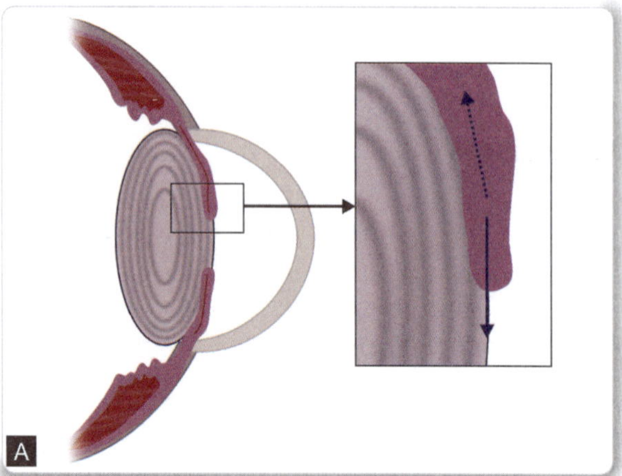

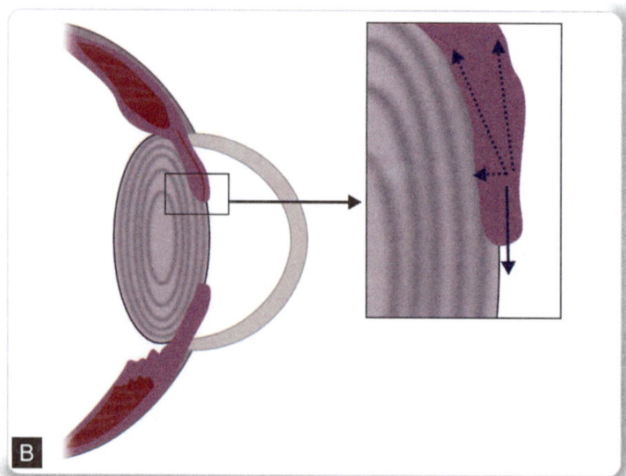

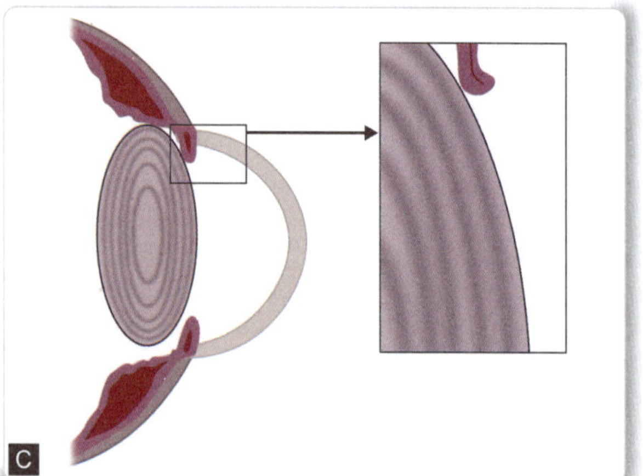

FIGURES 21.22A to C: Relative pupillary block mechanism. **A.** With pupil in its normal position the iris skims the surface of the lens and grips it to cause resistance to flow of aqueous; **B.** With pupil in mid-dilated position a little of the lens in a shallow anterior chamber juts into the pupil and is held by the pupillary muscles. Primarily by the sphincter pupillae and secondarily by the posterior component of the vector of force from the dilator. This causes a relative pupillary block to flow of aqueous through the pupil; **C.** With pupil in dilated positions the iris falls away from the lens and is unable to cause resistance to flow of aqueous.

chamber. Thus, the aqueous flow is blocked at the pupil. This is not an absolute block and hence is called relative pupillary block.

In this state of relative pupillary block, to overcome the increased resistance to the flow of aqueous from the posterior chamber to the anterior chamber through the pupil, the pressure gradient has to be higher than normal. The differential pressure pushes the iris forward and the peripheral anterior chamber is obliterated or closed (Figs 21.23 and 21.24). Because the peripheral iris is opposed firmly to the peripheral cornea obliterating the angle of the anterior chamber, the major route of outflow of fluid from the eye (anterior chamber) will be blocked. This will stop all aqueous outflow from the eye and the IOP can rise dramatically.

Plateau Iris

In plateau iris condition, there is abnormal insertion of the iris to the ciliary body. As a result, the root of iris is slanted abnormally forward. On ultrasound biomicroscopy, these patients are often noted to have anteriorly placed ciliary processes pushing the peripheral iris root forward. Central anterior chamber is relatively deep. When the pupil dilates, the peripheral iris bunches up and these rolls of iris in the periphery crowds the angle closed.

Lens Size (Phacomorphic Like)

Here the lens itself pushes the iris forward contributing to the closure of the angle of the anterior chamber. The lens is enlarging throughout the life as new lens fibers are laid down. Angle closure occurs when the lens reaches a critical size in comparison to the anterior chamber depth.

Ciliary Body

The ciliary body is attached anteriorly to the scleral spur. Beyond this there is no attachment to the outer coat of the eye (sclera). When the ciliary muscles contract, the circumference of the ciliary body decreases and the ciliary body tends to rotate anteriorly on its attachment at the scleral

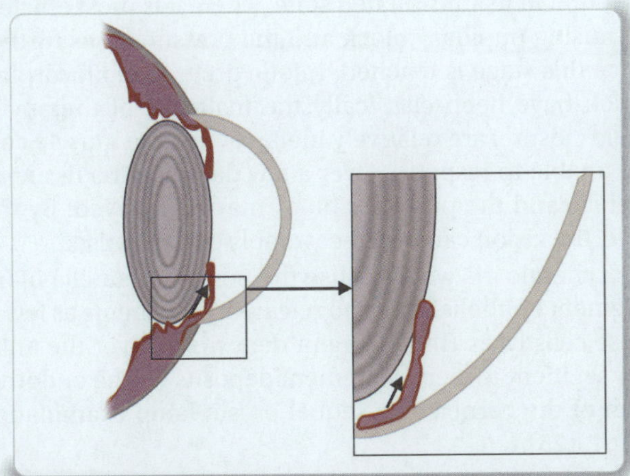

FIGURE 21.23: When aqueous flows into the posterior chamber, the pressure in the posterior chamber push the peripheral iris forward and obliterate the angle of the anterior chamber. This stops almost all outflow from the eye and the intraocular pressure (IOP) can rise dramatically.

spur. This would rotate the peripheral iris root, attached to it closer to the trabecular meshwork. This would also move the entire zonular ligament with it and hence the lens moves forward. An anterior rotation of the ciliary body would thus move the lens-iris diaphragm forward and narrow the angle of the anterior chamber. In cases where this mechanism contributes significantly, pilocarpine would worsen the angle closure as it causes contraction of ciliary muscles and consequent anterior movement of the same.

Pathophysiology

By combination of above mechanisms, the anterior chamber angle can close. Over time the lens thickness is marginally increasing. This means that the angle closure would worsen in a given patient as age advances. Initially, the angle closes for short spans of time. A tiny movement of the iris would relieve the angle closure long enough, opening the aqueous outflow channels and allows the IOP to reduce. Later on, the duration of angle being closed increases and the pressure can rise to higher levels and it can remain high for longer periods of time. At some point a sudden acute angle closure occurs with severe pain, constitutional symptoms like headache, nausea and vomiting, intense congestion, high IOP, corneal edema and mid-dilated pupil.

Effects of Angle Closure in Different Parts of the Eye

In the Cornea (Blurring and Halos)

When the IOP rises to approximately 30 mm Hg, a cornea with average endothelial function develops epithelial edema. Epithelial edema causes the epithelial cells to swell up and form multiple tiny elevations on the corneal surface, each of which acts optically like a prism capable of dispersion of light. Dispersion of light causes white light to split up into its spectrum of colors as in a rainbow. This causes formation of ring-shaped colored halos around light sources like an incandescent bulb with the red color

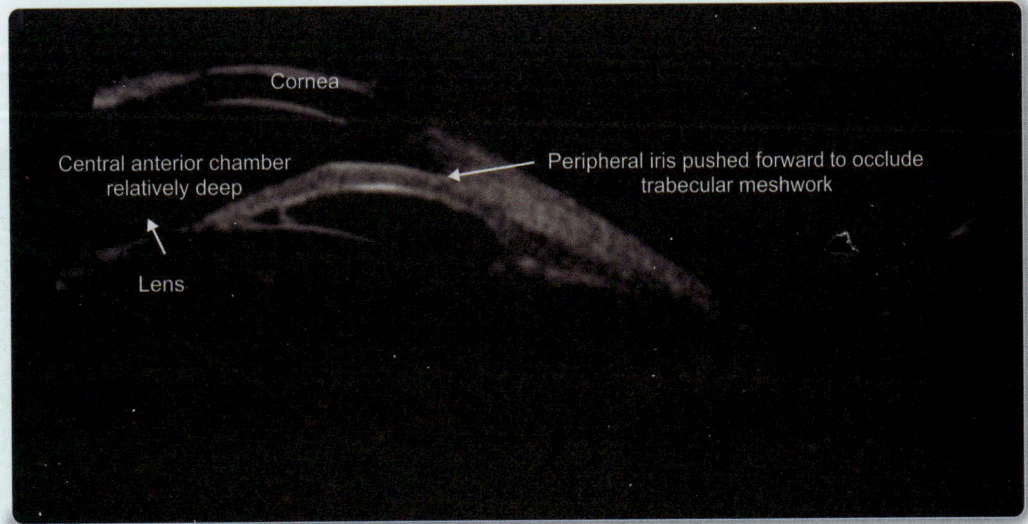

FIGURE 21.24: Ultrasound biomicroscopic (UBM) image of pupillary block causing angle closure

seen on the outside and blue on the inside of the ring (red light has a longer wavelength). At this stage there can be some degradation of quality of vision in the form of slight blurring, foreign body sensation and watering due to irregularity of the ocular surface.

Halos can also be seen in early stages of cataract and when mucus strands are present in the tear film. Halos arising from the lens are due to prismatic effect in the peripheral lens fibers near the lens equator. Thus lenticular halos would break up if a stenopaic slit is passed across the eye unlike a corneal edema halo as in a corneal edema the prismatic effect is present over a diffuse area. Halos due to mucus strands would vary with blinking and disappear if the eye surface is washed clear of mucus.

Scleral Stretch (Headache and Constitutional Symptoms)

Pressure rise would stretch the scleral fibers and ocular discomfort occurs as a dull ache (40 mm Hg approximately). Further pressure rise would convert this periorbital ache into a more severe headache, which is often felt all over the head as the stretch is increased. Additionally, the scleral stretch causes stimulation of the vagus nerve and symptoms expected in a vagal stimulation may supervene in the form of nausea, vomiting and prostration. In fact, often the patient reaches the internal medicine casualty with headache and vomiting as the predominant symptoms prior to recognition of the ocular cause by the internist.

Ischemia of Optic Nerve (Decreased Vision, CRA Occlusion and Optic Atrophy)

When the IOP raises further, the retinal and optic nerve functions get compromised as circulation of blood slows down. Further reduction in visual function results in loss of visual acuity. When the IOP goes above 60 mm Hg there is a significant risk of total cessation of blood flow in the central retinal artery (CRA). This can lead to a CRA occlusion itself. In such an acute event, one may see primary optic atrophy like picture in the sequel (cupping or cavernous optic atrophy occurs when the pressure rise is gradual and not acute, and so dramatic and the gradual reduction in blood circulation occurs).

Ischemia of Iris (Sphincter Paralysis Dilated Pupil, Pigment Dispersion and Iris Atrophy)

At pressures in the range of 40 mm Hg or so the iris also becomes ischemic. This causes a paralysis of the iris musculature, especially the sphincter pupillae. This freezes the pupil in its mid-dilated state, where it is most efficient at causing pupillary block and the pressure rises further. Once this stage is reached, miotic drugs like pilocarpine, which have been classically the mainstay of therapy of angle closure, are relatively ineffective as the muscle cells are unable to respond. Over a few days, the iris tissue atrophies and the pupillary block may be relieved. By this time, the vision can be irrecoverably compromised.

Ischemic iris would cause the posterior lamella of iris (pigment epithelial layer) to release iris pigments as few of these cells lyses. This pigment deposits all over the anterior segment is seen as pigment deposits on the endothelium of the cornea as a sequel on slit lamp examination (Fig. 21.25).

Lens (Anterior Subcapsular Cataracts)

As the outflow is compromised, ultrafiltration at the ciliary body slows down due to back pressure. In short, aqueous secretion comes to a standstill. The lens being avascular is totally dependent on the nutrients and oxygen supplied by the aqueous to it. Lack of the same causes formation of anterior subcapsular opacities in the lens called glaucomflecken (Figs 21.26A and B).

Vogt's Triad

Vogt's triad is a set of three findings such as iris atrophy, pigment deposits on the endothelium of the cornea and glaucomflecken that suggests previous occurrence of an acute congestive angle-closure attack. This once present, persists for life (refer Figs 21.26A and B).

Peripheral Anterior Synechiae

When the iris stays in contact with the angle structures in the periphery of the anterior chamber, it gets stuck to it

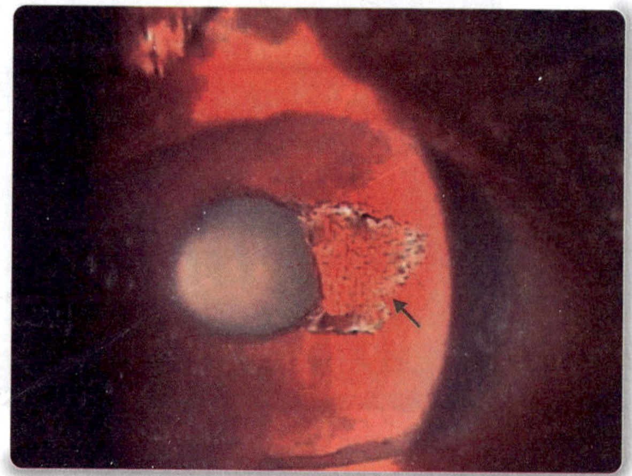

FIGURE 21.25: Patch of iris atrophy

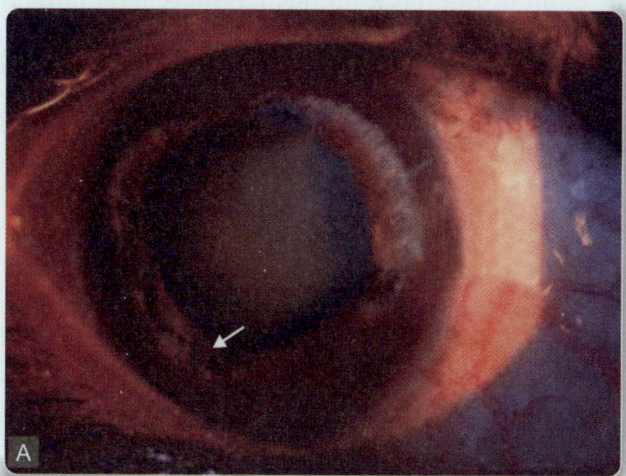

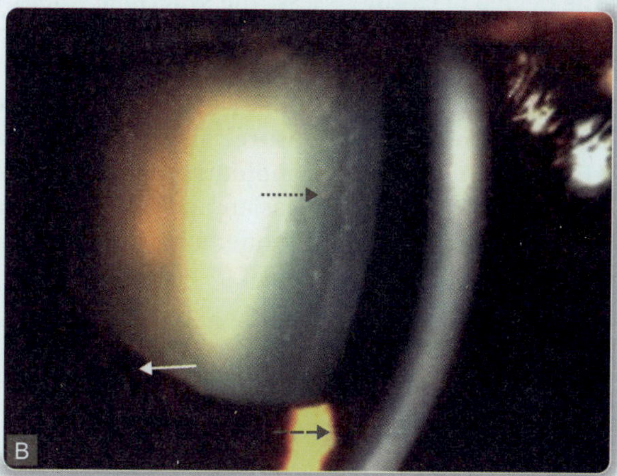

FIGURES 21.26A and B: Vogt's triad. Pigment deposits on back of the cornea (endothelium), iris atrophy and glaucomflecken (anterior subcapsular lens opacities) constitute the Vogt's triad. **A.** Diffuse illumination to show iris atrophy (solid arrows); **B.** Slit lamp picture to show anterior subcapsular opacities (dotted arrows) and pigment (dashed arrows).

permanently. This leads to blockage of outflow in that area permanently. When half the circumference of the angle is compromised, usually the IOP stays raised permanently.

Stages of Angle Closure

Classical Stages

Classically, angle closure has been staged with pupillary block as the mechanism of closure with a sequence as following. Not all patients follow all the stages and so the staging does not reflect the course of all patients.

1. Latent stage

In latent stage, the eye has a shallow anterior chamber on slit lamp examination and gonioscopy. The patient has no symptoms and the pressures are normal.

2. Prodromal stage

In prodromal stage, there are intermittent episodes of closure of the angle leading to transient rise in IOP to moderate levels enough to cause corneal epithelial edema. This happens when the pupil is mid-dilated, when the ambient light is dim (scotopic conditions), when the patient is in a movie theater or when they are tired at the end of the day, the pupil dilates physiologically. This causes a relative pupillary block in predisposed eyes, leading to pressure rise in the range of 30s. The patient now sees halos around lights with decrease in vision and some discomfort around eyes. At this stage, these episodes occur widely spaced and are spontaneously relieved, e.g. with sleep that induces miosis (pupillary constriction). If examined during this episode one would find pressures in the range of 30–40 mm Hg with corneal epithelial edema and gonioscopically appositionally closed angle.

3. Stage of constant instability/intermittent closure

The process is the same as in prodromal stage with increasing frequency and regularity. At this point of time the patient realizes that there is something amiss about their eye and seeks medical help.

4. Acute angle closure/acute congestive glaucoma

Now the pupillary block is more severe and the IOP raises high enough to make the sphincter pupillae ischemic and paralyzed temporarily in its mid-dilated position. The pressure rises markedly and there is marked loss of visual acuity. But the predominant symptom is headache caused by scleral stretch, associated with nausea and vomiting. The patient feels very sick and prostrate, and may land in medical casualty.

On examination, the vision is markedly reduced. There is circumcorneal congestion with hazy cornea (steamy) due to stromal edema along with epithelial edema. The pupil is mid-dilated, vertically oval and non-reactive. If one checks for a relative afferent pupillary defect, it is often present.

5. Chronic angle closure/chronic congestive glaucoma

Chronic glaucoma stage is characterized by the presence of peripheral anterior synechiae. These would compromise aqueous humor outflow in that area and the IOP rises above baseline. Usually, this happens by the time synechiae close half the angle. Now the baseline pressure is constantly elevated. The optic disk and field changes, as in POAG, will start to develop over time after this.

Though the stage of chronic angle closure can occur after an acute angle-closure attack, some patients develop peripheral anterior synechiae without going through a dramatic acute angle closure. The mechanisms are the same, but the degree of closure is less. The synechiae would develop slowly from posterior part of the angle and work its way anteriorly closing the angle progressively. A larger circumference is often involved. This slow process of closure is called **'creeping angle closure'.** These patients have POAG-like picture as far as symptoms go. Creeping angle closure is rarely seen in Caucasian and African populations, whereas this is the commoner form in the Mongoloid races and Indian subcontinent.

6. Absolute glaucoma

Absolute glaucoma is the end stage of any glaucoma, where all vision is lost and eye is stony hard, blind and often painful. This can occur in all types of glaucoma.

ISGEO Classification

As there are different mechanisms contributing in varying degrees in a given person, not all patients follow the classical stages in order. The stage of acute closure is often skipped. This means that in epidemiological studies it is difficult to classify closure in the classical scheme across various regions. So, a classification was developed only for epidemiological studies by the 'International Society for Geographic and Epidemiologic Ophthalmology' (ISGEO):

1. Primary angle-closure suspect (PACS): Iridotrabecular contact in the angle of anterior chamber in three or more quadrants.
2. Primary angle closure (PAC): PACS plus raised IOP or peripheral anterior synechiae on gonioscopy.
3. Primary angle-closure glaucoma (PACG): PAC plus disk and field changes typical of glaucoma (as in POAG).

Examination

As in any patient with glaucoma one should record visual acuity, pupillary responses (especially look for a relative afferent pupillary defect), IOP, appearance of the optic disk and visual fields.

Specific to angle-closure glaucoma, one should look for the Vogt's triad.

Shallow anterior chamber can be suspected on torchlight examination with the oblique flashlight test. Here the flashlight is shown with the light beam parallel to the iris plane from the temporal side. If the iris configuration is flat as in a normal anterior chamber, almost the entire circumference is lit up. But in an eye with closure (or predisposed to closure) the anterior chamber is crowded by the crystalline lens, pushing the central iris forward. This will cause a crescent-shaped shadow to fall on the nasal side of the iris. If the shadow obscures half the distance from pupil to the nasal limbus (corneoscleral junction), we consider the anterior chamber shallow. This is roughly the same as saying that with the oblique flashlight test; if the nasal collarette of the iris is in the shadow, the eye has a shallow anterior chamber.

van Herick's Test

van Herick's test is a method of estimation of depth of anterior chamber with the help of the slit lamp.

Method: To perform the van Herick's test, the slit beam is made very bright and thin. It is set at 60° temporally to the eye. The thickness of the cornea is compared to the depth of the peripheral anterior chamber. If the anterior chamber depth is as deep as the cornea is thick, then the angle is presumed to be wide open. If there is only a slit of aqueous then the angle is estimated to be dangerously narrow.

Gonioscopy

The definitive way of knowing what is happening in the angle of the anterior chamber is to visualize it using special lenses called gonioscopes (gonio means angle) (Fig. 21.27) along with the slit lamp (Figs 21.28A and B, 21.29A and B). With this technique, one can see if the anterior chamber angle is open or closed as well as note other features like peripheral anterior synechiae (adhesions between iris and anterior structures, viz. trabecular meshwork and cornea) (Figs 20.30A and B).

In the latent stage, the peripheral iris root is often noted to be close to the trabecular meshwork, though not apposed to it.

In angle-closure glaucoma, the angle is closed by apposition of iris root to the trabecular meshwork. Here, indentation on the cornea would open up a gap between the two tissues, as will pupillary constriction.

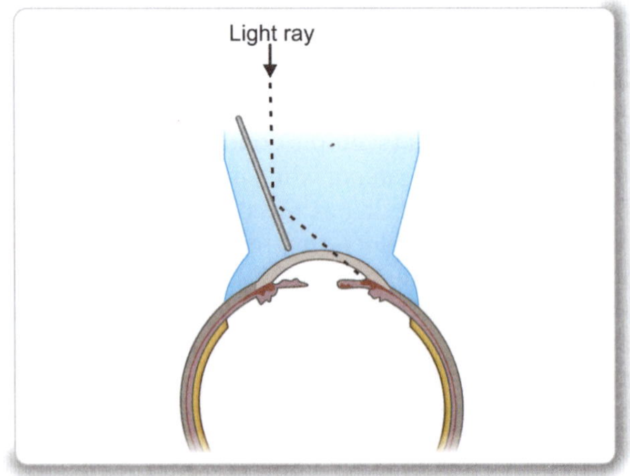

FIGURE 21.27: Gonioscopy

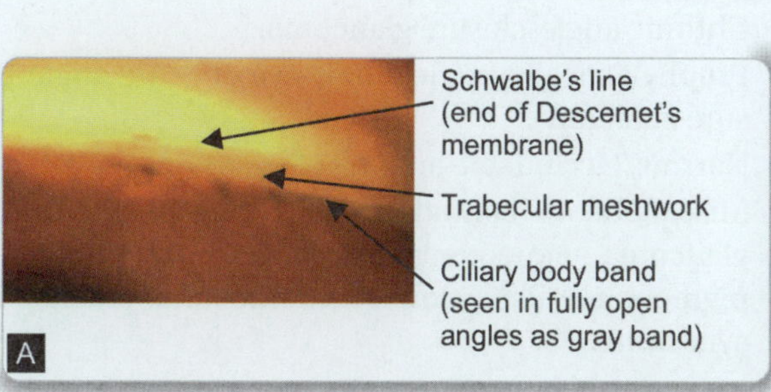

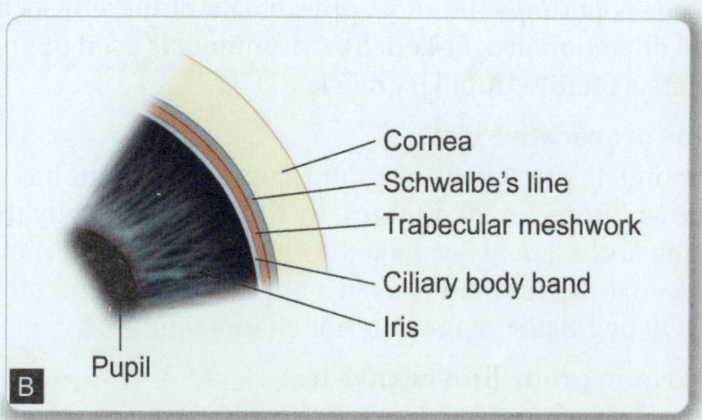

FIGURES 21.28A and B: Structure in angle of anterior chamber. **A.** Photograph; **B.** Diagrammatic representation.

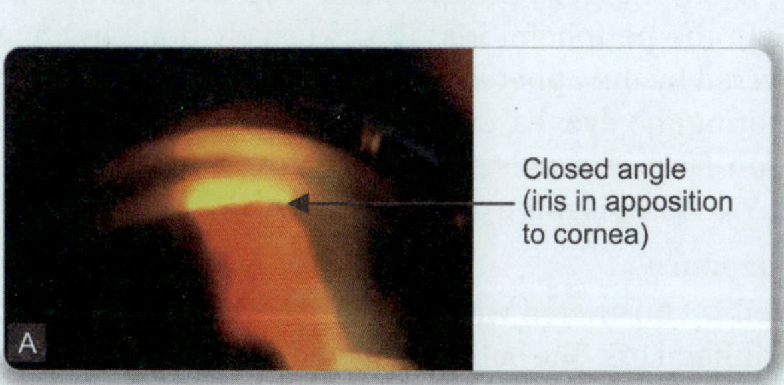

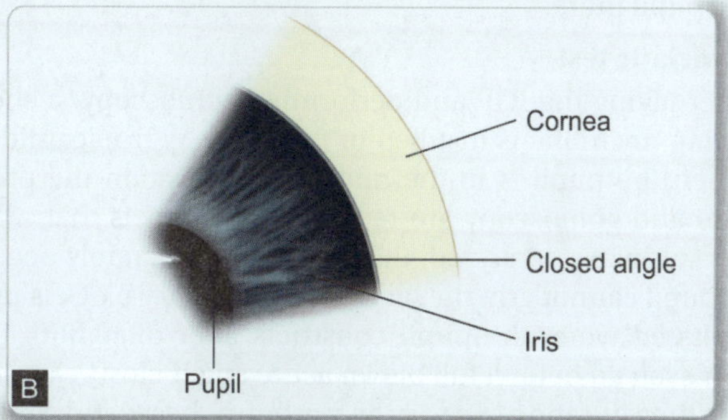

FIGURES 21.29A and B: Closed angle. **A.** Photograph; **B.** Diagrammatic representation.

At a later stage, when apposition has gone for some time, the tissues stick to each other structurally and cannot be separated and now it is called synechia (plural synechiae). Now the closure is in chronic angle-closure glaucoma stage.

Provocative Tests

Provocative tests were been used clinically in the past, but now they are rarely used as the test itself can precipitate an acute angle-closure glaucoma attack. These are of historical importance and one can learn a lot about pathogenesis of angle closure with these tests. In all these tests, pretest IOP and gonioscopy are done. Then the pupil is stressed to precipitate a relative pupillary block and look for the rise in IOP and pupillary block by repeating gonioscopy.

Darkroom test

Pretest IOP and gonioscopy are done. Then the patient is allowed to remain in a darkened room for 20 minutes and IOP is checked and pupillary block is looked for, by gonioscopy.

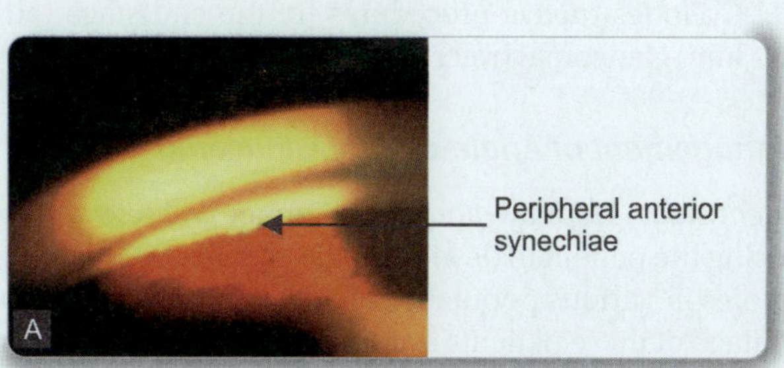

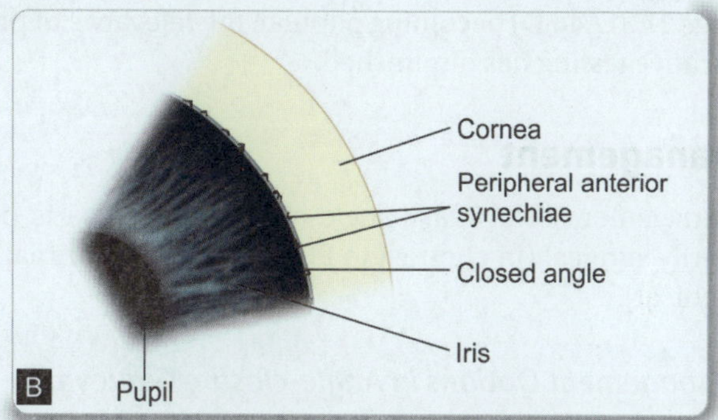

FIGURES 21.30A and B: Peripheral anterior synechiae. **A.** Photograph; **B.** Diagrammatic representation.

This is perhaps the most physiologic of these tests as pupil dilatation in a darkened environment is used to precipitate a relative pupillary block.

Prone provocative test

After pretest pressures and gonioscopy, the patient has to lie down prone for 20 minutes. By the effect of gravity the weight of the lens is expected to appose the pupil more firmly to it. This should worsen a pupillary block and raise the IOP by closure of the anterior chamber angle.

Darkroom prone provocative test

In the darkroom prone provocative test, the prone provocative test is done in a darkroom, i.e. both the darkroom test and the prone provocative tests are combined to stress the pupil more.

Mydriatic test

After taking the IOP and performing gonioscopy, a short acting mydriatic is instilled in the eye (e.g. tropicamide). When the pupil is in the mid-dilated position the pressure and gonioscopy are repeated. The flaw is that, with the sphincter paralyzed, the pupillary block rarely occurs as pupil cannot grip the lens. Often pupillary block is precipitated when the pupil constricts after dilatation and can even go in for a full blown acute angle-closure attack. The time duration can vary by few hours, because different persons would take different time durations to constrict after dilatation.

Mapstone test

Here the pupil is stressed purely pharmacologically. The 1% pilocarpine, which causes contraction of sphincter papillae, as well as 10% phenylephrine, which causes contraction of the dilator papillae is concomitantly instilled in the eye. Contraction of both the muscles can result in a pupillary block and the same is looked for.

If the result is positive in all these test, than the patient has to be treated. But a negative result does not mean that the patient is safe. They were thus relevant as one more evidence to proceed to open surgery in an era when that was the only option. Now with the less invasive laser iridotomy (Figs 21.31A to D) becoming popular, the relevance of provocative testing has diminished.

Management

Management of primary angle-closure glaucoma is primarily surgical (in contrast to POAG where it is primarily medical).

Management Options in Angle-closure Glaucoma

Laser iridotomy: An opening is made in the peripheral iris without loss of tissue with the help of a laser beam.

Indications

1. Acute angle-closure glaucoma.
2. Chronic angle-closure glaucoma.
3. Prophylactically in the fellow eye of acute angle-closure glaucoma.
4. Narrow/Occludable angle.
5. Miscellaneous conditions, including phacomorphic glaucoma, aqueous misdirection, nanophthalmos, pigmentary dispersion syndrome and plateau iris syndrome.

Principle

The resistance to flow of aqueous is at the pupil. So, if we bypass the pupil, the pathogenesis of glaucoma by relative pupillary block could be halted (refer Figs 21.31A to D).

Laser energy is used to create 100–150 micron opening in the peripheral iris. This is usually done in an area covered by the upper eyelid to prevent glare by stray light entering the eye. Lasers described for the procedure are argon laser and pulsed Nd:YAG laser. Nowadays pulsed Nd:YAG laser is more often used.

Procedure

Pupil is constricted with pilocarpine drops to stretch the peripheral iris. The patient is seated at the laser under topical anesthesia (proparacaine/lignocaine drops instilled). A laser iridotomy lens (Abram's lens) is placed on the eye to see the iris magnified. A suitable crypt (pit-like depression in the thin area of iris near iris root) in the peripheral iris is chosen aimed at and laser fired a few times to create an adequately sized peripheral iridotomy (PI) (Fig. 21.32).

Open surgical procedures: This is the another procedure of management.

Indications

1. When a laser PI alone is not sufficient to control IOP.
2. When other procedures fail to make an opening on the iris with laser.

Methods

1. A surgical peripheral iridectomy.
2. Drainage procedures like trabeculectomy.
3. Cyclodestructive procedures [in the end-stage (absolute) glaucoma] (refer Chapter 29 'Glaucoma Surgery').

Management of Angle-closure Glaucoma

Latent stage: Here the anterior chamber is shallow predisposing the patient to develop angle closure. Epidemiologic studies in various populations show that only a small percentage of these patients eventually develop angle-closure glaucoma. So, this group warrants no treatment. But this group is at risk compared to the general population and

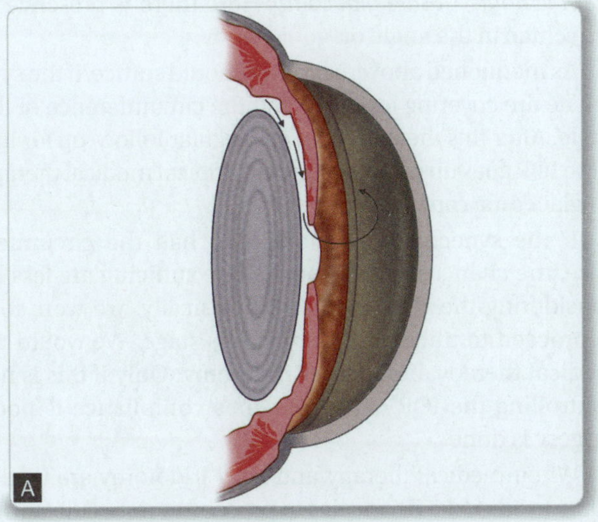

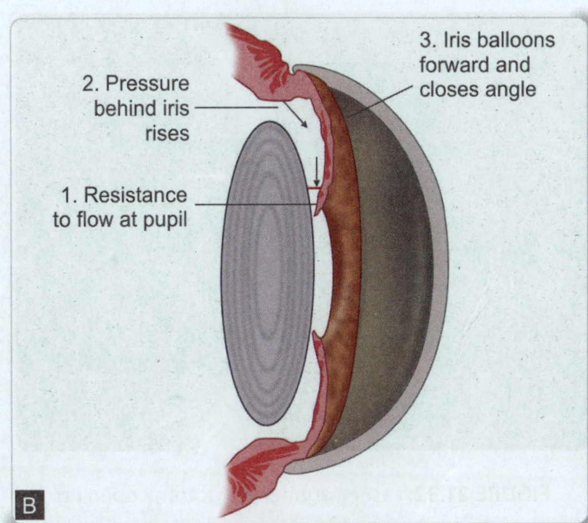

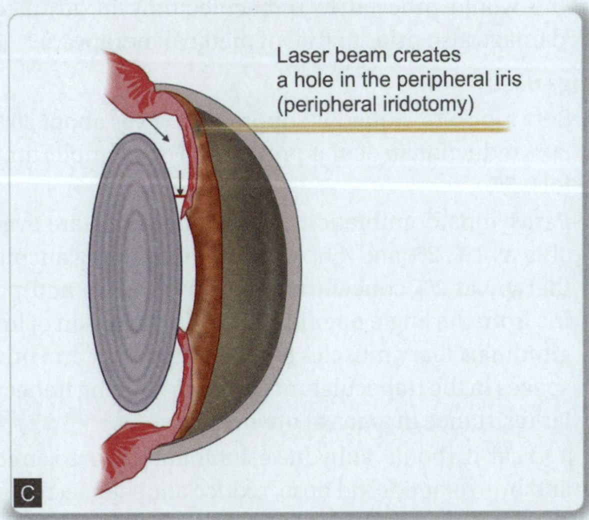

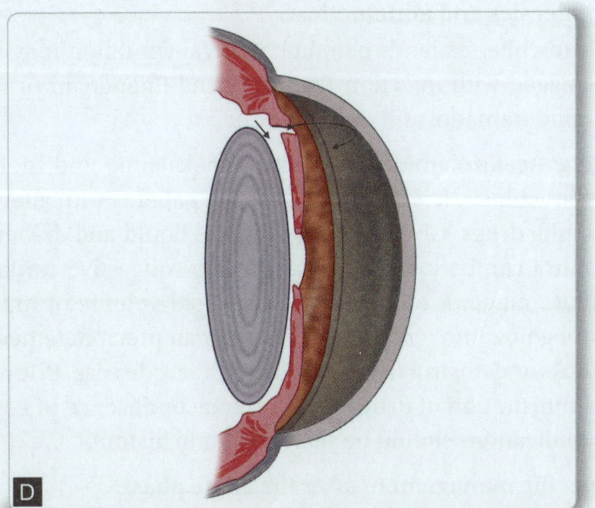

FIGURES 21.31A to D: Laser peripheral iridotomy. **A.** Normal aqueous flow from ciliary body to trabecular meshwork; **B.** Pupillary block causing closure of anterior chamber angle (trabecula); **C.** Nd:AG or argon laser is used to create an opening in peripheral iris; **D.** Aqueous now flows through the peripheral iridotomy, bypassing the pupil to reach the trabecular meshwork in the anterior chamber angle.

hence needs follow-up and education regarding angle-closure glaucoma symptoms.

At least once a year, they need follow-up including IOP measurement and gonioscopy.

Prodromal stage and stage of intermittent closure: Here there are symptoms suggesting a rise in pressure in addition to an occludable angle on gonioscopy. One can find a closed or occludable angle on gonioscopy. Here a laser PI would be enough to relieve a pupillary block. The patient should be maintained on follow-up.

Acute angle-closure glaucoma: This is a medical emergency and immediate measures are required to bring down the IOP and to relieve the pupillary block.

Once diagnosed, one should bring down the IOP with systemic medications medically as quickly as possible.

Antiglaucoma measures

Intravenous 20% mannitol 200 mL given rapidly over 20 minutes. Intravenous acetazolamide, if available is given.

Oral acetazolamide 500 mg immediately and 250 mg 6 hourly is started. Oral 50% glycerol 60 mL 8 hourly can be added.

But oral medications are rarely tolerated, since the patient will be having nausea and vomiting. Topical aqueous suppressant drug timolol 0.5% twice daily can be added. Pilocarpine 1%–2% four times daily is also useful (once pressure starts to come down and pupil can react) by causing miosis.

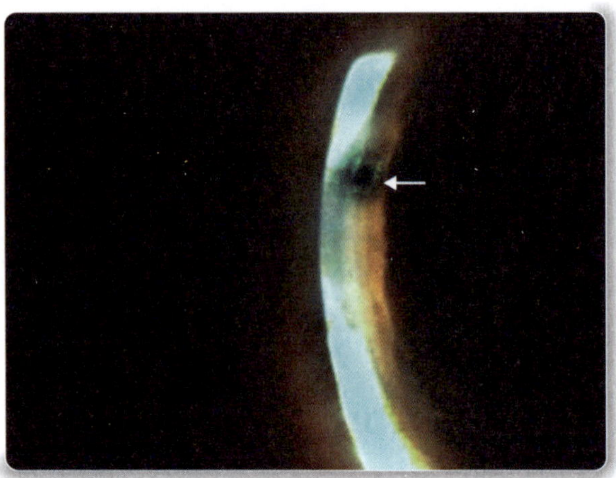

FIGURE 21.32: Laser peripheral iridotomy opening

Analgesics and antiemetics

Meanwhile, patient's pain and general condition may be managed with injection Pethidine and Phenergan or injection tramadol and domperidone.

Note: Acetazolamide can cause hypokalemia and metabolic acidosis. It is contraindicated in patients with allergy to sulfa drugs. Glycerol is high calorie liquid and diabetic control can be lost. Patients prone to congestive cardiac failure may not tolerate the large rapid volume of mannitol going into circulation. Timolol can precipitate heart blocks and obstructive pulmonary airway disease. Prior to administration of drugs, the presence or absence of contraindications should be searched for in history.

Specific management after the acute phase

Once the IOP is brought down and the corneal edema has decreased, the gonioscopy is done. If there is no synechial closure or if the synechiae are less than 180° or 6'O clock, then a PI should suffice. If the iris is too edematous and laser iridotomy is not possible on two or more attempts, one can opt for a surgical iridectomy.

If synechiae are more than half the circumference of the angle, one should proceed doing a trabeculectomy. This is undertaken only after the inflammation has subsided (to improve the chances of success of surgery) till then the IOP can be kept under control with topical and systemic antiglaucoma medications.

After this the patient needs regular follow-up for life. If the IOP goes up during follow-up, topical medical therapy for glaucoma can be instituted or repeat trabeculectomy may be contemplated if topical therapy is not successful in controlling the IOP.

Chronic angle-closure glaucoma: Here there is presence of synechiae in the angle on gonioscopy.

As mentioned above, a laser PI should suffice, if the synechiae are covering less than half the circumference of the angle. After this the patient needs regular follow-up for life. If the IOP goes up during follow-up, topical medical therapy for glaucoma can be instituted.

If the synechiae are more than half the circumference, the chances of iridotomy alone sufficing are less by considering the risks involved. Classically, we were told to proceed to trabeculectomy at this stage. We would try medical therapy after a laser iridotomy. Only if this is not controlling the IOP or the patient's compliance is poor, surgery is done.

When medical therapy and laser iridotomy are inadequate to control IOP, one has to proceed to trabeculectomy.

One would proceed to trabeculectomy in advanced disk damage also prior to trial of medical therapy.

Drugs used

1. Beta blockers: Aqueous suppressant gives about 20%–30% reduction in ocular pressures. For example, timolol 0.5%.
2. Parasympathomimetics: Pilocarpine drops are available as 1%, 2% and 4%. Most often used in glaucoma therapy at 2% concentration. Cause miosis and pull iris from the angle opening it. Also contraction of longitudinal ciliary muscles pull on sclera spur and open spaces in the trabecular meshwork, reducing trabecular resistance in areas of open angle.
3. Topical carbonic anhydrase inhibitors: Dorzolamide and brinzolamide, tid dose, reduce aqueous secretion.
4. Alpha-agonists: This increases outflow and decreases inflow. Prone to cause ocular surface side effects and drowsiness (contraindicated in infants, as they can cause sleep apnea), e.g. brimonidine.
5. Prostaglandin analogs: In presence of a fully closed angle their effect is not much and so unlike in open-angle glaucoma, these are the last choice in angle-closure glaucoma.

Absolute glaucoma: Here there is a blind eye with high pressure. If there is pain due to high pressure, one should proceed to cyclodestructive procedures to bring down the pressure and thus to make the patient comfortable.

Plateau iris configuration: Here again a laser PI is done. If the angle does not open up after the pupillary block component is removed, it is called plateau iris syndrome. These patients respond well to pilocarpine therapy, which pulls the peripheral rolls of iris out of the angle.

CONGENITAL AND DEVELOPMENTAL GLAUCOMA

Glaucoma occurring in the very young are different and there are certain features that make them stand apart from glaucoma in an adult:

1. The outer coats of the eye (sclera and cornea) are elastic in the first 3 years of life and hence can stretch with rise in pressures. As a consequence, glaucomatous eyes enlarge in this age group and are often described as 'buphthalmos' or bull's eye (Figs 21.33A to D).
2. The IOP also tend to be lower, when measured, for the same reason. A lowering of pressure tends to cause some degree of shrinkage also.
3. The optic nerve cup is often very large, as the sclera rim of the optic disk stretches. The cupping also comes down with control of pressures in the eye, in contrast to older-age glaucoma.
4. The change in size of the globes causes change in refractive errors rapidly (to myopia with high pressures and reversal of myopia when pressures come down).

Any visual impairment in childhood impairs development of vision (Box 21.1) and leads to amblyopia.

BOX 21.1: Causes of poor visual prognosis in congenital glaucoma

Corneal opacities
Subluxation of lens
Anisometropia and amblyopia
High risk for failure of surgeries to control intraocular pressure

CLASSIFICATION

Glaucoma in childhood can be thought of as three different groups:

1. **Primary congenital glaucoma:** Where a developmental anomaly of the angle of the anterior chamber causes resistance to outflow and it has no association with other ocular or systemic anomalies.
2. **Developmental glaucoma:** It is associated with ocular congenital anomalies, where the rise in IOP is caused by the congenital anomalies.

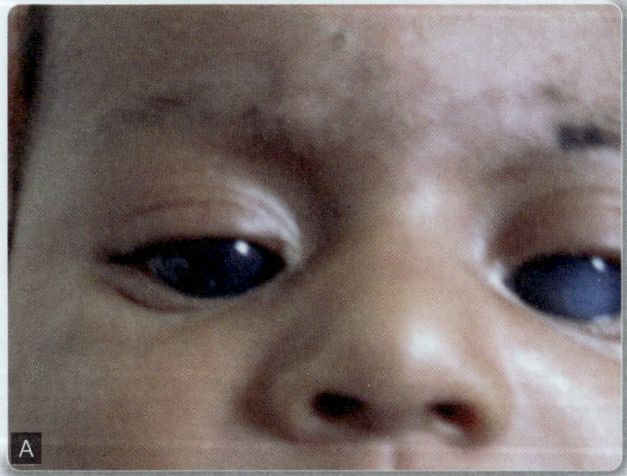

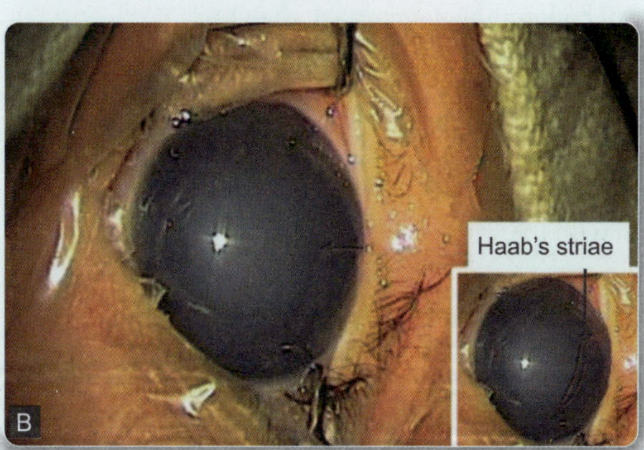

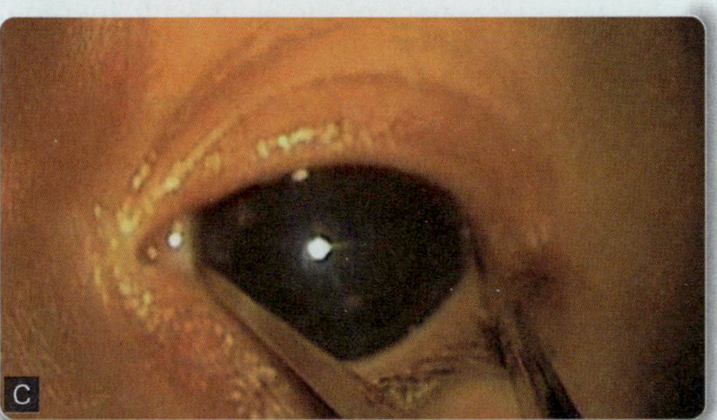

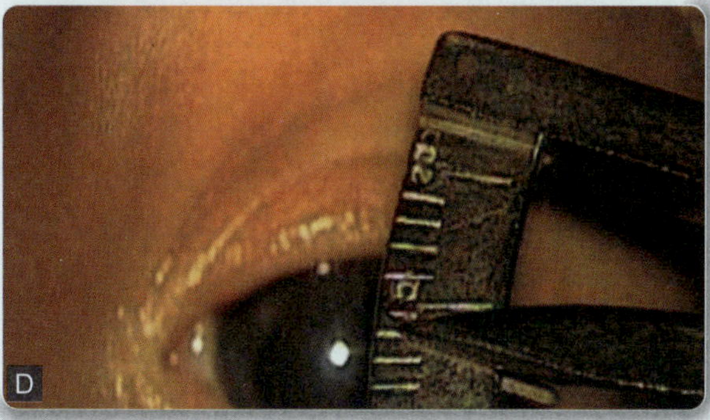

FIGURES 21.33A to D: Buphthalmos. **A.** Photograph; **B.** Congenital glaucoma eye with Haab's striae as shown in diagrammatic overlay in inset. Note the grossly enlarged eyeball with corneal haze due to edema; **C.** Corneal diameter measured from white to white limbus; **D.** Corneal diameter of 15.5 mm in a child.

3. **Secondary glaucoma in childhood:** The causes are same as in adults, but enlargement of globes and amblyopia complicates the situation.

Buphthalmos was a term used synonymous with primary congenital glaucoma by most and sometimes to include all childhood glaucoma, where the eye enlarged. To avoid confusion most experts now refer to childhood glaucoma under the above three headings, viz. congenital glaucoma (or primary congenital glaucoma), developmental glaucoma and secondary glaucoma.

PRIMARY CONGENITAL GLAUCOMA

Epidemiology

It is estimated that primary congenital glaucoma occurs in 1 out of 10,000 live births and represents 22.2% of all childhood glaucoma. About 80% of these patients have onset within the 1st year of life with 25% diagnosed at birth itself.

Open-angle glaucoma presenting after 3 years of age do not have buphthalmic features and are often classified as juvenile glaucoma (POAG presenting prior to age of 35 years. It is not yet clear as to whether the pathogenesis is that of congenital glaucoma or of POAG).

Most congenital glaucoma occurs as sporadic cases, though approximately 10% have a positive family history, suggesting an autosomal recessive inheritance with variable penetrance. It is assumed that parents of a child with congenital glaucoma have a 3% chance of having a second child with the same disease.

Clinical Features

Classic triads of symptoms suggesting congenital glaucoma are:

1. Epiphora (watering from eyes).
2. Photophobia (intolerance to light).
3. Blepharospasm (inability to open eyes in bright light).

   All these symptoms are caused by corneal edema and the consequent epithelial irregularities.
4. Additionally the large size of the cornea and corneal haze/opacification may be noted.

Examination Findings

Corneal Changes

Corneal edema: This is a direct result of IOP rise, producing diffuse corneal haze and sometimes localized stromal opacities. The stretched cornea may develop Descemet's membrane tears called Haab's striae (refer Figs 21.33A to D). These are typically a pair of parallel glassy lines at level of Descemet's membrane oriented horizontally or concentric to the limbus and can be single/multiple.

Differential diagnosis

Haab's striae: Tears in the Descemet's membrane can occur with trauma from a forceps delivery. The tears caused by forceps tend to be vertically oriented and more often in the left eye, due to the more common left occipitoanterior obstetric presentation.

Corneal opacification and haze: May be due to a variety of causes, viz. sclerocornea, corneal dystrophies, inflammation (e.g. interstitial keratitis), inborn errors of metabolism (mucopolysaccharidoses and cystinosis). Congenital endothelial dystrophy mimics glaucoma most, as these infants present with diffuse corneal edema.

Corneal diameter: Often the most striking feature is the large corneal diameters. A newborn's cornea has a horizontal diameter of 9.5–10.5 mm. This enlarges by another 0.5–1.0 mm in the 1st year of life. A corneal diameter more than 12 mm in the 1st year is suspicious (refer Figs 21.33A to D). At any age corneal diameter of 13 mm or more or an asymmetry between the two eyes are suspicious findings.

Differential diagnosis

Megalocornea: Here the corneal diameter is large (often 14 mm or more) and no other pathology is present in the eye (often X-linked recessive inheritance). High myopes also have large eyes with relatively large corneas. Both these situations have normal IOP and optic nerve cup (Fig. 21.34).

Anterior Chamber, Iris and Lens

Anterior chamber is uniformly deep. Iris often looks normal, but may have stromal hypoplasia with loss of crypts and iridodonesis. The lens is typically clear, but looks obviously flattened out and in late stages zonular dehiscence and subluxation are seen. These features are explained easily by the enlargement of the globe with consequent circumferential stretch.

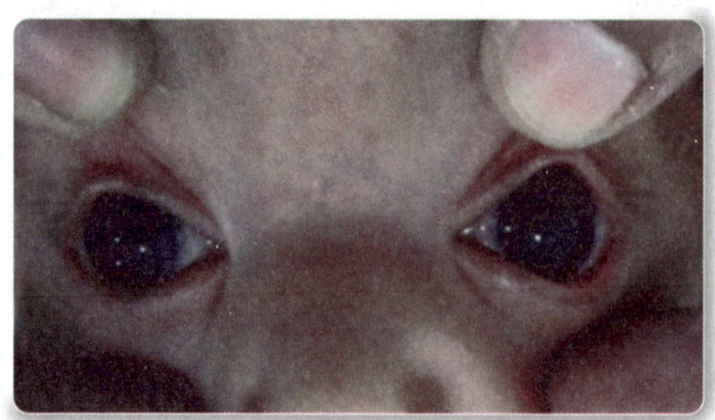

FIGURE 21.34: Megalocornea

Refractive Error

Progressive enlargement of the globe causes axial myopia due to sclera stretching. The stretching of the zonules due to the enlargement of the eye leads to a flattening and posterior displacement of the lens. This will compensate the myopia to some extent. Presence of Haab's striae can lead to astigmatism. Progressive myopic shift in the very young should alert one to the possibility of glaucoma.

Tonometry

Tonometry in an alert child is difficult. A struggling child would cause IOP estimation to be falsely high due to the child's Valsalva maneuver. One may achieve pressure measurements in a child under topical anesthesia when adequately distracted as when feeding from a bottle or nursing. Handheld tonometers like Perkins applanation tonometer or tonopen are the best implements to estimate IOP in children. Normal IOP in infants is less than in adults and are about 10 mm Hg. By about 7 years this becomes about 13 mm Hg as opposed to the adult mean IOP of 16 mm Hg. In congenital and infantile glaucoma, the pressures are usually in the range of 30–40 mm Hg.

Quite often IOP measurements need to be done under general anesthesia. Here one has to consider changes in pressure due to drugs used in anesthesia, e.g. halothane causes a significant reduction in pressures whereas ketamine and succinylcholine cause significant elevation of pressures.

Gonioscopy

Any goniolens may be used though gonioprisms like the Koeppe lens are easier to use in a supine child. Unlike adults the infant's trabecula is less granular in appearance and is non-pigmented. In a glaucomatous child the anterior insertion of iris in the angle ahead of the sclera spur is seen. The trabecula is glassy and looks like a membrane (this is called Barkan's membrane, which is not demonsatrated on histopathological examination). The peripheral iris may be concave and is seen to have a 'wrap around' configuration as it approaches the angle.

Fundus Examination

Estimation of the ONH cupping and its response to changes in pressures ar e the most important findings in diagnosis and assessment of response to therapeutic interventions.

Optic disk in a child is usually pink with very small cup. In congenital glaucoma the disk changes are similar to POAG, but do not indicate loss of tissue to the same extent as expected from the cupping. This is because the scleral rim in a child stretches and the disk size itself enlarges, adding to the empty space in the middle as cupping. The lamina cribrosa also stretches backwards and the cup looks very deeply excavated. With reduction in pressures the cupping reverses to a great extent and now the actual loss of nerve fibers in the optic disk will reveal as the remaining cupping.

Visual Fields

Being a psychovisual test requiring correct responses from the patient, visual field charting is often not possible in children. Once they are old enough to cooperate, this can be done and the field loss is similar to that in POAG. Typically automated perimetry can be reliably done by the age of 8 years. But sometimes children as young as 4 can cooperate for testing (one should let them try and practice on the field analyzer from a very young age).

Visual Acuity

Visual acuity needs to be recorded frequently. Good pressure control alone, even in the absence of optic atrophy does not guarantee good visual acuity. Corneal opacities, Haab's striae, refractive errors and subluxated lenses all can lead to loss of clear central vision. In addition, amblyopia would set in due to anisometropia (difference in refractive errors between the eyes) and strabismus (squint), which are often present.

Amblyopia is loss of visual acuity due to blurred images at the fovea or dissimilar images being projected on the two foveae during the age of visual development—less than 7–10 years. The loss is more profound at younger age than when the child is 10 year old.

As much information as possible, is obtained in the first examination itself and an examination under general anesthesia is planned when congenital glaucoma is suspected. Whenever, an examination under general anesthesia is planned it is to be done by the surgeon trained to operate on pediatric glaucoma and if required, the surgery is proceeded at the same sitting to reduce risk involved in general anesthesia.

CLINICAL FEATURES

The symptoms and signs of congenital glaucoma are given below.

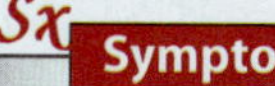

Symptoms

Triad of epiphora, blepharospasm and photophobia.

Signs

- Large eye with thin bluish sclera
- Corneal changes—increased corneal diameter, corneal edema, corneal opacities, Haab's striae
- Deep anterior chamber
- Subluxation of lens
- Moderate increase in intraocular pressure
- Deep cupping
- Myopic astigmatism
- Gonioscopy—abnormal tissue in angle of anterior chamber.

PATHOGENESIS

Barkan's Theory

The incomplete resorption of mesodermal tissue in the trabecular meshwork area led to a membrane covering the trabeculae being left behind (Barkan's membrane), obstructing flow of aqueous. Smooth appearance of visible trabecular meshwork seemed to confirm this on gonioscopy. Goniotomy and trabeculotomy are surgeries devised to incise into this membrane and they work well to reduce IOP. Unfortunately, histological studies failed to demonstrate such a membrane.

Now, most experts agree that there is an arrest of development of the anterior chamber cells derived from the neural crest in its angle (destined to form the trabecular meshwork and Schlemm's canal) leading to aqueous outflow obstruction. A high insertion of iris and ciliary body anterior to the sclera spur in the angle, may compress the trabecular meshwork and this compacted fibers cause resistance to outflow of aqueous (Figs 21.35A to C). Hence the resistance to aqueous flow is primarily between the anterior chamber and the Schlemm's canal in these children (occasionally the Schlemm's canal is segmented and not a complete ring, but the contribution to resistance to flow is less from this factor).

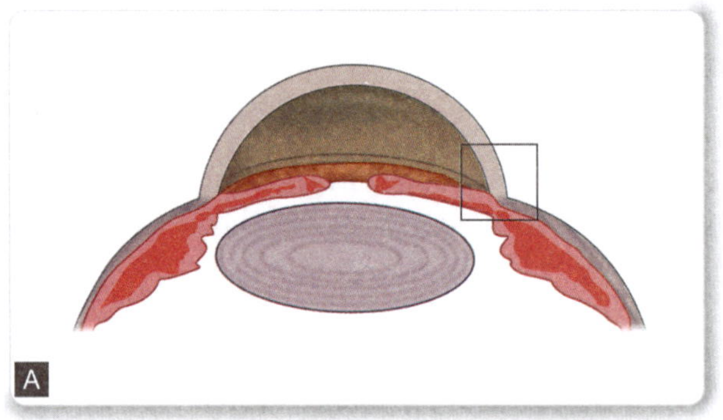

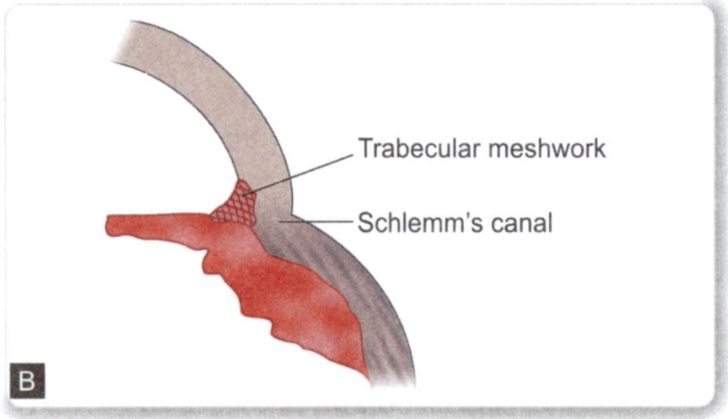

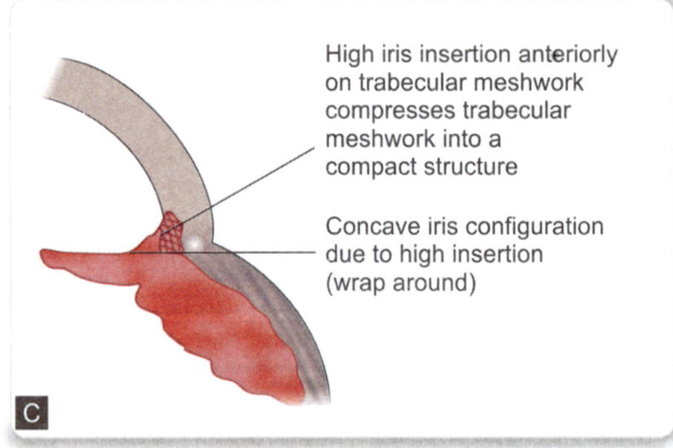

FIGURES 21.35A to C: A. Normal angle; **B.** Normal iris insertion; **C.** Shows a high insertion of iris and ciliary body anterior to the sclera spur in the angle may compress the trabecular meshwork and this compacted fibers cause resistance out flow of aqueous.

MANAGEMENT

Management of congenital glaucoma is primarily surgical. Once the diagnosis is established, either a goniotomy or a trabeculotomy is proceeded with, at the time of examination under anesthesia. Some surgeons add on a trabeculectomy at the primary sitting itself.

If the control of pressure is inadequate, a repeat surgery is done at a new site and another quadrant of trabecular meshwork is incised open. If pressure control by surgery is inadequate medical therapy is added on.

Medical Therapy Options

Surgery is the first option in management. Medical therapy is useful in the preoperative waiting period and to manage higher IOP after postsurgery if and when it occurs.

Medical management utilizes the same medications as in adults. The contraindications and side effects are the same as in adults. The α-adrenergic agonist brimonidine is usually avoided in infants as it causes central nervous system depression and can lead to sleep apnea.

Beta blockers are used in half strength to start with (timolol 0.25%) and are considered the first-line drugs in children. To reduce systemic side effects, all topical drugs are employed with punctal occlusion (after instilling drops the index finger of the parent is pressed on the medial canthus to occlude the canaliculi for 30 seconds to prevent systemic absorption from the nose via nasolacrimal drainage).

Prostaglandin analogs (latanoprost, bimatoprost, travoprost and tafluprost) can be used especially in older children. Experience in congenital glaucoma with these drugs is limited.

Topical carbonic anhydrase inhibitors (dorzolamide and brinzolamide) are well-tolerated and can be used in children as first or second line drug.

Miotics are rarely used now in pediatric glaucoma (except in immediate postoperative goniotomy and trabeculotomy).

Systemic acetazolamide can be given in a dose of 10–20 mg/kg body weight/day in the short term.

Surgical Management

Goniotomy and trabeculotomy are the primary surgical procedures for congenital glaucoma. If they fail or the cornea is too hazy for proper visualization, trabeculectmy is done (refer Chapter 29 'Glaucoma Surgery').

DEVELOPMENTAL GLAUCOMA

Developmental glaucoma, which are present in infancy or childhood, are associated with a definite developmental anomaly.

Axenfeld-Rieger Syndrome

Axenfelf-Rieger syndrome is characterized by a thickened and more anteriorly placed Schwalbe's line (edge of Descemet's membrane), which appears as a ridge called posterior embryotoxon. Iris strands come from peripheral iris to attach to this structure obscuring view of angle beyond it.

Rieger's Syndrome

Rieger's syndrome may have associated dental anomalies as well. A developmental arrest leading to incomplete anterior chamber cleavage is the postulated cause. Half the patients with this anomaly are expected to develop glaucoma.

Peters' Anomaly

Here there is a defect in the Descemet's membrane of central cornea and endothelium. There is a corresponding thinning and opacity. Iris may be adherent to this opacity and also to the lens. The lens can be cataractous. Half the patients develop glaucoma. Management involves keratoplasty and if required cataract surgery to clear the optics of the eye to allow visual development at an early age.

Aniridia

Aniridia is bilateral absence of 'normal' iris. It is a misnomer as there is always a rudimentary iris stump in the periphery all around, in variable width. This stump invariably rotates anteriorly and causes a 360° secondary angle closure and consequent glaucoma. This anomaly may be associated with Wilms' tumor of the kidney.

SECONDARY GLAUCOMA

Secondary Glaucoma in Childhood

Most of the secondary glaucoma can occur in childhood. A few need special mention as these are frequently encountered in children.

Glaucoma Following Trauma

Post-traumatic glaucoma are more common in children as they are more often engaged in sport activities prone to ocular trauma. Hyphema can cause acute glaucoma and angle recession can lead to chronic glaucoma.

Steroid-induced Glaucoma

Children are more prone to allergies (ocular and systemic, e.g. vernal conjunctivitis). This would entail use of steroids and consequent steroid-induced glaucoma in susceptible patients. This often happens when a patient goes on chronic self-medication (after the initial prescription). So, all patients who are on steroids need to be warned of this potentially blinding side effect.

Secondary Glaucoma (In General)

Secondary glaucoma is a group of conditions of raised IOP with its ocular effects occurring as a complication of some other ocular pathology.

It is important to understand secondary glaucoma as there are critical differences in their diagnosis and management. The secondary glaucoma can be differentiated according to the site of the main outflow resistance and the configuration of the chamber angle.

Classification

Secondary glaucoma can be classified based on the level of blockage to the drainage of aqueous.

Secondary Open-angle Glaucoma

1. Pretrabecular outflow resistance:
   a. Epithelialization of the chamber angle.
   b. Early ICE syndrome.
   c. Neovascular glaucoma stage II.
2. Trabecular outflow resistance:
   a. Pigmentary glaucoma.
   b. Pseudoexfoliation glaucoma (PEXG).
   c. Steroid-induced glaucoma.
   d. Inflammatory glaucoma.
   e. Phacolytic glaucoma.
   f. Posner-Schlossman syndrome.
   g. Fuchs' heterochromic cyclitis.
   h. Ghost cell glaucoma.
   i. Hemolytic glaucoma.
   j. Neurofibromatosis.
   k. Siderosis.
   l. Post-traumatic glaucoma with angle recession.
3. Post-trabecular outflow resistance:
   a. Sturge-Weber syndrome.
   b. Arteriovenous fistulas.
   c. Idiopathic.

Secondary Glaucoma with Narrow Angle

1. Anterior type with outflow resistance in chamber angle:
   a. Neovascular glaucoma stage III.
   b. Advanced ICE syndrome.
2. Posterior type with pupillary block and vitreociliary block mechanism:
   a. Glaucoma with pupillary block due to synechiae.
   b. Traumatic dislocation of the lens.
   c. Microspherophakia in Weill-Marchesani syndrome (ectopia lentis).
   d. Intumescent cataract.
   e. Iridoschisis.
3. Posterior type with anterior displacement of iris lens diaphragm:
   a. Glaucoma in association with:
      - Choroidal bleeding
      - Edema of ciliary body
      - Ciliary body cysts
      - Ciliary body tumors (malignant melanoma, leiomyoma)
      - Malignant glaucoma.
4. Glaucoma associated with contraction of retrolental tissue:
   a. Persistent hyperplastic primary vitreous (PHPV).
   b. Retinopathy of prematurity.

Iridocorneal Endothelial Syndrome

Iridocorneal endothelial or ICE syndrome is a spectrum of diseases in the eye, where the inner layer of the cornea appears abnormal. It is associated with corneal edema at moderate IOP level and a variety of pathological iris alterations. The disease is typically unilateral, especially in young women. It includes Cogan-Reese syndrome, Chandler's syndrome and essential iris atrophy.

The iris nevus syndrome (Cogan-Reese) is characterized by the presence of iris nodules. These are aggregates of melanocytic cells in the anterior iris stroma, surrounded by ectopic endothelial cells and abnormal basal membranes (Fig. 21.36).

The Chandler's syndrome is a variation of essential iris atrophy. Early in the disease, corneal edema is present even if the IOP is normal or only moderately elevated. Endothelial microscopy shows cells that resemble battered silver. Remarkable iris changes are not seen until the late stages of the disease.

Essential iris atrophy is a slowly progressive iris atrophy with hole formation, ectropion uveae and distortion of the pupil. The pretrabecular secondary open-angle glaucoma turns into secondary narrow-angle glaucoma with peripheral anterior synechiae in the late stages of the disease.

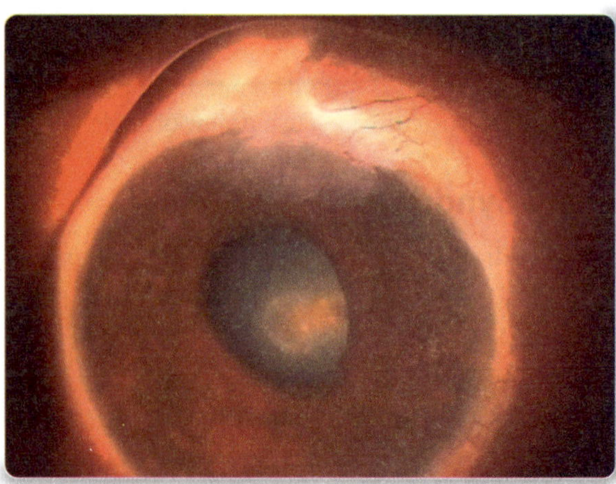

FIGURE 21.36: Cogan-Reese syndrome

Treatment

Treatment for early stages of glaucoma in ICE syndrome is with aqueous suppressants. In late stages, glaucoma filtering surgery is effective; although late failure may develop due to endothelialization of the fistula, which in some cases may be reopened with the Nd:YAG laser. The corneal problem will need keratoplasty.

Neovascular Glaucoma

The clinical sign of NVG is the rubeosis iridis with elevated IOP.

Causes

Retinal ischemia is the most important mechanism that results in the anterior segment changes causing NVG. This leads to liberation of VEGF, which leads to new vessel proliferation in the fundus as well as in the angle and surface of iris:

- Proliferative diabetic retinopathy
- Retinal vein occlusion together cause two third of cases
- Carotid artery occlusion
- Sickle cell retinopathy
- Eales' disease
- Retinopathy of prematurity
- Carotid-cavernous fistula
- Radiation retinopathy
- Severe intraocular inflammation
- Central retinal artery occlusion (rarely)
- Intraocular tumors.

In stage I, new vessels are found on the anterior surface of the iris (Fig. 21.37). These arise from the iris arteries and start at the pupillary border. The process of neovascularization progresses toward the chamber angle, but does not reach the outflow pathways in stage I.

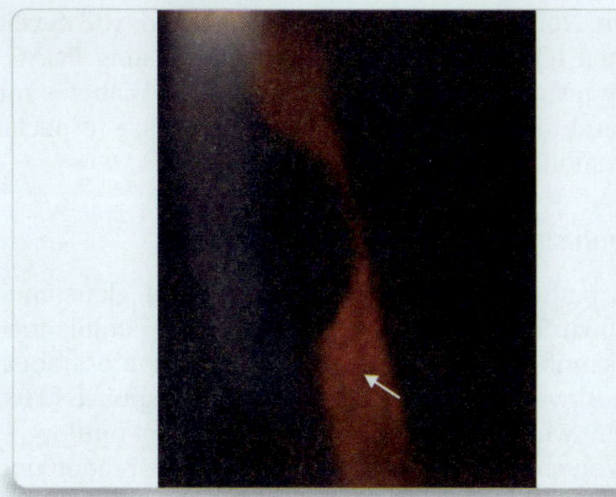

FIGURE 21.37: Iris new vessels

In stage II, the open chamber angle becomes covered with a fibrovascular membrane. Once this occurs, IOP may rise, resulting in secondary open-angle glaucoma.

The next stage (II–III) is a progressive closure of the angle. The formation of anterior synechiae pulls the iris forward, up to Schwalbe's line.

In stage III, the chamber angle is completely closed.

Management

Regression of the neovascularization, prior to the chamber angle coverage, may be induced by a panretinal laser photocoagulation.

Injection of anti-VEGF factors like bevacizumab, ranibizumab can lead to regression of new vessels.

In the end stages of the disease, where angle is closed with neovascular membrane trabeculectomy will not be able to control raised IOP. Filtering surgery with drainage implants can be done if there is visual potential or cyclodestructive procedures can be done, if there is no visual potential.

Pigmentary Glaucoma

Pigmentary glaucoma is characterized by deposition of pigment granules in the anterior segment and loss of iris pigment epithelium. This condition is typically seen in young male myopes.

Clinical Features

Iris depigmentation results in radial slits parallel to the zonules of the lens, which can be observed at the slit lamp using retroillumination. A vertically oriented pigment line at the center of the posterior cornea is known as a Krukenberg spindle. Pigment deposits are found in the trabeculae, the periphery of the lens and along the zonules. A classic sign is the concave iris configuration, with a deep anterior chamber. Medical and surgical treatment regimens are the same as for POAG. Nd:YAG laser iridotomy may be considered to overcome the postulated reverse pupillary block, in eyes with a posterior bowing of the iris root towards the zonules.

Pseudoexfoliation Glaucoma

Pseudoexfoliation glaucoma (PEXG) entity is characterized by flakes of granular material at the pupillary margin of the iris and throughout the inner surface of the anterior chamber (Fig. 21.38). It is also associated with secondary open-angle glaucoma, known as pseudoexfoliation glaucoma. Pseudoexfoliative material can be seen on the

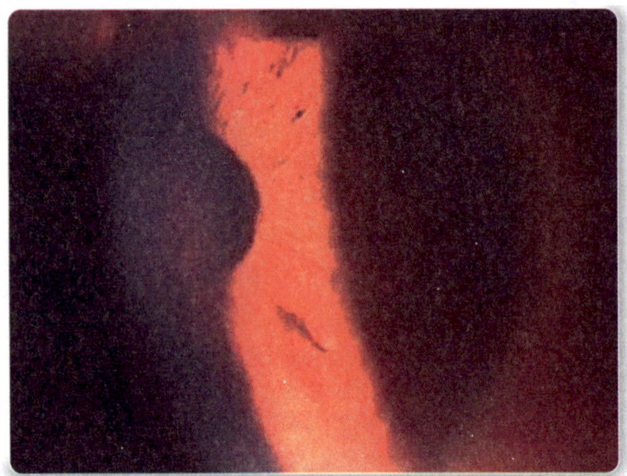

FIGURE 21.38: Pseudoexfoliation glaucoma

pupillary border of the iris without dilation. Gonioscopy shows a discontinuous pigmentation of the trabecular meshwork, usually less dense than seen in pigmentary glaucoma. Also, the pigment is characteristically deposited on the Schwalbe's line or anterior to the Schwalbe's line (Sampaolesi's line). Other signs of pseudoexfoliation syndrome are insufficient mydriasis, posterior synechiae, pigment deposition on the iris surface, deposition of pigment and pseudoexfoliation material on the corneal endothelium, pigment liberation after pupillary dilation and pseudoexfoliation material covering the ciliary processes and the zonules. Phacodonesis, lens subluxation and corneal endothelial decompensation can be present. An associated nuclear cataract is a common finding.

The treatment of PEXG is with topical medications in early stages. Because patients with PEXG have higher IOP, they tend to undergo glaucoma filtering surgery more frequently than patients with POAG. Cataracts occur more commonly in patients with pseudoexfoliation syndrome. Weakness of the zonular fibers, spontaneous lens subluxation and phacodonesis also can be present. Therefore, in these patients, cataract surgery alone or combined cataract surgery and glaucoma filtering surgery in the presence of pseudoexfoliation is associated with a higher incidence of intraoperative complications, most notably zonular dialysis, vitreous loss and lens dislocation.

Glaucoma Associated with Inflammation

Glaucoma can occur as a complication of uveitis.

Causes

In most cases of glaucoma associated with uveitis, the anterior chamber angle is open and the increase in IOP results from direct involvement of the trabecular meshwork. It can be due to local inflammation (e.g. secondary trabeculitis) or as a consequence of accumulation of inflammatory debris.

In the late stages, an increase in IOP can occur as a result of secondary angle closure following pupillary block.

Glaucoma can also occur as an effect of steroid therapy (steroid-induced glaucoma).

Very rarely, in patients prone for narrow-angle glaucoma use of mydriatics as part of treatment for uveitis can trigger an angle-closure attack.

Treatment

Includes the treatment of underlying cause of the uveitis, along with both anti-inflammatory (topical corticosteroids) and antiglaucoma medications (aqueous suppressants).

Cycloplegics are used to prevent or break already formed posterior synechiae and to decrease choroidal effusion.

Miotics are avoided because their use may exacerbate ciliary spasm, inflammation and increase the likelihood of synechia.

Prostaglandins are also avoided, as they may exacerbate the inflammatory component.

If the patient is found to be steroid responders, discontinue or change the steroid medication. If this is not possible, then more aggressive management of the IOP is needed until the steroid can be discontinued.

Steroid-induced Glaucoma

Causes

Steroid-induced IOP elevation typically occurs within a few weeks of beginning steroid therapy. More people respond from topically applied drops (including topically applied creams to the periorbital area) or intravitreal injection. Not all patients taking corticosteroids will develop elevated IOP. Risk factors include pre-existing POAG, a family history of glaucoma, high myopia, diabetes mellitus and history of connective tissue disease (especially rheumatoid arthritis).

Mechanism

Exact pathophysiology of steroid-induced glaucoma is unknown. The defect could be increased accumulation of glycosaminoglycans or increased production of trabecular meshwork-inducible glucocorticoid response (TIGR) protein, which could mechanically obstruct outflow. Patients on chronic corticosteroid therapy can remain undiagnosed with an elevated IOP, which can result in glaucomatous optic nerve damage.

Treatment

Includes discontinuation of corticosteroids or switching over to a lower potency steroid medication.

Antiglaucoma medications are also needed to control the high IOP till the effect of steroids wears off.

In the occasional cases in which the patient's IOP does not normalize by stopping steroid drops or in those patients, who must continue on corticosteroid medications, prolonged use of standard antiglaucoma medication will be required. Only rarely trabeculectomy is required.

Posner-Schlossman Syndrome (Glaucomatocyclitic Crisis)

Posner-Schlossman syndrome is a condition with self-limited recurrent episodes of markedly elevated IOP with mild idiopathic anterior chamber inflammation.

Clinical Features

1. Uniocular involvement.
2. Recurrent episodes of mild cyclitis with keratic precipitates (KPs) and aqueous flare.
3. Duration of attack varying from a few hours to several weeks.
4. A slight decrease in vision.
5. Elevated IOP with open angles.
6. Corneal edema with a few KPs.
7. Heterochromia with anisocoria and a large pupil in the affected eye.
8. Normal visual fields, normal optic disk, normal IOP and outflow facility.
9. All provocative tests are normal between episodes.

The presence of KPs on slit lamp examination gives the clue to the diagnosis.

Treatment

Treatment recommended include topical steroids, topical antiglaucoma drops, systemic carbonic anhydrase inhibitors, topical non-steriodal anti-inflammatory durgs (NSAIDs) and oral NSAIDs.

Fuchs' Heterochromic Iridocyclitis

Fuchs' heterochromic iridocyclitis (FHI) is a chronic, unilateral iridocyclitis characterized by iris heterochromia. The classic triad of FHI is heterochromia, cataract and KPs.

Clinical Features

1. Keratic precipitates are numerous, small, non-pigmented, translucent and star shaped (stellate) and are nearly pathognomonic. These are distributed over the entire posterior corneal surface.
2. There is minimal anterior chamber cells and flare.
3. Posterior synechiae are never present.
4. Many cases develop a posterior subcapsular cataract, which mature rapidly.
5. Whitish vitreous cellular infiltrates, varying from dust like to stringy veils are observed.

Any young male patient presenting with a unilateral cataract has to be examined in natural light for heterochromia and KPs.

Management

In general, treatment is not necessary for patients with the typical low-grade inflammation. Symptomatic flare-ups may require short-term topical corticosteroids.

Most secondary glaucoma associated with FHI can be controlled with antiglaucoma medications. Glaucoma filtering procedures in patients with FHI are less successful compared with that for patients with POAG. Glaucoma drainage implants may improve the outcome of glaucoma surgery for patients with uveitic glaucoma. Cataract surgery has good visual prognosis.

Traumatic Glaucoma

Traumatic glaucoma include:
1. Angle-recession glaucoma.
2. Acute glaucoma associated with hyphema.
3. Late onset ghost cell glaucoma.
4. Glaucoma associated with traumatic uveitis.
5. Phacolytic glaucoma.
6. Glaucoma associated with lens dislocation.

In the acute phase, the presence of blood in the anterior chamber (hyphema) or inflammation as a result of injury (e.g. traumatic iridocyclitis) may cause an increase in IOP that mandates treatment.

Since, acute increases in IOP due to blunt trauma may be only for a short duration, observation and careful follow-up may be all that is required (assuming the presence of a healthy optic nerve prior to injury). If treatment is indicated, aqueous suppressants (e.g. beta blockers, α-agonists) are the mainstay of treatment.

Angle-recession Glaucoma

Angle-recession glaucoma is a type of traumatic secondary open-angle glaucoma. In angle recession, there is variable degree of cleavage between the circular and the longitudinal fibers of the ciliary muscle.

On gonioscopy the ciliary band will be widened and in long-standing cases there will be hyperpigmentation of the angle and the widening will not be obvious due to scarring. It can present with and without glaucoma and it may take several years for the glaucoma to manifest.

Management: Long-term follow-up care of patients with recognized angle recession is warranted because of the risk of delayed asymptomatic onset. Of those eyes with known angle recession, 0%–20% subsequently glaucoma develops. Glaucoma after angle recession of less than 180° is unusual; recessions greater than 180° are associated with a 4%–9% incidence of glaucoma. Eyes with angle recession of greater than 240° appear to be at the highest risk of chronic glaucoma.

Treatment: In patients with an abnormal elevation of IOP aqueous suppressants or prostaglandin analogs are given.

Surgical intervention in angle-recession glaucoma is usually indicated when maximally tolerated medical treatment has failed. Filtration surgery has a success rate lower than that of POAG.

Ghost Cell Glaucoma

Ghost cell glaucoma is a secondary open-angle glaucoma caused by degenerated red blood cells (ghost cells) blocking the trabecular meshwork.

Mechanism

Following a vitreous hemorrhage episode, blood breakdown products may accumulate in the trabecular meshwork. Hemolyzed erythrocytes may obstruct aqueous outflow and lead to a secondary open-angle glaucoma known as ghost cell glaucoma. Ghost cells are generally 4–7 micrometers in size and less pliable than normal RBCs. As a result of their loss of pliability, ghost cells remain longer in the anterior chamber because their rigidity makes it difficult for them to escape through the trabecular meshwork.

Treatment

Aqueous suppressants are the first-line approach. Surgery might be required to clear the cell load from the trabecular meshwork. This can be accomplished by anterior chamber paracentesis and irrigation, pars plana vitrectomy (PPV) and/or a trabeculectomy.

Malignant Glaucoma

Malignant glaucoma describes an entity characterized by elevated IOP with a shallow or flat anterior chamber in the presence of a patent peripheral iridectomy.

Malignant glaucoma is rare, but one of the most serious complications of glaucoma filtration surgery in patients with narrow-angle glaucoma.

Mechanism

A blockage of the normal aqueous flow at the level of the ciliary body, lens and anterior vitreous face is believed to cause malignant glaucoma. Posterior misdirection of aqueous humor into the vitreous cavity occurs producing a continuous expansion of the vitreous cavity and increased posterior segment pressure. This accumulation of aqueous fluid in the vitreous cavity causes anterior displacement of the lens-iris diaphragm in phakic and pseudophakic eyes or forward displacement of the anterior hyaloid in aphakic patients. The resulting shallow or flat chamber is believed to exacerbate the condition because of the decreased access of aqueous to the trabecular meshwork.

Management

The first line of treatment should be medical:

1. Cycloplegic agents like atropine paralyze the sphincter muscle of the ciliary body, increasing zonular tension with flattening, posterior movement of the lens and deepening the anterior chamber.
2. Topical beta blockers, α-adrenergic agonists and topical and oral carbonic anhydrase inhibitors are effective in decreasing aqueous humor production and lowering IOP, presumably decreasing aqueous misdirection.
3. Osmotic agents help to decrease vitreous volume and include oral glycerol or isosorbide or intravenous mannitol.
4. The Nd:YAG laser can break the anterior hyaloid to allow free movement of fluid from the vitreous cavity to the anterior chamber.
5. If medical or laser treatment fails or if lens-corneal touch occurs, surgery should be considered. PPV with or without lensectomy, disrupts the impermeable anterior vitreous face and reduces the vitreous volume.

Lens-induced Glaucoma

Phacolytic glaucoma is the sudden onset of open-angle glaucoma caused by a leaking mature or hypermature cataract. It is cured by cataract extraction.

Phacomorphic glaucoma is the term used for secondary angle-closure glaucoma due to lens intumescence.

The increase in lens thickness from an advanced cataract, a rapidly intumescent lens or a traumatic cataract can lead to pupillary block. Laser iridotomy can temporarily stop an attack of acute pupillary block. But in most patients with phacomorphic glaucoma, cataract extraction is needed. Laser iridotomy should be performed first, as mydriasis before surgery can exacerbate the condition or osmotic agents such as mannitol or glycerine should be given before surgery to decrease vitreous volume and deepen the anterior chamber.

Phacotopic glaucoma is often due to a traumatic pathology causing anterior subluxation or dislocation of lens. It is very important to recognize the pathogenic mechanism for a proper treatment. It can be pupillary block and/or angular block or phacolytic glaucoma.

Management

Laser iridotomy may control the glaucoma in mild cases and lens removal with/without anterior vitrectomy will be required in severe displacement with severe glaucoma and significant drop in vision. Improvements in lens and vitreous surgery have changed the prognosis of these diseases.

Aphakic or Pseudophakic Glaucoma

Aphakic or pseudophakic glaucoma are secondary glaucoma occurring after cataract surgery. It is more common in children.

Mechanisms

A transient rise can be due to retained viscoelastics or blood in the eye or due to postoperative uveitis. It can be managed with topical and systemic antiglaucoma medications and corticosteroids. An anterior chamber intraocular lens (IOL) is more prone to produce secondary glaucoma.

A chronic rise in IOP can occur due to angle closure resulting from papillary block by posterior synechiae in uveitis. Mydriatics are used to break the synechiae and if that fails, Nd:YAG laser iridotomy is done to form alterative pathway for the aqueous.

An open-angle type of secondary glaucoma can occur due to vitreous in anterior chamber, retained lens materials or pigment dispersion. Transient cases can be managed with antiglaucoma medications. Prostaglandin derivatives are avoided to prevent cystoid macular edema. Removal of retained lens materials or anterior vitrectomy may be needed in some cases. In some chronic cases trabeculectomy with antifibroblastic agents like mitomycin may be needed.

In any case of raised IOP, it is essential to take a careful history of the problem and careful slit lamp examination to differentiate between primary and secondary glaucoma. Proper diagnosis will help to manage the problem in the correct way with a more successful outcome.

Intraocular Tumors

22

Girija Devi PS

Intraocular tumors comprise a broad spectrum of benign and malignant lesions that can sometimes lead to loss of vision and even loss of life. A thorough clinical examination and effective use of ancillary diagnostic tests aid the clinician in the accurate diagnosis and proper management of these conditions.

TUMORS OF UVEAL TRACT

TUMORS OF IRIS

Iris Nevus

Iris nevus, which is a common benign lesion appears as a darkly pigmented lesion of the iris stroma with minimal distortion of iris architecture. Iris nevi may present in two forms:

1. Circumscribed iris nevus—usually nodular and involving a discrete portion of iris.
2. Diffuse iris nevus—may involve an entire sector or rarely the entire iris (Fig. 22.1).

Iris nevi usually require no treatment. If diagnosed, suspicious lesions need close follow-up and photography to evaluate the growth.

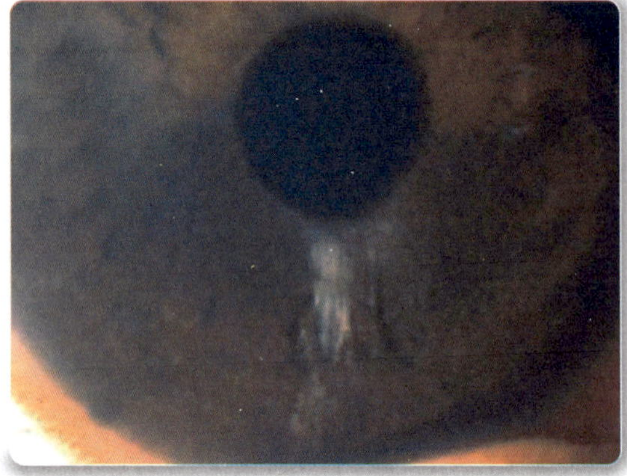

FIGURE 22.1: Diffuse iris nevus with iris atrophy

Iris Cysts

Primary Iris Cysts

Primary iris cysts are rare lesions arising from iris epithelium (epithelial cysts) or rarely iris stroma (stromal cysts).

Secondary Iris Cysts

Secondary cysts develop as a result of the following.

Implantation cysts: Due to deposition of surface epithelial cells following surgical or penetrating trauma. They can be pearl cysts or serous cysts (Figs 22.2A and B).

Drug-induced cysts: Prolonged topical use of long acting-miotics.

Parasitic cysts: They are rare. Cysticercosis or hydatid cysts can rarely involve the iris.

Malignant Melanoma of the Iris

Iris melanomas account for 3%–10% of all uveal melanomas.

Clinical Features

Malignant melanoma of the iris, usually appear as an isolated pigmented or amelanotic nodule that grows very rapidly, commonly involving the inferior iris. They may rarely assume a diffuse growth pattern resulting in a unilateral acquired hyperchromic heterochromia and secondary glaucoma. If untreated, it may perforate the globe.

Signs suggestive of malignancy include extensive ectropion iridis, prominent vascularity, secondary glaucoma, seedling of angle structures, extrascleral extension, increasing lesion size and documented progressive growth.

Investigations

Photographic documentation of tumor growth.

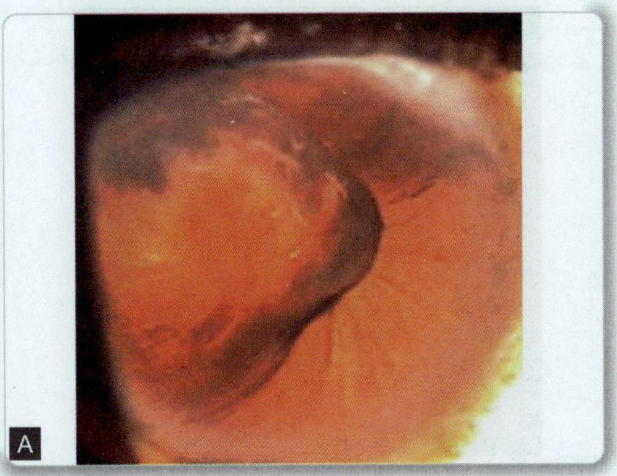

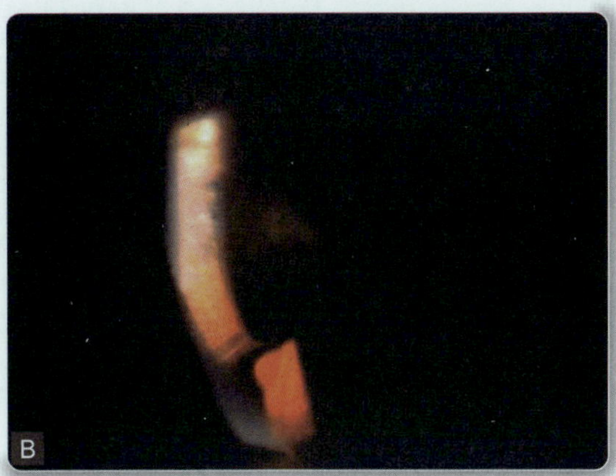

FIGURES 22.2A and B: Implantation cysts of iris. **A.** Pearl cyst; **B.** Serous cyst.

Ultrasound biomicroscopy: Tumor size and anatomical relationship to normal ocular structures can be accurately documented.

Treatment

Diagnostic and therapeutic excision of the mass:
- Iridectomy, if feasible
- Iridocyclectomy, if the lesion is involving the root of iris and ciliary body
- Brachytherapy with custom designed plaques in select cases
- If completely removed, the prognosis is excellent in most cases.

Differential Diagnosis of Iris Nodule

- Iris nevus
- Iris melanoma
- Iris nodules in chronic anterior uveitis—Koeppe and Busacca nodules
- Retained foreign bodies can become secondarily pigmented and it can also be associated with chronic inflammation
- Brushfield spots usually in Down syndrome
- Iris pigment epithelial cysts
- Epithelial invasion, serous cyst, pearl cyst or implantation cysts
- Juvenile xanthogranuloma—may be associated with spontaneous hyphema and secondary glaucoma
- Lisch nodules—hamartomatous lesions seen in neurofibromatosis (Fig. 22.3)
- Metastatic carcinoma—rare
- Retinoblastoma—iris invasion with or without pseudohypopyon.

CILIARY BODY TUMORS

Ciliary Body Melanoma

Ciliary body melanomas constitute 12% of the uveal melanomas (Figs 22.4 and 22.5).

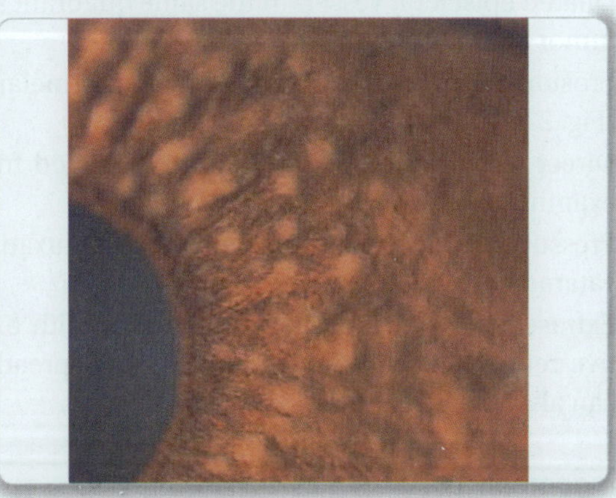

FIGURE 22.3: Lisch nodules in neurofibromatosis 1

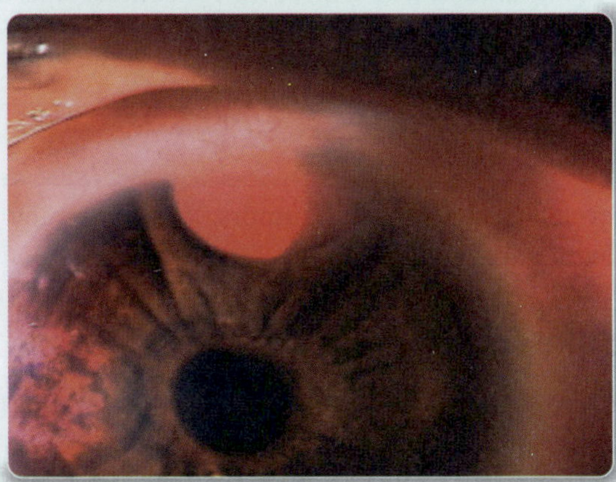

FIGURE 22.4: Hemangioma of iris and ciliary body

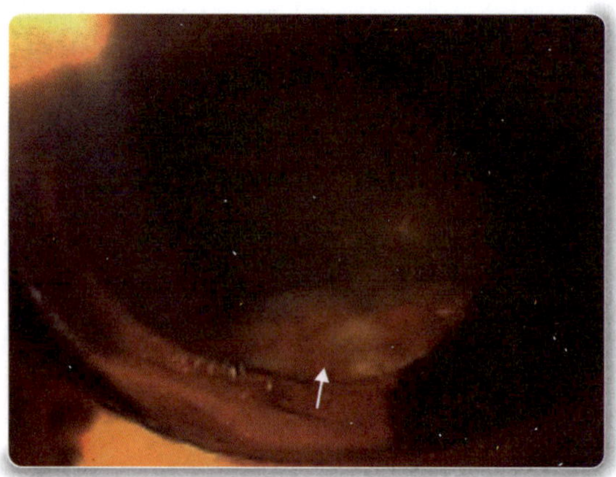

FIGURE 22.5: Ciliary body tumor seen through dilated pupil

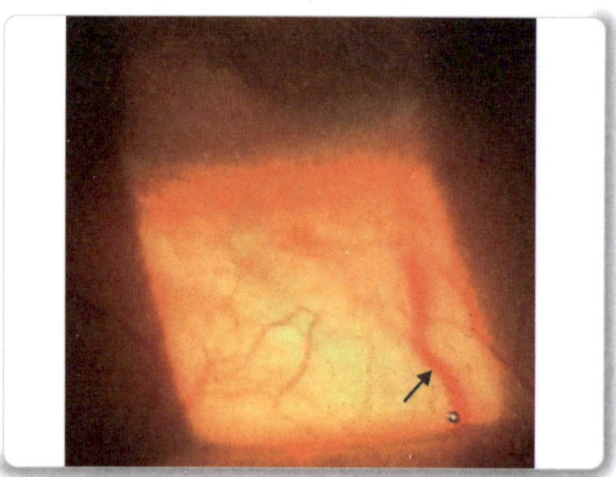

FIGURE 22.6: Sentinel vessel (black arrow) in ciliary body tumor

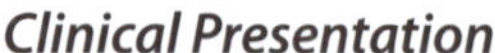

Clinical Presentation

Ciliary body melanoma usually present in the sixth decade with visual symptoms or sometimes detected incidentally.

Signs

1. Dilated episcleral vessels in the same quadrant as the tumor (sentinel vessels) (Fig. 22.6).
2. Erosion through iris root may mimic iris melanoma (Fig. 22.7).
3. Direct visualization of the tumor on dilated fundus examination.
4. Pressure on lens causing astigmatism, subluxation or cataract formation.
5. Extrascleral extension, posterior spread with exudative retinal detachment, circumferential spread, etc. can also occur (Fig. 22.8).

Management

Direct examination with a three mirror contact lens, ultrasound biomicroscopy (UBM), biopsy, etc. are employed to establish the diagnosis (Fig. 22.9).

Treatment

Iridocyclectomy for small tumors, brachytherapy and enucleation for large tumors.

Medulloepithelioma

Medulloepithelioma is a rare embryonal neoplasm (previously called diktyoma) occurring in the first decade of life. Malignant forms are fatal due to intracranial spread or metastatic disease.

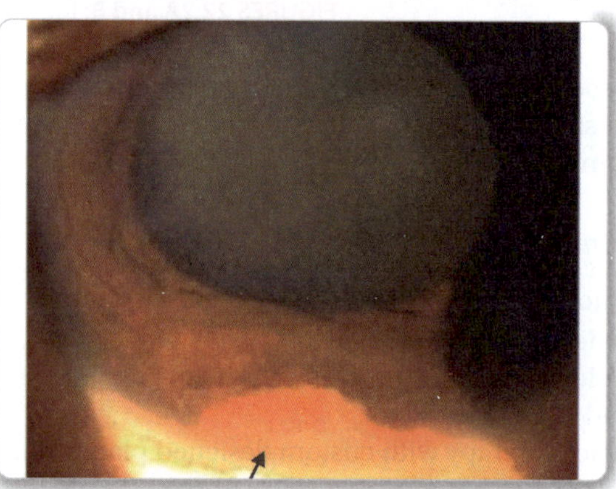

FIGURE 22.7: Ciliary body tumor eroding root of iris

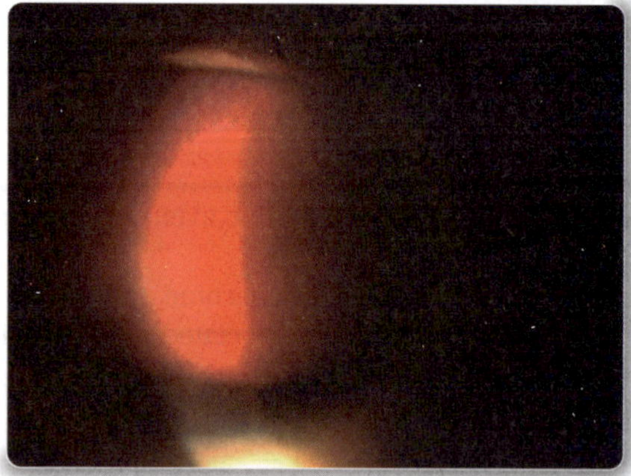

FIGURE 22.8: Ciliary body tumor protruding into anterior chamber (AC) through pupil

TUMORS OF CHOROID

Choroidal Nevus

Choroidal nevi are composed of benign proliferation of choroidal melanocytes, usually more common in the

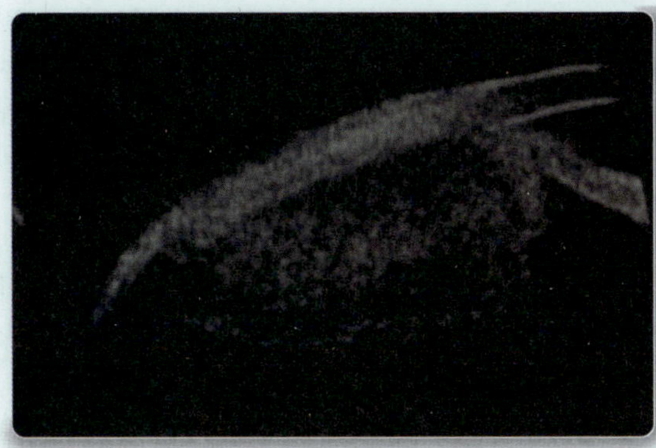

FIGURE 22.9: Ultrasound biomicroscopy (UBM) picture of CB mass

white races. They are usually asymptomatic and detected on routine fundus examination.

Typical choroidal nevus appears as an oval to circular, brown to slate gray lesion in the postequatorial fundus often with surface drusen.

Suspicious nevi are those with documented growth, those producing symptoms like blurring of vision, those showing presence of surface lipofuscin, etc. They should be kept on close follow-up, reclassified as small melanomas if needed and managed accordingly.

Choroidal Melanoma

Choroidal melanoma is the most common primary intraocular malignancy in adults and accounts for 80% of all uveal melanomas (Fig. 22.10).

Pathology

The tumor is composed of a malignant proliferation of choroidal melanocytes either as spindle cells or as epithelioid cells.

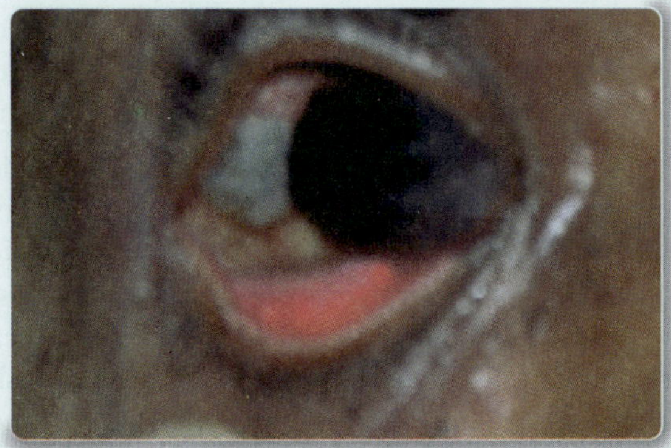

FIGURE 22.10: Choroidal melanoma with extraocular spread

Classification

1. Spindle cell melanomas (spindle A and spindle B)—formed exclusively of spindle cells.
2. Epithelioid cell melanomas—most malignant.
3. Mixed cell melanomas—formed of both spindle cells and epithelioid cells.

Patterns of Tumor Growth

The tumor can grow inwards, break through the Bruch's membrane and retinal pigment epithelium (RPE) into the subretinal space with the development of a collar stud appearance.

Invasion of scleral channels for blood vessels and nerves, and invasion of vortex veins resulting in orbital spread. Hematogenous spread to the liver, lungs, bone, skin and brain. Optic nerve invasion is rare.

Clinical Presentation

The tumor often presents in the fifth to sixth decade of life. It is usually primary, single and unilateral.

Sx Symptoms

Choroidal melanoma may be either detected incidentally on a routine fundus examination or may become symptomatic. The usual symptoms are decreased vision, metamorphopsia, floaters or photopsia (ball of light).

Signs

The tumor appears as a solitary, elevated, dome-shaped brown or grayish mass or less commonly as an amelanotic mass usually in the posterior pole.

Clumps of orange pigment, lipofuscin, is often seen in the RPE overlying the tumor.

Dilated blood vessels may be seen on the surface in amelanotic masses. Exudative retinal detachment occurs overlying the tumor.

Other signs—choroidal folds, intraocular inflammation, hemorrhage, rubeosis, secondary glaucoma and cataract.

Investigations

Ultrasound scan (USS): B-scan ultrasonography shows a dome or mushroom-shaped choroidal mass with internal homogeneity (acoustic hollowing), choroidal excavation and orbital shadowing; a collar stud configuration is almost pathognomonic (Fig. 22.11).

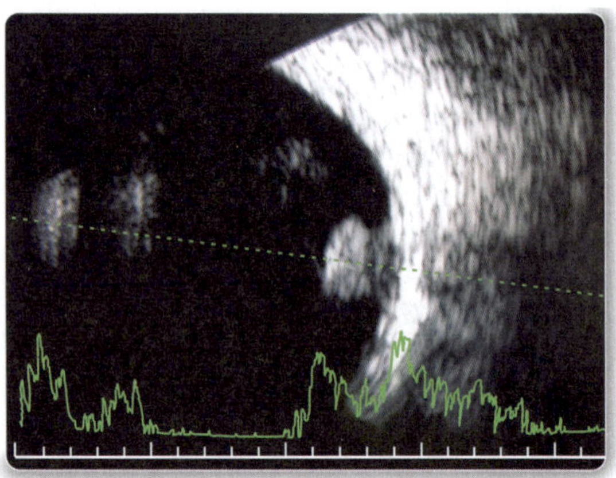

FIGURE 22.11: Ultrasound scan shows a mushroom-shaped mass in choroidal tumor

Fluorescein angiography: Most common findings are intrinsic tumor (dual) circulation, mottled fluorescence during the avenue vision phase and late diffuse leakage and staining.

Indocyanine-green (ICG) angiography: It shows hypofluorescence throughout the study.

Radioactive tracers: Neoplastic tissue has an increased rate of phosphorus (P) uptake as demonstrated by P^{32} uptake studies.

Magnetic resonance imaging (MRI): It shows hyperintensity in T1-weighted images and hypointensity in T2-weighted images.

Biopsy: It is useful when the diagnosis cannot be established by less invasive methods.

Systemic investigation: It is aimed at excluding a metastasis to the choroids most frequently from the lungs in both sexes and from the breast in women and detecting possible metastatic spread from the choroid. In cases with clinical suspicion of metastasis, ultrasound abdomen and chest radiography may be done.

Treatment

The primary aim of treatment is to avoid the development of a painful and unsightly eye, preferably conserving as much useful vision as possible. The following factors are considered in the treatment:

1. Size, location and extent of the tumor and its effect on vision.
2. Condition of the fellow eye.
3. Age and general condition of the patient.
4. Patient consent.

The main treatment options are detailed below.

Brachytherapy (plaque radiotherapy): This therapy with ruthenium 106 or iodine 125 applicator is employed in treatment of tumors less than 20 mm basal diameter in which there is a reasonable chance of salvaging vision.

External beam radiotherapy: Irradiation with charged particles like protons is usually done in those tumors, which are unsuitable for brachytherapy because of their large size or posterior location.

Transpupillary thermotherapy (TTT): This technique uses an infrared laser beam to induce tumor cell death by hyperthermia. It is a useful adjunct to radiotherapy.

Transscleral choroidectomy: It is a difficult procedure and not widely performed.

Enucleation: This technique is indicated in large choroidal melanomas, optic disk invasion, extensive involvement of the ciliary body or angle, irreversible loss of useful vision and poor motivation of patient to keep the eye.

Differential Diagnosis

- Pigmented lesions:
  - Large choroidal nevus
  - Melanocytoma
  - Congenital hypertrophy of the RPE
  - Subretinal/Suprachoroidal hemorrhage.
- Non-pigmented lesions:
  - Circumscribed choroidal hemangioma
  - Choroidal metastasis
  - Choroidal granuloma in tuberculosis
  - Posterior scleritis.

Choroidal Hemangioma

Circumscribed Choroidal Hemangioma

A circumscribed choroidal hemangioma is not associated with systemic disease. It is usually asymptomatic, but can give rise to symptoms due to overlying retinal detachment.

Clinical features: Circumscribed choroidal hemangioma usually presents in two to three decades of life as unilateral blurring of vision, field defect or metamorphopsia.

The lesion appears as an oval orange mass at the posterior pole with overlying subretinal fluid in symptomatic cases. Ultrasound reveals an acoustically solid lesion with sharp anterior surface and high internal reflectivity. Photodynamic therapy, TTT and radiotherapy are described in the treatment.

Diffuse Choroidal Hemangioma

Diffuse choroidal hemangioma occurs almost exclusively in patients with Sturge-Weber syndrome, ipsilateral to the nevus flammeus.

The tumor usually presents in the second decade. The fundus has a diffuse deep red 'tomato ketchup' color mostly in the posterior pole.

Optic Disk Melanocytoma

Melanocytoma is a rare, unilateral, heavily pigmented, congenital hamartoma usually seen at the optic nerve head. It is seen more commonly in the dark skinned and more in females. Most cases are asymptomatic.

It appears as a brown or black, flat or slightly elevated lesion with feathery edges that may extend over the edge of optic disk. Complications are optic nerve compression, central vein occlusion, tumor necrosis and rarely malignant transformation.

Choroidal Metastasis

The choroid is the most common site for uveal metastasis. The most frequent primary site is the breast in females and lungs in males. Other sites are gastrointestinal tract, kidneys and skin.

They appear clinically as creamy white placoid lesions with indistinct margins usually at the posterior pole. The deposits can be multifocal in 30% cases and bilateral in 10%–30% cases. They are usually associated with exudative retinal detachment (Figs 22.12A and B).

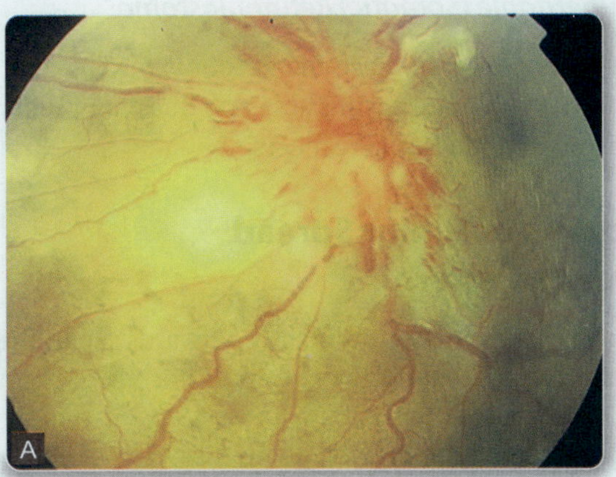

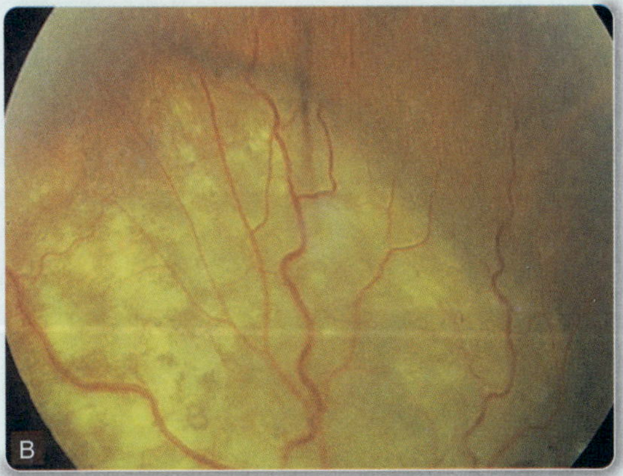

FIGURES 22.12A and B: Choroidal metastasis. **A.** Metastatic infiltration of ON head; **B.** Choroid with overlying exudative RD.

TUMORS OF RETINA

RETINOBLASTOMA

Retinoblastoma is the most common primary intraocular malignancy of childhood.

Epidemiology

The frequency of retinoblastoma ranges from 1 in 14,000 to 1 in 20,000 live births. About 90% of cases present before 3 years of age. It has no racial predilection and occurs equally in males and females. About 60%–70% cases are unilateral and 30%–40% cases are bilateral.

Genetics of Retinoblastoma

Retinoblastoma is caused by a mutation in the *RB1* gene on the long arm of chromosome 13q14. This is a tumor suppressor gene that controls retinal cell division. In children with retinoblastoma, retinal cell division continues unchecked causing retinal tumors. Both copies of the *RB1* gene must be mutated for the tumor to form. Retinoblastoma can be heritable or non-heritable.

Types

Heritable (Germline) Retinoblastoma

Heritable retinoblastoma accounts for 40% of cases. Here, one allele of *RB1* (tumor suppressor gene) is mutated in all body cells. When a further mutagenic event ('second hit') affects the second allele, the cell undergoes malignant transformation. Since all the retinal precursor cells contain the initial mutation, these children develop bilateral and multifocal tumors. They also have a predisposition to non-ocular malignancies like pineoblastoma (trilateral retinoblastoma) and secondary malignancies like osteosarcoma, melanoma, etc. About 15% of heritable cases can have unilateral presentation.

Non-heritable (Somatic) Retinoblastoma

Non-heritable retinoblastoma accounts for 60% of cases. It is unilateral, not transmissible and does not predispose to secondary non-ocular cancers.

Patterns of Tumor Spread (Growth Pattern)

Retinoblastoma may grow mainly outwards separating the retina from the choroids **(exophytic)** or inwards toward the vitreous **(endophytic)** with seeding of tumor cells throughout the eye (Figs 22.13A and B):

1. Optic nerve invasion with spread along the subarachnoid space to the brain.
2. Diffuse infiltration of the retina.
3. Metastatic spread to regional lymph nodes, lungs, brain and bone.

Clinical Presentation

Retinoblastoma usually occurs in infants and 90% cases occur within the first 3 years of life.

The most common clinical presentation is as a white pupillary reflex or leukocoria (amaurotic cat's eye), i.e. in almost 54%–62% cases (Figs 22.14 and 22.15).

Other modes of presentation include strabismus (18%–22%), ocular inflammation (2%–10%), pseudohypopyon, hyphema, heterochromia, secondary glaucoma with buphthalmos, cataract, anisocoria, orbital inflammation, orbital invasion in neglected cases, etc.

Diagnosis

The diagnosis of retinoblastoma is essentially clinical. Indirect ophthalmoscopy with scleral indentation must be performed on both eyes after full mydriasis in all suspected cases.

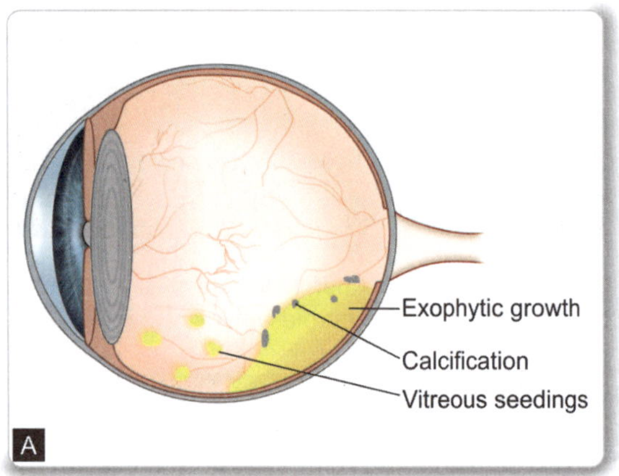

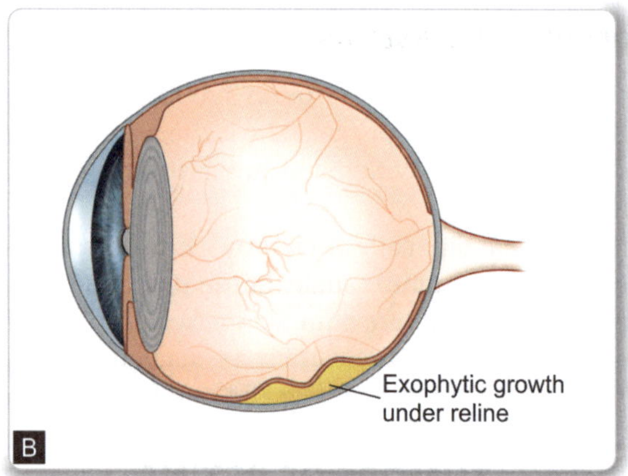

FIGURES 22.13A and B: Retinoblastoma. **A.** Exophytic growth; **B.** Endophytic growth.

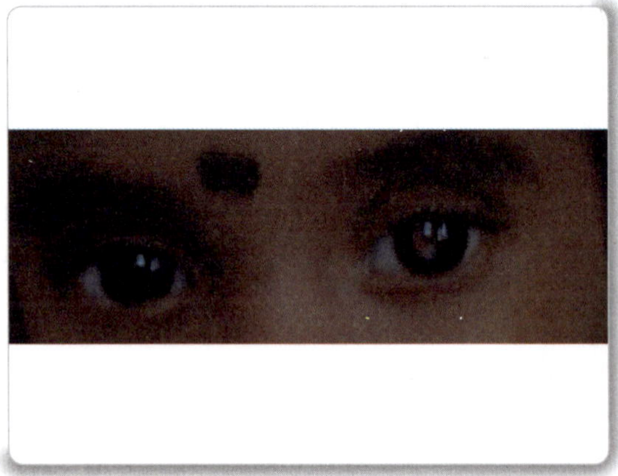

FIGURE 22.14: Leukocoria in retinoblastoma

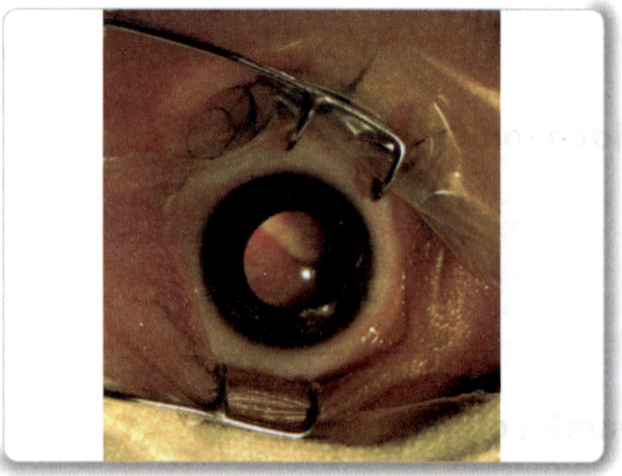

FIGURE 22.15: Leukocoria (magnified view in the same child)

An intraretinal tumor is a homogeneous, chalky white dome-shaped lesion often with whitish flecks of calcification. An endophytic tumor projects into the vitreous as a whitish mass with seeding into the vitreous. An exophytic tumor forms as subretinal, multilobular mass with overlying retinal detachment. Lesions may be often multiple.

Pathology

Retinoblastoma is composed of small cells with large hyperchromatic nuclei and scanty cytoplasm (retinoblasts). Undifferentiated tumors show no characteristic arrangement of these cells. Well differentiated tumors show characteristic arrangement patterns as following.

Flexner-Wintersteiner rosettes: Tall columnar cells arranged around a lumen, with their nuclei lying away from the lumen.

Homer-Wright rosettes (pseudorosettes): There is no lumen, but the cells are arranged around a mass of eosinophilic processes.

Fleurettes: Here the cells show some photoreceptor differentiation with long cytoplasmic processes of a group of cells projecting through a fenestrated membrane to appear like a wreath of flowers.

Tumor will show areas of necrosis and calcification.

Clinical Stages

1. **Quiescent stage:** The tumor is confined within the eye and presents as leukocoria or squint. The child is apparently healthy and symptomless.
2. **Stage of glaucoma:** The involvement of the angle of AC or the drainage channels will lead to rise in intraocular pressure (IOP). The child will develop buphthalmos and the child may be in distress due to the pain and discomfort of raised IOP.
3. **Stage of extraocular extension:** The child will present with proptosis (Fig. 22.16).
4. **Stage of metastasis**: This can be direct extension along the optic nerve to involve the brain. Bloodstream spread to cranial bones (most common), liver and lungs, and lymphatic spread to preauricular and submandibular lymph nodes.

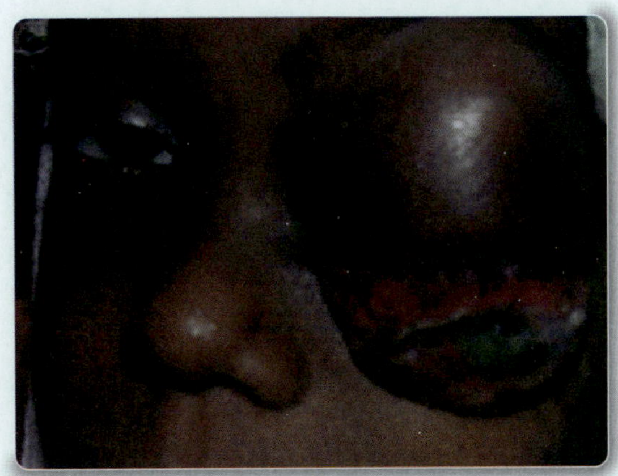

FIGURE 22.16: Extraocular and orbital invasion in a neglected case of retinoblastoma

Investigations

Examination under Anesthesia

Examination should be done in all suspected cases and should include tonometry, measurement of corneal diameter, axial length, anterior chamber examination with hand-held slit lamp, indirect ophthalmoscopy with 360° scleral indentation and documentation of all findings with color drawings or photography.

Ultrasound Scan

Ultrasound A- and B-scans are used to assess tumor size and calcification within the tumor. Calcification occurs in 75% of cases and is almost pathognomonic of retinoblastoma.

The B-scan ultrasound displays a cauliflower like mass arising from the retina, with or without a retinal detachment or vitreous seeds. A scan through the mass shows a characteristic V-Y pattern.

Computed Tomography of Brain and Orbit

Computed tomography (CT) can detect calcification, but confers significant dose of radiation to the child and hence routinely not preferred (Fig. 22.17).

Magnetic Resonance Imaging

Magnetic resonance imaging (MRI) is superior to CT in evaluation of optic nerve and for detection of extraocular extension or pinealoblastoma, but cannot detect calcification.

Systemic evaluation: It includes physical examination and MR scans of the orbit and skull, as a minimum in high risk cases. Bone scans, bone marrow study and lumbar puncture is done in all metastatic disease.

Genetic Studies

Tumor tissue from enucleated eyes and a blood sample can be taken for DNA analysis. Parents and siblings should be examined for untreated retinoblastoma or retinoma, which would provide evidence for a hereditary predisposition for the disease.

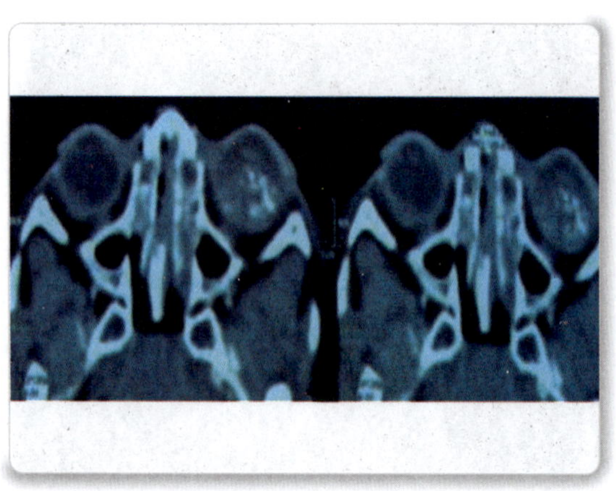

FIGURE 22.17: Computed tomography showing an intraocular mass with calcification suggestive of retinoblastoma

Differential Diagnosis

A number of lesions can simulate retinoblastoma. The differential diagnoses for a child presenting with leukocoria include the following.

Persistent Fetal Vasculature or Persistent Hyperplastic Primary Vitreous

Persistent fetal vasculature or persistent hyperplastic primary vitreous (PHPV) is typically recognized within days or weeks of birth. The condition is unilateral in two third of cases and may be associated with microphthalmia, shallow AC, iris hypoplasia and a retrolental fibrovascular mass that draws the ciliary process inwards. B-scan helps in diagnosis by showing the persistent hyaloid remnants arising from the optic nerve head associated with a closed funnel retinal detachment.

Coats' Disease

Coats' disease is almost always unilateral, more common in boys and tends to present later than retinoblastoma, i.e. in the first decade (Fig. 22.18).

Retinopathy of Prematurity

Advanced retinopathy of prematurity (ROP) can cause retinal detachment and leukocoria. There will be a history of prematurity and low birth weight in most cases.

Toxocariasis

Chronic toxocara endophthalmitis may cause cyclitic membrane and a white pupil. A granuloma at the posterior pole can mimic an endophytic retinoblastoma.

Vitreoretinal Dysplasia

Conditions like Norrie's disease, incontinentia pigment, etc. can be associated with a detached, dysplastic retina forming a retrolental mass with leukocoria.

Retinoma

Retinoma is a benign variant of retinoblastoma, which can undergo spontaneous involution and present as a calcified mass.

Retinal Astrocytoma

Retinal astrocytoma tumor appears as a small, smooth white tumor, which may be solitary or multiple, unilateral or bilateral. They are usually seen in patients with tuberous sclerosis.

Chronic Endophthalmitis

Chronic endophthalmitis can occur during intrauterine life or infancy due to septicemia and vitreous exudation will give a yellow reflex mimicking a retinoblastoma.

Classification of Retinoblastoma

The Reese-Ellsworth clinical classification is commonly used in categorizing intraocular retinoblastoma.

Reese-Ellsworth Classification

Group I: Very favorable:

1. Solitary tumor less than 4DD in size at or behind the equator.
2. Multiple tumors, none larger than 4DD in size, all at or behind the equator.

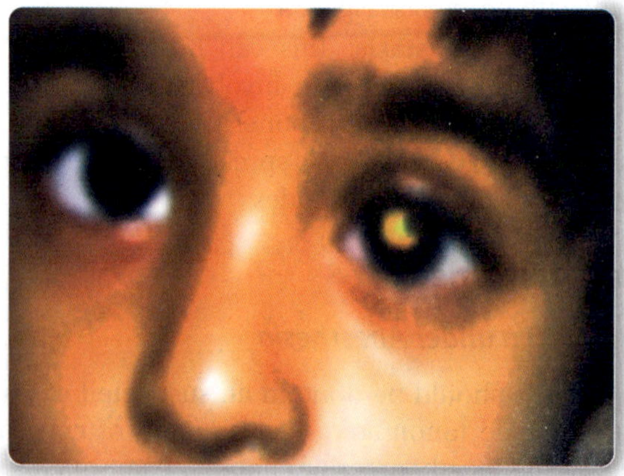

FIGURE 22.18: Advanced Coats' disease

Group II: Favorable:

1. Solitary tumor, 4–10DD in size at or behind the equator.
2. Multiple tumors, 4–10DD in size behind the equator.

Group III: Possible to maintain sight:

1. Any lesion anterior to the equator.
2. Solitary tumor, larger than 10DD in size behind the equator.

Group IV: Unfavorable:

1. Multiple tumors, some larger than 10DD in size.
2. Any lesion extending anteriorly to the ora serrata.

Group V: Highly unfavorable:

1. Massive tumors involving more than one half of the retina.
2. Vitreous seeding.

International Classification of Intraocular Retinoblastoma

Group A: Small tumors (< 3 mm) outside macula.

Group B: Bigger tumors (> 3 mm) or any tumor in macula or any tumor with subretinal fluid.

Group C: Localized seeds (subretinal or vitreous).

Group D: Diffuse seeds (subretinal or vitreous).

Group E: No visual potential or presence of any one or more of the following:

- Tumor in the anterior segment
- Tumor in or on the ciliary body
- Neovascular glaucoma
- Opaque media from hemorrhage
- Tumor necrosis with aseptic orbital cellulitis
- Phthisis bulbi.

Treatment of Retinoblastoma

Treatment of retinoblastoma is considered mainly under three headings, i.e. treatment of:

1. Small tumors.
2. Large tumors.
3. Extraocular extension.

Treatment of Small Tumors

Earlier the only method of treatment was enucleation and histopathological examination to confirm the diagnosis in unilateral cases. In bilateral cases, the worse eye is enucleated to confirm the diagnosis histopathologically and the second eye is treated with radiation. Nowadays the focus is to conserve the eye as far as possible if there is any chance for vision by treatment with photocoagulation, chemotherapy and radiotherapy:

1. Tumors not more than 3 mm diameter and 2 mm thickness may be treated with:
   a. Photocoagulation using argon or diode laser.
   b. Usually TTT as an adjunct, following chemoreduction.
   c. Cryotherapy for pre-equatorial tumors.
   d. Chemotherapy for small macular tumors to conserve as much vision as possible.
   e. Treatment of medium sized tumors.
2. Tumors up to 12 mm wide and 6 mm thick may be treated with:
   a. Brachytherapy using iodine 125 or ruthenium 106 for anterior tumors.
   b. Primary chemotherapy with intravenous carboplatin, etoposide and vincristine (CEV) for 3–6 cycles followed by local treatment with cryo or TTT.
   c. External beam radiotherapy generally avoided due to risk of secondary malignancies and also due to radiation-induced orbital growth retardation in young children.

Treatment of Large Tumors

Chemotherapy to shrink the tumor (chemoreduction) and make it amenable to local measures. This is especially useful in cases with bilateral tumor or pinealoblastoma.

Enucleation is indicated if tumor involves more than 50% of the globe, orbital or optic nerve invasion or anterior segment involvement with or without neovascular glaucoma. It should be performed with minimal manipulation and a long piece of optic nerve (12–15 mm) should be obtained. The cut end of the optic nerve is histopathologically examined to make sure that it is free of any invasion by the tumor.

Treatment of Extraocular Extension

1. Adjuvant chemotherapy is given after enucleation.
2. External beam radiotherapy is indicated in optic nerve invasion or extension through the sclera.
3. Metastatic disease is treated with high dose chemotherapy with hematopoietic stem cell rescue, but prognosis is poor.

Targeted Therapy

Gene therapy for treatment of retinoblastoma is currently undergoing clinical trials.

Follow-up

After radiotherapy or chemotherapy, tumor regresses to a cottage cheese calcified mass or a fish flesh like mass or an atrophic scar. Children who are treated conservatively are kept on regular follow-up till 10 years of age. Children with unilateral disease and who had enucleation of the involved eye should undergo regular periodic detailed evaluation of the second eye till 10 years of age.

Retinoblastoma can also undergo complete and spontaneous necrosis and regression, and phthisis bulbi can ensue.

Prognosis

The prognosis of retinoblastoma, if untreated is always bad. The prognosis is fair if extraocular extension is avoided. The prognosis for 5 year disease free survival in intraocular retinoblastoma is more than 90%. However, in extraocular extension, the 5 year disease free survival is less than 10%.

RETINAL ASTROCYTOMA

Astrocytoma of the retina and optic nerve head is a rare hamartoma, which does not usually threaten vision. They are most frequently seen in tuberous sclerosis and occasionally in neurofibromatosis 1.

Multiple and bilateral fundus astrocytomas occur in about 50% of patients of tuberous sclerosis. The tumor appears as large elevated mulberry like lesions, which may become calcified. They usually show fundus autofluorescence.

RETINAL HEMANGIOMA

Retinal capillary hemangioma is a rare vascular tumor of the retina usually seen in association with von Hippel-Lindau disease. It appears as a round orange-red mass in the retinal periphery or as an ill-defined juxtapapillary lesion. The tumor can be sight threatening due to macular edema, exudates or retinal detachment.

Retinal cavernous hemangioma is a rare, unilateral congenital hamartoma that can occur in combination with lesions of the skin and central nervous system (CNS). They appear as sessile clusters of saccular aneurysms resembling a bunch of grapes in the peripheral retina.

Racemose hemangioma or arteriovenous (AV) malformation of the retina is a sporadic congenital malformation involving direct communication between arteries and veins. Brain involvement with similar ipsilateral lesions can occur in Wyburn-Mason syndrome.

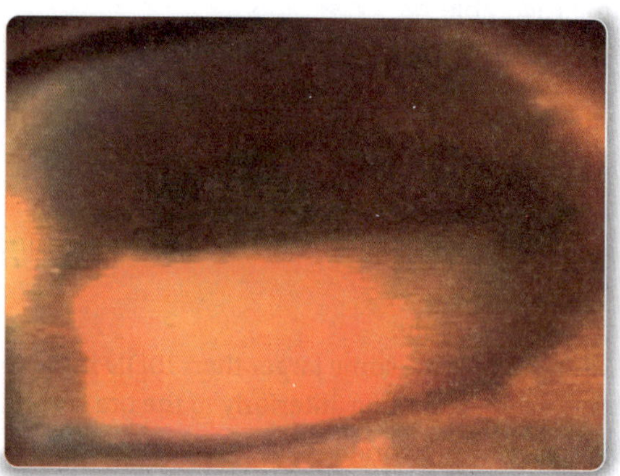

FIGURE 22.19: Anterior chamber invasion in advanced primary intraocular lymphoma (PIOL)

PRIMARY INTRAOCULAR LYMPHOMA

The PIOL is a subset of primary central nervous system lymphoma (PCNSL), which is a variant of extranodal non-Hodgkin lymphoma. The tumor arises from the brain, spinal cord and leptomeninges and has a very poor prognosis. About 20% of patients with PCNSL have ocular manifestations, which can precede or follow neurological involvement. The anterior chamber invasion in advanced PIOL is shown in Figure 22.19.

Ocular Features

Primary intraocular lymphome usually presents in the sixth to seventh decade with unilateral or bilateral floaters and blurring of vision. Vitritis is usually present with some mild anterior uveitis and presenting as a masquerade syndrome. Multifocal subretinal infiltrates, which can occasionally coalesce to form ring infiltrates, retinal vasculitis, exudative retinal detachment and optic atrophy are the other ocular findings. The absence of cystoid macular edema differentiates this from true uveitic conditions.

Neurological features include headache, personality changes, focal deficit, seizures, cranial nerve palsies, etc.

Treatment

Radiotherapy is the first line treatment for PIOL, but recurrence is common. Intravitreal methotrexate is useful in recurrent disease. Systemic chemotherapy can prolong survival in CNS disease. Biologic agents like rituximab is recently tried alternative.

Ocular Trauma

23

Girija Devi PS, Jasmin LB

Ocular trauma can be physical or chemical and they are medical emergencies. Injury is often a under-recognized health problem and unless promptly and correctly managed, it can cause permanent impairment of vision.

Even though the eye is protected by the bony orbit and the lids in front, no part of the eye can escape the effects of trauma. The majority of eye injuries occur in people below 30 years of age and statistics show that eye injury is a leading cause of monocular blindness in United States and one third of these are job-related accidents. The 90% of eye injuries are preventable. Proper safety precautions at the workplace, inside the house, as well as careful supervision of children's activities can prevent injuries to a considerable extent. Considerable advances have been achieved in the investigations and successful management of ocular trauma decreasing the visual impairment.

CHEMICAL INJURIES

Chemical injuries of the eye are real ocular emergency, which produce extensive damage to the ocular surface and lead to visual impairment. Most chemical injuries are due to alkali or acid compounds.

Alkalis

Alkali injuries occur more commonly than acid injury as they are frequently used in fertilizers, household cleaning agents, fire crackers and construction work. The most severe alkali injuries are usually due to ammonia. It has the potential to cause the most severe eye damage because of its characteristic of both lipid and water solubility. It penetrates the eye very quickly and can reach the anterior chamber in 1 minute. The most common alkali injury is due to cement falling in the eye, which usually happens in construction workers.

Pathogenesis

Alkali injury cause ocular damage by saponification and disruption of fatty acids in cell membranes leading to cell death. The lipid saponification associated with alkali injuries allows rapid penetration of alkali substance into tissue, in contrast to most acidic compounds. A pH of 11.5 or higher is associated with severe ocular damage.

Acids

Acidic compounds are found in household chemicals such as cleaners, rust removers and in car batteries. Sulfuric acid is the most common cause of acidic chemical injury to the eye. Lead batteries contain up to 25% sulfuric acid. During recharging of a battery, hydrogen and oxygen are produced by electrolysis and form an explosive mixture. Acid used in preparation of rubber sheets is a common cause for injury in places where rubber plantations are situated.

Pathogenesis

Acid injuries produce precipitation and coagulation necrosis of corneal epithelium, which forms a protective barrier to further penetration. This barrier may protect against weaker acids, but strong acids may continue to penetrate deeply.

The severity of ocular injury depends on:

1. Area of surface contact.
2. Depth of penetration.
3. Degree of limbal stem cell injury.

Classification

Classification of chemical injuries was first proposed by Hughes and then modified by Roper-Hall. This helps to guide prognosis and treatment.

Grade I: Involves little or no loss of limbal stem cells and presents with little or no evidence of ischemia (Fig. 23.1).

Grade II: Involves subtotal loss of limbal stem cells and presents with ischemia of less than one-half of the limbus.

Grade III: Involves total loss of limbal stem cells with preservation of proximal conjunctival epithelium and presents with ischemia of one-half of the entire limbus (Fig. 23.2).

Grade IV: Involves total limbus stem cell loss as well as loss of proximal conjunctival epithelium and extensive damage to entire anterior segment (Fig. 23.3).

Clinical Course

Immediate Phase

Clinically present as—conjunctival congestion, areas of necrosis that appear white, subconjunctival hemorrhages, large epithelial defects involving cornea, cloudy edematous and opaque cornea, elevated intraocular pressure (IOP), fibrin reaction in anterior chamber, cataract, hypotony due to ciliary body injury, etc.

Acute Phase (0–7 Days)

Mild injuries tend to heal during this period. Severe injuries show no re-epithelization.

Early Phase (7–21 Days)

Epithelial migration and regeneration occur in grade I and II injuries. Fibrovascular pannus, symblepharon and stromal ulceration can develop between 7 and 10 days.

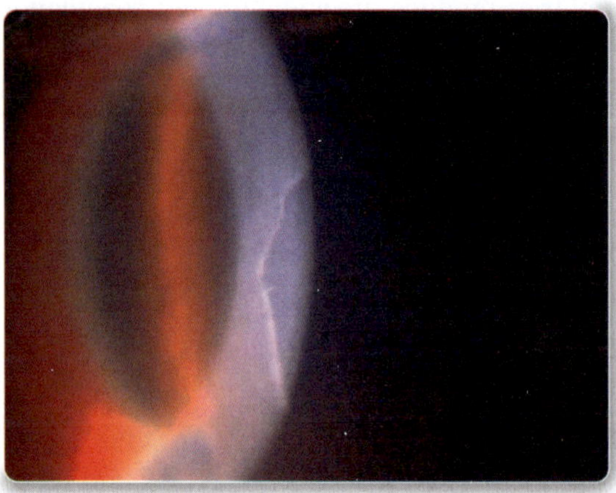

FIGURE 23.1: Grade I chemical injury with epithelial defect and no limbal ischemia

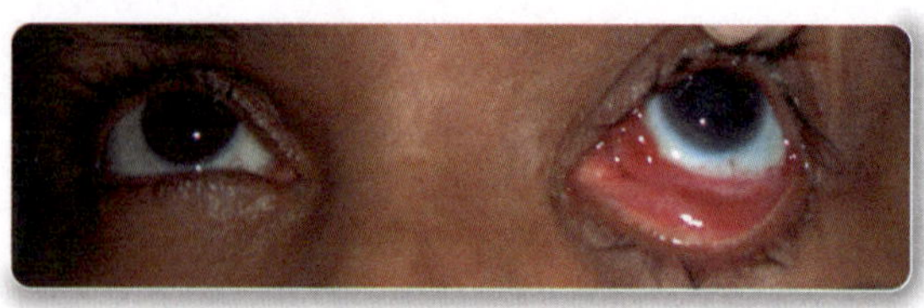

FIGURE 23.2: Grade IV chemical injury in left eye with 360° limbal ischemia hazy cornea and total cataract

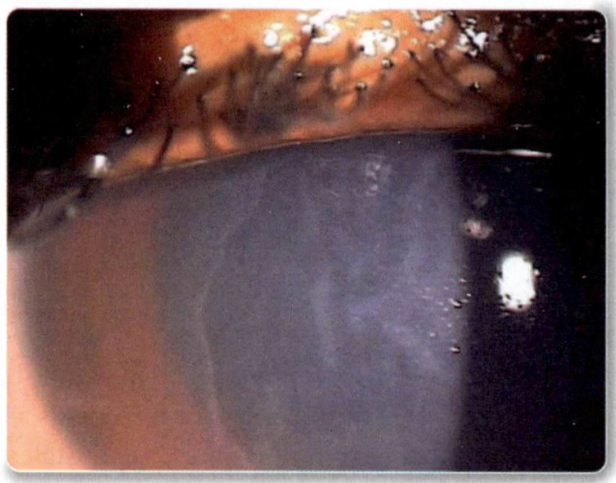

FIGURE 23.3: Extensive epithelial loss, corneal haze and Descemet's membrane (DM) folds

Late Repair Phase (> 21 Days)

Conjunctival scarring, trichiasis, cicatricial entropion and corneal scarring can progress. Tear deficiency develop due to loss of goblet cells or decreased aqueous production. Corneal sensation may be decreased.

Management

Immediate Treatment

1. Irrigation with normal saline/water/balance salt solution for at least 30 minutes or till pH turns neutral.
2. Eyelid immobilization with eyelid speculum or retractor.
3. Instillation of topical anesthesia.
4. Removal of particulate matter/debris after double eversion of lids.
5. Evaluation of the extent and depth of burn is done under slit lamp. Fluorescein staining is done. Limbal stem cell ischemia is looked for and graded by the newer classification.

Aim of treatment is to restore the cornea with normal epithelium and a clear stroma by decreasing the inflammation, and enhancing the healing.

Treatment after Irrigation

Treatment after irrigation is as follows:

1. Topical steroid 2 hourly inhibits polymorphonuclear proliferation and function.
2. Topical sodium citrate 10% 2 hourly inhibits polymorphonuclear degranulation by calcium chelation.
3. Tetracycline 1% ointment qid inhibits collagenase enzyme by chelating with zinc (Zn).
4. Oral sodium ascorbate 500 mg qid promotes collagen synthesis.
5. Topical sodium ascorbate 20% 2 hourly promotes collagen synthesis.
6. Tear substitutes 2 hourly promote epithelial healing.
7. Cycloplegics tds or bd relieves pain.
8. Topical/Oral antiglaucoma therapy, if needed.
9. Conjunctival/Tenons advancement for grade IV improves vascularization.

Healing Patterns of Chemical Burns

After 1st week

After 1st week, reassess the patient. The severity of injury will show the following healing patterns:

Grade I: Healed cornea with normal epithelium.

Grade II: Epithelial defect, smaller in size.

Grade III: No epithelization, inflammation.

Grade IV: Sterile corneal ulcer + conjunctival defect inflammation.

Management at this stage

1. Taper steroids in the next week.
2. Remaining same treatment is continued for 3 weeks.
3. Amniotic membrane transplantation in 2nd to 3rd weeks in grade III–IV to control inflammation and lessen symblepharon and vascularization of cornea.

After 3 weeks to several months

Grade I/II: Healed cornea/healed with pannus.

Grade III: No healing; finally heal as a scarred and vascularized cornea.

Grade IV: Sterile corneal ulcer or vascularized cornea after conjunctival advancement.

Management option

Grade I/II: Taper medical treatment.

Grade III/IV: Impending or actual perforation:

1. Tissue adhesives for less than 1 mm perforations.
2. Tectonic keratoplasty.

Vascularized Cornea

1. Limbal stem cell transplantation followed by:
   a. Penetrating keratoplasty (PK).
   b. Lamellar keratoplasty (LK) after 6 months.
2. Large PK or large LK.
3. Keratoprosthesis in bilateral cases.

For symblepharon/cicatrization of conjunctiva, amniotic membrane transplant/mucous membrane transplant can be done.

MECHANICAL INJURIES

Ocular trauma is the cause of blindness or partial loss of vision in more than half a million people worldwide. The National Eye Institute Trauma System Registry (NETSR) report on penetrating eye injuries noted that 83% of patients were men and the average age was 27 years. Posterior segment trauma is the most common cause of severe visual loss after eye trauma.

During the last several decades, the prognosis for patients with ocular injuries, especially those with open globe injuries has significantly improved. This has been attributed to the advent of enhanced microsurgical technique and instrumentation, along with an improved understanding of the pathophysiologic mechanism of ocular trauma.

Ocular Trauma Classification System

The ocular trauma classification group was organized to establish a system to classify mechanical injuries of the eye. This system provides unambiguous definition for each term and has become the common international language of ocular trauma terminology improving the accuracy in both clinical practice and research.

Birmingham Eye Trauma Terminology

Birmingham Eye Trauma Terminology (BETT) satisfies all criteria for unambiguous standard terminology by:

1. Providing a clear definition for injury types (Table 23.1).
2. Placing each injury type within the framework of a comprehensive system (Fig. 23.4).

The ocular trauma classification group has developed a classification system based on BETT and features of globe injury at initial examination. Mechanical trauma to the eye is subdivided into open and closed globe injuries because these have different pathophysiological and therapeutic ramifications. The system categorizes trauma by four parameters (Table 23.2).

Types of Injury

The following are the types of injury as given by the above criteria.

Visual acuity

As defined by the visual acuity measurement at the initial examination. Testing may be done with a Snellen acuity chart for distance and near. Visual acuity at initial examination has been demonstrated to be the most reliable prediction of functional visual outcome in open globe injury.

Relative afferent pupillary defect

The presence of relative afferent pupillary defect (RAPD) is measured by swinging flash light test, and it grossly measures optic nerve and retinal functions. If the affected eye is non-reactive for mechanical or pharmacologic reasons, observing the consensual response in the follow eye is advised.

Extent (zone) of the injury

Denotes wound location in open globe injuries or the posterior extent of damage in closed globe injuries.

Investigations

The imaging methods used are plain X-ray orbit, ultrasonography, computed tomography (CT), magnetic resonance imaging (MRI) and electrophysiological tests. Plain X-ray and ultrasonography give sufficient information in most of the cases.

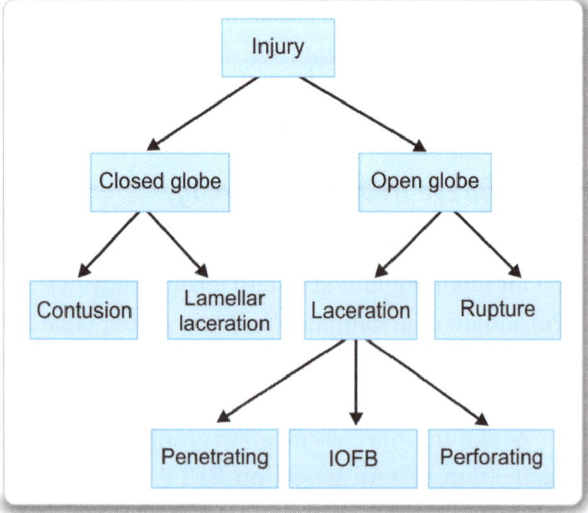

FIGURE 23.4: Mechanical injuries (IOFB, intraocular foreign bodies)

TABLE 23.1: Birmingham eye trauma terminology

Term	Definition and explanation
Eye wall	Sclera and cornea Although technically the eye wall has three coats, posterior to the limbus, for clinical and practical purposes, violation of only the most external structure is taken into consideration
Closed globe injury	No full-thickness wound of eye wall
Open globe injury	Full-thickness wound of the eye wall
Contusion	There is no (full-thickness) wound The injury is due to either direct energy delivery by the object (e.g. choroidal rupture) or the changes in the shape of the globe (e.g. angle recession)
Lamellar laceration	Partial-thickness wound of the eye wall
Rupture	Full-thickness wound of the eye wall, caused by a blunt object Because the eye is filled with incompressible liquid, the impact results in momentary increase in intraocular pressure (IOP) The eye wall yields at its weakest point (at the impact site) or elsewhere (e.g. an old cataract wound dehisces even though the impact occurred elsewhere); the actual wound is produced by an inside-out mechanism
Laceration	Full-thickness wound of the eye wall, caused by a sharp object The wound occurs at the impact site by an outside-in mechanism
Penetrating injury	Entrance wound If more than one wound is present, each must have been caused by a different agent
Retained foreign object(s)	Technically a penetrating injury, but grouped separately because of different clinical implications
Perforating injury	Entrance and exit wounds Both wounds caused by the same agent

Electrophysiological Test

Both, electroretinogram (ERG) and visual evoked potential (VEP), are used as valuable prognostic indicators, especially in opaque media. A non-recordable ERG means

TABLE 23.2: Classification of injuries

Open globe injury	Closed globe injury
1. Type	
Rupture	
Penetrating	Contusion
IOFB*	Lamellar laceration
Perforating	Superficial foreign body
Mixed	Mixed
2. Grade (visual acuity)	
> 20/40	> 20/40
20/50–20/100	20/50–20/100
19/100–5/200	19/100–5/200
4/200 to light perception	4/200 to light perception
NLP†	NLP
3. Pupil	
Positive, relative APD‡ in injured eye	Positive, relative APD in injured eye
Negative, relative APD in injured eye	Negative, relative APD in injured eye
4. Zone	
Cornea and limbus	External (limited to bulbar, conjunctiva, sclera, cornea)
Limbus to 5 mm posterior into sclera	Anterior segment (includes structures of the anterior segment and the pars plicata)
Posterior to 5 mm from the limbus	Posterior segment (all internal structures posterior to the posterior lens capsule)

*IOFB, intraocular foreign bodies; †NLP, no light perception; ‡APD, afferent pupillary defect.

a poor visual outcome. VEP is found to be the single best predictor of visual outcome. ERG also has a role in the assessment of metallosis bulbi.

X-ray

X-ray has limited use in the present scenario. It can show fractures and radiopaque foreign bodies (RFBs).

Ultrasonography

The most valuable tool for imaging a traumatized eye is ultrasonography. The main indications for ultrasound examination of traumatized eye include:

1. To assess the posterior segment of eye in closed globe injuries, e.g. dislocated lens, rupture of lens capsule, vitreous hemorrhage, retinal detachment and choroidal detachment.
2. In open globe injuries to detect occult scleral perforation, lens dislocation ruptured lens capsule, vitreous hemorrhage, retinal detachment, choroidal detachment, vitreous leak and intraocular foreign bodies (IOFB).

Computed Tomography

Generally 1.5-2 mm thick axial cuts and 2-4 mm thick coronal sections are used. To detect IOFB, smaller cuts can be specifically asked for.

Advantages: They are as follows:

- Superior to ultrasound imaging to detect size and site of IOFB
- No contact with eye
- Ideal for orbital fractures.

Disadvantages: They are as follows:

- Contraindicated in pregnant patients
- Intraocular structures are not well-imaged like ultrasound scan
- Cannot be performed in operating room or at the bed side.

Computed tomography findings suggestive of open globe injury (Fig. 23.5): They are as follows:

- Eye wall deformity
- Intraocular gas
- IOFB.

Magnetic Resonance Imaging

Magnetic resonance imaging investigation technique provides superior tissue definition and resolution. However, it cannot be used in the suspicion of a ferromagnetic IOFB, which could be dislodged and produce further damage to the eye. With its superior resolution, it helps in evaluation of occult scleral rupture, large hemorrhagic choroidal detachments and dense vitreous hemorrhage. It can be used to detect radiolucent substances like wooden, plastic

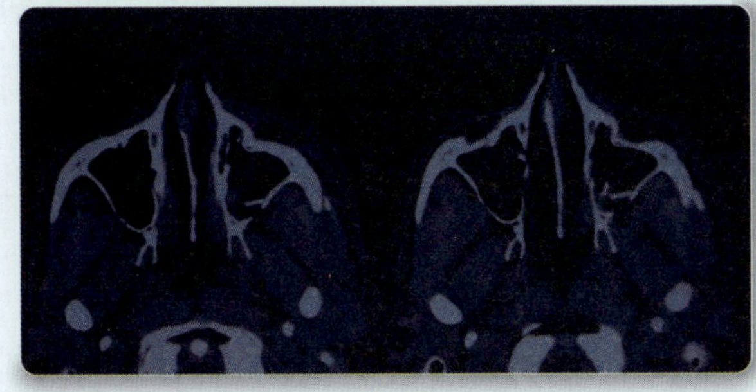

FIGURE 23.5: Computed tomography showing fracture of floor of orbit

and glass intraocular foreign (IOF) body. It can be used in pregnant patients and contraindicated in patients with pacemaker and cochlear implant.

Mechanism of Blunt Injury

Anteroposterior compression of the globe at the cornea result in equatorial expansion and shortening of the globe along the visual axis. The anteroposterior diameter of the globe decreases by, as much as, 41% leading to corneal contact with the lens and iris. As the anteroposterior diameter decreases, the equatorial diameter increases up to 128% of normal. The extreme stretching of the ocular tissue results in specific type of injury to the eye.

Application of force to the globe is said to cause coup injury at the site of force application and contrecoup injury to areas of the globe opposite to the site of force of application. Force waves transmitted through the globe may be the mechanism of contrecoup injury.

There are seven rings of tissues anterior to equator, which are to expand, because fluid in the eye cannot be compressed. The lens-iris diaphragm is forced posteriorly, due to the attachment of the structures to the scleral wall, which is moving in the perpendicular direction; a shearing strain is created, which may split the tissues at their roots.

The seven ring structures are:

1. Sphincter pupille: Tears can occur.
2. Anterior ciliary body, producing angle recession or ciliary body tear, typically the separation occurs between circular and longitudinal fibers. The longitudinal fibers remain attached to the sclera and form the new anterior boundary of the recessed chamber, which corresponds to the broad ciliary body band seen gonioscopically.
3. Attachment of the ciliary body muscle to the scleral spur resulting in cyclodialysis cleft. Aqueous is allowed to pass directly from anterior chamber to suprachoroidal. Hypotony is common.
4. Trabecular meshwork: A tear in the anterior portion of the meshwork resulting in a trabecular flap.
5. Attachment of zonules, resulting in subluxation and dislocation of the lens.
6. Attachment of retina to the ora serrata resulting in retinal dialysis and retinal detachment.

EFFECTS OF BLUNT TRAUMA ON THE EYE

Lesions of Conjunctiva

- Subconjunctival hemorrhage
- Foreign bodies
- Laceration (Fig. 23.6)
- Emphysema.

Subconjunctival Hemorrhage

Subconjunctival hemorrhage appears as a bright red patch of conjunctival tissue with distinct or feathered borders, which resolves spontaneously in 7–10 days.

Subconjunctival hemorrhage may be due to the tracking forward of the blood from the orbit following fracture of the orbital walls or the base of the skull. It should be differentiated from local bleeding. When a fracture is the cause, the densest and most extensive part of the hemorrhage is posterior, where no edge is seen. Anteriorly it may not reach the limbus. In case of local bleeding, the densest area is usually on the anterior part and it starts disappearing towards the equator. In bleeding from a fracture, the color of the hemorrhage is purplish and subconjunctival in site, whereas local bleeding is bright red and intraconjunctival moving with this membrane (Fig. 23.7).

The presence of subconjunctival pigmentation in association with a hemorrhage is very suspicious of occult scleral rupture (Fig. 23.8).

Foreign Bodies

Conjunctival foreign bodies are common. Most conjunctival foreign bodies are easily removed with a cotton-tipped applicator or 26 gauge needle.

Laceration

Laceration may be isolated injuries or indicates a deeper trauma. In case of conjunctival laceration a thorough examination is done to rule out an open globe injury. The scleral

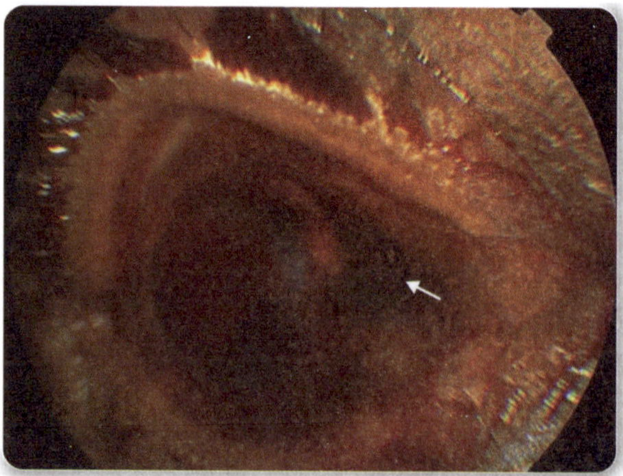

FIGURE 23.6: Rupture globe with hyphema and uveal tissue prolapse (white arrow)

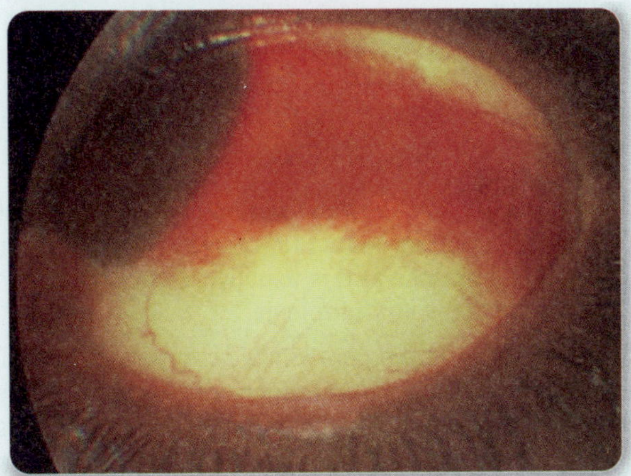

FIGURE 23.7: Subconjunctival hemorrhage

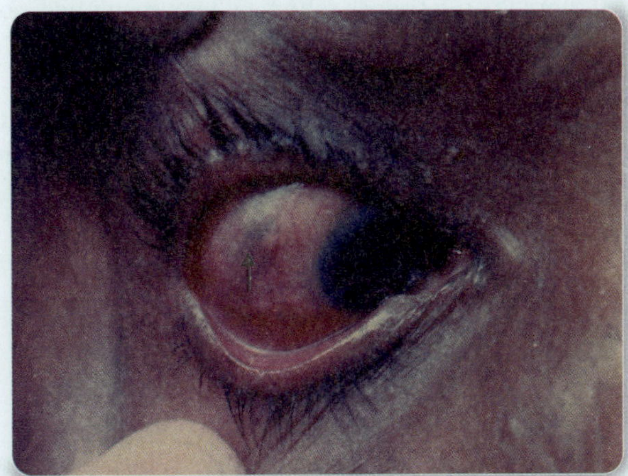

FIGURE 23.8: Subconjunctival pigmentation suggesting scleral rupture

The scleral defect may be from a significant distance from the site of the conjunctival injury. So examine the eye in a variety of gazes and if necessary conjunctival exploration should be performed under local anesthesia.

Larger lacerations may require closure using absorbable suture materials.

Emphysema

Emphysema occurs when air gets trapped under or in the conjunctiva. In orbital fracture, air from paranasal sinuses enter into the orbit and dissects anteriorly under and into the conjunctiva. Patients with orbital fractures should be advised against nose blowing or sneezing with a closed mouth so as to avoid orbital and subconjunctival emphysema.

Lesions of the Cornea

- Corneal abrasions
- Recurrent erosion
- Corneal foreign bodies
- Corneal lacerations.

Corneal Abrasions

Superficial corneal abrasions are frequently seen with minor trauma.

Clinical features: Due to the dense innervation of sensory nerves of the corneal epithelial surface, corneal abrasion causes intense pain, photophobia and lacrimation. Irregular corneal light reflex may indicate presence of an abrasion. On examination, a corneal abrasion stains with fluorescein dye and its borders are generally sharp.

Routine treatment of corneal abrasion includes the use of a broad-spectrum antibiotic drop for infection, prophylaxis and cycloplegic agent. A pad and bandage is generally applied to shield the epithelium.

Recurrent Erosion

Corneal abrasions caused by any shearing injury (e.g. finger nail, paper cut or vegetable matter) may damage epithelium—basement membrane adhesion complexes and consequently lead to recurrent or persistent epithelial defects. Predisposing conditions such as epithelial or stromal dystrophies may contribute to recurrent erosions.

Clinical features: Patients typically presents with acute onset of pain, redness and tearing on awakening. On examination, an irregular area of epithelium causing a focal breakup of the tear film to a full thickness epithelial defect with elevated gray margins is seen.

Treatment: Aim of the treatment is to maintain epithelial stability and integrity until the adhesion complex can form and hemidesmosomal anchoring fibers extend into the basement membrane to secure the epithelium firmly in place. The treatment for recurrent erosion are as follows:

1. A topical hyperosmotic agent, e.g. 5% sodium chloride ointment applied before sleep. During sleep, tear film becomes hypotonic due to lack of evaporation, which make the corneal epithelium edematous and easily damaged with the first blink and hyperosmotic agents help to reduce the corneal epithelial edema and this should be used for at least 8 weeks, which is the minimum period required for the formation of adhesion complex.

2. If there is no response to topical hyperosmotics, next step is extended wear bandage contact lens for a minimum of 6–8 weeks.
3. Debridement using a cotton-tipped applicator or using a blade will help regrowing of normal epithelium.
4. Stromal micropuncture with a straight 20 gauge needle is used to create a partial thickness penetration of the anterior corneal stroma.
5. Excimer laser ablating the basement membrane and the superficial bowman's layer.

Corneal Foreign Bodies

The symptoms caused by corneal foreign bodies are frequently out of proportion to the severity of the injury. Individuals with foreign bodies remaining on the corneal surface can be highly symptomatic; conversely, high speed objects that are embedded in or pass completely through the cornea may give rise to no or only minimal symptoms.

Ferrous foreign bodies: They oxidize and form rust deposits in cornea as easily as 3 hours after injury. Because rust can retard wound healing, its removal by scraping is recommended.

Caterpillar hairs: It may cause intense irritation and can migrate into the deep stroma.

Treatment

Removal with a cotton tipped applicator or a 26 gauge needle in the case of deeper foreign bodies, application of antibiotic drops or ointment till the wound heals and patching of the eye to promote healing as well as to relieve pain and irritation.

Corneal Lacerations

Bandage lenses are useful for non-displaced laceration less than 3 mm in length, particularly, if they are self sealing. Large lacerating wounds, displaced wounds, wounds with loss of corneal tissue and lacerations with accompanying iris or lens incarceration must be sutured.

Lesion of Iris and Ciliary Body

- Changes in pupil and accommodation
- Vascular changes
- Interstitial tears of the sphincter
- Tears at the pupillary border
- Partial or complete dehiscence at pigmentary layer
- Iridodialysis
- Irideremia
- Iridoschisis
- Traumatic cyclodialysis
- Pigmentary changes.

Changes in Pupil and Accommodation

Traumatic miosis and spasm of accommodation: A spastic miosis is a immediate sequel to trauma. The constriction of the pupil is intense and is usually transient, to be followed frequently by an iridoplegia.

Traumatic mydriasis and paralysis of accommodation: Dilation of the pupil is a very common sequel of a concussion of the globe and it is usually associated with a paralysis of accommodation coming after the intense miosis has passed. The pupil is moderately dilated, often eccentric, usually with diminished reaction to light and accommodation and this deformity is permanent.

Vascular Changes

Reactive hyperemia and exudation—concussion effect on uveal vessels comprise initially an ischemic spasm followed by a prolonged reactive vasodilatation. Clinically evident by circumcorneal injection and the vascular dilatation is associated with edema of the tissue. Slit lamp examination reveals the presence of increased protein in the anterior chamber.

If the reaction is severe, it leads to formation of microscopically visible masses of fibrin in the anterior chamber.

Interstitial Tears of the Sphincter

Tears of the sphincter muscle without external involvement of the tissues of the iris are usually small and may be multiple. They are difficult to see clinically, but are made obvious by transillumination in which case, the torn area appears as a reddish glow. There may also be changes in the contour of the pupil involving a minimal amount of notching.

Tears at the Pupillary Border

The tears at the pupillary border is common, the laceration may involve the anterior layers of the stroma of the iris and leave the sphincter intact, alternatively, the posterior pigmented layer and the sphincter may be implicated, while the anterior stroma remain intact. But much more commonly, the whole depth of the tissue anterior stroma, sphincter muscle and pigmentary epithelium is torn.

If the tear involves the posterior pigmentary epithelium and sphincter muscle, hyphema is common from the capillaries of the muscle. A complete tear, involving all the layers of the iris is the most common.

Dehiscence of the Pigmentary Layer of the Iris

Common sequel of concussion injuries, which are not visible ophthalmoscopically or by direct observation, but only by retroillumination they appear as bright red areas. The dehiscence is either single or multiple, round, oval or irregular and occurs preferentially near the root of the iris where this tissue is thinnest.

Iridodialysis

When the trauma is of considerable severity as from the direct blow by a stone, a ball or other flying object or from an explosion, the iris may be torn away from its insertion into the ciliary body to a greater or lesser extent (Fig. 23.9).

Clinical features: As follows.

A black linear crescentic slit at the periphery of the iris, through which the zonule and even the periphery of the lens and ciliary process may be visible and through which the vitreous may occasionally herniate.

D-shaped pupil: The papillary margin will be straightened at the site of the iridodialysis resulting in a D-shaped pupil [refer Fig. 23.9 (white arrow)].

This type of injury is accompanied by a hyphema of considerable size due to rupture of the large vessels supplying the iris. The deformity is permanent and the ciliary region atrophies. If the iridodialysis is large, uniocular diplopia will be a symptom. If visual confusion and diplopia distress the patient, operative measures may be indicated.

If the iridodialysis is very extensive, the detached portion sometimes becomes completely rotated, so that the pigmented back of the iris faces forward called anteflexion of the iris.

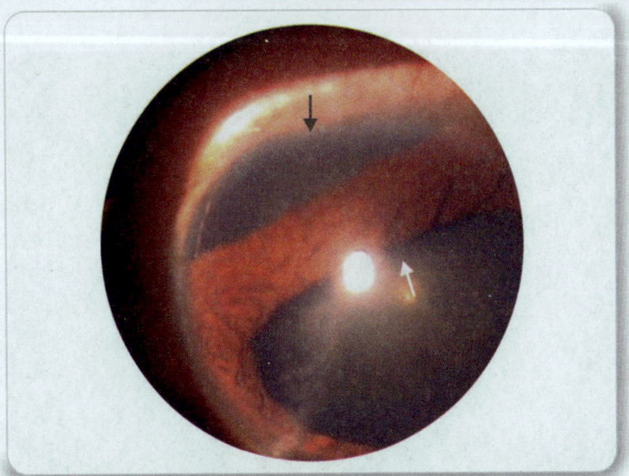

FIGURE 23.9: Iridodialysis (black arrow) with D-shaped pupil (white arrow)

Irideremia

The root of the iris is completely torn from its attachment, i.e. if the dialysis is complete, the condition of irideremia or traumatic aniridia results. It is completely detached and lies curled up into a little ball at the bottom of the anterior chamber where it eventually shrinks into a gray body.

Iridoschisis

A detachment of the anterior leaf of the mesodermal stroma of the iris from the deeper layers is a rare result of severe trauma.

The detached portion may float forward in the anterior chamber and may even simulate an anterior synechia.

Pigmentary Changes

Shortly after the injury, a powdering of uveal pigment on the surface of the iris, on the posterior surface of the cornea and on the anterior capsule of the lens is the rule. Following an atrophy of iris, the pigmentary layer may show an extensive ectropion, spreading widely over the anterior surface of the structure. Pigmentary change may occur as a long-term result of concussion injuries, partly due to migration of pigment and possibly new formation of pigment as a result of trauma or following iritis, i.e. the injured iris becomes darker than its follow—known as inverse heterochromia (hyperchromic), which is particularly evident in light-colored eyes.

CILIARY BODY

Dysfunction of the ciliary body may result in loss of the normal IOP. With the loss of IOP, phthisis invariably ensures, leading to a poor functional and cosmetic result.

Causes of Hypotony

Wound Leak

Wound leak is a common cause of hypotony after open globe injury. An anterior wound fistula may be detected using the Seidel test.

Posterior Scleral Rupture

B-scan ultrasonography is sometimes useful in identifying discontinuities in the posterior sclera. Leaking wounds must be surgically repaired because they have very low rate of spontaneous closure and have a significant risk for endophthalmitis.

Cyclodialysis

Cyclodialysis is separation of ciliary body from the sclera spur. Cyclodialysis creates free communication between the AC and the suprachoroidal space.

Presence of a cyclodialysis cleft should be suspected in any hypotonous eye that had recent surgery or trauma.

Diagnosis: The cleft between the ciliary body and the sclera spur can be identified by gonioscopy.

Ciliochoroidal Detachment

Ciliochoroidal detachment is commonly seen in presence of hypotony.

TRAUMATIC HYPHEMA

An accumulation of free blood in the anterior chamber is a common result of contusion (Figs 23.10A and B).

Primary Hyphema

Primary hyphema appears at the time of accident and it settles gravitationally, and varies in height from 1 to 2 mm to filling completely the anterior chamber. Such hemorrhages usually absorb rapidly and are particularly seen in case of children.

Secondary Hemorrhage

The picture may be complicated by the occurrence of a fresh bleeding usually on the 2nd or 3rd, or sometimes on the 4th or 5th post-traumatic day. The secondary type is seen most frequently in older patients.

Secondary hemorrhages tend to be more profuse than the primary hemorrhages.

Traumatic hyphema rapidly and permanently absorb in 1–7 days, leaving no trace, absorption is mainly through the anterior surface of the iris.

Complications

However, an iridocyclitis may develop with the formation of anterior and posterior synechiae. Secondary glaucoma is a complication, if the hemorrhage is massive.

When the hyphema is associated with rise in tension, development of blood staining of cornea is a permanent disability.

A long-term complication such as development of hematogenous pigmentation of the iris causes a heterochromia iridum wherein the iris of the injured eye becomes darker.

Treatment

A small hyphema gets absorbed by itself. Patient should be hospitalized and advised bed rest. Using mydriatics have is controversy. Since, absorption of blood is partly through the anterior surface of the iris, the greater the available surface, the more rapid is the process and mydriatics may retard this action. But, hyphema is associated with iritis and this warrants the use of mydriatics:

1. Patient should be hospitalized, advised bed rest and head end of the bed should bed elevated.
2. Place a shield over the involved eye, do not patch because this prevents recognition of sudden visual loss in the event of rebleed.

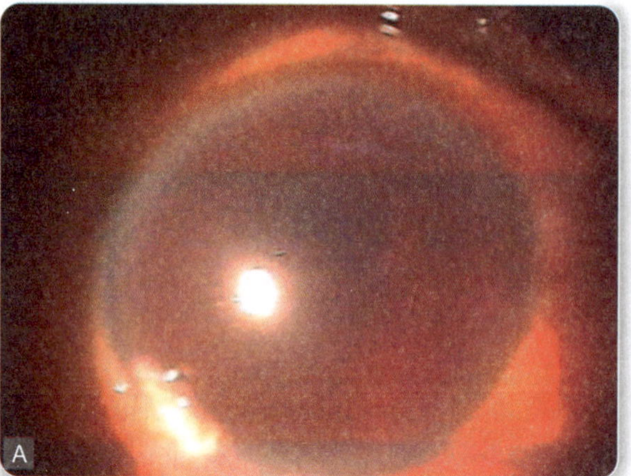

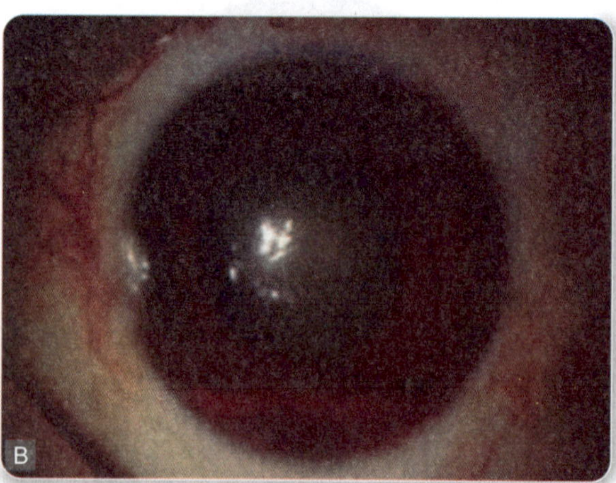

FIGURES 23.10A and B: Traumatic hyphema

3. Atropine 1% solution bid or tid to prevent contraction of ciliary body and pupil, and subsequent disruption of damaged blood vessels.
4. Use topical steroids to prevent iritis.
5. For increased IOP, start with a beta blocker, e.g. timolol, avoid prostaglandin analog and miotics since they may increase inflammation.

If topical therapy fails, add acetazolamide 20 mg/kg/day in divided dose/day or mannitol 1–2 g/kg intravenously over 45 minutes.

Surgical Measures

A controlled AC paracentesis is safe and this will remove blood from the AC as well as control the secondary glaucoma.

Indications for surgical evacuation of hyphema:

1. Corneal stromal blood staining.
2. Hyphema that does not decrease to less than 50% by 8 days [to prevent peripheral anterior synechiae (PAS)].
3. For IOP > 60 mm Hg for > 48 hours despite maximal medical therapy.
4. For IOP > 25 mm Hg with total hyphema for > 5 days (to prevent stromal blood staining).
5. For IOP of 24 mm Hg for > 24 hours (or any transient increase in IOP > 30 mm of Hg) in sickle cell trait/disease patients.

CONCUSSION EFFECTS ON THE LENS AND ZONULE

Vossius Ring

Vossius ring is an imprint of the pupillary border of iris upon the lens capsule corresponding to the extreme miosis, which develops on receipt of the injury. This annular deposition appears only in the young because the iris in the young possesses considerable elasticity to deposit the imprint and it serves as an indicator to prior blunt trauma.

Traumatic Cataract (Rosette-shaped Opacity or Stellate Cataract)

Two types of rosette-shaped opacity can follow trauma; those occurring very shortly after the injury (early rosette) and those appearing after sometime (late rosette).

Early Rosette

The early rosette opacity may appear sometimes in the anterior, sometimes in the posterior subcapsular region and sometimes in both region simultaneously, which appear within few hours, after the injury. In early rosette, the lines of opacity feather out from the suture, which themselves lie in the center of each petal (Fig. 23.11).

Late Rosette

Late rosette opacities are seen few years after the trauma and are usually found lying deep in the cortex or in the adult nucleus, separated from the capsule by a clear zone of varying thickness (Figs 23.12A to C).

In late concussion rosette; the lines of opacity feather out from the sutures in such a way that the petals are formed from adjacent suture, which themselves lie between the petals.

Subluxation and Dislocation of the Lens

In subluxation of lens, phacodonesis may be the initial clinical sign. Once the zonular attachment is damaged, lens become more spherical and myopic, sometimes astigmatism and impairment of accommodation is the visual result.

If the subluxation is greater, the lens may slip from its axial position and its equatorial edge may appear as a crescent in the pupillary aperture dividing it into phakic and aphakic parts and the AC will have unequal depth.

In complete traumatic luxation, the lens may follow different routes into the anterior chamber, the vitreous, the inter-retinal space, outside the eye if the globe is ruptured and comes to rest in the subconjunctival or Tenon's space.

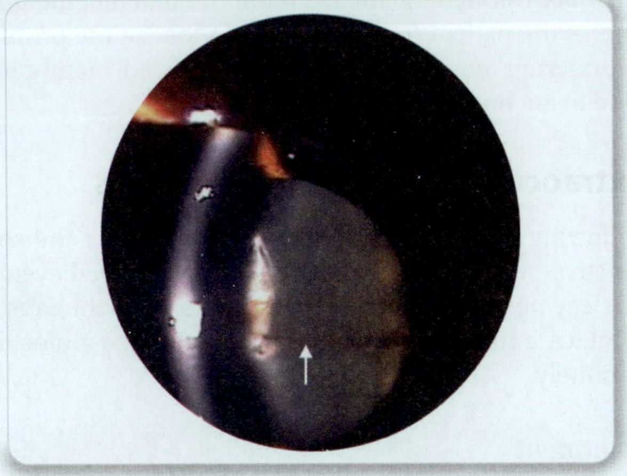

FIGURE 23.11: Traumatic cataract with capsular injury

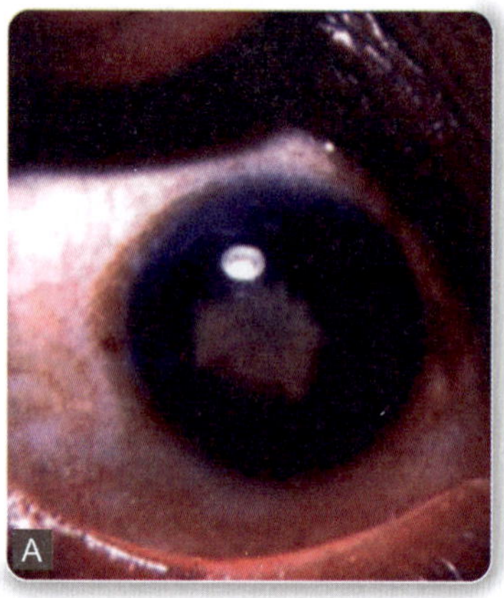

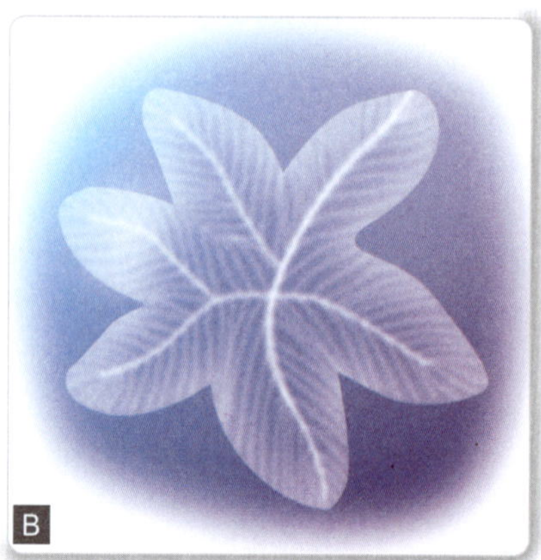

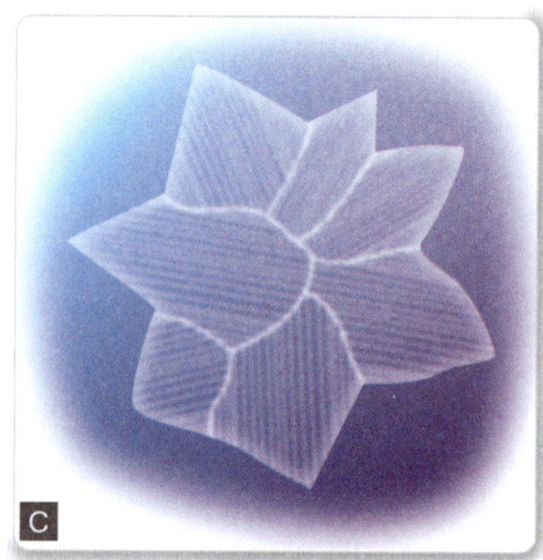

FIGURES 23.12A to C: Rosette cataract. **A.** Photograph; **B and C.** Diagrammatic representation of early and late rosette, respectively (*Courtesy:* Eye rounds online Atlas of Ophthalmology).

Dislocation into the Anterior Chamber

The lens lies in front of the iris as a transparent body, sometimes almost filling the anterior chamber, sometimes lying in its lower part with its rim showing a golden luster so that it resembles a large globule of oil in the aqueous with the pupil spasmodically contracted.

Complications

A sudden onset fulminating glaucoma due to pupillary block of an intractable iridocystitis and endothelial damage can follow in AC dislocation.

Dislocation into vitreous is twice as common as anterior dislocation. In this position of lens, eye may remain quiet, but severe iridocystitis and secondary glaucoma can occur.

At first, the lens is mobile in the vitreous (lens natans) and may even travel from the vitreous into the anterior chamber through the dilated pupil by changing the position of the patient from the prone to the supine position (wondering lens), but eventually organized membranes tend to anchor it (lens fixata).

Extraocular Dislocation of the Lens

Following rupture of globe, lens may lie under the conjunctiva (lenticule phacocele) and gets absorbed eventually leaving some by calcareous deposits. But if the capsule is intact, it may remain practically unattended almost indefinitely.

Treatment

A traumatic cataract is soft and can be aspirated through the large aspiration port of the phaco tip especially in a young patient. Ophthalmic viscosurgical device (OVD) tamponade of vitreous can be used for areas of zonular incompetence.

If vitreous has migrated into the anterior chamber, the surgeon should perform an anterior vitrectomy before starting phacoemulsification or cortical aspiration in order to avoid vitreous aspiration with resulting retinal traction.

If there is no enough capsular support to allow phacoemulsification, a capsular tension ring (CTR) can be inserted into the capsular bag. This device provides adequate support for nuclear and cortical removal, as well as for in-the-bag intraocular lens (IOL) insertion.

When the nucleus is markedly subluxed or dislocated and vitreous fills a substantial part of the anterior chamber, the surgeon should consider removing the lens through a pars plana approach.

An anterior chamber IOL or transclerally fixated posterior chamber lens may be necessary in case of inadequate capsular support for a posterior chamber lens.

Anterior dislocation of lens is an ophthalmic emergency and lens removal after medical control of secondary glaucoma is needed to prevent decompensation of cornea due to endothelial touch of the lens and permanent secondary glaucoma due to PAS.

Concussion Changes in the Vitreous

Changes in vitreous body after a concussion injury are disruption of the framework and liquefaction of gel (syneresis).

Vitreous hemorrhage following tearing of the retina with or without detachment.

Detachment of the vitreous and herniation of vitreous into anterior chamber.

CONCUSSION EFFECTS ON THE RETINA

Damage to the retina after concussive injuries to the globe, affecting particularly the macula and periphery is common.

Commotio Retinae (Berlin's Edema)

Clinical Features

A milky white area of transient cloudiness with an ill-defined margin extending over the posterior region of the fundus due to the development of retinal edema is a common sequel of concussions of the globe. It occupies a considerable area usually surrounding the optic disk and particularly always involving the macula, which shows a bright red spot in center in brilliant contrast to the gray back ground as cherry red spot. The cloudiness increases progressively for 24 hours after the injury, thereafter it slowly fades away. The central vision is lowered considerably and with the disappearance of edema, the vision may again become normal, but unfortunately the lesion may be followed by the appearance of pigmentary deposits, cystoids formation at the macula and even a hole. The macula is most frequently affected because of the richness of the underlying capillary network and because of the anatomical peculiarities of the structure of the retina in this region.

Traumatic Macular Cyst and Hole

Postcontusion necrosis may result in cystoid macular edema and the development of cystic space that coalesce to produce a large cyst. Rupture of inner layer of a larger macular cyst may produce a macular hole. If both the inner and outer walls of a macular cyst disappear a full thickness hole may develop.

Peripheral atrophic retinal changes seen after ocular concussion as localized retinal atrophic change as well as widespread change. These atrophic and pigmentary changes resemble those seen in myopia or congenital and acquired syphilis.

Diffuse Pigmentary Changes

The posterior region of the fundus is affected with migration of pigments. Sometimes pigments are fine and dust, and at other times it is corpuscular or arranged in clumps, being arranged without reference to blood vessels.

Vascular Change in Retina

Vascular lesions include hemorrhages, vascular occlusions and the formation of traumatic aneurysms.

Small hemorrhages from the retinal vessels, usually single, but sometimes multiple are common after ocular contusions. The most common are intraretinal hemorrhage usually small round extravasation in the outer retinal layers or flame-shaped extravasations in the nerve fiber layer, but preretinal hemorrhages either subhyaloid or extravasation into the vitreous are not unusual.

Traumatic Aneurysms

Traumatic aneurysms in the retina are rare sequel of contusion of the globe.

Peripheral Retinal Tears

Peripheral retinal tears are common source of post- traumatic retinal detachment. These tears tend to be large, more irregular and located at the site of direct ocular contusion. They can subsequently lead to retinal detachment for a variable period after the trauma.

In most cases, contusion related retinal tears are located inferotemporally, probably because the bony orbit affords less protection at this location.

Retinal Dialysis

Retinal dialysis is defined as a break or separation occurring at the anterior edge of the ora serrata. Retinal dialysis is the most frequent traumatic retinal break. It almost always occurs at the time of the injury. The most common location is the inferior temporal quadrant.

CONTUSION EFFECTS ON THE CHOROID

Choroidal Hemorrhage

Hemorrhages in the choroid are frequent sequel of injuries. It appears as a rounded dark blotch with blurred edges over which the retinal vessels course. It slowly tends to absorb leaving considerable pigmentation and usually some degree of atrophy.

Rupture of Choroid

The choroid is prone to rupture from the effects of blunt trauma applied to the globe and the rupture may occur directly at the site of application of the force or indirectly on the opposite side of the globe. The choroid is susceptible to rupture because of the inelastic characteristic of Bruch's membrane (Fig. 23.13).

Direct Rupture of the Choroid

A large, broad and usually irregular lesion lies near the periphery exposing the white sclera, bordered initially by hemorrhage and eventually by heavy pigmentary changes.

Indirect Rupture of the Choroid

Indirect rupture of the choroid is more common and initial appearance is usually obscured by hemorrhages. When multiple tears occur, the central one is usually the largest and the most peripheral smallest.

The rupture is usually crescentic in shape and runs concentrically with the margin of the disk. As a rule, it is broadest in its middle and narrows toward each end. Over the rupture, the retina usually remains structurally intact and the vessels course over the rent in the choroid without any break in their continuity. When choroidal rupture is accompanied by retinal rupture it is called retinitis sclopetaria or chorioretinitis sclopetaria, or chorioretinitis plastic sclopetaria.

Eventually the overlying retina becomes atrophic and degenerated showing neuroglial proliferation, wandering of pigment and the new formation of vessels. After sometime it becomes adherent to and is incorporated in the fibrous tissue, which fills the gap in the choroid.

Traumatic Choroiditis

Lesions may be small and discrete, round or oval and sharply defined or they may be diffused and widespread, assuming the irregular and map-like shapes and are always associated with a considerable degree of pigmentary proliferation and subsequent atrophy.

Ciliochoroidal detachment (Fig. 23.14) is commonly seen in presence of hypotony.

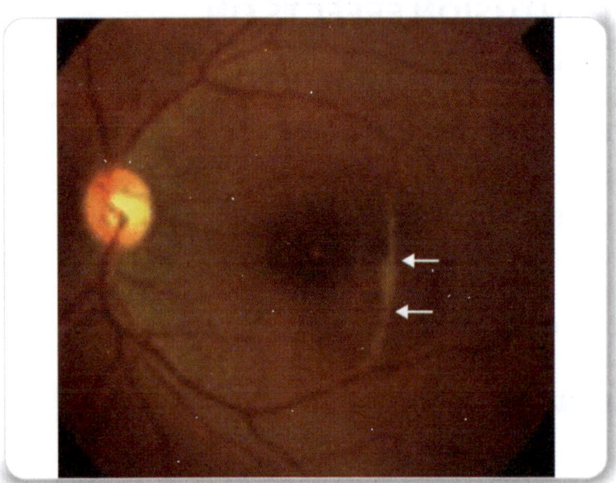

FIGURE 23.13: Choroidal rupture

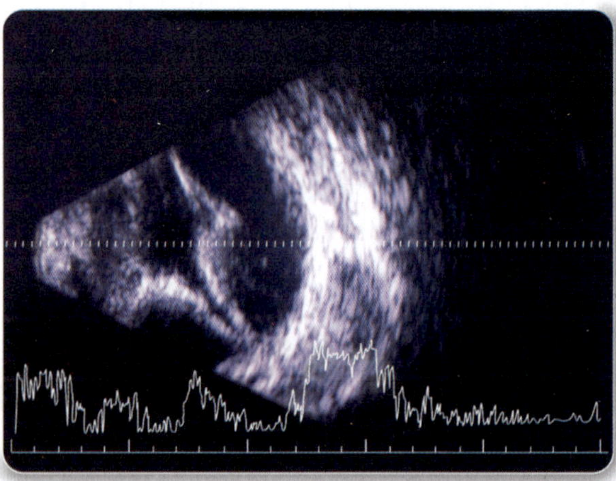

FIGURE 23.14: B-scan choroidal detachment

CONCUSSION EFFECTS AT THE OPTIC DISK

Papillitis: Causing considerable swelling of the disk may be associated with ocular contusion.

Optic atrophy: It may be a sequel to widespread retinal or choroidal damage.

Rupture and Avulsion of the Optic Nerve

The most common cause of a rupture and avulsion of the optic nerve is a penetrating injury of the orbit.

CONCUSSION EFFECTS ON REFRACTION

Traumatic Hypermetropia

Traumatic hypermetropia causes are paralysis of accommodation due to an injury of the ciliary nerves or in more severe cases to organic lesions in the ciliary muscles, raising of retina with organized material after a rupture of the choroid or posterior dislocation of the lens with an increased depth of the anterior chamber.

Traumatic Myopia

Traumatic myopia is the commonest refractive change following a concussion injury. An increase in myopia of

1D–6D can occur and starts disappearing within a week or two and becomes normal within a month.

Ciliary Spasm

Ciliary spasm can occur in majority of cases due to irritation of muscle fibers or the III nerve, sometimes to paresis of cervical sympathetic.

Damage to the Suspensory Apparatus

Damage to the suspensory apparatus of the lens cause an increase in lenticular curvature. If the zonules are ruptured and the lens remain in the place, the myopia may amount from 5D to 6D and be permanent, while a higher degree may be caused by an anterior dislocation of lens.

TRAUMATIC GLAUCOMA

Glaucoma Associated with Closed Globe

Glaucoma associated with closed globe injuries are:
- Early onset
- Delayed onset.

Early-onset Traumatic Glaucoma

Early-onset traumatic glaucoma is due to inflammation, trabecular meshwork disruption and hyphema.

Inflammation: It can induce high IOP due to outflow obstruction by the inflammatory debris, cells or protein in the anterior chamber and possibly due to inflammation at the trabecular meshwork. Inflammation is usually self-limiting and close monitoring along with aqueous suppressants, topical steroids and cycloplegic should be used.

Trabecular meshwork rupture: The meshwork can be superficial or full thickness. Gonioscopy is the most useful technique for diagnosis.

Hyphema: It is caused by the tear in the iris root and bleeding from the small branches of the arterial circle of the iris. High IOP results from RBC obstruction, inflammation and disruption of the outflow pathway.

Delayed-onset Glaucoma

Delayed-onset glaucoma include angle recession, ghost cell, hemolytic, hemosiderotic, lens subluxation, phacomorphic, lens particle and lens induced.

Angle recession: In the presence of hyphema, angle recession is found in 71%–100% of eyes. Only 7%–9% patients with angle recession develop glaucoma. Risk of development is greater, if more than 180°–240° are affected. Increased outflow resistance is caused by either growth of membrane covering the angle or scarring. Gonioscopic examination shows broad ciliary body band, torn iris processes and an abnormally white scleral spur.

Ghost cell glaucoma: In the presence of vitreous hemorrhage, ghost cell glaucoma develops within 1–3 weeks post injury. It is caused by old and degenerated RBCs obstructing the aqueous outflow pathway because they are more rigid to pass through.

Hemolytic glaucoma: It occurs after several days to weeks of intraocular hemorrhage produced by hemoglobin laden macrophages, free hemoglobin remnants of lysed RBCs and clogging the trabecular meshwork.

Hemosiderotic glaucoma: Tissues of eye-like trabecular meshwork, endothelial cells absorb iron liberated from the lysed RBCs. If the normal ferritin-apoferritin system is saturated, toxic granules of inorganic iron accumulates within the cells and cause hemosiderosis and obliteration of intertrabecular spaces.

It is a rare condition associated with prolonged history of intraocular bleed.

Lens related glaucoma: Injury to zonules result in subluxation or dislocation. In anterior displacement, lens may cause papillary block and result in reduced visual acuity, myopia, closed angle on gonioscopy. Treatment is relieving the pupillary block by removal of subluxated lens.

In posterior displacement, pupillary block by vitreous occur leading to secondary glaucoma.

Phacomorphic glaucoma: There will be swelling of lens due to disruption of lens capsule leading to rapid hydration of lens and pupillary block or angle block result. The clinical features are irregular AC, dense cataract and increased lens thickness measured by a scan compared to the follow eye. Treatment is cataract extraction.

Lens particle glaucoma: Lens particle released into AC obstruct trabecular meshwork and cause glaucoma. It is commonly seen in open globe injury.

Glaucoma Associated with Open Globe Injury

Inflammation Glaucoma

Inflammatory cells may block the trabecular meshwork and peripheral anterior synechia.

Flat Anterior Chamber

Aqueous loss may cause flat anterior chamber. Prolonged flat anterior chamber leads to peripheral anterior synechia and angle closure. Prevention is the best option by meticulous wound reconstruction, intraoperative reformation of anterior chamber and postoperative mydriasis and topical steroids.

Epithelial Down Growth

Epithelial down growth is caused by epithelial or fibrous down growth due to delayed or improper wound repair resulting in obliteration of trabecular meshwork.

Associated with IOFB

Iron foreign body leads to siderotic glaucoma, copper foreign body leads to tissue damage due to aseptic inflammation.

EXTRAOCULAR FOREIGN BODIES

The most common accident in ophthalmology is retention of foreign body on the surface of eye. Common foreign bodies, which enter eye are pieces of metal and stone, in industrial workers, while husks, pieces of straw, grain, thorns, leaves, insects or their wings are common in agricultural surroundings.

Foreign bodies particularly if sharp and metallic and travelling at high speed, get embedded themselves more deeply in the tissues of the cornea or the episclera or sclera, while others with sufficient momentum penetrate the coats of the eye and enter the globe (Fig. 23.15).

If the cornea is affected by a superficial foreign body, symptoms present as sharp burning pain, reflex gush of tears with momentary blindness and the lids close in blepharospasm. On the other hand, if particles penetrate deeply and remain impacted or perforate the globe, less symptoms are produced. In all these cases there is evidence of uveal irritation as shown by circumcorneal injection and miosis.

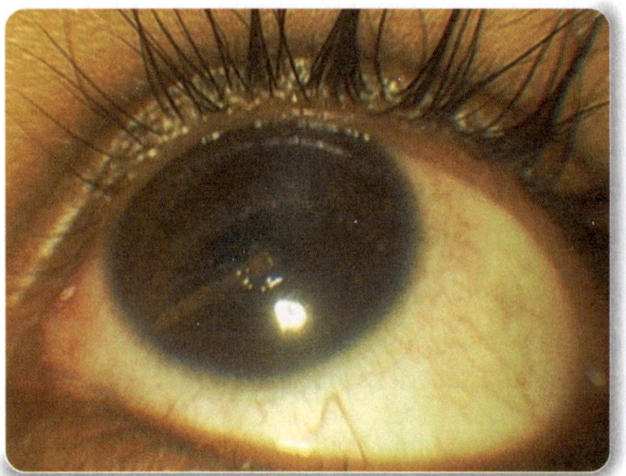

FIGURE 23.15: Corneal foreign body penetrating into the anterior chamber

In any case with corneal abrasion in the upper half of cornea, the upper lid has to be everted and examined for the presence of any foreign body.

In the conjunctiva, sharp gritty particles adherent to the inner surface of the upper lid, particularly those lying in the subtarsal fold, continuously abrade the cornea in the movements of blinking and cause symptoms more severe than results from those impacted on the corneal surface.

In the sclera, the impaction of foreign bodies is rare. They are usually found in the palpebral aperture.

Complication of Extraocular Foreign Bodies

Important complications of extraocular foreign bodies are the introduction of infection at the time of the injury, the formation of corneal ulcers leading to corneal opacity and traumatic implantation cyst.

Treatment of Extraocular Foreign Bodies

Superficial Foreign Bodies

A superficial foreign body is removed by a moist cotton-tipped applicator after putting topical anesthesia.

Embedded foreign bodies: Removed with ordinary stainless steel hypodermic needle supported on the syringe.

Deeply embedded foreign bodies: Removal of deeply embedded foreign bodies should be undertaken in the operating theater as a major surgical procedure. Severe complications such as corneal perforation and pushing of the particle into the anterior chamber should be anticipated and managed immediately.

Intraocular Foreign Bodies

Intraocular foreign bodies (IOFBs) are common problem in ocular injuries. IOFB most commonly affect young men, while hammering, shooting a shot gun, witnessing an explosion or using a machine tool. The majority occur in the workplace.

Retained IOFB represents a true emergency and can lead to severe vision loss caused by endophthalmitis, retinal detachment and metallosis and even loss of the eye despite the best efforts at treatment. Visual prognosis is best when the IOFB is removed during the initial wound repair surgery or as soon as possible.

The majority of IOFBs are small, sharp projectile produced in hammering metal or stone, up to 90% of IOFBs are metallic and 55%–80% of these are magnetic. Most frequently they enter the eye through the cornea (65%). Other common locations include the sclera (25%) and the limbus (10%). The IOFBs most frequently lodges in the vitreous cavity (Fig. 23.16) (61%), but can also be located within the anterior chamber (Fig. 23.17) (15%), retina (14%), lens (8%) or subretinal space (5%).

Clinical Features

The presence of an IOFB is to be suspected in any penetrating injury until it is excluded by investigations like CT, MRI, etc. The probabilities are high in injuries caused due to breaking stones with a metallic hammer. An IOFB has to be suspected if there is a through wound track in the cornea or iris.

Management

Investigations such as CT, MRI and X-ray of skull has to be done to confirm the presence as well as to locate the exact site of the foreign body.

Management of an IOFB injury requires immediate closure of the globe and removal of IOFB. Delay in removal of IOFB for more than 24 hours in primary repair and delay in IOFB removal, produces a 4-fold increase in the risk of endophthalmitis and severe vision loss.

Timing of IOFB removal depends on the factor such as; size of foreign body, amount of intraocular reaction, material of the IOFB on duration between injury and reporting time.

Treatment Methods

If a small magnetic IOFB, clear media, easily accessible anterior location and no associated ocular damage, then primary magnetic extraction is done.

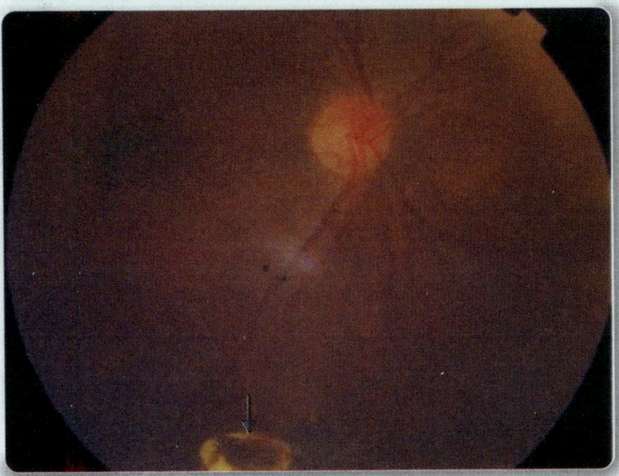

FIGURE 23.16: Intraocular foreign body in the vitreous

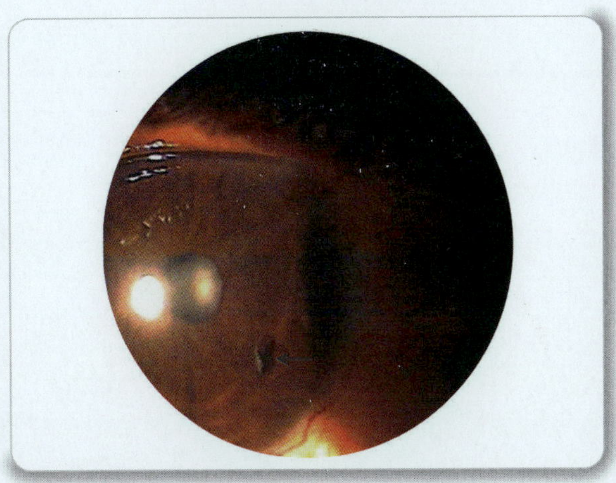

FIGURE 23.17: Intraocular foreign body in the anterior chamber (black arrow)

A pars plana vitrectomy is indicated in case of opaque media, associated retinal detachment or vitreous hemorrhage, endophthalmitis, non-magnetic foreign body, incarcerated foreign body and failed magnetic extraction.

Complication

Complications of IOFB injuries include endophthalmitis, retinal detachment with proliferative vitreoretinopathy, siderosis bulbi and chalcosis.

Siderosis

Siderosis is a tissue reaction caused by a retained iron foreign body. Electrolytic dissociation of iron and combination with tissue proteins result in cellular death (Fig. 23.18).

There will be gradual loss of vision due to development of secondary glaucoma and retinal atrophy if the iron foreign body is not removed.

The iris will take a rusty brown color and this discoloration is often the first indication that the eye is harboring an iron foreign body (Fig. 23.19). The lens will also show rusty brown discoloration and slowly turn cataractous. The retina will show retinitis pigmentosa like changes. There will be gradually rise in IOP and the eye will slowly become blind, if left untreated.

TRAUMATIC ENDOPHTHALMITIS

Endophthalmitis following intraocular trauma is different from other forms of endophthalmitis because of several reasons. Firstly disorganization of the normal anatomy due to trauma may cause difficulty in assessing

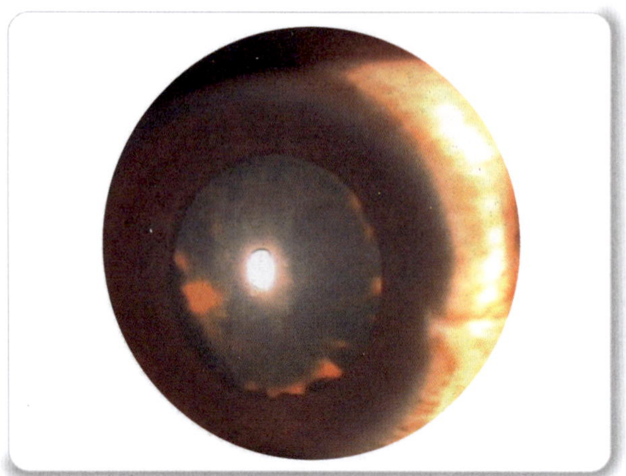

FIGURE 23.18: Siderosis bulbi

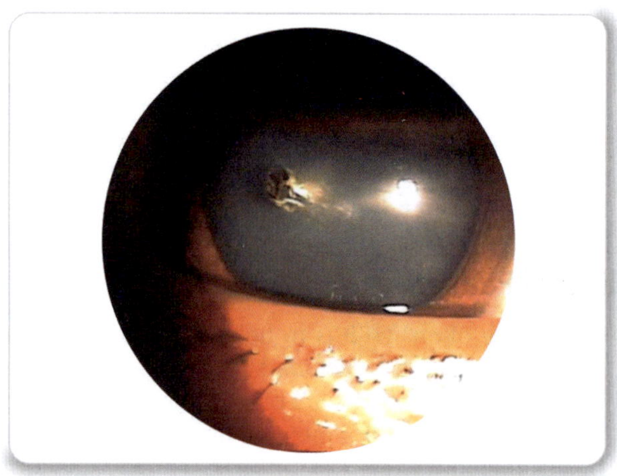

FIGURE 23.19: Foreign body in the lens

the clinical features and in making an accurate diagnosis in early stage. Secondly, the organism producing the infection is more virulent. Thirdly, the protocol for management remains ill defined (Fig. 23.20).

Ocular trauma has been reported to contribute 17%–40% of all cases of culture positive endophthalmitis.

Onset of endophthalmitis is about 1–2 days in fulminant cases caused by *Bacillus cereus* and streptococci, 3–4 days in acute cases caused by *Staphylococcus epidermidis* and gram-negative organisms and about 5–7 days for chronic endophthalmitis caused by fungi.

Infection caused by *Bacillus cereus* is characteristic, usually there is a history of trauma with a metallic foreign body lodged within the eye. The patient develops severe orbital pain within 24 hours of the injury and this is associated with a significant proptosis, chemosis and periorbital inflammation. A corneal ring infiltrates and ring abscess occur frequently. Most patients become febrile with a moderate polymorphonuclear leukocytes. The only other endophthalmitis producing organism capable of causing similar constitutional symptoms is *Clostridium.*

Collection of intraocular samples for laboratory investigations is necessary as in cases of postsurgical endophthalmitis. The procedures adopted are paracentesis, vitreous aspiration and vitreous biopsy.

Treatment should not be delayed for want of diagnostic specimens, start systemic antibiotics (e.g. ciprofloxacin, 400 mg IV12 hourly and cefazolin, 1 g IV qid).

Topical antibiotics (e.g. fortified gentamicin and fortified cefazolin or fortified vancomycin 1 hourly).

Intravitreal antibiotics (e.g. amikacin 0.4 mg in 0.1 mL and vancomycin 1 mg in 0.1 mL or clindamycin 1 mg in 0.1 mL) these may be repeated every 48–72 hours as needed.

The benefit of pars plana vitrectomy is unknown for traumatic endophthalmitis. However pars plana vitrectomy reduces infectious load and provide sufficient material for diagnostic culture and pathologic investigation.

Early vitrectomy has been advocated in all cases with retained IOFB. Steroids should not be used until fungal organisms are ruled out.

FRACTURES OF THE ORBIT

Most of the serious injuries of the ocular adnexa involve fractures in the region of the orbit. Common causes for fracture of the orbit are fall from a height, road traffic accidents and blow with a fist. High incidence of multiple and serious injuries is associated with head and facial trauma has been noted. So as a general rule immediate examination of all systems are necessary.

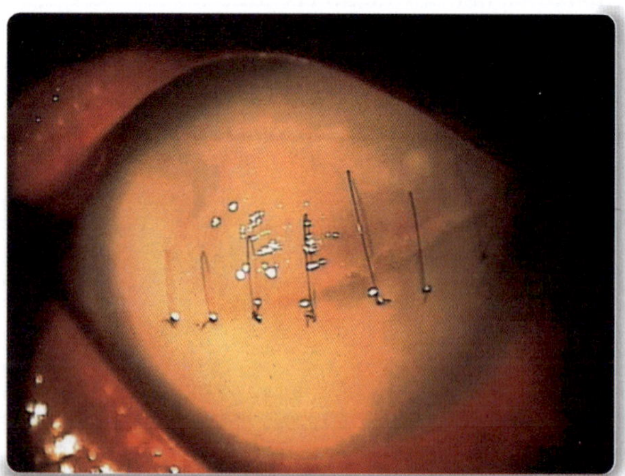

FIGURE 23.20: Traumatic endophthalmitis following penetrating injury

From the ophthalmological point of view injuries may be divided into two types: direct and indirect. Direct injury is due to blunt violence falling directly upon the orbit and the indirect injury results from an involvement of the orbital bones, in a radiating fracture of the vault of the skull or the bones of the face.

Blow Out Fractures (Fig. 23.21)

Blow out fractures result from a sudden increase in intraorbital pressure, secondary to a blow to the eye and soft tissues of the orbit from a non-penetrating convex object such as Tennis ball, a fist or other bodies of greater diameter than the orbital margins.

The tissue of the orbit is suddenly compressed and the increased pressure is transmitted to the walls of which the more delicate portions are fractured and blown outwards. Floor is the usual site of fracture, bony fragments and orbital soft tissue may be displaced downwards into the maxillary antrum, usually giving rise to a hemorrhage. Sometimes blow out fractures involve the medial orbital wall in the area of the lamina papyracea and the orbital plate of the ethmoid, resulting in the medial displacement of the bony fragments and orbital soft tissue with local hemorrhage in the plane of the ethmoid air cells (Fig. 23.22).

Clinical Picture

Displacement of Globe

Either proptosis due to intraorbital hemorrhage or exophthalmos due to fracture of floor with herniation of orbital contents into the maxillary antrum or nasal cavity, or vertical displacement that may be upward by the presence of bony fragments in the orbit, downward due to loss of supporting action of the ligament of Lockwood, which stretches like a hammock from the medial to the lateral bony margins of the orbit. When the exophthalmos is gross following downward displacement of orbital contents, a pseudoptosis of the upper lid and deepening of the supratarsal fold will occur.

Diplopia

Usually due to restriction of vertical movements and main factors responsible are incarceration within the fracture-line of the extraocular soft tissues, particularly inferior rectus and oblique muscles, displacement of the suspensory ligament of Lockwood, the periorbital, the muscle sheaths and their connections. While in fracture of medial wall, the medial rectus muscle and its sheath get involved resulting in limitation of horizontal movement of the globe.

Forced Duction Test

The muscle is gently grasped with a forcep after anesthetizing the eye and the eye is moved in the direction of action of the muscle. There will be limitation of movement if there is entrapment of the muscles in the fracture. Inferior rectus is usually involved due to its midline position over the infraorbital canal where such fractures most frequently occur, but as there is some fibrous connection between the inferior rectus and inferior oblique muscle both muscles are usually affected.

Sensory Loss

Infraorbital anesthesia over to the region of skin and oral mucosa supplied by the infraorbital nerve support

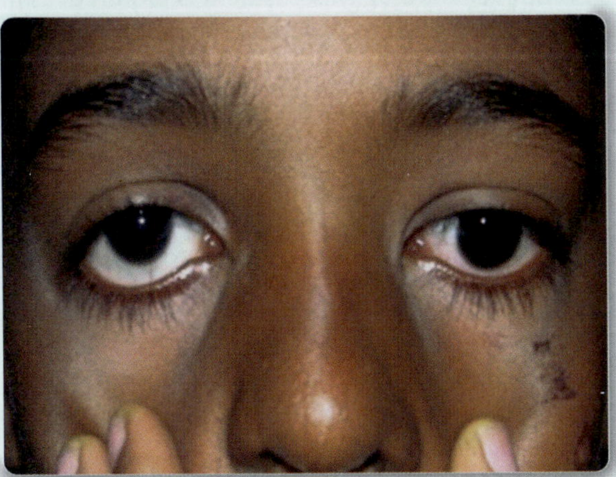

FIGURE 23.21: Movement of left eyeball is restricted on elevation

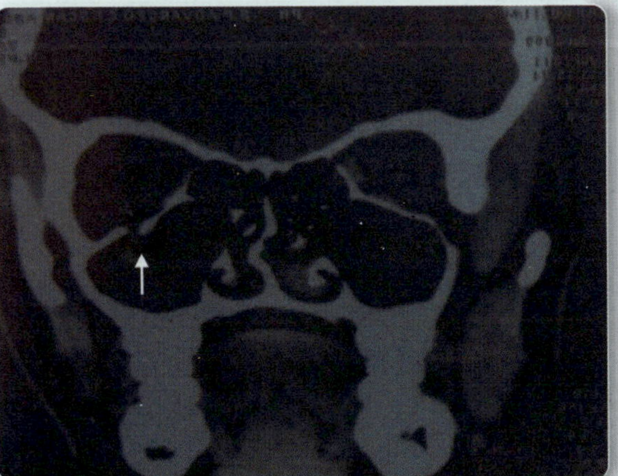

FIGURE 23.22: Coronal cut CT showing orbital floor fracture with soft tissue entrapment

a fracture in the central part of the floor of the orbit. The absence of such sensory loss in the presence of other signs of fracture of the orbital floor indicates that the injury may be either medial or lateral to the infraorbital canal. In case of lateral orbital floor fracture sensory loss occur in the distribution of the zygomatic nerve.

Epistaxis

Epistaxis occurs in nasomaxillary injury or a fracture of medial orbital wall.

Cerebrospinal Rhinorrhea

Clear watery discharge from the nose or ear following an injury to the head indicates that a communication exists between the subarachnoid space and the exterior. In all such cases the advice of a neurosurgeon should be sought at an early stage.

Management

Antibiotics and anti-inflammatory drugs are given to control the inflammation and to prevent infection.

If there is significant diplopia and exophthalmos, surgery is indicated. The periosteum is elevated from the floor of the orbit and all entrapped orbital contents are separated and the defect in the bone is repaired using silicone or teflon mesh.

TRAUMATIC OPTIC NEUROPATHY

Trauma may affect any segment of visual pathway. Optic nerve is about 47–50 mm in length and can be divided into four parts as intraocular (1 mm), intraorbital (30 mm), intracanalicular (6–9 mm) and intracranial (10 mm).

The intracanalicular part is the most vulnerable to external blunt trauma. It is immobilized in the canal, which is fixed to the surrounding periosteum and bone.

Intraorbital optic nerve injury rarely occurs because of the laxity of the optic nerve in this area and is cushioned by surrounding orbital fat. Intracranial optic nerve is rarely damaged indirectly due to its mobility within the cranium and it is cushioned by the surrounding cerebrospinal fluid.

Classification

Traumatic optic neuropathy can be classified into three types:

1. Optic nerve avulsion where the optic nerve is partially or completely separated from the globe.
2. Direct injury caused by the impact on the optic nerve or nerve sheath from a penetrating foreign body, a displaced bone fragment or a retro-orbital hematoma.
3. Indirect injury, here forces are transmitted to the optic nerve within the optic canal.

Optic Nerve Avulsion

Visual acuity is reduced to a variable degree in partial avulsion. In total avulsion, the vision is reduced to no perception of light. The fundus changes with time. Immediately after the injury, the disk is often obscured by overlying vitreous hemorrhage. Overtime in cases of total avulsion the sclera canal is seen devoid of optic disk and this defect is gradually filled with glial tissue, which may extend into the vitreous. Associated ocular finding include dilated and amaurotic pupil.

Visual acuity ranges from a minimal decline to no perception of light.

Apart from defective vision, signs include relative afferent papillary defect, defective color vision and field defect. Disk pallor develops within 3–4 weeks after injury.

Electrophysiology

The VEP may be used to document conduction delays in comatose patients and the initial VEP may correlate with the final visual acuity.

High resolution CT: Both the coronal and axial cuts should be performed to detect facial and optic canal fractures.

MRI: Although inferior to CT in the detection of bone defects, MRI is an adjunct to CT in imaging the intracranial segment of the optic nerve for disruption or hematoma.

Complete neurologic assessment is required, as many of these patients have associated brain injuries.

Management

Medical therapies with intravenous high dose of corticosteroids have been reported to be effective in some cases. Methylprednisolone 20–30 mg/kg/day or dexamethasone 3–5 mg/kg/day. Treatment should be instituted within 24–48 hours and if improvement occurs, oral steroid therapy can be started and tapered off over the next 2 weeks.

If an obvious compressive lesion is present on imaging studies (e.g. bone fragment, hematoma) decompression should be considered.

If there is no visual impairment within 48 hours or the patient's vision worsens despite steroids, optic nerve decompression should be considered.

Optic Canal Decompression

Decompression of optic nerve within the optic canal may be performed through various approaches (e.g. transcranial, transorbital, transethmoidal). The goal of surgery is to reverse any component of compression (edema, hematoma, bone fragment) of the intracanalicular portion of the optic nerve.

Optic Nerve Sheath Decompression

The goal of surgery is to decompress the orbital portion of the optic nerve.

SYMPATHETIC OPHTHALMIA

Sympathetic ophthalmia is a rare, bilateral diffuse granulomatous uveitis that presents insidiously after open globe injury or surgery. The injured eye is known as the exciting eye and the follow eye developing inflammation weeks to years later known as the sympathizing eye.

Incidence

The exact figures are difficult to ascertain due to delayed presentation, lack of histopathological confirmation in clinical sympathetic ophthalmitis and absence of clinical evidence in histopathologically positive cases of sympathetic ophthalmitis. Due to meticulous suturing techniques, prompt repair of corneoscleral wounds and use of steroids, the incidence of sympathetic ophthalmitis is now reduced drastically.

Clinical Features

The average onset is 3 months after injury. About 90% occurs in 1 year, but can occur as early as 2 weeks and as late as 50 years. Onset is never earlier than 2 weeks since this is a hypersensitivity reaction.

The clinical features comprises of a spectrum ranging from mild to severe. The patient first seeks advice for photophobia and lacrimation or transient defective near vision due to weakness of accommodation in the uninjured eye.

The first sign may be the presence of keratic precipitates on the back of the cornea or the presence of retrolenticular flare and cells, which are noticed at early stage.

Typical features are granulomatous bilateral uveitis, mutton fat keratic precipitates (KPs), vitreous cells, yellow-white choroidal infiltrates and Dalen-Fuchs nodules.

The exiting eye may show traces of old iridocyclitis and still possess useful vision or may have shrunken completely.

The B scan often reveals choroidal thickening, fluorescein angiography shows early hyperfluorescent sites of choroidal leakage. Indocyanine green is an important additional test and shows multifocal hypofluorescent dots, which become prominent with time.

Differential Diagnosis

- Phacoanaphylactic endophthalmitis
- Vogt-Koyanagi-Harada syndrome: Absence of history of trauma/surgery.

Histopathology

- Diffuse granulomatous infiltrates throughout uveal tissue
- Dalen-Fuchs nodules: These are epithelial granulomas seen between the Bruch's membrane and the retinal pigment epithelium
- Choroidal thickening
- Absence of uveal necrosis
- Choriocapillaris and retina being spared
- Immunohistochemical studies show histolytic cells with degenerating retinal pigmented epithelium (RPE) cells and lymphocytes
- Predominant CD4 in early stage and CD8 lymphocytes evident in late stage.

Etiopathogenesis

Sympathetic ophthalmia is an autoimmune disorder. Release of uveoretinal antigen following penetrating injury exposes it to conjunctiva. It is then processed through the lymphatic channels, which act as immune stimulants. The normal suppressor mechanism is bypassed and an autoimmune uveitis results in genetically susceptible individuals. Genetic predisposition to sympathetic ophthalmia is evidenced by increased frequency of human lymphocytic antigen-A11 (HLA-A11) in histologically proven sympathetic ophthalmitis.

Prevention

The best way to prevent sympathetic ophthalmia is early enucleation of a badly damaged eye before the sensitization occurs. But the decision to enucleate an eye is difficult and controversial. The need to remove a traumatized eye is very remote in present times. Other measures include meticulous and prompt closure of corneoscleral wounds, trauma to uveal tissue should be minimized and prolapsed tissue should be excised or reposited. The role of prophylactic steroids is controversial.

Management

Early detection and prompt initiation of high-dose steroids holds the key to a good outcome.

Topical steroids and mydriatics can be used to control anterior uveitis. Systemic corticosteroids in high doses, at least 1–1.5 mg/kg of prednisolone should be promptly commenced, followed by a slow taper to a maintenance dose for several months, up to at least a year.

Treatment may sometimes be commenced with pulsed steroids, three infusions of intravenous methylprednisolone 1 g over 3 days, followed by oral steroids. Relapse has been noted commonly on taper of corticosteroids.

Other Immunomodulators

Cyclosporine has been used as a second line drug in the treatment of sympathetic ophthalmia in case with poor response to corticosteroids. Cyclosporine 5 mg/kg/day helps in inhibition of T-cell production in this T-cell mediated disease. Other agents used in addition to steroids include Azathioprine, Methotrexate and Chlorambucil with varying success.

Outcome

Early diagnosis and aggressive therapy are correlated directly with better visual outcome. Other causes of poor vision include glaucoma, cataract, macular scarring, cystoids macular edema. Due to relapsing nature of this disease, long-term follow-up is required, even in patients who are symptom free for years.

After resolution the fundus may appear normal, but pigment migration and optic atrophy can occur.

Section 5

Diseases of the Adnexa

Lids

24

Girija Devi PS, Lekshmi P Moorthi

The lids are the movable folds provided in front of the eye. Their main function is protection of the eyeball, a mere touch or even a loud noise will cause reflex closure of the lids. The lid movements are essential to spread the tears over the eyeball and also to wash away any dust, foreign bodies, debris, etc. into the lacrimal sac by the action of the lid closure. Unknowingly, the eyes are continuously washed with tears by the lid movements.

APPLIED ANATOMY

The lids are covered by skin in front and mucous membrane behind (Fig. 24.1). The junction between the skin and the mucous membrane is the 'intermarginal strip' the transitional zone lining the lid margins. In between the skin and the mucous membrane there are muscles, the fibrous plate called tarsus, the blood vessels and nerves. The detailed anatomy is described in Section 1 'Anatomy and Physiology of the Eye'.

The skin of the lids has many anatomical peculiarities. It is the thinnest in the body and it has no subcutaneous fat. Being very elastic and loosely attached to the underlying structures, it can get easily distended with fluid or blood, which can gravitate to it from the scalp or neighboring structures.

It has fine hairs and it is well lubricated with fine sebaceous glands, but has only small sweat glands. At the lid margin these structures undergo modification. The hair is modified into eyelashes—curved short strong hairs usually in two or more rows. The sebaceous glands supplying these eyelashes are also suitably modified to form the Zeis' glands. The sweat glands are also modified into large glands at the lid margin to form the Moll's glands. The ducts of the Moll's glands open into the hair follicles of the lashes or into the ducts of the Zeis' glands. The fibrous tissue near the lid margin is strong and almost like cartilage. This is called tarsal plate. The tarsal plates contain vertically arranged large sebaceous glands called meibomian glands or tarsal glands. Their ducts open along a straight line at the lid margin.

There is a fine gray line immediately anterior to the openings of the meibomian glands. This is an important anatomical landmark of the lids. The lids can be split into two layers at the gray line—the anterior and posterior lamellae.

The anterior lamella consists of the skin and orbicularis muscle. The posterior lamella consists of the tarsal plate, conjunctiva and the eyelid retractors. The eyelid retractor in the upper lid is the levator palpebrae superioris. The lower lid retractor is a fascia extending from the inferior rectus muscle, which splits to enclose the inferior oblique muscle and then reunite to form a fibrous sheet, which attaches to the inferior border of the tarsal plate.

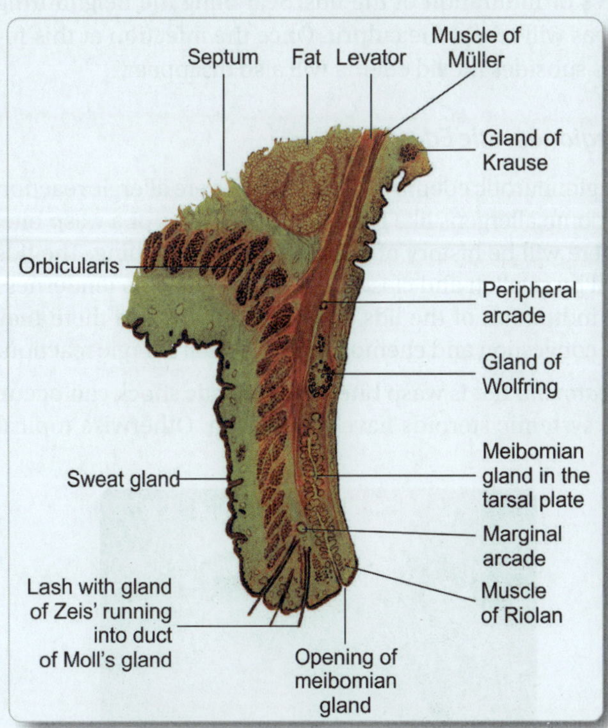

FIGURE 24.1: Anatomy of upper lid

The lids are richly supplied by blood vessels. Hence wounds of the lids heal well even if heavily contaminated. Even small tags of tissue, however devitalized it may appear, will survive and no tissue of the lid need be sacrificed in repair of lacerated wounds of lids.

DISEASES OF THE LIDS

Lid Edema

Since the skin of the lids is very elastic and loosely attached to the underlying tissue, fluid can easily collect in the lid. Many conditions can lead to lid edema.

Inflammatory Lid Edema

Edema of the lids is common in any inflammation of the lids, adnexa or eyeball. The extent of edema depends on the severity of the inflammation.

Reactionary Lid Edema

In any inflammation of the surrounding structures like an infected wound on the scalp or a boil on the forehead a reactionary lid edema can occur. The lids may get so swollen that it is difficult to examine the eyeball. But on retracting the lids, the eye will be normal. There will be no tenderness or induration of the lids. Searching the neighboring areas will reveal the culprit. Once the infection at this focus subsides the lid edema will also disappear.

Angioneurotic Edema

Angioneurotic edema (Fig. 24.2) is a severe allergic reaction to some allergens like medicines, cosmetics or a wasp bite. There will be history of sudden onset and itching. The lids will be swollen and closed, but there will be no tenderness or induration of the lids. On retracting the lids there may be congestion and chemosis, if it is a local allergic reaction.

Treatment: If it is wasp bite, anaphylactic shock can occur. So systemic steroids have to be given. Otherwise topical steroids and/or antihistamines and removal of the offending allergen are sufficient to control the problem.

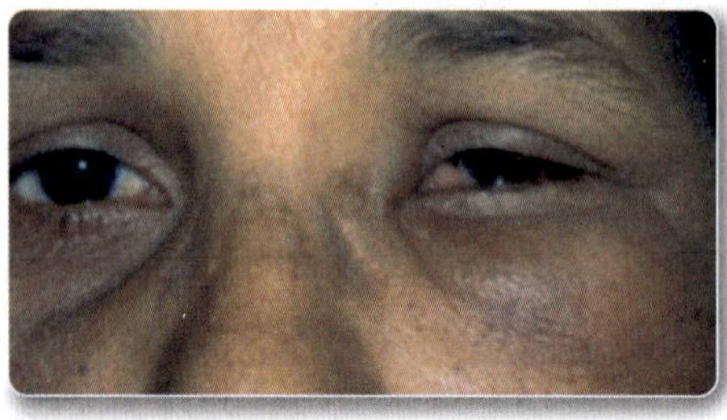

FIGURE 24.2: Angioneurotic edema

Passive Lid Edema

A puffiness of the lid can appear, especially in the morning on waking up in conditions of generalized fluid collection due to renal disease or cardiac failure. Passive lid edema can occur in local circulatory obstruction as in cavernous sinus thrombosis.

Ecchymosis or Black Eye

Since lids are highly vascular and tissues are lax, any contusion injury can lead to bleeding into the subcutaneous tissue. The subcutaneous blood will give a bluish color to the lids and the lid swelling will depend on the extent of the bleed. This condition is called 'black eye'. This bluish discoloration can disappear within 1–3 weeks depending on the amount of blood. Bleeding need not be from the lid itself. Any blood from the neighboring structures like bleeding under the scalp or even the blood from the other eye can gravitate to the lids due to the looseness of the tissue. In this situation the black eye will appear only 1–2 days after the trauma.

Treatment

No treatment is required. This blood will get absorbed in 1–3 weeks. If the bleeding is massive serratiopeptidase can be given to facilitate reabsorption of the blood.

Inflammations of the Lid

Blepharitis

Anterior blepharitis

Seborrheic blepharitis: It is similar to seborrhea or dandruff of the scalp. Patients, usually complain of itching of the lid margins. The lid margins are usually hyperemic and there are tiny scales in between the lashes. The lashes fall off frequently, but they are replaced without any distortion (Table 24.1).

TABLE 24.1: Blephiritis

Anterior blepharitis	Posterior blepharitis
Squamous/seborrheic blepharitis	Meibomian seborrhea
Ulcerative blepharitis	Meibomianitis

Treatment: Clean the lashes with baby shampoo or warm 3% sodium bicarbonate solution regularly. In acute exacerbations steroid ointments can be applied after cleaning.

But their use must be kept to the minimum due to the complications associated with prolonged steroid ointment.

Ulcerative blepharitis: This condition is due to chronic inflammation of the follicles of the lashes usually due to *Staphylococcus aureus*.

The presenting complaints will be mild swelling of the lid margins, irritation and crusting of the lid margins. The symptoms will be aggravated with redness, lacrimation and photophobia when the infection spreads to the ocular surface to produce blepharoconjunctivitis (Fig. 24.3).

On removal of the crusts, small ulcers can be seen in between the roots of the lashes. There will be redness and swelling of the lid margins. The lashes will fall off and do not grow again leading to areas with no lashes on the lid margin (madarosis). The scarring produced by prolonged inflammation can lead to distortion of the lashes and trichiasis (lashes rubbing on the ocular surface). Conjunctivitis and toxic marginal keratitis can occur.

Treatment: Clean the lid margin with baby shampoo or warm sodium bicarbonate solution and apply antibiotic ointment. The antibiotic treatment has to be continued for 2-3 weeks or longer, since organisms can survive deep in the hair follicles and lead to recurrence. In resistant cases a C and S study must be done to decide on the antibiotic needed. The toxic keratitis may require weak steroids like fluorometholone drops 2-3 times daily for control.

Sequele: If not properly managed, the infection can become chronic and lead to serious sequelae. The lid margin abnormalities like madarosis and trichiasis can occur.

The lid margin can become thickened leading to drooping of the lids—tylosis. If the lower lid is involved it can lead to eversion of the lower punctum and epiphora, and ectropion.

Posterior Blepharitis

Posterior blepharitis is characterized by abnormal and excessive meibomian secretion.

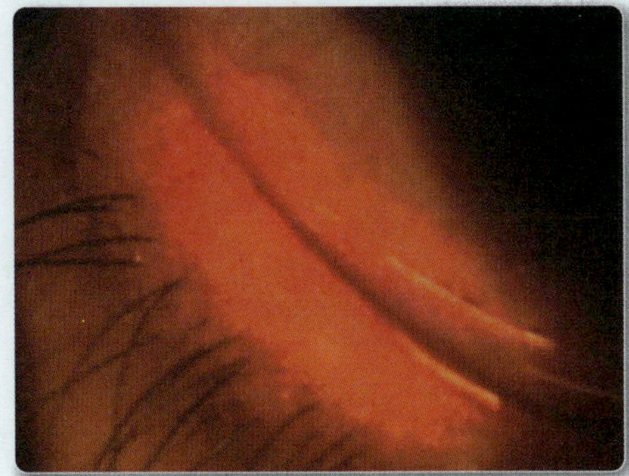

FIGURE 24.3: Ulcerative blepharitis

Meibomian seborrhoea: The excessive and abnormal meibomian secretion leads to froth in the precorneal tear film and there will be oil droplets at the openings of the meibomian glands. These abnormalities can cause tear film instability and irritation, burning and soreness of the eyes.

Meibomianitis: The conjunctiva on the tarsal surface will be congested and prominent meibomian glands will be seen through the tarsal conjunctiva as pale yellow streaks. Lid massage will lead to thickened cheesy secretions coming out from the ducts. Obstruction of the ducts of meibomian glands with this thickened secretions lead to multiple chalazia formation.

Treatment

Warm compresses to melt the secretion and mechanical expression by lid massage. Antibiotics applied topically will help to control secondary infection. Doxycycline or tetracycline for 6–12 weeks will help to correct the abnormal secretions of the meibomian glands. This will control the infection also.

Sequelae: Multiple chalazia, tear film instability and marginal corneal infiltrates.

Phthiriasis palpebrarum (Fig. 24.4): It is an infestation of the eyelashes with the pubic louse (*Pthirus pubis*). The infection usually spreads in people living in unhygienic and overcrowded surroundings as in overcrowded hostels.

The infestation produces irritation and itching. The crab-like lice and its nits can be seen attached to the roots of the lashes.

Treatment:

1. Trimming of the lashes at their roots to remove all the lice and its nits.
2. Touching the lashes with petrol (after application of plenty of antibiotic ointment to protect the eye) 1% mercuric oxide ointment or cryotherapy.
3. Delousing of the patients by removing all body hair and the cleaning of the clothes in power laundry or by boiling is essential to prevent recurrence.
4. Treatment of all infested family members or the people in the hostel is also required.

Infections of the Glands of the Lids

Hordeolum Externum

Hordeolum externum (HE) is a suppurative inflammation of a Zeis' gland. Commonly it is staphylococcal infection. Since, Zeis' gland opens into a lash follicle an abscess forms at the root of the lash (Fig. 24.5).

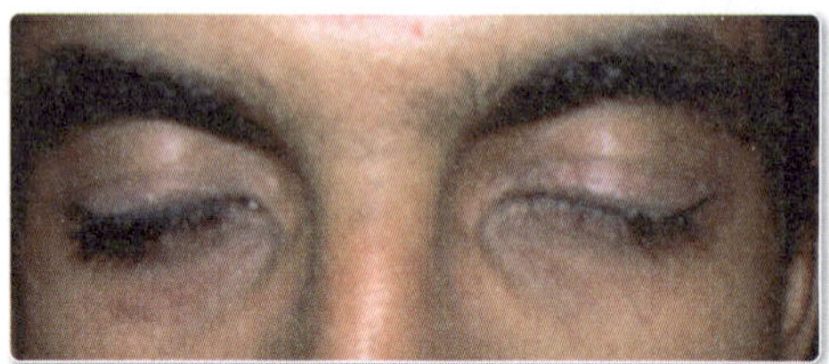

FIGURE 24.4: Phthiriasis palpebrarum

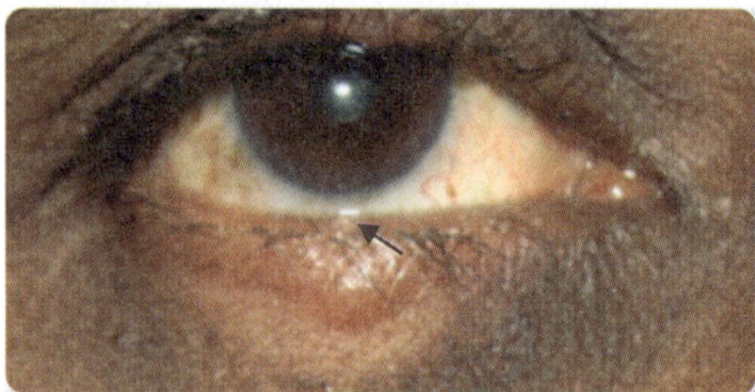

FIGURE 24.5: Hordeolum externum (HE) with pus pointing at lid margin

Symptoms: Children are more commonly affected. Pain and swelling of the affected lid will be the main complaint of the patient.

Sign: The affected lid will show edema. No definite visible or palpable swelling is present. Tender swelling is seen at the lid margin with pus pointing at the root of a lash.

Treatment: In the initial stages before an abscess is formed, hot compresses and antibiotic ointment application will control the inflammation.

If pus points, it can be evacuated by pulling out the affected lash or incision and curettage can be done, if the infection has spread to the surrounding tissues and a larger abscess has formed.

In recurrent attacks, an uncorrected refractive error or an undetected diabetes (especially in an adult with HE) has to be ruled out or a generalized poor health with diminished resistance to *Staphylococcus* infection may be the reason. A course of systemic antibiotics combined with hot fomentation and topical antibiotics for 2–3 weeks may eradicate the persistent *Staphylococcus* infection.

Complications: As follows:

1. Spread of infection to the surrounding tissues leading to preseptal cellulitis or orbital cellulitis.
2. Rarely, even cavernous sinus thrombosis can occur since the infection is in the danger zone of the face.

Hordeolum Internum

Hordeolum internum (HI) is a suppurative inflammation of the meibomian gland. Since, it is a much larger gland the inflammatory signs and symptoms are much more than in HE (Figs 24.6A and B).

Symptoms: Patient usually complaints of pain, worse on lid movements and swelling of the lids.

Signs: On examination, there will be some lid edema and tenderness at the site of the affected gland. But there will not be any palpable swelling, since the inflamed gland is confined within the tarsal plate. On examination of the palpebral conjunctiva, initially there will be localized congestion at the site of the involved gland and later, as pus forms yellow spot will be visible through the palpebral conjunctiva. The pus may burst spontaneously through the pointed spot and the inflammation will subside. Sometimes the infection will spread to the surrounding tissues, and a palpable and tender swelling will appear and the pus may burst through the skin surface also.

Treatment: Hot compresses and topical antibiotic ointment or drops may control the infection.

If pus points on the conjunctival surface a small incision will be sufficient to drain the pus.

Incision and curettage is needed, if a localized abscess has formed.

Complications: Lid abscess, preseptal cellulitis and cavernous sinus thrombosis.

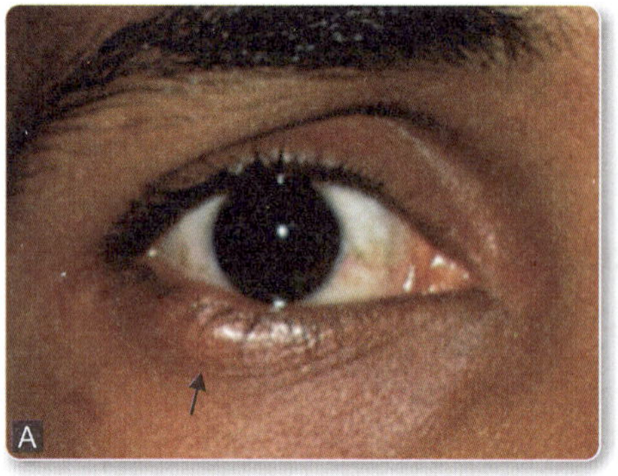

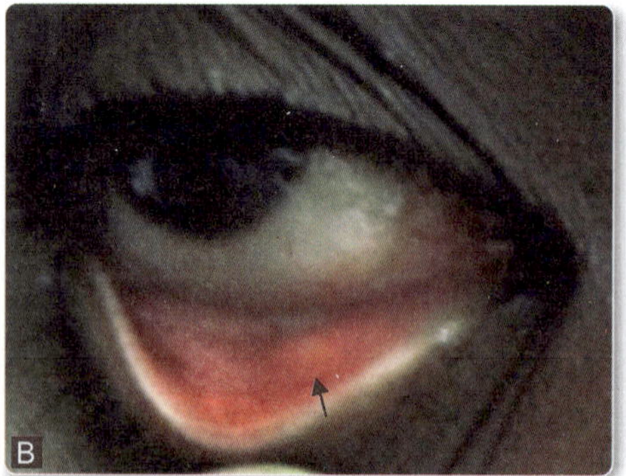

FIGURES 24.6A and B: Hordeolum internum with pus pointing on palpebral conjunctiva

Chalazion (Tarsal Cyst or Meibomian Cyst)

Chalazion (tarsal cyst or meibomian cyst) is a chronic inflammatory granuloma of the meibomian gland (Fig. 24.7). It is common in children than adults. People with chronic meibomianitis, seborrheic dermatitis and acne rosacea are prone to developing chalazion, which is often multiple.

Obstruction of the duct of the gland with thickened secretion may lead to accumulation of giant cells, plasma cells and histiocytes. The swelling is usually encapsulated and gradually increases in size (Table 24.2).

Clinical Features

Symptoms: The usual complaint will be a disfiguring swelling on the lids, which has been present for a few weeks to months. There will not be any pain or discomfort.

Sign: A visible and palpable non-tender firm swelling will be seen on the lids in the area of the tarsal plate. Smaller chalazia are more palpable than visible. The tarsal conjunctiva over the swelling will be showing some grayish or muddy discoloration, but pus will not be seen. The skin over the swelling will be freely mobile. The swelling does not usually extend to involve the lid margin and does not extend beyond the posterior edge of the tarsal plate.

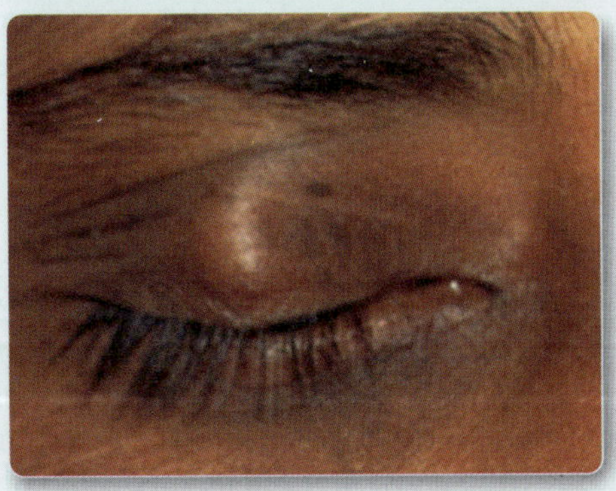

FIGURE 24.7: Chalazion

Rarely the chalazion will get resolved spontaneously. This usually happens in small chalazia in children. Usually an incision and curettage is required for its resolution.

Sometimes small amount of granulation will be seen protruding through the duct of the gland this is called marginal chalazion.

The granuloma will burst spontaneously through the conjunctival surface to form a papillomatous fleshy mass at the site, this is called **chalazion granuloma**.

Treatment

1. **Triamcinolone acetonide injection:** 0.1 mL diluted with equal quantity of lignocaine given into the chalazion may result in spontaneous resolution. The injection can be repeated after 2 weeks.
2. **Incision and curettage (I and C) method:** The lid is anesthetized with injection of xylocaine (Fig. 24.8A). A chalazion clamp is applied to the lesion so as to fix and evert the lid (Fig. 24.8B). Chalazion clamp also helps in hemostasis. With a sharp knife like a BP blade a small vertical incision is made over the chalazion at the conjunctival side without extending to the lid margin (Fig. 24.8C). Any fluid filling the cavity will flow out. A chalazion scoop is used to scoop out all semisolid granulation inside (Fig. 24.8D). The vertical incision is important to prevent damage to other glands because of the vertical arrangement of the meibomian glands.

   After all materials have been curetted out, a firm pressure dressing is given for 1–2 hours to control bleeding. If the chalazion is large and pointing more on the skin surface, an incision may be put on the skin surface also for complete removal of all material. On skin surface the incision is made horizontally along a skin crease to minimize scarring.

   After removing the dressing topical antibiotics are applied for a few days.

   If there is a chalazion granuloma, the protruding granulation should be excised before doing the incision. If there is a marginal chalazion, the duct of the gland should be curetted out.

TABLE 24.2: Differential diagnosis of hordeolum internum, hordeolum externum and chalazion

	Hordeolum internum (HI)	Hordeolum externum (HE)	Chalazion
Pain	++	+	–
Tenderness	+	+	–
Swelling	Lid edema only	Swelling at root of lashes	++
Palpable swelling	–	–	++
Conjunctival surface	Pus points	Mild congestion	Muddy discoloration over the swelling
Duration	Short	Short	Long

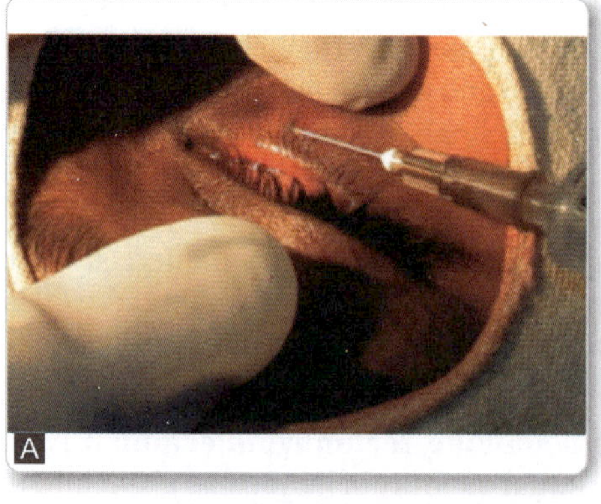

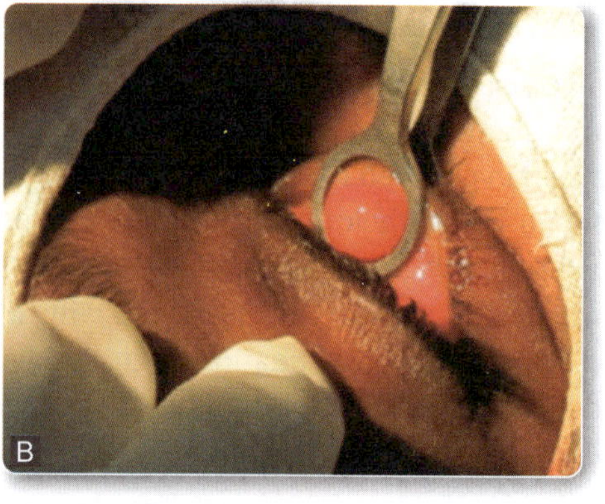

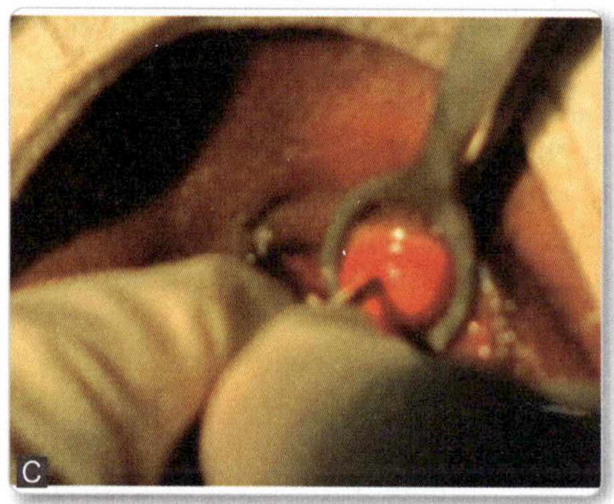

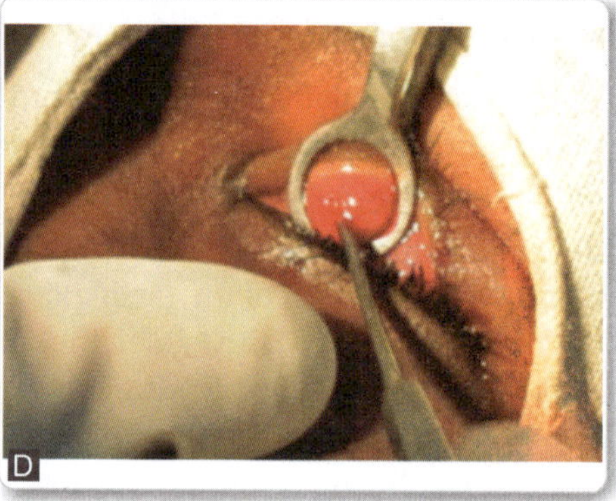

FIGURES 24.8A to D: Steps of incision and curettage. **A.** Local anesthesia infiltrated; **B.** Chalazion clamp applied and lid everted; **C.** Curettage done with a chalazion scoop; **D.** Vertical incision put with a Bard-Parker (BP) blade.

3. **Systemic tetracycline:** In patients with chronic meibomianitis and multiple chalazia, tetracycline or doxycycline has to be given for 4–12 weeks to prevent recurrence.

Complications:

1. Bleeding after I and C.
2. Persistence of the swelling, if the curetting is incomplete.
3. Recurrence of the swelling. Usually, it is a chalazion arising from a neighboring gland. If it is a true recurrence at the same site, an adenocarcinoma of the meibomian gland has to be suspected, especially if the patient is elderly. An excision biopsy has to be done to exclude or confirm adenocarcinoma by histopathological examination.

ANOMALIES IN THE POSITION OF THE LIDS AND LASHES

Congenital Anomalies

Distichiasis

Distichiasis is an extra row of lashes in all the four lids occupying the position of the meibomian glands. They may rub on the cornea and has to be removed by cryotherapy or radiofrequency epilation needle.

Epicanthus

There is a semilunar fold of skin extending from the upper lid to the lower one covering the inner canthus. It is normal in Mongolian races. This fold makes the distance between the two eyes appear wider than normal and gives an appearance of a pseudoconvergent squint. This fold may disappear as the child grows or it can be surgically corrected.

Blepharophimosis

Blepharophimosis (Fig. 24.9) is a congenital condition where the patient has bilateral ptosis with reduced lid size both in the vertical and horizontal dimensions. In addition to narrow palpebral fissure, there is epicanthus inversus, flat nose, ptosis and telecanthus. Epicanthus inversus means the fold of skin arises from the lower lid and goes upwards. This condition usually runs in families.

Treatment: Plastic reconstruction of the lids done in multiple stages at early childhood will correct the deformity to some extent.

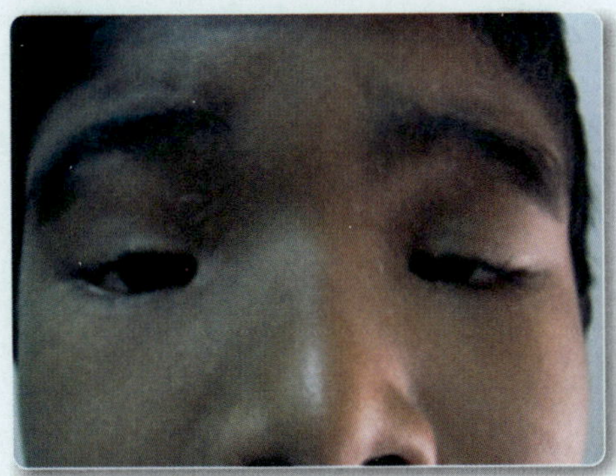

FIGURE 24.9: Blepharophimosis syndrome

Telecanthus

Telecanthus is characterized by widely separated medial canthus due to an abnormally long medial canthal tendon. It can occur alone or as part of blepharophimosis syndrome. It has to be differentiated from hypertelorism where the eyes are widely separated due to widening of the distance between the bony orbits.

Coloboma of the Lids

Coloboma of the lids (Figs 24.10A to F) is a congenital defect in the lid. It can be partial or full thickness defect and can be unilateral or bilateral. It may be associated with other congenital anomalies of the eye and there may be a dermoid cyst at the limbus in the area of the coloboma. Coloboma can lead to exposure of the cornea on lid closure. So the surgical correction has to be done as early as possible after birth.

Epiblepharon

There is an additional horizontal fold of skin close to the lid margin, which covers the lid margin and the lashes especially on the medical aspect of the lid. On pulling the skin of the lids away from the lid margin, the normal lid margin becomes visible and the lashes assume normal position temporally. Thus epiblepharon can be differentiated from congenital entropion. Spontaneous correction occurs in most of the cases as the infant grows up. If not, it has to be surgically corrected. Mean while antibiotic ointments can be prescribed to be applied frequently to protect the cornea.

Hypertelorism

Hypertelorism is a rare congenital condition where the distance between the two medial canthi are increased due to abnormally widely separated bony orbits. It will give an appearance of pseudoconvergent squint. In telecanthus, a similar appearance can be produced by abnormally long medial canthal tendons.

Cryptophthalmos

Here, there is no palpebral fissure. The skin of the forehead is continuous with the skin of the cheek and the eyes are hidden. It is often associated with severe congenital anomalies of the eye and orbit.

Congenital or Acquired Anomalies

Ptosis

Ptosis is a drooping of the upper eyelid. It can be congenital or acquired and also unilateral or bilateral.

Classification:

1. Congenital ptosis:
   a. Simple.
   b. Complication associated with other anomalies like:
      - Blepharophimosis syndrome
      - Marcus Gunn jaw-winking
      - Ocular motor anomalies.
2. Acquired ptosis:
   a. Neurogenic:
      - III nerve palsy
      - Horner's syndrome
      - III nerve misdirection syndrome.
   b. Myogenic:
      - Myasthenia gravis
      - Myotonic dystrophy
      - Ocular myopathy.
   c. Aponeurotic:
      - Involutional
      - Postoperative.
   d. Mechanical:
      - Tumors of the lid
      - Dermatochalasis
      - Symblepharon.

Pseudoptosis

Pseudoptosis (Figs 24.11A and B) is an apparent appearance of ptosis, but the levator function will be normal.

Causes:

1. Lack of support to the lid due to a small eye as in phthisis bulbi and enophthalmos or an empty socket after enucleation.
2. Contralateral lid retraction may give an apparent appearance of ptosis in the normal eye.

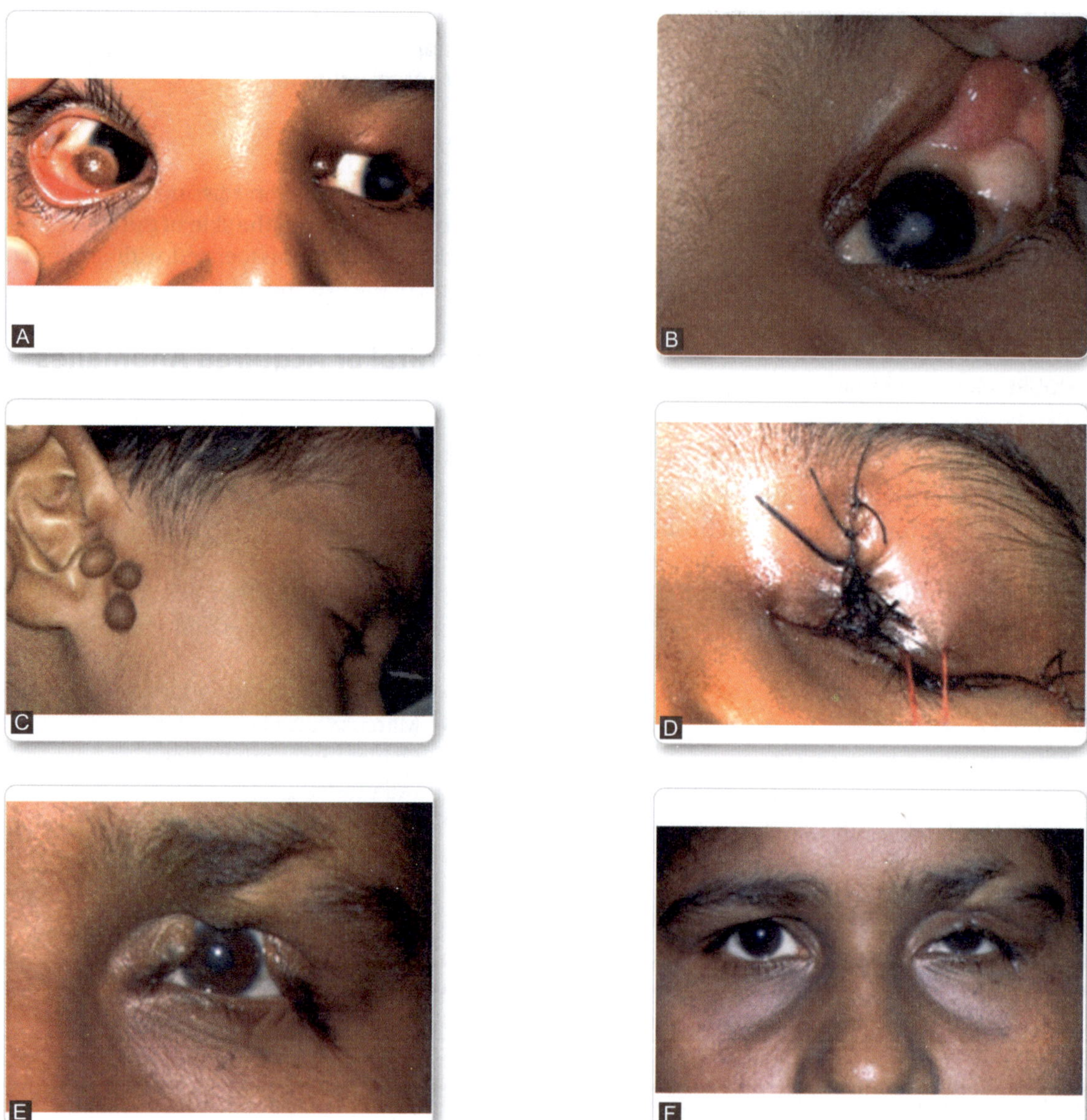

FIGURES 24.10A to F: Coloboma of the lids. **A.** Congenital dermoid and coloboma; **B.** Dermoid in the eye with coloboma; **C.** Accessory auricles in the child (Goldenhar syndrome); **D.** After coloboma repair; **E.** Traumatic coloboma; **F.** Traumatic coloboma after repair.

3. Brow ptosis: Brow is at a lower position leading to a narrow palpebral fissure, usually caused by VII nerve palsy.
4. Dermatochalasis: This condition is seen in middle or old age, there is an abundance of skin in upper lid with herniation of orbital fat, which hangs as loose folds over the palpebral fissure.

Pseudoptosis can be differentiated from a true ptosis by demonstrating normal levator action in cases of pseudoptosis.

Congenital ptosis

Congenital ptosis is the commonest type of ptosis and it can be unilateral or bilateral. It has a hereditary tendency and many people in a family will be affected (Figs 24.12A to C).

Clinical features: In severe weakness of the levator the upper lid fold will be absent. This may be the only sign that can be elicited in an uncooperative small child. There will be compensatory wrinkling of the forehead and brow elevation as well as elevation of the chin.

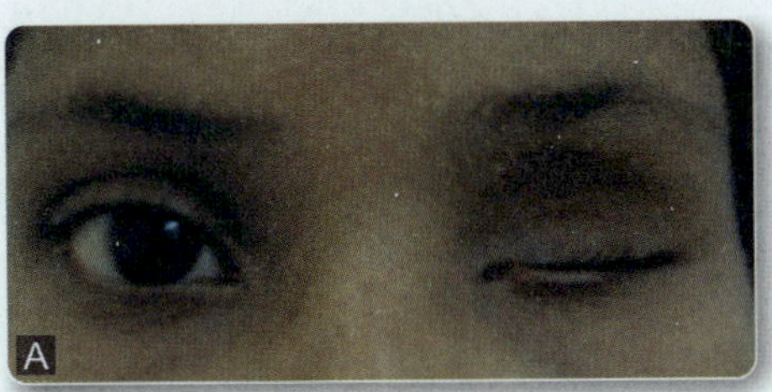

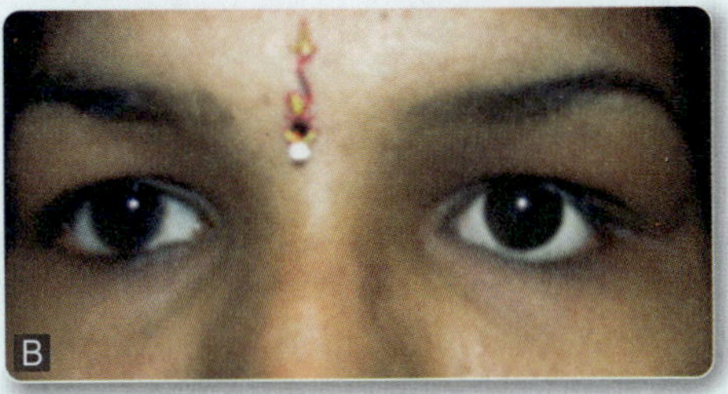

FIGURES 24.11A and B: Pseudoptosis. **A.** In an empty socket; **B.** Corrected when using artificial eye.

Usually congenital ptosis may be associated with weakness of the superior rectus muscle, since both muscles develop as a single block. If the lids are covering the pupil there is risk of development of amblyopia and surgery has to be done early. If the pupils are not covered, the child can be followed up till the preschool age since some spontaneous improvement will occur as the child grows. Surgery may be done before starting school.

Treatment: The treatment is surgical. The time of surgery depends on the severity of the problem.

Time of surgery: If the ptosis is severe enough to occlude the pupil this can result in amblyopia. If the child is constantly keeping the chin elevated to clear the visual axis, this can lead to permanent structural changes in the neck. In both these situations surgery has to be done before the age of 2 years. Otherwise surgery is ideally done before starting school.

Type of surgery: The type of surgery depends on whether it is unilateral or bilateral and whether the levator action is poor, fair or good. The aim is to obtain symmetrical look between the two eyes.

In eyes with fair and good levator action, levator muscle resection will gives good cosmetic appearance. In ptosis with poor levator action, frontalis sling operation has to be done. In this surgery the lid is mechanically lifted up by suspension at the brow from the frontalis muscle using various materials such as fascia lata, non-absorbable sutures or silicone band. This will give good appearance in primary gaze, but on looking down there will be limited lid movement and lid closure during sleep may be defective. In unilateral cases, the cosmetic appearance is generally unsatisfactory.

In such unilateral cases with poor levator function, it is better to give crutch spectacles, which will mechanically lift up the upper lid.

In patients with Marcus Gunn jaw-winking phenomenon, if the cosmetic problem is significant the surgical plan has to be suitably modified. The levator muscle has to be disinserted from the tarsal plate and frontalis sling surgery has to be done to manage both ptosis and jaw-winking together. In severe unilateral cases, bilateral levator disinsertion and frontalis sling surgery will be needed to produce a symmetrical look between the two eyes.

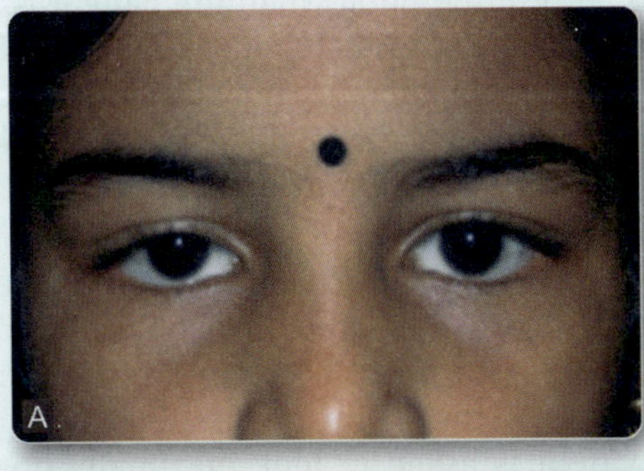

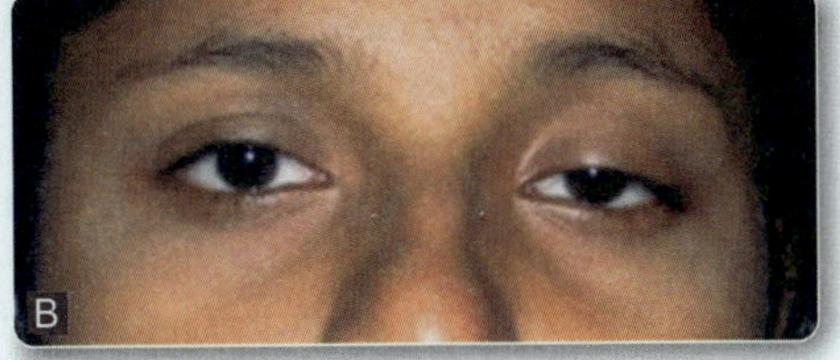

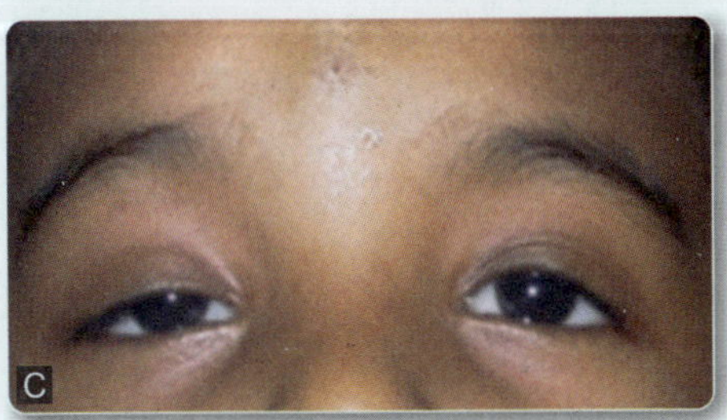

FIGURES 24.12A to C: **A.** Minimal ptosis right eye (RE) with good levator palpebrae superioris (LPS) function; **B.** Moderate ptosis in LE; **C.** Bilateral congenital ptosis with poor LPS action and compensatory frontalis overaction.

Acquired ptosis

Neurogenic ptosis

Neurogenic ptosis is due to III nerve palsy or due to sympathetic palsy as in Horner's syndrome. In III nerve palsy the motility of other muscles supplied by III nerve will be affected and the pupil may be affected or spared. On elevating the ptotic lid, the patient will experience diplopia. In ptosis due to Horner's syndrome other features of Horner's syndrome will be present.

Myogenic ptosis

Myogenic ptosis is bilateral. In myasthenia gravis, there will be variation in the ptosis in different times of the day. Ptosis will be more when the patient is tired or toward the evening. The Tensilon test will be positive.

Aponeurotic ptosis

Cause

Aponeurotic ptosis is due to weakness of the aponeurosis of levator muscle. There will be stretching, disinsertion or dehiscence of the aponeurosis, which makes lifting of the lid difficult when the levator muscle contracts. This can occur after some surgeries, trauma or in old age. If it is due to old age, which is the most common type, it will be bilateral (Fig. 24.13).

Clinical features: The upper eyelid crease will be at a higher level or absent in severe cases of aponeurotic ptosis. The upper sulcus will be deep and the lid above the tarsus will be thin. This is due to the disinsertion of the attachments of the levator aponeurosis to the tarsus and at the same time the skin attachments remain intact.

Mechanical ptosis

There will be a mechanical restriction to the movements of the lids as in upper lid tumors, edema of the lids or adhesion of the lids to the globe (symblepharon) (Figs 24.14A and B).

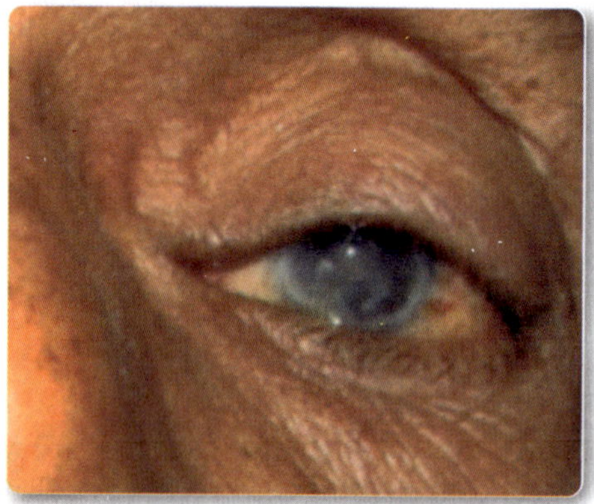

FIGURE 24.13: Aponeurotic ptosis with upper eyelid crease at a higher level

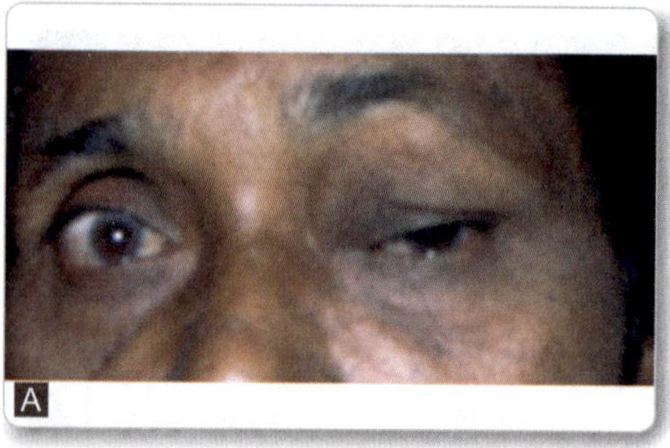

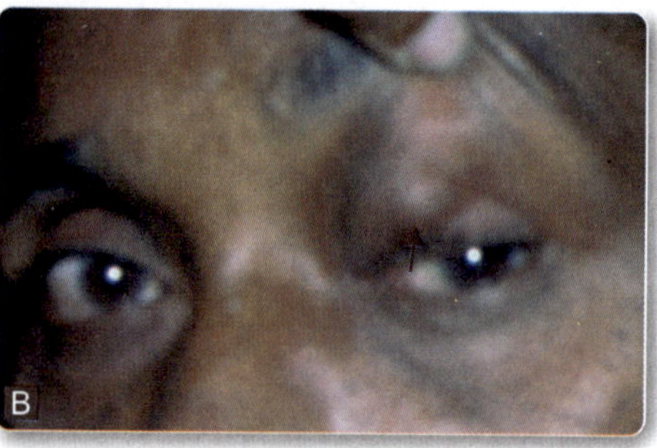

FIGURES 24.14A and B: Mechanical ptosis. **A.** Shows ptosis; **B.** Lid tumor, which is the reason for the mechanical ptosis is visible an elevating the lid.

Investigations:

1. **Margin reflex distance:** This is the distance between the center of the pupil and the upper lid margin.
   Normally it is 4–4.5 mm. In ptosis it will be less and it may be negative in severe ptosis (the lid line is below the pupil).
2. **Measurement of the palpebral fissure height:** This is the distance between the upper lid and lower lid at the level of the pupil when the patient is looking straight. Normally it is 7–10 mm in men and 8–12 mm in women. If the difference between the two eyes is 2 and 4 mm, the ptosis is mild, 4–7 mm, it is moderate and when more than 7 mm it is severe.
3. **Measurement of levator action:** The lid movement is measured with a transparent ruler held vertically before the eye in the pupillary plane. The compensatory action of the frontalis is prevented by firm pressure on the eyebrow with the thumb of the examiner. The patient is asked to look maximally down and then upwards as far as possible without moving the head. The difference in the reading on the rule at extremes of gauze gives the levator function. Normally it is around 15 mm. If the measurement is 4 mm or less, it is poor levator action, 5–7 mm it is fair and if it is more than 8 mm it is good levator action. In infants these measurements may not be possible. If the lid

fold is present, it can be taken that fair levator action is present and if the lid crease is absent, it denotes poor levator function.

4. **Measurement of action of associated muscles:** Like frontalis, orbicularis, superior rectus and other external ocular muscles must be done. In people with myasthenia frontalis over action and wrinkling of the forehead will be absent. The orbicularis action may be weak in myopathies.
5. **Bell's phenomenon:** It is tested by asking the patient to close the lid, while the lids are kept open by the fingers of the examiner. If the Bell's phenomenon is good, the eye will role upon attempted closure of the lids. If Bell's phenomenon is weak, there is greater risk for developing exposure keratitis after frontalis sling surgery. Absent Bell's phenomenon will lead to exposure of the cornea during sleep, if the lid closure is defective after surgery.
6. **Marcus Gunn jaw-winking phenomenon:** It has to be looked for in all congenital ptosis patients. It is seen in 5% of congenital ptosis. There is elevation of the eyelid on stimulation of the ipsilateral pterygoid muscle by chewing or opening the mouth. In severe form it can be very embarrassing to the patient.

Treatment of acquired ptosis

Neurogenic ptosis: The underlying neurological problem, if possible has to be treated. The patient has to be regularly followed up for spontaneous recovery. When the defect becomes stabilized and no more recovery is taking place, surgery has to be contemplated. In III nerve palsy, the squint has to be surgically corrected before ptosis is taken up. Otherwise diplopia will occur on elevation of the lid by surgery. If there is residual levator action levator surgery can be done. Otherwise frontalis sling surgery has to be done.

Myogenic ptosis: The ptosis is usually bilateral. The underlying condition has to be treated. In myasthenia gravis, steroids, immunosuppressants or thymectomy will give good results. In conditions like myopathies crutch spectacles can be used to lift the lid.

Aponeurotic ptosis: The aponeurosis may be reattached to the anterior surface of the tarsus and this may be combined with levator resection to get optimum results.

Mechanical ptosis: Treat the underlying pathology.

Surgeries for ptosis

Fasanella-Servat operation

Fasanella-Servat operation is done in:

1. Mild degree of congenital ptosis (2 mm).
2. Horner's syndrome.
3. Mild or moderate degrees of myogenic ptosis.

Technique: The upper lid is everted and a curved artery forceps is applied to include conjunctiva, 2–3 mm of the upper edge of the tarsus and corresponding amount of Müller's muscle. The clamped tissue is removed by cutting with scissors and the wound is sutured with absorbable sutures.

Levator resection

Levator resection is done when there is fair to good levator function. This can be done from the conjunctival or skin surface. The conjunctival approach is used when the amount of levator resection needed is 10 mm or less. The skin approach gives better exposure and this approach is used when larger resections have to be done.

On an average, levator resection of about 3–4 mm corrects 1 mm ptosis. For congenital ptosis the minimum amount of resection should be 10 mm. For a ptosis of 4–7 mm, the average resection is 15–22 mm.

A horizontal skin incision is put near the upper border of the tarsus. The orbicularis muscle is split to expose the aponeurosis of the levator. The muscle is separated from the upper tarsal border and the muscle is dissected out from the surrounding structures. The orbital septum is carefully separated from the muscle to expose the desired amount of muscle. The desired amount of muscle to be removed is marked. The lateral attachments of the muscle are also cut for free mobilization of the muscle. Then 3 mattress catgut sutures are passed above the level of excision of the muscle, then the amount of muscle is excised and the three preplaced mattress sutures are anchored to the anterior surface of the tarsal plate. The orbicularis and skin are sutured in layers (Figs 24.15A to C).

Frontalis Sling Surgery

Frontalis sling surgery (Figs 24.16A and B) is done when the levator action is poor. Materials used for suspension are fascia lata from the patient himself, 5-0 prolene suture or silicon band.

Three incisions are made on the upper lid skin parallel to the lid margin till the tarsal plate is exposed. Two incisions are put just above the eyebrow deep up to the frontalis muscle. Three strips of fascia lata or silicon bands are fixed to the tarsal plate. If prolene suture are used, bites are taken from the tarsal plate and the suture is fixed to the tarsal plate. A fascia lata introducer is passed from the incision above the eyebrow to reach the lower incisions and the strips of fascia are pulled up to the upper incision through a tunnel underneath skin and orbicularis muscle. A curved artery forceps can be used, if silicon band or prolene suture is used. The sling material is pulled up to give the desired lift to the eyelid and the material is primarily anchored to the frontalis muscle above the eyebrow with sutures. The skin incisions are then closed.

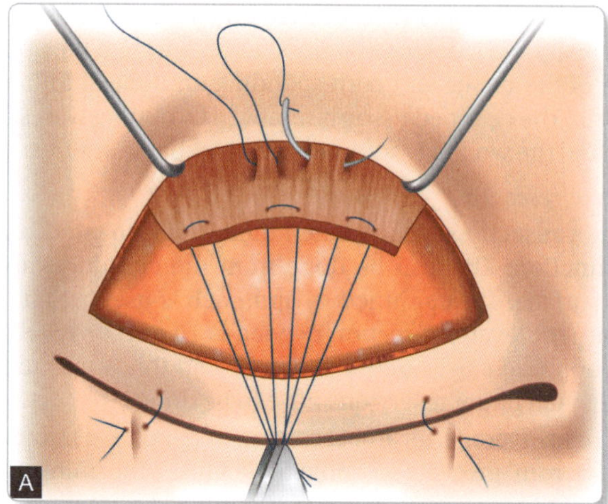

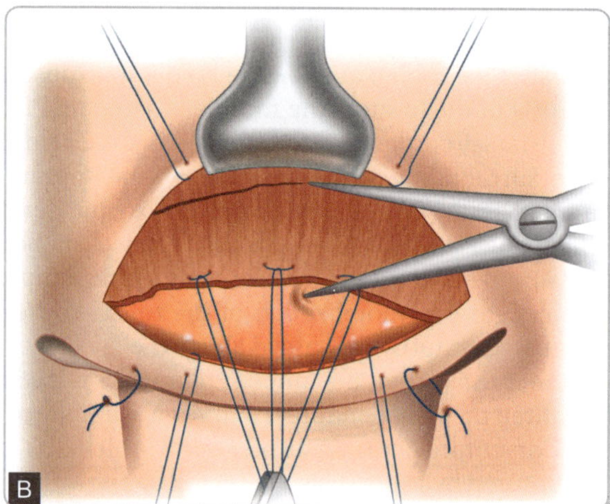

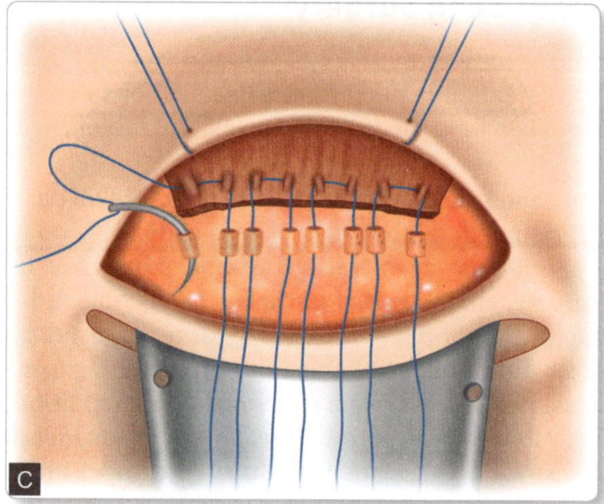

FIGURES 24.15A to C: **A.** Levator muscle disinserted from the tarsal plate; **B.** Levator to be resected is measured with calipers; **C.** Mattress sutures are passed through the cut end of levator palpebrae superioris (LPS) and the upper part of the anterior surface of tarsal plate (*Courtesy:* Stallard's eye surgery).

Lagophthalmos

Lagophthalmos is an incomplete closure of the palpebral aperture when an attempt is made to close the eye.

Causes:

1. Abnormalities of the lids:
    - Paralysis of the orbicularis
    - Symblepharon and scarring
    - Coloboma—congenital or traumatic
    - Severe ectropion.
2. Abnormal protrusion of the eyeball:
    - Thyrotoxicosis
    - Orbital tumor
    - Acute orbital cellulitis
    - Carotid—cavernous fistula
    - Buphthalmos.
3. Absence of reflex blinking:
    - In patients in coma or under anesthesia
    - Terminally ill patients
    - It can result in exposure keratitis.

In these conditions improper lid closure will lead to drying of the corneal epithelium, keratinization of corneal epithelium and exposure keratitis.

Treatment:

1. Treat the underlying pathology, if possible.
2. Keep the cornea well lubricated with frequent instillation of lubricant drops or ointments.
3. If proper protection of the cornea is impossible or exposure keratitis sets in, a lateral tarsorrhaphy is done

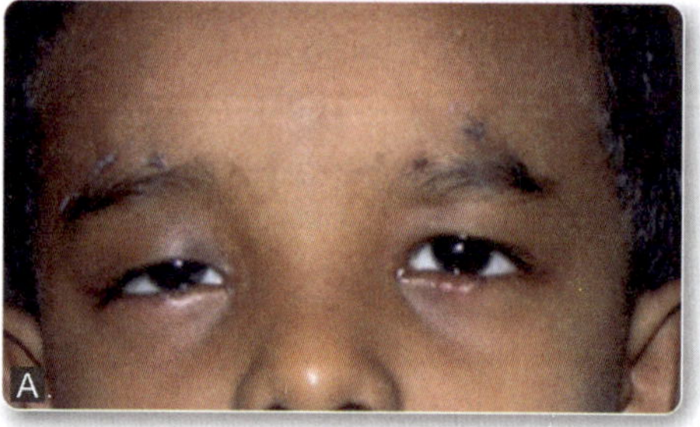

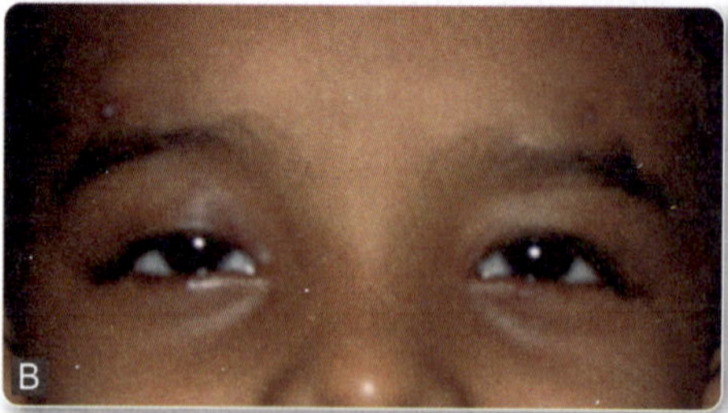

FIGURES 24.16A and B: Frontalis sling surgery. **A.** In the immediate postoperative; **B.** Late picture.

in lagophthalmos. In neuroparalytic keratitis a paramedian tarsorrhaphy is done.

Method: Two raw surfaces 6 mm in length are produced in corresponding position of the upper and lower lid margins by removing a strip of intermarginal strip of conjunctiva. The two raw surfaces are brought together and kept in approximation with sutures so that adhesions develop between the raw surfaces of the lid margins. The sutures will be removed after 2 weeks (Figs 24.17A to C).

ECTROPION

Ectropion is an eversion or rolling out of the lid margin away from the eyeball.

Types

1. Congenital.
2. Acquired:
   a. Involutional or senile.
   b. Cicatricial.
   c. Paralytic.
   d. Mechanical.

Congenital Ectropion

Congenital ectropion is a very rare condition. It is usually associated with other congenital anomalies like coloboma of the lids and microphthalmos.

Acquired Ectropion

Involutional ectropion

Involutional ectropion (Fig. 24.18) is the commonest type of ectropion. It usually affects the lower lid.

Mechanism: Horizontal lid laxity combined with laxity of the medial and lateral canthal tendons lead to this condition. Horizontal lid laxity can be demonstrated by the snap test. Pull the central part of the lower lid away from the eye. On releasing, the lid should snap back into position without blinking. If the lid takes time to go back to normal position or needs blinking to bring it back to position, horizontal lid laxity is present.

Involutional entropion and ectropion

Both conditions have almost similar etiological factors. There is horizontal lid laxity in both conditions.

People who develop ectropion have an atrophied or smaller than normal tarsal plate and a normal or increased tone of the preseptal/pretarsal orbicularis and the mechanical effect is a rolling out of the lids.

People who develop entropion have a normal or larger than normal tarsal plate and normal or decreased tone of the pretarsal orbicularis and the vector forces mechanically pull the lid margin inwards.

Management

Management depends on the cause for the ectropion. The surgical procedure depends on the severity of the problem and the portion of the lid where the malposition is most pronounced.

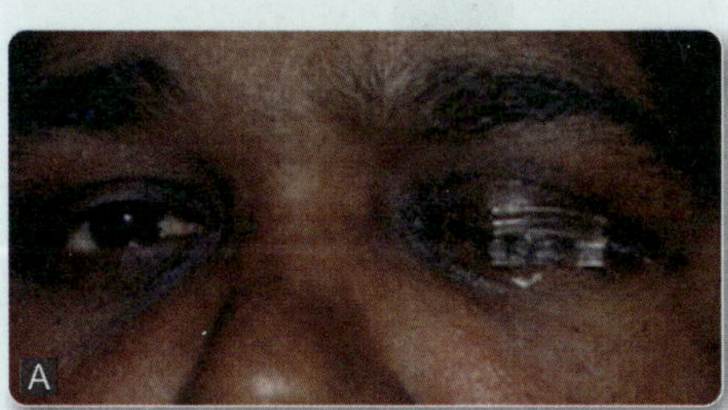

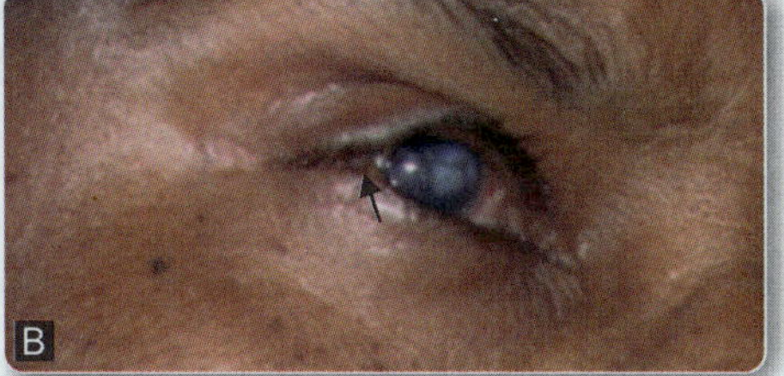

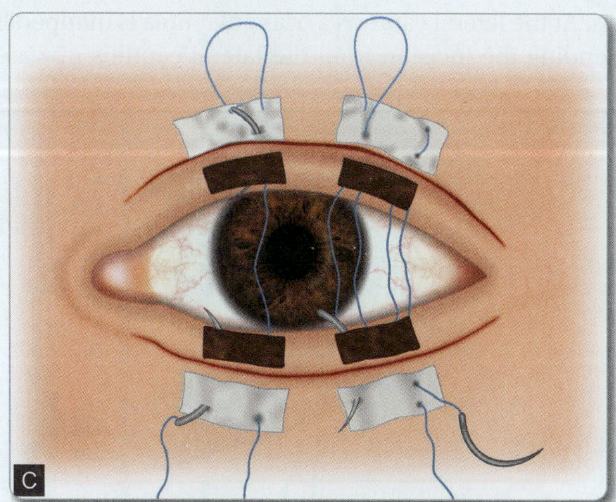

FIGURES 24.17A to C: Tarsorrhaphy. **A.** Immediately after surgery; **B.** Late picture; **C.** Diagrammatic representation (*Courtesy:* Stallard's textbook of surgery).

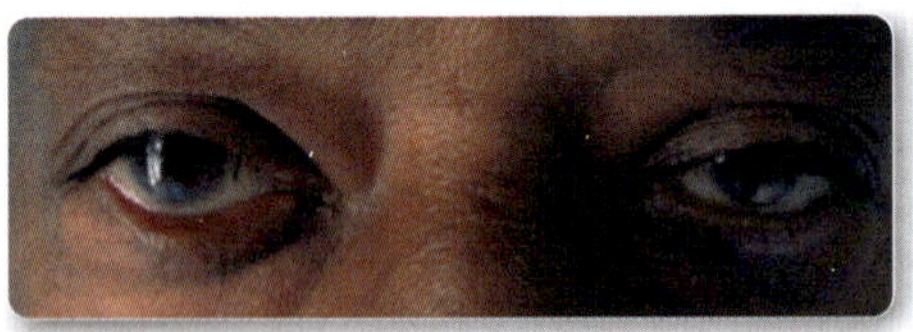

FIGURE 24.18: Involutional ectropion

Electrocautery puncture: In mild degree of senile ectropion especially involving the medial canthus, a row of electric cautery burns are applied to the conjunctival surface below the lower punctum. The contraction produced by the scarring will pull the lid inwards at the medial end and the punctum close to the globe.

Excision of a tarsoconjunctival spindle (Fig. 24.19): In moderate degrees of senile ectropion involving the medial end of the lower lid, excision of a horizontally oval area of tarsus and conjunctiva parallel with and inferior to the lower punctum and suturing the wound edges can be done. This will produce an inward pull on the inferior punctum.

Full thickness lid shortening: In generalized ectropion a wedge- or V-shaped full thickness area from the lower lid with the broader side of the wedge at the lid margin is excised. The site is selected at the area where the lid is maximally everted. The lid is closed in layers. Sometimes the medial canthus tendon laxity also has to be corrected.

Kuhnt-Szymanowski procedure (Fig. 24.20): This is done when there is severe ectropion with redundant skin.

Method: The lid is split along the gray line from the junction of the medial and central one thirds to the lateral canthus. At the lateral canthus a triangular area is mapped by extending the incision from the lateral canthus upwards and outwards for an appropriate length depending on the excess skin. From the lateral canthus a vertical incision downwards is made, which is twice the length as the horizontal extension. The ends of the two incisions are joined by a third incision to complete the triangle. The skin and muscle in this triangle is removed. A wedge flap with its base at the lid margin is excised from the inner lid flap. The outer split lid flap is pulled up and outwards to cover the defect formed by the excision of the triangle of skin and muscle, and sutured (Figs 24.21A to C).

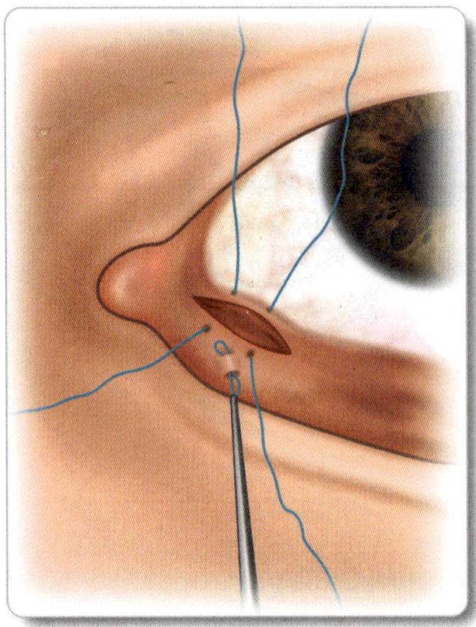

FIGURE 24.19: Excision of tarsoconjunctival spindle

Cicatricial ectropion

Cicatricial contracture of the skin of the lids and surrounding area of the face will pull the lid outwards and cause ectropion (Fig. 24.22A).

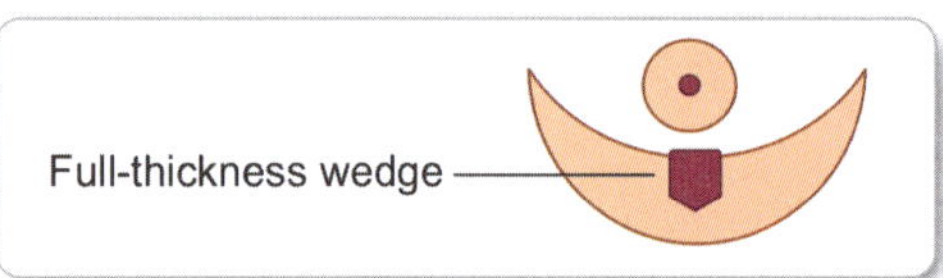

FIGURE 24.20: Diagrammatic representation of wedge resection

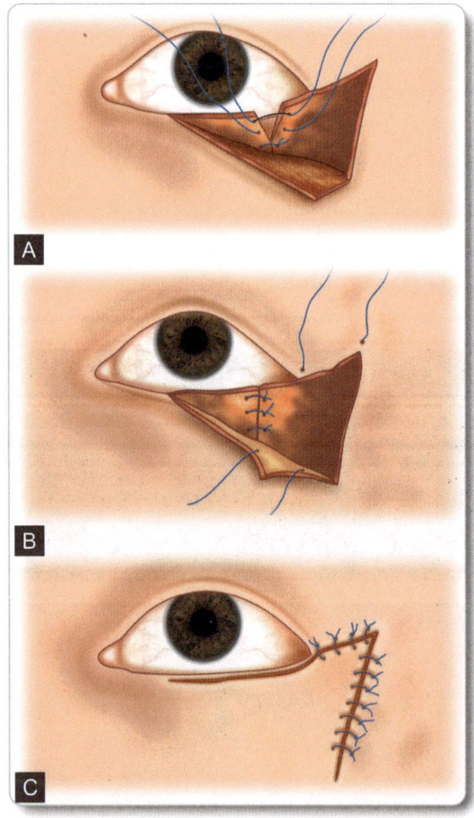

FIGURES 24.21A to C: Modified Kuhnt-Szymanowski procedure. **A.** Lid is split along the gray line and a wedge-shaped place is excised from the posterior lamella; **B.** The wedge is sutured and a triangular flap of skin is removed at lateral canthus; **C.** Skin edges are sutured (*Courtesy:* Stallard's eye surgery).

Causes: Burns of the face, scarring from injuries, congenital ichthyosis, etc.

Management: To correct the cicatricial ectropion all scar tissue has to be carefully excised to make the lid freely mobile. A full thickness or partial thickness skin graft may be used to cover the raw area created by the excision of the scar tissue. A temporary tarsorrhaphy may be done to prevent contracture during the healing stage (Fig. 24.22B).

Paralytic ectropion

Paralytic ectropion is due to paralysis of the VII nerve as in Bell's palsy, tumors like acoustic neuroma, parotid tumors, trauma, etc. Lack of muscle tone will pull the lower lid away from the globe due to the effect of gravity. There will be associated lagophthalmos and brow ptosis (the brow at a lower position compared to the normal side).

Clinical features: The ectropion of the lower lid leads to loss of contact of the lower punctum with the globe. So the tears will not be able to drain into the lacrimal sac when the orbicularis contracts and this will lead to epiphora. Frequent wiping of the eye will lead to aggravation of ectropion and epiphora. The exposed conjunctiva will undergo keratinization and will develop a raw beefy appearance. There will be chronic conjunctivitis, which will aggravate the epiphora. The skin of the lid becomes eczematous due to constant wetting and this will aggravate the ectropion, and the whole events become a vicious cycle.

Management

In minimal degrees a lateral tarsorrhaphy will be sufficient. In long standing cases with severe ectropion and lid laxity a lid shortening procedure by excision of a full thickness wedge from the lid has also be done. The medial and lateral canthal tendons will have to be strengthened by fascia lata suspension anchoring to the periosteum of the orbital rim.

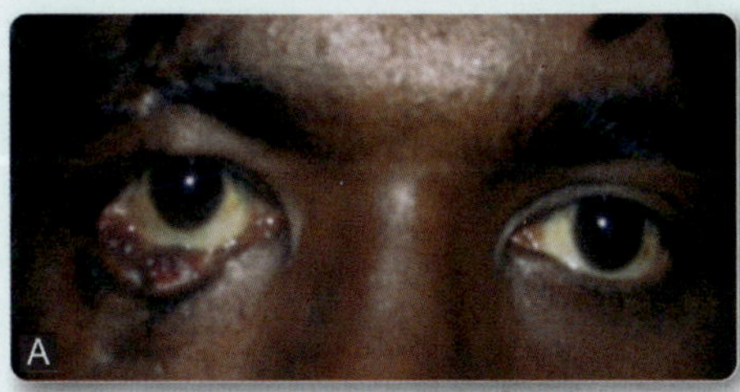

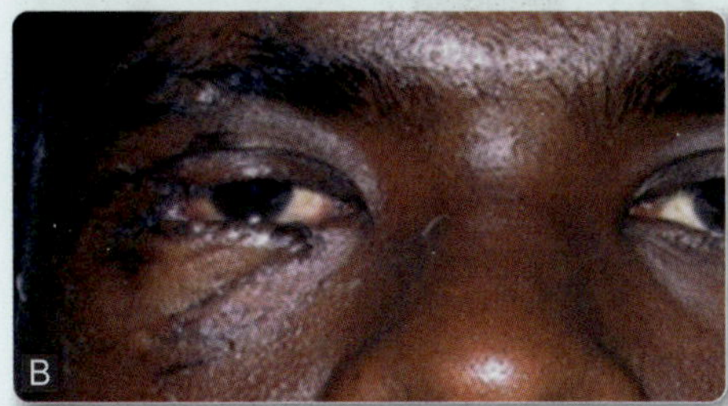

FIGURES 24.22A and B: Cicatricial ectropion. **A.** Cicatricial ectropion; **B.** After repair.

Mechanical ectropion

Mechanical ectropion is caused by tumors of the lids, which mechanically evert the lid. Management of the underlying cause will solve the problem.

ENTROPION

Entropion is a rolling of the lid margins. This will lead to a misdirection of the lashes and they will rub against the cornea—'trichiasis.' This in turn can lead to epithelial erosion and corneal ulcer.

Classification

Entropion can be:

1. Congenital.
2. Involutional or senile.
3. Cicatricial.

Congenital Entropion

Congenital entropion is a rare condition. The cause is a vertical shortening of the posterior lamella of lid. A curved fold of skin extends from the medial canthus to lateral canthus. This fold rides up and turns the lashes inwards. The lashes in babies are fine and they rarely cause any abrasion of the cornea. As the baby grows, this entropion gets corrected spontaneously. If not, surgery may be done.

Management: The rare condition often corrects itself. Surgery is done in cases, which fail to get corrected spontaneously or corneal problems are produced.

Technique: A horizontally oval strip of skin and orbicularis muscle is excised 3 mm below the lid margins and extending from the level of lower punctum to the lateral canthus. The skin and muscle are sutured with absorbable sutures.

Involutional (Senile) Entropion

Involutional entropion (Fig. 24.23) involves the lower lid. The upper lid, which has a broader tarsus, often remains in normal position. This turning in of the lower lid leads to trichiasis (Fig. 24.24), corneal erosion, ulceration and vascularization.

Causes

1. The horizontal lid laxity caused by stretching of the tarsal plate and the canthal tendons lead to weak apposition of the lower lid to the eyeball.

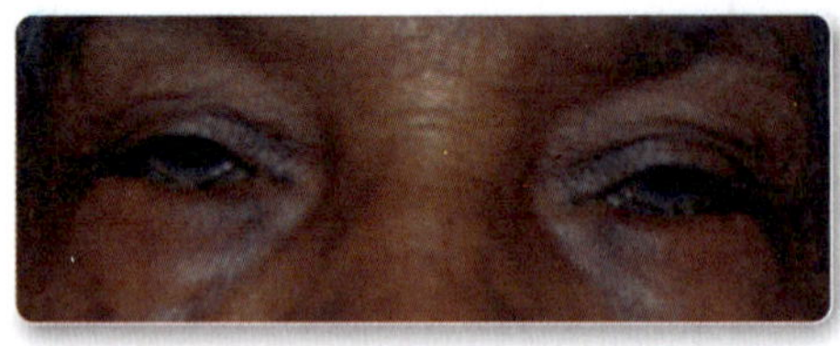

FIGURE 24.23: Involutional entropion

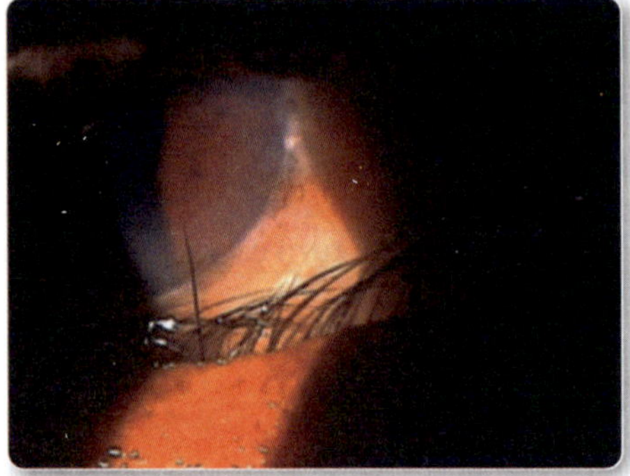

FIGURE 24.24: Trichiasis in entropion

2. Overriding of the preseptal portion of the orbicularis over the pretarsal portion of the orbicularis leads to inward turning of the lid margin during lid closure.
3. Laxity of the lower lid retractors and short postlamella of the lid allow the lower border of tarsal plate to move away from eyeball.

Treatment

Jone's procedure: This procedure is done for cases in which horizontal lid laxity is minimal and weakness or dehiscence of the lower lid retractors is the primary pathology. In this procedure the lower lid retractors are tightened and reattached to the lower border of the tarsal plate.

Technique: A horizontal skin incision is done 4 mm below the lash line in the lower lid. The incision is deepened and the orbicularis muscle is split to expose the lower border of the tarsal plate and the orbital septum below the tarsal plate. The orbital septum is cut transversely below the lower border of the tarsal plate and the orbital septum and the orbital fat beneath it are displaced downwards to expose the capsulopalpebral fascia. Three sutures are passed through the lower border of the tarsal plate and through the exposed capsulopalpebral fascia and tightened. Then the skin and muscles are sutured in layers. If there is redundant skin and muscle, an elliptical area of skin and orbicularis is resected before suturing.

In eyes with horizontal lid laxity as revealed by 'the snap back test,' 'modified Wheeler's procedure' or 'modified Fox procedure' is done.

Modified Fox procedure

The lower lid is split along the gray line to anterior and posterior lamellae. A triangle of tarsal plate and conjunctiva with its apex at the lid margin and base at the lower border of the tarsus is resected (Fig. 24.25).

A triangle of skin and orbicularis muscle is excised temporal to the lateral canthus with its base near the lateral canthus and slanting upwards. The edge of the resected tarsus and conjunctiva are sutured with absorbable sutures. Similarly the cut ends of the orbicularis and the skin are also sutured.

Modified Wheeler's procedure

An incision is done along the whole length of the lower lid just below the lid margin. A 3 mm band of underlying orbicularis muscle is dissected free from the skin and the tarsal plate and cut vertically in the middle. From the exposed tarsal plate a triangular piece with its apex toward the lid margin is excised as in Fox procedure. The tarsal plate is sutured. The cut ends of the orbicularis are pulled over one another till the lid is tightened and the overlapped edges of the muscle are sutured and a bite is taken from the lower border of the tarsal plate before the sutures are tightened. The skin is then closed with interrupted silk sutures (Figs 24.26A and B).

Spastic Entropion

In this condition there is spasm of the orbicularis muscle leading to the overriding of the preseptal portion of the orbicularis over the pretarsal portion and thus results in rolling of the lower lid margin. Any condition leading to severe photophobia and corneal irritation can lead to spastic entropion, especially in the elderly. Causes can be corneal ulcers, postoperatively following ocular surgery, etc. The condition may revert back to normal when the cause for photophobia subsides. It may result in permanent

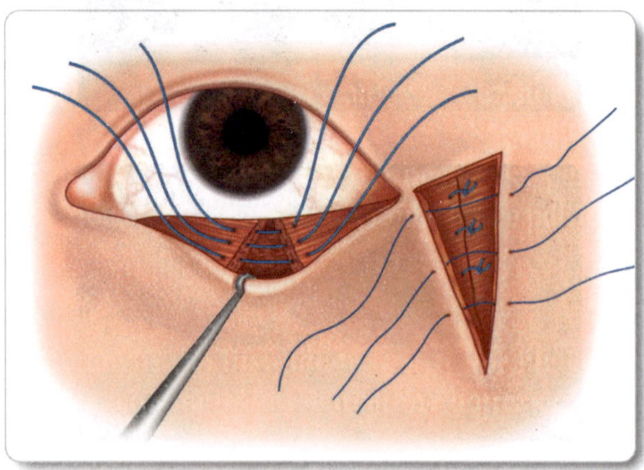

FIGURE 24.25: Modified Fox procedure

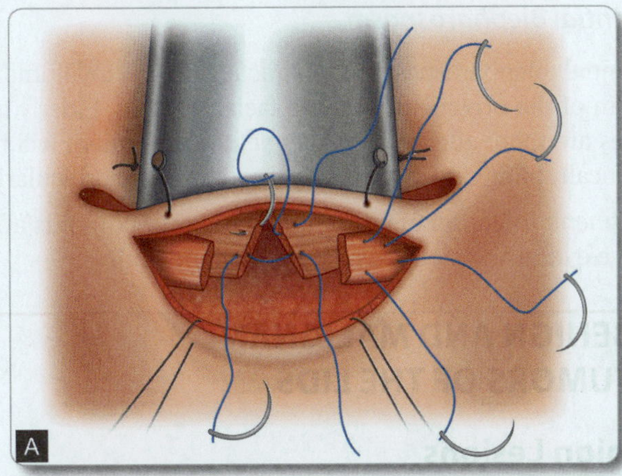

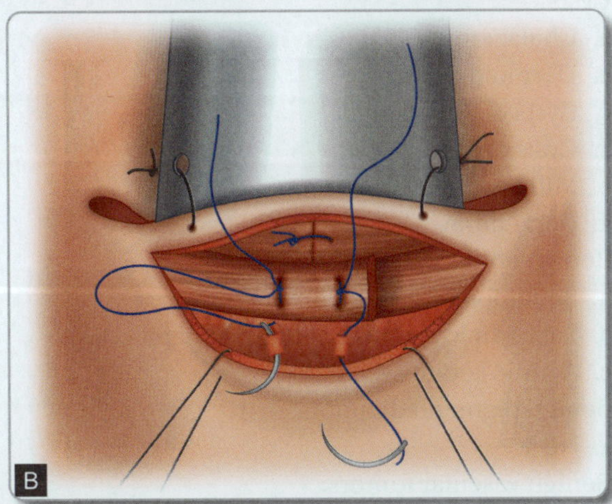

FIGURES 24.26A and B: Modified Wheeler's operation. **A.** Tarsus and the strip of orbicularis cut; **B.** Cut ends of tarsus sutured and the orbicularis overlapped and sutured (*Courtesy:* Stallard's eye surgery).

involutional entropion, especially if there is associated weakness or dehiscence of capsulopalpebral fascia (lower lid retractors).

Treatment

1. Lubricants to lessen irritation of the cornea by the rubbing lashes.
2. Temporary measures:
   a. Keep the lid in normal position by traction on the skin by a strip of adhesive tape stretching from the lower lid to the cheek.
   b. Injection of botulinum toxin into orbicularis muscle in severe cases—3 doses of 5 units medially, centrally and laterally. The effect lasts for 6 months.

Once the cause for photophobia is corrected, the lid may revert back to normal position. If there is involutionary changes in lower lid retractors, the entropion will persist. In this situation surgical correction will be required.

Cicatricial Entropion

Causes: As follows:

1. Severe scarring and contracture of the palpebral conjunctiva due to thermal or chemical injury.
2. Cicatricial inflammations like trachoma, Stevens-Johnson (SJ) syndrome.

The lid margin is pulled inwards and this involves both upper and lower lids (Fig. 24.27).

Treatment: This can involve both lids and the management depends on the severity of the problem, and the extent of scarring and adhesions on the conjunctival surface.

Mild cicatricial entropion

Skin and muscle operation is done for mild entropion of the medial end of the upper eyelid. An elliptical area of skin and orbicularis muscle is excised from the upper lid 3–4 mm above the area of localized entropion. Interrupted sutures, which pass through the underlying tarsal plate are used to close the defect. This will evert the lid margin and keep the lashes away from the cornea.

In moderate cases where the tarsus is not thickened or deformed complete dissection and excision of all scarred conjunctiva and subconjunctival scar tissue is done and the raw surface is covered with a conjunctival graft from the other unaffected eye or a thin mucous membrane graft or amniotic membrane graft in bilateral cases.

In severe cases where the tarsus is deformed. The surgical correction can be by:

1. Tarsal paring and eversion.
2. Tarsal rotation operation.

Tarsal rotation operation

In this operation, a strip of tarsus with the conjunctiva is rotated outwards to form a new intermarginal strip so that the lashes are directed outwards away from the cornea (Fig. 24.28).

After putting three traction sutures at the upper lid margin, the lid is everted and an incision is made through the full thickness of the tarsus, 3 mm from the lid margin. This strip of tarsus is freed from the orbicularis by careful dissection and is rotated through 90°.

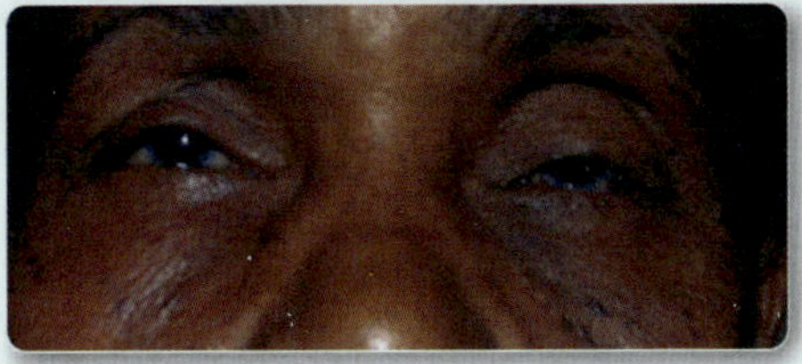

FIGURE 24.27: Cicatricial entropion of upper lids in trachoma

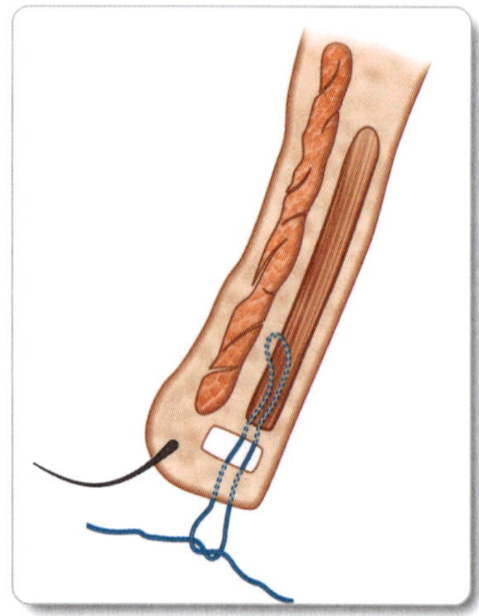

FIGURE 24.28: Tarsal rotation operation

Three mattress sutures are passed through this strip of tarsal plate in this rotated position and they are tied at the lid margin and these sutures ends are then brought out through the skin of the lid 5 mm from the lid margin and tied and cut.

Tarsal paring and eversion

An incision is made 3 mm above the lid margin though the skin and orbicularis to expose the tarsal plate. With a sharp knife, the tarsus is pared down along its entire length from its upper edge toward the incision. Three mattress sutures are then passed from the upper lid margin and the orbicularis and then the pared tarsal plate to come out through the lower edge of the incision and the skin of the lids just above lashes. On tying these sutures, the lid margin is bent outwards (Fig. 24.29).

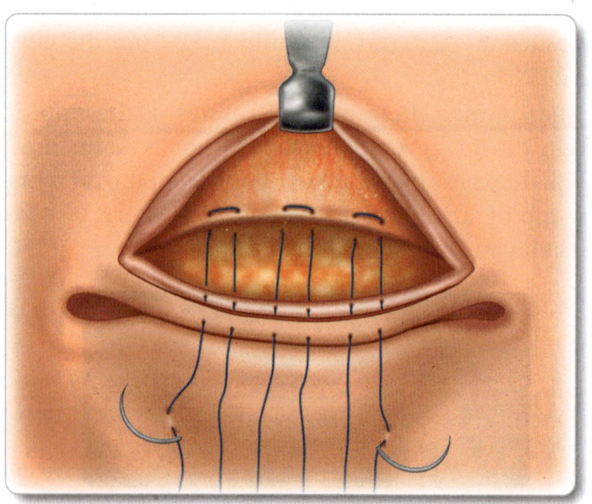

FIGURE 24.29: Sutures passed after pairing of the tarsal plate

Essential Blepharospasm

Essential blepharospasm is characterized by involuntary spasm of the orbicularis and the facial muscles. Elderly females are more affected. In severe cases the patient will be practically blind due to the continuous spasms of orbicularis.

Treatment: Injection of botulinum toxin into both lids and above eyebrow. Injections have to be repeated.

BENIGN AND MALIGNANT TUMORS OF THE LIDS

Benign Lesions

1. Cysts:
   a. Chalazion.
   b. Dermoid cysts.
   c. Cysts of Zeis' glands.
   d. Cysts of Moll.
   e. Milia.
   f. Comedone.
2. Benign epidermal tumors:
   a. Squamous cell papilloma.
   b. Seborrheic keratosis (basal cell papilloma).
   c. Actinic keratosis.
3. Benign pigmented tumors:
   a. Nevi.
4. Benign vascular tumors:
   a. Capillary hemangioma.
   b. Cavernous hemangioma or port-wine stain.
5. Miscellaneous benign lesions:
   a. Pyogenic granuloma.
   b. Xanthelasma.
   c. Neurofibroma.

Malignant Tumors

1. Basal cell carcinoma.
2. Squamous cell carcinoma.
3. Keratoacanthoma.
4. Sebaceous gland carcinoma.
5. Melanoma.
6. Kaposi sarcoma.

Benign Lesions

Cysts

Chalazion: Commonest cystic lesion of the lids arising from the meibomian glands (already described).

Dermoid cysts: Typically appear as congenital subcutaneous cystic lesions in the outer aspect of the upper lid. It may be attached to the periosteum of the orbit. If cosmetically disfiguring, the lesions can be excised.

Cyst of Zeis' glands: Small non-translucent cysts seen in the anterior lid margin.

Cysts of Moll: They are small translucent cysts at the anterior lid margin.

Milia: They are tiny white papules, often multiple, seen on the skin of the lids. They are retention epidermal cysts containing keratin.

Comedones: They are black heads seen in crops on the skin of lids, in people with acne vulgaris or elderly persons. They are dilated orifices of hair follicles plugged with sebum and keratin.

Benign Epidermal Tumors

Squamous cell papilloma: They appear as pedunculated reddish growths or as a sessile lesion (Figs 24. 30A and B). *Treatment:* Excision of the growth.

Basal cell papilloma or seborrheic keratosis: They are composed of proliferation of the basal cells of the epidermis. They appear as brown plaques with a verrucous surface and a 'stuck-on' appearance (Fig. 24.31), usually seen in elderly persons. Similar lesions will be seen on other parts of the face, neck and upper limb.

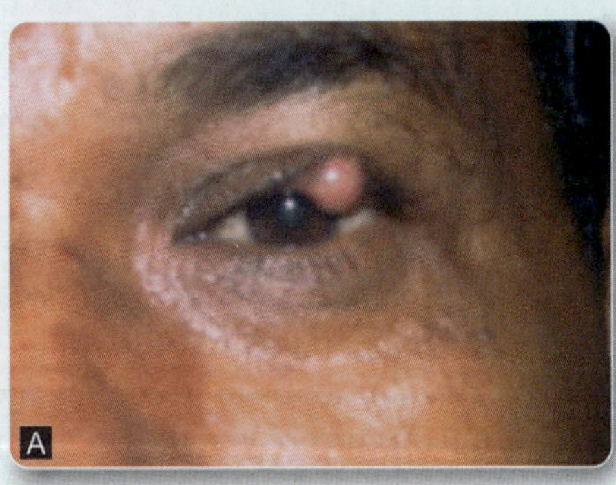

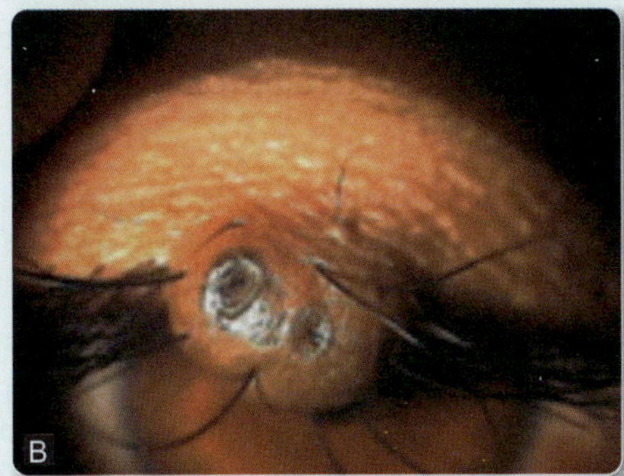

FIGURES 24.30A and B: A. Squamous cell papilloma; **B.** Benign wart at lid margin.

Treatment: Simple excision and biopsy to rule out basal cell carcinoma or melanoma.

Actinic keratosis: Commonly seen in elderly white skinned persons living in tropical countries and exposed to excessive sunlight. Appear as nodular or wart like lesions with a scaly surface and may show cracks and fissures. Similar lesions will be seen in other parts of the body exposed to sunlight. There is a risk of transformation into squamous cell carcinoma.

Treatment: Simple excision and histopathological examination to rule out malignancy.

Benign Pigmented Tumors

Nevus

Nevus (Figs 24.32A to D) can be congenital or acquired.

Congenital nevus: It can be small or involve extensive areas of the body and contain hairs (Fig. 24.32A). They can involve corresponding areas of both upper and lower lids called kissing or split nevus (Fig. 24.32B). The large lesions have a risk of developing malignant transformation.

Treatment: Surgical excision of larger lesions with skin grafting, if required.

Acquired nevus: They can have different clinical features and histopathological features depending on the level of involvement.

Junctional nevus: Appear as light brown macules or papules. The nevus cells are located at the junction of the epidermis and dermis. The risk of malignant transformation is low.

Compound nevus: These are raised lesions with uniform light brown to dark brown color (Fig. 24.32D). The nevus cells extent to the dermis from the epidermis and the potential for malignant transformation is low.

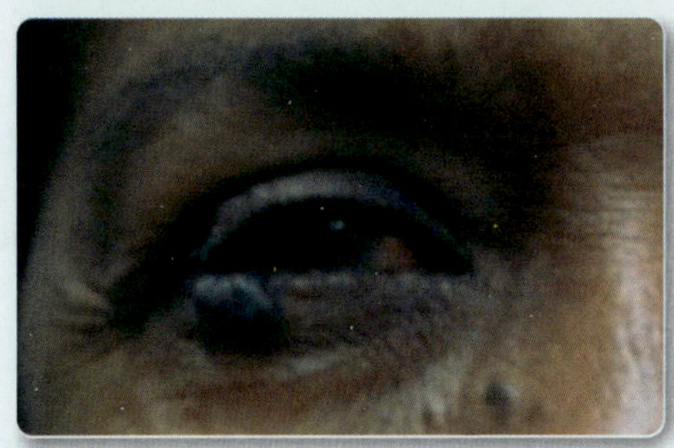

FIGURE 24.31: Seborrheic keratosis

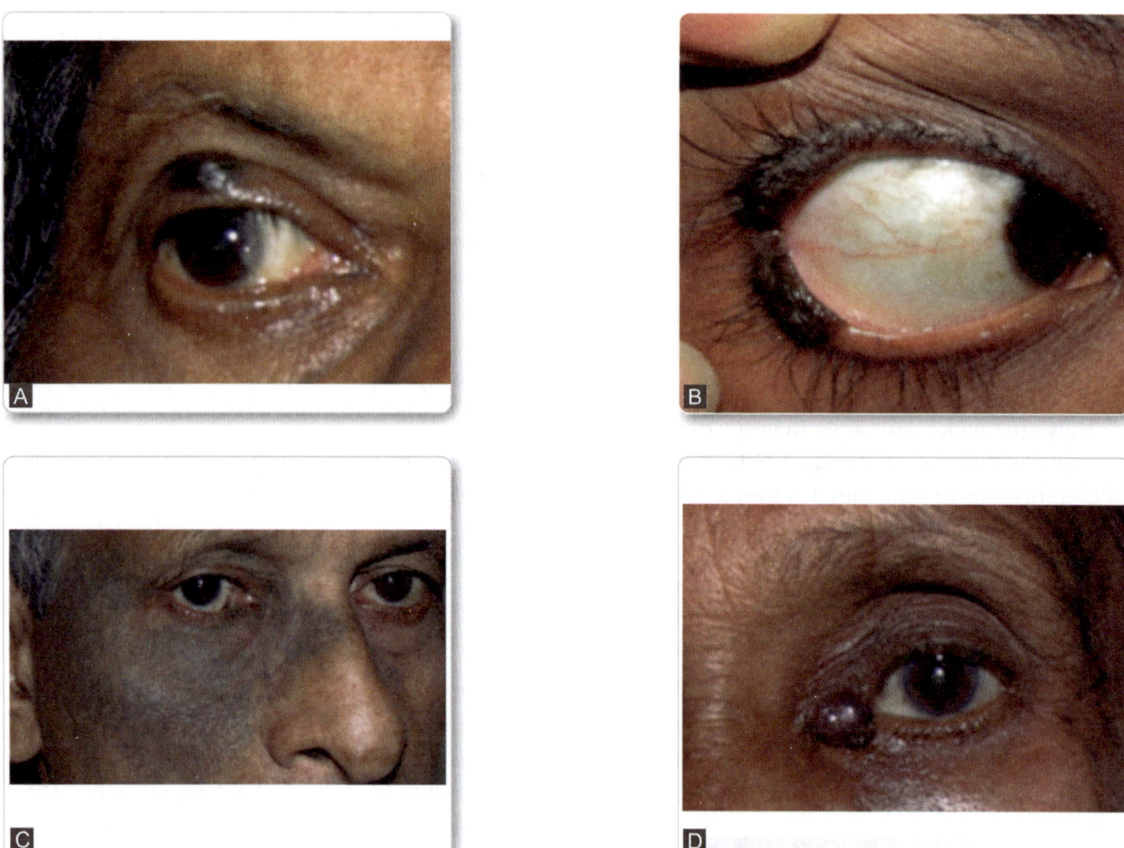

FIGURES 24.32A to D: Nevus. **A.** Congenital nevus; **B.** Kissing or split nevus; **C.** Nevus of Ota with heterochromia iridum; **D.** Compound nevus.

Intradermal nevus: This is the commonest type and usually seen in elderly persons. The nevus cells are situated in the dermis and the lesions are papillomatous with little or no pigmentation. There is no risk of transformation to malignancy.

Treatment: Excision, if it is disfiguring or suspicion of malignancy is aroused by increase in growth or vascularity. Excision must be complete or there is risk of recurrence.

Benign Vascular Tumors

Capillary hemangioma or strawberry nevus: They appear soon after birth as raised bright red lesions on the lids. It may extend to the skin of the face or into the orbit. It may also be associated with hemangiomas of internal organs. Large lesions on the upper lid can cause mechanical ptosis and block the pupil and result in amblyopia. Capillary hemangiomas blanch on pressure and this sign differentiates it from cavernous hemangioma.

Cavernous hemangioma or port-wine stain: It is a congenital subcutaneous lesion, which consists of a well demarcated patch, which consists of blood spaces of varying caliber. Some of them are form part of the Sturge-Weber syndrome.

Since they are subcutaneous lesions they appear bluish in color. The color tends to become darker with age due to spontaneous atrophy and thickening of the overlying skin. In course of time the overlying skin becomes thickened and nodular.

Cavernous hemangioma does not blanch with pressure and this feature differentiated it from capillary hemangioma.

Treatment

Capillary hemangioma: Small capillary hemangiomas usually disappear in 3–4 years. If they are large and cause mechanical ptosis, this can lead to amblyopia and require treatment. Treatment may be undertaken, if they are large and disfiguring. Local injections of triamcinolone plus betamethasone into the tumor may show resolution. Large diffuse lesions can be treated with systemic steroids. High doses for several weeks to months may be required. Superficial radiotherapy may also be useful.

Cavernous hemangioma: Laser therapy, early in life may help in decreasing the skin discoloration. Photodynamic therapy can be tried in large lesions.

Miscellaneous Benign Lesions

Pyogenic granuloma: It is a rapidly growing mass of vascularized granulation tissue (Fig. 24.33). They usually appear following surgery, trauma or infection, or sometimes with no specific cause.

Clinically they appear as reddish polyps that bleed readily following trivial trauma. Histologically, they consist of granulation tissue containing many vascular channels and inflammatory cells.

Treatment: Simple excision.

Xanthelasma: It is a common condition seen in middle aged or elderly persons, often associated with hypercholesterolemia. Yellowish raised plaque-like lesions is seen on the medial aspects of the lids, often bilateral and both lids are involved. Histologically, it consists of accumulation of lipid laden histiocytes in the dermis.

Treatment: Excision can be done, if the patient finds these patches are disfiguring. CO_2 or argon laser therapy is also useful. Patients with xanthelasma have to be investigated for high cholesterol levels. If there is hypercholesterolemia, it has to be controlled. Otherwise xanthelasma will recur after excision.

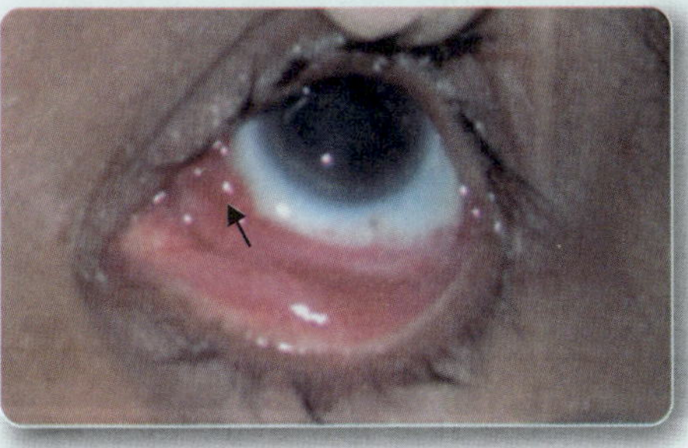

FIGURE 24.33: Pyogenic granuloma

Neurofibroma: Plexiform neurofibroma can involve the lids along with the surrounding areas of the face in people with neurofibromatosis type 1 (Figs 24.34A and B). The lid will be considerably swollen and has a feeling of bag of worms due to the hypertrophied nerves in the swelling. It can lead to mechanical ptosis and amblyopia, in addition to the gross disfigurement. The orbit may also be involved along with the lids.

Treatment: Simple excision is difficult in diffuse lesions.

Malignant Tumors

Basal Cell Carcinoma

Basal cell carcinoma (BCC) is the commonest malignancy in the lids.

Risk factors: Caucasians are more affected. Exposure to sunlight for long periods increases the risk.

Clinical features: The lower lid especially near the medial canthus is preferably affected. Usually starting as a small nodule it soon ulcerates and the ulcer has a raised, rolled out indurated edges. The ulcer spreads slowly and invade the surrounding structures including the orbit and bones, hence the name rodent ulcer (Fig. 24.35). The spread is local and the lymph nodes are not usually affected. Incomplete removal can lead to recurrence and the growth tends to be more aggressive.

Histology: The malignancy arises from the basal layer of the epidermis and proliferates as large palisades into the dermis.

Clinical types:

1. Nodular type: Slow growing nodule with dilated vessels over it.
2. Noduloulcerative type: This is the typical rodent ulcer.
3. Sclerosing type: It is rare and appears as an indurated plaque and sometimes look like chronic blepharitis.

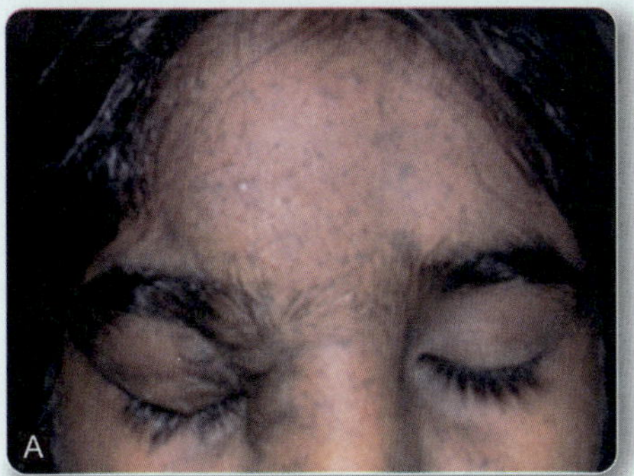

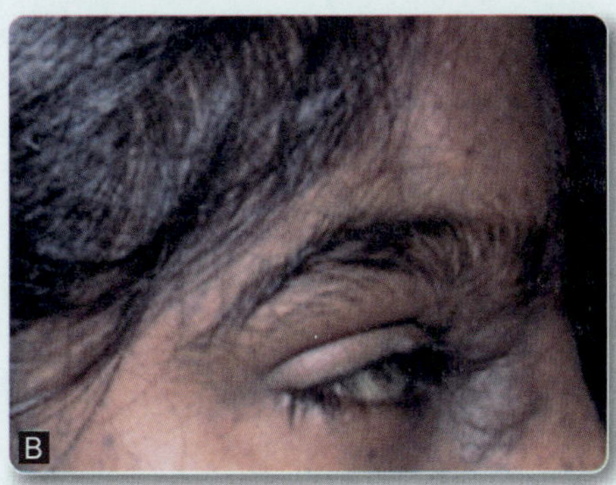

FIGURES 24.34A and B: Plexiform neurofibroma. **A.** Front view; **B.** Lateral view.

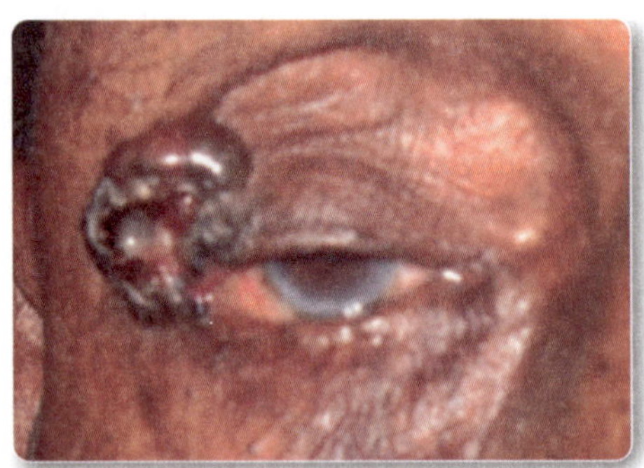

FIGURE 24.35: Basal cell carcinoma

Treatment:

1. Excision with normal surrounding area and reconstruction of the lids is the best treatment.
2. It is sensitive to radiation also. Radiation is preferred for large tumors where surgical reconstruction is difficult or for recurrence. The results of radiation treatment can be misleading. It may show remission superficially, but continue to spread deeply.
3. Exenteration is indicated for tumors involving the sclera or extraocular muscles.

Squamous Cell Carcinoma

Squamous cell carcinoma (SCC) in this lids is less common than BCC, but tends to be more aggressive with spread to the preauricular or submandibular lymph nodes. It may arise from preexisting ca-in situ or actinic keratosis or arise without any pre-existing conditions. SCC preferentially arises from sites where the character of the epithelium shows a transition. So, in the lids, the lid margins are preferentially affected (Figs 24.36A to C).

Clinical features: Since it can arise from pre-existing conditions or denovo it has no specific clinical features. It can arise as a hyperkeratotic nodule or as ulcerative type, which is difficult to differentiate from BCC and the diagnosis is often confirmed by histopathological examination. The rapid growth, the surrounding feeder vessels and the involvement of the regional lymph nodes favor a clinical diagnosis of SCC.

Histology: It arises from the squamous cell layer of the epidermis. It is composed of groups of malignant epithelial cells with prominent nuclei within the dermis. Well differentiated tumors will show the characteristic 'keratin pearls.'

Treatment: As follows:

1. Wide excision complete excision is often difficult due to ill-defined margins of the lesion.
2. Photodynamic therapy is emerging as a treatment with reasonable efficacy and gives good cosmesis for large or multiple SCC.
3. Radiotherapy or cryotherapy can also be tried.

Keratoacanthoma

Keratoacanthoma is a rare tumor found in fair-skinned people exposed to sunlight for long periods. Histologically it is considered to be a variant of SCC. Clinically it appears as a rapidly growing pink hyperkeratotic lesion. It may show a period of regression after rapid growth for a few months. During this period it may appear as a keratin filled crater.

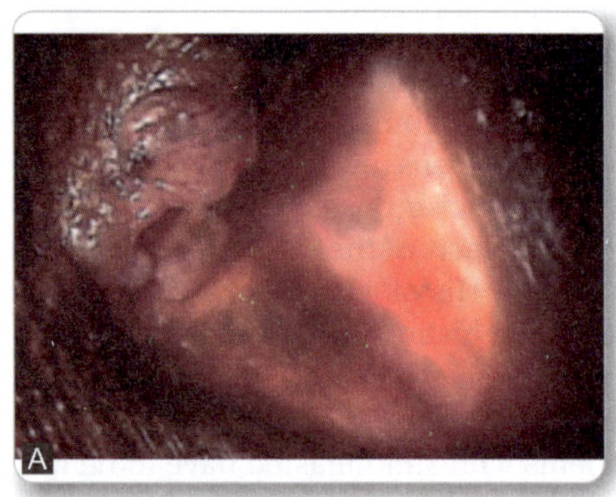

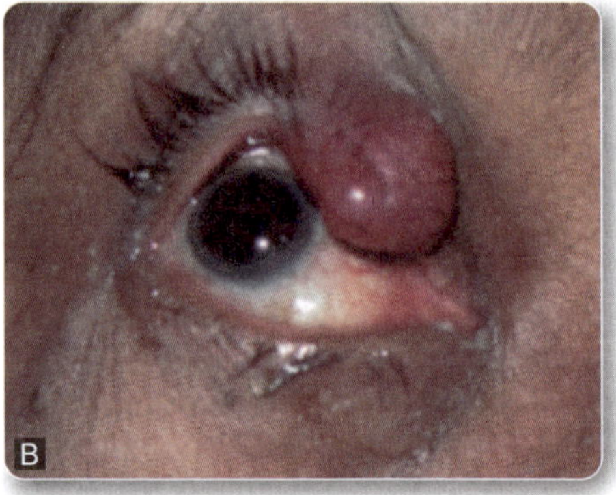

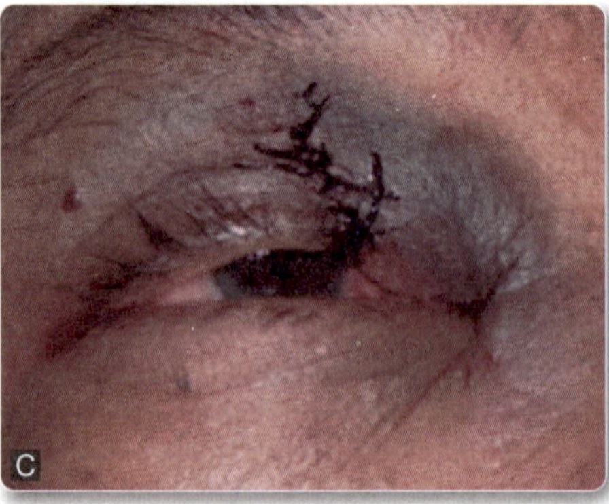

FIGURES 24.36A to C: Squamous cell carcinoma (SCC). **A.** Ulcerative type on lid margin; **B.** Nodular type; **C.** After excision.

Treatment: Complete excision, radiotherapy or cryotherapy. Intralesional 5-fluorouracil can also be tried.

Sebaceous Gland Carcinoma

Sebaceous gland carcinoma (SGC) the lids it usually arises from the meibomian glands. It is more common in the upper lid. Rarely it can arise from the Zeis' glands or sebaceous glands in the caruncle:

1. In the 'nodular type' in the early stages it appears as a chalazion (Figs 24.37A and B). Unlike a simple chalazion, which usually occurs in children or young adults, this chalazion like tumor arises in elderly people—females are more affected. Yellowish lobules of cells on I and C or recurrence after I and C should arise suspicion.
2. Rarely it can appear as a spreading SGC, which may simulate chronic blepharitis.
3. Rarely a 'pagetoid spread' can occur where it spreads into the fornices or bulbar conjunctiva and may look like an inflammatory condition (Figs 24.38A to C).

Treatment: Wide excision with 3–4 m normal surrounding tissue and reconstruction of the lids. In deeply spreading type, excenteration is indicated or intralesional mitomycin can be tried. There is a high risk of recurrence and 10% cases show lymph node involvement.

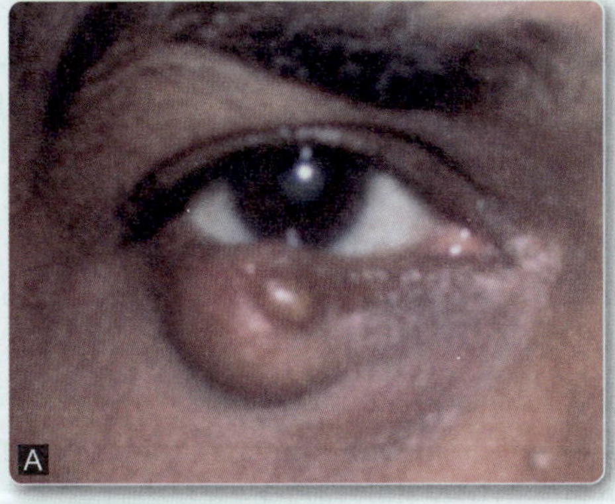

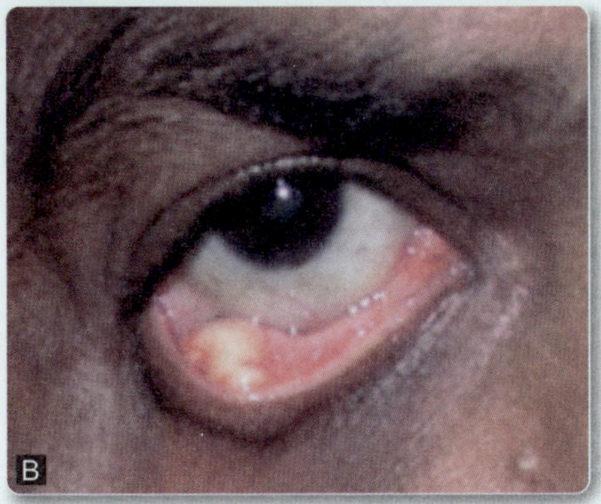

FIGURES 24.37A and B: Meibomian carcinoma simulating a chalazion; **A.** Appearance from skin side; **B.** Appearance on everting the lid.

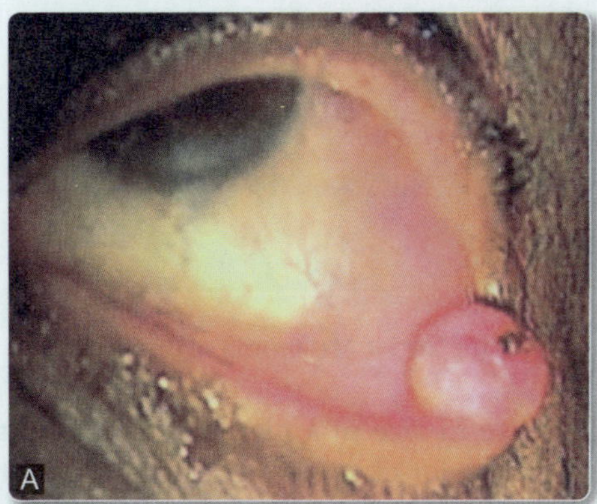

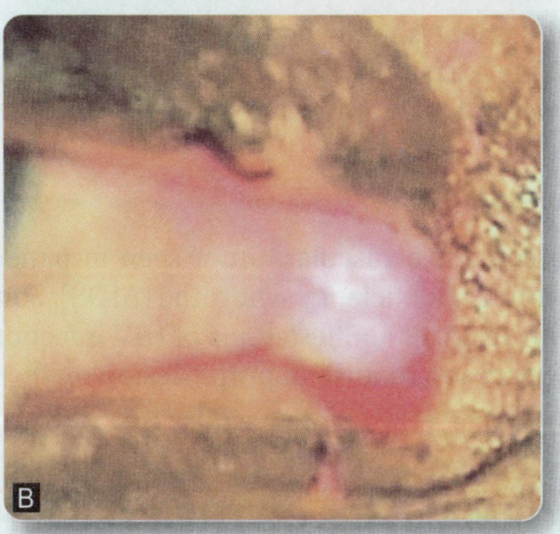

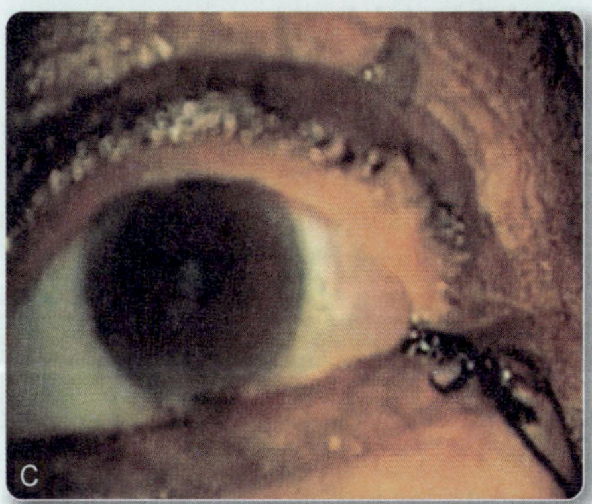

FIGURES 24.38A to C: **A.** Meibomial carcinoma (nodular type); **B.** After wide excision; **C.** After suturing.

Melanoma

Melanoma is a rare tumor and is less than 1% of eyelid tumors. It can be variably pigmented. Half the cases are non-pigmented and diagnosis is arrived by histopathological examination (Fig. 24.39).

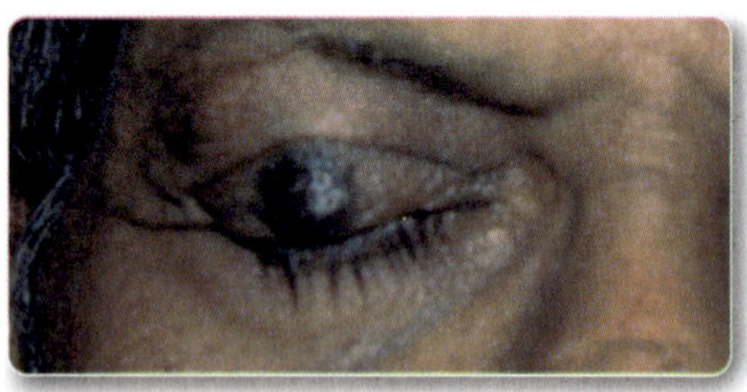

FIGURE 24.39: Melanoma of upper lid

Any increase in size of a pigmented lesion, irregular margins, recent color change or presence of multiple tumors should arouse the suspicion of melanoma.

Treatment: Patient should be evaluated for any systemic spread. Wide excision with local lymph node removal is the best method of treatment.

Kaposi Sarcoma

Kaposi sarcoma is a vascular tumor seen in patients with acquired immunodeficiency syndrome (AIDS). Sometimes it is the only clinical manifestations of HIV infection. Clinically it appears as a reddish or purple lesion on the lids.

Treatment: Excision or radiotherapy.

ABNORMALITIES OF THE EYELASHES

Congenital Distichiasis

Congenital distichiasis is a rare congenital abnormality where the meibomian glands will form a complete hair follicle containing unit and the person will have an extra row of lashes. These lashes are usually thinner and shorter and rarely cause damage to the cornea.

Treatment

In cases where it is causing problem the extra row of lashes can be destroyed by cryotherapy after splitting the lid into anterior and posterior lamellae along the gray line or by application of radiofrequency waves.

Acquired Distichiasis

Differentiation of the meibomian glands to hair follicles can occur in chemical injuries, SJ syndrome and ocular cicatricial pemphigoid.

Treatment: Cryotherapy on epilation.

Madarosis

Madarosis is an absence or decrease in lashes. It can be congenital or acquired. Common causes for acquired madarosis is burns, infiltrating lid tumors, radiation treatment, lepromatous leprosy, hypothyroidism, etc.

Poliosis

Poliosis is a premature localized whitening of hair, which can involve the eyebrows and lashes also. Vogt-Koyanagi-Harada syndrome, Waardenburg syndrome, vitiligo and chronic anterior blepharitis are the common causes.

Trichomegaly

Trichomegaly is an excessive eyelash growth. The common cause is the use of topical prostaglandin analogs like latanoprost, porphyria or AIDS and rarely it can be familial.

Trichiasis

Trichiasis is a posterior misdirection of the lashes where it can traumatize the cornea. This can lead to epithelial erosions, ulceration, pannus formation and opacification of the cornea.

The common causes are scarring of the lid margin due to chronic blepharitis, trachoma, herpes zoster ophthalmicus (HZO), SJ syndrome, etc.

Treatment: Management options for trichiasis:

1. Simple epilation with forceps—the lash will grow again and irritate the cornea.
2. Electroepilation: This is useful if the in turned lashes are few. The electrolysis needle is introduced 2-3 mm along the root of the cilia under operating microscope and low current is passed to destroy the hair follicle permanently.
3. Cryosurgery of lashes and follicles.
4. Radiofrequency ablation of lashes.
5. Argon laser ablation.
6. Wedge resection of the segment of the lid.

Lacrimal Apparatus

25

Girija Devi PS, Sahasranamam

ANATOMY

The lacrimal apparatus (Fig. 25.1) of the eye consists of essentially two parts:

1. Secretory system (tear production).
2. Excretory system (drainage of tears).

Secretory System

Secretory system consists of the lacrimal gland and its ducts and the accessory lacrimal glands. The lacrimal glands start functioning fully only by about 6 weeks after birth. So, the newborn infants do not produce tears, when crying.

Excretory System

Excretory system is composed of the lacrimal puncta, the lacrimal canaliculi, the lacrimal sac and the nasolacrimal duct (NLD) draining into the inferior meatus of the nose.

Lacrimal Glands

Lacrimal glands are tubuloracemose glands situated at the upper and outer angle of the bony orbit in the fossa of the lacrimal gland. It is made up of lobules, resembling the structure of the parotid gland. It is composed of secretory epithelial cells. The gland is divided into two parts—the superior orbital part and the inferior palpebral part. The ducts of the lacrimal gland, which are about 10–12 in number, open in the lateral part of the superior fornix. The glands secrete tears composed of water, electrolytes and lysozyme.

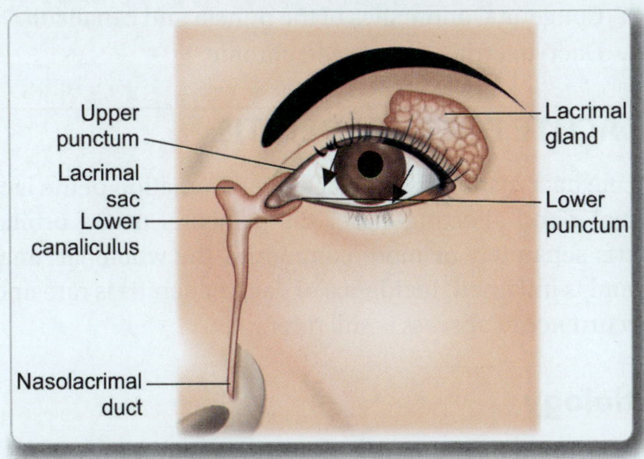

FIGURE 25.1: Lacrimal apparatus

Accessory Lacrimal Glands

Accessory lacrimal glands are small glands, which secretes tears and maintain the basal secretion of tears. They are glands of Krause and Wolfring.

Glands of Krause

The glands are about 20 in number in the upper lid and about 8–10 in the lower lid, situated within the stroma of the conjunctiva, mainly near the fornix.

Glands of Wolfring

The glands are few in number situated near the upper border of tarsal plate.

Lacrimal Puncta

Lacrimal puncta are two small round or oval openings situated on a small elevation called lacrimal papilla, about 8 mm from the inner canthus on each lid margin. Punctual region appears paler than the surrounding area. The puncta are in line with the openings of the meibomian glands. The puncta are slightly inverted and opposed to the lacrimal lake and are visible only if the lid is everted.

Lacrimal Canaliculi

The upper and lower canaliculi in either lid are narrow tubular passages, which pass medially to enter the lacrimal sac.

The two canaliculi may open separately in the lacrimal sac or may join to form a common canaliculus. The puncta and canaliculi are surrounded by fibers of orbicularis oculi, the action of which on blinking helps in tear drainage.

Lacrimal Sac

The lacrimal sac is situated in the anterior part of the medial wall of orbit, in the lacrimal fossa. The lacrimal fossa is formed by the lacrimal bone and the frontal process of the maxilla. The lacrimal sac is about 15 mm in length and 5 mm width. The portion of the sac above the opening of the canaliculi is known as the fundus of the sac, the portion below is called body of the sac. The sac is continuous with the NLD inferiorly.

Nasolacrimal Duct

Nasolacrimal duct is a membranous tubular structure approximately 15–20 mm long, extending from lower part of the sac to the inferior meatus of the nose. The direction of the NLD is downwards, posteriorly and laterally. The direction can be drawn as a line joining the medial canthus of the eye to the first upper molar. The valve of Hasner is a mucous membrane fold, present at the lower end of the nasolacrimal duct. It prevents air from the nasal cavity, entering the lacrimal sac during sneezing or blowing of the nose.

Blood Supply of the Lacrimal Gland

The arterial supply is by the lacrimal branch of the ophthalmic artery and infraorbital branch of the maxillary artery. The venous drainage is by the lacrimal vein, which drains into the superior ophthalmic vein.

Lymphatic Drainage

The lymphatics from the lacrimal gland join the conjunctival and palpebral lymphatics and drain to the preauricular nodes.

Nerve Supply

Sensory supply is through the lacrimal branch of the ophthalmic division of the trigeminal nerve, sympathetic supply is derived from the carotid plexus from the cervical sympathetic and the secretomotor fibers, i.e. the greater superficial petrosal nerve is derived from the facial nerve via the sphenopalatine ganglion.

The arterial supply of the sac and duct is derived from the superior and inferior palpebral branches of the ophthalmic artery, the angular artery and infraorbital artery. Venous drainage is into the angular vein, infraorbital veins and nasal veins.

Nerve supply to the lacrimal sac and NLD comes from infratrochlear and anterior, superior alveolar nerves.

Secretion of Tears

Normally, the rate of secretion of tears is such that there is normal wetting of the ocular surface. The basal secretion is mainly from the accessory lacrimal glands. When a foreign body or other irritant enters the eye, the secretion of tears is greatly increased and the mucus in the tear film coats the foreign body to prevent damage to the ocular surface. Secretion of tears is also increased in emotional states. The reflex secretion is from the main lacrimal gland.

Almost 25% of the tears are lost by evaporation. The remaining 75% is carried into the nasal cavity via the lacrimal drainage system. The lacrimal pump mechanism (contraction of the orbicularis oculi pulls on the lacrimal sac and draws tears into it) should function normally for drainage of tears into the nose.

Disease of the Lacrimal Gland

Common diseases of the lacrimal gland include:

1. Acute dacryoadenitis.
2. Dacryops.
3. Mikulicz's syndrome.
4. Tumors.

Disease of the Lacrimal Passages

Common diseases of the lacrimal passages include:

1. Epiphora.
2. Congenital anomalies of the puncta and canaliculi.
3. Dacryocystitis—acute and chronic.

ACUTE DACRYOADENITIS

Acute dacryoadenitis is an acute inflammation of the lacrimal gland affecting either the palpebral or the orbital parts separately or more commonly, the whole lacrimal gland is inflamed. Incidence of dacryoadenitis is rare and occurrence of abscess is still rarer.

Etiology

1. Acute dacryoadenitis is a rare condition occurring in association with viral infections like mumps or

influenza and also infectious mononucleosis, etc. sometimes leading to suppuration and fistula formation.
2. Orbital cellulitis, erysipelas of the face, etc. may also lead to this disease.
3. Primary acute dacryoadenitis may occur without any obvious cause.

Symptoms

There is marked pain, redness and swelling in the upper and outer part of the orbit along with mechanical ptosis.

Signs

1. Palpation will reveal a tender swelling at the outer part of the upper lid, spreading toward the temple and cheeks.
2. There is congestion and chemosis of the conjunctiva in upper and outer part with mucoid or mucopurulent discharge.
3. Abduction of the affected eye will be painful and sometimes restricted.
4. The preauricular glands may be enlarged and tender.
5. On lifting the upper lid and looking down and in, the inflamed gland can be visualized.

Complications

1. Suppuration can lead to abscess and fistula formation, if not promptly treated.
2. Rarely, the gland may undergo degeneration and atrophy, resulting in dry eye.

Differential Diagnosis

Acute dacryoadenitis should be differentiated from lid abscess, hordeolum internum, hordeolum externum, acute purulent conjunctivitis with chemosis and orbital cellulitis by the focus of inflammation on the outer and upper quadrant of the orbit and painful limitation of abduction of the eye.

Treatment

Treatment consists of systemic broad-spectrum antibiotics and anti-inflammatory agents and hot fomentation. Incision and drainage is done in cases of lacrimal abscess formation.

DACRYOPS

Dacryops is a cystic swelling of the lacrimal gland (palpebral lobe), due to retention of lacrimal secretion due to blockage of one of the lacrimal ducts. It presents as a nontender, mobile and fluctuant swelling in the upper lid on the lateral aspect.

Treatment

Treatment is excision through conjunctival approach.

MIKULICZ'S SYNDROME

Mikulicz's syndrome presents with a classical clinical picture with symmetrical enlargement of the lacrimal and/or salivary glands (parotid glands), usually with lymphoid tissue hyperplasia. The etiology is unknown, but it is seen in uveoparotid inflammations (Fig. 25.2).

TUMORS

Benign Tumor

The most common tumor is pleomorphic adenoma [mixed tumor (Figs 25.3A to C)]. The tumors are basically arising from the ducts of the gland. The benign mixed tumor usually occurs at around 30–50 years of age. It presents as a slowly progressive painless palpable mass in the upper lid. It may result in mechanical ptosis.

Treatment

Treatment is excision of the tumor.

Malignant Tumors

The malignant tumors can be:
1. Pleomorphic adenocarcinoma.
2. Adenoid cystic carcinoma.
3. Lymphoreticular tumors (bilateral as in leukemias, Hodgkin's disease and lymphosarcomas).

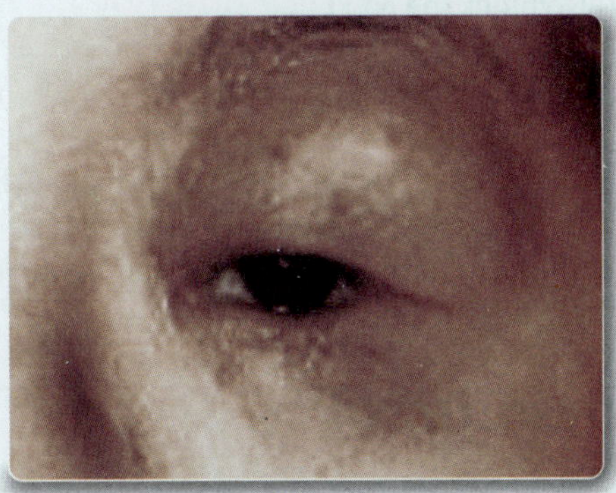

FIGURE 25.2: Mikulicz's syndrome

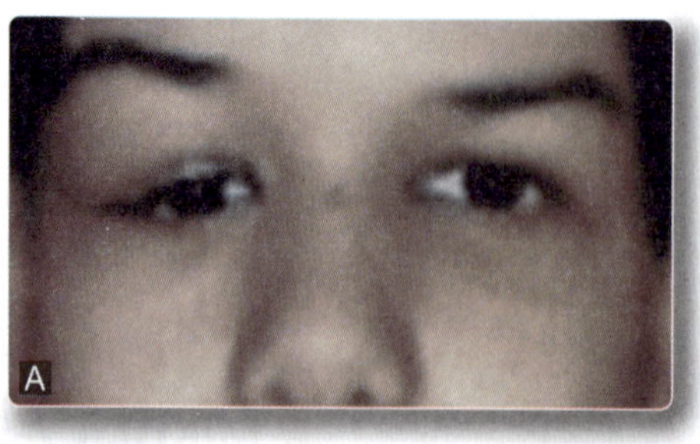

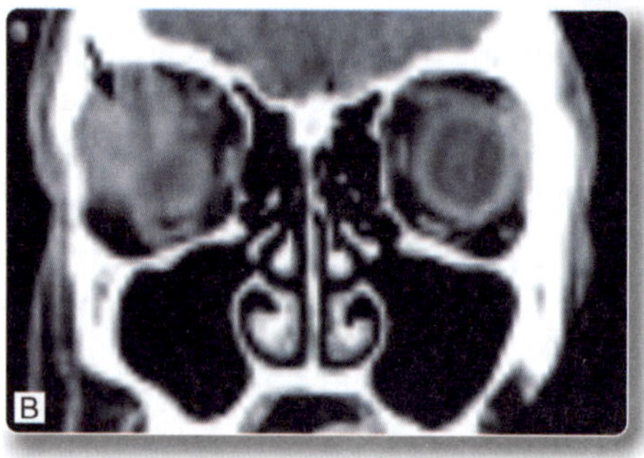

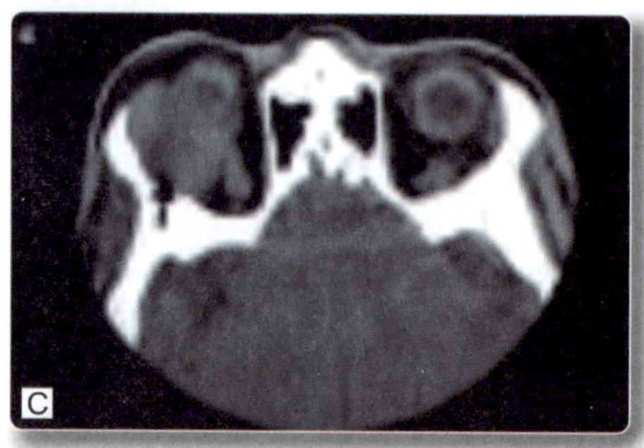

FIGURES 25.3A to C: Pleomorphic adenoma (mixed tumor). **A.** Photograph; **B and C.** Scanned pictures.

Treatment

Treatment for adenocarcinomas is radical excision followed by radiotherapy, if needed. Lymphoreticular tumors need systemic treatment for the respective disease, local radiotherapy for the lacrimal gland and if the size of the tumor is large, it needs excision.

EPIPHORA

Epiphora is excessive tearing of the eyes due to imperfect drainage through the lacrimal drainage system.

It may be due to lacrimal punctal abnormalities like congenital absence of puncta, punctal stenosis or ectropion. It may be due to obstruction at the level of canaliculus, lacrimal sac or NLD. It may occur in the form of atresia (non-canalization) canaliculitis, dacryocystitis, trauma, etc. Nasal pathologies may also block the NLD.

Treatment

Treatment is directed toward the specific cause. Excessive tearing due to hypersecretion of tears is called lacrimation. The difference between hypersecretion and defective drainage is given in Table 25.1.

CANALICULITIS

Canaliculitis is an inflammation of the canaliculi and will be associated with epiphora (Fig. 25.4).

Causes

Trachomatous canaliculitis occurs in areas where trachoma is rampant. Infection by *Actinomyces israelii,* anaerobic gram-positive bacteria is a common cause in nonendemic areas.

Clinical Features

There will be chronic conjunctivitis with pouting and inflammation of the lacrimal puncta. The chronic conjunctivitis will not be responding to conventional treatment

TABLE 25.1: Hypersecretion vs defective drainage

Hypersecretion	Defective drainage
Ocular inflammations like conjunctivitis, keratitis and uveitis, acute congestive glaucoma, etc.	Malposition of the puncta as in ectropion, eversion of the puncta
Emotional states	Obstruction of lacrimal drainage system
Reflex hypersecretion due to irritants, foreign bodies, etc.	Punctal stenosis Canaliculitis Nasolacrimal duct obstruction
Sympathetic stimulation elsewhere	Lacrimal pump failure Lower lid laxity Lower motor neuron (LMN) facial palsy

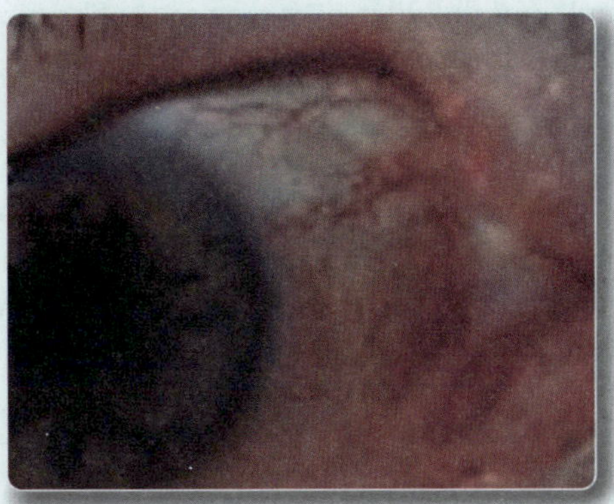

FIGURE 25.4: Canaliculitis with inflamed pouting punctum

of conjunctivitis. The pouting and inflamed canaliculus will lead to the diagnosis. Pressure over the canaliculus will express mucopurulent discharge and sometimes concretions. Aggregates of the organism will produce granular concretions.

Treatment

The treatment of *Actinomyces* canaliculitis consists of slitting the canaliculus, expressing out the contents and topical antibiotics. The organism is sensitive to penicillin drops or levofloxacin drops.

Canaliculitis may be difficult to eradicate and the patient should be warned regarding the chronic nature of the disease and treatment over multiple sittings.

DACRYOCYSTITIS

Dacryocystitis is the inflammation of the lacrimal sac. It may be congenital or acquired.

Congenital Dacryocystitis (Dacryocystitis Neonatorum)

Inflammation of the lacrimal sac in the newborn may present with an acute or chronic clinical picture.

Etiology

There may be failure in canalization of the NLD or its lumen may be blocked by epithelial debris or a membrane may be blocking the lower part of NLD. It may be a bilateral or unilateral. Many obstructions open spontaneously within 4–6 weeks after birth.

Clinical Features

There is epiphora, usually evident from 2nd week of life. Normally, the tears are secreted 3–4 weeks after birth. There may be purulent discharge in infected cases and may be mistaken for conjunctivitis. Mucopurulent discharge and persistent epiphora are two important signs of the disease. There may be regurgitation of mucopurulent discharge on pressure over lacrimal (the sac area), which confirms that there is obstruction below the level of the lacrimal sac.

Treatment

Conservative treatment is indicated in early cases. This includes observation, lacrimal sac massage and topical antibiotics.

Massage over the lacrimal sac area and clean the discharge as and when it occurs. Educate the mother/ parents regarding the illness and teach the mother to apply pressure over the lacrimal sac area by the thumb. Then bring the thumb downward, pressing toward the ala of the nose (Figs 22.5A and B). This is repeated many

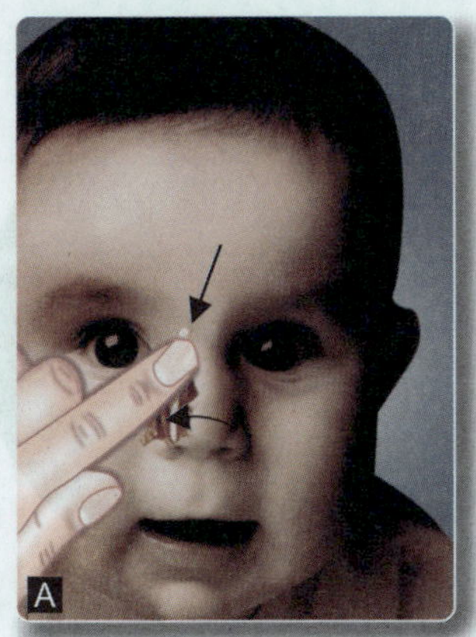

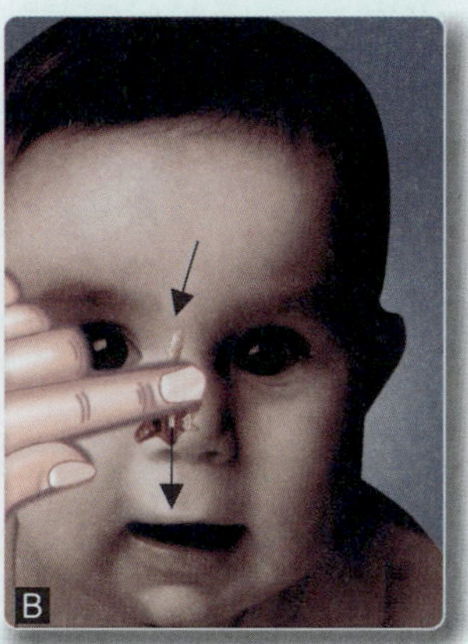

FIGURES 25.5A and B: Direction of massaging over the lacrimal sac

times daily. Massage helps to increase the pressure inside the sac and helps to open up the membranous occlusions in many cases. But make sure that it is done properly. Broad-spectrum antibiotic eyedrops are instilled frequently after expressing out the contents of the sac, by pressure over the sac area. 80%–90% cases may be cured by this treatment. Conservative treatment may be continued up to about 1 year of age in many cases.

Diligent medical management for 3–4 months is given deciding on surgical treatment. Diligent medical management cures the problem in majority of cases.

Aim: To open up or recanalize the NLD. If conservative methods fail, we have to resort to surgical modalities. This includes:

1. Probing of the NLD.
2. If repeated probings fail, intubation with silicone stent (e.g. Crawford stent) may be performed. The silicone tubing may have to be kept in the NLD for about 6 months.
3. Balloon dilatation of the duct (balloon dacryoplasty) is another modality of surgical intervention, which can be adopted. Since the equipment and procedure is expensive, it is limited to complicated cases.
4. Dacryocystorhinostomy (DCR) may have to be done when the other measures fail and the child is 3–4 years old.

Probing of Nasolacrimal Duct

If there is persistent epiphora and discharge after 3 months of conservative treatment, probing of the NLD may have to be performed. Ideally it should be done within the 1st year of life, before permanent structural damage of the canaliculus occurs. Care should be taken to avoid injury to the walls of canaliculi and the duct, as it may cause fibrosis or pericanalicular inflammation (Fig. 25.6).

Procedure

The procedure is done under general anesthesia. The upper canaliculus is usually probed. This is to avoid damage to the lower punctum and canaliculus, which is more important in drainage of tears. The punctum and canaliculus are dilated with a Nettleship dilator. A small probe No. 1 or 2 is inserted vertically downwards into the canaliculus for 2 mm. It is gently, but firmly passed inwards until bony stop of lacrimal fossa is felt. The probe is then rotated toward the midline and pushed down the NLD, till it reaches the floor of the nose. The whole procedure will take only a few minutes and if performed in the right way, will cure many cases of congenital dacryocystitis.

Complications

Failure to open the NLD, creation of a false passage and spread of infection to surrounding tissues leads to orbital cellulitis.

ACUTE DACRYOCYSTITIS

Acute dacryocystitis is an acute suppurative inflammation of the lacrimal sac.

Etiology

Acute dacryocystitis can occur as an acute exacerbation of a chronic dacryocystitis or it may occur without previous history of watering from the eye (Fig. 25.7).

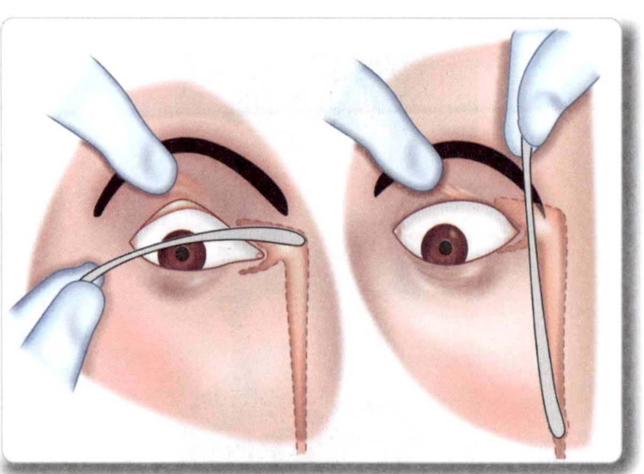

FIGURE 25.6: Probing of nasolacrimal duct

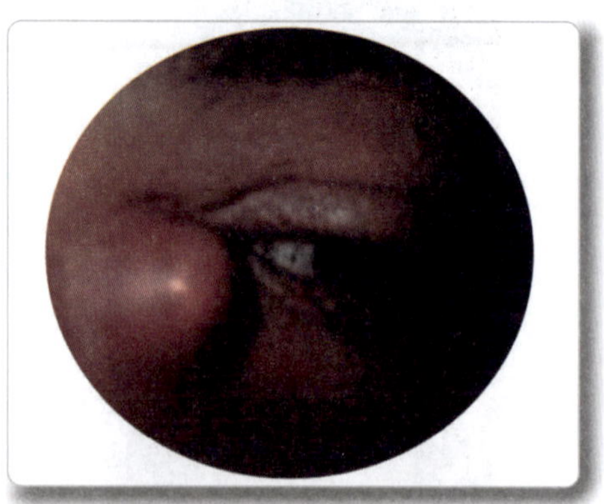

FIGURE 25.7: Acute dacryocystitis

Clinical Features

The patient presents with an acute onset of swelling, redness, pain and tenderness of the skin over the lacrimal sac area. No regurgitation may be present, as the canaliculi are blocked due to edema. Conjunctival congestion, mucopurulent discharge from the eye and submaxillary lymph node enlargement may be present. Fluctuant swelling may be present on palpation over the sac area, when there is abscess formation. But this may be difficult to elicit, due to severe tenderness.

Complications

1. Lacrimal fistula may result, if the abscess bursts open or if it is incised repeatedly.
2. Osteomyelitis of the lacrimal bone.
3. Orbital cellulitis.
4. Cavernous sinus thrombosis (not very common).

Treatment

1. Hot compresses, systemic broad-spectrum antibiotics, analgesics and anti-inflammatory drugs are effective.
2. In case of lacrimal abscess, a vertical incision can be made over the sac area in the lower part.
3. In case of lacrimal fistula, fistulectomy and removal of lacrimal sac is done.
4. Once the acute inflammation is over, DCT or DCR is done to prevent recurrence.

CHRONIC DACRYOCYSTITIS

Chronic dacryocystitis is a chronic suppurative inflammation of the lacrimal sac that usually results from obstruction of the NLD.

Etiology

Chronic dacryocystitis is usually due to stricture of the NLD as a result of chronic inflammation of the nasal mucosa or obstruction by nasal polyps, grossly deviated nasal septum or a hypertrophied inferior turbinate bone. The stagnant tears in the lacrimal sac may get infected by pyogenic bacteria.

Another cause for chronic dacryocystitis is rhinosporidiosis, which may be seen in people who take bath in stagnant water, like ponds.

The disease is more common in females, probably due to narrow bony canal in females.

Clinical Features

The disease may present with chronic epiphora or mucopurulent discharge from the eye. It may also present as a swelling (mucocele) of the lacrimal sac. Regurgitation of mucopurulent fluid by pressure over the sac area may be present.

If the common canaliculus is also blocked, a firm cystic swelling will be seen in the lacrimal area (**encysted mucocele**) and there will be no regurgitation on pressure over the sac.

Complications

1. Non-healing corneal ulcer or hypopyon corneal ulcer may occur due to spread of infection from the sac to a corneal abrasion.
2. Postoperative endophthalmitis after intraocular surgery.
3. Lacrimal abscess may occur as a result of infection by pyogenic organisms.
4. A lacrimal fistula (Fig. 25.8) may form following spontaneous bursting of the lacrimal abscess or following incision and drainage of a lacrimal abscess.

Investigations

1. A thorough nasal examination by an ENT surgeon is important to exclude deviation of septum, polyps, any abnormal mucosal growth and atrophic rhinitis.
2. Radiological examination to visualize the lacrimal passage though not commonly done include the following:
   a. Dacryocystography is done using Lipiodol, Urografin, etc. which outlines the lacrimal drainage system. X-ray films are taken to find out the size of the sac and site of obstruction.

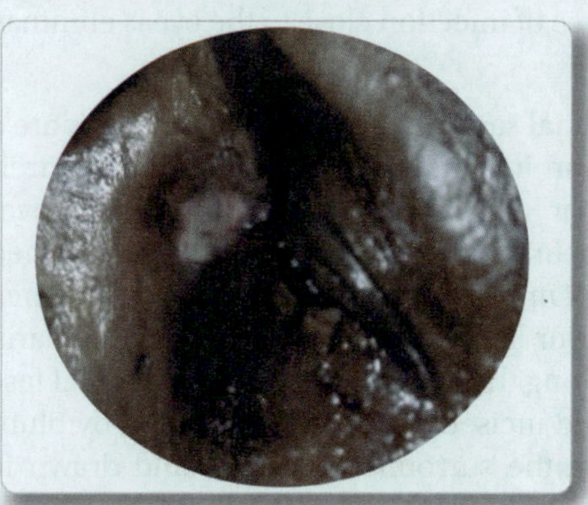

FIGURE 25.8: Lacrimal fistula

b. Subtraction macrodacryocystography with canalicular catheterization gives better results.
c. Lacrimal scintigraphy with radioactive technetium-99 (^{99}Tc) instilled into the eye as a drop, can be traced with a gamma camera.

These tests are now done infrequently because of better methods of evaluation including endonasal evaluation, computed tomography (CT) scan, magnetic resonance imaging (MRI), etc.

Treatment

Surgery is the treatment of choice and includes:

- Dacryocystectomy (DCT)
- Dacryocystorhinostomy (DCR)
- Canalization with special tubes like the Lester Jones tube.

Dacryocystectomy

A complete excision of the lacrimal sac is done in this procedure.

Indications: This is not the surgery of choice, but may be done in cases of an atrophic, fibrous sac, atrophic rhinitis, etc. It is preferred in elderly patients who may be having associated dry eye also.

Advantage

1. Dacryocystectomy is the ideal surgery in rhinosporidiosis, since DCR may result in the spread of infection to the nasal cavity.
2. It is the surgery indicated in tumors of the sac and specific infections of the sac-like TB.

Disadvantage

1. The disadvantage of this surgery is that the natural lacrimal drainage system is abolished.
2. Epiphora may persist though it may become lesser. But recurrent sac infections and the danger of a source of infection close to the eye is eliminated.

Method

The lacrimal sac and the area surrounding it are anesthetized by an injection of 2% Xylocaine with adrenaline. A curvilinear incision is made starting 2 mm above the medial palpebral ligament, 3 mm medial to the medial canthus and 4 mm downwards and outwards. It coincides with the anterior lacrimal crest (Fig. 25.9). Orbicularis muscle is split along the line of incision. The lacrimal fascia is exposed and incised. Lacrimal sac is freed by blunt dissection from the surrounding tissues and drawn forwards. The sac may be excised close to the NLD. The upper end of the NLD may be curetted. Orbicularis muscle is sutured with catgut and the skin is sutured with continuous subcuticular sutures after attaining hemostasis (Fig. 25.10).

Dacryocystorhinostomy

The usual DCR done is a traditional external DCR (transcutaneous). The surgery is usually done under local anesthesia, especially in adults. General anesthesia or monitored sedation may be used in some cases.

In this surgery, an anastomosis is made between the medial wall of the lacrimal sac and the nasal mucosa in the middle meatus. This is done after making an opening in the bone, which forms the floor of the lacrimal sac.

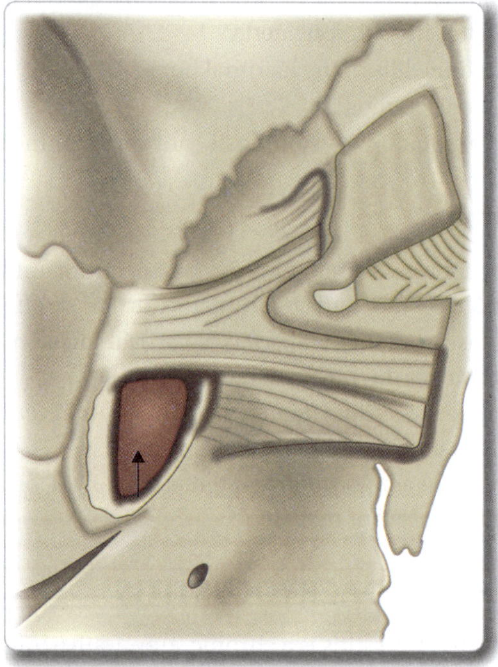

FIGURE 25.9: Lacrimal sac in the lacrimal fossa under the medial palpebral ligament

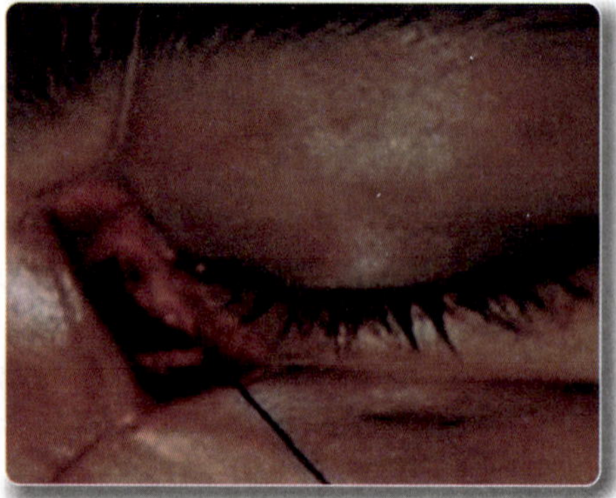

FIGURE 25.10: External dacryocystectomy in progress

Procedure

1. The nasal cavity of the same side is packed with gauze soaked in Xylocaine and adrenaline. Local anesthesia with 2% Xylocaine and adrenaline is used for local skin infiltration.
2. The canaliculi are dilated and lacrimal sac is irrigated with saline.
3. The initial steps are same as for DCT.
4. The lacrimal sac is carefully separated from the lacrimal fossa and displaced laterally to expose the bone.
5. The periosteum over the lacrimal crest is incised and lacrimal bone is exposed.
6. The bony crest is removed with a bone gouge and hammer and an opening, roughly 1 cm diameter, is created in the lacrimal fossa extending from the anterior to the posterior crest and downwards up to the opening of the NLD. The underlying nasal mucosa is exposed.
7. A vertical incision is put in the exposed nasal mucosa to create an anterior and posterior flap. Similarly, the sac is also slit vertically to produce two flaps.
8. The nasal mucosa of the middle meatus is anastomosed with the sac by suturing the anterior flap of the sac to the anterior flap of the nasal mucosa. The posterior flap of the mucosa of the lacrimal sac and nasal mucosa are also sutured together.
9. Syringing is done to test the patency of the passage.

Complications

1. Hemorrhage from the nasal mucosa, which is usually very vascular is a common complication. To prevent this, nasal packing may be maintained for a day.
2. Failed DCR may occur following an improper bony ostium, improper suturing of the flaps or persistent nasal pathology like a polyp.

Advantages of external DCR

1. The lacrimal sac is fully exposed and intrasac pathology identified.
2. The rhinostomy is large (at least 10 mm) and the mucosal flaps are sutured.
3. Success rate is higher compared to newer techniques.

Disadvantages of external DCR

1. More hemorrhages intraoperatively.
2. Occasional incision scar.
3. Interference with lacrimal pump function because of medial canthal changes.

Modification to conventional DCR includes: transcanalicular endolaser DCR, endonasal DCR, etc.

Transcanalicular endolaser DCR

The procedure is performed under general anesthesia. The nasal mucosa is anesthetized and an endoscope is used for examination of the lacrimal pathways. The site of osteotomy is determined with transillumination of the lateral nasal wall. By applying laser energy via an optic fiber passed through the canaliculi, an opening is created from the sac into the nasal mucosa. A bicanalicular silicone stent can be inserted as the last step. Success of procedure is absence of epiphora (subjective) or patency of the lacrimal drainage system on irrigation (objective).

Endonasal DCR

This is performed under local or general anesthesia by direct visualization of the nasal mucosa using endoscope. Lignocaine with adrenaline is injected under the nasal mucosa at the proposed site of osteotomy. The endoscope gives magnification as well as illumination. The opening into the lacrimal sac from the nasal mucosa is made manually or with laser. Mainly the thin lacrimal bone is removed in endonasal laser DCR and no sutures are put.

Advantages of an endonasal DCR (internal DCR):

- Lack of visible scar
- Shorter recovery time
- Less discomfort.

For this surgery either the ophthalmologist should have special training in endonasal surgery or he may take help of an ENT surgeon.

Orbit

26

Girija Devi PS, Sija S

ORBIT

Orbital cavity is a small area containing many important blood vessels and nerves in addition to eyeball and any pathological process here has serious consequences.

Infectious Inflammatory Disorders

Infections can be of various types depending on the tissue involved. It can be classified as:

1. Orbital cellulitis:
   a. Preseptal cellulitis.
   b. True Orbital cellulitis.
2. Dacryoadenitis.
3. Subperiosteal abscess.
4. Tenonitis.

BACTERIAL INFECTIONS OF THE ORBIT

Orbital Cellulitis

The most common cause of cellulitis is bacterial infections of the orbit or periorbital soft tissues (Fig. 26.1). It occurs from three primary sources:

1. Direct spread from an adjacent sinusitis or surrounding structures.
2. Direct inoculation following trauma or skin infection.
3. Bacteremic spread from a distant focus (otitis media, pneumonia).

Although periorbital infections are typically classified as being either preseptal or orbital cellulitis, they often represent a continuum with common underlying cause, requiring similar treatment regimens. It must be emphasized that infectious cellulitis, whether preseptal or orbital, is most commonly caused by underlying sinusitis, if no obvious source of inoculation is noted.

Preseptal Cellulitis

Infectious preseptal cellulitis is defined as inflammation and infection confined to the eyelids and periorbital structures, anterior to the orbital septum. The orbital structures posterior to the septum are not infected, but may be secondarily inflamed.

Clinical features

Eyelid edema, erythema and inflammation may be severe. Swollen closed lids will be tender and indurated and proper examination of the eye will be difficult. Usually the globe is uninvolved, but the swollen closed lids give an apparent appearance of proptosis. On examining the eyes, usually with the help of lid retractors, eyeball will appear normal. Pupillary reaction, visual acuity and ocular motility are not disturbed. Pain on eye movements and chemosis are absent. If an abscess forms, pus will be pointing at some part of the lids.

Causes

Although preseptal cellulitis in adults is usually due to penetrating trauma or a cutaneous source of infection like hordeolum internum or externum, in children, the most common cause is underlying sinusitis.

Management

Computed tomography (CT) evaluation of orbit and sinuses is essential, if eyelid swelling is profound enough to

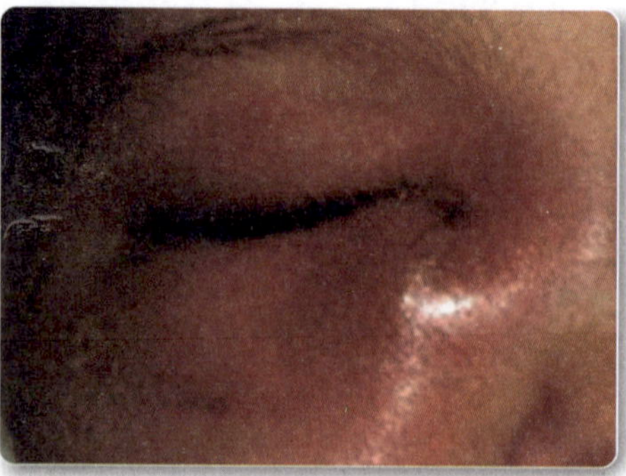

FIGURE 26.1: Orbital cellulitis

preclude examination of the globe and thereby excluding orbital cellulitis is difficult. The patient should be treated in consultation with primary care physician.

Oral antibiotics and nasal decongestants, in cases of associated sinusitis are typically effective therapy. Hospitalization and intravenous antibiotics are indicated if the cellulitis progresses despite outpatient therapy, as cases of preseptal cellulitis can progress to orbital cellulitis.

In teenagers and adults, preseptal cellulitis usually arises from a superficial source (e.g. traumatic inoculation, infected chalazion or epidermal inclusion cyst), and responds quickly to appropriate oral antibiotics and warm compresses.

Surgical drainage may be necessary, if preseptal cellulitis progresses to a localized abscess. Incision and drainage can usually be performed directly over the abscess, but care should be taken to avoid damage to levator aponeurosis. To avoid contaminating the orbital soft tissues, the surgeon should not open the orbital septum.

Complications

- Lid abscess
- Orbital cellulitis
- Cavernous sinus thrombosis.

True Orbital Cellulitis

In infectious orbital cellulitis, disease is present posterior to the orbital septum.

Etiology

In more than 90% of cases, orbital cellulitis occurs as a secondary extension of infection from surrounding structures:

1. Acute or chronic bacterial sinusitis is the common source of infection.
2. In children, it can be from the teeth.
3. Other sources can be deep injuries of orbit including surgeries like retinal detachment (RD) or squint surgery.
4. Spread of infection can be from the eye itself as in panophthalmitis or perforated corneal ulcers.
5. Infection can come from distant foci by septicemia or bacteremia.

Clinical features

1. General symptoms like fever and malaise.
2. Lid edema with tense indurated lids and marked chemosis.
3. Proptosis, which is usually axial.
4. Restriction of ocular movements and pain with ocular motility.

Vision will be normal in the early stages, but decrease in visual acuity, color vision and visual field abnormalities as well as pupillary abnormalities suggest compressive optic neuropathy, demanding immediate investigation and aggressive management.

A significant percentage of adult cases of orbital cellulitis proceed to abscess formation, which may present as progressive proptosis or globe displacement. Abscesses usually localize in the subperiosteal space, adjacent to the infected sinus, but may extend through the periosteum into the orbital soft tissues. Such abscesses should be suspected, if patients on IV antibiotics do not show daily improvement (Fig. 26.2).

Management

Early diagnosis and aggressive management is required.

Investigations

A CT scan of the head and orbit is mandatory to localize the source of infection as well as to look for any abscess formation and complications like cavernous sinus thrombosis.

Treatment

IV broad-spectrum antibiotics

Patient should be hospitalized and intravenous broad-spectrum antibiotics should be started. Antibiotic therapy should provide broad-spectrum coverage because, infection in adults usually includes multiple organisms that may include gram-positive cocci, *Haemophilus influenzae, Moraxella catarrhalis* and anaerobes.

Surgical management

Early surgical intervention to drain the involved sinus is usually indicated, especially if orbital findings progress during IV antibiotic therapy. In contrast, orbital cellulitis in children is more often caused by a single gram-positive organism and is less likely to require surgical drainage of the infected sinus.

Computed tomography scan will help to identify and localize the abscess. Pus obtained can be sent for

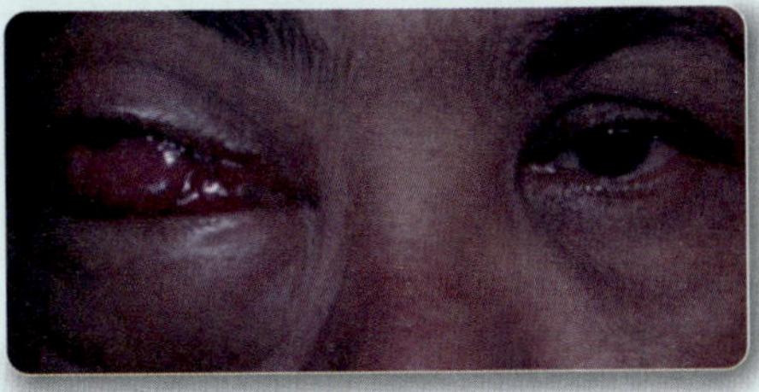

FIGURE 26.2: Orbital cellulitis with abscess formation below the eyeball

microbiological studies and the antibiotics can be suitably modified.

Not all subperiosteal abscesses require surgical drainage. Isolated medial or inferior subperiosteal orbital abscesses in children younger than age 9 with underlying isolated ethmoid sinusitis, intact vision and moderate proptosis typically respond to medical therapy.

Surgical drainage coupled with appropriate antibiotic therapy is recommended in older patients or more severe presentation and usually leads to dramatic clinical improvement within 24–48 hours. Concomitant sinus surgery is indicated, if sinusitis is present.

Delay in treatment may result in blindness, cavernous sinus thrombosis, cranial neuropathy, brain abscess and death.

Complications

1. Cavernous sinus thrombosis: Orbital infections rarely spread posteriorly to the cavernous sinus. Cavernous sinus thrombosis is heralded by the rapid progression of proptosis and by anesthesia in both the first and second divisions of the trigeminal nerve. There will be worsening of the general condition and lateral rectus palsy may develop in the other eye also.
2. Meningitis and brain abscess may develop.
3. Optic nerve compression, spread of infection to the optic nerve, central retinal artery CRA or vein occlusion can lead to rapid drop in vision and even blindness.
4. Spread inside the eye can lead to panophthalmitis or endophthalmitis.
5. Bacteremia and septicemia can develop leading to distant infections.

FUNGAL INFECTIONS OF ORBIT

Mucormycosis and aspergillosis can cause rapidly progressing and fatal infection of the orbit and should be managed on an emergency basis (refer Section 'Systemic Diseases and Eye').

PARASITIC INFECTIONS OF ORBIT

The common parasitic infestations of the orbit are:

- Trichinosis
- Cysticercosis
- Echinococcosis or hydatid cyst.

Parasitic infestations are more common in tropical countries and in areas where these infestations are common, any case of proptosis or orbital inflammation has to be investigated by ultrasonography (US) and CT scan to exclude their presence.

Trichinosis

Trichinosis is caused by the round worms of the species *Trichinella spiralis*. Eating undercooked pork meat or sausages containing the trichinosis larvae lead to human infestation.

Clinical Features

Constitutional symptoms like fever and headache, gastrointestinal (GI) symptoms like abdominal cramps, diarrhea and vomiting, joint and muscle pains will be present. Larval encystment can occur in the lids, conjunctiva or ocular muscles leading to lid edema, proptosis, pain and diplopia on ocular movements. Rupture of the cysts can produce severe inflammatory symptoms.

Treatment

Systemic steroids combined with albendazole 25 mg/day or mebendazole 200–400 mg/day for 10 days may be effective. Steroids will control the inflammation, but elimination of the adult worm is difficult and larvae will continue to be produced resulting in recurrence of symptoms.

Cysticercosis

Cysticercosis is an infestation by the pork tapeworm, *Taenia solium*. Human beings are the carriers and the infestation is spread through water and food contaminated with the eggs passed in the feces of an infected person. The eggs hatch once they reach the stomach and the larvae can reach any part of the body via bloodstream and lead to cyst formation. One or more cysts may form in the conjunctiva, ocular muscles, vitreous or retina. It can lead to proptosis, limitation of ocular movements and diplopia. Death and rupture of the cysts can lead to severe inflammatory reaction.

Management

Orbital US and CT scans are essential to confirm the diagnosis. The cystic lesion with the central hyperechoic spot formed by the scolex is diagnostic.

Treatment

Removal of the cyst by orbitotomy is the treatment of choice. Cysticidal therapy with praziquantel (50 mg/day, three times daily for 14–30 day) or albendazole (15 mg/day, three times daily for 8–15 day) combined with systemic steroids is also effective. Before starting medical therapy a detailed fundus evaluation to rule out intraocular cysts and a central nervous system (CNS) evaluation to rule out intracranial cysts is essential, since death of the cysts can lead to severe intraocular inflammation and loss of vision.

Echinococcosis or Hydatid Cysts

Hydatid cysts is the cyst formed by the larvae of *Echinococcus granulosus*, which lives in the intestine of cats and dogs.

Hydatid cysts can form in the orbit leading to progressive proptosis.

Management

Diagnosis is confirmed by CT and US scan and by Enzyme-linked immunosorbent assay (ELISA) test for Echinococcus antibodies.

Treatment

Treatment is excision of the cyst without rupturing its wall. Rupture of the cyst can lead to severe inflammation.

NON-SPECIFIC ORBITAL INFLAMMATION (ORBITAL PSEUDOTUMOR)

Non-specific orbital inflammation (NSOI) also known as orbital pseudotumor, is currently defined as an idiopathic tumor like inflammation consisting of a pleomorphic cellular response and a fibrovascular tissue reaction. NSOI is usually confined to the orbit, but may extend to the sinuses and the intracranial space. It has a variable, but generally self-limited course. Both children and adults may be affected (Figs 26.3A and B).

The subclassification of NSOI is made on the basis of the anatomical target:

1. The inflammation can primarily affect the lacrimal gland (dacryoadenitis).
2. One or more extraocular muscles (myositis).
3. The sclera and posterior tenons (scleritis).
4. The optic nerve sheath (inflammatory optic neuritis).
5. It can be restricted to the superior orbital fissure and cavernous sinus (Tolosa-Hunt syndrome).

Sx Symptoms

- Deep-rooted boring pain
- Visual acuity may be impaired
- Conjunctival inflammation and eyelid erythema
- Orbital imaging may confirm the diagnosis.

Signs and Symptoms

Depend on the involved tissue, however deep-rooted boring pain is a typical feature of the process. Extraocular movement restriction, proptosis, conjunctival inflammation and chemosis are common and eyelid erythema and soft tissue swelling may be present. Visual acuity may be impaired, if the optic nerve or posterior sclera is involved.

On the whole, there will be some signs of inflammation, but not so acute or severe as in orbital cellulitis, but also some features of a tumor, clinically or radiologically evident mass-like lesion, but biopsy or fine-needle aspiration cytology (FNAC) shows some non-specific cellular reaction.

A typical clinical presentation is often diagnostic and orbital imaging may confirm the diagnosis. A thorough systemic evaluation should be undertaken, if there is any uncertainty regarding the diagnosis. Not all patients with NSOI present with the classic signs and symptoms. There may be a typical pain, limited inflammatory signs or a fibrotic presentation termed sclerosing NSOI. Such lesions more commonly require biopsy for diagnosis.

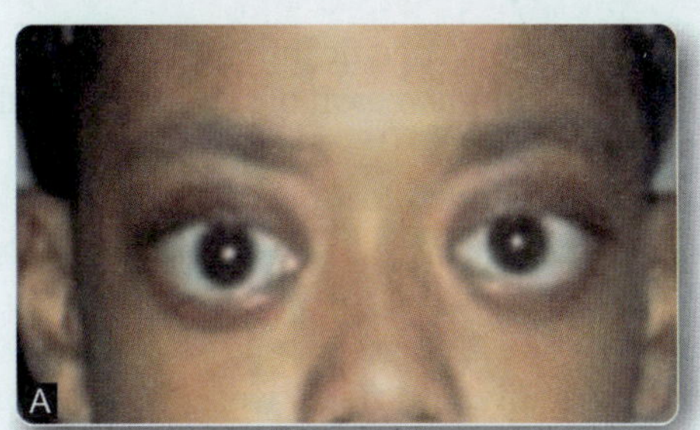

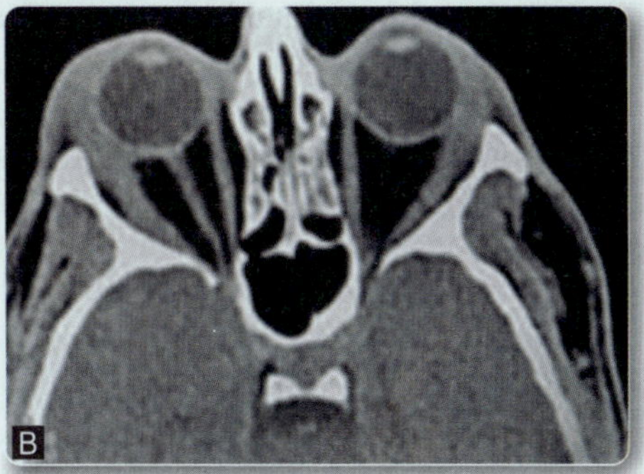

FIGURES 26.3A and B: Orbital pseudotumor. **A.** Clinical picture; **B.** CT scan showing thickening of muscles including tendon.

Investigations

Biopsy is not necessary in all cases because the findings on clinical, ultrasonographic and radiologic examination may be sufficiently diagnostic to institute therapy. Biopsy is reserved for cases that fail to respond rapidly to corticosteroids or for those with recurrence, after treatment is discontinued. Simultaneous bilateral idiopathic inflammation in adults suggests the possibility of systemic vasculitis. In children, however approximately one third of cases of NSOI are bilateral and are rarely associated with systemic disorders.

Histopathologically: NSOI is characterized by a pleomorphic cellular infiltrate consisting of lymphocytes, plasma cells and eosinophils with variable degrees of reactive fibrosis. The sclerosing type demonstrates a predominance of fibrosis with sparse inflammation.

Computed tomography scan: In dacryoadenitis, CT scan reveals diffuse enlargement of the lacrimal gland. In myositis, the extraocular muscle tendons of insertion may be thickened in up to 50% of patients with NSOI in contrast, thyroid-associated eye disease (TED) typically spares the muscle insertions.

An inflammatory infiltrate of the retrobulbar fat pad is commonly seen and contrast enhancement of the sclera may be caused by tenonitis (producing the ring sign).

B-scan ultrasonography often shows an acoustically hollow area corresponding to an edematous Tenon's capsule.

Treatment

Initial therapy consists of systemic corticosteroids. Acute cases generally respond rapidly with an abrupt resolution of the associated pain. The use of steroids can be tapered as soon as the clinical response is complete, but this tapering should be done slowly. Rapid reduction of systemic steroids may cause a recurrence of inflammatory symptoms and signs.

An incomplete therapeutic response or recurrent disease suggests the need for orbital biopsy, which can provide histopathologic confirmation and exclude specific inflammatory diseases.

After the diagnosis is confirmed, orbital irradiation, antimetabolites or alkylating agents such as methotrexate or cyclophosphamide and continued steroid therapy may be useful for controlling the disease.

Rarely orbital decompression is necessary, if optic nerve compression is progressive.

Tumor necrosis factor alpha (TNF-α) blockers have been used in recurrent cases or for those patients in whom corticosteroids are contraindicated.

Sclerosing NSOI is a distinct subset of disease with predominant fibrosis and minimal cellular inflammation. It responds poorly to steroids and to low-dose radiotherapy and typically requires more aggressive immunosuppression with cyclosporine, methotrexate or cyclophosphamide.

Cavernous Sinus Thrombosis

The cavernous sinus has several tributaries connecting it to the eyes, ear, face, sinuses and most part of the cerebrum. Infection in any of these areas can reach cavernous sinus and produce inflammation and thrombosis. *Staphylococcus aureus* is the causative organism in 70% of cases.

Clinical Features

Cavernous sinus thrombosis is closely simulates an orbital cellulitis, but the constitutional symptoms are much more severe. There will be high fever, headache and cerebral symptoms. The second eye will also be involved in 50% of cases and a lateral rectus paresis will be the earliest sign. A swelling behind the ear due to involvement of the mastoid emissary vein is another early sign.

Unlike in case of orbital cellulitis there will be severe neuralgic supraorbital pain due to involvement of the ophthalmic division of the trigeminal. Disk edema with engorgement of the retinal veins may be present.

Investigation

Computed tomography scan will confirm the diagnosis.

Treatment

Aggressive management is required to prevent loss of vision as well as life. Broad-spectrum antibiotics and anticoagulants should be administered. Though the signs and symptoms are mainly in the eye, it is primarily an intracranial problem, and it has to be managed by the neurologist and the ophthalmologist together.

Tolosa-Hunt Syndrome

The syndrome is a non-specific inflammatory process with granulation tissue in the region of superior orbital fissure. It is characterized by:

1. Recurrent unilateral retro-orbital pain.
2. Palsies of the extrinsic ocular muscles involving the III, IV and VI cranial nerves, the sympathetic and the V nerve.
3. The visual acuity and fields were usually normal although the optic nerve might be affected.
4. The pupils are relatively spared.

Males and females are equally affected. It is more common in the 5th decade. The symptoms last for some days or weeks with spontaneous remissions lasting some months or years.

Treatment

Dramatic response to systemic steroid therapy within a very short time is seen, which is another important characteristic.

PROPTOSIS

Proptosis is an abnormal protrusion of the eyeball. Exophthalmos is a term conventionally used for proptosis seen in TED (Box 26.1).

BOX 26.1: Causes of Proptosis

- Congenital conditions
  - Crouzon syndrome
  - Apert syndrome
  - Orbital dermoid
- Inflammatory conditions
  - Orbital cellulitis
  - Mucormycosis
  - Dacryoadenitis
  - Tolosa-Hunt syndrome
  - Wegener's granulomatosis
  - Orbital pseudotumor
- Vascular conditions
  - Cavernous hemangioma
  - Caroticocavernous fistula
  - Orbital varices
- Tumors
  - Lacrimal gland tumors
  - Optic nerve glioma
  - Meningioma
  - Lymphoma
  - Neurofibroma
  - Metastatic tumors
  - Frontal and ethmoidal mucocele
- Endocrine diseases
  - Thyroid exophthalmos
- Traumatic conditions
  - Orbital fractures
  - Orbital hemorrhage
  - Orbital emphysema

Proptosis can be:

- Unilateral or bilateral
- Acute or chronic
- Axial or eccentric
- Pulsatile or non-pulsatile
- Static, intermittent or progressive.

Pseudoproptosis

Pseudoproptosis is an apparent appearance of proptosis.

Causes

1. Severe enlargement of one eye alone as in unilateral high myopia or buphthalmos.
2. Unilateral lid retraction.
3. Facial asymmetry.
4. Enophthalmos or ptosis of one eye, which makes the uninvolved eye more prominent.

Thyroid-associated Eye Disease

Thyroid eye disease is the most common cause for unilateral as well as bilateral proptosis. So, thyroid function tests have to be done in the investigations of all cases of proptosis.

Unilateral Proptosis

Unilateral proptosis can be due to:

- Thyroid eye disease
- Orbital cellulitis
- Parasitic infestations
- Benign or malignant tumors
- Cavernous sinus thrombosis in the early stages.

Bilateral Proptosis

Bilateral proptosis can be due to:

- Thyroid eye disease
- Caroticocavernous fistula and cavernous sinus thrombosis in late stages
- Parasitic infestations
- Bilateral orbital tumors as in lymphomas, secondary deposits or orbital extension of bilateral retinoblastoma
- Pseudotumor in children
- Craniofacial synostosis like Crouzon syndrome.

Acute Proptosis

Acute proptosis usually appears within a few hours to few days. It can be due to:

- Orbital cellulitis
- Orbital hemorrhage
- Orbital emphysema
- Caroticocavernous fistula.

Axial Proptosis

A condition (Figs 26.4A and B) where the eye is pushed straight forward is seen in:
- Thyroid eye disease
- Orbital cellulitis
- Intraconal mass lesions.

Eccentric Proptosis

A condition where the eye is displaced sideways is seen in extraconal mass lesions.

Pulsatile Exophthalmos

The condition is seen in:
- Caroticocavernous fistula
- Meningoencephalocele with bony defects of orbit
- Highly vascular tumors.

Static Proptosis

Static proptosis condition is rare and seen in congenital conditions like dermoid cysts and craniofacial synostosis with shallow orbits.

Intermittent Proptosis

The condition is seen in orbital varices.

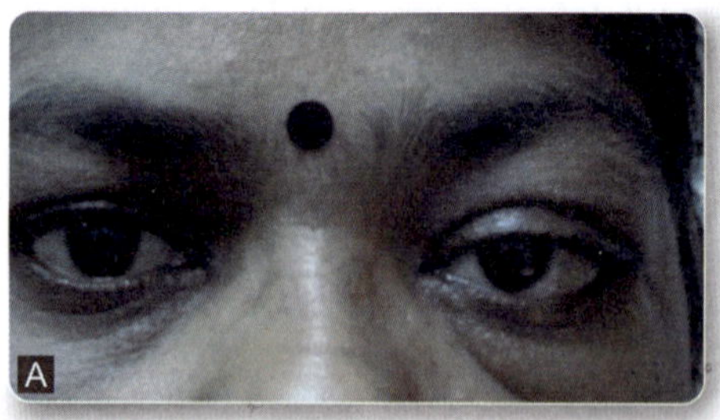

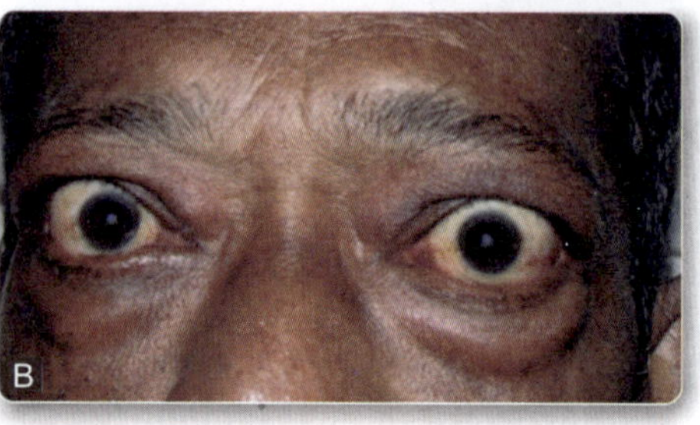

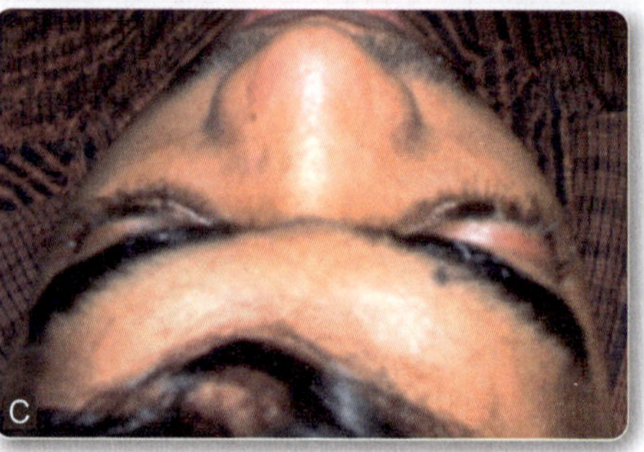

FIGURES 26.4A to C: Proptosis. **A.** Left axial proptosis; **B.** Bilateral axial proptosis with lid retraction in thyrotoxicosis; **C.** Naffziger's sign with prominent right eye.

Investigations in a Case of Proptosis

1. Exophthalmometry: A simple instrument called Hertel exophthalmometer is used to measure the displacement of the globe. Normal measurement is 18–21 mm and a measurement of more than 21 mm or a difference of more than 2 mm between the two eyes is significant.

   If exophthalmometer is not available, a transparent ruler held at the lateral canthus, parallel to the nose can be used to make an approximate measurement.

   Naffziger's sign—look down at the patient from above and behind, so that you are looking down at the patient's eyebrow and nose from above. Any proptosis can be made out (Fig. 26.4C).
2. Thyroid function tests to rule out any thyroid eye disease.
3. Plain X-ray of skull and orbit to highlight any fractures or erosions of the bones. Special view like water's view is required to visualize the optic foramen. With the advent of CT scan and MRI, the importance of X-rays has come down.
4. Ultrasonography scan easily delineates the size and location of a space occupying lesion.
5. Computed tomography scan gives useful clue regarding the anatomical nature of the mass lesions, especially those arising from the bones and also helps to visualize calcification and any extension to the sinuses or intracranial areas.
6. Magnetic resonance imaging helps better anatomical identification of soft tissue masses than CT scan, but it is contraindicated in the presence of a metallic foreign body.

Magnetic resonance imaging angiogram is indicated in special situations like orbital varices, any vascular anomalies and to identify the feeder vessels in highly vascular tumors.

Treatment

1. This depends on the underlying cause. So, all investigations have to be done to make a correct etiological diagnosis.

2. If it is thyroid exophthalmos, thyrotoxicosis has to be treated. Antithyroid drugs have to be monitored carefully so as to avoid going in for hypothyroidism, since this can aggravate the protrusion of the eyeball.
3. If it is due to a tumor, surgery is required.

General Measures

1. Artificial tears have to be instilled frequently to avoid drying of the cornea.
2. If there is corneal exposure, lateral tarsorrhaphy is indicated to protect the cornea.
3. Systemic steroids can be given in addition to antithyroid drugs to decrease the inflammatory infiltration and control the protrusion in severe cases.
4. If all these measures fail and optic nerve compression or exposure keratitis sets in, surgical decompression of the orbit has to be done.

Enophthalmos

Enophthalmos is an inward displacement of the eyeball. It has to be differentiated from microphthalmos—a congenitally small eye or phthisis bulbi, a disorganized eyeball due to disease. In enophthalmos, the abnormality is in the orbital walls or its contents and the eye is normal.

Causes

1. A blowout fracture of the orbit: This is a fracture of the orbital walls without involving the orbital margins, usually caused by a blunt trauma of considerable force. The inferior or the medial wall of the orbit is involved. There will be herniation of orbital soft tissue into the sinuses and entrapment of the ocular muscles in the fracture. This will lead to enophthalmos and limitation of ocular movements.
2. Atrophy of orbital fat due to extreme malnutrition, radiation treatment or repeated steroid injections into the orbit.
3. Sclerosing orbital lesions like metastatic scirrhous carcinoma and sclerosing orbital pseudotumors.

ORBITAL NEOPLASMS

Congenital Orbital Tumors

Dermoid Cyst

Dermoid and epidermoid cysts are among the most common orbital tumors of childhood. These cysts are present congenitally and they enlarge progressively as the child grows. The more superficial cysts usually become symptomatic in childhood, but deeper orbital dermoids may not become clinically evident until adulthood. Orbital dermoid cysts are lined by epidermis only and are usually filled with keratin, and they do not contain dermal appendages.

Preseptal orbital dermoid cysts occur most commonly in the area of the lateral brow adjacent to the frontozygomatic suture. Dermoid cysts commonly present as palpable smooth, painless, oval masses that enlarge slowly. They may be freely mobile or they may be fixed to periosteum at the underlying suture (Figs 26.5A and B). Medial lesions in the infant should be distinguished from congenital encephaloceles and dacryoceles.

Dermoid cysts that do not present until adulthood are often not palpable because they are situated posteriorly in the orbit, usually in the superior and temporal portions, adjacent to the bony sutures. The globe and adnexa may be displaced causing progressive proptosis and erosion or remodeling of bone can occur. Less commonly, the clinical presentation may be orbital inflammation, which is incited by leakage of oil and keratin from the cyst.

Management

Dermoid cysts are usually removed surgically. Superficial dermoids can be excised through an incision placed in the upper eyelid crease or directly over the lesion. If possible,

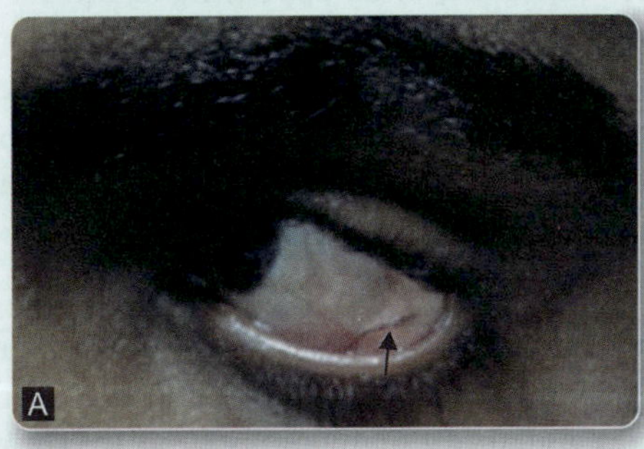

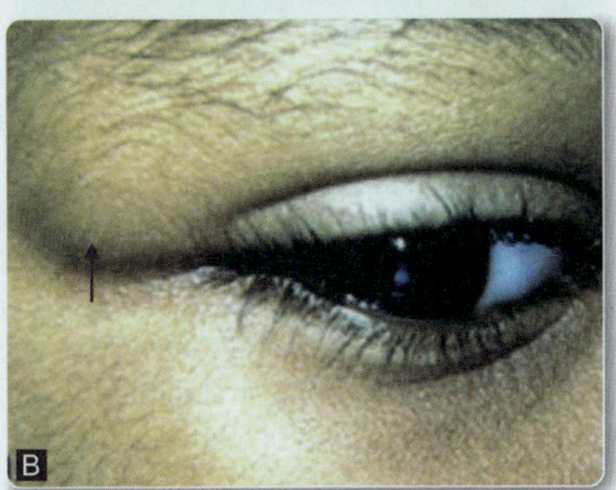

FIGURES 26.5A and B: Dermoid cyst. A. Dermoid with hair; B. Orbital dermoid.

the cyst wall should be maintained during surgery. Rupture of the cyst can lead to an acute inflammatory process, if part of the cyst wall or any of the contents remains within the eyelid or orbit. If the cysts wall is ruptured, the surgeon should remove the entire wall and then thoroughly irrigate the wound to remove all cyst contents.

Teratoma

Teratomas are rare tumors that arise from all three germ layers. These tumors are usually cystic and can cause dramatic proptosis at birth. The globe and optic nerve may, as a consequence, be maldeveloped. Exenteration is sometimes performed because of the fear of malignancy. Some cystic teratomas can be removed and ocular function preserved.

Vascular Tumors

Capillary Hemangiomas

Capillary hemangiomas are common benign primary tumors of the orbit in children. They should be distinguished from cavernous hemangiomas, which are the most common benign orbital tumors in adults (Figs 26.6A and B).

Capillary hemangiomas are seen primarily in children in the first year of life, often appearing in the 1st week or 2 weeks after birth, enlarging dramatically over the first 6–12 months of life. They are more common in girls and premature newborns. After the first year, these vascular tumors begin to involute, 75% of lesions resolve during the next 4 years of life.

Clinical features

The clinical appearance of a periorbital capillary hemangioma depends on the depth of tumor under the skin. Superficial capillary hemangiomas produce an elevated red discoloration with a dimpled texture (refer Fig. 26.6A). Deeper ones cause a bluish discoloration or may present merely as a progressively enlarging mass without any overlying skin change.

Periocular hemangiomas are commonly associated with hemangiomas on other parts of the body. Common sites of involvement are superonasal quadrant of the orbit and medial upper eyelid. Capillary hemangiomas of the eyelids and orbit may cause anisometropia, strabismus or deprivation amblyopia. Cosmetic deformity is often significant.

Management

1. Magnetic resonance imaging demonstrates the characteristic fine intralesional vascular channels and also defines the speed of blood flowing within the lesion. Capillary hemangiomas usually have high blood flow derived from multiple fine feeder vessels.
2. Ophthalmic indications for treatment of capillary hemangiomas are anisometropia, strabismus and amblyopia.
3. Radiation therapy, pulsed dye laser therapy and high-potency topical corticosteroids has been used in the treatment of capillary hemangiomas.

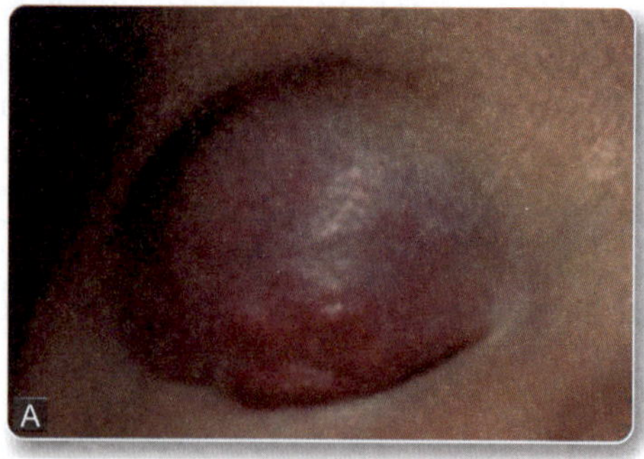

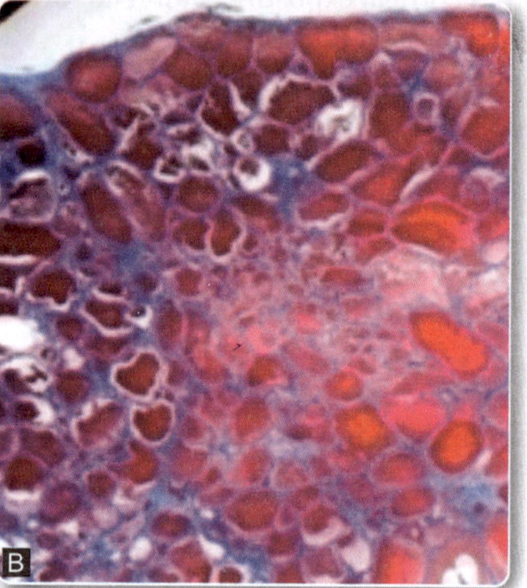

FIGURES 26.6A and B: Capillary hemangioma. **A.** Gross anatomy; **B.** Histopathology showing vascular channels.

Cavernous Hemangioma

Cavernous hemangiomas are the most common benign neoplasms of the orbit in adults (Figs 26.7A and B). Middle-aged women are most commonly affected. Proptosis is usually slowly progressive, although growth may accelerate, if the patient is pregnant.

Complications

Retinal striae, hypermetropia, optic nerve compression, increased intraocular pressure and strabismus may develop:

1. Histopathologically, the lesions are encapsulated and are composed of large cavernous spaces containing

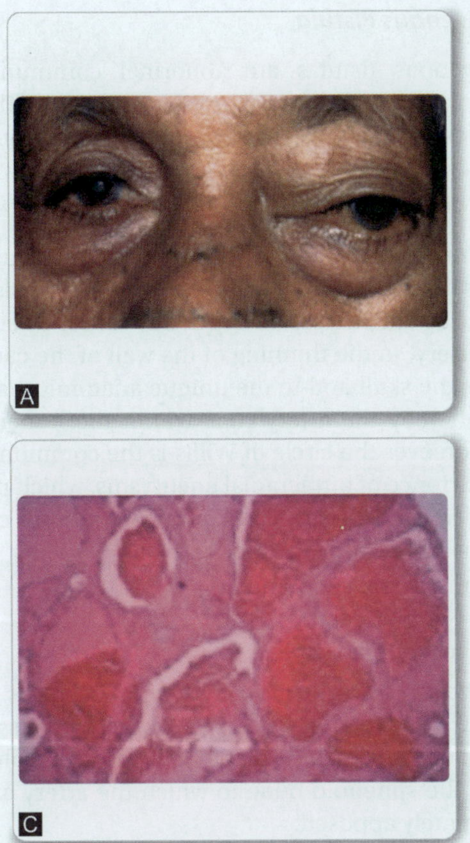
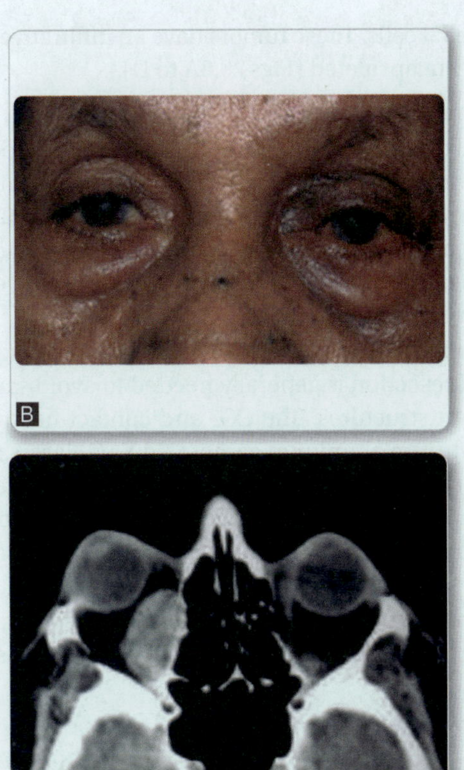

FIGURES 26.7A to D: Cavernous hemangioma. **A.** Before surgery; **B.** After surgery; **C.** Histopathology; **D.** CT scan in cavernous hemangioma.

red blood cells and the walls contain smooth muscle (Fig. 26.7C).

2. MRI demonstrates an enhancing lesion with small intralesional vascular channels containing slowly flowing blood.
3. Arteriography and venography has no much role because the lesion has a very limited communication with systemic circulation.
4. Computed tomography shows a homogeneously enhanced well-encapsulated mass (Fig. 26.7D). Old lesions may contain radiodense phleboliths.

Management

Treatment consists of surgical excision of the lesion comprising ocular function. These tumors rarely undergo spontaneous involution.

When therapy is indicated, initial treatment consists of local steroid injection, usually an equal mixture of 0.5 mL betamethasone and 0.5 mL triamcinolone. Adverse effects include necrosis of the skin overlying the hemangioma, subcutaneous fat atrophy, systemic growth retardation and embolic visual loss.

Systemic steroids have also been used, especially in lesions that extend more deeply into the orbit. Injecting deep orbital lesions carries a higher risk of orbital hemorrhage and retinal emboli.

Lesions that are smaller, those that are subcutaneous and nodular, and those refractory to steroids can be managed with surgical excision. The use of systemic interferon-α has been reported, but poorly tolerated in most cases.

Lymphangioma

A lymphangioma is a relatively uncommon tumor that usually becomes apparent in the 1st decade of life. It may occur in the conjunctiva, eyelids, orbit, oropharynx or sinuses. Lymphangiomas often enlarge during upper respiratory tract infections, probably because of the response of the lymphoid tissues within the lesion. They may present with sudden proptosis caused by spontaneous intralesional hemorrhage.

Histologically, these tumors are characterized by large serum-filled spaces that are lined by flattened, delicate endothelial cells. These tumors have an infiltrative pattern and not encapsulated (Figs 26.8A to D).

Management

In blood cysts associated with lymphangiomas, spontaneous regression is common. Surgical intervention should be deferred unless vision is affected. If optic neuropathy or corneal ulceration threatens vision, aspiration of blood through a hollow-bore needle or by open surgical exploration can be attempted.

Because of the infiltrating nature of lymphangioma, a subtotal resection is generally needed to avoid sacrificing important structures. The CO_2 and contact neodymium-doped yttrium aluminum garnet (Nd:YAG) lasers are useful adjuncts for surgery, which improves hemostasis and can be used to cause shrinkage and scarring of some unresectable areas of tumor. Bipolar cautery can also be applied to shrink the tumor during surgical excision.

In more extensive diffuse lesions of the orbit, a transcranial approach may allow total or subtotal excision.

Arteriovenous Malformations

Arteriovenous malformations are developmental anomalies composed of abnormally formed anastomosing arteries and veins without an intervening capillary bed.

Arteriovenous Fistula

Arteriovenous fistulas are abnormal communications between previously normal arteries and veins. These acquired lesions may be caused by trauma or degenerations.

Caroticocavernous Fistula

The common occurrence of a caroticocavernous fistula (CCF) is due to the partly fixity of the vessels in this area to the bone so that, a fracture frequently causes direct injury to the artery, to the thinning of the wall of the carotid, as it enters the skull and to the unique anatomical arrangement whereby the artery runs within the lumen of the vein. Moreover the circle of Willis is the common site for the occurrence of intracranial aneurysms, which provides point of weakness (Fig. 26.9). Caroticocavernous communications can be divided into:

- Traumatic and spontaneous
- Direct or indirect
- Low flow or high flow.

Traumatic cases: Occur most frequently in males, constituting 80% of the total cases. 75% of these are associated with a fracture of the base of the skull, mostly involving the body of the sphenoid bone to which the artery and vein are intimately apposed.

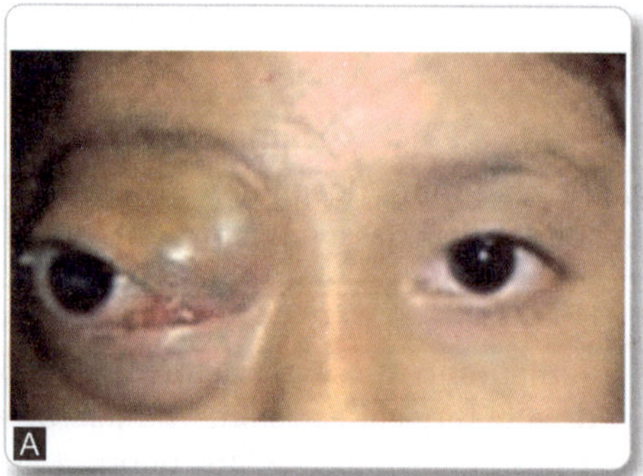

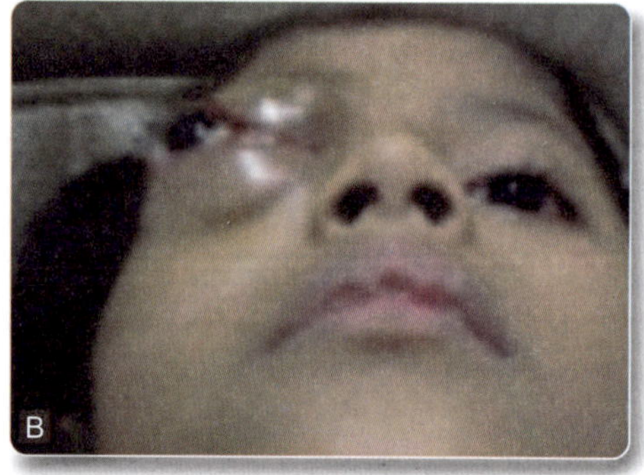

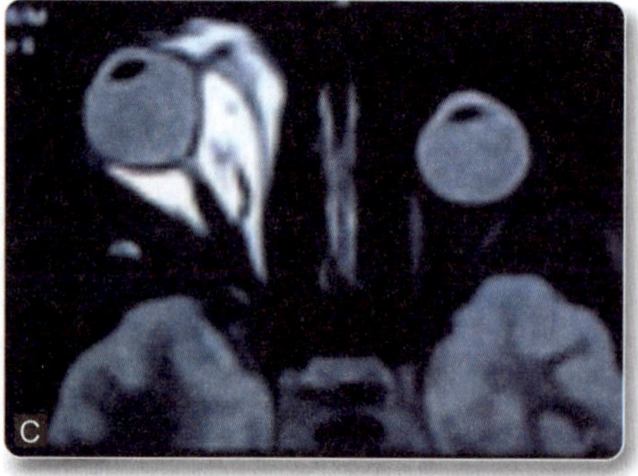

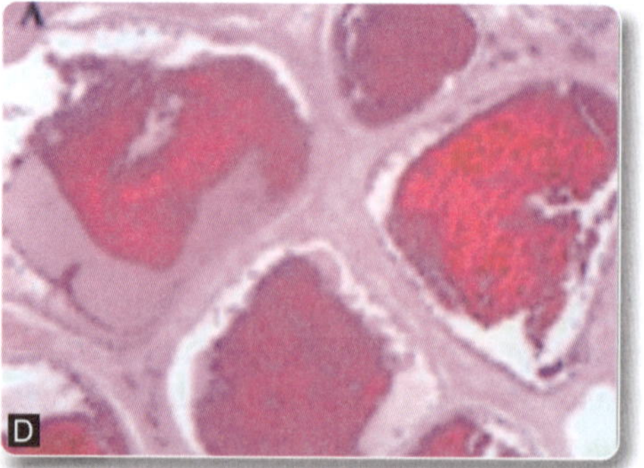

FIGURES 26.8A to D: Lymphangioma. **A and B.** Clinical pictures; **C.** CT scan in lymphangioma; **D.** Histopathology.

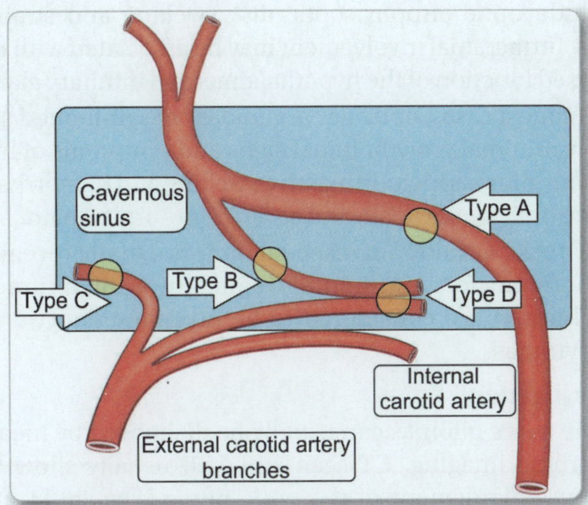

FIGURE 26.9: Types of caroticocavernous fistula

Spontaneous fistulas: Occur due to the communication between the carotid and sinus, an event, which usually presumably results from the bursting of an aneurysm or a weakness of the wall of the vessel. Majority of spontaneous fistulas occur in females with systemic hypertension and atherosclerosis.

Direct CCF: Occurs when the communication is between the internal carotid artery and the cavernous sinus.

Indirect CCF: Occurs when a branch of internal carotid or the external carotid artery communicates with the cavernous sinus.

Mechanism of the symptomatology of the condition is clear. Rupture of the carotid allows direct escape of arterial blood under high pressure into the cavernous sinus, the venous pressure is increased and the flow of blood reversed. Ophthalmic veins are dilated, causing stasis and edema in the orbit producing pulsatile proptosis synchronous with the systolic beat. Arterial pressure is lowered and venous pressure is raised resulting in acute reduction in the perfusion pressure of the circulation and hypoxia. Usually the ipsilateral orbit and eye are affected, but the proptosis may be bilateral or become evident on the other side or even alternate between the two. This is due to the communication channels between the two cavernous sinuses.

Clinical feature

Clinical feature is usually typical. Frequently, the onset is sudden either on recovering consciousness from a head injury or without apparent cause. A swishing noise in the head, considerable pain and usually diminution of vision, and a marked unilateral pulsating proptosis are the characteristic features (Figs 26.10A and B).

Signs in a high-flow fistulas: Tortuous epibulbar and forehead vessels, bruit that may be audible to the examiner, a pulsatile proptosis and paralysis of cranial nerves III, IV or most commonly VI with associated muscle palsies.

Fundus examination reveals engorged veins, disk edema, choroidal effusions and vitreous hemorrhage may occur. Increased episcleral venous pressure will lead to a secondary glaucoma.

Investigations

Computed tomography scan show diffuse enlargement of all the extraocular muscles resulting from venous engorgement and a characteristically enlarged superior ophthalmic vein (refer Fig. 26.10A).

Low-flow fistulas: It often close spontaneously. Recent data suggest that patients with low-flow fistulas are at a higher risk of intracranial hemorrhage because of the arterialization of the venous system.

Selective arteriography is used to evaluate the arteriovenous fistulas of the orbit and cavernous sinus.

Treatment

Embolization using coils to obstruct the fistula is generally accomplished through an endovascular transarterial route.

Orbital Varix

An orbital varix can occur primarily as dilatations of preexisting venous channels. It can be:

1. Primary varices due to a congenital venous malformation in the orbit.
2. Secondary varices due to an arteriovenous shunt either intracranially or within the orbit itself.

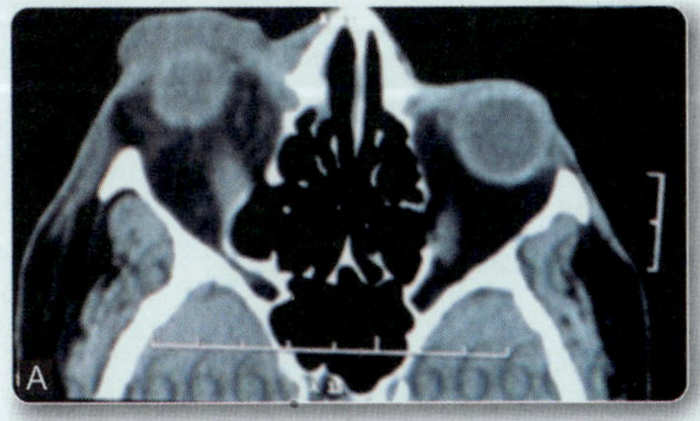

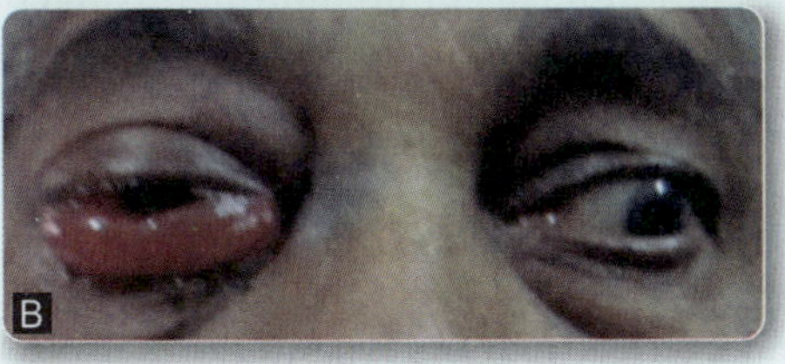

FIGURES 26.10A and B: Caroticocavernous fistula. **A.** MRI scan; **B.** Photograph.

Clinical features

Clinical feature presented by a case of orbital varix is dramatic and typical; the significant sign is a transient proptosis, which may last a few seconds, a few hours or a few days. It is always unilateral and usually left sided due to the narrowness of the jugular foramen on that side. Proptosis increases when the patient's head is dependent or after a Valsalva maneuver. Patients may exhibit enophthalmos at rest, when the varix is not engorged due to pressure atrophy of the orbital tissue resulting from recurrent attacks. Vision is usually unimpaired. Mydriasis in the affected eye is common and venous engorgement of the retina is the rule.

Investigations

The diagnosis can be confirmed via contrast-enhanced spiral CT scan. Rapid spiral CT scan during the Valsalva maneuver or other means of decreasing venous return shows characteristic enlargement of the engorged varix. Phleboliths can sometimes be seen on plain film radiographs. If the diagnosis is suspected, biopsy should be avoided because significant bleeding can be anticipated.

Treatment

Treatment is usually conservative. Surgery is reserved for relief of significant pain or for cases in which the varix threatens vision, because of compressive optic neuropathy. Complete surgical excision is difficult, as the varix is intertwined with normal orbital structures and directly communicates with the abundant venous reservoir in the cavernous sinus. Intraoperative embolization of the lesion aids surgical removal followed by excision. Embolization with coils inserted through a distal venous cut down has also been reported to diminish symptoms.

Neural Tumors

Neural tumors include:

- Optic nerve glioma
- Neurofibromas
- Meningiomas
- Schwannomas.

Optic Nerve Glioma

Rare benign tumors occur predominantly in children in the 1st decade of life. Malignant optic nerve gliomas are very rare and tend to affect adult males. Approximately, 25%–50% of optic nerve gliomas are associated with neurofibromatosis.

Clinical features

The chief clinical feature is gradual, painless, unilateral, axial proptosis associated with loss of vision and an afferent pupillary defect. Other ocular findings may include optic atrophy, optic disk swelling and strabismus. Intracranial involvement may be associated with decreased function of the hypothalamus and pituitary gland.

In most cases, optic nerve gliomas are self-limited and show minimal growth. Initial signs and symptoms of malignant gliomas include massive swelling and hemorrhage of the optic nerve head, and severe retro-orbital pain.

Gross pathology of resected tumors usually reveals a smooth, fusiform intradural lesion. The benign tumors in children are considered to be juvenile pilocytic astrocytomas.

Investigation

Optic nerve gliomas can usually be diagnosed by means of orbital imaging. CT scan and MRI usually show fusiform enlargement of the optic nerve (Figs 26.11 and 26.12A and B). MRI may be more accurate in defining the extent of an optic canal lesion and intracranial disease.

Treatment

1. Treatment of optic nerve glioma is controversial. Presumed optic nerve glioma particularly with good vision on the involved side may be carefully followed up, if it is confined to the orbit.
2. Excision is considered in situations like rapid growth, intracranial optic nerve involvement, increase in intracranial pressure and massive proptosis with corneal exposure.
3. Radiation therapy is considered, if the tumor cannot be resected and if symptoms progress.
4. Combination chemotherapy using actinomycin D and vincristine has also been reported to be effective in patients with progressive chiasmatic/hypothalamic gliomas.

Meningioma

Meningiomas are invasive tumors that arise from arachnoid villi and usually originate intracranially along

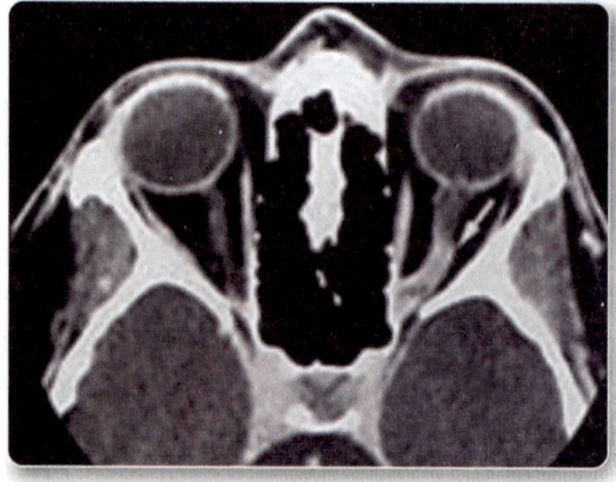

FIGURE 26.11: Optic nerve glioma

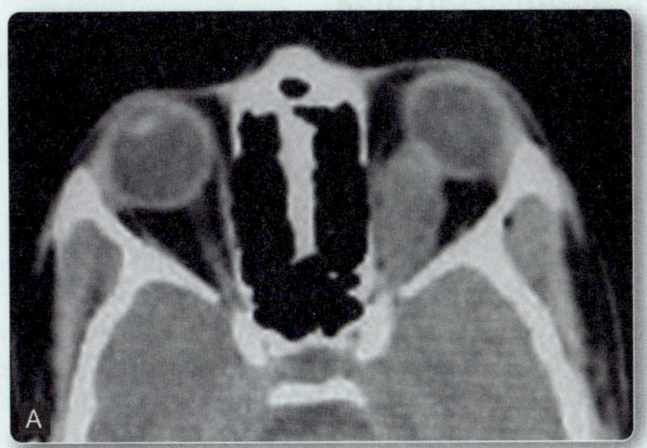

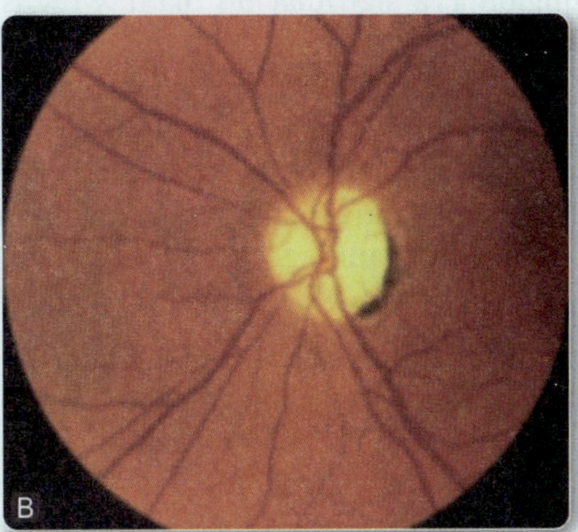

FIGURES 26.12A and B: Optic nerve glioma; A. CT scan; B. Optic atrophy.

sphenoid wing with secondary extension into the orbit through the bone, the superior orbital fissure or the optic canal. Ophthalmic manifestations are related to the location of the primary tumor. Meningiomas arising near the sella and optic nerves cause early visual defects and papilledema or optic atrophy. Tumors arising near the pterion often produce a temporal fossa mass and proptosis. Primary optic nerve meningiomas can produce early profound vision loss without any proptosis (Fig. 26.13A).

Sphenoid wing meningiomas produce hyperostosis of the involved bone and hyperplasia of associated soft tissues.

Primary orbital meningiomas usually originate in the arachnoid of the optic nerve sheath. They occur commonly in women in their 3rd and 4th decades of life. Symptoms include gradual, painless, unilateral loss of vision. Relative afferent pupillary defect and decreased visual acuity are the typical signs. Proptosis and ophthalmoplegia may be present at presentation. The optic nerve head may appear normal, atrophic or swollen and optociliary shunt vessels may be visible (Figs 26.13B and C).

Computed tomography and MRI show diffuse tubular enlargement of the optic nerve with contrast enhancement. In some cases, CT scan shows calcification within

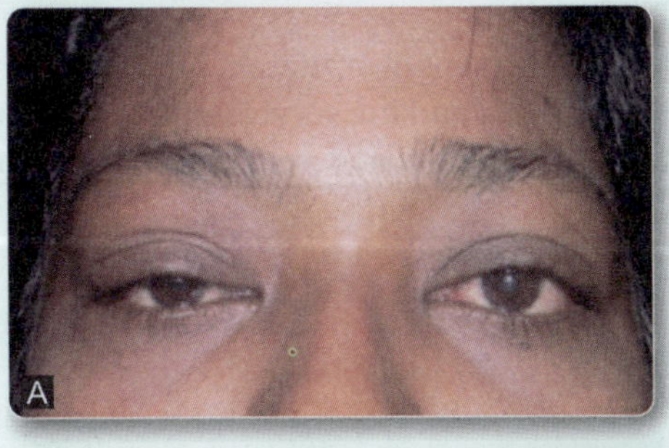

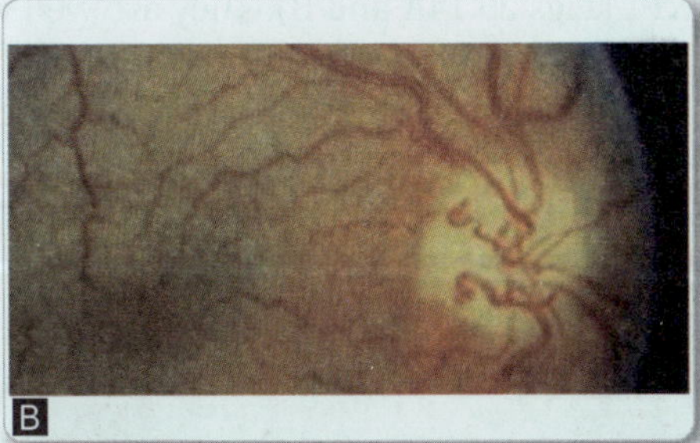

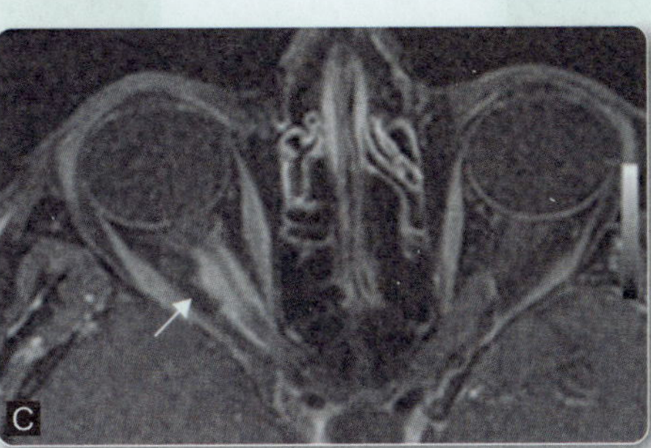

FIGURES 26.13A to C: Optic nerve meningioma. A. Clinical picture; B. Optociliary shunt vessel; C. CT scan.

the meningioma, a sign that on plain X-ray is termed tram-tracking.

Malignant meningioma is rare and results in rapid tumor growth that is not responsive to surgical resection, radiotherapy or chemotherapy. Both the extent of visual loss and the presence of intracranial extension are important factors in treatment planning.

Treatment

Treatment of optic nerve sheath meningiomas must be individualized, if minimally affected and no intracranial extension is present. If the tumor is confined to the orbit and visual loss is significant or progressive, radiation therapy should be considered. Surgery is reserved for patients with severe visual loss and profound proptosis.

Schwannomas

Schwannomas (also known as neurilemmas) are proliferations of Schwann cells that are encapsulated by perineurium. Hypercellular schwannomas sometimes recur even after what is thought to be complete removal, but they seldom undergo malignant transformation. These tumors are usually well encapsulated and can be excised with relative ease.

Neurofibromas

Neurofibromas (NF) are tumors composed chiefly of proliferating Schwann cells within the nerve sheaths. Plexiform neurofibromas are infiltrative tumors that usually occur in NF1 (Figs 26.14A and B). They are well vascularized and can seldom be completely removed by surgical excision. Discrete neurofibromas can usually be excised surgically without recurrence.

Rhabdomyosarcoma

Rhabdomyosarcoma is the most common primary orbital malignancy of childhood. The average age of onset is 8–10 years (Fig. 26.15A).

Clinical Features

The classic clinical features are one of a child with sudden onset and rapid evolution of unilateral proptosis. There is often a marked adnexal response with edema and discoloration of eyelids. Ptosis and strabismus may also be present. A mass may be palpable particularly in the superonasal quadrant of the eyelid.

If a rhabdomyosarcoma is suspected, the workup should proceed on an urgent basis. CT and MRI can be used to define the location and extent of the tumor (Figs 26.15B and C). CT is particularly helpful, if the tumor has caused bony destruction, although the orbital walls remain intact in most cases. A biopsy should be undertaken, usually through an anterior orbitotomy.

Rhabdomyosarcomas arise from undifferentiated pluripotent mesenchymal elements in the orbital soft tissues and not from the extraocular muscles.

They may be grouped into four categories:

- Embryonal
- Alveolar
- Pleomorphic
- Botryoid.

Treatment

The standard treatment of orbital rhabdomyosarcoma was orbital exenteration and the survival rate was poor. But recently, radiation therapy and systemic chemotherapy has

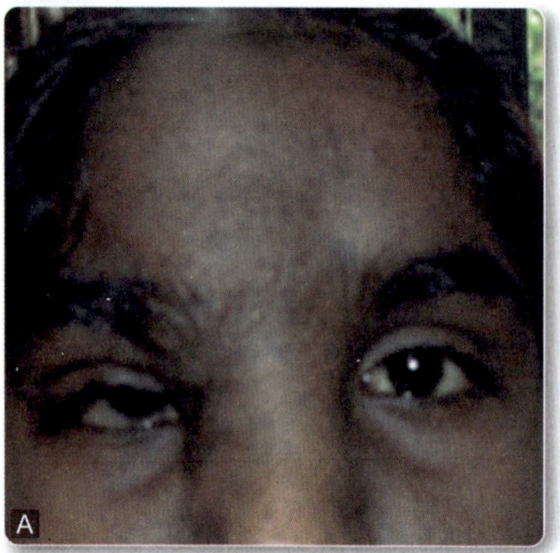

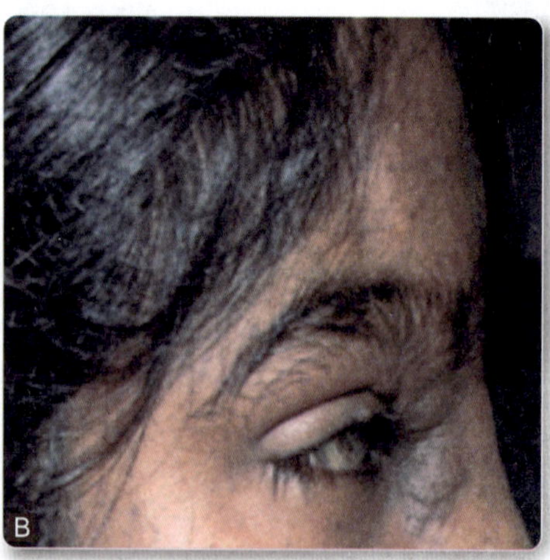

FIGURES 26.14A and B: Plexiform neurofibroma. **A.** Frontal view; **B.** Lateral view.

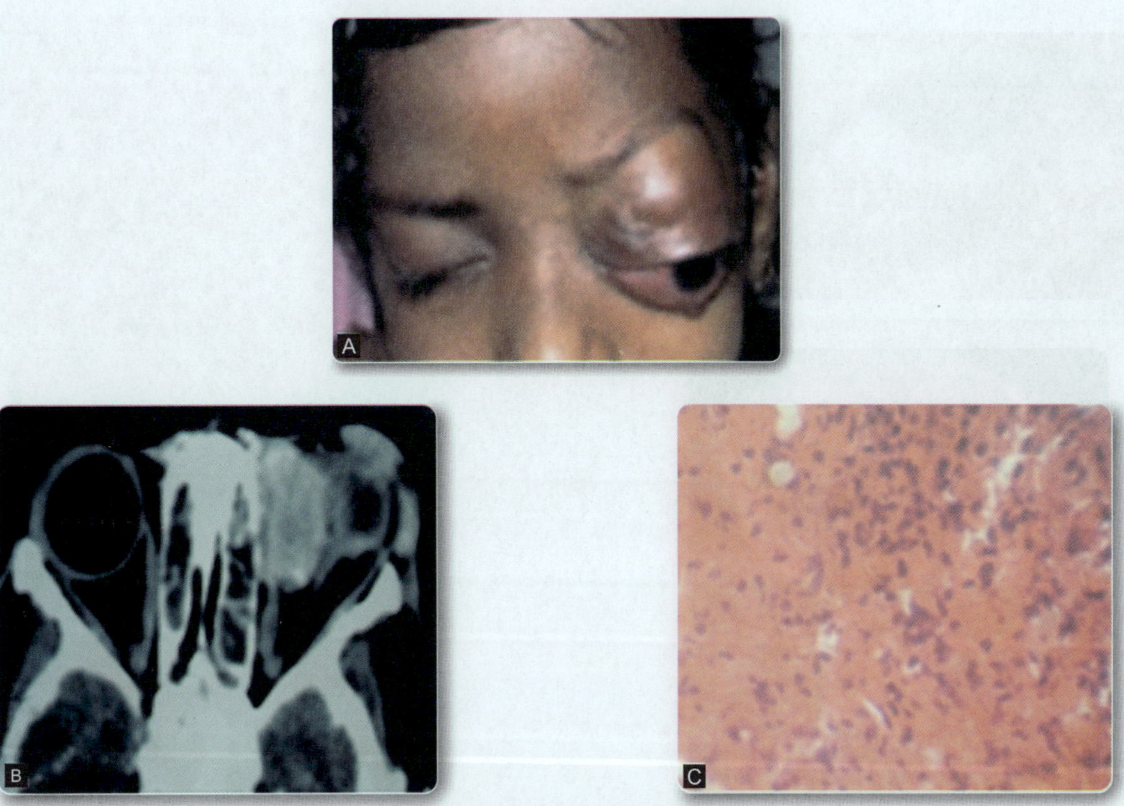

FIGURES 26.15A to C: Rhabdomyosarcoma; A. Clinical picture; B. CT scan findings; C. Histopathological findings.

become the mainstay of primary treatment. Survival rate is better than 90%, if the orbital tumor has not evolved or extended beyond the bony orbital walls.

Lymphoproliferative Disorders

Lymphoproliferative lesions of the ocular adnexa constitute a heterogeneous group of neoplasms that accounts for more than 20% of all orbital tumors. Most are non-Hodgkin lymphomas.

The vast majority of orbital lymphomas (Figs 26.16A to D) are B-cell derived. T cell lymphoma is rare and more lethal. Based on the revised European-American lymphoma classification (REAL), the following represent the four most common orbital lymphomas:

1. Mucosa-associated lymphoid tissue (MAT).
2. Chronic lymphocytic lymphoma (CLL).
3. Follicular center lymphoma.
4. High-grade lymphomas include large cell lymphoma, lymphoblastic lymphoma and Burkitt's lymphoma.

The typical lymphoproliferative lesion presents as a gradually progressive painless mass. These tumors are often located anteriorly in the orbit or beneath the conjunctiva, where they may feature the typical salmon-patch appearance. Lymphoproliferative lesions, whether benign or malignant, usually mold to surrounding orbital structures rather than invade them. Disturbances of extraocular motility or visual function are unusual. Orbital imaging reveals characteristic putty-like molding of tumor to normal structures up to 50% arise in the lacrimal fossa.

Management

Although systemic corticosteroids are useful in idiopathic orbital inflammation (pseudotumor), they are not recommended in the treatment of lymphoproliferative lesions.

Radiotherapy is the treatment of choice for patients with localized ocular adnexal lymphoproliferative disease. A surgical cure, usually, cannot be achieved because of the infiltrative nature of lymphoid tumors.

Secondary Orbital Tumors

Tumors from the neighboring structures can extend to the orbit and can result in proptosis. Tumors of the lids or intraocular tumors like retinoblastoma can extend to the orbit and lead to proptosis.

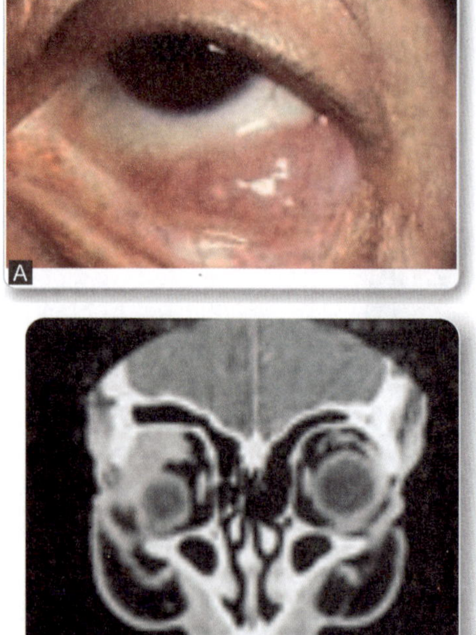

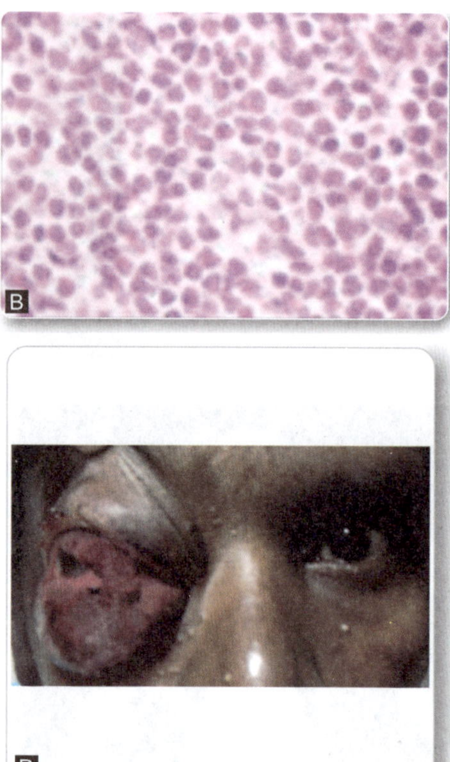

FIGURES 26.16A to D: Lymphoma. **A.** Clinical picture; **B.** Histopathological findings; **C.** CT scan findings; **D.** Lymphoma advanced stage.

Mucoceles of Paranasal Sinuses

The openings of the paranasal sinuses can get blocked and they can get distended with secretions. The frontal and ethmoidal sinuses are separated only by thin bones from the orbit and the frontal and ethmoidal mucoceles can bulge into the orbit to form bulging in the upper and outer quadrant of the orbit displacing the eye downwards and upwards (Fig. 26.17).

Malignant Nasopharyngeal Tumors

More than one third of the cases of nasopharyngeal tumors can produce orbital symptoms. Paresthesia or numbness on the area of distribution of the infraorbital nerve on the lower lid and cheek may be an early symptom. Extension of the tumor into the orbit will cause proptosis with displacement of the globe upwards.

ORBITAL SURGERIES

Surgical Spaces

There are five surgical spaces within the orbit, which are shown in Figures 26.18A and B:

1. The subperiosteal surgical space, which is the potential space between the bone and the periorbital.
2. The extraconal surgical space (peripheral surgical space), which lies between the periorbital and the muscle cone with its fascia.
3. The intraconal surgical space (central surgical space), which lies within the muscle cone.

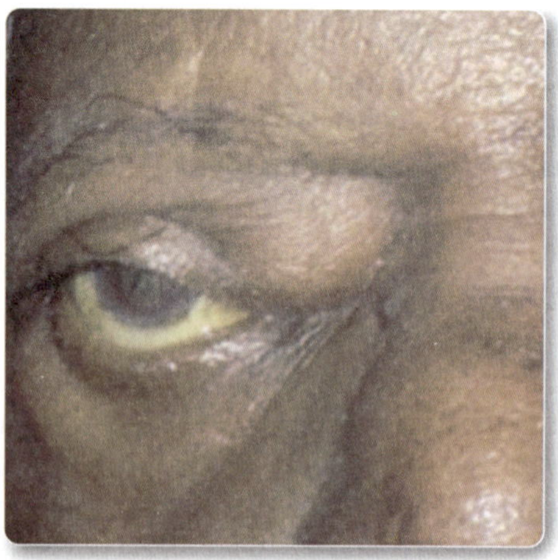

FIGURE 26.17: Frontal mucocele

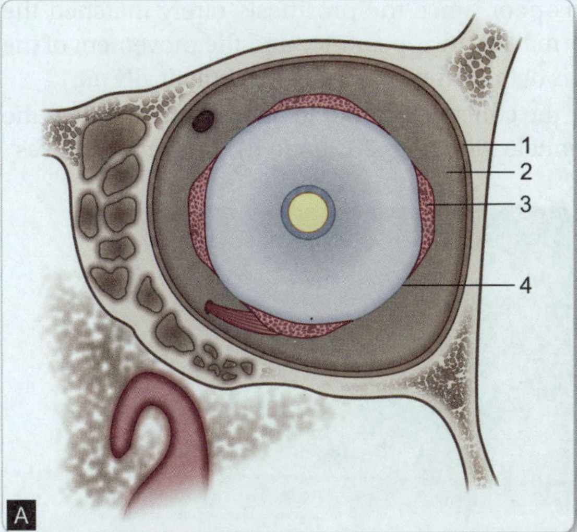

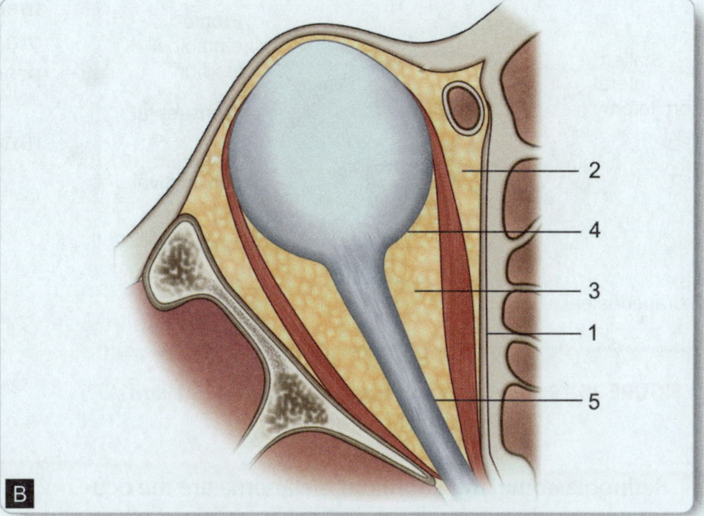

FIGURES 26.18 A and B: Surgical spaces of the orbit. **A.** Anteroposterior view; **B.** Crosssectional view. **1.** Subperiosteal space; **2.** Peripheral orbital space; **3.** Intraconal space; **4.** Sub-Tenon's space; **5.** Subarachnoid surgical space.

4. The episclera (sub-Tenon's) surgical space, which lies between Tenon's capsule and the globe.
5. The subarachnoid surgical space, which lies between the optic nerve and the nerve sheath.

Orbitotomies

A myriad of clinical disorders can affect the orbit. The timing and approach of surgical intervention are based on the nature of the orbital disease process defined by clinical and imaging study.

Basic indications for orbital surgery are:

- Incisional biopsy
- Excision of a cyst or mass
- Repair and reconstruction
- Abscess drainage
- Decompression
- Exenteration.

The common surgical approaches to the orbit include anterior, lateral or superior orbitotomy.

The location of the mass within the surgical space and its extent, its relation to the extraocular muscles and optic nerve and the character of the lesion determine the specific choice.

Anterior Orbitotomy

Anterior orbitotomy techniques are used for the incisional biopsy of palpable orbital tumors or the excision of anteriorly located well-defined lesions.

Lateral Orbitotomy

Lateral orbitotomy with or without removal of lateral wall gives excellent approach to the intraconal and extraconal spaces of the orbit, lateral to the optic nerve. The two most popular approaches are the Berke-Reese incision and the Stallard-Wright incision (Fig. 26.19).

The Berke-Reese incision involves a 3–5 mm horizontal incision after a complete lateral canthotomy.

The Stallard-Wright incision is curvilinear extending from lateral half of the eyebrow, toward the lateral bony orbital rim. Stallard-Wright incision gives a better access to lacrimal gland fossa tumors and does not require reconstruction of the lateral canthus.

Orbital Decompression

The goal of orbital decompression is to allow the enlarged muscles and orbital soft tissue to expand into periorbital spaces, to relieve optic neuropathy and to decrease proptosis. It is done usually in thyroid ophthalmopathy.

Enucleation

Enucleation is the removal of the entire globe, while preserving other orbital tissues.

Indications

1. Enucleation is indicated for primary intraocular malignancies; not amenable to alternative modes of therapy.

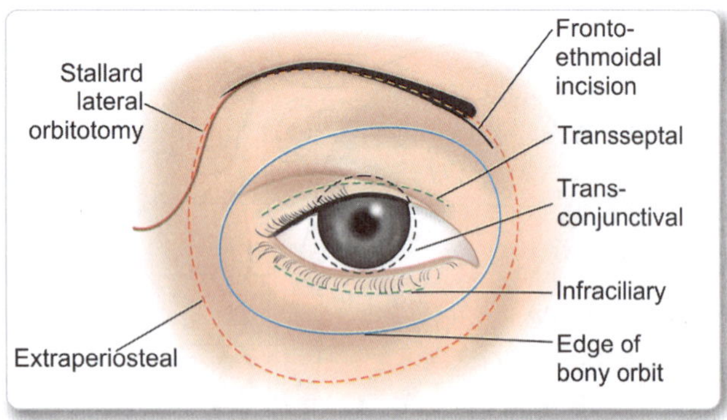

FIGURE 26.19: Incisions for orbitotomy (*Courtesy*: Stallard's Textbook of Surgery)

Retinoblastoma and choroidal melanoma are the ocular tumors that most commonly require enucleation. Evisceration should not be performed in cases of suspected intraocular malignancy. Surgeon must take care to avoid penetrating the globe during surgery and he/she must handle the globe gently to minimize the risk of disseminating tumor cells. In case of suspected retinoblastoma, the surgeon should obtain a long segment of optic nerve with the enucleation specimen to increase the chance of completely resecting the tumor.

2. Blind eyes with opaque media, suspected of harboring an occult neoplasm unless another cause of ocular disease can be surmized. Ultrasonography is useful in evaluating these eyes and planning proper management.
3. In severely traumatized eyes, enucleation within first 14 days of the injury may be considered, if the risk of sympathetic ophthalmia and harm to the remaining eye is judged to be greater than the likelihood of recovering useful vision in the traumatized eye. Although there is some conflicting evidence, removal of an eye that has already stimulated sympathetic ophthalmia is unlikely to prevent progression of the disease.
4. Painful blind eyes as in neovascular glaucoma, when conservative measures fail and unsightly eyes as in huge anterior staphyloma. Enucleation with an orbital implant will relieve the symptoms and give good cosmetic appearance. Evisceration can also be done in these situations, but enucleation is better, if the chance of an intraocular malignancy is not completely ruled out.
5. For endophthalmitis, evisceration is not possible if there is scleral abscess or scleromalacia.
6. For eye donation in a dead person.

Guidelines for enucleation

Earlier the eye was removed leaving an empty socket. After 30–45 days, when the healing has completed, a readymade artificial eye is fitted. The cosmetic improvement was poor, since the prosthesis rarely matched the other normal eye in appearance and the movement of the prosthesis on ocular movements was practically nil.

Now, the concept is to put in an orbital implant at the time of enucleation (Figs 26.20A to E). This implant gives

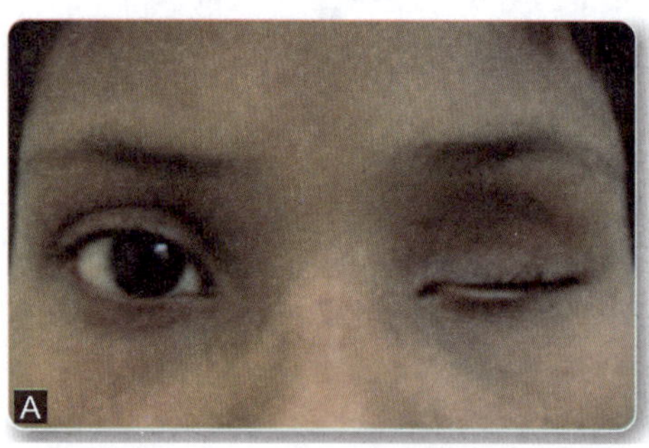

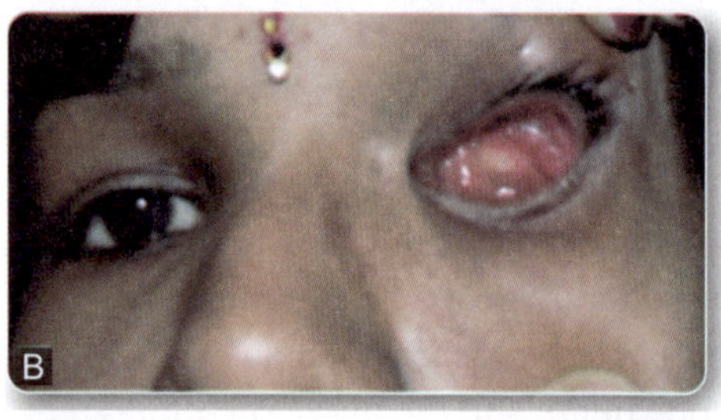

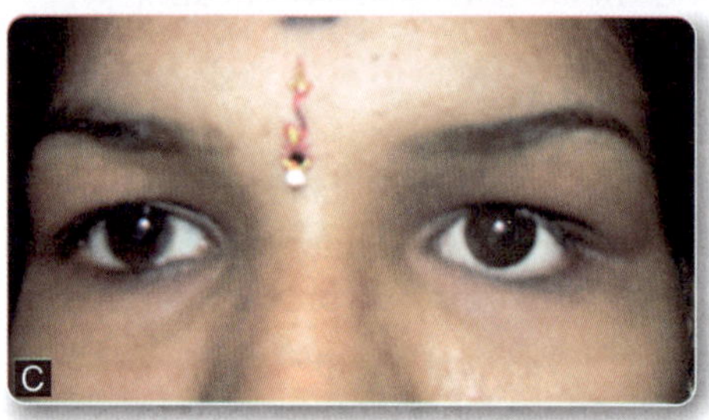

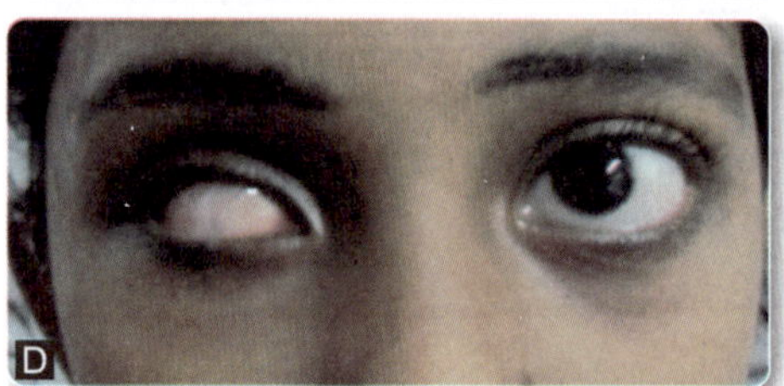

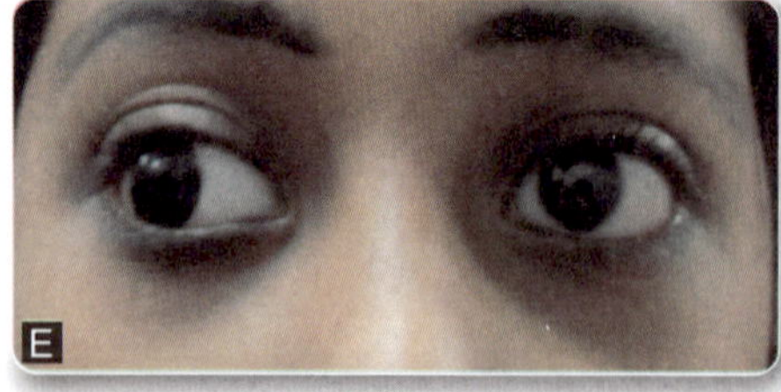

FIGURES 26.20A to E: Enucleation with and without an implant. **A and B.** Enucleation without implant; **C.** Same eye with artificial eye; **D.** Enucleation with implant; **E.** Appearance with prosthesis in place with fair motility.

volume to the orbital contents and fixing the ocular muscles to the implant gives some mobility to the prosthesis worn over it.

Muscles sutured into the normal anatomical locations, either directly to the implant or to homologous sclera or autologous fascia surrounding the implant, allow superior motility and prevent migration.

Volume loss in the adult anophthalmic socket may be adequately replaced by a 20–22 mm sphere implant.

The prosthesis is now custom made to match the other eye and with the mobility given by the implant, the cosmetic appearance is excellent.

A functionally and aesthetically acceptable anophthalmic socket must have the following components:

1. An orbital implant of sufficient volume centered within the orbit.
2. A socket lined with conjunctiva or mucous membrane with fornices deep enough to hold a prosthesis.
3. Eyelids with normal appearance and adequate tone to support prosthesis.
4. Good transmission of motility from the implant to the overlying prosthesis.
5. A comfortable ocular prosthesis that looks similar to the normal eye.

Enucleation in Childhood

Enucleation in early childhood, as well as congenital anophthalmos or microphthalmos, may lead to underdevelopment of the involved bony orbit with secondary facial asymmetry. When enucleation is necessary in childhood, a large implant should be used to replace orbital volume. Autogenous dermis-fat grafts are used successfully as anophthalmic implants in children, as they appear to grow along with the expanding orbits.

Enucleation Technique

Prior to performing enucleation surgery, it is crucial that the patient be advised of the advantages and disadvantages of enucleation surgery, implant migration or extrusion and the need for fitting of an ocular prosthesis, 6–8 weeks postoperatively.

The correct eye is marked immediately before surgery.

Anesthesia

Either general anesthesia or local anesthesia is given with conscious sedation. In either case, a retrobulbar block using a 50:50 mixture of 2% lidocaine with epinephrine and 0.75% bupivacaine provides vasoconstriction intraoperatively, as well as sustained analgesia postoperatively.

Procedure

1. A lid speculum is placed to retract the lids.
2. A 360° conjunctival peritomy is created with scissors. Tenon's capsule is bluntly dissected off the globe in all four quadrants.
3. One by one, the four recti muscles are secured with a muscle hook and a 5-0 polyglactin suture is passed through the muscle near the insertions and the muscles are cut from the globe.
4. The globe is rotated laterally with the traction sutures and a clamp is inserted medially and applied to the optic nerve to crush the central retinal artery. The nerve is then cut with curved scissors and the eye is removed. Every attempt should be made to obtain as long a section of optic nerve as possible.
5. Bleeding can be controlled by digital pressure or with bipolar cautery.
6. The appropriate size implant is chosen and soaked in antibiotic solution. The extraocular muscles can be sutured directly to a porous polyethylene implant either by passing the suture needles through the implant material or through the predrilled suture tunnels.
7. Tenon's capsule is closed with interrupted 6-0 polyglactin sutures and conjunctiva is closed with a running 6-0 polyglactin suture.
8. A conformer is placed and the lids are closed. A pressure patch is applied.
9. Avoid excessive dissection near the orbital roof and apex to reduce the chance of damaging the extraocular muscles or their innervation and resulting in ptosis.

Complications

1. Bleeding intraoperatively or in the immediate postoperative period.
2. Infection.
3. Extrusion or the implant.
4. Socket granuloma.

Evisceration

Evisceration is the removal of the contents of the eye leaving the sclera and the extraocular muscles intact.

Evisceration should be considered only if the presence of an intraocular malignancy has been ruled out.

Indications

1. Panophthalmitis.
2. Bleeding anterior staphyloma.

3. Painful blind eye (for better cosmesis compared to enucleation, since an implant placed within the sclera will have better motility).

Contraindication

Any blind eye is suspected to have malignant growth inside.

Advantages

1. Less disruption of orbital anatomy.
2. Better motility of the prosthesis.
3. Better treatment of endophthalmitis because subsequent orbital cellulitis or intracranial extension of infection is reduced.
4. A technically simpler procedure.
5. Lower rate of migration, extrusion of the implant and reoperation.

Disadvantages

1. Evisceration should never be performed, if a tumor is suspected.
2. Sympathetic ophthalmia is rarely caused by a reaction to uveal tissue in the eviscerated socket.
3. Evisceration affords a less complete specimen for pathologic examinations.

Techniques

Evisceration can be performed either with retention of the cornea or with excision of the cornea. The cornea can be retained, if it is of normal thickness and shows no active corneal disease.

After insertion of the speculum, the eye is fixed by forceps. A cataract knife enters the cornea, just anterior to the limbus. With a few snips of the scissors, the cornea is detached and removed. A scoop of appropriate size is inserted between the sclera and uveal tract and is swept circumferentially to separate the ciliary body from the scleral spur, the choroids from the sclera and posteriorly to tear through the intraocular portion of the optic nerve. The intraocular contents are scooped out. All uveal tract must be thoroughly removed. Retained fragments are potentially danger for sympathetic ophthalmitis.

A very satisfactory cosmetic result may be achieved by including an implant within the scleral cup. Tenon's capsule is sewn over this with horizontal line of interrupted sutures and the conjunctiva is closed separately.

Exenteration

Exenteration involves the removal of the soft tissues of the orbit including the globe (Figs 26.21 and 26.22A and B).

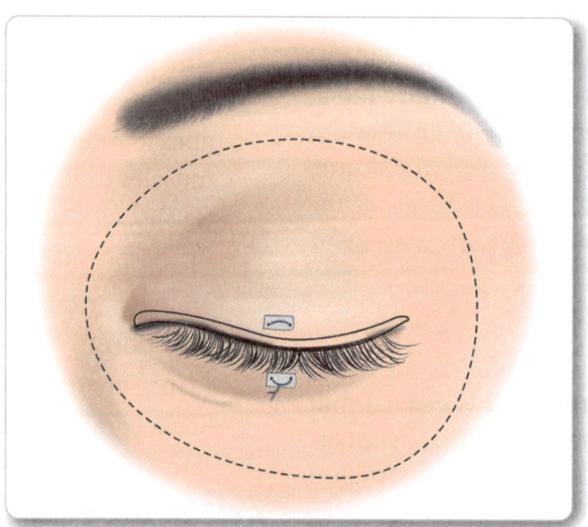

FIGURE 26.21: Incision for exenteration

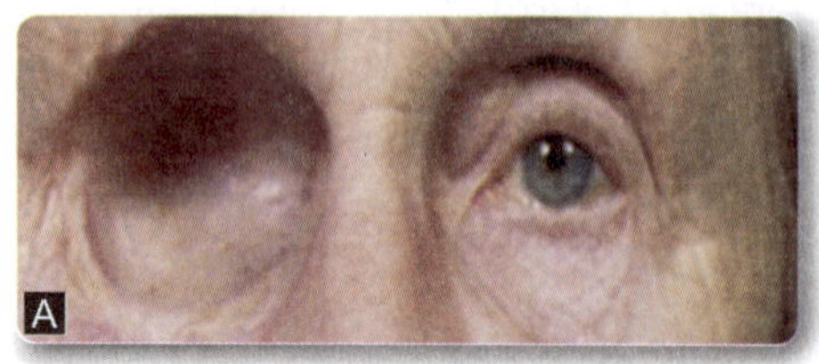

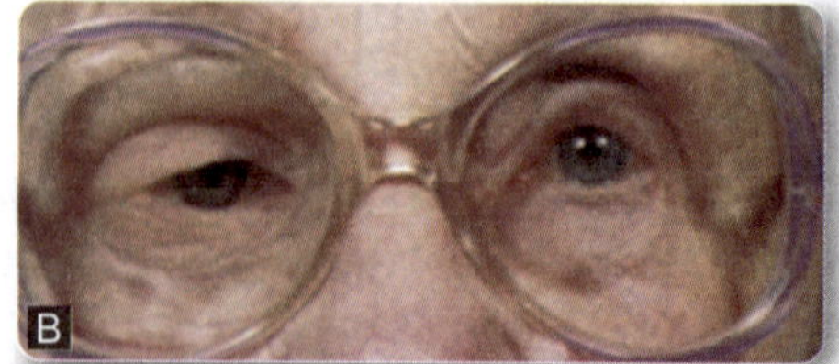

FIGURES 26.22A and B: Exenteration. **A.** Postexenteration. **B.** With spectacle attached prosthesis (*Courtesy:* www.medicalartprosthetics.com).

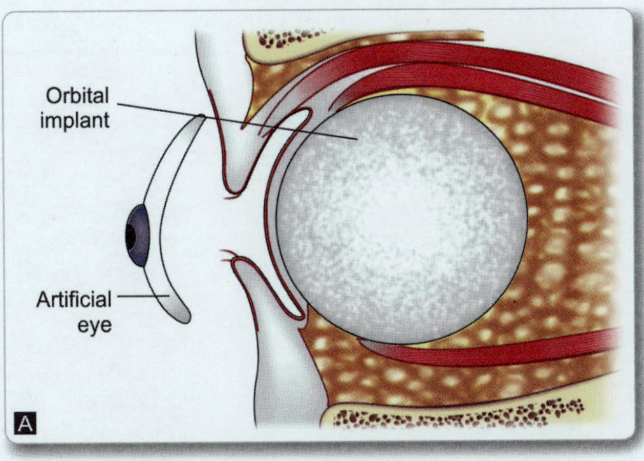

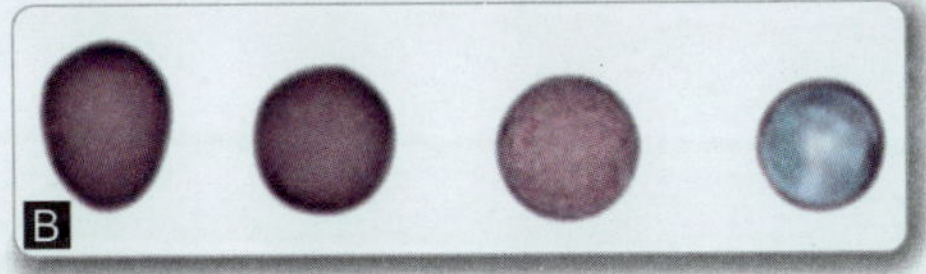

FIGURES 26.23A and B: Implants after enucleation

Indications

1. Destructive tumors extending into the orbit from the sinuses, face, eyelids, conjunctiva or intracranial space.
2. Intraocular malignant melanomas or retinoblastoma that has extended outside the globe.
3. Malignant epithelial tumors of the lacrimal gland.
4. Sarcomas and other primary orbital malignancies that do not respond to non-surgical therapy.
5. Orbital phycomycosis.

Types

Subtotal: The eye and adjacent intraorbital tissues are removed, so that the lesion is locally excised (leaving periorbital and part or all of eyelids). This technique is used for some locally invasive tumors for debulking of disseminated tumors or for partial treatment in selected patients.

Total: All intraorbital soft tissues including periorbita are removed with or without the skin of the eyelids.

Extended: All intraorbital soft tissues are removed, together with adjacent structures (usually bony walls and sinuses).

Following removal of the orbital contents, the bony socket may be allowed to spontaneously granulate and epithelialize or may be covered by a split thickness skin graft, which may be placed onto bare bone or over a temporalis muscle or temporoparietal fascial flap.

Orbital Implants

Prosthesis

An ocular prosthesis is fitted within 4–8 weeks after enucleation. The ideal prosthesis is custom fit to the exact dimension of the orbit after postoperative edema has subsided (Figs 26.23A and B).

Section 6

Disorders of Ocular Motility

Strabismus

27

Anitha Balachandran, Girija Devi PS

INTRODUCTION

The term strabismus is derived from the Greek word 'strabismos' meaning 'to squint, to look obliquely or askance'. Strabismus means ocular misalignment, whether caused by abnormalities in binocular vision or by anomalies of neuromuscular control of ocular motility.

Orthophoria is the ideal condition of ocular balance. In reality, orthophoria is seldom encountered; a small heterophoria can be documented in most persons.

Heterophoria is an ocular deviation kept latent by the fusional mechanism (latent strabismus).

Heterotropia is a deviation that is manifest and not kept under control by the fusional mechanism (manifest strabismus).

PREFIXES

Eso: The eye is rotated so that the cornea is deviated nasally because the visual axes converge. This is also called convergent strabismus (Figs 27.1A and B).

Exo: The eye is rotated so that cornea is deviated temporally because the visual axes diverge. This is known as divergent strabismus (Figs 27.2A and B).

Hyper: The eye is rotated so that cornea is deviated superiorly. This is also called vertical strabismus (Figs 27.3A and B).

Hypo: The eye is rotated so that the cornea is deviated inferiorly. This is also called vertical strabismus.

SUFFIXES

Phoria: A latent deviation.

Tropia: A manifest deviation.

CLASSIFICATION

No classification is perfect or all inclusive and several methods of classifying eye alignment and motility disorders are used.

According to Fusional Status

1. **Phoria:** A latent deviation in which fusional control is always present.
2. **Intermittent tropia:** A deviation in which fusional control is present part of the time (Figs 27.4A and B).
3. **Tropia:** A manifest deviation in which fusional control is not present (Fig. 27.5).

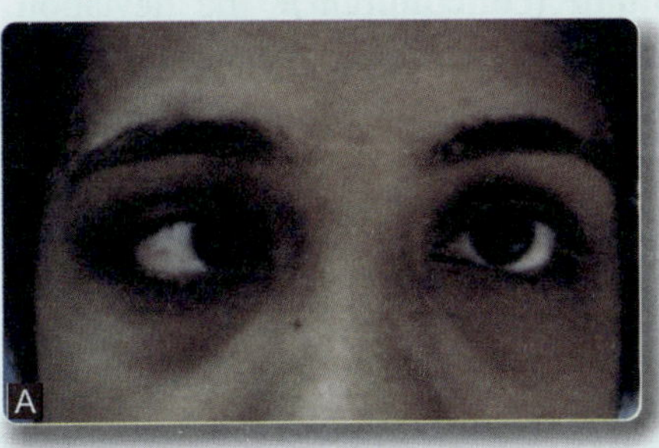

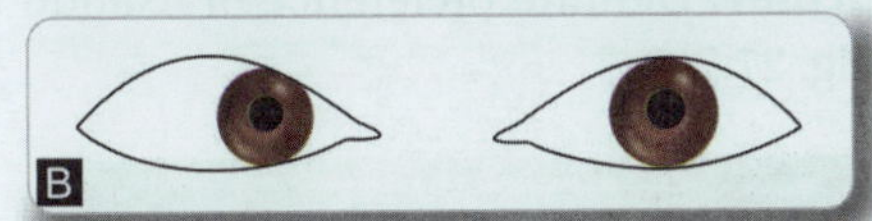

FIGURES 27.1A and B: Esotropia. **A.** Clinical picture; **B.** Diagrammatic representation.

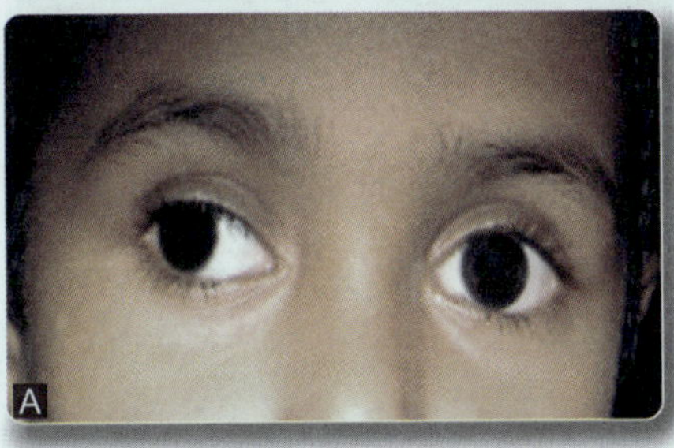

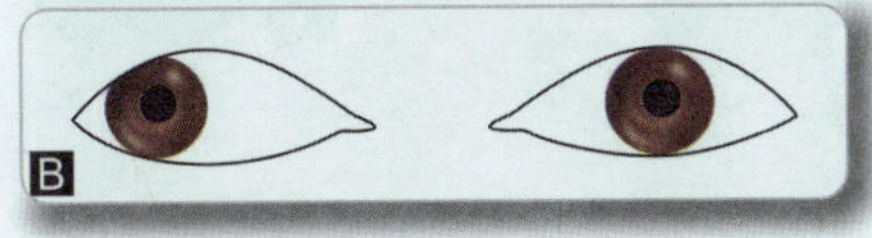

FIGURES 27.2A and B: Exotropia. **A.** Clinical picture; **B.** Diagrammatic representation.

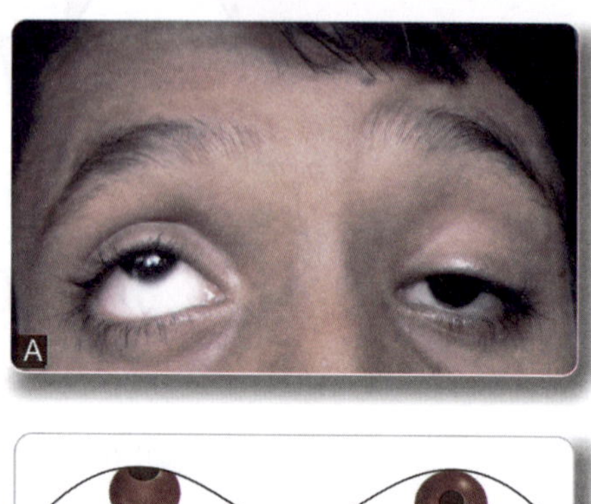

FIGURES 27.3A and B: Hypertropia. **A.** Clinical picture; **B.** Diagrammatic representation.

According to Variation with Gaze Position or Fixating Eye

1. **Comitant (concomitant):** The deviation does not vary in size with direction of gaze or fixating eye.
2. **Inconcomitant (non-comitant):** The deviations vary in size with direction of gaze or fixating eye.

According to Fixation

1. **Alternating:** Spontaneous alternation of fixation from one eye to other (Figs 27.6A and B).
2. **Monocular:** Definite preference of fixation with one eye (Fig. 27.7).

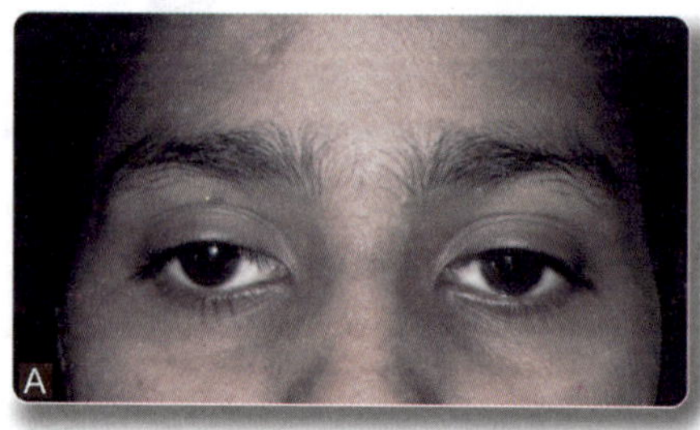

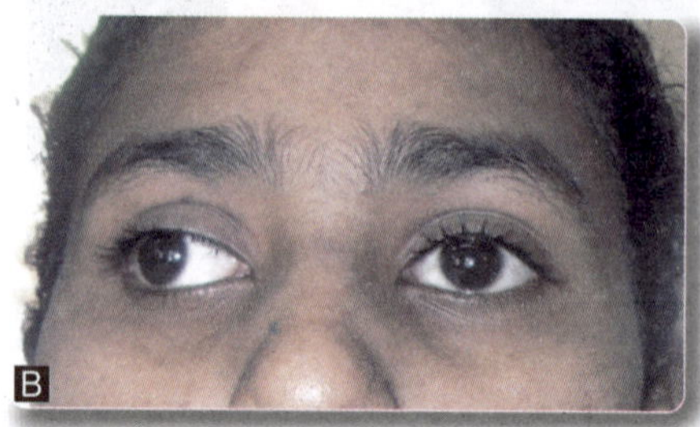

FIGURES 27.4A and B: Intermittent exotropia. **A.** No deviation; **B.** Deviation of right eye is present.

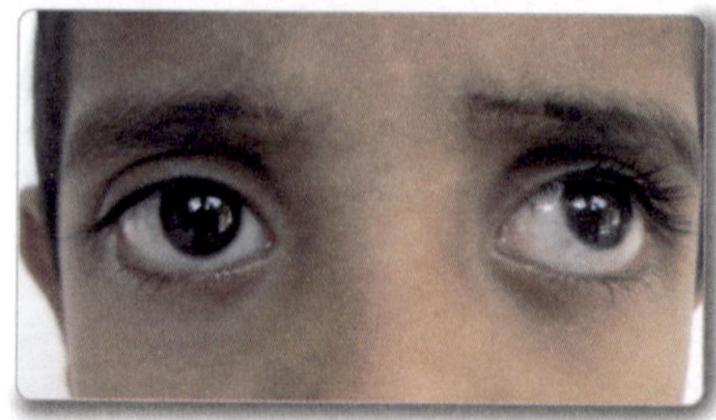

FIGURE 27.5: Constant exotropia

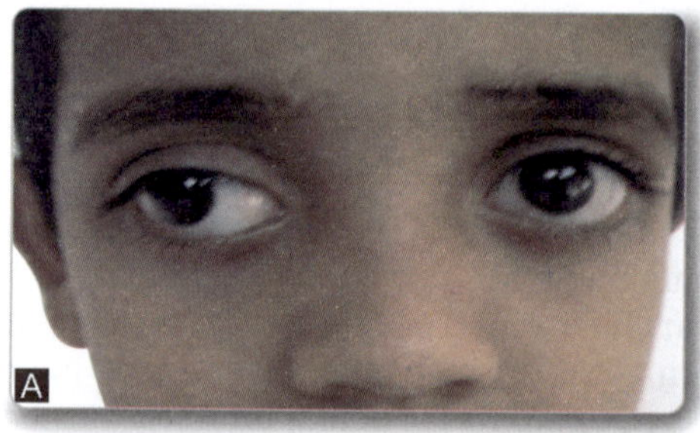

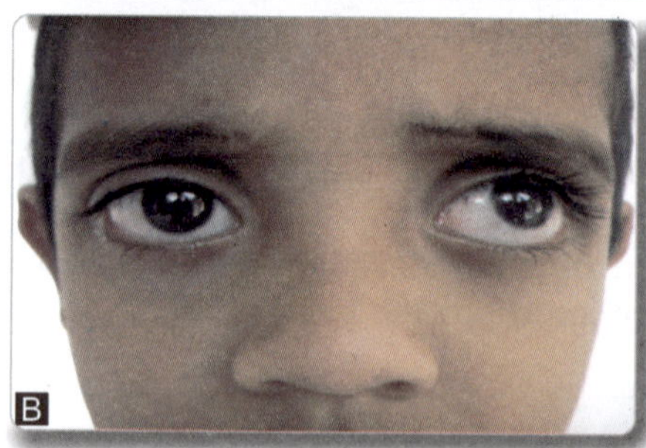

FIGURES 27.6A and B: Alternating exotropia. **A.** Right eye is diverting; **B.** Left eye is diverting.

According to Age of Onset

Congenital/infantile: For a deviation documented prior to 6 months, the term infantile may be more appropriate.

According to Type of Deviation

1. **Horizontal:** Esodeviation or exodeviation.
2. **Vertical:** Hyperdeviation or hypodeviation.
3. **Torsional:** Incyclodeviation or excyclodeviation.
4. **Combined:** Horizontal, vertical, torsional or any combination.

HETEROPHORIA

Heterophoria is a condition where there is a tendency for misalignment of visual axes, but remains latent and can be corrected by the fusional capacity. This ability is shared between the two eyes. But the tendency for deviation becomes manifest by dissociation test.

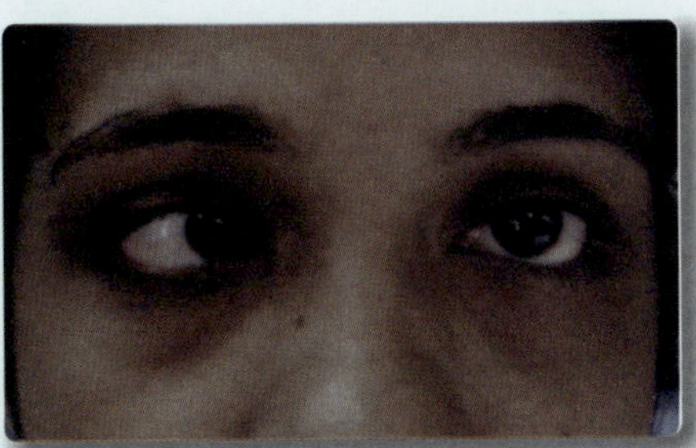

FIGURE 27.7: Monocular (right) esotropia

If the latent deviation is one of convergence, it is called esophoria, if it is divergence, exophoria and if vertical, hyperphoria. It is impossible to be sure whether there is absolute hyperphoria of one eye or hypophoria of other. If the deviation is torsional, the condition is cyclophoria.

Predisposing Factors

1. Ill health, fatigue of eyes due to eyestrain, certain occupation like computer workers/tailors, painters, etc.
2. Age:
   a. In infancy, binocular reflexes are only developing, so there is a tendency for divergence or exophoria.
   b. In childhood, accommodation and convergence reflexes are powerful, so there is a tendency for deviation inwards or esophoria.
   c. In presbyopic age, as the near point of distant version recedes, the convergence becomes weaker and there is tendency for deviation of eye outwards.
3. Influence of refraction:
   a. In hypermetropia there is a tendency for esophoria due to excessive use of accommodation to correct hypermetropia.
   b. In myopia there is a tendency for exophoria, since they are not using accommodation to see near objects clearly.
4. Anatomical defects of muscles, ligaments or fascia in orbit.

Sx Symptoms

Since the parallelism of visual axes is maintained by tonic contraction of appropriate muscles, symptoms of eyestrain are encountered in higher degrees of phoria (asthenopic symptoms). For the same reason cyclophoria is the most symptomatic.

Blurring of vision, while reading, the letters seem to run together.

Intermittent diplopia due to intermittent phases of manifest squint, when overstrained muscles relax and assume position of rest.

Diagnosis

The diagnosis of heterophoria depends on abolishing fusion by dissociation test, so that without fusional control, the eyes assume their natural position of rest.

Cover Test

Cover test is the simplest test, which gives valuable information.

Principle: In phorias the parallelism of the eye is maintained by the power of fusion. When the image to one eye is blocked, the fusional mechanism will not be acting and the covered eye goes to its natural position. When the cover is removed and the stimulus for fusion comes back, the eye will resume parallelism.

When a distant or near object is regarded and both eyes are uncovered, there is no deviation. One eye is covered, while other eye continues to fix at the object. If there is heterophoria, the eye under cover deviates. The cover is then quickly removed and the eye under cover is observed. As soon as the cover is removed, the eyes under cover move back and corrects the deviation and regain the position of binocular fixation. The speed of movement of recovery shows the amount of ability of the fusional control. The other eye reacts similarly when the test is repeated by covering the other eye and the deviation in both remain the same. Cover test should be done with spectacles for both near and distant objects (Figs 27.8A to D and 27.9).

Both eyes are straight, but on covering right eye it deviates under cover, which is revealed immediately on removing the cover. Both eyes become straight again. On covering the other eye, the covered eye also deviates under cover and the eyes become straight again on removing the cover.

If the eye deviates outwards under cover and moves inwards on removing the cover, the patient is having exophoria or latent divergent squint. Similarly, in esophoria, the eye moves outwards on removing the cover. So, the deviation is opposite to the movement of the eye on removing the cover.

Maddox Rod Test

The test depends on altering the appearance of retinal image in one eye, so that no stimulus is given for fusion. Of these, the simplest is the Maddox rod.

The patient is placed at 6 mm from a bright spot of light. Maddox rod consists of four or five cylinders of red glass joined side-by-side within a supporting frame. A Maddox rod is now placed in a trial frame in front of one of the eyes. The eye with the Maddox rod sees the spot light as a red straight line at right angles to the axis of rod. If the

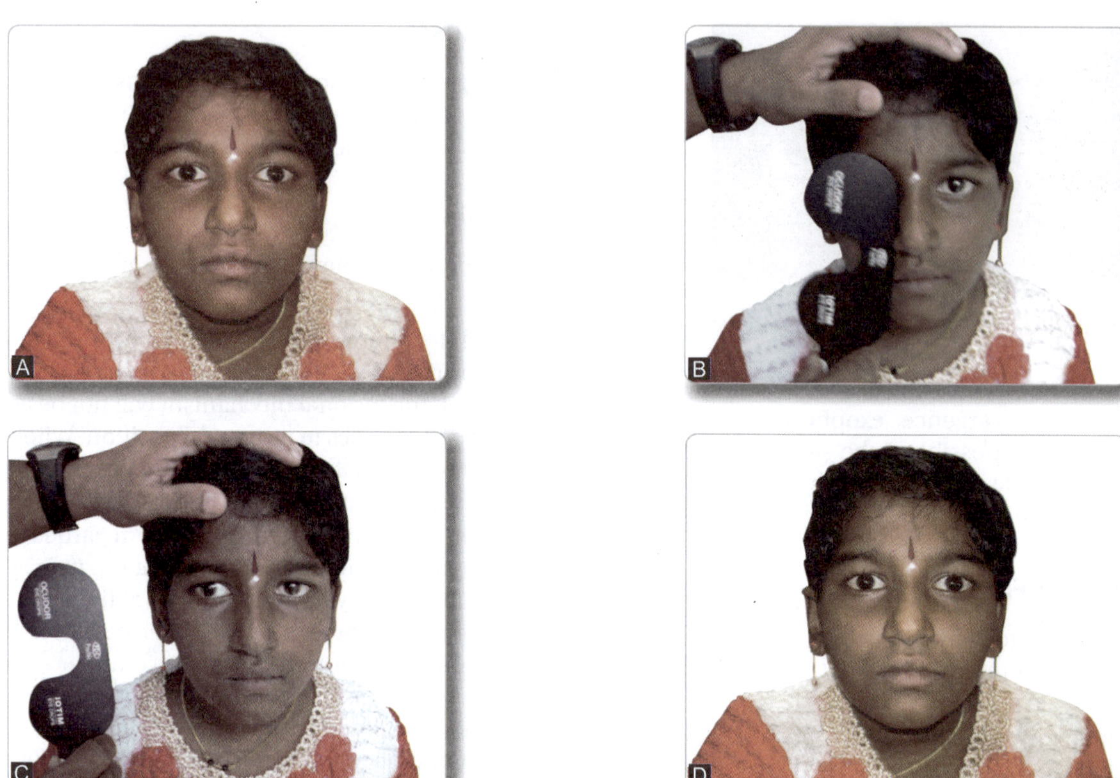

FIGURES 27.8A to D: Latent squint. **A.** Eyes straight ahead in normal situation; **B.** Covering one eye leads to dissociation; **C.** Note that the eye has deviated outwards under cover, which is revealed immediately after removal of the cover; **D.** Once fusional mechanism is activated by removal of the cover, eyes will become straight ahead again.

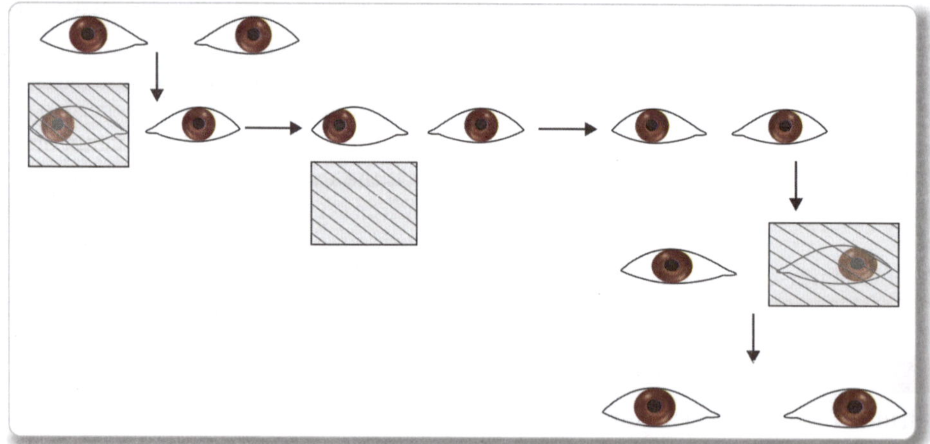

FIGURE 27.9: Cover-uncover test to detect heterophoria

Maddox rod is placed with the axes horizontal, the red line is vertical. Thus, the images of spotlight in the two eyes become dissimilar and fusion becomes dissociated. If there is orthophoria (Figs 27.10A to D), the bright spot will appear to be in the center of vertical red line, if there is eso or exophoria red line will be to one side of the spot. Maddox rod is then rotated so that cylinders are vertical; the red line will be below or above the spot. If there is hyperphoria. In each case, amount of deviation is measured by the strength of prism required to correct it or it is measured on a Maddox tangent scale set on wall. Maddox rod test can be done for near and distance (Figs 27.11A to C).

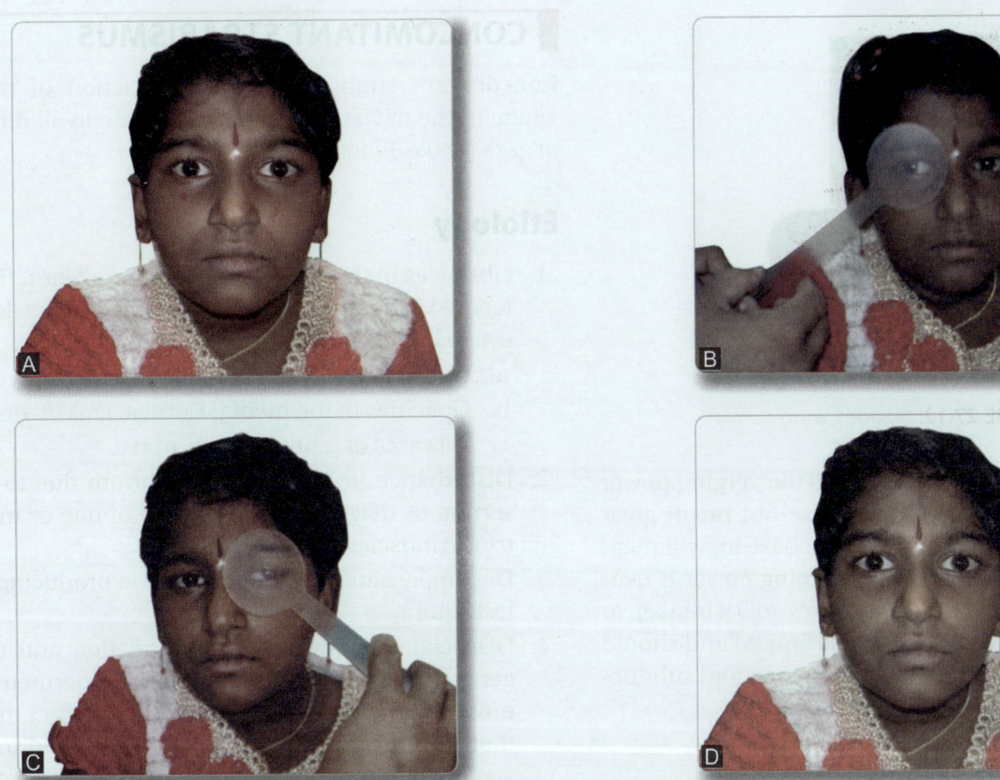

FIGURES 27.10A to D: A. Orthophoric in normal situation; B and C. In heterophoria, both eyes deviate under cover; D. On removing the cover, both eyes resume fixation.

Maddox Wing Test

The deviation in latent squint is often different in near vision and distant vision. An exophoria appearing more for near is regarded as insufficiency of convergence, which gives rise to symptoms when much near work is undertaken. The deviation in near is tested using a Maddox wing test (Fig. 27.12). At 33 cm from eye, when viewed through the two slit holes of the instrument, the fields, which are exposed to each eye is separated by a diaphragm. The right eye sees a white arrow pointing vertically upwards and a red arrow pointing horizontally to left. The left eye sees a horizontal row of figure in white and vertical row is red. These are calibrated to read the deviation in degrees. In orthophoria, the white arrow pointing to white horizontal line and the red arrow pointing to red vertical line should be at zero. Any deviation indicates eso or exo, the amount of which can be read off on the scale.

Prism Vergence Test

Besides the actual measurement of heterophoria the vergence power for fusional control of the phoria can also be measured. For this, prism vergence tests are done with the patient seated at 6 m from light. Prisms deviate the direction of light rays toward its base and a person looking through the prism will see it toward its apex. Highest prism,

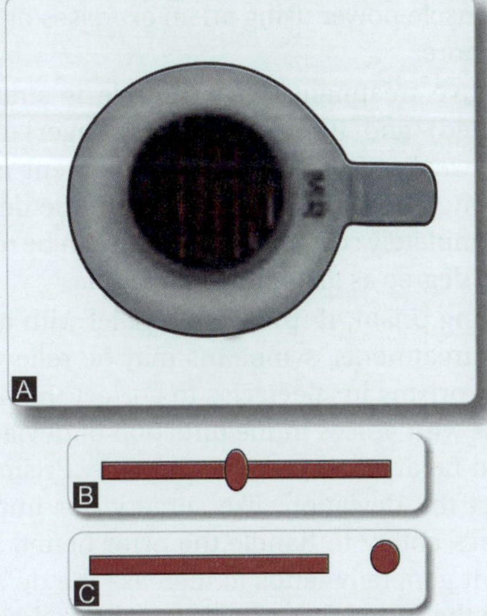

FIGURES 27.11A to C: Maddox rod test; A. Maddox rod; B. Retinal image with no heterophoria; C. Retinal image with heterophoria.

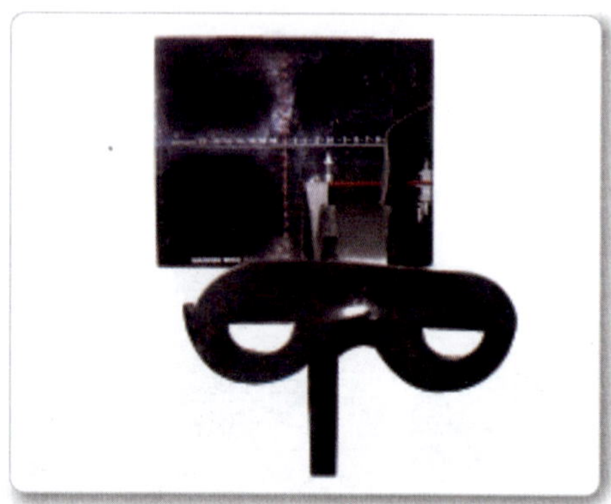

FIGURE 27.12: Maddox wing

which can still give single vision, gives the verging power for the particular direction tested. Base-out prism gives the converging ability and the one with base in, will measure the divergence power. The converging power is usually 40–45 diopters (D) and if it falls below 20D it is taken to be insufficient. The diverging power is limited and should be 4D–5D and normal limits of superduction and subduction (vertical vergence) are from 2D–3D.

Treatment of Heterophoria

The lower degrees of esophoria and to a less extent of exophoria are almost universal. These cause no symptoms and need no treatment. In larger degrees of phorias and symptoms producing phorias:

1. The refractive error must be corrected.
2. Orthoptic treatment to increase the fusional range and muscle power using prism exercises or with synoptophore.
3. Operative treatment: Weak muscle is strengthened (resected) and its antagonist (stronger) muscle is made weaker (recessed). This treatment is considered when deviation is large. Even if the deviation is not completely corrected, deviation can be reduced to such a degree as to abolish asthenopia.
4. Relieving prism: If there is no relief with any of the above treatments, symptoms may be relieved by ordering prisms in spectacles to correct the defect, i.e. prisms with apices in the direction of deviation. This should be avoided as far as possible. Prisms neither correct the deviation, like surgery nor improve the person's ability to handle the error better, like exercises. It generally tends to increase the defect by relaxing the fusional mechanisms. Hyperphoria in less degree should unhesitatingly be treated in this way since in this condition, the fusional power is limited and hence exercises are useless.

CONCOMITANT STRABISMUS

Concomitant strabismus is a dissociation of the eyes where in the deviation remains the same in all directions of gaze (Duke-Elder).

Etiology

1. Obstacles in the sensory path of binocular reflex: Defective vision in one eye makes it easy for the defective eye to lose fixation:
   a. Uncorrected errors of refraction.
   b. Opacities in the media: Cornea, lens or vitreous.
   c. Diseases of retina or optic nerve.
2. Disturbance in muscular equilibrium due to malinsertion or defective development of one or more extrinsic muscles.
3. Decompensation of a heterophoria producing manifest squint.
4. Dissociation between accommodation and convergence relationship. For example, in hypermetropia as more accommodation is exerted to correct the error there is more tendency for convergence and so a convergent squint may develop. Similarly, in myopia, as accommodation is not exerted to correct the error or for near work, convergence is weak and there is tendency for divergent squint.
5. Central causes:
   a. Defective development of fusional faculty.
   b. Hyperexcitability of central nervous system (CNS): As in seizure disorders, mental retardation, etc.

Sx Symptoms

Usually, there is no symptom and the deviation of eyes is detected by the parents or relatives. Although the image of an object does not fall on the fovea in the squinting eye there is no diplopia. The reason is that this image is automatically suppressed. The main feature of concomitant squint is failure of binocular single vision.

Signs

There are two important signs for concomitant squint:

1. The primary deviation is equal to the secondary deviation: The primary deviation is the angle of deviation of the squinting eye, when the normal eye fixes an object. The secondary deviation is the angle of deviation of the normal eye, when the squinting eye is made to fix the object. The amount of deviation also remains the same in all directions of gaze.

2. There is no limitation of movements of eyeball in any direction.

Age Incidence

Usually, concomitant squint develops during the periods when reflexes governing binocular vision are established, i.e. within 5 years of age.

Types of Concomitant Squint

Depending on Deviation

- Convergent: Esotropia
- Divergent: Exotropia
- Vertical: Hypertropia or hypotropia.

Depending on Fixation Preference

Unilateral strabismus

If one eye habitually fixes and other eye squints, the case is one of unilateral strabismus. This leads to decreased usage of the squinting eye and leads to decreased vision of that eye and amblyopia (Fig. 27.13).

Alternating strabismus

In alternating strabismus when one eye fixates, the other eye deviates either inward or outward, depending on the type of squint, but either of the eyes can take up fixation. One important feature of altering squint is normal vision in each eye.

Investigations of Strabismus

History

1. Age of onset of squint: Squint due to congenital paresis appears at very early age. Accommodative type of convergent squint manifests at about 2–5 years of age, when accommodative mechanism is stronger. Infantile esotropia is a convergent squint manifesting at about 6 months of age. In general, older the age of onset and shorter the squinting period, better is the prognosis.
2. Any history of illness, fatigue, trauma or delayed developmental milestones.
3. Is the squint intermittent or constant?
4. Which eye is deviating predominantly?
5. Family history of squinting or poor eyesight in the family.

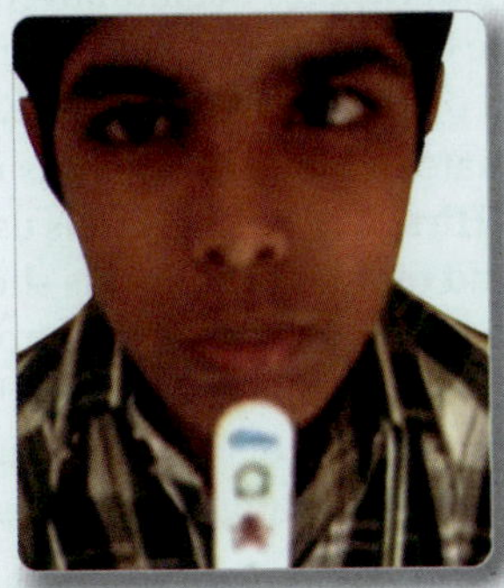

FIGURE 27.13: A left constant esotropia

Examination of Patient

1. Inspection: The first step is to ensure that the apparent deviation is indeed real.

   An apparent squint or pseudostrabismus is due to the configuration of palpebral aperture, e.g. in children with telecanthus or epicanthal fold, medial canthi approach the corner eccentrically and the appearance of a convergent squint results. More commonly such an appearance is due to the divergence between visual axis and optic axis. In emmetropic eye, the visual axis cuts the optic axis nasally, since the macula is temporal to the optic disk. So, angle formed between them called angle gamma is positive. In hypermetropic eyes angle gamma is also positive, but greater than emmetropia; in myopia since visual axis and optic axis coincides or latter even cuts temporal to it, the angle gamma is negative. Neither of these can be seen and direction of line is judged by position of reflex at pupil. A light shone onto cornea will cause a reflex just nasal to center of cornea. This is termed positive angle kappa. Greater the size of positive angle, eye appear to look divergent. If angle kappa is negative, eye appear to look convergent. So in high hypermetropia, there is an apparent divergent squint and in high myopia there is an apparent convergent squint.

   Unilateral ptosis gives the appearance of pseudohypertropia. Asymmetry of face is a cause for pseudo vertical squint.
2. Which eye is deviated, right or left?
3. Is the deviation inwards, outwards or vertical?
4. Any opacity in cornea lens or reaction of pupil.
5. The next step is to confirm the presence of deviation, identify the direction of deviation, to differentiate a unilateral from alternating type and to differentiate a concomitant from a paralytic squint (Table 27.1).

   All these can be analyzed by a cover-uncover test (Figs 27.14A and B).

   True or apparent squint: When the supposedly fixating eye is covered, while when the patient fixes at a target, there is movement of the squinting eye to

TABLE 27.1: Distinguishing features of non-paralytic and paralytic strabismus

Non-paralytic (concomitant) strabismus	Paralytic (inconcomitant) strabismus
Primary deviation is equal to secondary deviation	Secondary deviation is greater than primary deviation
Ocular movement shows no limitation	There is limitation in the direction of action of paralyzed muscle
No diplopia	Diplopia is present
Normal head posture	Abnormal head posture
False projection is absent	False projection is present
No vertigo or vomiting	Symptoms like vertigo, nausea and vomiting

take up fixation, if there is a true squint. In apparent deviation, there is no movement of the supposedly deviating eye to take up fixation.

Type of squint: Depending on the deviation of movement of the eye to take up fixation, the nature of strabismus is confirmed. That is, eye moves inwards to take up fixation in a divergent squint and outwards in a convergent one (Figs 27.15A to E).

Uniocular or alternating: In uniocular squint it is one eye, which is always maintaining fixation. Only during the cover test the deviating eye take up fixation, but goes back to the deviated position when the cover is uncovered. In alternating squint, both the eyes take up fixation alternately.

In concomitant deviation, the primary deviation is equal to the secondary deviation unlike in inconcomitant where primary deviation is less than secondary deviation.

6. Ocular motility is tested in all direction of gaze to find out any limitation of movement in any direction.
7. Recording of the visual acuity to find out any error of refraction. If so, refractive error has to be assessed by complete cycloplegic retinoscopy.
8. The anterior and posterior segments of the eye has to be examined in detail to rule out any sensory cause for the deviation.

Measurement of the Angle of Deviation

Measurement of the angle of deviation is important in all cases of concomitant squint as a guide to treatment. The following methods are used.

Neutralization method by prism: Handheld prisms are placed in front of deviating eye with the base of prism placed in the direction opposite to deviation or in other words, apex of prism in the direction of deviation, e.g. in convergent squint, prism is held base out. Cover test is then performed. Stronger prisms are used till the end point is reached when prism negates ocular movements to take up fixation. The angle of deviation is read from the strength of the prism. A set of prism bar is shown in Figure 27.16.

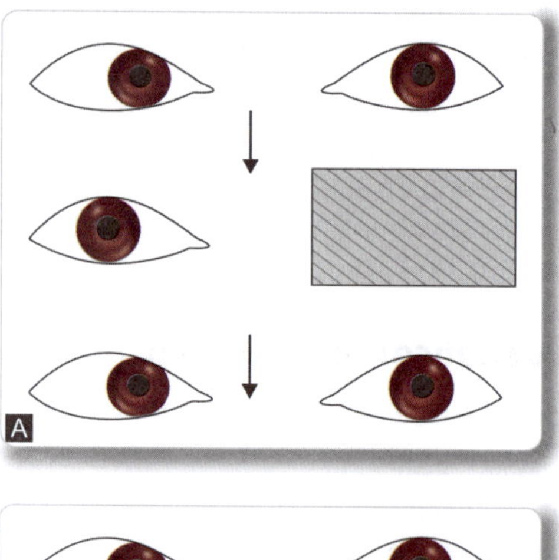

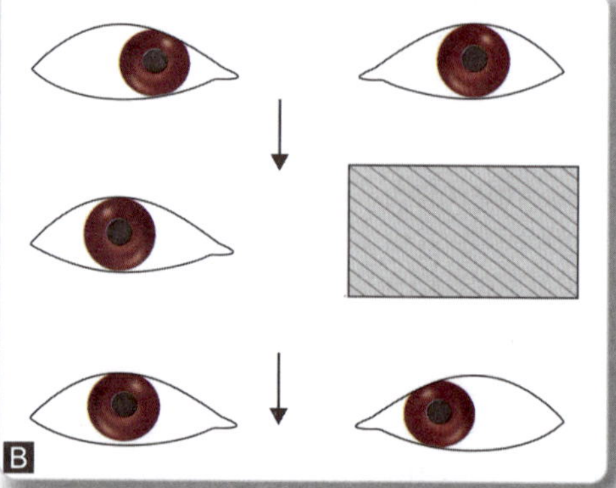

FIGURES 27.14A and B: Cover-uncover test to detect true squint. **A.** On covering the apparently fixing eye, the deviating eye becomes straight. On removing the cover, the deviating eye moves back to its original deviated position. **B.** Cover test in alternating squint. Right eye appears to have convergent squint. After occluding the left eye, right eye becomes straight. On removal of the cover, the covered left eye shows convergent squint and the right eye is straight.

A rough estimate of angle of squint is obtained by the **reflection test of Hirschberg.** This test is useful in uncooperative patients and in infants. A light is shone into the eye and the deviation of corneal light reflex from the center of the pupil is noted in the squinting eye. If the reflex is situated at the temporal border of the pupil angle is about 15% and if it is at the limbus, the angle measures about 45%.

By synoptophore: The angle of squint measured with this equipment is very accurate.

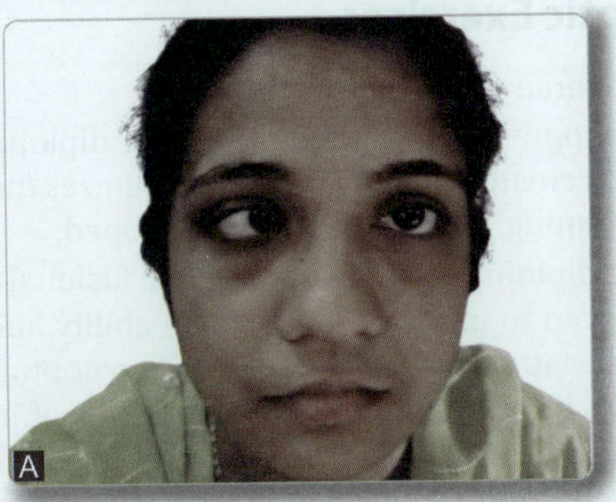

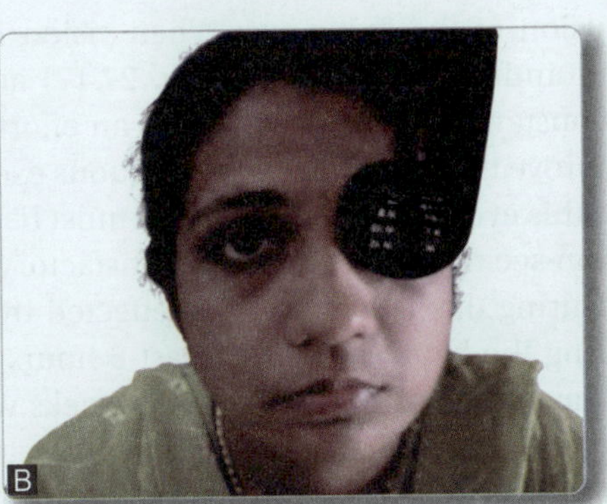

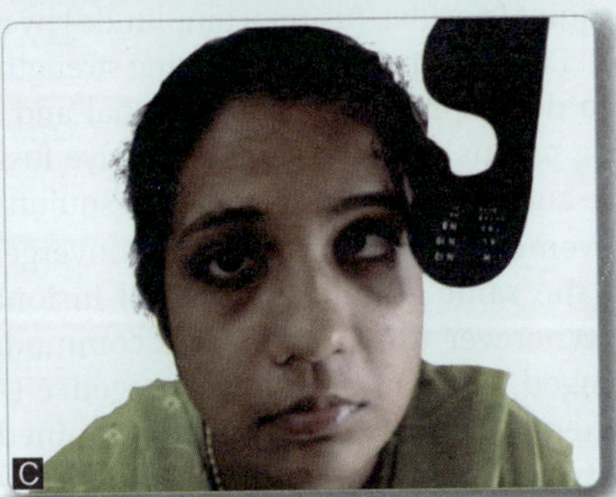

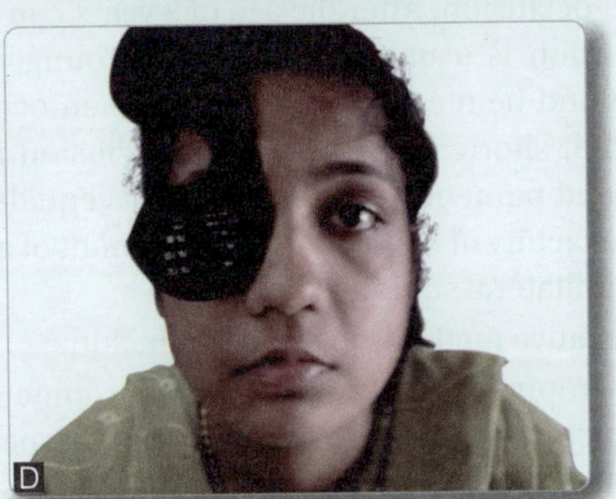

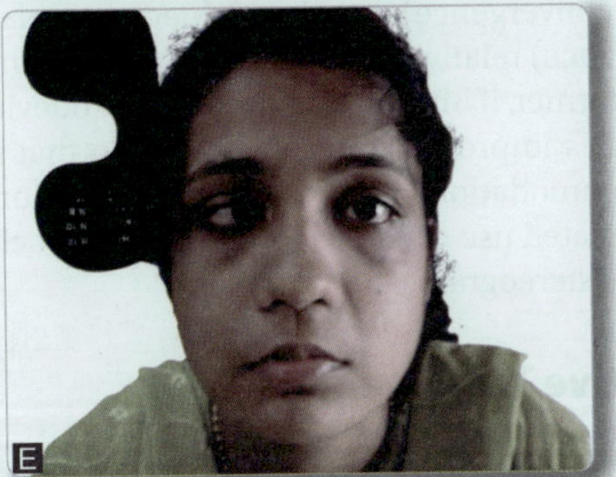

FIGURES 27.15A to E: Cover-uncover test to detect the types of squint. **A.** Note that right eye is convergent; **B.** On occluding the left eye, right eye moves to take up fixation; **C.** On removing the cover note that left eye is convergent; **D.** Now on covering the right eye, left eye takes up fixation; **E.** The right eye goes back to the convergent position.

Treatment of Concomitant Squint

1. Correction of any error of refraction by suitable spectacle correction for constant use, after complete cycloplegic retinoscopy:
   a. **Spectacles:** These help in forming a sharp retinal image, which helps in fusing the two images. It also helps in achieving the balance between accommodation and convergence in hypermetropia and myopia. A convex lens will decrease the increased accommodation in hypermetropia and thereby convergence. A concave lens will stimulate accommodation and thereby convergence, and helps in controlling the divergence in myopia. The patient should be re-examined in a month's time.
   b. **Bifocals:** If there is no significant refractive error and eyes are straight for distance, but esotropia is present for near, bifocals with +3D should be presented. The most satisfactory form is the executive type of bifocals where intersection cuts the lower portion of pupil.

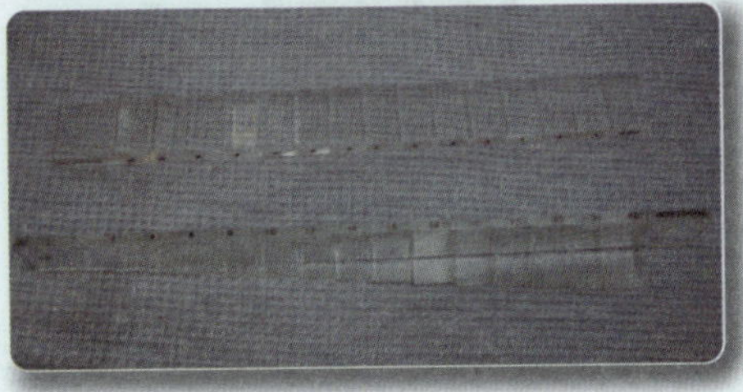

FIGURE 27.16: A set of prism bar

2. Occlusion of the fixing eye: When vision is tested, the squinting eye is usually (Fig. 27.17) amblyopic in a constant unilateral squint and an effort is made to improve the vision in it by continuous exercise. To make this eye being used, the other must be prevented from seeing clearly. The only satisfactory method of ensuring this is by occlusion effected by a patch covering the better eye for at least 6 hours a day. It may have to be continued for 6–12 weeks when improvement is found to occur. It may be discontinued, if no improvement has occurred after 6 months of strict occlusion. After the age of 9 years conventional occlusion is usually unsuccessful. Younger the patient and better the visual acuity, when occlusion is started, shorter the duration of occlusion required. The end point of occlusion therapy is equalization of visual acuity of two eyes or development of alteration in a unilateral squint.
3. Alternative methods to occlusion include:
   a. Atropine penalization—where atropine eye ointment 1% is used to blur the vision, especially for near in the better eye. It is found to be useful only if vision in amblyopic eye is good and hence this modality is useful mostly for mild-to-moderate amblyopia. When properly done this technique is found to be equally effective as occlusion for amblyopia treatment.
   b. Manipulation of glasses: This is most effective for high myopia. The correction in amblyopic eye is not changed, but correction in better eye is replaced by plane lens and thus, the child is forced to use the affected eye.
   c. Stripe therapy [complementary and alternative medicine (CAM) therapy]: This consists of viewing of rotating high contrast gratings of varying widths before the amblyopic eye. In this way, entire population of visual neurons in the visual cortex is activated.

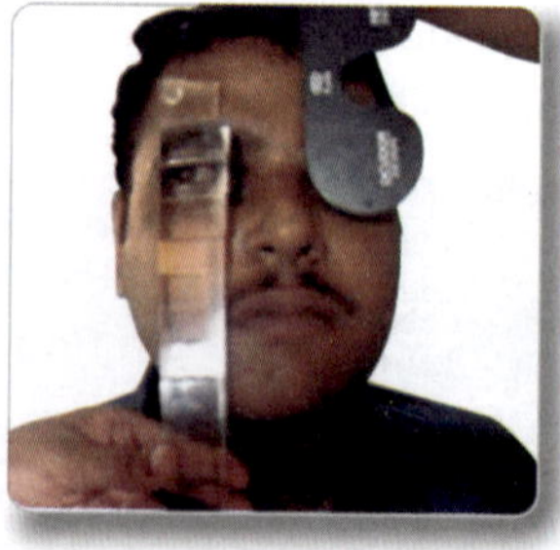

FIGURE 27.17: Prism is kept with apex toward the direction of deviation. Base in and apex out in exotropia.

Orthoptic Exercises

There are three stages of exercises:

1. Antisuppression exercises in which diplopia awareness is created and the patient recognizes that he/she is squinting, when diplopia is developed.
2. Once diplopia awareness is created, fusional exercises are given to improve the fusional ability and control the deviation. This can be through synoptophore exercises or exercising prisms. The prisms of increasing strength placed base out in front of the eye will increase the converging ability and help in controlling a divergent squint (positive fusional amplitude) by adducting prism). Likewise, prism of increasing strength base will help in developing divergent potential and help (abducting prisms) to improve the negative fusional amplitude and in controlling convergent squints.
3. Improvement of relative fusional convergence: This is not the same as improvement of fusional amplitude. Wherever the amount of accommodation (A) is changed, accommodative convergence (AC) is either exerted or relaxed by a predetermined amount (the AC/A ratio), but if accommodation is constant, fusional convergence can be exerted (positive relative convergence) or relaxed (negative relative convergence) relative to that amount of accommodation. The former, if improved, can control exodeviation; the latter is improved in esodeviation, so that sufficient accommodation can be used for clear vision without associated use of convergence. These are achieved by using stereogram card exercises.

Operative Treatment

Surgical treatment of concomitant unilateral squint is indicated when the angle of squint is 10° or more when wearing correcting lenses and in children, when orthoptic training has failed to correct the deviation within a reasonable time.

As a general rule, if indicated, it should be undertaken early and as soon as possible before the child develops irrevocable vision loss due to amblyopia. Postponement until the child is 10 years or more of age usually results in permanence of amblyopia and failure to establish binocular vision. The surgery in those cases is purely cosmetic.

Surgical treatment of alternating concomitant squint without error of refraction is purely cosmetic; as fusion does not develop in this type, unless the case is seen when the patient is very young or immediately after the squint has been first noticed. Both the eyes have to be operated to correct the deviation, since it is usually large.

Type of Surgery

The overacting muscle is weakened by recession: The muscle is detached from its insertion and reattached at a position behind the site of insertion. This will weaken its action.

The weak muscle is strengthened by resection: The muscle is detached from its insertion, the required amount of muscle is cut and removed, and the shortened muscle is reattached at its original position:

1. In unilateral convergent squint:
   a. The medial rectus is weakened or recessed by shifting its insertion backwards. About 1 mm of recession of medial rectus corrects about 2°–3° of angle of squint, though this may vary with each surgeon. The medial rectus should not be recessed more than 5 mm. If so, weak convergence occur leading to discomfort in reading and near work, and to headaches.
   b. The lateral rectus (LR) is strengthened or resected (Figs 27.18A to D), if a portion of the muscle is removed and reattached to the original insertion such that muscle becomes straightened and taut. About 1 mm of resection of lateral rectus corrects 1°–2° of angle.
   c. Similarly, in a uniocular divergent squint, the lateral rectus is recessed and medial rectus resected.
   d. In hypertropia, the superior rectus is recessed and inferior rectus is resected.
   e. In hypotropia, the inferior rectus is recessed and superior rectus resected. Always recession is done before resection.
2. In alternating convergent squint: Bilateral medial rectus recession in patients with equal vision is both eyes and in which the deviation for distance is greater than that for near.
3. In alternating divergent squint: Bilateral lateral rectus recession is done in patients with equal vision is both eyes and in which the deviation for distance is greater than that for near.

The recession and resection types of squint surgeries are shown in Figures 27.19A and B.

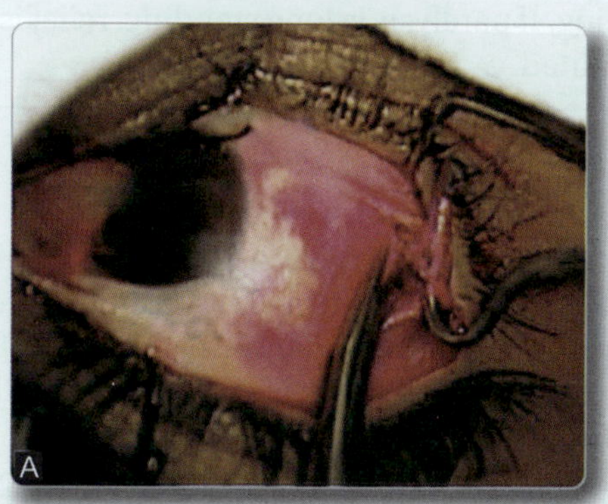

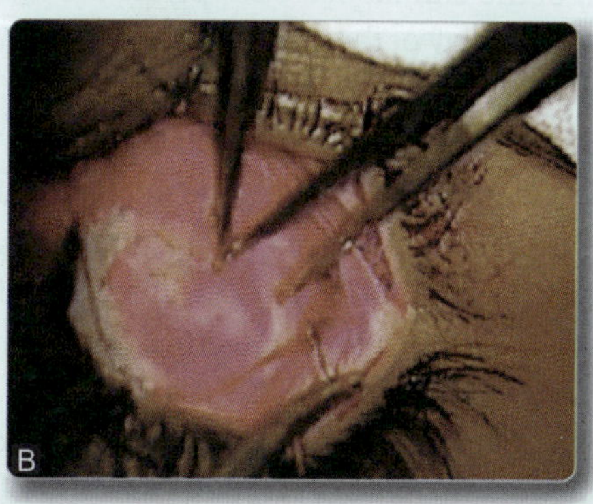

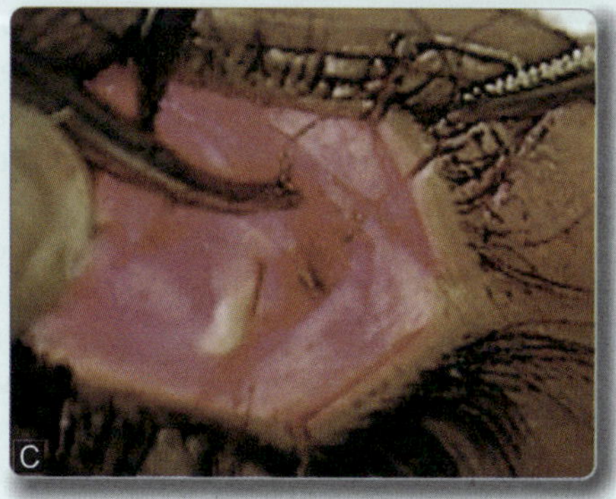

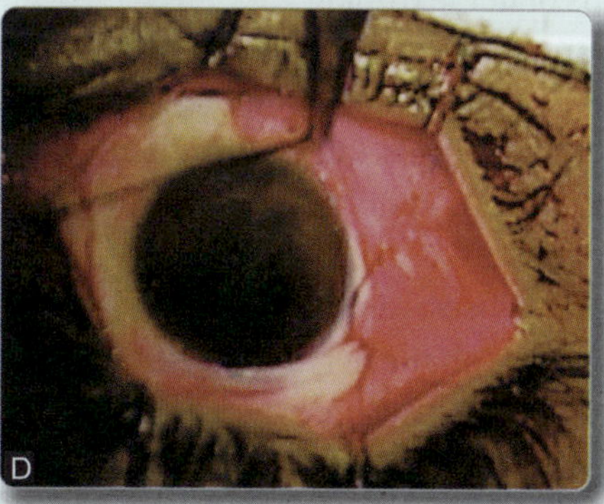

FIGURES 27.18A to D: Unilateral convergent squint surgery. **A.** Lateral rectus (LR) isolated and pulled up with muscle hook and cut with scissors; **B.** The amount of recession measured with calipers; **C.** The LR reattached with sutures at the recessed position; **D.** Conjunctiva sutured back.

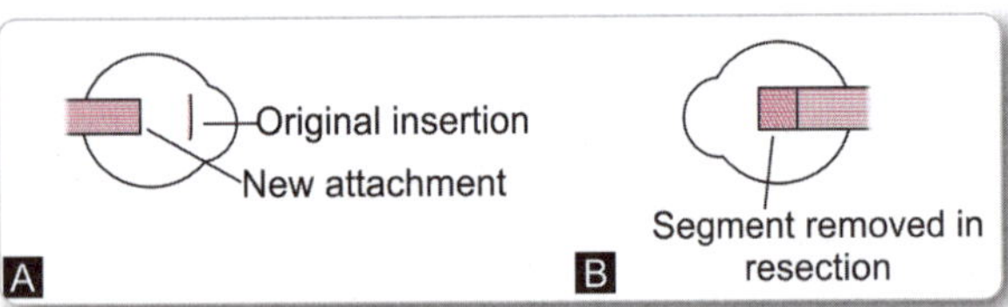

FIGURES 27.19A and B: Squint surgery. **A.** Recession; **B.** Resection.

NON-COMITANT OR PARALYTIC SQUINT

Definition

Non-comitant squint is a deviation caused by paralysis or restriction of extraocular muscles and it is a condition in which deviation of eye varies in different directions of gaze.

Etiology

Any lesion of the cranial nerve supplying the muscle. The lesion may be at any of the following locations:

1. Lesion of motor nerve nucleus:
   a. Congenital, absence of nucleus.
   b. Vascular causes affecting the nucleus (midbrain).
   c. Toxic causes like endogenous (diphtheria), exogenous (alcohol, lead, botulism, thiamine deficiency).
   d. Inflammatory lesion affecting muscles, e.g. encephalitis, neurosyphilis.
2. Lesions of the nerve root just beyond the nucleus: Inflammation, neoplasm, vascular cause.
3. Lesions of nerve trunk:
   a. Trauma: Direct injury to trunk, pressure on the nerve by hematoma, stretching of nerve due to cerebral edema or intracranial hemorrhage.
   b. Neuritis: As in diabetes, vitamin deficiency or lead poisoning.
   c. Toxic causes: Alcohol.
   d. Pressure on the nerve by aneurysm or neoplasm.
4. Lesion of muscle itself:
   a. Congenital absence or maldevelopment of muscle.
   b. Injury to muscle.
   c. Disease of muscle or myopathy, as in thyrotoxic myopathy, ocular myopathy.

Signs and Symptoms

Sx **Symptoms**

Diplopia: It is the chief complaint. It is most marked in the direction of action of the paralyzed muscle. Binocular diplopia results; diplopia is present when both eyes are open. Diplopia may be crossed (heteronymous) or uncrossed (homonymous). If the eyes are divergent (uncrossed) diplopia is crossed as in III nerve paresis. If the horizontally acting muscles are affected, the two images are seen side by side, if vertically acting muscles are affected one image appears at a lower level than other. If oblique muscles are affected, one of the images appears tilted.

Vertigo and nausea: These symptoms are due to diplopia and false projection of images. These unpleasant symptoms are counteracted partially by altering the position of head or completely by shutting or covering the affected eye. In congenital strabismus, these symptoms are not obtrusive since the vision in one eye is suppressed. In acquired cases, they are at first very distressing. If paralysis is long standing, relief is gradually obtained.

Signs

Limitation of extraocular movement: In paralysis of an ocular muscle, the ability to turn the eye in the direction of normal action of muscle is diminished or lost. Limitation is tested roughly by fixing patient's head and telling him/her to follow the movements of surgeon's finger. The finger should be held vertically to test horizontal movements and horizontally in testing vertical movements.

Primary deviation is less than the secondary deviation: Primary deviation is the deviation of the squinting eye and secondary deviation is the deviation of the unaffected eye when the deviating eye is forced to take up fixation (Figs 27.20A and B). The relative movements of the two eyes when each is used for fixation are of importance. For example, if the right lateral rectus is paralyzed and the left eye is covered, then on attempting to fix an object situated to right with the paralyzed eye, left eye will deviate very much to the right under cover. The deviation in the left eye is the secondary deviation; the deviation of right eye when the left eye fixates is the primary deviation. The reason for this difference is due to the fact that equal motor energy goes to the synergic muscles of both eyes in any ocular

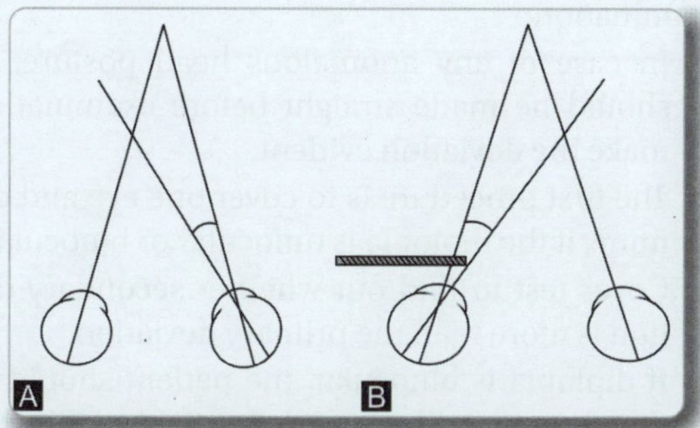

FIGURES 27.20A and B: Primary and secondary deviation. **A.** Deviation of the squinting eye when the normal eye is used for fixing; **B.** When the normal eye is occluded and the squinting eye is forced to take up fixation, the normal eye undercover is deviating more due to the increased nervous energy exerted for making the paralyzed eye to work.

movement. When the paralyzed muscle tries to fix an object in the field of action of the affected muscle (an object on the right side in a case of right lateral rectus palsy), extra motor energy is necessary to fix with the squinting eye and this will be shared by the normal eye and so it deviates more.

Visual acuity: This is normal in each eye and there is no amblyopia.

False orientation: This is a necessary accompaniment of binocular diplopia. Suppose a patient whose right lateral rectus is paralyzed, shuts the left eye and attempts to fix an object situated to the right. When the patient is asked to point at the object with the extended index finger, the finger will pass considerably to the right of object. This is called false projection. It depends on some principle as increase of secondary deviation. The object is projected according to amount of nervous energy exerted. As this is greater than that exerted normally, the object is projected too far in the direction of action of paralyzed muscle. As soon as he realizes that the finger has overshot the target, suitable adjustment will be made.

Anomalous/compensatory head postures: The patient holds the head so that the face is turned in the direction of action of paralyzed muscle. For example, in paralysis of right lateral rectus the patient keeps his head turned to the right. This is to decrease the need for looking toward the right side and thus, to lessen the diplopia and its attendant unpleasant consequences as much as possible. The position is unconsciously adopted. Any anomalous posture may mask an underlying deviation.

Ocular torticollis is a term applied to tilling of head to compensate for defective vertical movements of one eye. It is distinguished from true torticollis due to contraction of sternomastoid muscle. In that, there is simple tilling of head without rotation of the chin toward the opposite shoulder and sternomastoid is not unduly contracted. It occurs in cases of congenital origin, but it also follow traumatic fractures, if binocular single vision can be obtained by adjusting head posture. The vertical squint is made manifest by placing the head straight when diplopia is also elicited.

Sequelae of external ocular muscle palsy: If the paralysis is of some duration, certain changes occur in the muscles. These are:

1. Overaction of contralateral synergist.
2. Contracture of the direct antagonist.
3. Secondary inhibitional palsy of the contralateral antagonist.

For example, in a case of right lateral rectus palsy there is overaction of left medial rectus (contralateral synergist), contracture of right medial rectus (direct antagonist) and secondary palsy of left lateral rectus (contralateral antagonist). Similarly, in case of left superior oblique palsy there are overaction of right inferior rectus, contracture of left inferior oblique and secondary inhibitional palsy of right superior rectus.

Varieties of ocular paralysis: If one muscle alone is affected, it is generally the lateral rectus or superior oblique, since each of these is supplied by an independent nerve. Affliction of several muscles are due to paralysis of III nerve.

Total Ophthalmoplegia

Total ophthalmoplegia is the condition when the entire motor apparatus of the eye, including the intrinsic muscles (ciliary muscle, sphincter and dilator pupillae), the extrinsic muscles and the levator palpebrae superioris, is paralyzed.

External Ophthalmoplegia

External ophthalmoplegia is the condition when only the extrinsic muscles including the levator are paralyzed sparing the ciliary muscle, sphincter and dilator pupillae:

1. Paralysis of lateral rectus: This is the commonest. The clinical signs are:
   a. The eyeball is rotated inwards.
   b. There is restriction of movement of eyeball outwards.
   c. There is face turn toward the paralyzed side.
   d. Homonymous (uncrossed) diplopia occurs on looking to paralyzed side.

2. Paralysis of superior oblique:
   a. The eyeball is deviated upwards and inwards; there is limitation of movement downward and toward the sound side.
   b. The face is turned downwards (chin depressed) and toward the sound side. Head is tilted toward the sound side.
   c. Homonymous diplopia in looking down and in, the false image is lower with upper end tilted toward true image. The patient has great difficulty in going downstairs and vertigo is the particular symptom.

      When the eyes are crossed, the diplopia is uncrossed and vice versa.
3. Paralysis of III nerve: In complete paralysis of III nerve there is ptosis, which prevents diplopia. On raising the lid with a finger, the eye is seen to be deviated outwards and rotated internally owing to the tone of two unparalyzed muscles, viz. lateral rectus and superior oblique:
   a. Limitation of movements in all directions except outwards.
   b. Pupil is mid-dilated and inactive.
   c. Accommodation is completely lost.
   d. Paralysis of III nerve is often incomplete and individual muscles may occasionally be affected alone.

Misdirection in regeneration of III cranial nerve is common after total interruption of function usually by head trauma. The ocular signs are:
1. Pseudo-Graefe lid sign: As eye attempts to move downwards, upper lid retracts.
2. Pseudo-Argyll Robertson pupil: There is a slow light reflex, but better constriction of pupil to the near reflex.
3. Horizontal-gaze lid dyskinesis: The upper lid retracts as eye is adducted and falls as the eye is abducted.
4. Adduction on attempted vertical gaze.

Investigations of a Case of Paralytic Squint

1. History:
   a. Regarding the onset and associated illness that may be a precipitating factor.
   b. History of symptoms like vertigo, vomiting.
   c. History of diplopia, which is the most common complaint.
   d. History of trauma/head injury.
   e. History of any anomalous head posture.
2. Examination:
   a. In case of any anomalous head posture, head should be made straight before examination to make the deviation evident.
   b. The first procedure is to cover one eye and determine, if the diplopia is uniocular or binocular.
   c. Cover test to find out whether secondary deviation is more than the primary deviation.
   d. If diplopia is binocular, the patient should fix at the surgeon's finger and the field of fixation of each eye is tested. The limitation of movements in each deviation is carefully documented.
   e. In such cases diplopia must be investigated by more specific tests.

Diplopia Charting

A spectacle containing a red glass for the right eye and a green glass for the left eye is worn by the patient to distinguish the images (Fig. 27.21). In the darkroom a bar of light through a stenopaic slit in a handheld torch is moved in the field of binocular fixation at a distance of 4 ft (120 cm) from the patient, patient's head being kept stationary. The position of the images is accurately recorded on a chart with nine squares showing the nine gaze positions. The following data are derived:
- Areas of single vision and diplopia
- Distance between two images in the areas of diplopia
- Whether the images are on the same level or not
- Whether the image is inclined or both are erect
- Whether the diplopia is crossed or uncrossed (Fig. 27.22).

These data, if concordant, are sufficient to diagnose the paralysis. The false image, which is frequently tilted, is the fainter of two. Find the position of gaze when the separation of the image is maximal. In that position the farthest displaced image belongs to eye with muscle palsy. By covering one eye, it can be shown as to which eye this image belongs.

There are other methods to find out exactly, which muscle is affected by testing using a Hess chart, Les screen

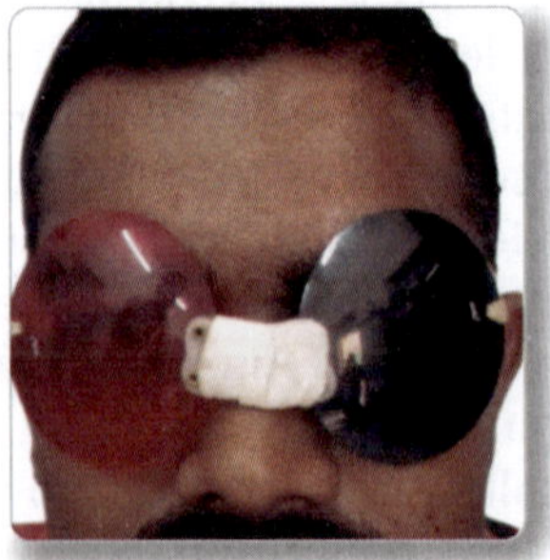

FIGURE 27.21: Patient wearing red-green goggles

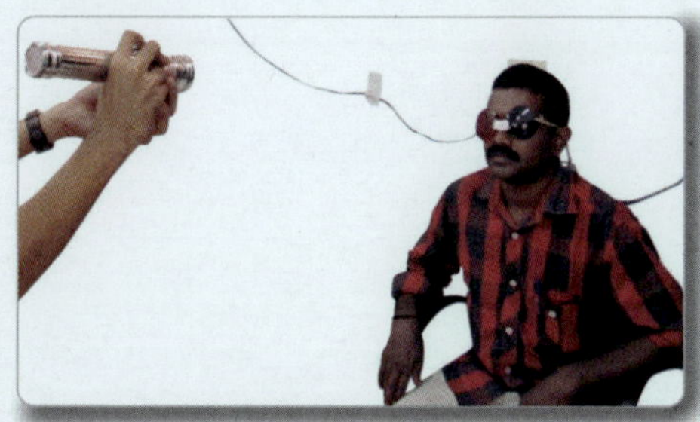

FIGURE 27.22: Testing diplopia

or Lancaster screen. Synoptophore examination can also be done in different position.

Treatment of Paralytic Squint

1. Etiological treatment should be directed to the cause of palsy.
2. To avoid diplopia, occlusion of the better eye may be done, so that movement to the paralyzed side may be initiated by the affected eye without diplopia and contracture of the antagonist of the paralyzed muscle does not develop.
3. Relieving prisms may be given, but this treatment is rarely of much use, since there is variation in amount of deviation in different gaze position and variation over time.
4. Surgery: Sufficient time should be allowed for recovery before decisions on surgery is taken. It is indicated when the deviation has become stabilized and no more spontaneous recovery is taking place, and before permanent structural changes like contracture develop in the synergic muscles. The operative measures consist of weakening the antagonistic muscles by recession and strengthening the synergic muscles by resection.

SECTION 7

Ophthalmic Surgeries

Surgery for Cataract 28

Girija Devi PS

EVOLUTION OF CATARACT SURGERY

Cataract surgery has a long and interesting history dating from the medieval period. The first documented cataract surgery was done in the 5th century BC by the renowned Indian physician of that period 'Sushruta'. At that time the lens was supposed to be occupying the center of the eyeball and 'cataract' is some bad 'humor' that flowed in front of the lens.

COUCHING

The surgery practiced at that period was 'couching'. The aim was to displace the so called abnormal humor from its position in front of the lens. The patient was restrained by someone, while the surgeon sits in front of the patient and a small incision is made inferiorly just behind the corneoscleral junction. A couching needle is introduced through this wound, and the cataractous lens is pushed backwards and inferiorly leaving the pupillary area aphakic, and thus giving a momentary improvement in vision to a person blind due to cataract.

Due to lack of asepsis and the inflammation induced by the lens material liberated into the eye, very few people retained the vision.

EARLY PHASE (EXTRACAPSULAR CATARACT EXTRACTION)

By 17th century, the correct position of the lens was identified and cataract was recognized as the opacification of the lens.

Jacques Daviel is the Father of Modern Cataract surgery. He developed instruments with which incision was put through the inferior cornea, which was then extended with scissors. The cornea is lifted up, the interior capsule is incised, the nucleus expressed out and the anterior chamber (AC) was also washed out. The concept was correct, but the lack of fine instruments of modern era and fine suture material to close the wound, and lack of knowledge about aseptic precautions lead to a high rate of postoperative complications. But this technique was widely accepted. The von Graefe's cataract knife developed by von Graefe in 19th century created a better incision, which reduced the incidence of infection and iris prolapse. Even then, since the wound is not sutured, the patient has to lie down in a supine position without moving the head for at least 2 weeks for the wound to heal satisfactorily without complications.

CATARACT

Even with a better incision using the von Graefe's knife, the retained cortical matter produced increased inflammation and interference with regaining satisfactory vision. This led the surgeons to search for methods for removing the opaque lens in its entirety. Samuel Sharp first performed a successful intracapsular cataract extraction (ICCE) in 1753. How to rupture or lyse the suspensory ligament to release the lens was a problem. Sir Henry Smith, an English Surgeon, who was working in Punjab in India started using a muscle hook to apply pressure externally at the inferior limbus to 'tumble' the lens out through a limbal incision made at superior limbus. His technique came to be known as the **'Smith Indian technique'** and gained wide popularity. The next improvement was the use of a toothed lens forceps to gently grasp the anterior capsule, and rock it side to and to rupture the zonules. The next device to be introduced was 'erysiphake', which is a small suction cup applied to the anterior lens capsule to create a vacuum and suction force, and the lens is removed.

MODERN CATARACT SURGERY

Modern Intracapsular Cataract Surgery

The introduction of cryoapplication started the modern era of ICCE. A cryoprobe, which is cooled with nitrous oxide to temperatures below 0°C, is applied to the anterior capsule. An ice ball forms fixing the anterior capsule to the tip of the cryoprobe and the zonules are ruptured with gentle rocking movements, and the lens attached to the tip of the cryoprobe is removed. Lens extraction became easy with this equipment.

With modern sterilization techniques, fine suture material to suture the incision and operation microscopes, which increased the precision of the surgery, ICCE became a successful operation for cataract.

This surgery is still in practice in many parts of the developing countries where large volume of blind population has to the treated without the recent sophisticated equipments for today's cataract surgery.

It is still useful in the management of subluxated cataractous lens.

Though a successful procedure, ICCE had certain limitations:

1. Not useful in young people who have strong zonules, which are not easily torn and firm adhesion of the vitreous to the posterior capsule, which can lead to vitreous loss. Zonules can be lysed with enzymes like α-chymotrypsin, but due to the strong attachment of the vitreous to the posterior capsule vitreous loss with all its complication will follow ICCE in children or young adults.
2. The patient is still dependent on strong convex lenses for visual rehabilitation after ICCE. The vision through the high convex lens is associated with several problems and patients are usually not happy with aphakic spectacle correction. Many of them refuse to wear the aphakic spectacles and hence have no functional visual improvement.
3. The ICCE requires a fairly large incision, which is associated with complications like delayed wound healing, iris prolapse, vitreous loss and most importantly, significant astigmatism even in uncomplicated cases.
4. Loss of barrier between the posterior and anterior segment leads to anterior movement of the vitreous. This plays a role in the high incidence of postoperative complications like cystoid macular edema and rhegmatogenous retinal detachment.

These problems associated with ICCE led to the renaissance of extracapsular cataract extraction (ECCE).

Extracapsular Cataract Extraction in Modern Era

The ECCE has come back with modern sophisticated equipments and the intraocular lenses (IOLs), it has become a surgery with minimum complications and adequate visual rehabilitation. The surgery, which was done sutureless earlier, because fine sutures and were not available, has become sutureless again because the decrease in the size of the incision and the valve-like technique of making the incision made suturing unnecessary. Once it was done without anesthesia because no local or systemic anesthetic was available. Now it can be done with no anesthesia, only local anesthetic drops are required. ECCE of the modern era can be:

1. The conventional ECCE with suturing of the wound.
2. Manual small incision cataract surgery (MSICS) where the nucleus is removed manually through a valve like sclerocorneal incision followed by aspiration of all residual lens matter.

   The introduction of many new instruments made the new ECCE a safer technique. These include:

   a. Cystitomes that can be fashioned from 26 gauge needles to do controlled capsulotomy (opening in the anterior capsule).
   b. Irrigation and aspiration cannula, which infuse fluid into the eye and aspirate the cortical matter simultaneously.
   c. The introduction of ophthalmic viscoelastic surgical devices (OVDs), which help to maintain the AC, and protect the corneal endothelium during manipulations inside the eye, increased the success rate and decreased the complications.

      The added advantage that highly expensive equipments like phacoemulsifier are not required for MSICS, made it highly suitable for developing countries like India and this surgery is very popular here.
3. Phacoemulsification: In MSICS, the incision has to be big enough to manipulate the nucleus out of the eye. In phacoemulsification, ultrasound waves are used to fragment the nucleus into microscopic particles and they are aspirated, while fluid is infused into the eye—all done through a single small handpiece of the phacoemulsifying equipment. This allowed cataract surgery to be done through a small incision 2.8 or even lesser in size. The IOLs are also suitably modified foldable or injectable type to introduce through this small incision. Smaller the incision size, lesser the postoperative astigmatism and earlier the return to normal routine for the patient.

Intraocular Lens Implantation

The visual rehabilitation after ICCE using high-powered convex lens is very unsatisfactory due to the image magnification and distortion of images, while looking through the side of the glasses. This led people to search for better alternatives to spectacles, especially methods to replace an artificial lens for the God-given lens, which is removed.

Harold Ridley was the first surgeon who introduced IOLs made of polymethyl methacrylate, into the posterior chamber after ECCE. The initial attempts for IOL implantation met with high rate of complications due to poor lens shapes and chemical reactions produced by the methods of sterilization of the lenses. Continued research in this field led to improvements in lens design and its sterilization techniques, and now IOL implantation is hardly associated with any complication in the hands of an experienced surgeon.

The introduction of foldable and injectable lenses allows implantation of IOL through the small incision of phacoemulsification surgery.

The visual rehabilitation with IOLs is excellent except for one factor, i.e. lack of accommodation. Even little children who have to undergo cataract surgery for congenital or traumatic cataract have to wear bifocal spectacles to facilitate near vision. Now multifocal and accommodative lens are available, which help to see clearly at all distances with less dependence on glasses. These lenses are not as perfect as God-given lenses and with the continuing research near perfect lenses can be expected in future.

The cataract surgery now has come to full circle. From the days of couching, which was done through a 2 mm incision without anesthesia, it has come to the days of phacoemulsification done through 2 mm or less incision with only topical anesthetic drops. The modern cataract surgery has now become a simple and almost outpatient procedure for the patients, but demands a high level of skill and precision, and consequently a long and steep learning curve for the surgeon.

EVALUATION FOR CATARACT SURGERY

When to do Surgery?

In the era of ICCE, surgery was done only when the lenticular opacity has progressed to mature cataract stage. The reason was that the rupturing of the zonular fibers to remove the lens intact was easier when the cataract has reached maturity. So, patients have to remain partially blind for a variable period of time waiting for the right time for surgery. With the advent of modern techniques, this scenario has completely changed. Cataract surgery and the replacement of the lens with artificial lens can be done even in the early stages of lenticular opacification. The time of surgery depends on the visual requirements of the patient and the interference in the activities of daily living by the visual disturbance caused by the cataract.

Indication for Surgery

Visual Disability

If the reduced visual acuity caused by the cataract is interfering with daily activities, surgery is indicated. This will vary from person to person depending on education, job requirements, routine activities, etc. All posterior subcapsular cataracts (PSCs) can grossly interfere with the visual acuity especially the near vision and reading and an office worker will require early surgery to continue his/her official activities. Similarly PSC and anterior cortical cataract will produce glare during night driving, and a person who is a driver by profession will require surgery to continue the profession even before significant drop in vision has occurred. At the same time an old illiterate person leading a sedentary life or a manual laborer will be able to continue routine activities till the visual acuity is considerably decreased. So the right time for cataract surgery is a decision to be taken by the patient and the doctor together, depending on the interference in routine activities and the desire to improve the vision.

Professional Requirements

Certain professions like that of a pilot will require perfect vision and surgery has to be done if the best corrected visual acuity (BCVA) is less than normal, and cataract is the reason for the decrease in vision.

Cosmetic

A total cataract in an eye with long-standing retinal detachment or glaucomatous optic atrophy will have to be surgically removed for cosmetic purpose even though there is no chance of improving vision by surgery.

Medical Indication

1. Condition like phacolytic glaucoma, phacomorphic glaucoma or dislocation of the lens into the AC demand lens removal to cure the secondary glaucoma.
2. In patients requiring posterior segment surgeries like retinal detachment surgery or vitrectomy, cataract surgery is indicated if the opacification of the lens is interfering with clear visualization of the posterior segment.

Preoperative Evaluation

A patient with some decrease in vision and some cataractous changes in the lens has to be properly evaluated to solve the following issues:

1. Is the drop in vision solely due to cataract or is there some other pathology?
2. Even in patient with other ocular problems affecting vision, e.g. glaucoma, is cataract surgery going to produce a significant improvement in vision?
3. Is the lens capacity secondary to some systemic or ocular problem?
4. Whether the general condition is fit for undergoing cataract surgery?
5. Is there any local ocular problem that can adversely affect the procedure, e.g. chronic dacryocystitis, dry eye, etc.

The preoperative evaluation is done to get satisfactory answers to the above questions.

Clinical History

A proper and careful elicitation of history is important in:

1. Determining the type of cataract.
2. Whether there are other ocular problems affecting the vision as well as the outcome after surgery.
3. Any systemic problem that has to be taken care of before surgery.

Nature of Visual Loss

Cataract is the most common cause for gradual loss of vision. But all patients having gradual loss of vision are not suffering from cataract. Other common causes for gradual loss of vision like primary open angle glaucoma, uncorrected refractive error or macular degeneration may be the reason for defective vision, or these problems may be coexisting with cataract.

History of any sudden loss of vision or sudden drop in vision at some point in the course of gradual loss of vision is important and may point toward some other pathology like retinal detachment, vascular occlusion or exudative type of macular degeneration.

Possibility of any posterior segment problem—then patients have to be clearly evaluated for deciding whether there are any co-existing posterior segment problems and whether the lenticular opacity is sufficiently advanced so that cataract surgery will give some visual benefits in spite of the other ocular diseases. This is particularly important in people with diabetes who may have diabetic retinopathy.

A past history of recurrent attacks of redness and pain, which subsided with or without treatment is important since this may indicate the presence of chronic anterior uveitis, and the cataract may be a complicated cataract.

A history of previous trauma to the eye is important for two reasons. This may mean that:

1. The cataract is of traumatic origin.
2. The patient may have other damage to the eye due to trauma like secondary glaucoma, macular degeneration or retinal detachment, which may adversely affect the postoperative visual recovery.

A careful elicitation of clinical history is important in all uniocular cataracts and cataracts in young people to rule out a traumatic, complicated or metabolic cataract.

Medical History

A complete medical history is an important part of the preoperative evaluation:

1. A careful history is important regarding medical problems like diabetes mellitus (DM), hypertension (HT), coronary artery disease, chronic obstructive pulmonary disease (COPD), bleeding disorders or any general medical problems, which necessitate long-term steroid therapy.
2. Any history of taking any immunosuppressants or anticoagulants is also important since drug modification is necessary during the time of surgery.
3. Any history of drug allergy is also important since this necessitates careful drug allergy testing for all medicines and local anesthetics that have to be used at the time of surgery.

Preoperative Clinical Examination

Systemic Examination

The general health of the patient should be assessed to determine whether he/she can safely undergo cataract surgery. If the patient is suffering from DM, HT, coronary heart diseases, chronic airway obstruction or psychiatric disorder, these illnesses have to be medically controlled before surgery. A general medical check-up, and routine blood and urine examination are essential to rule out any of the systemic problems.

Ocular Examination

A careful ocular examination is essential to rule out any ocular problem that may adversely affect the visual recovery (e.g. macular degeneration), as well as adversely affect the natural course of cataract surgery (e.g. chronic dacryocystitis, which can lead to postoperative infection).

Visual acuity and refraction: The distance as well as the near visual acuity should be measured both unaided as well as with the most suitable spectacle correction decided by refraction (BCVA).

Lids and ocular adnexa: Look for any lid abnormalities like lagophthalmos, ectropion or entropion. They have to be corrected before cataract surgery. Any infection like hordeolum internum or externum, or blepharitis has to be controlled before under taking surgery. Dacryocystitis, if present, can lead to postoperative endophthalmitis. Syringing of nasolacrimal ducts should be done to rule out chronic dacryocystitis. If dacryocystitis is present a dacryocystectomy (DCT) or dacryocystorhinostomy (DCR) should be done before undertaking cataract surgery.

Ocular motility: A pre-existing squint means the patient may be having amblyopia in the squinting eye. A cataract surgery in that eye cannot be expected to give good visual improvement.

Conjunctivitis: If present should be treated and controlled before planning surgery.

Cornea: Careful examination of the cornea under slit lamp is essential to rule out any increase in corneal thickness or corneal edema, which denotes a compromised endothelial layer. The surgical trauma can aggravate this problem and hamper visual recovery. If the patient had undergone a previous refractive surgery, the corneal thickness and clarity have to be assessed. Special techniques for IOL power calculation has to be made in these patients.

Any keratic precipitates, old or new is a warning sign about the presence of uveitis. The cataract in this situation may be a complicated cataract due to uveitis. All inflammation has to be controlled before surgery and the surgery is usually undertaken under cover of systemic steroids.

Anterior chamber: A shallow AC indicates narrow angle or an intumescent lens and gonioscopy should be done to rule out narrow angle glaucoma. Gonioscopy is essential to rule out angle abnormalities or abnormal vessels in the angle if an AC IOL is planned. Look for any cells or flare in the AC, which means an active anterior uveitis, which is a contraindication for cataract surgery.

Iris: Look for posterior synechiae, which indicates a coexisting or previous anterior uveitis. Inflammation has to be controlled before planning cataract surgery. Look for any exfoliative material on iris, which mean weak zonules or secondary glaucoma, which can accompany pseudoexfoliative glaucoma with cataract.

Pupil: Examination of the pupil is very important in the preoperative evaluation of cataract. The pupillary reaction will be brisk even in hypermature cataract. A swinging flash test should be done to rule out any relative afferent pupillary defect.

Look for any iris shadow, while examining the pupil. Throw the light from one side so that the light falls obliquely on the lens near the edge of the pupil. If the lens is partially opaque, as in an immature cataract, the clear lens matter will act as a mirror with the opaque lens fibers underneath simulating the silvering at the back of a mirror and a crescentic shadow of the iris will be seen at the edge of the pupil on the same side as the light (Fig. 28.1). If the lens is totally opaque (mature cataract) no shadow will be seen.

Crystalline lens: The lens has to be examined under the slit lamp to assess the level of opacity whether posterior subcapsular, nuclear or cortical cataract. Assess whether the lenticular opacity correlates with the decrease in vision. If the cataract is insignificant and the decrease in vision is considerable, the patient has to be carefully evaluated for some other problem affecting vision.

Look for any subluxation or phacodonesis of the lens, which mean the zonular integrity is compromised.

Fundus evaluation: The evaluation of fundus after dilatation by both direct and indirect ophthalmoscope is essential to evaluate the optic disk (for any cupping or pallor), the retinal vessels (for any evidence of fresh or old vasculitis or vascular occlusion), macula (for any macular degeneration) and the peripheral retina for any peripheral retinal degeneration or retinal detachment.

In patients in whom the cataract is too dense for proper visualization of the fundus, special investigations like B scan must be done in addition to clinical tests like:

1. Projection of light.
2. Gross color vision like identifying the red or green color of a fairly large object.
3. Macular function tests to access the functional integrity of the retina.

Electroretinography (ERG) and visually evoked potential (VEP) may be indicated in specific circumstances.

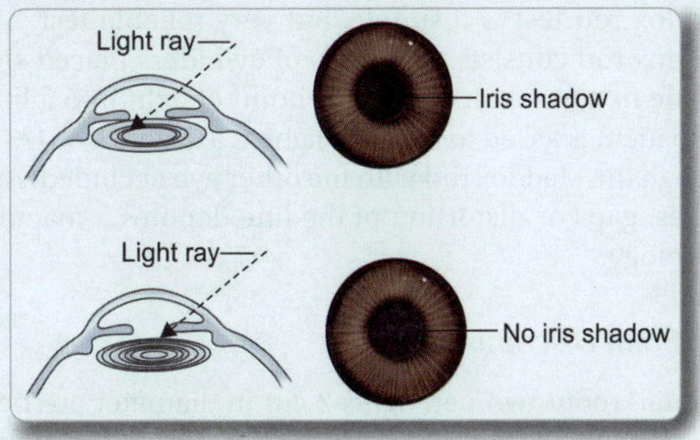

FIGURE 28.1: Demonstration of iris shadow

Routine Investigations

1. Checking intraocular pressure (IOP) is mandatory in all patients to undergo cataract surgery. If there is any suspicious optic disk cupping or elevation of IOP, further tests are indicated to rule out glaucoma. If glaucoma is detected or already existing, it is important to decide whether:
   a. Cataract and glaucoma surgery may be done as a combined procedure.
   b. Glaucoma surgery is done first and cataract surgery later.
   c. Cataract surgery alone is done and glaucoma managed by topical antiglaucoma medications.
2. Projection of light: This test is important in all patients with advanced cataract, so that visual acuity is reduced to PL or HM. If projection of light is inaccurate, a posterior segment problem like glaucoma or optic atrophy has to be suspected.
3. Gross color vision: Even in the presence of advanced cataract, the patient will be able to identify primary colors like red, green or blue.
4. Visual field testing by confrontation method should be done in all cataract patients. If there is a visual field loss, patient has to be evaluated for glaucoma, optic nerve disease or retinal detachment.

Special Tests

Macular Function Tests

The visual recovery after surgery depends to a large extent on the functional integrity of the macula. So a series of special tests are designed to assess the macula, especially in cases where the lenticular capacity is dense enough to prevent proper visualization of retina.

Maddox Rod Test

Maddox rod test is a simple, but very reliable test. The Maddox rod consists of a series of cylinders placed side by side in a frame. It converts a point of light into a line. The patient is asked to look at a light at a distance of 1/3 m through the Maddox rod with the other eye occluded. Any brakes, gaps or distortion of the line denotes a macular pathology.

Two Point Discrimination Test

In a darkroom two pen lights 2 cm in diameter are held close together 60 cm away from the eye and gradually separated until the patient can perceive two lights.

With HM vision—two lights are perceived when they are 12 cm apart:

- CF to 3/60–7 cm apart
- More than 3/60–5 cm apart.

Color Perception Test

The patient wears red-green goggles and a light is shown through the spectacle. Blue color is tested with the blue light of a blue field endoscope. If the patient can perceive at least one color that indicates a good macular function.

Blue Field Entoptic Phenomenon (Flying Corpuscle) Test

The retina is uniformly illuminated with the blue light of an endoscope held close to the eye. The number of white corpuscles moving in the parafoveal capillaries will be visualized as an entoptic phenomenon if the photoreceptors and capillaries at the macula are intact. A normal response is 15 or more corpuscles moving in a pulsatile manner. Many patients will find difficult to understand this test.

Purkinje Vascular Entoptic Test

Like blue field test this test, is also subjective. A bright source of light is shined through the patient's closed eyelids. If the patient can perceive images of the retinal vasculature, the retina is probably attached and healthy.

Estimation of Potential Visual Acuity

The possible postoperative visual acuity can be measured by two methods.

Laser interferometry: In this method monochromatic helium-neon laser light from two sources produce a fringe pattern on the retina. The transmission of these patterns is not affected by the lenticular opacity. By gradually decreasing the spacing of the pattern, the potential visual acuity is estimated. The limitation of this technique is that a small foveal lesion that can considerably diminish the visual acuity may go undetected.

Potential acuity meter: A miniature Snellen's chart is projected into the eye and the patient is asked to read the letters on the chart. PAM tends to be most accurate in eyes with visual acuity of 6/60 or better.

Electroretinography and Visually Evoked Potential

When other tests are inconclusive, electroretinography or visually evoked potential testing can be done to evaluate retinal and optic nerve functions.

Preoperative Measurements

Biometry is done to calculate the IOL power. Corneal power is first detected using keratometry or corneal topography equipment. The actual length of the eye is measured using A scan—ultrasonography. From these two measurements (keratometry reading and axial length of the eye) IOL power can be calculated. All ultrasound machines have built in software to calculate the IOL power if the corneal keratometry value is also given to the machine. Accurate IOL power calculation is essential for proper visual rehabilitation after cataract surgery.

Corneal pachymetry is the method to measure the corneal thickness. If there is endothelial dysfunction the central corneal thickness will be more than 640 μ and these patients are at a higher risk for developing postoperative endothelial decompensation and corneal edema. Specular microscopy is used to determine the endothelial cell density per millimeter square as well as its morphological abnormalities like polymegathism (increase in size) or pleomorphism (irregular shape). Eyes with such abnormalities are at increased risk for developing postoperative endothelial decompensation.

Preoperative Patient Preparation

Before surgery the patient and their family members should be informed about the procedure, the pre- and post-operative care, the visual improvement that can be expected and the risk for any complication, sight threatening as well as life-threatening. A written informed consent should be obtained from the patient before surgery.

Any medical problem like DM, HT, COPD, any cardiac condition, etc. should be well-controlled before surgery.

Any ocular or periocular infections like blepharitis, conjunctivitis, chronic dacryocystitis should be treated and cured in advance before deciding on the surgery. Patients with chronic dacryocystitis should undergo DCR or DCT and postoperative inflammation should subside before cataract surgery. If the patient has glaucoma this should be medically controlled before cataract surgery.

The preoperative medications and preparation of the eye will vary from center to center and from one surgeon to another. Patient is usually started on a broad spectrum systemic antibiotic on the previous day of surgery. Some surgeons do not use any systemic antibiotics at all. Some surgeons like to give acetazolamide tablets 250 mg on the previous night and the morning before surgery, to keep the IOP low. Again, many surgeons do not use this. Patient is asked to apply some broad spectrum topical antibiotic drops starting from the previous day of surgery. Since non-steroidal anti-inflammatory drops may prevent intraoperative pupillary constriction, this may be started 2–3 days before surgery. On the day of surgery, the pupils are dilated with tropicamide phenylephrine drops and sometimes cyclopentolate drops are also applied. The eye- lashes may be clipped before surgery or they are left alone and kept away from the surgical field with the help of adhesive surgical eye drapes. Povidone-iodine eyedrops are instilled just before surgery because they have a broader spectrum of action against bacteria, fungi and virus than any antibiotic drops.

Anesthesia for Cataract Surgery

Cataract surgery has evolved from surgery without any anesthesia in the historical era through retrobulbar anesthesia, peribulbar and sub-Tenon's anesthesia to today no anesthesia technique, i.e. no anesthetic injection is given, only topical anesthesia drops are used.

Retrobulbar anesthesia: The local anesthetic solution is xylocaine 2% injection mixed with 1 in 1,000,000 adrenaline and hyaluronidase 150 units in 20 mL of xylocaine. 2–4 mL of this mixture is injected inside the muscle cone either through the lower lid at the junction between the lateral and inferior walls of the orbit or through the lower fornix. The retrobulbar block may be supplemented with facial block injected near the temporomandibular joint. The facial block is to paralyze the orbicularis muscle and prevent squeezing of the lids, which can increase the IOP, and can cause vitreous loss during surgery. Good anesthesia and akinesia are obtained with retrobulbar injection.

Complications: Retrobulbar hemorrhage, accidental globe perforation or optic nerve injury.

Accidental intravenous (IV) injection of xylocaine can lead to cardiac arrhythmias and inadvertent intradural injection is associated with seizures and respiratory arrest.

Peribulbar anesthesia

To lessen the complications of retrobulbar anesthesia, peribulbar anesthesia was introduced. Here the anesthetic injection is given outside the muscle cone into the peripheral orbital space from where it will slowly diffuse into the muscle cone and produce anesthesia and akinesia.

The disadvantages are the longer time interval between the injection and the onset of action, peribulbar swelling and slightly less effectiveness than retrobulbar anesthesia.

The advantages are lesser incidence of complications compared to retrobulbar anesthesia, but the risk of globe perforation is not totally eliminated.

Sub-Tenon's infusion or injection of xylocaine

Here the anesthetic drug is injected or given as repeated bolus through a cannula introduced into the sub-Tenon's space. It provides good anesthesia, but only moderate akinesia during surgery. The complications are almost absent.

Topical anesthesia

Using proparacaine drops—this requires good cooperation from the patient, and can be used only in intelligent and cooperative patients. It is not useful in anxious and apprehensive patients. Topical anesthesia is supplemented with the use of preservative-free xylocaine injected into the AC (intracameral xylocaine) once the AC is entered into.

General anesthesia

General anesthesia is required in young children and in adults whose cooperation cannot be expected as people with mental retardation or psychiatric disorders.

TYPES OF CATARACT SURGERY

Intracapsular cataract surgery is practically obsolete in modern times, but it is still practiced in some remote areas of undeveloped countries where the facilities for surgery are minimal. It is still useful in cases of subluxation or dislocation of lens.

Method

Intracapsular cataract extraction is usually done under retrobulbar anesthesia. After giving the retrobulbar injection, cleaning the eyelids and surrounding skin is done with povidone-iodine solution, and draping is done with sterile towels. A disposable plastic drape if available can be used, which will minimize the exposure of the skin and also help to keep the lashes away from the surgical field.

Separation of the lids can be done with sutures put on the upper and lower lids or using a wire speculum.

A suture is passed underneath the superior rectus muscle and this is fixed to the surgical drapes using an artery forceps. This superior rectus bridle suture helps to steady the globe and rotate it downwards so that the superior limbus is well-exposed to put the incision.

A fornix-based conjunctival flap is fashioned using a conjunctival forceps and scissors. Since a fornix-based flap tends to retract and expose the sutures, some surgeons prefer a limbus-based flap. A limbus-based flap will interfere with proper visualization of the AC and in putting the sutures, but it will keep the sutures nicely covered in the postoperative period. After the flap is made, bleeding vessels are cauterized with the thermal cautery or wet-field cautery.

Incision

The incision is made at the superior limbus and extends up to 180° (9 O'-3 O'clock). A large incision is required to remove the whole lens intact. An initial groove is made with a sharp Bard-Parker knife or razor blade fragment. AC is entered into with the sharp point of the number 15 BP knife or razor blade fragment, usually at 12 O'clock position. The initial entry wound is extended to either side using corneal scissors. This is an 'ab externo' incision. In the earlier days when von Graefe's knife was used, the incision was 'ab interno'. The knife enters the eye at 3 O'clock or 9 O'clock and comes out at the opposite limbus, and it is slowly moved upward till it is completely out of the AC, meanwhile making a limbal incision from 3 O' to 9 O' clock position. This 'ab interno' incision is difficult to make correctly and likely to injure the cornea, iris or lens.

A suture is placed into the cornea at 12 O'clock meridian with 8-0 black silk or 10-0 prolene. By pulling this suture the cornea can be lifted up and folded back to expose the lens. The cryoprobe is applied to the anterior lens capsule and an ice ball is formed, which attach the capsule to the tip of the probe. With gentle rocking movements the zonules are ruptured, and the lens is lifted up and out through the limbal incision. A small peripheral iridectomy is done after lens removal. The purpose is to make an alternate passage for the aqueous from posterior to the AC if the pupil gets blocked with the vitreous. The AC may be reformed with an air bubble or balanced salt solution. If IOL is to be placed it has to be an anterior chamber IOL, which is supported at the angle. Then AC is formed with air or viscoelastic material and the IOL is placed in the AC with the supporting haptics in the horizontal meridian. It is made sure that the pupil is round and the iris is not caught in the haptic of the lens. The limbal wound is then closed with interrupted or continuous 8-0 black silk or 10-0 nylon. If viscoelastic was used it has to be removed before wound closer is completed. If viscoelastics is left behind this can lead to secondary glaucoma in the immediate postoperative period (viscoelastics and IOLs were not available in the era of ICCE. They are part of modern times and used if ICCE is done now).

A subconjunctival injection of 0.5 mL of gentamicin and dexamethasone is given by many surgeons at the end of the surgery to counter postoperative infection as well as inflammation.

Enzymatic Zonulolysis

In patients below 50 years the zonules will be stronger and difficult to rupture. Enzymatic zonulolysis can be done before lens removal by injection of α-chymotrypsin into the AC.

Postoperative Care

Topical antibiotic and steroid drops are given at frequent intervals initially and slowly tapered off within 6–8 weeks. In ICCE usually a mydriatic like homatropine or atropine is also given 2–3 times daily. The sutures can be removed after 6–8 weeks.

VISUAL REHABILITATION AFTER ICCE

Conventional ICCE is done without IOL implantation. Simple removal of the cataractous lens alone is not going to benefit the patient significantly as far as vision is concerned. Without the crystalline lens, only the corneal refraction will be taking place and the light rays will be coming to focus considerably behind the retina and the **eye will be strongly hypermetropic**. In a previously emmetropic person the uncorrected visual acuity will be around CF at half meter. If the patient was previously myopic, the myopia will compensate the hypermetropia to some extent and the vision will be better, depending on the degree of myopia.

The methods of visual rehabilitation include:

1. Spectacle correction.
2. Contact lens.
3. A secondary IOL implantation done at a later date after all postoperative inflammation has subsided. This can be a ACIOL (Fig. 28.2) supported at the angle of AC iris clip lenses supported by the haptics clipping the iris or a scleral fixated IOL, which is placed behind the pupil after anterior vitrectomy, and kept in place with sutures through the ciliary body and sclera fixing the haptic of the lens in the ciliary sulcus.

Spectacle Correction

An aphakic person will require strong convex lenses to correct the hypermetropia.

Disadvantages of Aphakic Spectacle Correction

1. Magnification of the image size: The strong convex lenses increase the image size by 25%–30%. This produces two problems:
   a. If the other eye has good vision the difference in the size of the images between the two eyes will produce diplopia. Binocular vision is impossible unless the other eye also undergoes cataract surgery.

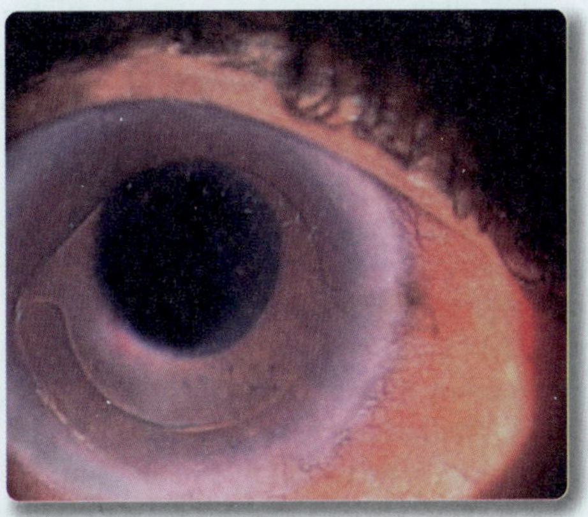

FIGURE 28.2: Anterior chamber intraocular lens (ACIOL)

   If this is not done and the other eye has good vision, the aphakic spectacle has to be abandoned, and the patient has to depend on the vision of the unoperated eye alone, until the vision in that eye decreases due to cataract or some other pathology, or cataract surgery is done in that eye also.

   What happens if a patient who is aphakic in one eye undergoes cataract surgery with IOL implantation in the other eye?

   The problem of diplopia sets in due to the difference in the size of the images, if he/she wears aphakic glasses. Either the patient has to abandon aphakic glasses and use the pseudophakic eye alone or a secondary IOL implantation has to be done in the aphakic eye also.

   b. If the other eye has poor vision due to cataract, or some other problem or both eyes are aphakic, the magnification of the images produce another problem. We assess the distance of objects by the size of the images formed on the retina and the magnification produces a false spatial orientation. Even simple tasks like picking up a piece of paper or pouring tea into a cup becomes a difficult task and all movements become clumsy. There is a long learning curve before the patient can adjust to the new spatial orientation. Some people never learn to adjust to this and go about without wearing glasses. They prefer the blurred uncorrected image to the clearer magnified images of an unfamiliar world.
2. Loss of accommodation: Once the lens is removed all power of accommodation is lost. For near and intermediate vision, the person is totally depend on glasses whatever be the age of the patient. This is

more relevant in young children who have to undergo cataract surgery for congenital cataract. The benefit of retaining accommodation with blurred vision has to be weighed against clearer vision with no accommodation before embarking on surgery.

3. Spherical aberration: The spherical aberration of the thick convex lens gives a pincushion effect to the visual field. Straight lines appear curved and the whole world is converted into a parabola and every eye movement make the objects move like a writhing snake. The patient can see clearly only by looking straight through the center of the lens, and he/she has to turn the head and not the eye to see to the sides.
4. Restriction of visual field: With spectacle correction the visual field is restricted due to:
   a. Small size of the aphakic lenses due to the heaviness of the thick lens and spherical aberrations of the periphery, the aphakic glasses are given as small lenticular lenses. This leaves a large portion of the peripheral field uncorrected.
   b. Roving ring scotoma—due to the prismatic effect of the periphery of a spherical lens there is a ring of scotoma extending from 30° to 50°. When the eye moves to one side the scotoma moves in the opposite direction and hence some objects, which were previously invisible (Fig. 28.3) become suddenly visible and other objects, which were previously visible disappear. This is called **'Jack-in-the-box phenomenon'** (Fig. 28.4). This is very disturbing to some patients and they feel giddy and nauseated, and refuse to wear aphakic glasses. The peripheral field from 65° to 80° goes unrefracted since this is outside the spectacles.

These various disadvantages of aphakic spectacle correction led to research for better options.

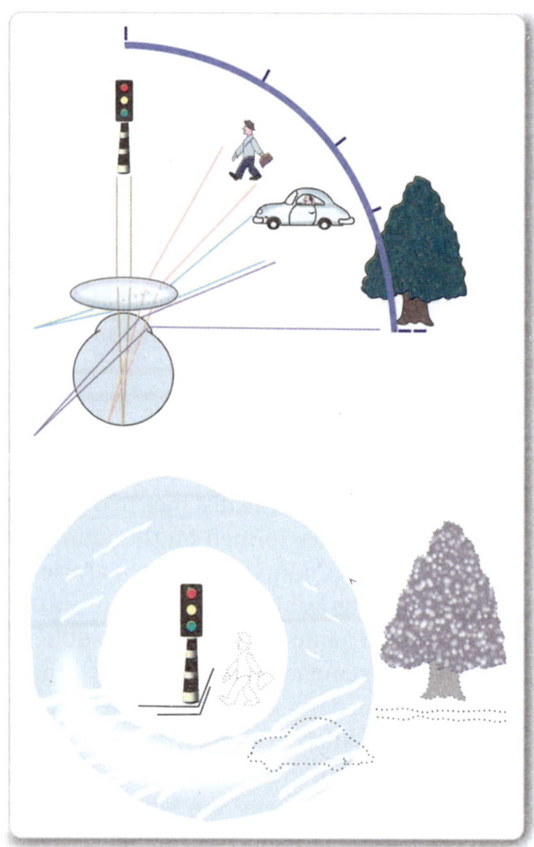

FIGURE 28.3: Aphakic spectacle corrected vision in straight ahead gaze. Rays from 50° to 65° fail to enter the eye producing a ring scotoma. The car in this area is invisible. Rays from 65° to 90° are unrefracted by spectacle glasses (*Courtesy:* Cataract surgery and its complications by Norman S Jaffe).

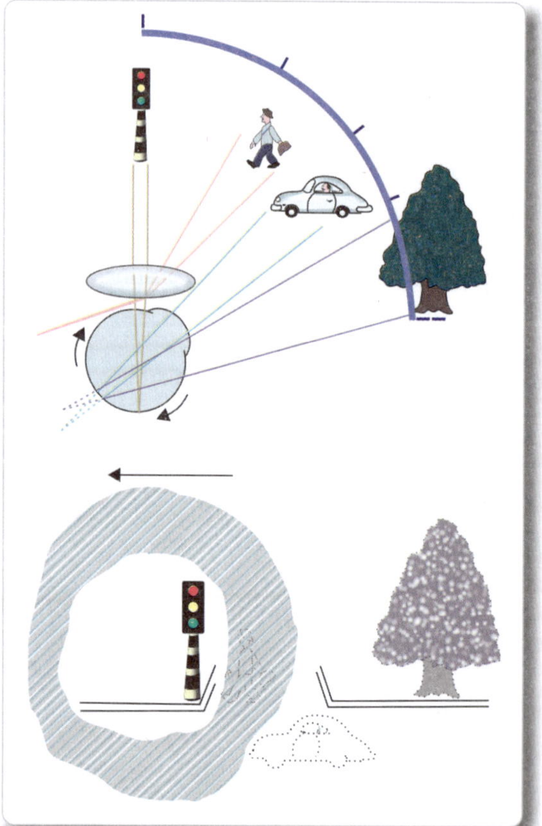

FIGURE 28.4: Demonstration of roving ring scotoma. When the gauze is directed laterally, lateral rays from 30° to 50° fail to enter the eye. Rays from 50° to 90° are unaffected. Due to the central shift of the scotoma, the man disappears and the car suddenly comes into view (Jack-in-the-box phenomenon).

Contact Lenses

Contact lenses are better option than glasses. The magnification with contact lens is only 5%, which is tolerated by our visual mechanism. There is no spherical aberration, distortion of images or restriction of fields with contact lenses.

But many of the patients undergoing cataract surgery are elderly patients who often lack the finger dexterity to insert and remove the contact lenses themselves. So, the use of contact lenses is often limited to younger patients.

In short, the logical solution for the removal of the natural crystalline lens is the replacement by an artificial lens.

COMPLICATIONS OF INTRACAPSULAR CATARACT EXTRACTION

Higher incidence of complications is associated with ICCE compared to ECCE and its various modifications.

Preoperative Complication

Associated with retrobulbar injection, retrobulbar hemorrhage, accidental globe perforation, etc. (mentioned earlier).

Intraoperative Complications

Inadequate Incision

A large incision 160º–180º in size is required for ICCE for easy delivery of the whole lens. A smaller incision can lead to endothelial damage, Descemet's membrane stripping, difficulty in delivery of the lens leading to capsule rupture and vitreous loss.

Irregular Incision

Often occurs from inexperienced hand. It will lead to delayed wound healing, iris prolapse, marked astigmatism, epithelial ingrowth, etc.

Excessive Bleeding from the Corneal Wound and Iris

Excessive bleeding from the corneal wound and iris can occur especially in people on anticoagulants or drugs like Aspirin, which prevents clotting of blood.

Iridodialysis

Iridodialysis can occur when the initial entry wound is extended with corneal scissors. This can lead to hyphema. If the dialysis is large, it can displace the pupil or cause uniocular diplopia in the postoperative period. Large iridodialysis should be sutured.

Inadequate Pupillary Dilatation

Inadequate pupillary dilatation can occur in people on long-term pilocarpine therapy for glaucoma, pseudoexfoliation and senile miosis. This will cause difficulty in delivering the lens leading to sphincter tear or capsule rupture. This can be avoided by doing a sector iridectomy.

Vitreous Loss

Vitreous loss can occur if the IOP is not kept low preoperatively with acetazolamide or mannitol.

Intraoperative rise in IOP can occur:

1. In short-necked people on lying down.
2. If too much xylocaine is injected during retrobulbar block.
3. If the lid suture or speculum is applying pressure on the eyeball.
4. If the patient is anxious and restless.

Problems caused by vitreous loss

Vitreous loss per se is not the problem. Vitrectomy is done as a surgical procedure in many vitreoretinal disorders. The space left behind by the removed or lost vitreous will be filled up with aqueous humor.

But the vitreous loss during surgery can lead to a series of complications due to forward movement of the vitreous through the pupil and the incarceration in the incision.

Vitreous loss leads to problems by two mechanisms:

1. Vitreous incarceration in the wound unless a very meticulous vitrectomy is done.
2. The moving forward of the vitreous exerts traction at its attachments to the retina mainly at the vitreous base at pars plana, and also at its posterior attachments at macula and the edge of the optic disk.

   The adverse effects of vitreous loss are due to these sequelae.

Vitreous incarceration in the incision leads to delayed wound healing, iris prolapse, epithelial and fibrous downgrowth onto the posterior surface of the cornea, and iris and marked astigmatism. Vitreous touch on the corneal endothelium can lead to corneal decompensation and corneal edema.

Updrawn pupil: The vitreous coming through the pupil and getting incarcerated in the wound leads to this phenomena.

Pupillary block by the vitreous: It can occur leading to shallow AC and secondary glaucoma.

Secondary glaucoma: It can occur due to the pupillary block as well as the blockage of the angle by the vitreous filling the AC.

Chronic iritis: The vitreous in the AC can cause irritation to the iris and lead to mild chronic anterior uveitis and persistently irritable eye.

Cystoid macular edema (CME): The traction exerted on the macula as well as the release of prostaglandins can lead to CME.

Retinal detachment (RD): The traction exerted at the retinal periphery at the vitreous base can lead to retinal degeneration, hole formation and subsequent retinal detachment.

Even if there is no vitreous loss at the time of surgery, the loss of barrier between the posterior and the anterior compartment after the lens removal will lead to a gradual moving forward of the vitreous into the AC, and this can lead to cystoid macular edema and RD. ECCE retain the barrier between the two compartments, and decrease the incidence of CME and RD.

Management of vitreous loss

All the problems related to vitreous loss can be prevented to a large extent by meliculous removal of all vitreous in front of the papillary plane manually by cutting with a Vanna's scissors or with the help of anterior vitrectomy machine.

Suprachoroidal or Expulsive Hemorrhage

In people with high IOP or high blood pressure (BP) in the preoperative period and people with atherosclerosis, the sudden lowering of the IOP at the time of the entry into the AC can lead to rupture of the choroidal vessels and massive intraocular bleeding.

All intraocular contents, i.e. retina, vitreous, lens and uveal tissue will be thrown out by the blood gushing out of the eye. An expulsive hemorrhage will lead to loss of the eye and vision unless an early drainage of the blood through a scleral incision is made (suprachoroidal drainage) and the wound is closed immediately to give a tamponade effect as soon as the choroidal bleeding is suspected. Once well-established, this massive bleeding can be controlled only by evisceration of the eye.

Lens Capsule Rupture

Lens capsule rupture can occur, while attempting to remove the lens with the cryoprobe or the capsule forceps. The surgery will then have to be converted into ECCE.

Nucleus Drop

Nucleus drop complication is more common in ECCE than ICCE.

A capsule tear extending to the posterior capsule can lead to lens matter and even the nucleus falling into the vitreous cavity. The soft cortical matter in the vitreous will slowly get absorbed even though it can lead to secondary glaucoma or uveitis. But the nucleus will not get absorbed and it has to be removed by a second surgery with the help of the vitrectomy machine by the vitreoretinal surgeon. A nucleus left behind in the vitreous cavity can lead to intractable secondary glaucoma, uveitis and RD, and finally loss of vision.

Postoperative Complications

Early Phase

1. Postoperative shallow AC can occur due to wound leak, if the corneoscleral incision is irregular and not sutured properly. It can also occur associated with choroidal detachment and malignant glaucoma.
2. Iris prolapse is due to inadequate wound closure or due to rise in IOP in the immediate postoperative period or due to restlessness of the patient. If detected within 24 hours after surgery, the prolapsed iris may be repositioned and resuturing of the incision is done. If detected later, repositioning can lead to infection since the prolapsed iris may be contaminated with microorganisms. So the prolapsed iris is cut off (iridectomy) and the wound is resutured.
3. Hyphema—bleeding can occur from iris vessels or the incision into the AC, if the patient is restless or the suturing is not proper. This blood will get absorbed. Patient may be given acetazolamide tablets to control any rise in IOP due to the blood in AC.
4. Endophthalmitis: Can be acute or chronic or sterile (Fig. 28.5):

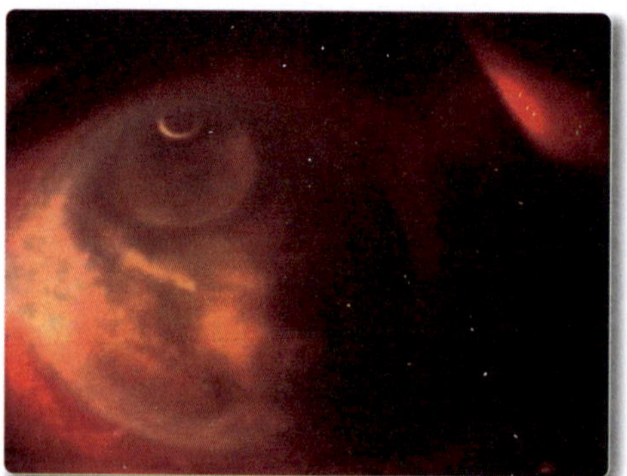

FIGURE 28.5: Postoperative endophthalmitis

a. **Acute endophthalmitis** develops in 2–5 days after surgery.

Patient presents with pain, redness, loss of vision and photophobia. On examination this will be corneal edema, exudates on the iris or pupillary area and hypopyon. The pupil will give a yellow reflex due to vitreous exudation. The pathogen is often bacterial organisms and the source is contaminated instruments or fluids used during surgery or the commensals from the skin of the lids or neighboring structures.

Treatment: Immediate vitreous or aqueous tap should be done to isolate the organism by smear and culture. At the same time intravitreal injection of 0.4 mg in 0.1 mL amikacin and vancomycin (1 mg in 0.1 mL) is also given. These antibiotics are also given IV or as subconjunctival injection or as fortified drops. If vision is considerably reduced, vitrectomy is done to remove all the exudates and toxic material in the vitreous early before toxic damage to the retina occurs.

b. **Chronic endophthalmitis** may present a few weeks after surgery. The inflammation is less acute and drop in vision will be the main complaint of the patient. The pathogenic organism is usually fungus.

c. **Sterile endophthalmitis or toxic anterior segment syndrome (TASS)** is a sterile inflammation that appear within 12–24 hours after surgery due to introduction of toxic material as a contaminant on the instruments or fluids used in surgery.

Treatment: To control the inflammation with intensive topical and systemic steroid therapy.

5. Secondary glaucoma can occur due to pupillary block by the vitreous, especially if an iridectomy has not been performed. If viscoelastics used during surgery are not completely removed (rarely used in the era of ICCE and commonly used in modern extracapsular surgery) this can lead to transient rise in IOP in the postoperative period.
6. Malignant glaucoma: This is due to a posterior misdirection of aqueous, which collects in the posterior part of the vitreous cavity pushing the vitreous forward. This will lead to shallowing of the AC, pupillary block and rise in IOP. Shallow AC is usually associated with wound leak and decrease in IOP. When shallow AC is associated with increase in IOP, malignant glaucoma should be suspected.

   Treatment: Atropine eyedrops four times daily may cure mild cases. Relaxation of the ciliary muscles by atropine stretches the suspensory ligament and pulls the lens backwards. Aspiration of the fluid through the pars plana or a pars plana vitrectomy may be needed in intractable cases.
7. Choroidal detachment: Persistent wound leak and chronic uveitis can lead to exudation into the suprachoroidal space leading to bullous elevation of the choroid. In mild cases choroidal folds will be seen as radiating folds around the optic disk. When bullous elevations occur they will be seen as dark swellings through the pupil.

   Management: If there is wound leak and hypotony, resuture the wound to correct the hypotony. The uveal inflammation, if present, should be controlled by systemic steroids.

Late Complications

1. Filtering cicatrix: If there is wound leak, healing will be delayed leading to the development of cystoid spaces at the incision through which aqueous will pass into the subconjunctival space. This will appear like the filtering bleb produced by trabeculectomy.

   Management: The cystoid cicatrix should be excised and resuturing is done.
2. Epithelial ingrowth: Epithelial down growth can occur if the wound apposition is not proper and/or associated with iris prolapse. Epithelial cells from the ocular surface will grow inwards lining the posterior surface of the cornea, angle and the anterior surface of the iris. The epithelial down growth will be seen as a translucent membrane on the back of the cornea with a horizontal advancing edge. The membrane blocking the angle will lead to secondary angle closure glaucoma. The eye will remain persistently irritable. Sometimes the epithelial cells will form cystic swelling inside the AC (Fig. 28.6).
3. Chronic uveitis: It can sometime follow cataract surgery.
4. Secondary glaucoma: It can be pre-existing open angle glaucoma or secondary glaucoma due to secondary angle closure or as a complication of chronic uveitis.

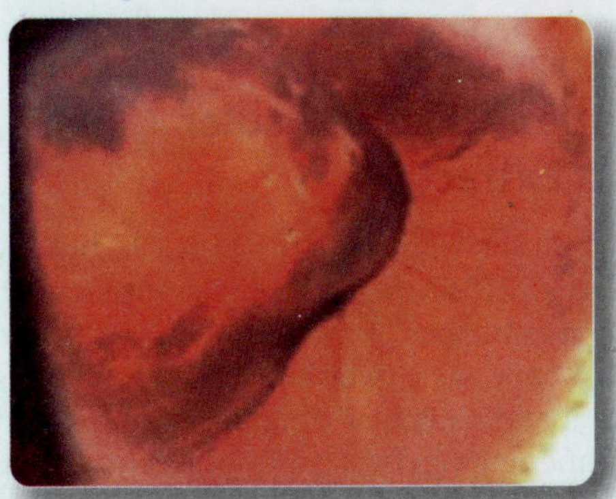

FIGURE 28.6: Postoperative implantation iris cyst

Secondary angle closure glaucoma may be due to:

- Peripheral anterior synechiae formation due to persistent postoperative shallow AC
- Due to epithelial down growth
- Secondary to pupillary block with vitreous.

5. Cystoid macular edema (Irwin-Gauss Syndrome). This is the most common posterior segment complication after cataract surgery. The incidence is higher after ICCE than ECCE and the incidence is higher if there is vitreous loss after surgery. The release of prostaglandins and vitreoretinal traction at the macula following vitreous loss are the reasons. The CME will lead to decrease in visual acuity.

   Treatment: Topical and systemic steroidal and nonsteroidal anti-inflammatory drugs.
6. Retinal detachment: The risk for development of RD is higher after ICCE than ECCE, higher in people with vitreous loss at the time of surgery and also in people with high risk for RD like high myopes.

EXTRACAPSULAR CATARACT EXTRACTION

Extracapsular cataract extraction (ECCE) can be the conventional type or manual small incision cataract surgery (SICS).

The high rate of complications associated with ICCE revived the interest in extracapsular extraction.

Main advantage of ECCE over ICCE:

1. The 'posterior capsule zonular complex' retains the normal anatomical compartments of the eye. So the complications like vitreous loss and its sequelae—CME and RD are comparatively less after ECCE.
2. The incision required in ECCE is smaller compared to ICCE and hence lesser the amount of astigmatism.
3. There is the added advantage that the IOL can be placed in the normal anatomical position behind the iris supported by the posterior capsule and the zonules.

Conventional Extracapsular Cataract Extraction

Corneoscleral incision is put as in ICCE, but the size is smaller about 120° since only a smaller incision is required to remove the nucleus. A cystitome or a 26 gauge needle (with its tip bent twice to fashion a disposable cystitome) is used to make a circular opening on the anterior capsule. This opening can be a continuous curvilinear capsulorhexis (CCC) or can opener capsulorhexis. Since ECCE require lot of manipulations inside the AC, viscoelastics are injected into the AC after entering into the AC. These viscoelastics helps to maintain the AC with the iris and the lens in the normal anatomical position, as well as protect the corneal endothelium.

After capsulorhexis, about 0.1–0.5 mL balanced salt solution is gently injected into the lens between the cortex and the nucleus, and also between the capsule and the cortex. This helps the separation of the nucleus from the cortex and the cortex from the capsule (hydrodissection), and allows easy removal of the nucleus and the cortex. After hydrodissection the nucleus is eased into the AC using a Synsky's hook or the disposable cystotome. The nucleus is delivered out of the eye using a vectis attached to a syringe or an IV line. After the removal of the nucleus, the cortex is aspirated out using the 'Simcoe irrigation aspiration cannula' attached by an IV line to a bottle of Ringer's lactate or balanced salt solution. The Simcoe cannula allows simultaneous irrigation of the fluid into the eye and the aspiration of the cortex. This helps to maintain the AC and protect the endothelial layer during these manipulations. In the absence of this, an aspiration cannula attached to a 5 or 10 mL syringe containing fluid can be used to irrigate and aspirate alternatively to remove the cortex. The viscoelastics can be injected as and when required to maintain the AC. Once the entire cortex is removed, the posterior capsule with the peripheral rim of anterior capsule is left behind. The IOL is now introduced into the AC. The posterior chamber IOL can be put inside the capsular bag or kept in front of the capsule with the haptics of the IOL supported at the ciliary sulcus. After the insertion of the IOL, all viscoelastics are removed by irrigation and aspiration. The AC can be maintained with fluid or an air bubble (which will get absorbed in a few days) and the wound is closed with interrupted or continuous 10-0 nylon or 8-0 black silk.

Manual Small Incision Cataract Surgery

Manual small incision cataract surgery is a very popular and widely practiced surgery in developing countries like India. The advantage of this technique is that it is a small incision sutureless surgery that can be done without any expensive equipment like the phacoemulsification unit. Careful construction of the entry wound results in minimal induced astigmatism, early visual rehabilitation and return to routine life for the patient.

The valve like self-sealing wound consists of an initial vertical incision on the sclera, sclerocorneal tunnel and again a vertical internal incision in the cornea to enter the AC. The external incision can be of various shapes—straight, V shaped, frown or curved incision (Fig. 28.7) made on the sclera 2–3 m behind the limbus. Its length varies from 5.5 to 6.5 mm. The sclerocorneal tunnel is dissected forward

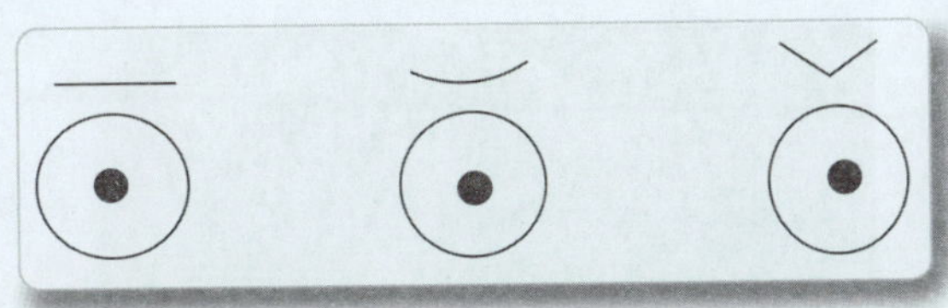

FIGURE 28.7: Incisions in small incision cataract surgery (SICS)—straight, frown or 'V' shaped

from this external incision until it reaches 1 mm into clear cornea. The AC is entered about 2 mm from the limbus with a 3.2 m keratome by dipping it toward center of the AC. Thus this incision has an initial vertical component in the sclera, a horizontal tunnel through the sclera and cornea, and a final vertical component through the cornea to reach the AC. This valve-like incision is self-sealing, and the lip of the wounds are kept in opposition by the normal IOP and does not require any sutures.

After the entry into the AC, the surgery is continued and completed as in conventional ECCE. Since all manipulations have to be done through a smaller valvular incision, there is a learning curve to master this technique.

Some surgeons use an AC maintainer introduced into the AC through a small incision put in the lower part of the cornea. It is connected by an IV line to a bottle of balanced salt solution. With the self-sealing valve-like incision the continuous irrigation through the AC maintainer keeps the anterior segment structures in their natural position and maintains normal IOP. The use of the AC maintainer reduces the need for viscoelastics during surgery. The steps of SICS are given in Figures 28.8 A to P.

Advantages of SICS

1. No suturing required.
2. Minimal induced astigmatism.
3. Marked low incidence of postoperative iris prolapse and hyphema.
4. Better control of expulsive hemorrhage by spontaneous closure of the wound.
5. Early ambulation of the patient from the day of surgery itself.
6. It can be done without any expensive equipments like phacoemulsification unit (Fig. 28.9).

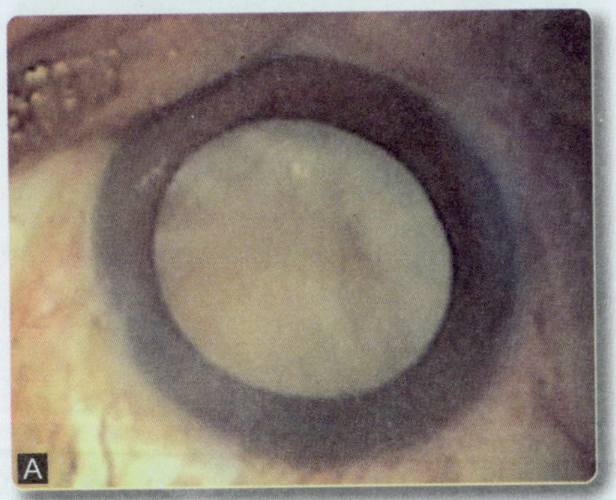

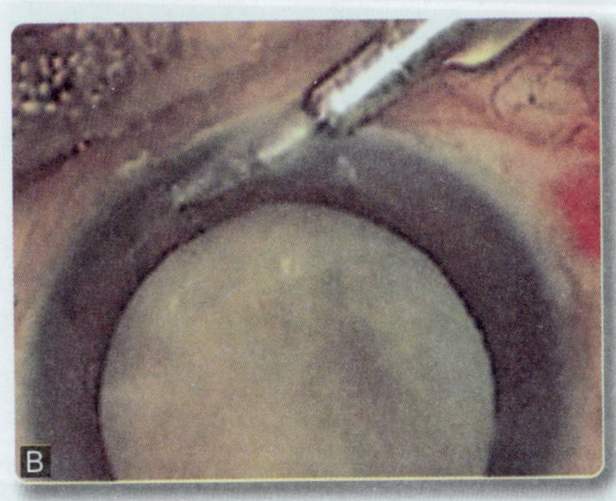

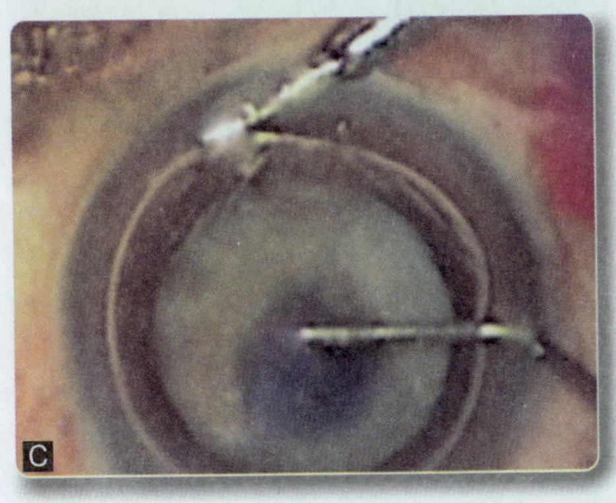

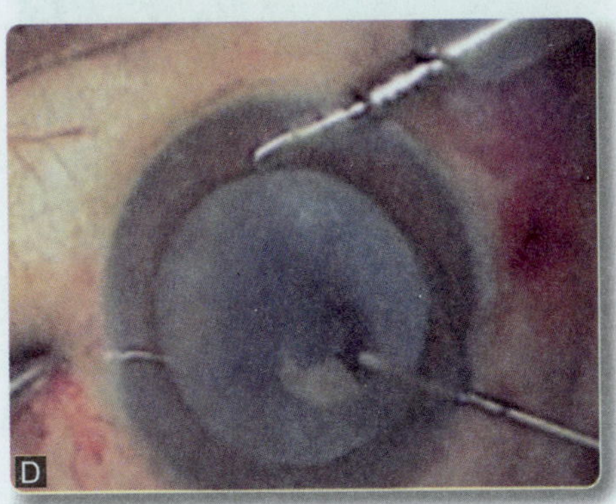

FIGURES 28.8A to D: Steps of cataract surgery (SICS). **A.** Eye exposed with speculum; **B.** Anterior chamber (AC) maintainer introduced at lower limbus; **C.** Trypan blue dye injected under air bubble through the side-port incision; **D.** Capsulorhexis started.

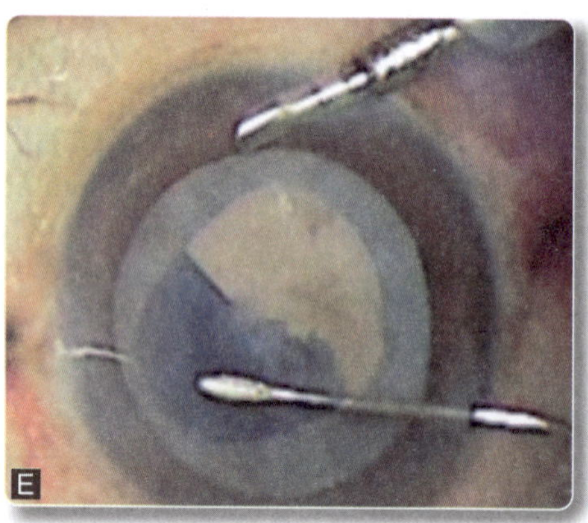

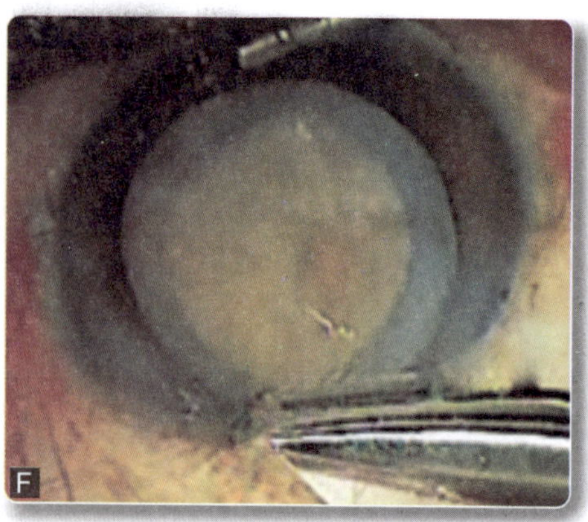

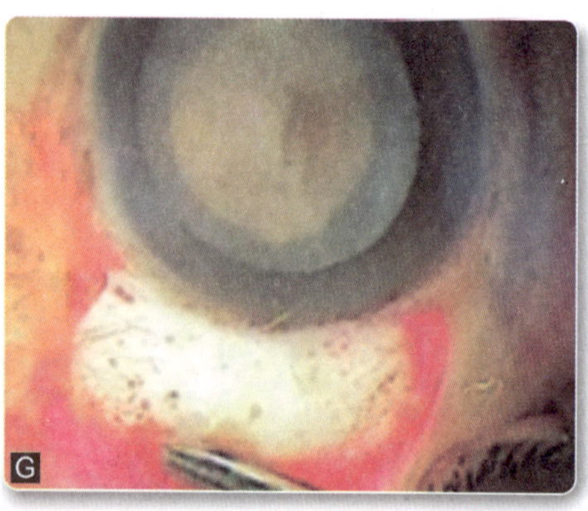

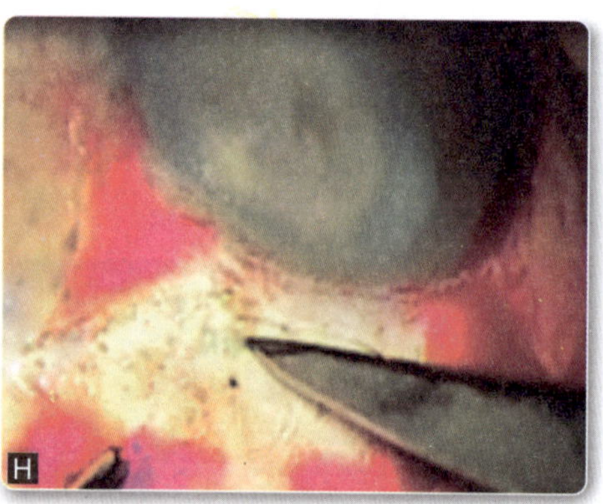

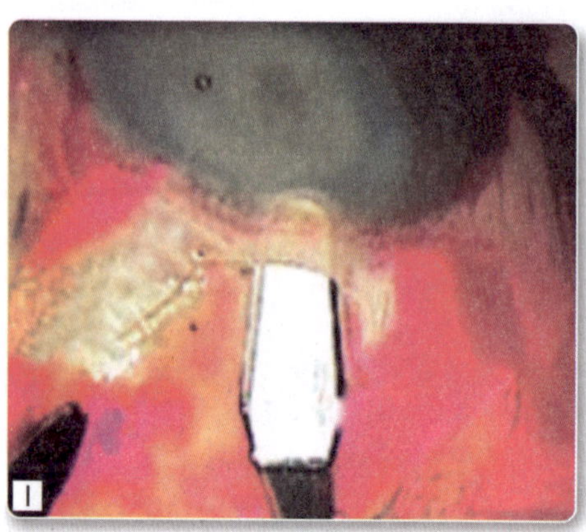

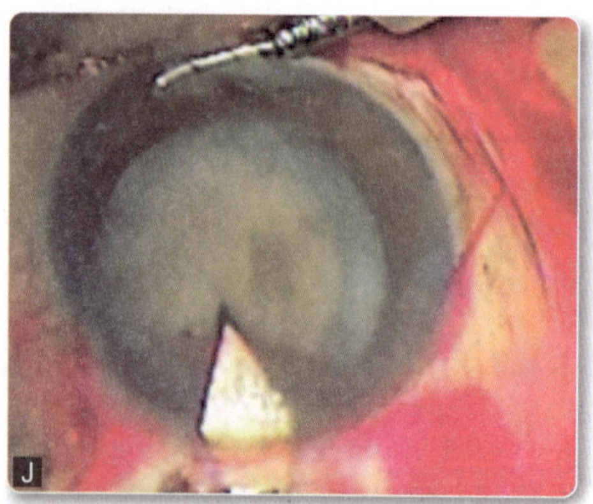

FIGURES 28.8E to J: Steps of cataract surgery (SICS). **E.** Capsulorhexis continued; **F.** Limbus based conjunctival flap cut with scissors after completion of capsulorhexis; **G.** Cautery applied to bleeding spots; **H.** Incision put with Bard-Parker (BP) blade; **I.** Tunnel incision put up to clear cornea with crescent knife; **J.** Anterior chamber (AC) entered with keratome.

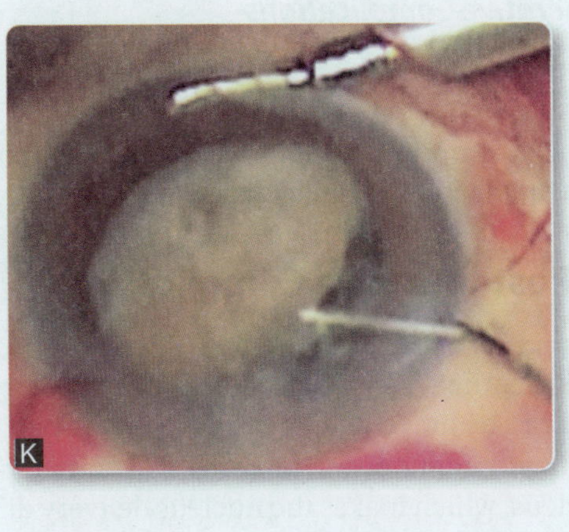

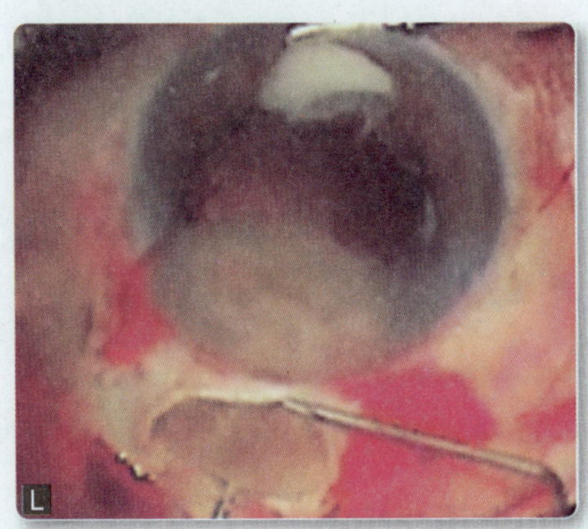

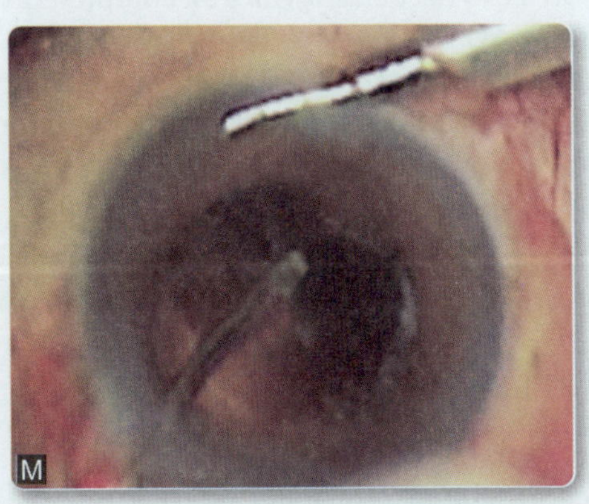

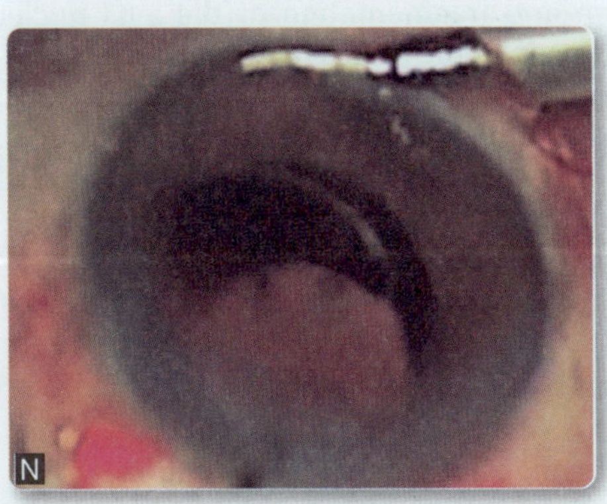

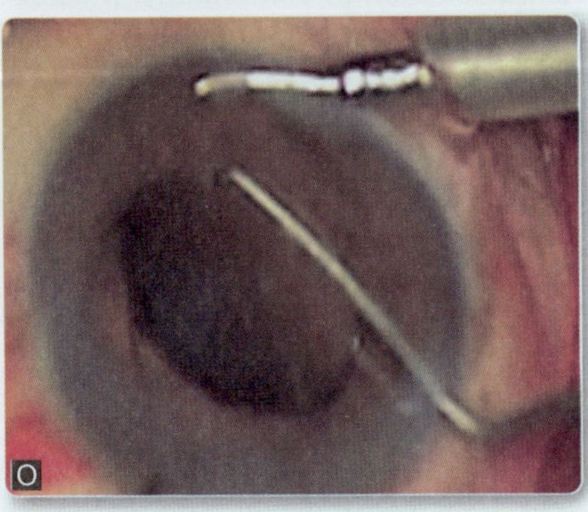

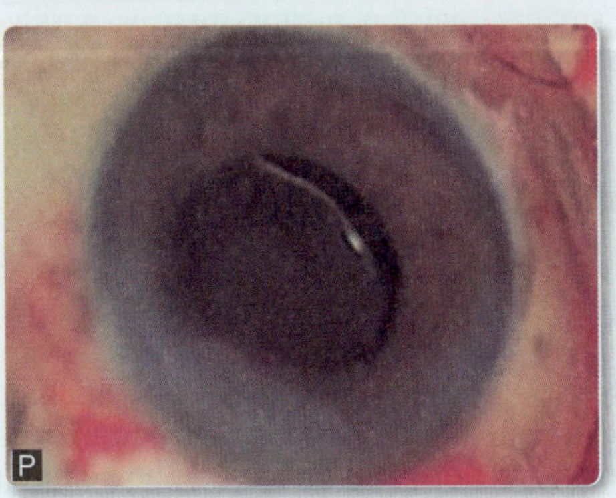

FIGURES 28.8K to P: Steps of cataract surgery (SICS). **K.** Nucleus delivered into anterior chamber (AC); **L.** Nucleus removed with two instruments; **M.** Cortex aspirated with Simcoe cannula; **N.** Posterior chamber intraocular lens (PCIOL) introduced into the eye; **O.** Intraocular lens (IOL) rotated with the dialer into place; **P.** IOL in position on posterior capsule.

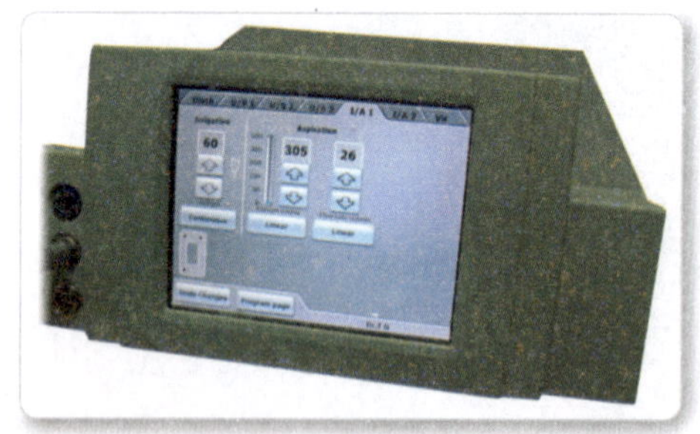

FIGURE 28.9: Console of phacoemulsification unit

Phacoemulsification

The introduction of phacoemulsification by Kelman in 1967 revolutionized cataract surgery. With this instrument the nucleus is fragmented to fine particles by ultrasound energy and aspirated. In phacoemulsification, irrigation, aspiration and fragmentation of the lens nucleus takes place at the tip of the phaco handpiece (Fig. 28.10), which can be introduced into the eye through an incision 2.8 m in size. With modern phacoemulsifying equipments, emulsification can be done through an incision 1 mm in size, while irrigation and manipulations of the nuclear fragments are done through another small incision with a second instrument (irrigating chopper). This is called microincision cataract surgery (MICS).

The three operations at the tip of the handpiece are:

- Irrigation alone
- Simultaneous irrigation and aspiration
- Ultrasound fragmentation and aspiration. All these operations are controlled by three positions of a foot switch.

The IOL that has to be introduced into the eye through the small incision is also suitably modified—foldable lenses or injectable lenses, or lenses preloaded into an injector are used, which can be introduced through the small incision.

The smaller incision means there is hardly any induced astigmatism and the patient can return to normal activities quickly.

Complications of ECCE

Many complications of ICCE like wound related problems, expulsive hemorrhage, CME and RD are less in SICS and phacoemulsification. But both SICS and phacoemulsification surgeries involve a lot of intraocular manipulations, which require a lot of skill and precision from the surgeon. Phacoemulsification is the most complex of all types of cataract surgeries and there is a steep learning curve. This can lead to a high rate of complications, specific to these keyhole cataract surgeries in the initial learning phase, which tend to come down as the skill and experience of the surgeon increases.

Intraoperative Complications

1. Posterior capsular rupture and vitreous loss (discussed earlier).
2. Nuclear drop into vitreous (an important complication of phaco, especially in the early learning period).

Early Postoperative Complications

1. Wound leak and shallow AC. This can occur if the sclera-corneal tunnel incision is not properly made. This can be prevented by suturing the wound.
2. Corneal edema occur in cases with large and hard nucleus, which makes the nucleus delivery difficult in SICS and increased ultrasound fragmentation time in phacoemulsification leading to corneal burns.
3. Rise in IOP can occur in the immediate postoperative period if the viscoelastics are not completely removed from the AC.
4. IOL decentration (Fig. 28.11): This can occur if some parts of the zonules are weak or ruptured during surgical manipulations or if there is a posterior capsular tear.

   Management: The IOL may be repositioned and fixed with 10-0 or 9-0 prolene suture to a scleral wound or the iris. If the IOL is totally unstable it may be removed and replaced with a scleral fixated or AC IOL.
5. Postoperative uveitis can occur if the cortical matter is not completely removed.
6. Endophthalmitis, which can be sterile or infective (already discussed).

Late Postoperative Complications

1. Pseudophakic bullous keratopathy: It can occur due to endothelial decompensation due to surgical trauma. Penetrating keratoplasty is required to manage this problem (Fig. 28.12).
2. Posterior capsular opacification: The posterior capsule tends to become translucent and the vision will be decreased (Fig. 28.13).

   This can be managed by posterior capsulotomy using yttrium-aluminum garnet (YAG) laser. This can be done as an OP procedure. If the laser machine is

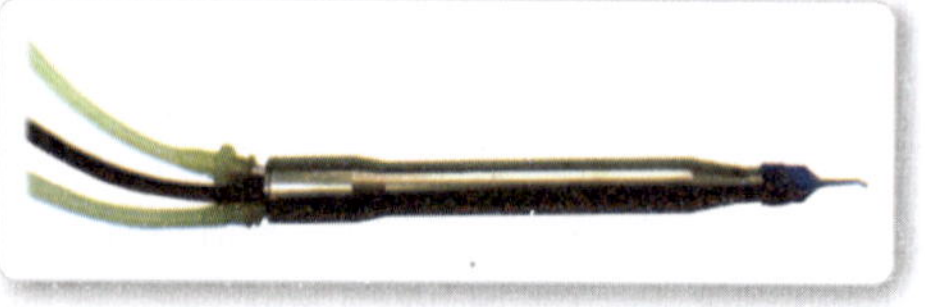

FIGURE 28.10: Phaco handpiece

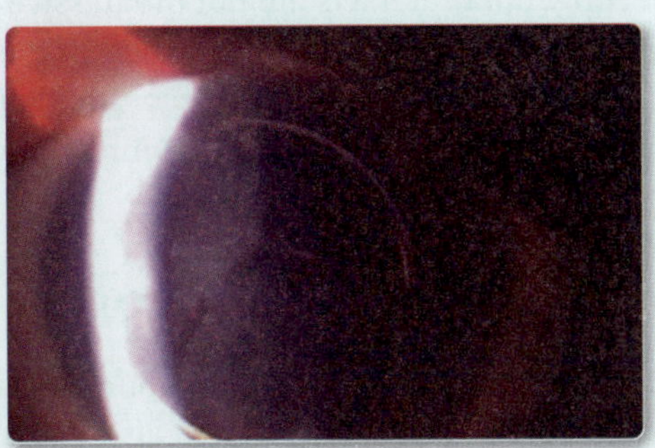

FIGURE 28.11: Intraocular lens (IOL) decentration

not available, surgical posterior capsulotomy has to be done.

3. Pupillary capture of the IOL: Part of the optic is seen anterior to the papillary margin. Usually caused by postoperative iritis and there is a higher incidence of this problem in children undergoing cataract surgery (Fig. 28.14).
4. Glaucoma it may be a pre-existing primary open angle glaucoma or pupillary block glaucoma or secondary glaucoma due to chronic uveitis.
5. Decentered IOL: A mild decentration in the immediate postoperative period may increase as time passes:
   a. Wind shield wiper syndrome: This happens when the IOL is too small for the eyes (usually a myopic eye) and the lens is placed in the sulcus. The lens moves like a wind shield wiper with each ocular movement.

      Management: Lens may be made more stable with sutures or replace it with a larger lens.
   b. Sunset syndrome: Due to inferior zonular dialysis the IOL slowly sinks toward the 6 O'clock meridian, so that the upper part of the pupil is aphakic and the lower part is phakic and the edge of the optic portion of the IOL is seen through the pupil (refer Fig. 28.11).
6. Intraocular lens drop into the vitreous: This can occur if there is a zonular dialysis or a posterior capsular tear, which was undetected at the time of surgery and a posterior chamber IOL was inserted or zonular rupture can occur later due to some trauma.

   Management: The IOL has to be removed by vitrectomy and a scleral fixated IOL or AC IOL may be placed.
7. The uveitis glaucoma hyphema (UGH) syndrome: This UGH syndrome is usually seen in eyes, in which AC IOL is placed. The haptic placed in the angle leads to chronic irritation and recurrent uveitis, glaucoma and hyphema.
8. CME and RD: The incidence is lower compared to ICCE.

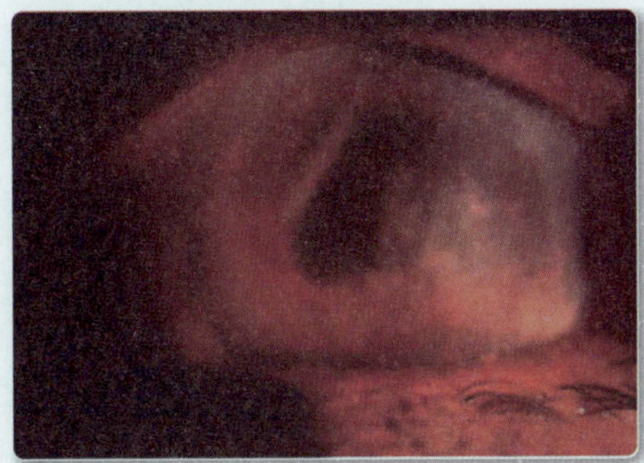

FIGURE 28.12: Pseudophakic bullous keratopathy

CATARACT SURGERY IN CHILDREN

Problems of Cataract Surgery in Children

The cataract and its surgery in children differ from that done in an adult in many aspects:

1. The capsule of a pediatric lens is thicken and more elastic. So a circular capsulorhexis is often difficult. The capsulorhexis often tends to extend to the periphery.
2. The lens does not have a hard nucleus and so no phacofragmentation is required. The whole lens matter can be removed by irrigation and aspiration.
3. The epithelium living the posterior capsule is more active and tends to multiply rapidly, and hence there is invariably posterior capsular opacification. To avoid this, a small posterior capsulorhexis and anterior vitrectomy is done at the end of lens matter aspiration to maintain a clear visual axis.
4. The sclera is less rigid than that of an adult and so the incision, even if made in a self-sealing valvular fashion, has to be sutured to keep it watertight.
5. In children less than 1–1½ years of age, cataract surgery alone is usually done and a secondary IOL

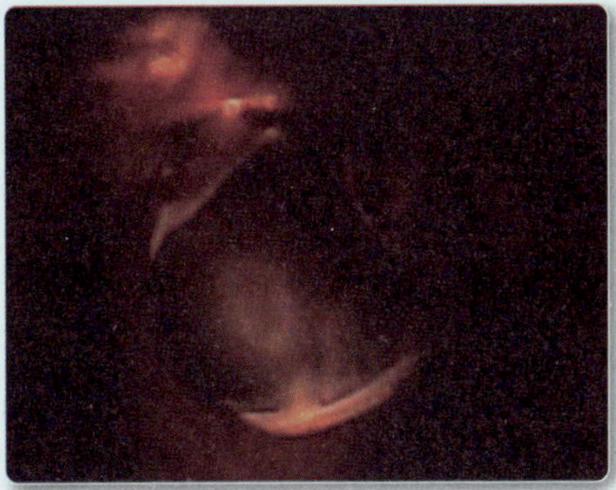

FIGURE 28.13: Posterior capsular opacification

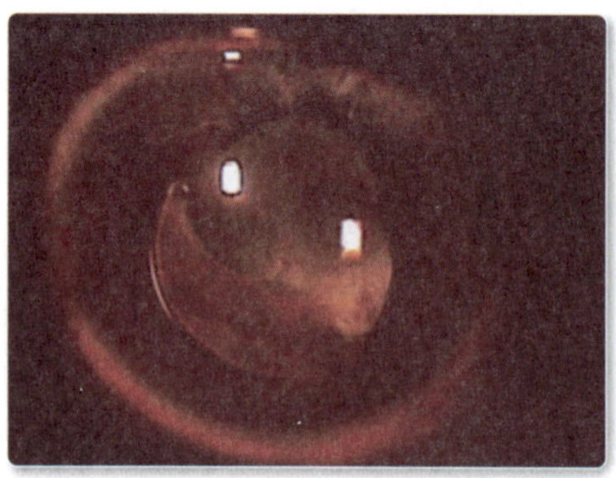

FIGURE 28.14: Pupillary capture of intraocular lens (IOL) with posterior capsular opacification (PCO)

implantation is done later after the child has become older. Till then spectacle correction or contact lens is given. In children older than 1½ years, IOL implantation can be done as a primary procedure.

6. Postoperative complications:
   a. The postoperative inflammation is often more severe than in an adult and often require systemic steroids to control it. Due to the active proliferation of the capsular epithelium and the postoperative inflammation, there is a high incidence of IOL displacement and pupillary capture.
   b. There is also an increased risk of glaucoma in the postoperative period. This may be a coexisting congenital glaucoma associated with congenital cataract or a secondary glaucoma. So the patient has to be closely watched for any rise in IOP.
   c. The RD CME and corneal problems are rare in children.

Time of Surgery

The risk of development of amblyopia is an important factor in deciding the time of surgery. Unilateral cataracts are at the highest risk for developing amblyopia and so a unilateral cataract, which is sufficiently dense as to interfere with vision should be removed as early as 6 weeks after birth or should be ideally done before 10 weeks.

In older children with congenital cataract, surgery should be done if it is interfering with near vision and reading, even if the distant visual acuity is fairly adequate. In bilateral cataracts with fairly good vision and it is not interfering in studies the surgery can be delayed, till the child is older when the problems in IOL power calculation will be lesser. Another advantage is that accommodation will be retained.

Most congenital cataracts are not progressive and decision regarding surgery depends on whether it is preferential to have clearer vision with no accommodation than slightly poorer vision with retained accommodation.

INTRAOCULAR LENS IMPLANTATION IN CHILDREN

The child's eye tends to grow throughout the first 8–10 years of life and the refractive power also changes. The correct selection of IOL power in children is very difficult. The measurement of IOL power by biometry in small children is difficult. The future change in refraction is often variable.

If a child is made emmetropic with an IOL at the age of 1 year, as the child grows there will be gradual development of myopia and at the age of 10 years the child may require -7D or -8D spectacle connection to see normally.

So the IOL power selection depends on its effect on vision immediately after surgery and also the power that is expected to be required in adulthood. Some surgeons calculate and select the IOL power depending on the power expected to be required in adulthood. The child will have to wear hypermetropic spectacle correction, the power of which can be decreased gradually till emmetropia is achieved in adulthood. Some surgeons aim for emmetropia at the time of IOL implantation and any future change in refraction (usually myopia) will be corrected with spectacles. This is done more in unilateral cataracts to decrease the risk of amblyopia by providing equally good vision in both eyes in early childhood. Some surgeons prefer to take a midway.

Amblyopia management is important and should begin immediately after surgery. Aphakic children should be given spectacles or contact lens. Extended wear contact lens can be given in unilateral cataracts in small children and aphakic spectacles are enough in bilateral cataracts. Since the power changes rapidly in young children frequent change of spectacles and contact lens (CL) are required at 3–6 monthly intervals in children up to 2–3 years of age.

Part time occlusion of the better eye should be done in all cases of unilateral cataract to overcome amblyopia.

Even in children in whom IOL implantation has been done it is essential to give adequate spectacle connection, especially for near vision and regular follow-up for any change in refraction.

Long-term follow-up for any change in refraction and treatment for amblyopia are essential for proper visual rehabilitation after congenital cataract surgery.

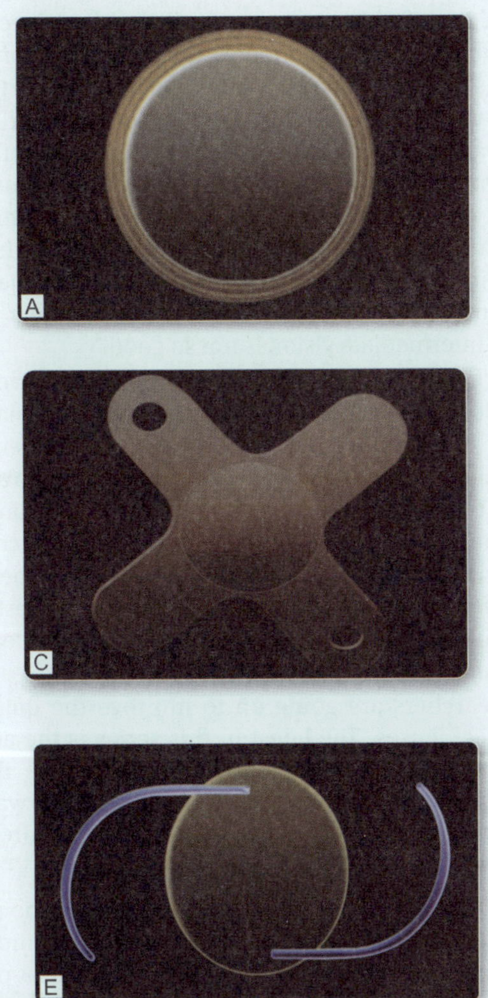

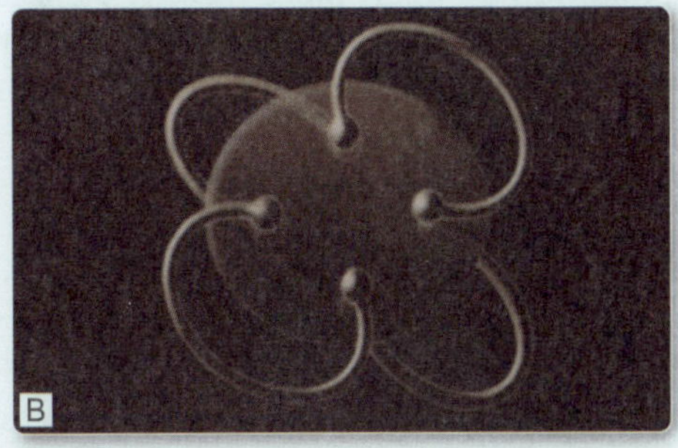

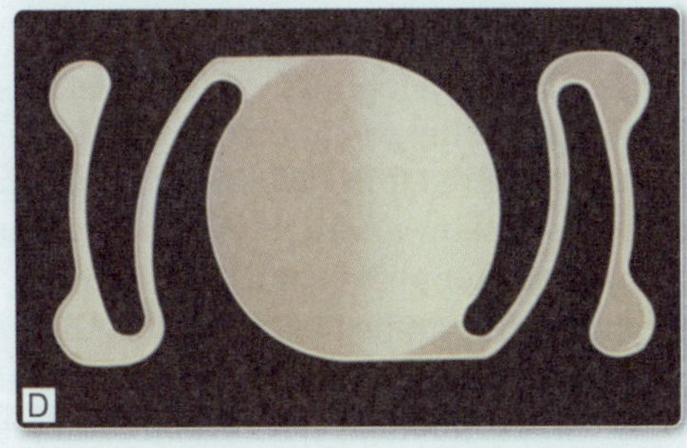

FIGURES 28.15A to E: Various models of intraocular lenses (IOLs). **A.** Original Ridley IOL first implanted by Sir Harold Ridley; **B.** Iris fixated IOL designed by Fyodorov; **C.** Iris supported IOL for intracapsular cataract extraction (ICCE) with two opposing haptics placed anterior and posterior to iris; **D.** Modern anterior chamber IOL with flexible four point angle support; **E.** Modern posterior chamber IOL.

Intraocular Lenses

Brief History

Sir Harold Ridley did the first intraocular lens implantation in 1949. He was inspired by the fact that polymethyl methacrylate (PMMA) windshield fragments in the AC were well-tolerated by the pilots of World War II. His lens was a biconvex disk made of PMMA inserted in the posterior chamber after ECCE. His idea had firm scientific basis, but the ECCE at that time was a crude surgery, and IOL was also heavy and had problems from its sterilization. This resulted in many complications and limited the use of his lenses.

The surgeries at that time were mostly ICCE and the need for better alternatives to aphakic correction led to the development of several lenses, which required fixation to the iris by suture through loops, struts or holes. The AC IOL was the next lenses to come, which were supported at the angle with rigid haptics. The exact fitting of size of the lens to that of the AC was often a problem. If the lens was too big this led to tenderness of the eye and pupillary distortion and UGH syndrome. If the lens was small for the eye this can cause lens decentering, poor vision and endothelial damage. Flexible loop AC IOLs were subsequently developed, which lessened the complications of AC IOLs. Closed flexible loops were replaced with open flexible loops and these types of lenses are still used today when there is posterior capsular tear or for secondary IOL implantation in aphakic patients. With the dawn of the modern era of ECCE, AC IOLs has lost their importance and focus was shifted to the development of posterior chamber IOLs.

Posterior Chamber Intraocular lenses

The earlier versions were three piece lenses with prolene haptics and the lenses were of planoconvex design. This was soon followed by single piece biconvex lenses. Many modifications were made in the shape of the posterior surface and edge of the lenses to decrease the development of posterior capsular opacification.

Special Purpose Lenses

Scleral-fixated lenses: Lenses with eyelets in the haptics were introduced to be used in aphakic patients as scleral-fixated lenses by passing sutures through the eyelets.

Aniridia lenses: Another type of special lens is lenses with opaque flanges to be used in aniridia or iris coloboma.

Foldable lenses: The development of foldable lenses was the next major step in the evolution of IOLs. Most foldable lenses are manufactured from silicone or acrylic material. The foldable lenses allow insertion of the lens through the small incision made for phacoemulsification.

The acrylic lenses can be hydrophobic or hydrophilic. Hydrophobic lenses have less water content and are thinner, but they can produce greater reaction in eyes prone to develop uveitis. Hydrophilic lenses are more biocompatible and better tolerated by eyes with less chance for uveitis, but the chances of development of posterior capsular opacification is higher.

Most IOLs contain chromophores that give UV protection. Some lenses contain blue light filters also, which lessen the damage to the retina.

Aspheric optics: Some IOLs have aspheric optic, which overcome the spherical aberration and improve the quality of vision especially in medium intensity lighting.

Heparin-coated lenses: This coating reduces the adhesion of inflammatory cells and such lenses are useful in eyes with uveitis undergoing surgery.

Multifocal lenses: The main disadvantage of IOLs compared to natural lens is that they are of fixed focal length and give clear vision only at a specific distance. Usually, when the IOL power is calculated, surgeons aim for correction of distant vision and suitable spectacles are given for correction of near vision, irrespective of the age of the patient. Multifocal lenses are developed for overcoming this problem. In the first models, the central portion of the lens was designed for near vision and the outer portion for distant vision. The main disadvantage of these earlier designs was poor distant vision in bright light when the pupil constricts in bright light. Modern multifocal lenses are of two types—diffractive or refractive type. The diffractive lenses have a series of blended diffractive zones, which focus light from distant, intermediate and near objects on the retina. These lenses give good distant and near vision, but the intermediate vision is not so good.

The refractive type has five zones, which give fairly good distant, intermediate and near vision. The main advantage of multifocal lenses is the less dependence on spectacles, and hence most suitable for ladies who are unwilling to wear glasses and do not do much driving. The disadvantage of multifocal lenses is reduction in contrast sensitivity and visual acuity, and patients may experience some glare and colored halos. These lenses are best tolerated if implanted bilaterally and there is a short learning phase to adjust to the new visual sensations.

Researchers are going on to improve the quality of multifocal lenses. The latest in this series is the accommodative IOL. The lens optic has supportive flanges with hinges, which allow the lens to move forward on attempting accommodation and backwards on relaxing accommodation.

Adjustable IOL: It is another one in this series. The refractive power can be adjusted with UV light after implantation done 1 week after surgery. The UV light causes polymerization of the molecules with precise correction of the spherical and astigmatic power.

Toric IOLs: These they are lenses with a cylindrical correction also, used in patients with high astigmatic error. The axis of the cylinder is also marked on the lens and the lens has to be positioned in the capsular bag with the axis in the correct meridian.

Lot of research is going on to improve the quality of vision with the lenses and we can expect lenses with near perfect vision in the market soon.

Glaucoma Surgery

29

Girija Devi PS, Thomas George T

PREPARATION OF PATIENT

Preparation of patient is common to all intraocular surgical procedures.

Preoperative Preparations

1. Preoperatively one has to rule out/control systemic diseases like diabetes mellitus, hypertension, heart disease, pulmonary disease and allergies to drugs as with any surgical procedure.
2. Local foci of infection would predispose to postoperative endophthalmitis and need to be looked out for and treated, especially chronic dacryocystitis by syringing the nasolacrimal ducts. If there is a dacryocystitis it has to be dealt with by a dacryocystorhinostomy/dacryocystectomy surgery. Hordeolum internum/externum as well as conjunctivitis if present, need treatment.
3. Complete blood count screen for systemic infections that can spread to the eye compromised by surgical wound, by a bacteremia (e.g. osteomyelitis, dental caries, etc.). Erythrocyte sedimentation rate is a general screening for inflammation in the body, some of which can predispose to severe postoperative inflammation in the eye (e.g. rheumatoid arthritis).
4. Most centers would cover the surgery with perioperative broad-spectrum systemic antibiotics (e.g. a fluoroquinolone started 1 day prior and continued for 2 days after surgery). The patient is put on preoperative topical antibiotics and anti-inflammatory drops.
5. To avoid sudden decompression during surgery, the intraocular pressure (IOP) is reduced preoperatively by medical therapy (with acetazolamide tablets). If required, topical antiglaucoma medications and intravenous mannitol can be given (pilocarpine and prostaglandins are generally not used preoperatively as they cause uveal inflammation).
6. On the day of surgery, the eye to be operated is prepared by cleaning with povidone-iodine solution (5%) instilled in both eyes and periocular skin surface wipe (7.5% or 10%).
7. Local anesthesia is given in the form of regional block (peribulbar injection of 2% lidocaine and bupivacaine) for anesthesia of eye with akinesia of muscles of ocular motility and orbicularis oculi muscles.

After the operative procedure the eye dressed for about 6–12 hours.

Postoperative Preparations

Topical steroids and antibiotic drops are instituted and tapered over 6–8 weeks.

SURGICAL PERIPHERAL IRIDECTOMY

Surgical peripheral iridectomy also creates a peripheral iris defect that bypasses the pupil in a pupillary block to aqueous flow.

Indications

1. Nowadays surgical peripheral iridectomy done as part of other surgeries, e.g. trabeculectomy, cataract surgery with vitreous loss and when using anterior chamber (AC) intraocular lenses.
2. Sometimes, the iris is too thick or edematous due to inflammation that laser iridotomy is not possible. Then surgical iridectomy is done.
3. Non-glaucoma indications are foreign bodies on the iris, tumors of the iris, for optical purposes (optical iridectomy used to be done in the past in central stationary opacities, usually in the lower nasal segment to facilitate reading), etc.

Procedure

The pupil should not be dilated. All precautions for an intraocular surgery are to be taken. After preparation and anesthesia the eye is draped and opened with a speculum. A superior rectus tendon bridle suture is taken to expose more of the superior corneoscleral junction or limbus. A 3–4 mm beveled incision is made in the cornea close to the limbus. The peripheral iris is grasped with a fine-toothed forceps (e.g. Lims' forceps) and cut with scissors (e.g. de Weckers' scissors). This creates a triangular opening in the iris at the periphery with the apex toward the pupil. The corneal wound is sutured with 10-0 nylon suture. Subconjunctival injection of steroid antibiotic can be administered.

TRABECULECTOMY

Trabeculectomy is the most commonly done antiglaucoma surgery.

In the past, the full thickness filtration procedures were done like iridencleisis, trephining, thermal sclerostomy, etc. A filtering surgery done with a partial thickness scleral flap, e.g. trabeculectomy gives some resistance to aqueous outflow and helps to maintain the IOP at physiological level.

Principle

Here an alternate pathway for aqueous drainage is created from the AC to the subconjunctival space bypassing the pupil (as peripheral iridectomy is part of the procedure) and the trabecular meshwork via the ostium created (Figs 29.1 to 29.3). Aqueous from the subconjunctival space gets absorbed by the episcleral veins. It is done in almost all types of glaucoma where medical therapy is inadequate to control IOP.

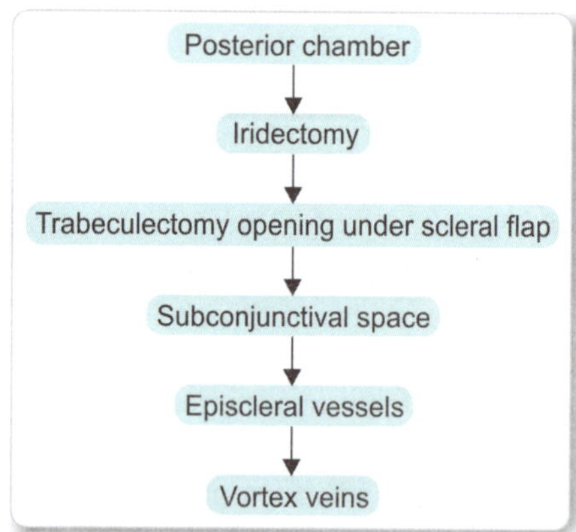

FIGURE 29.1: Pathway for drainage of aqueous after trabeculectomy

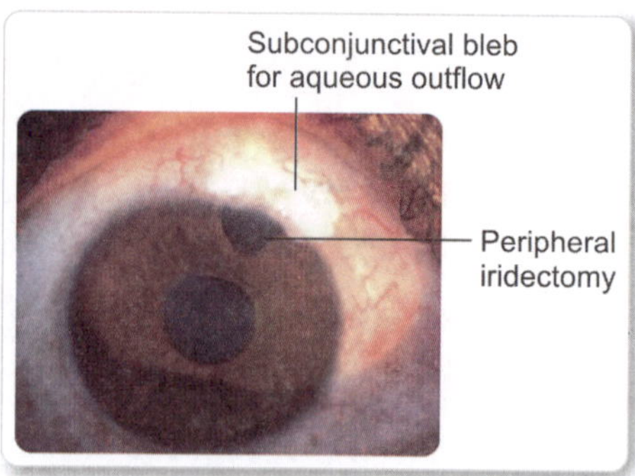

FIGURE 29.2: A post-trabeculectomy eye

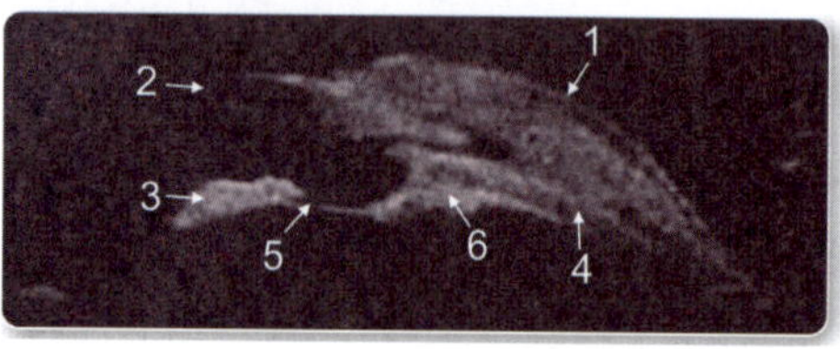

FIGURE 29.3: Ultrasound biomicroscopic image of a post-trabeculectomy eye to show normal tissues. **1.** Conjunctiva; **2.** Cornea; **3.** Iris; **4.** Sclera; **5.** Anterior lens capsule; **6.** Ciliary body.

Procedure

The pupil should not be dilated. All precautions for an intraocular surgery are to be taken. After preparation and anesthesia, the eye is draped and opened with a speculum. A superior rectus tendon bridle suture is taken to expose more of the superior corneoscleral junction or limbus. A slow-controlled 20 G paracentesis (stab incision through clear cornea into the AC) is made to decompress the AC. A limited peritomy (conjunctiva disinserted at the limbus) is done in one of the superior quadrants (this is a fornix-based conjunctival flap). Some surgeons may prefer a limbus-based flap, where the conjunctiva is opened near the superior rectus tendon and dissected anteriorly up to the limbus. The Tenon's capsule is opened to expose the episclera below. Wet field bipolar diathermy or cautery is done in this exposed area of episclera. A triangular or rectangular flap 3–4 mm wide is marked out and dissected from posterior to anterior with a Bard-Parker (BP) knife. This scleral flap (Fig. 29.4) is one-fourth to one-third thickness of sclera. The dissection is carried till the limbus, so that clear cornea is visible under the flap. The flap is not cut at the limbal end (i.e. it is left hinged at the limbus). Now a rectangular window is made in the sclera bed under the flap anterior to the scleral spur with a sharp blade or a trabeculectomy punch (this full thickness window is the trabeculectomy ostium into the AC and the size of the same in comparison to the overlying scleral flap decides the resistance to outflow postoperatively). The peripheral iris under the trabeculectomy ostium is grasped with a fine-toothed forceps and cut with scissors to create a peripheral iridectomy. Now the scleral flap is reposited and

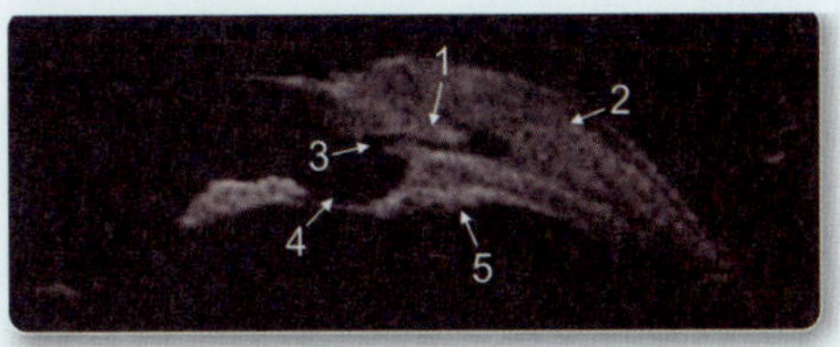

FIGURE 29.4: Ultrasound biomicroscopic image shown in Figure 29.3 with specific features of trabeculectomy marked out. The peripheral iridectomy allows aqueous to bypass the pupillary block. Flow through the trabeculectomy ostium under the sclera flap takes aqueous to the subconjunctival space, bypassing the trabecular meshwork resistance also. **1.** Scleral flap; **2.** Subconjunctival bleb; **3.** Trabeculectomy ostium; **4.** Peripheral iridectomy.

the edges sutured loosely with 10–0 nylon interrupted sutures. The conjunctiva is reposited and sutured to the limbus with 10-0 nylon interrupted sutures. The AC is reformed via the paracentesis with balanced salt solution and a small air bubble. Subconjunctival injection of steroid and antibiotic can be administered.

Measures to Increase Aqueous Drainage

Postoperative subconjunctival fibrosis is one of the main reasons for failure of trabeculectomy. This can be reduced by the following methods:

1. Preoperative use of antimitotic agents subconjunctivally (mitomycin C and sometimes 5-fluorouracil, especially).
2. Releasable sutures.
3. Laser suture: Lysis may be used to control aqueous drainage and corresponding IOP in the immediate postoperative period.

Steps of Trabeculectomy

The steps of trabeculectomy are shown in Figures 29.5 to 29.13.

Complications

Complications of filtering surgery include the following:

1. Hypotony due to excessive drainage.
2. Hyphema.
3. Suprachoroidal hemorrhage or effusions.
4. Blebitis/Endophthalmitis.
5. Encapsulation of the bleb with resultant transient IOP elevation.
6. Loss of one or more lines of visual acuity.
7. Increased risk of cataract formation.

Vision loss may be a serious complication after trabeculectomy, especially in patients with advanced optic disk damage, with severe and ongoing unexplained loss ('snuff-out') experienced by as many as 2% of patients.

Drainage Implant

Indications

When chances of failure are high as in failure of repeated trabeculectomy or neovascular glaucoma.

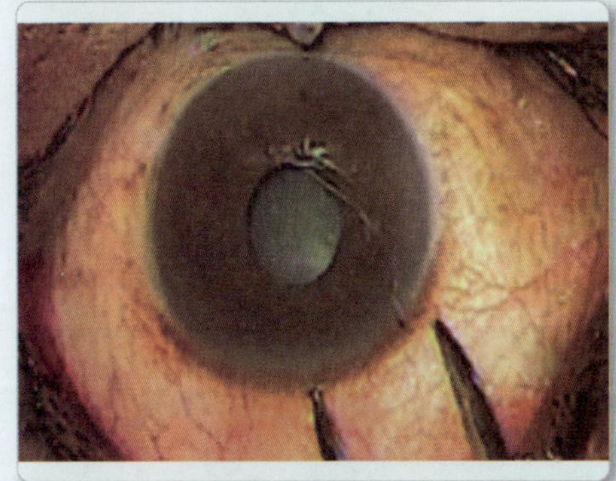

FIGURE 29.5: Conjunctival flap to be dissected is measured with calipers

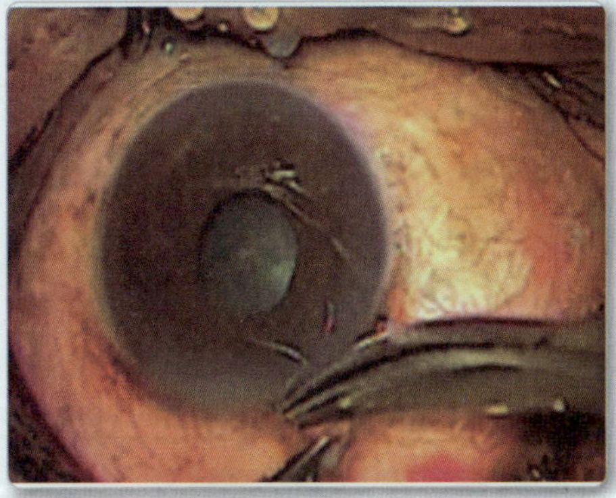

FIGURE 29.6: Fornix-based conjunctival flap dissected

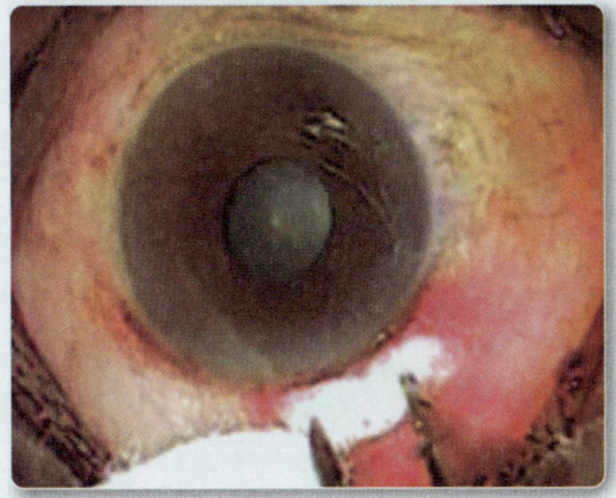

FIGURE 29.7: Lamellar scleral flap to be dissected is measured with calipers

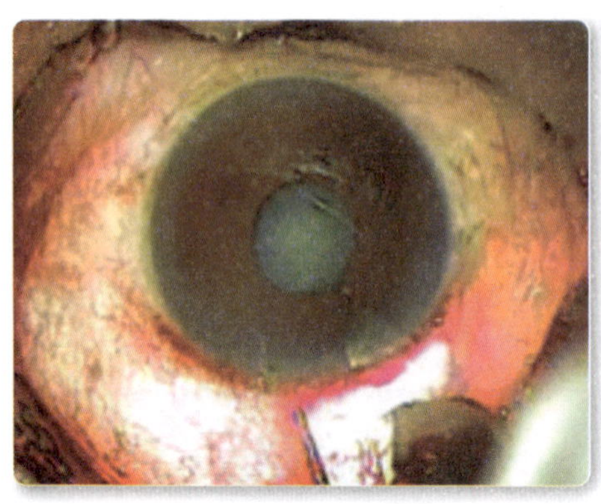

FIGURE 29.8: Incision put with Bard-Parker (BP) knife

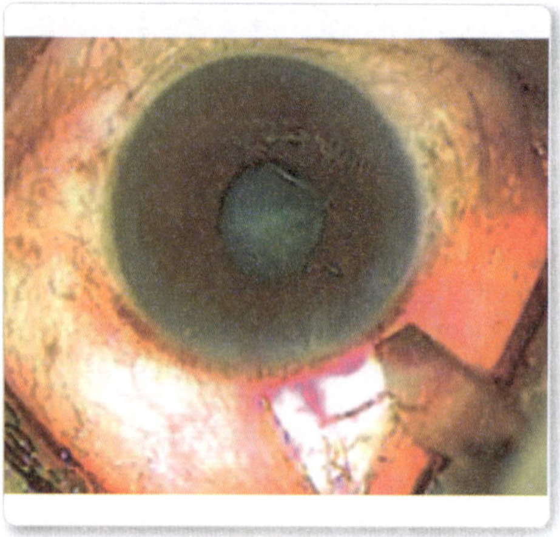

FIGURE 29.9: Incision completed

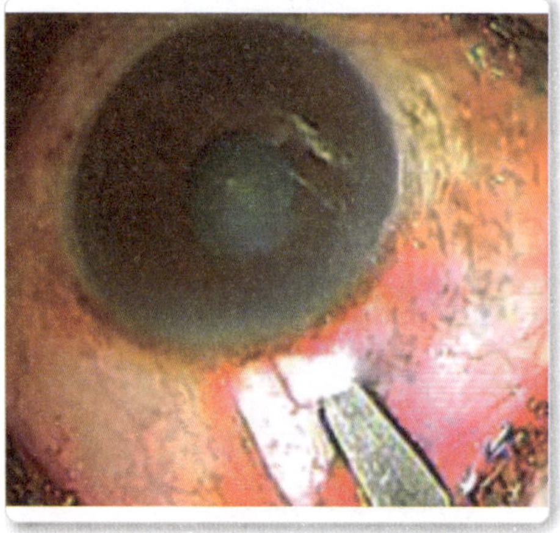

FIGURE 29.10: Lamellar flap dissected with crescent knife

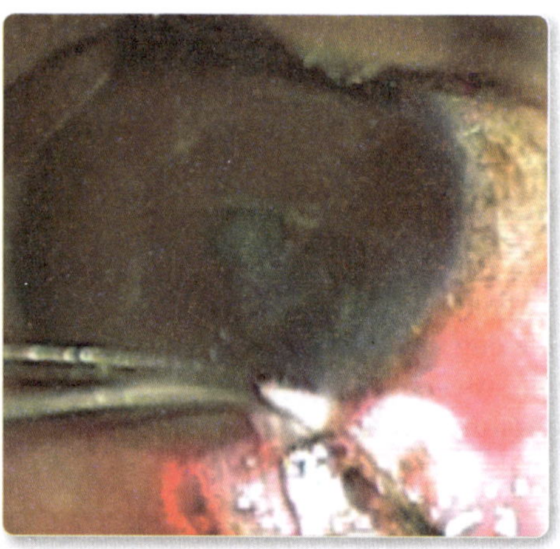

FIGURE 29.11: Lamellar scleral flap dissected and lifted up

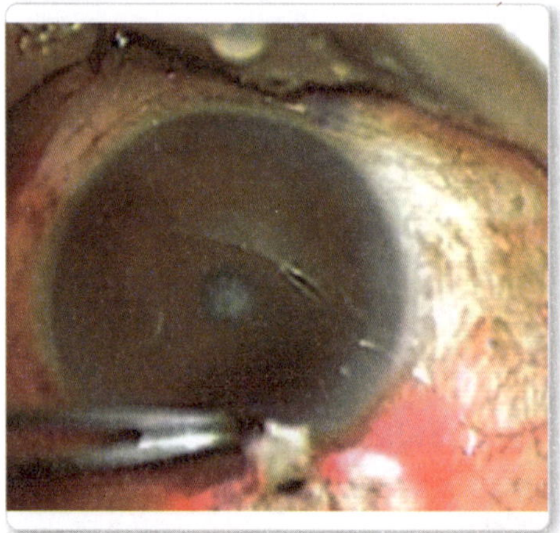

FIGURE 29.12: A rectangular block of trabecular tissue is removed exposing the underlying iris

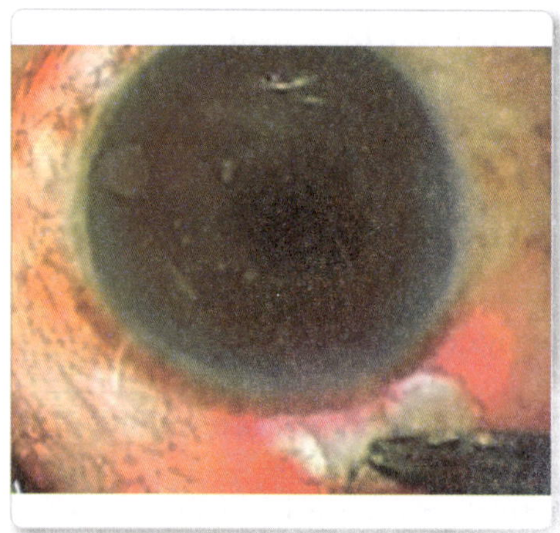

FIGURE 29.13: Scleral flap sutured after an iridectomy is done

Method

The implant has a silicon drainage plate with a flexible plastic tube attached to it.

The tip of the tube is placed in the AC to shunt aqueous to an equatorial reservoir and then posteriorly to be absorbed in the subconjunctival space.

After creating a conjunctival flap the drainage plate is fixed with sutures between two recti muscles 8–10 mm behind the limbus. After the plate is attached to the globe, the tube is laid across the cornea and cut with a sharp scissors to create a beveled edge with the opening toward the cornea. The tube should extend approximately 2.5–3 mm into the AC to minimize the risk of tube-cornea touch or retraction out of the AC. A 23-gauge needle is used to create a track through which the tube is inserted into the AC just anterior and parallel to the iris. The tube may be secured to the sclera a few millimeters anterior to the plate with 7-0 or 8-0 Vicryl suture. This suture helps to stabilize the tube and should not be tight; otherwise, it will restrict flow in valved devices.

The tube is covered to prevent its erosion through the conjunctiva. Preserved sclera or cornea can be used for this purpose. After the patch graft has been placed, the conjunctiva and Tenon's layers are pulled over the plate, tube and patch graft, and sutured into place with 8-0 Vicryl suture. If patch graft is not available the procedure can be done under a lamellar scleral flap. The needle track and tube entry are done under this flap. The flap is then sutured with 10-0 nylon sutures.

Aqueous drains through the tube to the area below the plate, which acts as a reservoir from where episcleral veins absorb the aqueous.

Types of Implants

Baerveldt implant: It is available with larger plates with increased reservoir size. The Seton (tube) connected to the reservoir, usually is tied off with an absorbable suture, allowing flow to initiate 4–6 weeks postoperative once some conjunctival wound remodeling has taken place, thereby reducing the risk of immediate postoperative hypotony (Fig. 29.14).

Ahmed and Krupin implants: These have one way valves, which are designed to maintain pressure above 8 mm Hg. These implants may reduce the risk of hypotony, a complication of non-valved shunts in the early postoperative period (Fig. 29.15).

Molteno implant: It consists of a silicone drainage tube, which is connected to 1 or 2 acrylic plates that are sutured to the sclera (Fig. 29.16).

CYCLODIALYSIS

Here the ciliary body is surgically detached from the scleral spur using a special instrument called cyclodialysis spatula. After entering the AC, the tip of this instrument is swept across the opposite angle to separate the ciliary body from the scleral spur. This opens a channel to the suprachoroidal space from the AC for egress of aqueous. Hypotony often results and results are unpredictable. In the past, it was commonly used for management of aphakic glaucoma.

CYCLODESTRUCTIVE PROCEDURES

Indications

Indication is to reduce pain in an eye with little or no useful vision.

These can be used in eyes with vision also when all other means fail, but then one is cautious and small areas are treated (say 1 quadrant) and its effect observed for 3–6 weeks before more treatment is done.

Principle

Principle of all these procedures is to reduce inflow of aqueous by destruction of ciliary processes. Options are:

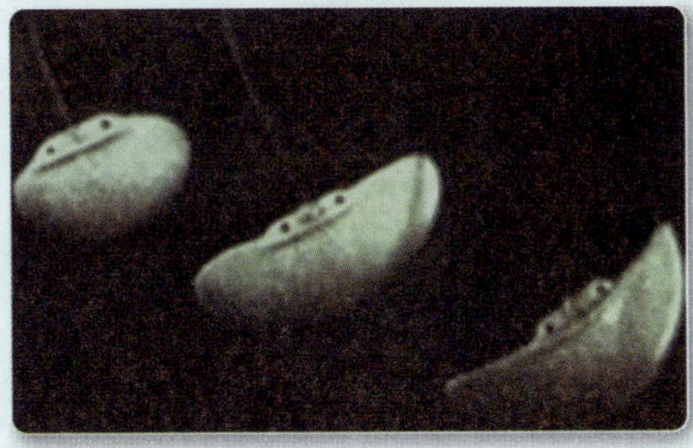

FIGURE 29.14: Baerveldt implant

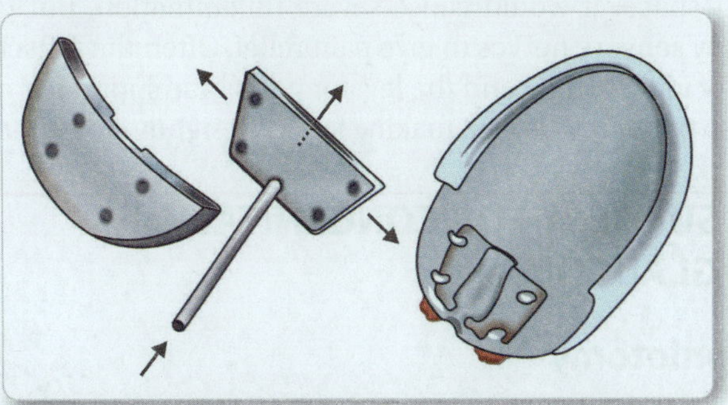

FIGURE 29.15: Ahmed glaucoma valve

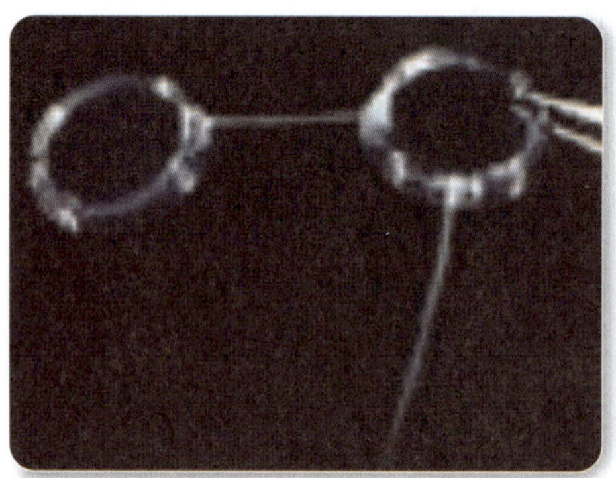

FIGURE 29.16: Molteno implant

1. **Cyclocryotherapy:** Here a CryoProbe, which freezes the ciliary body transsclerally, is used. It achieves -80°C at its tip by the Joule Thomson effect (sudden expansion of a compressed gas).
2. **Cyclophotocoagulation:** It can be done by direct visualization of ciliary processes during surgery with endolaser probes (surgically) or through the pupil in aphakic eyes. The lasers used are the same as in retinal photocoagulation, e.g. Argon, frequency doubled Nd:YAG 532 nm and infrared diode 810 nm. Cyclophotocoagulation can be achieved transsclerally with infrared lasers like the continuous wave Nd:YAG thermal laser (1,064 nm wavelength) and infrared diode 810 nm. This requires a fiberoptic contact probe.
3. **Cyclodiathermy:** Destruction of ciliary processes by diathermy probe (needle).
4. **Cycloanemization:** Rarely done nowadays, but it was considered in past. Surgically deprive ciliary body of its blood.

RETROBULBAR ALCOHOL INJECTION

In an absolute glaucoma, where the eye is blind and painful, one can inject 4 cc of absolute alcohol in the retrobulbar space. It would cause severe inflammation, but destroy sensory nerves to give pain relief. Often the muscles of ocular motility and the levator palpebrae superioris are also paralyzed as well making for an unsightly side effect.

SURGERY FOR CONGENITAL GLAUCOMA

Goniotomy

The prerequisite for this procedure is a reasonably clear cornea for visualization of the angle (quite a few of the patients with congenital glaucoma have opacities and corneal edema, which would not allow for this procedure).

Under general anesthesia the angle of the AC is visualized with a surgical gonioscope like the Barkan's lens and through a paracentesis the opposite angle is approached with the knife (e.g. Swan goniotomy knife). The anterior portion of the trabecular meshwork is incised circumferentially to allow the trabecular fibers and iris to fall back, and relieve resistance to outflow into the canal of Schlemm (Figs 29.17 and 29.18).

Trabeculotomy

Principle

Trabeculotomy is an ab externo procedure where the canal of Schlemm is dissected into a probe passed into the same and rotated into the AC to disrupt the trabecular meshwork to establish connection with the canal (Figs 29.19A to G).

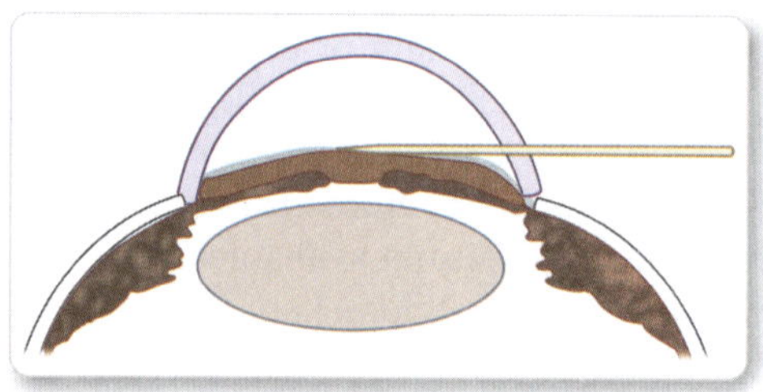

FIGURE 29.17: Goniotomy involves incising the anterior trabecular meshwork under direct gonioscopic visualization, allowing the trabecular meshwork and iris to fall back. This relieves resistance to aqueous flow into the canal of Schlemm.

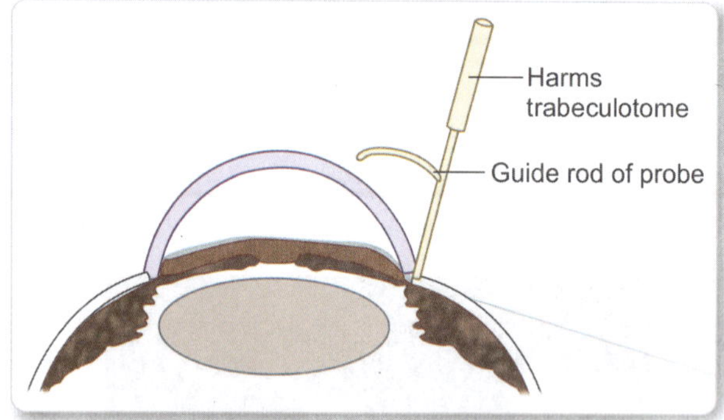

FIGURE 29.18: In trabeculotomy, the canal of Schlemm is identified externally and a probe passed through it and swung into the AC creating a tear in the trabecular meshwork. There is a guide rod parallel to the probe seen outside the eye to let the surgeon know the position of the probe. This allows the trabecular meshwork and iris to fall back and relieves resistance to aqueous flow into the canal of Schlemm.

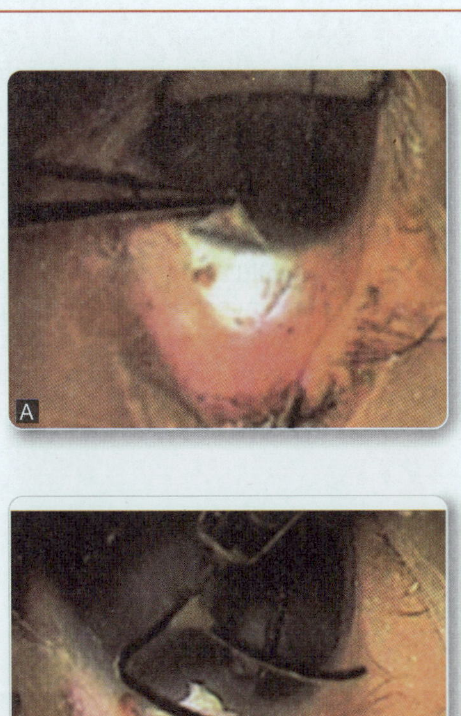

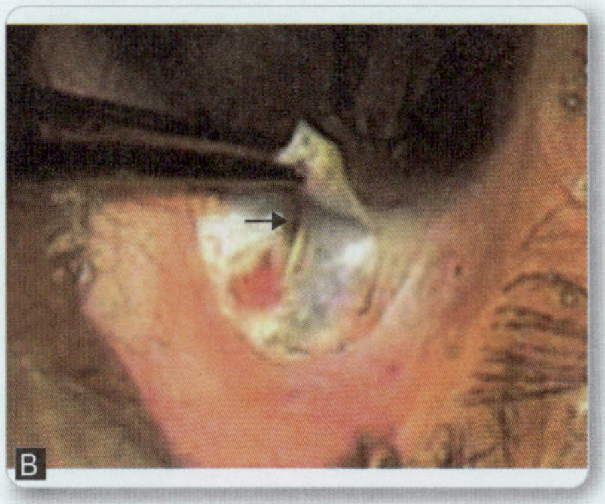

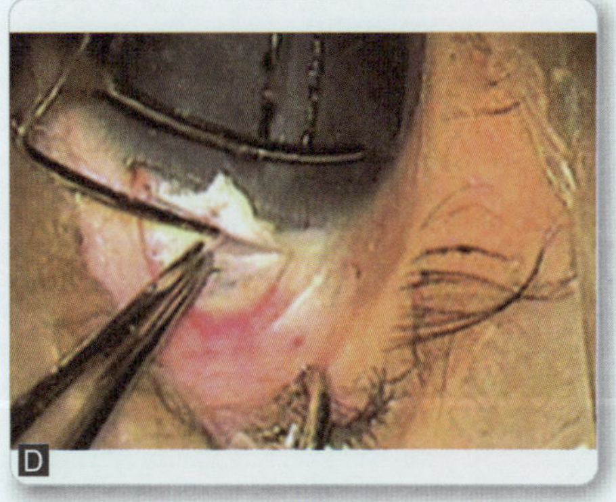

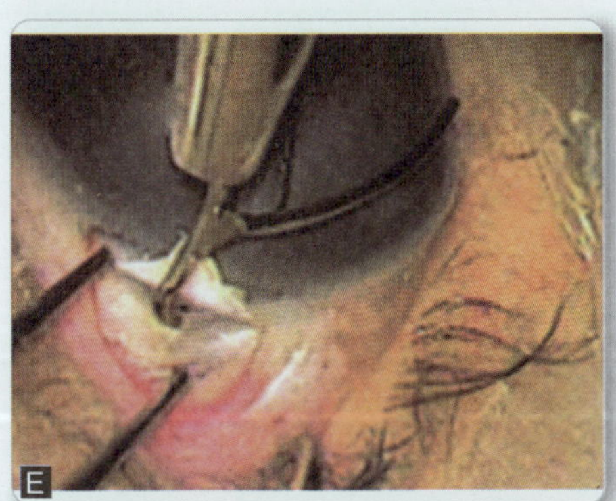

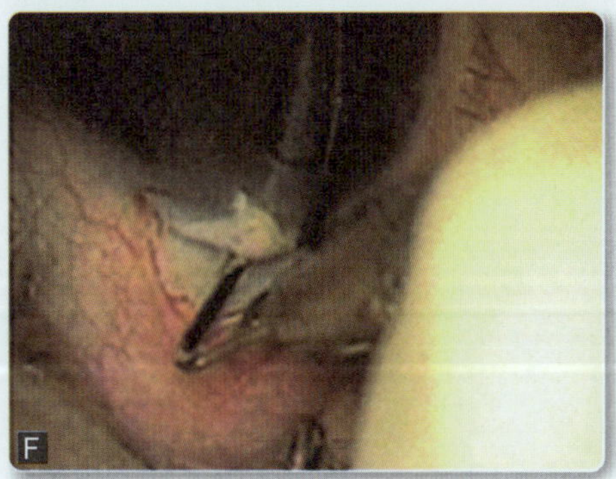

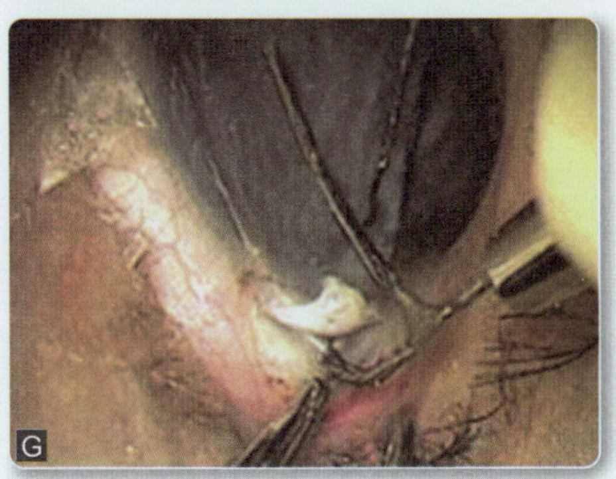

FIGURES 29.19A to G: Trabeculotomy. **A.** A partial thickness scleral flap is raised; **B.** Under the scleral flap a radial incision is made and deepened till Schlemm's canal is opened (arrow); **C.** Harms trabeculotome. Note the two parallel rods, the lower probe and the higher guide rod; **D.** The trabeculotome is inserted into the Schlemm's canal; **E.** Once inserted fully the direction of the probe is judged with the direction of guide rod; **F.** Now the probe is rotated into the anterior chamber (AC); **G.** The probe is inserted and rotated into AC on the left-hand side also.

Method

After a limited peritomy, a partial thickness scleral flap is raised. At the posterior end of the blue limbus a radial incision is placed straddling the scleral spur. This is deepened till the canal of Schlemm is opened (a drop of aqueous from the AC or blood from the episcleral veins would reflux often). Now, Harms trabeculotomy probe is passed into the right-hand side segment of the Schlemm's canal and rotated into the AC to tear open the trabecular meshwork and establish communication to the canal of Schlemm. During the rotation the surgeon knows the probe orientation based on the direction of the guide rod on the probe (otherwise one can easily damage nearby tissues like Descemet's membrane, iris, lens and ciliary body). The same is done on the left-hand side also and the scleral flap and conjunctiva are closed with sutures.

Postoperatively the child is kept on close follow-up for life. All congenital glaucoma cases need lifelong follow-up. The glaucoma may go out of control even very late and may require medical therapy (and if it fails resurgery with a trabeculectomy or drainage surgery added on).

Keratoplasty and Refractive Surgeries

30

Girija Devi PS

The structural integrity of the cornea is essential for vision. Any injury or infection that destroys the Bowman's membrane or the underlying layers will leave a permanent opacity. The relative dehydrated state of the cornea is essential for optical transparency and this is maintained by the endothelial cell pump. The endothelial layer is a non-dividing layer of cells and any injury or disease that damage or decrease the corneal endothelial density can lead to corneal edema and loss of transparency. There is a group of conditions called corneal dystrophies where abnormalities in the corneal structure lead to loss of transparency.

The only treatment for all these conditions causing loss of transparency is replacement of the damaged cornea with a donor button of similar size from a donor cornea. This is called **keratoplasty**.

Cornea is the major refractive surface of the eye. Any change in the refractive power can be produced by procedures that change the refractive power of the cornea. These procedures are called **refractive surgeries**.

EYE BANKING

Eye banks retrieve and store eyes for cornea transplantation. Each country has its own rules and regulations controlling the functions of an eye bank.

An eye bank should have the following facilities:

1. Storage space for storing instruments, supplies, registers, etc.
2. A refrigerator for storing eyes, blood samples and preservative media.
3. Facilities for autoclaving instruments.
4. Eye bank should have round-the-clock telephone and ambulance service for receiving information regarding the death of the potential donor.
5. Services of qualified personnel to retrieve the eye.

Corneal Retrieval

Cornea can be removed only after death. No living person can donate their eyes, unlike certain other organ transplantation like kidney, etc. The eye has to be removed within 4–6 hours after death. In bodies requiring autopsy, consent should be obtained from the forensic specialist doing the autopsy that the eyes are not essential for their autopsy investigations.

Consent for Eye Donation

According to the corneal transplantation act of India, the eyes can be received from any person after death, provided their first-line relatives give their consent and the dead person has not expressed any unwillingness for donating his/her eyes after death. Many people pledge their eyes, while they are alive. But this consent form is not essential for removing the eyes. But, if any one of the first-line relatives refuses permission, the eyes of the dead person cannot be removed, even if the person has given written consent for eye donation, while he/she was alive. So the awareness and willingness of the relatives are of paramount importance for eye donation.

Age for Eye Donation

The ideal age for eye donation is 16–60 years. In a country like India, where the availability of eyes is scarce, eyes from people of advanced years are also used.

Contraindications for Eye Donation

1. Any death of unexplained cause.
2. Eyes of a person suffering from infectious diseases like syphilis, tuberculosis, hepatitis, human immunodeficiency virus (HIV), poliomyelitis, rabies, slow virus diseases of central nervous system (CNS), etc. since there is a risk of spread of these infections through the donor cornea.
3. Eyes of a person dying of disseminated malignancy or eyes with intraocular tumors, since there is a slight risk of malignant cells reaching the recipient through the donor cornea.

Donor Material

The whole eyeball or the cornea with a rim of sclera is removed from the dead person under all aseptic precautions like any surgical procedure. If a whole eyeball is removed, an artificial eyeball is placed in the place of the removed eye and in the case of a corneoscleral button, a plastic corneal shield is placed in the place of the removed tissue and the lids are closed with a black silk suture. This is done to avoid any disfigurement to the dead body.

Preservation

Short-term preservation

Short-term preservation is done using the moist chamber method or with McCarey-Kaufman (MK) medium.

Moist chamber method: The whole eyeball can be preserved by moist chamber method. The whole eyeball is placed with the cornea on the upper side in a special stand inside a sterilized glass chamber. The air inside the glass chamber is kept humid with cotton gauze moisturized with sterile saline kept inside the glass chamber. The bottle is packed with ice around it in a transportation box and taken to the eye transplantation center where it is stored in a refrigerator at 4°C. An eye preserved by moist chamber method has to be utilized for transplantation within 48 hours.

MK medium: The corneoscleral button can be preserved in the MK medium for 4–7 days. The advantage of preserving the cornea in the MK medium is that the surgery can be done as a planned procedure.

Intermediate-term preservation

Optisol-GS and Eusol-C are the media that can help to preserve cornea up to 2 weeks.

Long-term preservation

Long-term preservation is done using tissue culture method. The cornea can then be stored at room temperature.

Suitability of the Donor Material

Suitability of the donor material for penetrating keratoplasty depends on the viability of the endothelium. The endothelial cell morphology and count can be measured with cadaver specular microscope. But this expensive equipment may not be available in all eye transplantation centers. But the assessment of the corneal thickness, clarity and the presence or absence of Descemet's membrane (DM) folds can help to decide whether the eye is suitable for penetrating keratoplasty. If the viability is doubtful it can be used for anterior lamellar keratoplasty where the DM and endothelium are not used.

Blood group matching or human leukocyte antigen (HLA) typing is not necessary for corneal transplantation.

Recipient eye factors

Recipient eye factors required for a successful corneal grafting:

1. Normal lid function—with no lagophthalmos, entropion, ectropion, trichiasis, etc.
2. Normal precorneal tear film. dry eye reduces the chances of success of a corneal graft.
3. Normal corneal sensation.
4. Absence of corneal vascularization. Vascularization of the cornea increases the risk of graft rejection. A normal avascular cornea is considered to be an **'immunologically privileged area'.** This advantage is lost once the cornea is vascularized.
5. There should not be any active infection in the eye or adnexa. The exception is a therapeutic graft, which is done for a non-healing corneal ulcer.
6. No limbal stem cell deficiency. The donor corneal surface epithelium has to come from the limbal stem cells. If they are permanently destroyed as in chemical or thermal injuries, Stevens Jonson syndrome, etc. graft survival is doubtful.
7. Secondary glaucoma—is the commonest cause for graft failure after penetrating keratoplasty (PKP). It should be controlled medically or surgically before undertaking corneal grafting.

Indications for Corneal Grafting

1. Optical—done for improving vision.
2. Therapeutic—in non-healing corneal pathologies like corneal ulcer, Mooren's ulcer.
3. Structural—to replace lost corneal tissue after surgery for pterygium, in corneal fistulas, descemetocele, etc.
4. Cosmetic—done in an eye with a corneal opacity, but no visual potential, to remove the disfigurement due to an opaque cornea.
5. Refractive—to alter the refractive power of the cornea so as to decrease the need for wearing spectacles or contact lens.
6. Preparatory keratoplasty—a lamellar graft as a preparation for a subsequent central penetrating graft done in vascularized corneas.

CORNEAL SURGERIES

1. Keratoplasty:
   - Penetrating keratoplasty
   - Lamellar keratoplasty (LKP).
2. Refractive surgeries.

PENETRATING KERATOPLASTY

Penetrating keratoplasty (Fig. 30.1) is otherwise called full thickness keratoplasty. Here, a full thickness corneal button is removed from the recipient's cornea and an equal sized or slightly larger corneal button from a donor cornea is sutured into its place.

Indications

1. Pseudophakic bullous keratopathy: Here, surgical trauma during cataract surgery causes damage and/or loss of the endothelial cells leading to failure of the endothelial pump mechanism. It is now coming up as the leading indication for penetrating keratoplasty.
2. Corneal opacities following injuries or ulceration.
3. Corneal dystrophies and degenerations.
4. Keratoconus that is too advanced and cannot be corrected with spectacles or contact lens.
5. Therapeutic indications like a non-healing corneal ulcer, which fails to respond to medical treatment.
6. Ectasias and thinning of the cornea.
7. Congenital opacities.
8. Chemical and thermal injuries.
9. Regrafting after a failed graft.

Evaluation for Keratoplasty

1. The patient has to be evaluated for the need for keratoplasty, i.e. whether the corneal opacity is producing significant visual loss (6/24 or less) or there is considerable pain and visual loss due to pseudophakic bullous keratopathy, whether all medical measures available have been tried for a corneal ulcer, etc.
2. The patient has to be evaluated for any posterior segment problem that may adversely affect visual recovery like a long standing retinal detachment, glaucomatous optic atrophy, etc. B-scan, electrophysiological tests, checking intraocular pressure (IOP), etc. may be required to rule out posterior segment problems in a patient with an opaque cornea.
3. Look for any associated problems that have to be corrected before undertaking keratoplasty like secondary glaucoma, canaliculitis dacryocystitis, etc.
4. Assess the factors that may decide the visual prognosis like presence or absence of dry eye problem, corneal vascularization, secondary glaucoma, etc.
5. Decide whether the patient is medically fit for undergoing keratoplasty.
6. Decide whether the patient is psychologically adjusted for the unpredictable outcome of keratoplasty and the long-term regular postoperative care and follow-up.

Surgical Procedure

Preparation of Donor Tissue

The donor button may be taken from a whole eyeball preserved by moist chamber method or a corneoscleral tissue kept in preservative medium. Depending on the extent of corneal pathology in the recipient's eye the size of the trephine is decided; 7–9 mm size trephines are commonly used. If it is a whole eyeball, it is fixed to a Tudor Thomas stand and trephination is done from the epithelial side. If it is a corneoscleral button, it is cut from the endothelial side using modern mechanized punch devices. The donor button is kept safe till the host cornea is ready.

Preparation of the Host Cornea

The eye is prepared as for a cataract surgery. The surgery is done under general anesthesia (GA) or local anesthesia (LA). The eye is cleaned and draped, and lid speculum is applied. The center of the pupil is marked with sterile methylene blue dye. The host trephine selected is usually 0.25 m smaller than the donor trephine (Fig. 30.2). The donor cornea is marked and cut to half thickness by gentle rotation of a vertically applied trephine centered on the mark on the cornea. A sharp blade is used to enter the anterior chamber (AC) at some point at the upper limbus. The pupil is constricted with pilocarpine injected into AC. Viscoelastics is injected through the entry wound to maintain the AC. Corneal scissors is used to complete the incision and the host button is removed. The donor button is placed in position by gently grasping with a fine forceps. Four interrupted radial 10-0 nylon cardinal sutures are put at 12, 6, 3 and 9 O'clock positions with the needle bites going approximately to 90% of the depth of corneal tissue. Additional 10-0

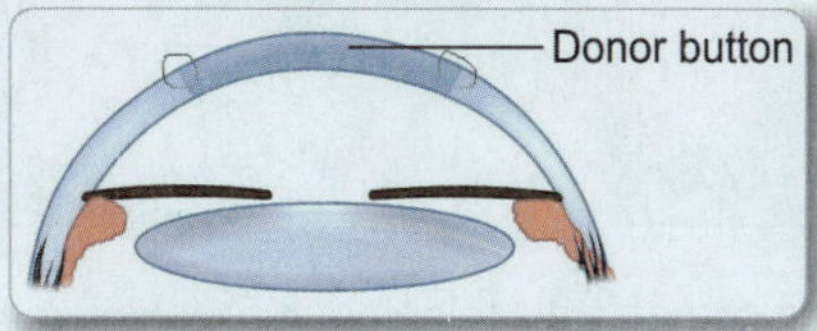

FIGURE 30.1: Penetrating keratoplasty

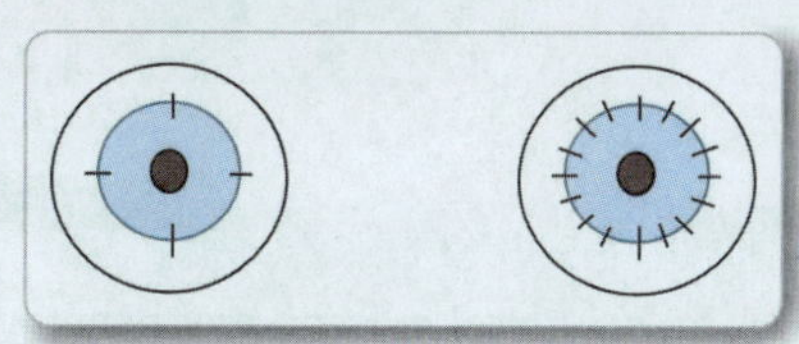
FIGURE 30.2: Graft on the host bed

continuous or interrupted sutures are put to get watertight closure. The suture knots are buried into donor tissue. The sutures are finally adjusted to minimize distortion of the tissue and thus reduce astigmatism (Figs 30.3A to F).

Combined Surgeries

In patients with significant cataract, a cataract surgery is also performed after removing the donor button and an intraocular lens (IOL) is put in the position. In patients with secondary glaucoma trabeculectomy may be combined with keratoplasty.

Postoperative Care

Systemic antibiotics are given both pre- and post-operatively to prevent infection. Topically antibiotic and steroid drops are given. Systemic steroids are indicated in high-risk cases like vascularized corneas, regraft, etc. to prevent graft rejection.

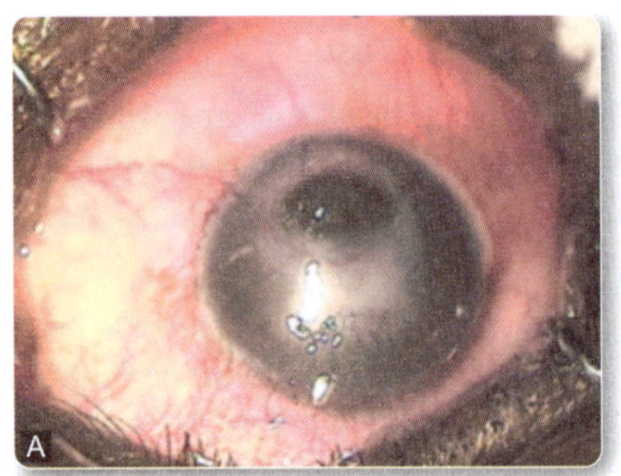
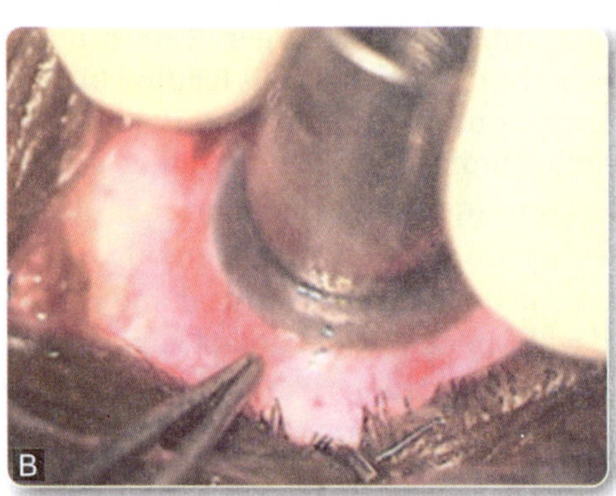
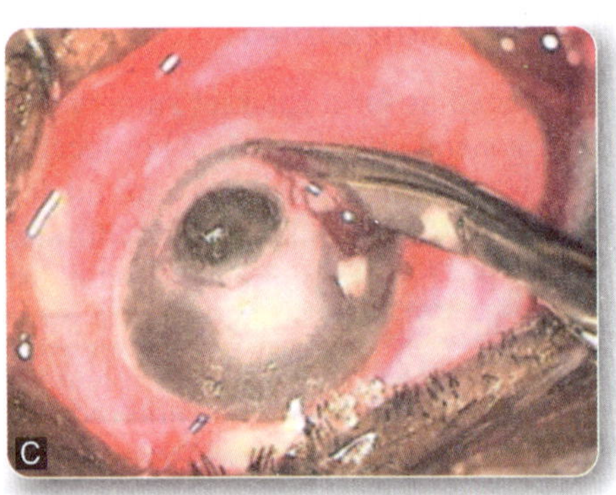
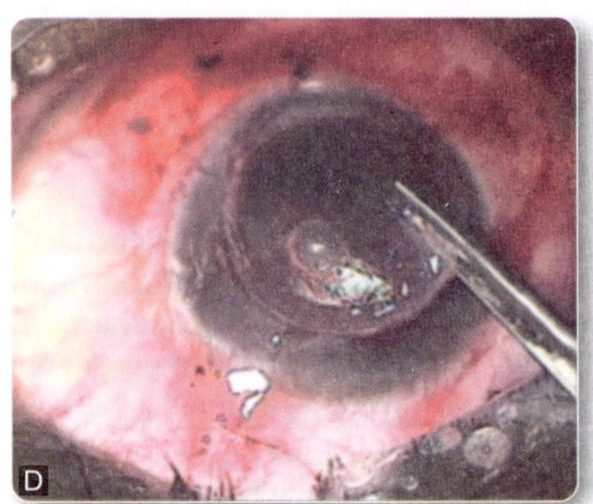
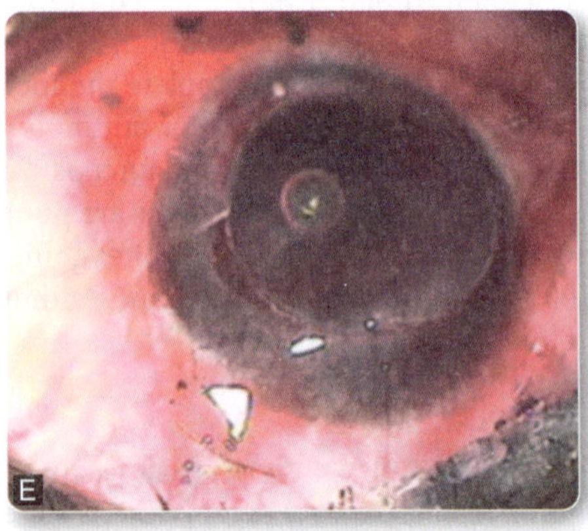
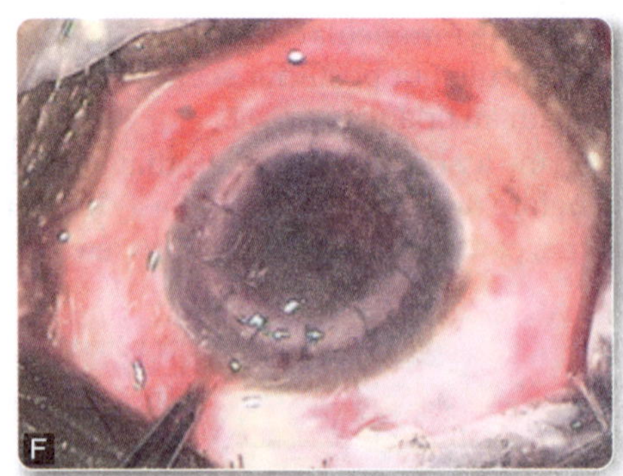

FIGURES 30.3A to F: Surgical procedure of penetrating keratoplasty. **A.** Opaque cornea with thinning; **B.** Trephining done with a disposable trephine; **C.** Incision completed with corneal scissors; **D.** Donor button placed on the eyeball; **E.** First cardinal suture put at 12 O' clock position; **F.** The picture at the completion of suturing.

The patient has to be closely followed up at close intervals for any graft infection or rejection, loosened or infected sutures and any sign of graft rejection or secondary glaucoma.

The frequency of follow-up is initially at weekly intervals and this can be gradually decreased depending on the progress of healing. The patient has to be followed up to 12–18 months. The sutures are removed as and when they show signs of healing and get loosened. This is usually done within 12–18 months. Appearance of the eye before and after keratoplasty is shown in Figures 30.4A and B.

Complications

Intraoperative

- Expulsive hemorrhage
- Loss of donor button.

Immediate Postoperative Period

- Wound leak and shallow AC
- Suture-related infection
- Secondary glaucoma
- Postoperative uveitis
- Pupillary block
- Ulcer on the graft.

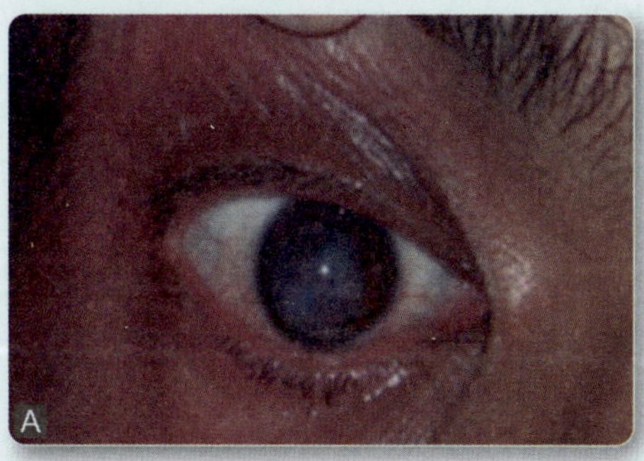

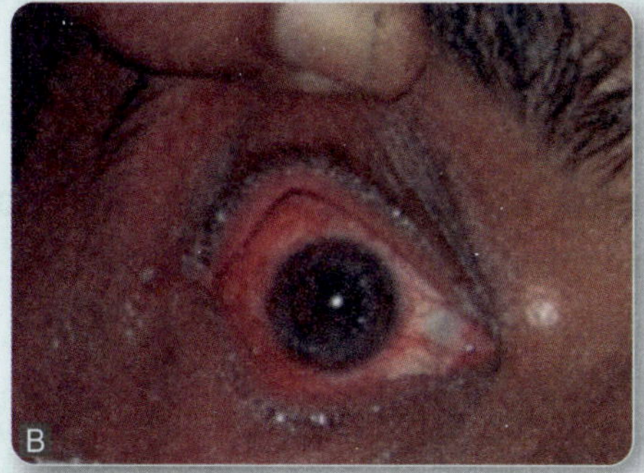

FIGURES 30.4A and B: Appearance of the eye. **A.** Before keratoplasty; **B.** After keratoplasty.

Late Postoperative Period

- Allograft rejection
- Secondary glaucoma
- Graft failure
- Infections on the graft.

In large extents, the success of keratoplasty depends on careful postoperative follow-up for any complications and their prompt management.

LAMELLAR KERATOPLASTY

In conventional LKP a superficial layer of the cornea is removed and a lamellar corneal disk of same size from a donor cornea is sutured into place. This is usually done in superficial corneal opacities or superficial epithelial dystrophies. Interface scarring is the main disadvantage of LKP. This reduces the expected visual acuity after LKP and also produces some glare. Lamellar keratoplasty is shown in Figure 30.5.

With advanced instruments and surgical techniques in lamellar keratoplasty, only the structurally abnormal layer of the cornea is now replaced, be it anterior or posterior component of the cornea. So, lamellar keratoplasty is now no longer a single surgery, but a series of different types of surgery called **selective tissue corneal transplantation or component surgery of the cornea**.

The various types of lamellar keratoplasty include:

1. Anterior automated lamellar keratoplasty (ALK).
2. Deep anterior lamellar keratoplasty (DALK).
3. Deep lamellar endothelial keratoplasty (DLEK).

Anterior Automated Lamellar Keratoplasty

Anterior automated lamellar keratoplasty is done for pathologies confined to the epithelium, basement membrane (BM) and the most superficial layers of the cornea, e.g. epithelial dystrophies, superficial diffuse corneal opacities.

In the anterior stroma, the corneal lamellae are shorter and more firmly intertwined, and manual dissection will lead to cutting of a lot of lamellae and consequently denser interface opacification. If the anterior lamellar disk is cut with a microkeratome used for refractive surgeries, a clear graft with less interface scarring will be obtained and a similar disk cut from a donor cornea is sutured in place.

Deep Anterior Lamellar Keratoplasty

Deep anterior lamellar keratoplasty can be done for any corneal pathology, which spares the DM and endothelium.

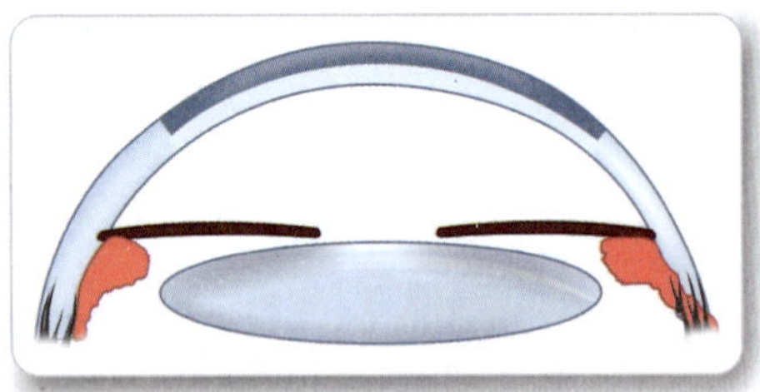

FIGURE 30.5: Lamellar keratoplasty

It can be done even for a leukomatous corneal opacity following a corneal ulcer, provided perforation has not occurred because the DM and endothelium will be normal even if the ulcer has extended deeply into corneal tissue, but no perforation has happened.

Preparation of the Donor Disk

The donor disk is cut with a punch from a donor tissue with the endothelial side up. The DM is stained with trypan blue and it is stripped off.

Preparation of the Host Eye

The epithelium, BM and 90% of the stroma are removed. In the posterior part of the stroma, the corneal lamellae are longer and more parallel in arrangement and hence it is easier to split the cornea mechanically. A 0.25–0.5 mm smaller trephine is used for making a partial thickness cut on the host cornea. The cornea is split into two layers along a plane just anterior to the DM by two methods:

1. Injecting air through a needle introduced into the deep stroma through the trephine incision (big bubble technique).
2. Instead of air, viscoelastic substance like hydroxy methyl cellulose can be injected into deep stroma to split the cornea at the desired level. The separated corneal disk is cut into four parts by a cruciate incision and removed by cutting with corneal scissors. The previously prepared donor disk is sutured into place.

Complication

Accidental posterior perforation can occur, while splitting the cornea. If the perforation is large, the LKP will have to be converted into PKP.

Deep Lamellar Endothelial Keratoplasty

In disorders involving the endothelial cell layer like pseudophakic bullous keratopathy and endothelial dystrophies, the malfunctioning is limited to the endothelium and the DM. The corneal edema resulting from this leads to corneal haze. If the DM and endothelium are replaced with a healthy DM and endothelium from a donor eye, before permanent structured damage has occurred to corneal stroma, corneal clarity can be regained.

The DM is too fragile a tissue and need careful handling. The donor button is fixed to an artificial AC and DM is carefully cut and folded using special instruments.

Using a technique similar to the capsulorhexis in cataract surgery, a circular cut is made in the host corneal DM through a scleral tunnel incision. The donor DM disk is removed. The folded DM from the donor cornea is introduced carefully into the AC of the host eye; it is gently unfolded and retained in position by an air bubble in the AC.

LAMELLAR VERSUS PENETRATING KERATOPLASTY

Deep Anterior Lamellar Keratoplasty versus Penetrating Keratoplasty

Disadvantages

Lamellar keratoplasty is technically more difficult than PKP. In anterior lamellar procedures, the interface haze will give slightly lesser vision compared to PKP.

Advantages

Anterior lamellar surgery has some definite advantages:

1. It is an extraocular surgery and hence lesser chances for intraoperative and postoperative complications of an intraocular surgery like endophthalmitis, expulsive hemorrhage, etc. So, LKP is safer in one-eyed persons.
2. Shorter postoperative care and earlier suture removal in LKP makes it a better choice for patients with poor compliance.
3. Chance of graft rejection is less in anterior lamellar procedures, since endothelium is the main source of antigen for allograft reaction.

Deep Lamellar Endothelial Keratoplasty versus Penetrating Keratoplasty

Posterior lamellar keratoplasty does not have the advantages of anterior lamellar procedure, since it is an intraocular procedure and the chances of graft rejection are the same as in PKP. But irregular astigmatism, which is one of the common causes for poor visual recovery after PKP, is not there in DLEK since there are no sutures on corneal surface and the normal anterior corneal curvature is maintained. It has faster recovery period compared to PKP.

Rotational Autograft

Rotational autograft is done in cases with a small eccentric opacity occupying the pupillary area. A circular graft is cut and it is rotated, so that the opacity is shifted from the pupillary area and sutured in this position (Fig. 30.6).

Advantages

Since this is an autograft, no need for a donor tissue and no risk of graft rejection.

Keratoprosthesis

In patients with severe ocular surface problems and severe dry eye as Stevens-Johnson syndrome, pemphigoid, chemical and thermal injuries, the chances of success of keratoplasty are very poor. In such patients, if the retina and optic nerve are functioning, an artificial optical device can be placed in the center of the cornea after removing the lens and anterior vitreous also. This is called keratoprosthesis. This will give some useful vision in bilaterally blind people with very poor chance of regaining vision after keratoplasty.

REFRACTIVE SURGERIES

Refractive surgeries are surgeries done to change the refractive power of the cornea so as to correct the refractive errors and lessen the dependence on spectacles or contact lens for good visual acuity. It has undergone considerable advances in the last few decades and every year the number of people undergoing these surgeries is increasing.

Keratomileusis

Keratomileusis is the first refractive surgery, which was introduced by Barraquer. A lamellar disk of cornea is removed from the patient's eye and it is frozen and cut on a micro lathe on the stromal side to alter the curvature. This disk of cornea is now gently thawed and sutured back into place. This is the precursor to modern laser in situ keratomileusis (LASIK) surgery.

Radial Keratotomy

Radial keratotomy is the next refractive surgery popularized by Fyodorov of Russia (Fig. 30.7). In this procedure 11-16 equally distanced radial cuts are made into the corneal stroma reaching up to 90% of depth. A central zone is left clear. The healing of these radial cuts and contracture will lead to flattening of the central zone. This will correct myopia.

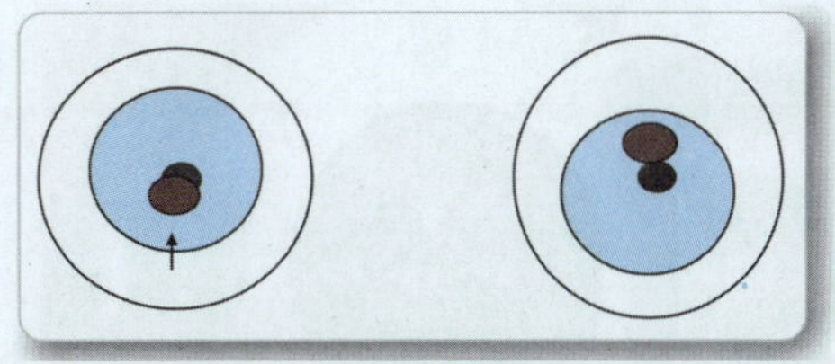

FIGURE 30.6: Rotational autograft

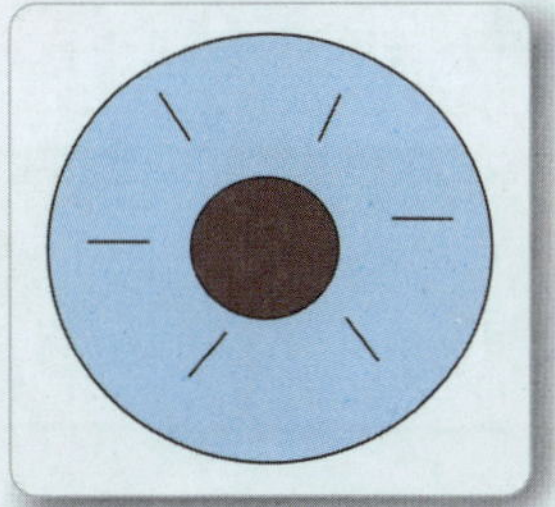

FIGURE 30.7: Radial keratotomy

REFRACTIVE SURGERIES USING LASER

The introduction of lasers revolutionized refractive surgery. Different lasers have different uses.

Photorefractive Keratectomy

Photorefractive keratectomy (PRK) is the first refractive surgery done with excimer laser. In this technique, laser energy is applied on the corneal surface and removes Bowman's membrane and a few microns of tissue from the corneal stromal surface in such a way as to alter the curvature and thus the refractive power of the cornea. The amount of tissue removed depends on the degree of myopia.

Re-epithelialization of the surface quickly occurs, but many patients experienced considerable pain in the immediate postoperative period till healing was complete. The surface scarring produced glare and halos, and interfered with night driving.

The shortcomings of photorefractive keratectomy led to more research and to overcome it LASIK was developed.

Laser In Situ Keratomileusis

In LASIK technique, a microkeratome is used to produce a hinged flap and laser is applied on the exposed stromal surface (Figs 30.8A to E). The flap is repositioned after laser therapy is completed.

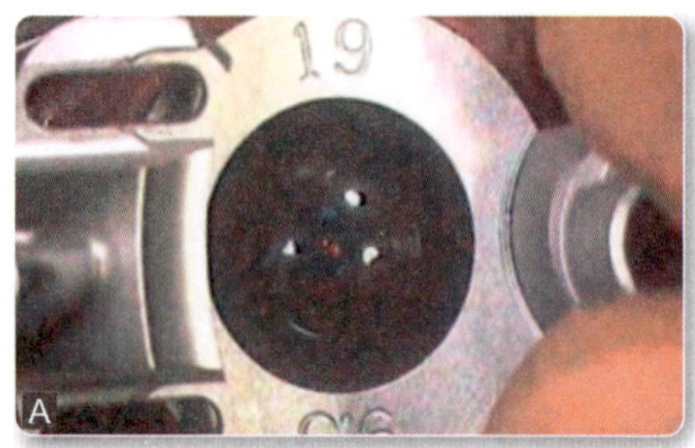

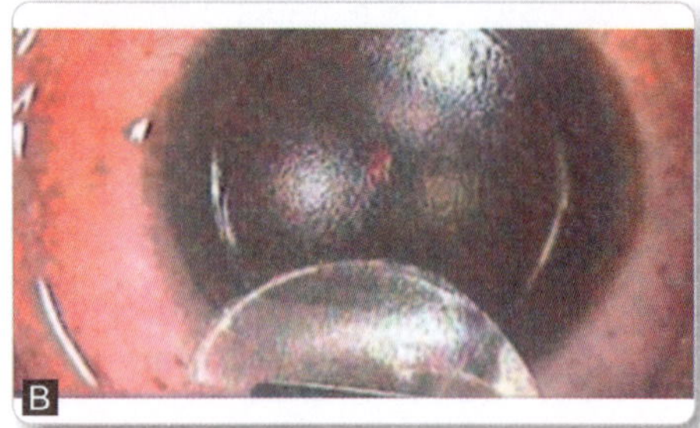

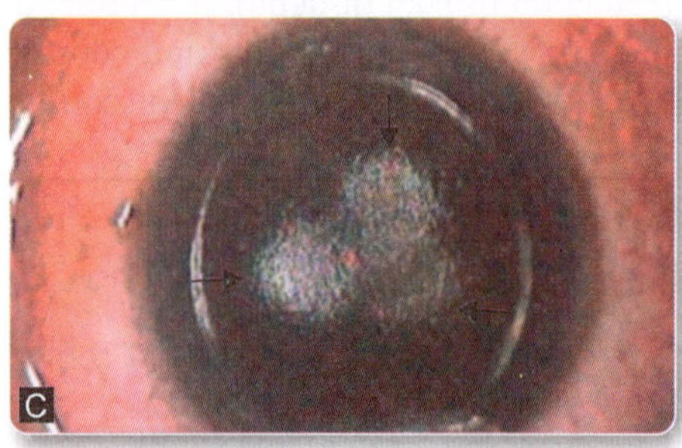

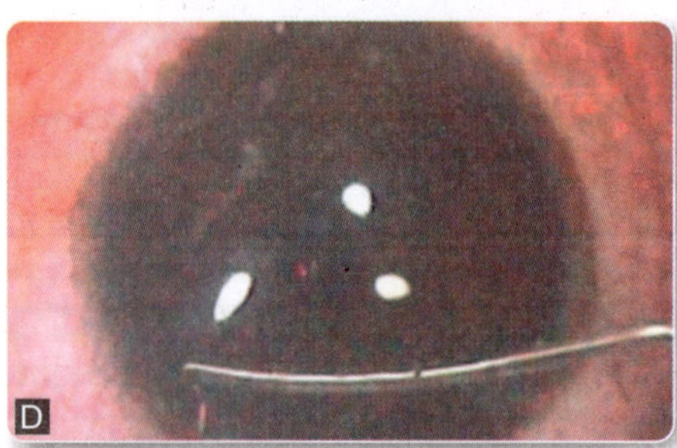

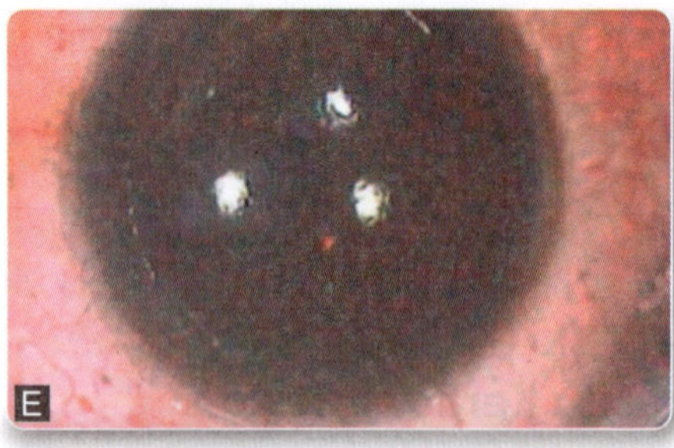

FIGURES 30.8A to E: Steps of LASIK. **A.** Microkeratome fixed on the cornea to cut the hinged flap; **B.** Hinged flap is folded back to expose the stromal bed; **C.** Laser ablation of the cornea done; **D.** Hinged flap is stroked back into place; **E.** Appearance at the end of LASIK.

Advantages

In LASIK there is less pain and visual recovery is faster. The stromal haze is less and hence glare and halos around light during night driving are less. Also the visual recovery after LASIK is more stable than that obtained after PRK, which shows some regression over the years.

Disadvantages

1. Flap-related complications such as incomplete or irregular cut, buttonholing of flap, loss of flap, etc. can occur.
2. Progressive corneal ectasia can occur, if LASIK is done on thin cornea.
3. Severe dry eye can also occur.
4. So, careful patient selection is important to get good results with LASIK. This should not be done in cornea with central thickness less than 490 micrometers or eyes with significant dry eye problems.

Laser Epithelial Keratomileusis

In laser epithelial keratomileusis (LASEK) technique, the epithelium is loosened by the application of dilute alcohol. It is scrolled back to expose BM and after laser ablation the epithelium is replaced and a bandage contact lens is applied. Thus, it can be considered as having advantages of both PRK and LASIK. It has less discomfort than PRK and less scarring and glare. At the same time flap-related complications are avoided and it can be done in thinner corneas where LASIK is contraindicated.

Improvements in refractive surgery are occurring every day. Instead of microkeratome femtosecond laser energy can be used to produce cleavage in corneal tissue. More precision and less flap-related complications occur when femtosecond laser is used for creating the flap.

Aberrometry and Customized LASIK

Wavefront technology is used to calculate the refractive error more accurately than the usual subjective methods used in routine LASIK. Here a thin infrared laser beam is projected onto the retina and the pattern formed on the retina is captured by a charge-coupled device (CCD) camera by indirect ophthalmoscopy. This image is analyzed to calculate the various aberrations in the optical system of the eye and the extent of ablation is decided by higher precision and a better visual outcome is obtained by this customized LASIK.

The refractive surgery is gaining popularity all over the world and better techniques with lesser complications and better vision can be expected to come out in future also.

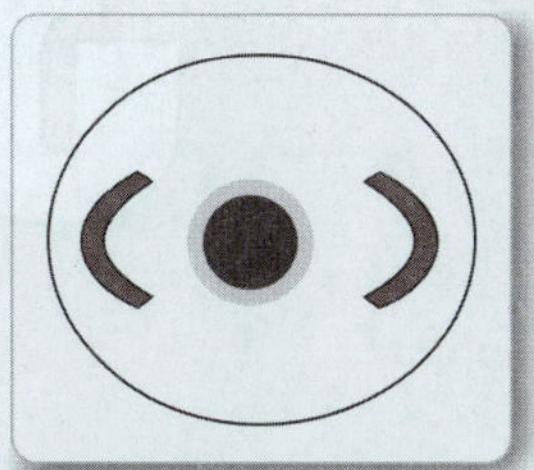

FIGURE 30.9: Intracorneal rings (INTACS) in the cornea

Miscellaneous Surgeries

Miscellaneous surgeries for correcting refractive errors are explained below.

Phakic Intraocular Lens or Implantable Collamer Lens or Implantable Contact Lens

Implantable contact lens (ICL) is a thin IOL made up of collagen copolymer material. Traditional IOLs are placed inside the eye after removing the natural lens. In phakic IOL surgery, IOL is placed in addition to the natural lens to correct the refractive error. The lens is placed behind the iris tissue to the center of the pupil and in front of the natural lens. This surgery is usually done in high myopic patients who cannot tolerate contact lens and have thin cornea not suitable for LASIK. In course of time patient may develop some lenticular opacities, which is not visually significant in majority of patients.

Intracorneal Rings

There are two crescent or semicircular-shaped rings made of polymethyl methacrylate (PMMA) implanted intrastromally, on each side of the pupil. These implants flatten the central cornea and charge the refraction. Initially they were used for connecting myopia. With the advent of wavefront LASIK and ICL, intracorneal rings are mainly used for the treatment of keratoconus. An advantage of this procedure over LASIK is that it is reversible. The implants can be removed or replaced with different rings to change the amount of correction. The procedure has low side effects. Infection and distortion of vision and glare at night can rarely occur (Fig. 30.9).

Collagen Cross-linking of Cornea

Collagen cross-liking of cornea is a new method of treatment for arresting the progression of keratoconus. Here, ultraviolet light (UVA 365 nm) along with riboflavin as photosensitizer is used to produce changes in the intrinsic biomechanics of the cornea. Cross-linking of collagen fibers occurs, which increases the rigidity of the cornea and arrests or slows down progression of keratoconus.

To do this procedure, patients should have progressive keratoconus, minimum corneal thickness of 400 microns and no other corneal pathology, and the age should be above 16 years.

Method

Riboflavin eyedrops are applied to the cornea after removing the central epithelium and the cornea is exposed to UV radiation, 365 nm for 30 minutes. Studies have shown that this treatment arrests progression of keratoconus in 100% of cases and some regression of keratoconus in 15%–20% of cases over a period of 1 year.

Ophthalmic Microsurgical Instruments

31

Girija Devi PS, Susan Thomas

Today most of the surgeries in ophthalmology are microsurgical procedures and an ophthalmic surgical instrument needs to be precise, efficient and well-controlled for a given surgical task. Instrument's design, intended use, technique, care and sterilization are all important aspects. The length of most of the instruments is dropped to about 14 cm in concordance with the working distance of the microscope. The instruments are made of either titanium or stainless steel. Titanium is lighter than steel, resists corrosion, non-magnetic and can have matte finish, so that it does not produce glare. However, titanium cannot maintain a sharp edge and are more expensive than stainless steel, but have a much longer lifespan. Stainless steel is still used for cutting instruments, since it holds a sharp edge, but is prone to corrosion especially, if not kept clean and dry.

GENERAL MICROSURGICAL INSTRUMENTS USED FOR OPHTHALMIC SURGERY

Speculum

Lid Speculum

A lid speculum is essential in ophthalmic surgery, for visualization and surgical access in extraocular and intraocular procedures. Their main purpose is to retract the lids and hold the eye open during surgery. They have a self-retaining action and are of varied designs that cater to different needs.

Barraquer Wire Speculum

Barraquer wire speculum is used for intraocular procedures, as they are lightweight and transmit little pressure to the eye (Fig. 31.1). Barraquer wire speculum with solid blades helps to keep the eyelashes away from the surgical field (Fig. 31.2).

Universal Eye Speculum

Full bladed, larger, rigid speculum, which is used for strabismus and other extraocular surgeries. It has two limbs and spring mechanism with a screw to adjust the limbs and the screw allows the palpebral fissure to be maintained as wide as desired. It is called universal because it can be used for both eyes—right and left (Fig. 31.3). Routinely used for extraocular surgeries such as:

- Squint surgery
- Pterygium excision
- Removal of corneal and conjunctival foreign body
- Enucleation and evisceration
- Examination of eye in a patient with blepharospasm.

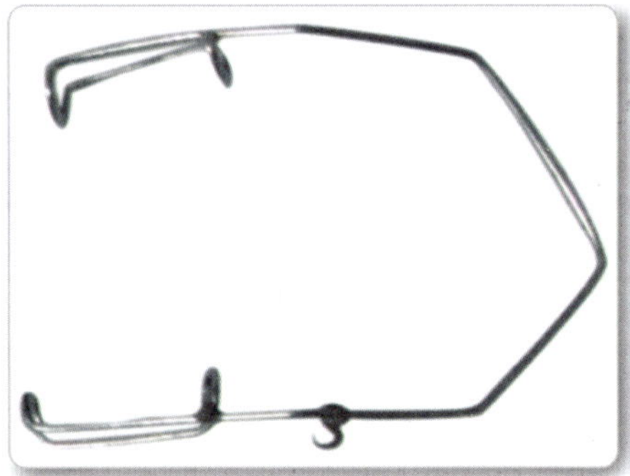

FIGURE 31.1: Barraquer wire speculum

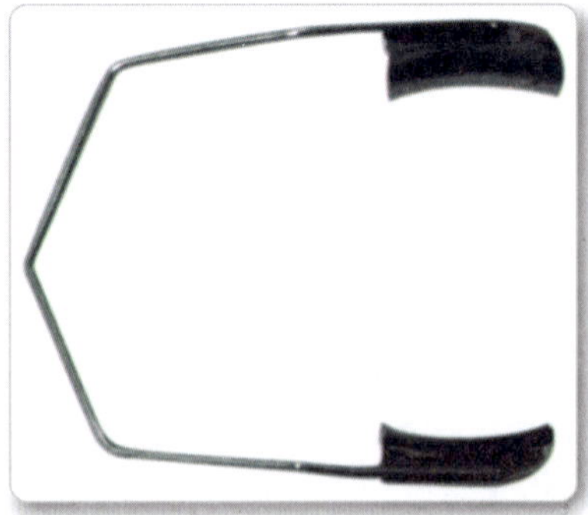

FIGURE 31.2: Barraquer wire speculum with solid blades

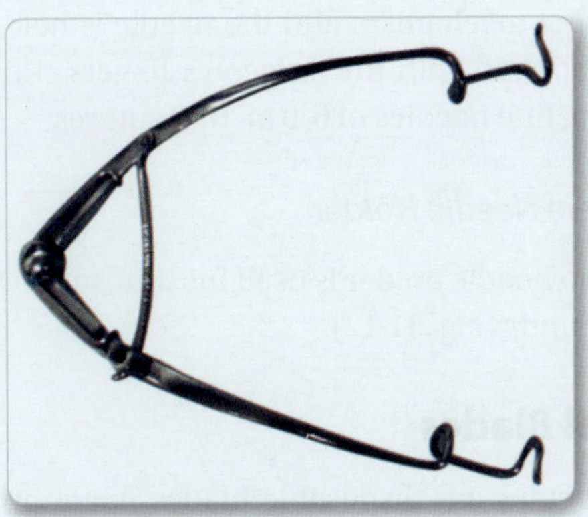

FIGURE 31.3: Universal eye speculum

It is not used in intraocular surgeries such as cataract surgeries, since this speculum applies some external pressure on the eyeball and can lead to vitreous loss. A smaller pediatric speculum is used for both examination and surgery of the children.

Forceps

Forceps are designed for catching and holding tissues or sutures and consists of a lip, shaft and a handle.

Superior Rectus Holding Forceps

Superior rectus holding forceps are toothed forceps (1 × 2 teeth) with shaped double curve near the tip (Fig. 31.4):

1. It is used to hold the superior rectus muscle, while passing a bridle suture under it (stay suture).
2. It is used to rotate the globe downwards to expose the upper limbus in cataract and glaucoma surgery.

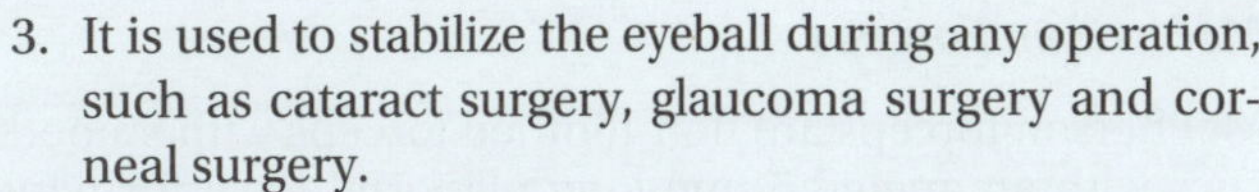

3. It is used to stabilize the eyeball during any operation, such as cataract surgery, glaucoma surgery and corneal surgery.

Globe Fixation Forceps

Globe fixation forceps are toothed and are used for grasping the conjunctiva and episcleral tissues at the limbus because, here the conjunctiva is firmly attached to the sclera and it is 4–5 layers thick. It has 2 × 3 or 3 × 4 teeth at the tip (Fig. 31.5).

Uses: As follows:

1. Fixing the eyeball during incisions of cornea to facilitate surgical maneuvers like pterygium surgery, paracentesis and excision of swellings or growths on the eyeball.
2. They are used to hold the eyeball during forced duction test as in blowout fracture, Duane's retraction syndrome or superior oblique sheath syndrome.

Corneoscleral Forceps

Corneoscleral forceps have toothed tip and a flat platform just behind the tip to facilitate both holding of the tissues and tying of the sutures. For example, Lims (Fig. 31.6) or colibri forceps (Fig. 31.7).

A forward angulation of the tip permits easier manipulation of ocular tissues. They are used to hold the corneal or scleral edge of incision for suturing during cataract, glaucoma, repair of corneal or scleral tears and keratoplasty operations.

Saint Martin's Forceps

Saint Martin's forceps are fine tooth forceps. It is useful for holding delicate tissues like cornea without crushing (Fig. 31.8).

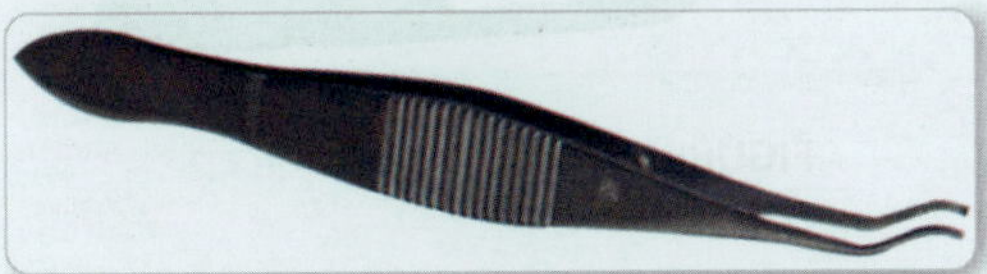

FIGURE 31.4: Superior rectus holding forcep

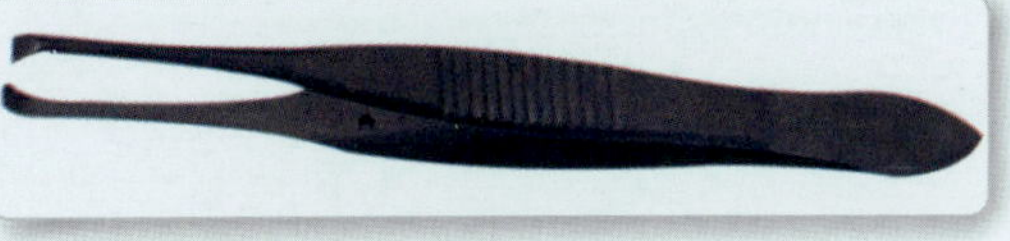

FIGURE 31.5: Globe fixation forcep

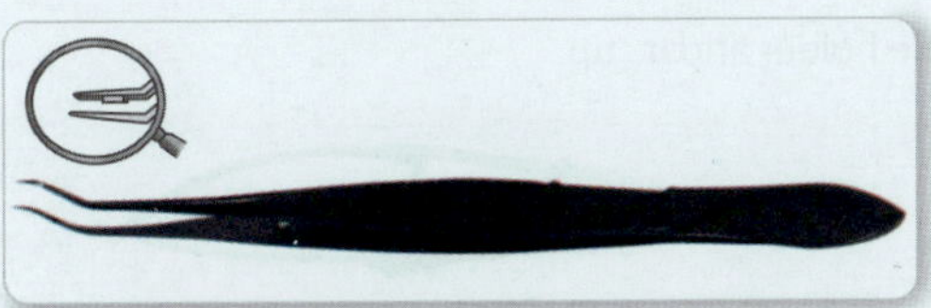

FIGURE 31.6: Lims forcep and its tip

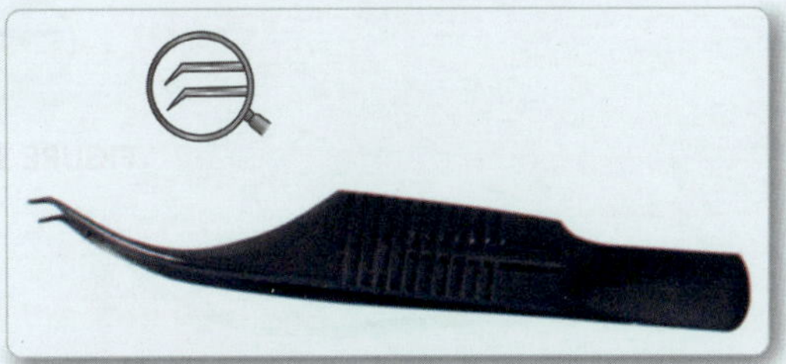

FIGURE 31.7: Colibri forcep and its tip

McPherson Forceps

McPherson forceps are non-toothed forceps with smooth jaws with an angled 5 mm long platform, ideal for tying 8-0 to 11-0 sutures. They are also useful for tearing the lens capsule and handling the intraocular lens (IOL) during implantation (Fig. 31.9).

Holders

Needle Holders

Needle holders grasp needles for suturing and therefore vary with both the thickness of the needle as well as the procedure performed.

Uses: As follows:
- Suturing cornea, sclera and conjunctiva
- Extraocular muscle as in squint
- Nasal mucosal flap in dacryocystorhinostomy (DCR)
- Skin suturing and eyelid repair.

Arruga Needle Holders

Arruga needle holders are used for extraocular procedures like lid surgery, for putting lid stay suture in ptosis surgery, for passing superior rectus bridle suture in cataract surgery and lid suture in cataract surgery. This needle holder has locking mechanism, which allows firm grasping of the needle (Fig. 31.10).

Barraquer Needle Holder

Barraquer needle holder (Fig. 31.11) is used for suturing conjunctiva, extraocular muscles and sclera. They do not have locking mechanism and the needle is held with the pressure applied with the surgeon's fingers. This is used for holding fine needles of 8-0 or 10-0 sutures.

Castroviejo Needle Holder

Castroviejo needle holder is used for suturing corneal and scleral wounds (Fig. 31.12).

Surgical Blades

Surgical blades are disposable blades made of stainless steel and are most commonly used. They are attached to reusable handle made of stainless steel called Bard-Parker (BP) handle (Fig. 31.13). Diamond knives and blades are extremely sharp with excellent cutting quality, but they are expensive.

Keratome

Keratome is a thin, diamond-shaped blade with sharp apex and two cutting edges. Straight, as well as angled keratomes are available in various sizes (2.8, 3, 3.5, 5.5 mm). Presently, disposable, angled keratomes of 2.8, 3 or 3.2 mm are commonly used (Fig. 31.14).

Uses: Used to make valvular corneal incision enter into anterior chamber (AC) for all modern techniques of cataract surgery like phaco, small incision cataract surgery (SICS) and other intraocular surgeries such as iridectomy and paracentesis.

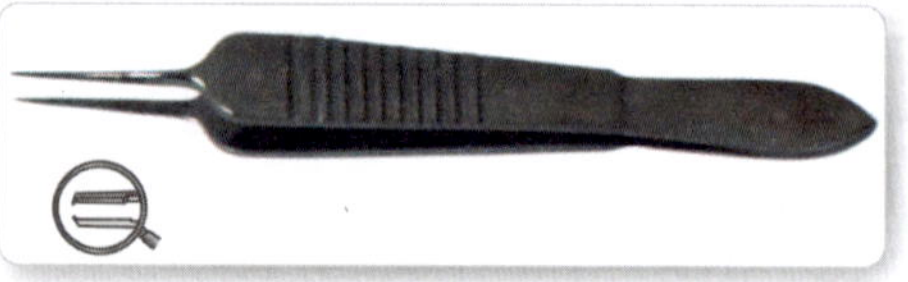

FIGURE 31.8: Martin's forcep and its tip

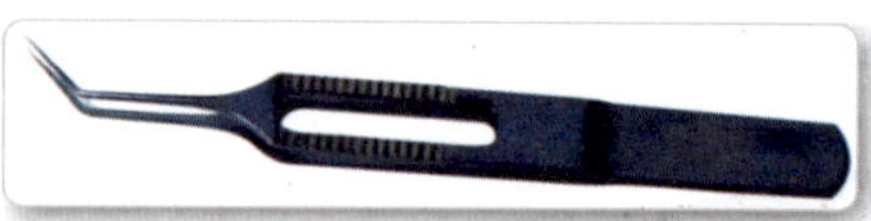

FIGURE 31.9: McPherson forcep

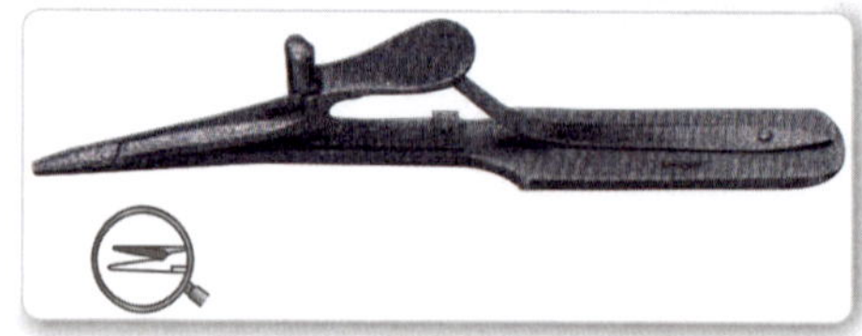

FIGURE 31.10: Arruga needle holder and its tip

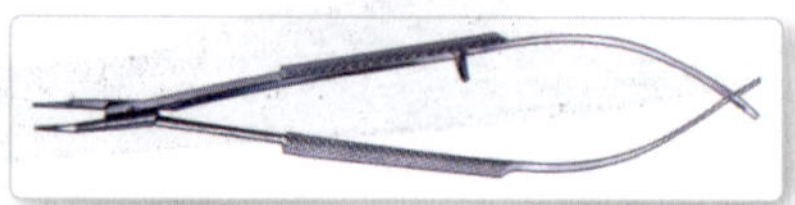

FIGURE 31.11: Barraquer needle holder

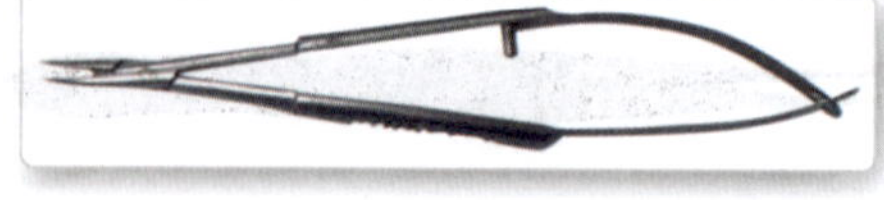

FIGURE 31.12: Castroviejo needle holder

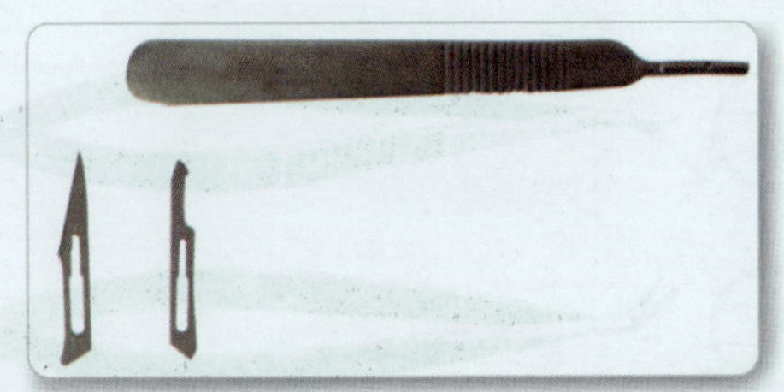

FIGURE 31.13: Bard-Parker handles for disposable slot blades (No. 11 and No. 15)

Crescent Knife

Blunt tip, bevel up knife having cut-splitting action at the tip and both the sides. Its blade is curved and either mounted on a plastic handle or can be fixed with a reusable handle (Fig. 31.15).

Uses: To make tunnel incision in the sclera and cornea for phacoemulsification, SICS and trabeculectomy.

Stiletto or Microvitreoretinal or V-lance Blade

Stiletto or microvitreoretinal (MVR) or V-lance blade (Fig. 31.16) is available as a disposable lancet-shaped knife mounted on a plastic handle. The blade is designed to make a slit-shaped self-sealing incision, which is a 20 gauge opening, 9–1.0 mm wide at the limbus into the AC or in the sclera. Also used in three-port sclerotomy incision in vitrectomy.

15° Side Port Entry Blade

The 15° side port entry blade is a fine, straight knife with a sharp pointed tip and cutting edge on one side, to make a small valvular clear corneal incision called side port, as in phaco, SICS and other intraocular surgery including pars plana vitrectomy (Fig. 31.17).

Scissors

There are various types of scissors used for different types of surgeries. The size of the handle and blades vary in size depending on how strong or delicate the targeted tissues are.

Castroviejo Corneoscleral Scissors (Universal Type)

The scissors are finely curved and their cutting blades are kept apart by spring action. There are right and left corneoscleral scissors designated for the two sides, identified by their concave side up. The universal corneoscleral scissors can be used for both sides (Figs 31.18A and B).

Uses: As follows:

- For dissecting the host button in keratoplasty
- To enlarge corneoscleral incision for extracapsular cataract extraction (ECCE)
- To cut the sclera and trabecular tissue in trabeculectomy.

de Wecker Iris Scissors

de Wecker iris scissors are unique in having the blades at right angle to the shaft and have a special, quick cutting in spring action (Fig. 31.19).

Uses: As follows:

- To perform iridectomy along with other surgeries like keratoplasty, cataract and trabeculectomy
- Iridectomy
- To cut prolapsed iris and formed vitreous
- To cut pupillary membrane
- To cut postoperative iris prolapse
- Iris excision (impacted, foreign body in iris, tumors of iris).

Vannas Scissors

Vannas scissors are fine multipurpose scissors useful for cutting iris, lens capsule, fine sutures, lamellar corneal tissue and harvesting limbal stem cells (Fig. 31.20). It is a fine delicate scissor with small cutting blades kept apart by spring action. The blades may be straight or curved.

Uses: As follows:

- For cutting anterior capsular tag after capsulotomy
- For cutting iris in performing iridectomy

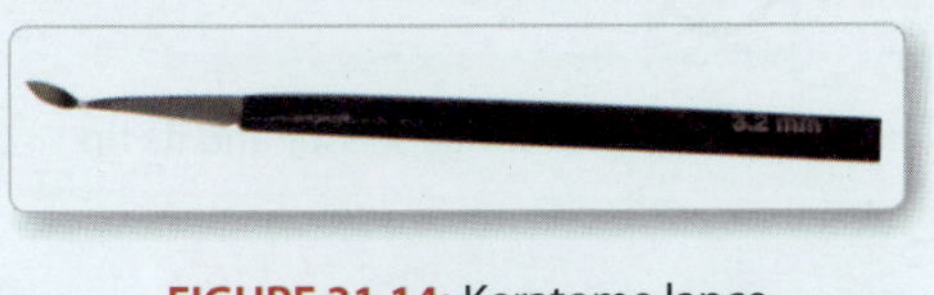

FIGURE 31.14: Keratome lance

FIGURE 31.16: Microvitreoretinal (MVR) blade

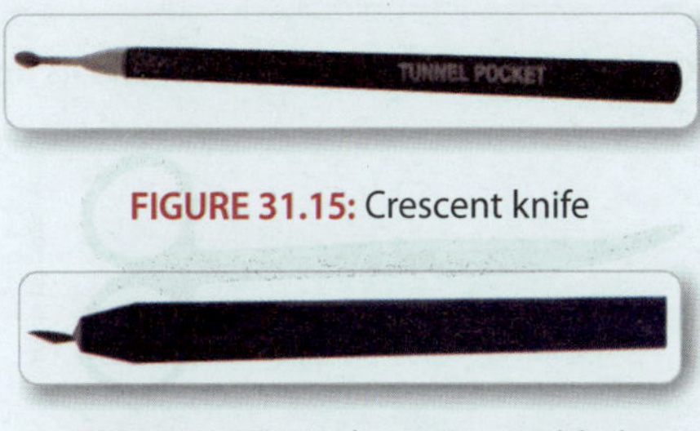

FIGURE 31.15: Crescent knife

FIGURE 31.17: Side port entry blade

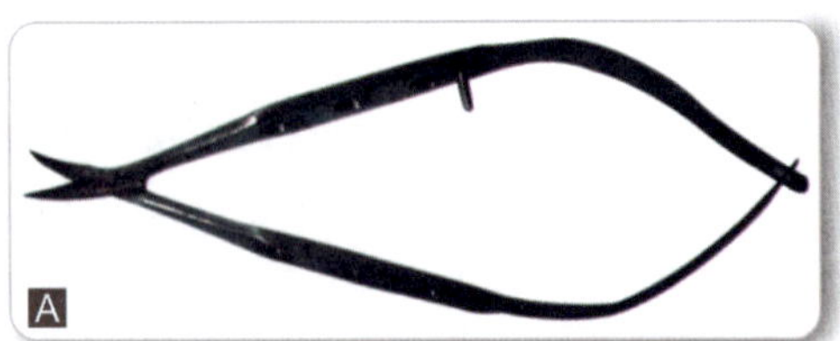

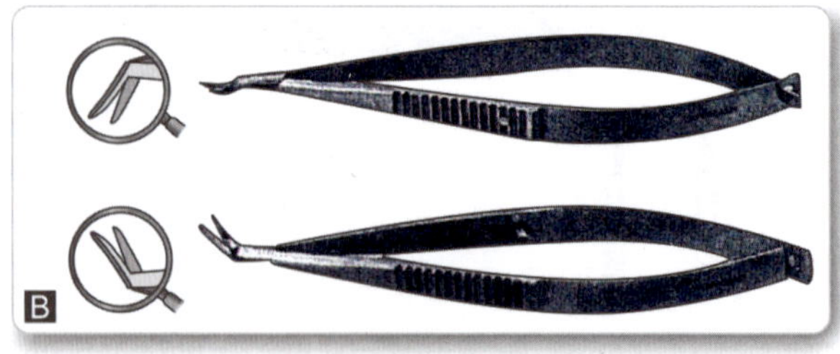

FIGURES 31.18A and B: Scissors. **A.** Castroviejo corneoscleral scissor (universal type); **B.** Castroviejo scissors (right and left) with their tips.

- For doing pupillary sphincterotomy (in sphincter rigidity with non-dilating pupil)
- For cutting prolapsed formed vitreous
- For cutting postoperative iris prolapse
- For cutting pupillary membrane (surgical membranectomy)
- For cutting trabecular meshwork in trabeculectomy
- For cutting fine sutures
- For harvesting limbal stem cells.

Enucleation Scissors

Enucleation scissors are large, stout and strong scissors having curved, sharp blades with blunt ends. They are used to cut the optic nerve during enucleation operation (Fig. 31.21).

Iris Repositor

Iris repositor is a smooth, spatulated instrument with a rounded tip, useful for repositioning iris into AC in any intraocular surgery (Fig. 31.22). It is also used for breaking synechiae at the pupillary margin.

Wire Vectis

Wire vectis is a wire loop attached to a metallic handle (Fig. 31.23).

Uses

1. It is used to remove dislocated and subluxated lens.
2. Nucleus delivery in ECCE (wire vectis is used to apply pressure in the sclera superiorly depressing the lip of wound posteriorly to facilitate nucleus delivery by sliding technique for ECCE.
3. In SICS, to sandwich the nucleus out from the AC. Serrated vectis is used in SICS to sandwich the nucleus out the other instrument used along with this is a dialer.

Lens Spatula

Lens spatula is a flat metallic handle with tiny spoon-shaped end. It is used to apply counter pressure at the 12 O' clock position, during expression of lens nucleus in ECCE (Fig. 31.24).

Cystotome

Cystotome is used for making an opening on the anterior capsule. Ordinary cystotome is a bent 26–27 gauge needle bent at the tip and close to the hub. Irrigating cystotome is connected to a bottle of Ringers lactate by an intravenous (IV) infusion set to give continuous irrigation during capsulotomy. Capsulotomy can be completed with bent needle or cystotome or by using a capsulorhexis forceps (Fig. 31.25).

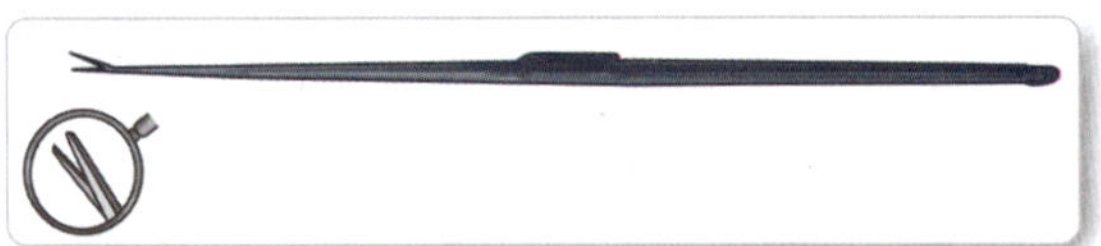

FIGURE 31.19: De Wecker iris scissor and its tip

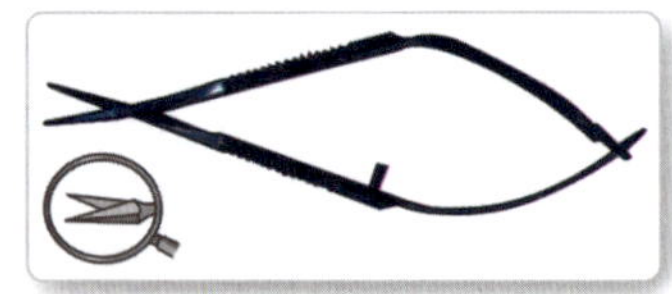

FIGURE 31.20: Vannas scissor and its tip

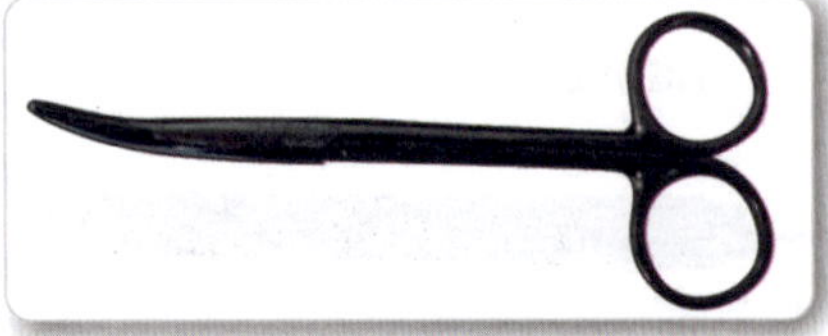

FIGURE 31.21: Enucleation scissor

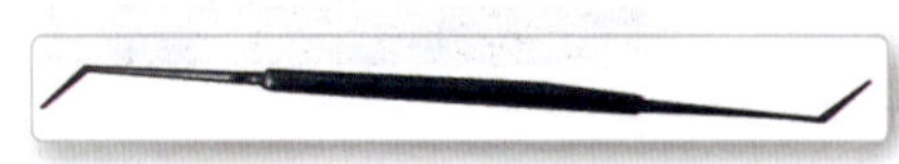

FIGURE 31.22: Iris repositor

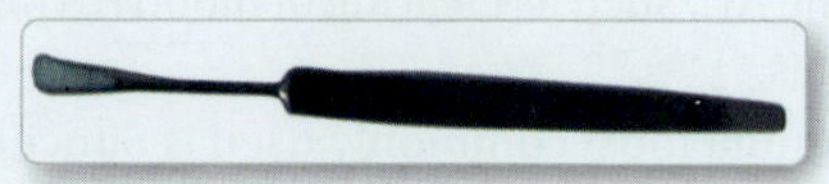

FIGURE 31.23: Wire vectis

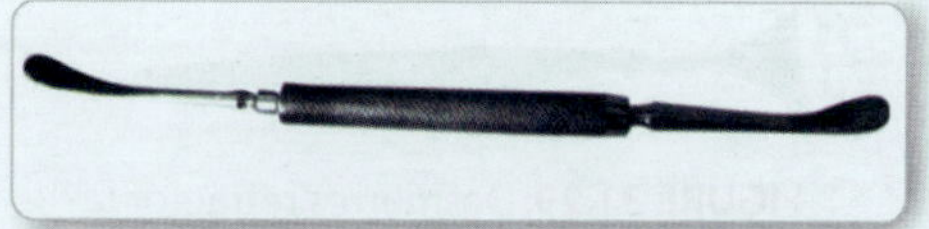

FIGURE 31.24: Lens spatula

Utrata Capsulorhexis Forceps

The forceps have very delicate grasping tips and extremely thin, long straight shanks. They are useful for holding the lens capsule, after a flap has been raised with cystotome or bent 26 gauge needle to perform a continues curvilinear capsulotomy (Fig. 31.26).

Hook

Smith Lens Expresser or Lens Hook

Smith lens expresser or lens hook has a flat metal handle and the handle is at right angles to the curvature of hook and the tip of curve is knobbed. It has a rounded tip with a gentle curve at the angulated elbow or knee, to apply gentle pressure at the limbus inferiorly at 6 O' clock position facilitating the delivery of lens nucleus in ECCE (Fig. 31.27). It can also be used as a muscle hook, if the latter is not available.

Muscle Hook

Muscle hook is similar to lens expresser in appearance, but has blunt guarding knob at one end to prevent muscles damage. The plain of the handle is same as that of the curvature of the hook (Fig. 31.28).

Uses: The muscle hook is used to pull the extraocular muscles during surgery for squint, enucleation and retinal detachment.

Desmarres Retractor

Desmarres retractor is saddle-shaped instrument folded at one end. It is available in two sizes, small pediatric and large adult (Fig. 31.29).

Uses

- Used to retract the lids during examination of the eyeball
- In case of blepharospasm and in children
- In case with marked swelling and ecchymosis
- Removal of corneoscleral sutures
- For double eversion of upper lid to examine the superior fornix.

Castroviejo Calipers

Castroviejo calipers is a divider-like instruments with a graduated scale (in mm) attached to one arm. Its other arm can be moved by a screw over the scale and measures the distance between the two tips of the instrument (Fig. 31.30).

Uses

1. Used to measure the length of extraocular muscles to be recessed or resected during squint surgery.
2. In ptosis, to measure the length of levator to be resected.
3. In retinal detachment (RD) surgery, to mark the site of detachment for external localization.

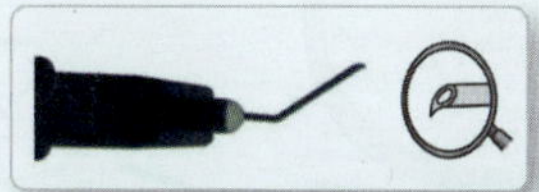

FIGURE 31.25: Irrigating cystotome made by bending 26 G disposable needle and its tip

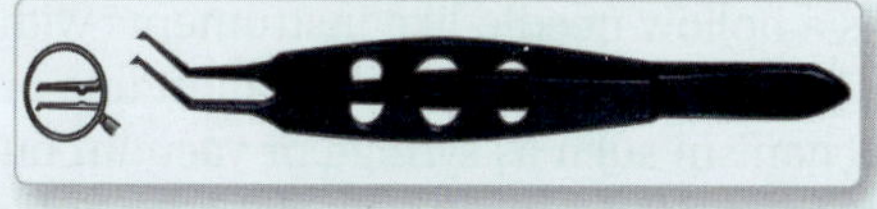

FIGURE 31.26: Utrata capsulorhexis forcep and its tip

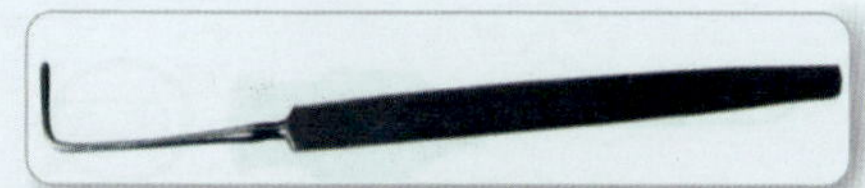

FIGURE 31.27: Smith lens expresser or lens hook

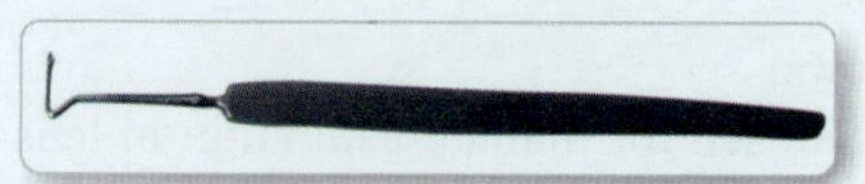

FIGURE 31.28: Muscle hook

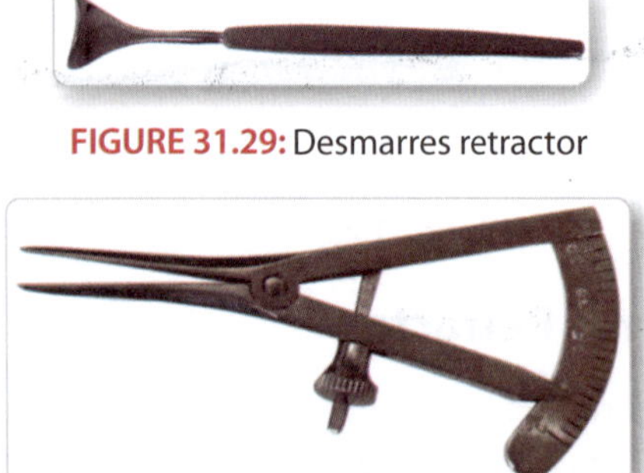

FIGURE 31.29: Desmarres retractor

FIGURE 31.30: Castroviejo caliper

4. In pars plana vitrectomy, to measure and identify the pars plana.
5. To measure the site of incision for removing retained intraocular foreign bodies (IOFB).
6. To mark the extent of incision in SICS.
7. To measure the size of the lamellar scleral flap in trabeculectomy.
8. To measure corneal diameter in buphthalmos and megalocornea.
9. To measure corneal opacity in keratoplasty.

Irrigating Vectis

Irrigating vectis is a modified vectis in which the loop is made of a thick, hollow wire. The anterior end of the loop has three 0.3 mm openings. The posterior end of the loop is continuous with a hollow handle (Fig. 31.31). The posterior end of the hollow handle has a hub, similar to that of a hypodermic needle to which a syringe or infusion set is attached. The size of the loop of the vectis is variable. In commonly used vectis, the loop is 4 mm wide and 8–9 mm length. The superior surface of the loop has a slight concavity to accommodate lens nucleus.

Cannula

Cannula is a hollow needle-like instruments with blunt or rounded tip that are fitted to an irrigation line or an aspiration mechanism such as syringe or vacuum bulb, either irrigate or aspirate fluid or soft material, such as lens cortex.

Simcoe Two Way Irrigation Aspiration Cannula

Uses: As follows:

1. Simcoe is used for manual aspiration of lens cortex and has the dual function of irrigation and aspiration (Fig. 31.32).
2. It can also be used for aspiration of other materials from the AC, such as clearing of blood (hyphema) and exudates.

The cannula most commonly used is Simcoe cannula. This is available in two different designs.

Direct Simcoe: Where aspiration is through the silicon tube and irrigation through the main hub. The surgeon holds the syringe attached to the silicon tube, which is used to generate suction for aspiration in the left hand and irrigation line is attached to the main central hub.

Reverse Simcoe: Where irrigation is through the silicon tube and aspiration through the main hub. Surgeon uses the syringe attached to the main hub to generate suction for aspiration of lens cortex. Cannulas are available in different sizes namely 21, 22 and 23 gauges, which have an aspiration size of 0.5, 0.35 and 0.3 mm respectively. The narrow bore ports are useful for aspiration of fine cortical fibers and get a better purchase on tissue, and larger cannulas are useful for faster aspiration of bulky lens cortex.

Hydrodissection Cannula

Hydrodissection cannula is a single bore 25, 27 or 40 G cannulas with a 45° angulation at about 10–12 mm from the free end. The tip of the free end may be flattened or beveled (Fig. 31.33).

Uses: Hydrodissection cannula is used to perform hydrodissection (separation of posterior capsule from the cortex) and hydrodelineation (separation of cortex from nucleus in

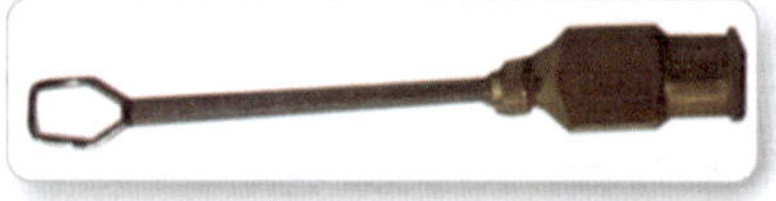

FIGURE 31.31: Irrigating vectis

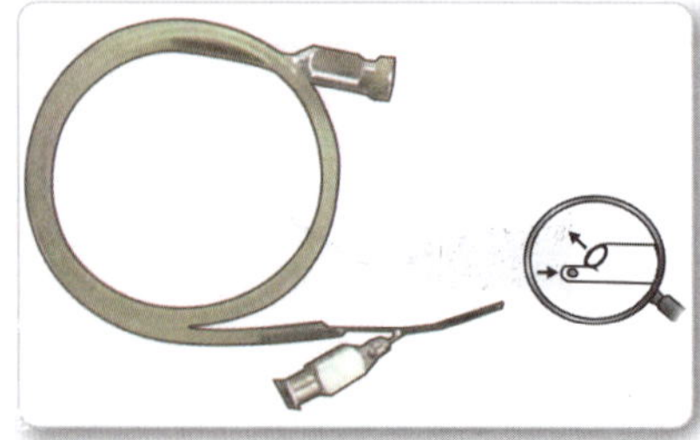

FIGURE 31.32: Simcoe cannula and its tip

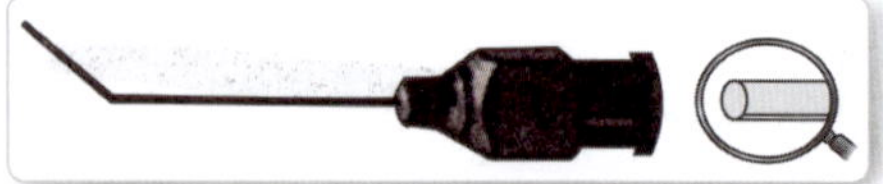

FIGURE 31.33: Hydrodissection cannula and its tip

phaco and SICS. This cannula is attached to a syringe carrying the irrigating fluid. For hydrodissection, its tip is introduced beneath the anterior capsular margin after capsulorhexis and fluid is injected to obtain subcapsular dissection.

Anterior Chamber Maintainer

Anterior chamber maintainer are self-retaining, short, fine cannulas that are connected at one end to irrigation infusion line, while the tip inserted into the AC is well infused with fluid to maintain the depth of the AC during surgery (Fig. 31.34).

Lewicky AC maintainer: It is a 20 gauge, 3.50 mm self-retaining cannula with 200 mm long silicone tubing and an adaptor.

Intraocular Lens Holding Forceps (Lens Holding Forceps)

Intraocular lens holding forceps (lens holding forceps) is a spring action forceps with short, blunt and curved blades having smooth edges and tips with platform (no teeth at serrations). Used to hold the optic of non-foldable polymethylmethacrylate (PMMA) IOL during implantation (Fig. 31.35).

Sinskey Hook

Sinskey hook or IOL dialer is fine, but stout instrument with a blunt tip. The tip engages the dialing holes of IOL (Fig. 31.36).

Uses

1. It is used to dial the PMMA non-foldable IOL for proper positioning in the capsular bag or ciliary sulcus.
2. It can be used to manipulate nucleus in phaco.
3. It can also be used to sandwich the nucleus out from the AC with the help of vectis and dialer.

Chopper

Chopper is a fine instrument resembling sinskey hook in shape. The inner edge in the bent tip is cutting and may have different uses. It is used to split or chop the nucleus into smaller pieces and also for the nucleus manipulation in phaco (Fig. 31.37).

Chalazion Clamp

Chalazion clamp consists of two limbs like a forceps, which can be clamped with the help of a screw. The tip of the one limb is flattened in the form of round disk, while the tip of the other arm has a small circular ring. Usually the flat disk is applied on the skin side and ring on the conjunctival side of the chalazion. It is used to fix the chalazion and achieve hemostasis during incision and curettage.

Chalazion Scoop

Chalazion scoop is a small cup with sharp margin, attached to a narrow handle (Fig. 31.38).

Used to scoop the contents of chalazion during incision and curettage.

Lid Spatula

Lid spatula is a simple metal plate, slightly concave surface at either end. Used to protect the globe and support the lid during entropion, ectropion, ptosis and other lid surgeries (Fig. 31.39).

Lid Clamp or Entropion Clamp

Lid clamp or entropion clamp consists of a D-shaped plate opposed by a U-shaped rim, which when tightened with the help of a screw, clamps the tissues. Two clamps are required; one can be used for right upper and left lower lid and the second for right lower and left upper lid (Fig. 31.40).

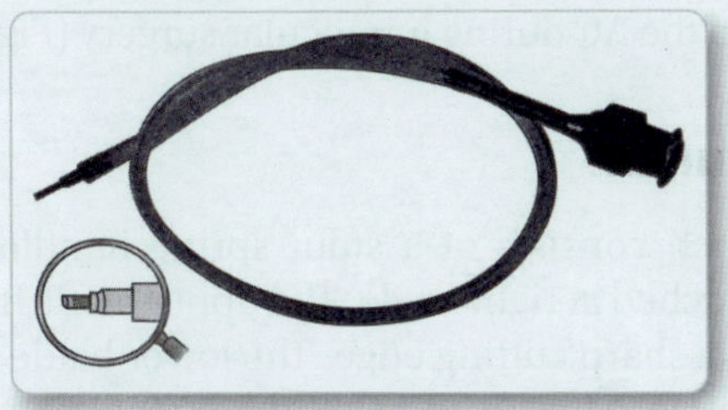

FIGURE 31.34: Anterior chamber (AC) maintainer and its tip

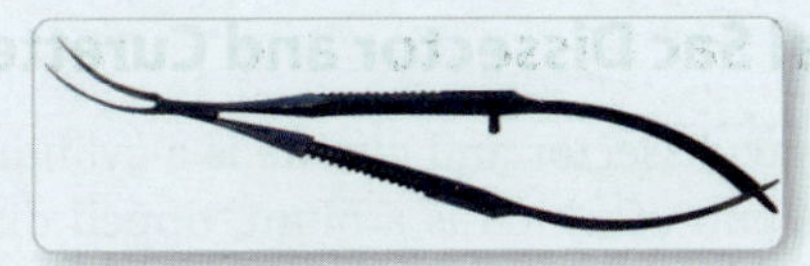

FIGURE 31.35: Intraocular lens (IOL) holding forcep

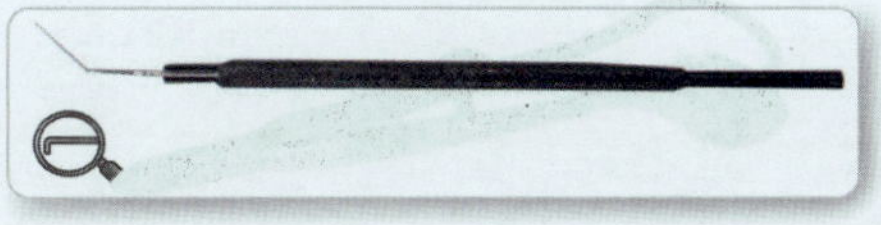

FIGURE 31.36: Intraocular lens (IOL) dialer and its tip

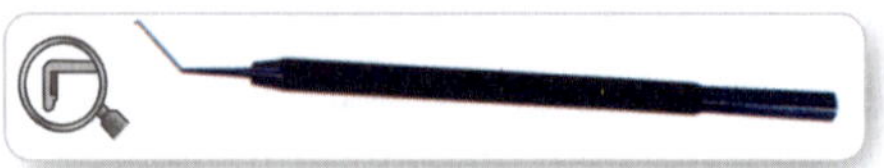

FIGURE 31.37: Chopper and its tip

Disadvantage

Operative field is less. Pressure necrosis can occur, if fitted tightly.

Ptosis Clamp

Ptosis clamp is like a forceps with J-shaped ends having internal serrations. The clamp has a locking mechanism. It is used to hold levator palpebrae superioris muscle during ptosis surgery (Fig. 31.41).

Muller's Self-retaining Hemostatic Lacrimal Retractor

Muller's self-retaining hemostatic lacrimal retractor is made up of two limbs with three curved pins on each for engaging the edges of the skin incision. The limbs are kept in a retracted position with the help of a fixing screw. It is used to retract the skin during surgery on the lacrimal sac (DCR or DCT) (Fig. 31.42).

Punctum Dilator (Nettleship)

The punctum dilator (Nettleship) has a cylindrical corrugated metal handle with a conical pointed tip. It is used in dilating the punctum and canaliculus during syringing, probing, dacryocystography, DCT and DCR procedures (Fig. 31.43).

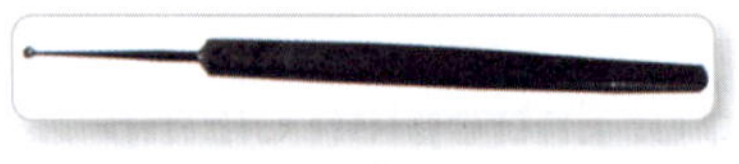

FIGURE 31.38: Chalazion scoop

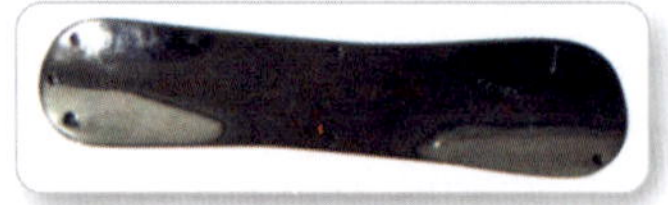

FIGURE 31.39: Lid spatula

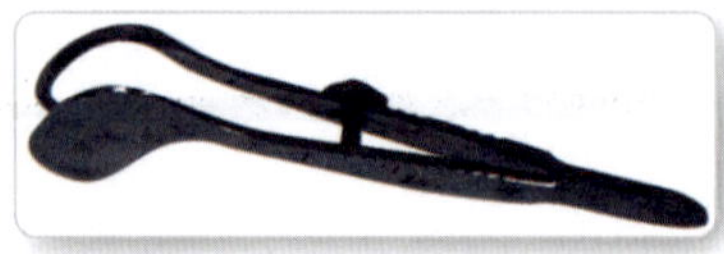

FIGURE 31.40: Entropion clamp

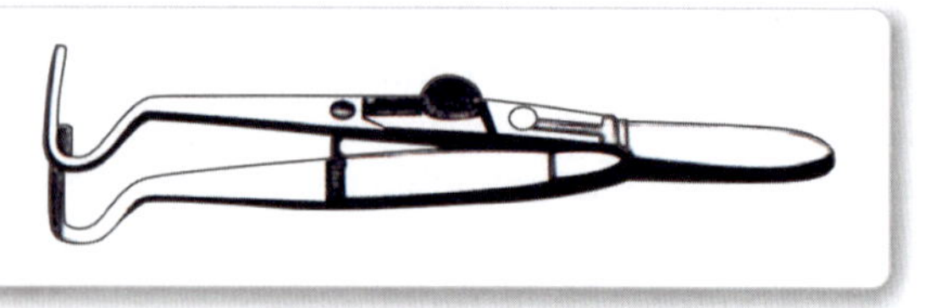

FIGURE 31.41: Ptosis clamp

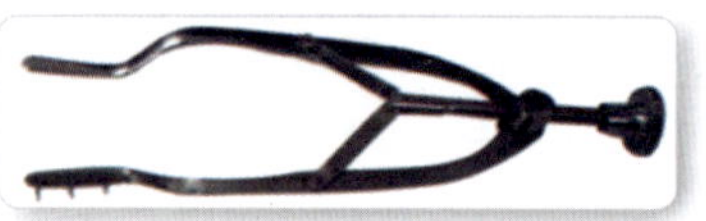

FIGURE 31.42: Muller's lacrimal retractor

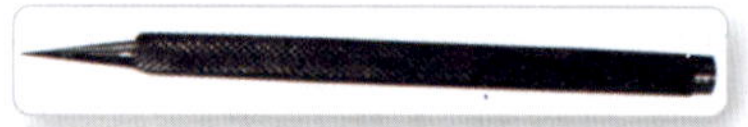

FIGURE 31.43: Nettleship's punctum dilator

Lacrimal Probes (Bowman)

Lacrimal probes (Bowman) are a set of straight metal wires of varying thickness with blunt, rounded ends and flattened central platform (Fig. 31.44).

Uses

- These are used to probe the nasolacrimal duct (NLD)
- In congenital NLD obstruction
- To identify lacrimal sac during DCT and DCR operations.

Lacrimal Cannula

Lacrimal cannula is a long, curved hypodermic needle with blunt tip. It is used for syringing the lacrimal passages. It can also be used as AC cannula for putting air or balanced salt solution in the AC during intraocular surgery (Fig. 31.45).

Bone Punch

Bone punch consists of a stout spring handle and two blades attached at right angle. The upper blade has a small hole with a sharp cutting edge. The lower blade has a cup like depression. It is used to cut the bones of the lacrimal fossa during DCR operation (Fig. 31.46).

Lacrimal Sac Dissector and Curette

Lacrimal sac dissector and curette is a cylindrical instrument, one end of which is a blunt, tipped dissector and the other end is curved. It is used in lacrimal sac surgery (Fig. 31.47).

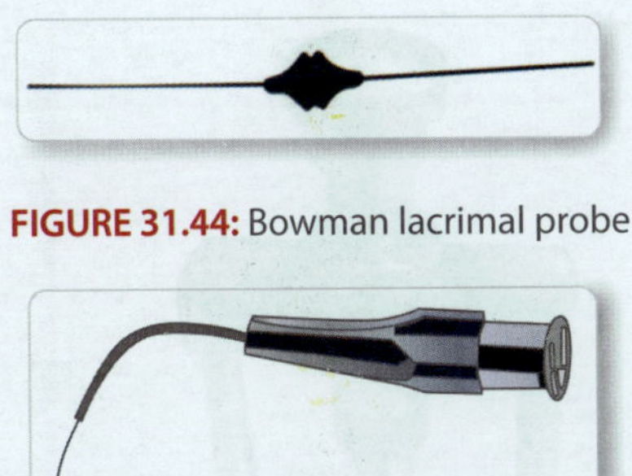

FIGURE 31.44: Bowman lacrimal probe

FIGURE 31.45: Lacrimal cannula

Optic Nerve Guard

Optic nerve guard is a spoon-shaped instrument with a central cleavage. It is used to engage the optic nerve during enucleation. The spoon is passed behind the eyeball. The optic nerve is engaged in the central cleavage of the spoon and it is lifted up. Then the enucleation scissor is passed from behind the spoon and the optic nerve is cut (Fig. 31.48).

Uses

Optic nerve guard is used to cut longer stump of optic nerve for enucleation of eyeball in retinoblastoma.

Evisceration Curette

Evisceration curette consists of an oval or rounded shallow cup with blunt margins attached to a stout handle. It is used to curette out the intraocular contents during evisceration operation (Fig. 31.49).

Castroviejo Corneal Trephines with Adjustable Stop

Castroviejo corneal trephines with adjustable stop are cylindrical in shape and have different sizes. It has got inner body and an outer shell, the circular end of which is sharp. There are marking on the inner body for adjusting the depth.

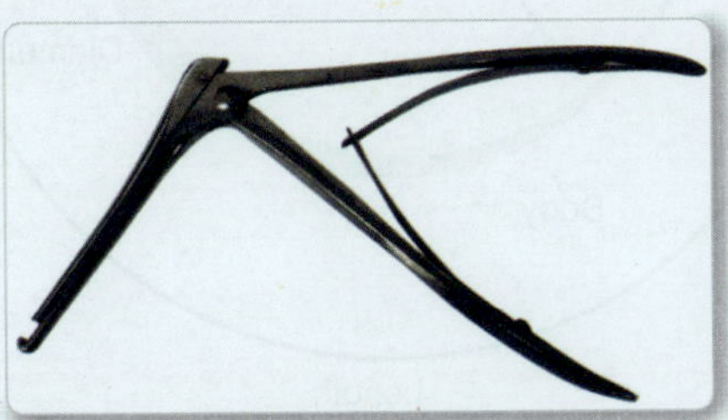

FIGURE 31.46: Bone punch

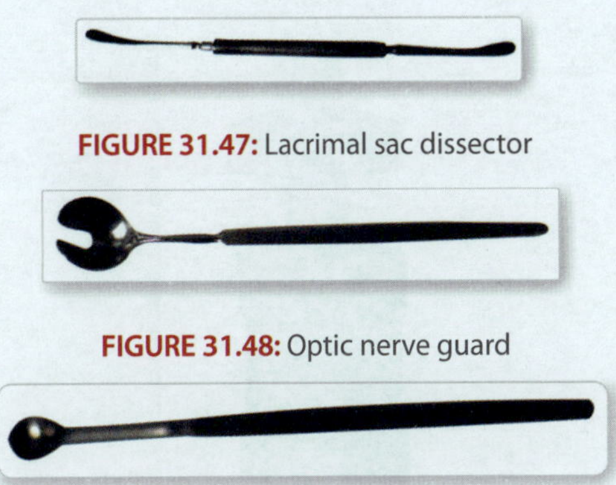

FIGURE 31.47: Lacrimal sac dissector

FIGURE 31.48: Optic nerve guard

FIGURE 31.49: Evisceration curette

The trephine is adjusted to the required depth in millimeter (mm) and the corneal button is made by rotating cutting motion of the trephine. After use of trephine the cutting end is withdrawn, so that it does not get damaged (Fig. 31.50).

Uses

Used for trephining the recipient and donor cornea in corneal grafting operation (keratoplasty).

Howard Punch

Howard punch is used with Howard universal trephine handle. The Howard punch has a self-aligning mechanism for easy insertion of Howard universal trephine handle. The base plug is Teflon block, which is used to support the donor corneoscleral rim (Fig. 31.51).

Tooke Corneal Knife

Tooke corneal knife is straight blade with curved cutting edge. Used for lamellar dissection on the cornea. It is a short blade with a semicircular blunt dissecting edge, which is beveled on both surfaces like a chisel (Fig. 31.52).

Uses

1. Used to separate corneal lamellae in lamellar keratoplasty.
2. To separate pterygium head or limbal dermoid from underlying corneal lamellae.
3. To separate partial thickness of lamellae of sclera during trabeculectomy.
4. To separate conjunctival and subconjunctival tissue from the sclera and limbus, when limbal-based flap is made for trab.

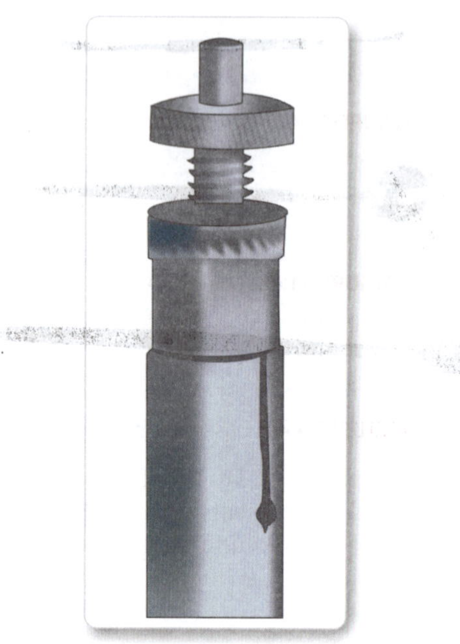

FIGURE 31.50: Castroviejo corneal trephine

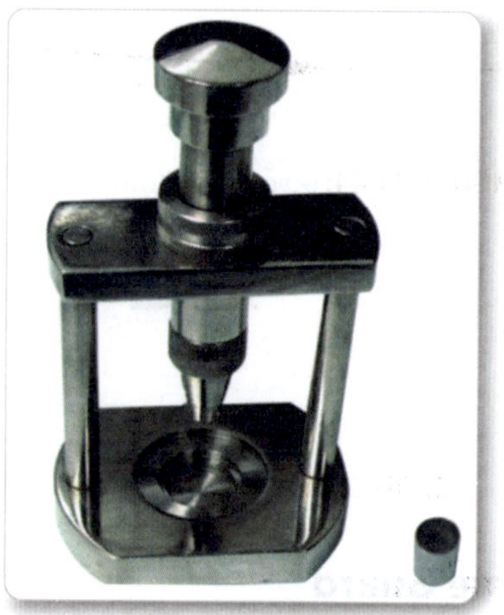

FIGURE 31.51: Howard punch and disposable trephine

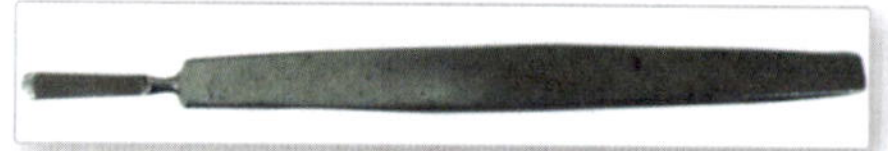

FIGURE 31.52: Tooke corneal knife

Needle and Sutures Used in Ophthalmology

Needles are made of stainless steel and come in many designs, each suited to specific purposes. Spatulating needles cut with both the tips and the sides and stay within a tissue plane. These are the most commonly used needles for corneoscleral, retinal and strabismus surgeries. Round bodied needles have a circular tapering point, which is relatively atraumatic and are preferred for conjunctival and iris suturing. Reverse cutting needles have a superior cutting edge and are used in procedure involving the skin. Needles are commercially available bonded to the sutures as atraumatic needles and are convenient to use.

For some procedures, such as application of surgical traction bridle sutures, fornix-forming sutures or for performing tarsorrhaphy, larger needles, which are reusable after sterilization and require to be threaded with silk or synthetic sutures or sterile cotton thread, can be used as an economic alternative.

Sutures used for extraocular and intraocular surgery can be of different materials and thickness. Gamma-irradiated sterile sutures are available as singular or double armed with one or two needles attached at each end, respectively. Sutures can be categorized as absorbable or non-absorbable, which can be relatively slowly biodegradable or permanent and can be available as a monofilament or braided. Silk and catgut are biologically-derived absorbable sutures, while Vicryl (polygalactin), which is a copolymer made from glycolide and L-lactide is a synthetic absorbable braided suture. Nylon, Mersilene, polypropylene and surgical stainless steel are synthetic, non-absorbable suture materials of which nylon slowly degrades with time and steel is truly permanent and non-biodegradable. The thickness of the sutures (Fig. 31.53) used, varies in a range from 4-0 to 5-0 thick sutures for extraocular surgery and fine 10-0 to 11-0 sutures for intraocular surgery.

Cautery

Episcleral and conjunctival blood vessels can be cauterized using electrically operated bipolar diathermy

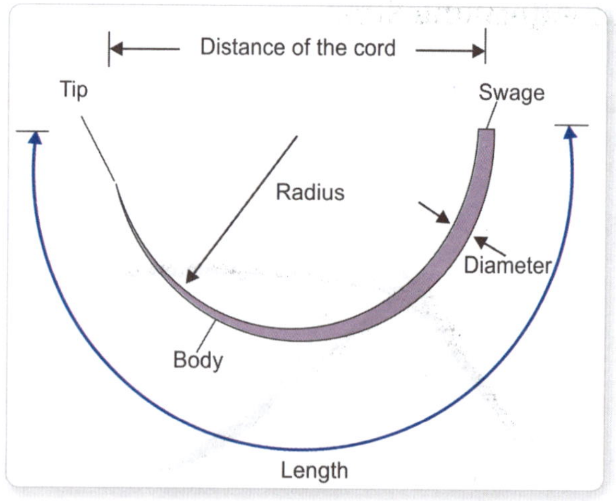

FIGURE 31.53: Needles and sutures used in ophthalmology

(electrocautery) or heat cautery. The probe used for bipolar cautery is designed to be used in a moist field and is called wet-field cautery. Heat cautery is applied by heating a heat cautery probe, which is made of stainless steel with a heat-retaining ball, which is made of copper. The instrument is simply heated with the ball held within the flame of a spirit lamp and the heat transmitted to the tip, achieves hemostasis on direct contact with the bleeding vessels. The copper ball helps to retain the heat for a longer time. The handle is so designed that the heat is not transmitted to the tip and achieves hemostasis on direct contact with the handle and vessels. The instrument can be reheated and reapplied as required.

Wet-field cautery allows controlled application of heat in a moist filed to coagulate bleeding vessels. Radio frequency cutter field cuts tissues and it is useful in tissue dissection and surgeries in vascular tissues like lids.

CONCLUSION

Since ophthalmic surgeries are fine microsurgical procedures, the instruments are delicate that need careful handling and cleaning to avoid damage and prolong their lifespan. They are cleaned with ultrasound cleaners to remove tissue debris and the tips are covered with silicon sleeves and packed in perforated trays lined with silicon sheets before sterilizing them in the autoclave.

Section 8

Pharmacology

Ocular Pharmacology

32

Girija Devi PS, Sunil

ANTIBACTERIALS

Antibacterials commonly used in ophthalmology are:

- Aminoglycosides
- Fluoroquinolones
- Chloramphenicol
- Cephalosporins
- Vancomycin.

Aminoglycosides

Aminoglycosides used in ophthalmology are:

- Gentamicin
- Tobramycin
- Amikacin.

Mechanism of Action

By binding to 30S ribosomal subunit of the bacteria, it inhibits its protein synthesis. They are active against aerobic gram-negative bacilli and *Staphylococcus aureus*. Gentamicin and tobramycin are available as 0.3% drops.

Both gentamicin and tobramycin can be used as fortified solutions in combination with cephalosporins for the treatment of severe corneal ulcers, especially those caused by *Pseudomonas*.

Side Effects

Corneal epithelial toxicity and pseudomembranous conjunctivitis are the adverse effects of topical fortified preparation. Nephrotoxicity and auditory or vestibular toxicity are the most serious adverse events and are characteristic of all the aminoglycosides.

Fluoroquinolones

Ciprofloxacin 0.3%, levofloxacin 0.5% and 1.5%, gatifloxacin 0.5%, ofloxacin 0.3% and moxifloxacin 0.5%.

Fluoroquinolones are bactericidal agents that act by inhibiting DNA replication. They are active against most gram-negative bacteria and some gram-positive bacteria and have good ocular penetration. Levofloxacin is the L-isomer of ofloxacin and has demonstrated increased activity against gram-positive bacteria, but less potent activity against *Pseudomonas aeruginosa* and certain enterobacteriaceae. Gatifloxacin and moxifloxacin are the most recently approved quinolones targeted both DNA gyrase and topoisomerase IV, but older generation fluoroquinolones target only DNA gyrase. Although all the quinolones have broad-spectrum activity, gatifloxacin and moxifloxacin have demonstrated enhanced activity against gram-positive organisms, especially *S. pneumoniae.* All quinolones are generally active against gram-negative rods such as *P. aeruginosa*. Gatifloxacin and moxifloxacin have increased activity against *S. aureus* and *S. epidermidis.* Bacterial resistance does not commonly develop during treatment with quinolones for ocular infections. Newer quinolones target two enzymes and so bacterial resistance develops slower with respect to newer quinolones. The quinolones are well absorbed after oral or intravenous administration. Ciprofloxacin, ofloxacin and gatifloxacin are available in 0.3% solution. Levofloxacin is available in both 0.5% and 1.5% solution, while moxifloxacin is available as 0.5% solution.

Chloramphenicol

Chloramphenicol is used as 1% applicaps or 0.5% eyedrops. The drug is a bacteriostatic agent that inhibits protein synthesis by binding reversibly to the peptidyl transferase component of 50S ribosomal subunit.

It is active against many gram-negative bacteria, *Chlamydia*, *Mycoplasma* and *Rickettsia*. *Pseudomonas* is usually resistant to chloramphenicol. It has good ocular penetration on topical application, but it is not systemically absorbed in any significant amount when applied topically.

But orally administered chloramphenicol is significantly absorbed. It is effective in bacterial conjunctivitis.

Adverse effects are dose-related bone marrow suppression and idiosyncratic aplastic anemia.

Cephalosporins

Cephalosporins are mainly used as fortified drops prepared from injection (50 mg/mL) in bacterial corneal ulcers. It can be given as intravitreal injection (2.25 mg/0.1 mL) in endophthalmitis. Topical preparations are not available commercially. Fortified drops are prepared by dilution in artificial tear drops. It should be used with caution in patients with history of allergic reaction to penicillins.

Ceftriaxone and Ceftazidime

Main use in ophthalmology is to give intravitreal injection in endophthalmitis (2 mg in 0.1 mL). It is repeated after 48 hours. It can be given parenterally in panophthalmitis and also as surgical prophylaxis in high-risk patients like those with valvular heart disease.

Vancomycin

Vancomycin is used in endophthalmitis (1 mg in 0.1 mL as intravitreal injection) by reconstituting from parenteral preparation or in severe corneal ulcers (50 mg/mL).

ANTIFUNGAL AGENTS

The major classes of antifungal agents used in ophthalmology are:
- Polyenes
- Imidazoles
- Pyrimidines.

Polyenes

Polyene antibiotics are produced from *Streptomyces* species. Polyenes have the ability to bind to mammalian cell membrane cholesterol (ergosterol).

Mechanism of Action

There are two mechanisms of action for polyene antibiotics. Short-chain polyenes bind to sterols in the fungal cell wall, forming blisters and causing lysis of the cell wall. This is a concentration-dependent action. Long-chain polyenes act by producing pores in the cell wall allowing small ions such as potassium to leak out causing imbalance in the osmotic gradient and lead on to cell lysis.

Types

Polyenes are classified into two groups:
1. Short-chain polyenes, e.g. Natamycin.
2. Long-chain polyenes, e.g. Amphotericin B.

Natamycin: For ophthalmic purpose 5% suspension is used. It has decreased penetration through intact epithelium, so repeated surface debridement may be necessary in the treatment of fungal corneal ulcer. It has broad spectrum of sensitivity and is the drug of choice in infections by *Fusarium* species. Subconjunctival and intravitreal administration are not recommended because of significant toxicity. Intravenous administration does not render significant levels in the eye.

Amphotericin B: It is more effective against yeasts than filamentous fungi.

Uses

1. Topical concentration of 2.5–10 mg/mL given every 30–60 minutes for the first 48–72 hours appears to deliver the optimal dose. This concentration is achieved by mixing the powdered amphotericin with sterile water. This should be stored in a dark bottle and refrigerated to maintain drug stability.
2. Intravitreal injection of 5 μg of amphotericin in 0.1 mL is used in endophthalmitis.
3. Intravenous amphotericin is given in orbital mucormycosis and fungal endophthalmitis. For intravenous use, test dose of 1 mg of amphotericin in 150 mL of 5% dextrose is given. Once the test dose is tolerated, 1–5 mg is given over 4–6 hours as an IV infusion.
4. The dose is increased daily until the desired dose of 0.5–1 kg/day is reached.

Side Effects

Hypokalemia and nephrotoxicity are the side effects.

Azoles

Most common azoles are imidazoles and triazoles. Imidazoles are mainly clotrimazole, miconazole, ketoconazole, thiabendazole and econazole. But triazoles are more commonly used for topical application.

Triazoles

The triazoles are fluconazole 0.3%, itraconazole 1% eye ointment and voriconazole 1% drops. Triazoles have wide spectrum of activity compared to imidazoles.

Voriconazole: In fungal endophthalmitis and orbital fungal infections, 200–400 mg bd is given. Now voriconazole drops are used in the management of resistant fungal corneal ulcers and they can also be given as intrastromal injections around the ulcer in resistant deep infections.

Fluconazole: It is the most widely used member of the triazoles. It has been used in the treatment of *Candida* species. It can penetrate intact corneal epithelium due to its lower molecular weight. Oral fluconazole is given in the dose of 200 mg/day. Topical 1% solution in sterile water can be prepared. Triazoles have wide spectrum of activity compared to imidazoles.

Itraconazole: It has a wider spectrum of activity than the imidazoles. It is effective against *Candida* and *Aspergillus*. Itraconazole has been used in its oral preparation as an adult dose of 200 mg/day.

Pyrimidines

Main drug in pyrimidines is flucytosine. Flucytosine (FC) is a fluorinated pyrimidine that might alter fungal RNA and DNA synthesis. It enters the cytoplasm by the action of cytosine permease and is then deaminated by cytosine deaminase into 5-fluorouracil (5-Fu). It is then phosphorylated and incorporated into uracil. In the nucleus, 5-Fu forms 5-fluoro-2′-deoxy uridylic acid (FdUMP), which inhibits thymidylate synthetase and thus, DNA synthesis.

ANTIVIRAL DRUGS

The DNA virus consists of a DNA core surrounded by a protein capsid coat and lipid envelope. After entering into the host cell, virus loses its lipid coat and passes into the cell nucleus. Therapy for intracellular DNA virus is based primarily on disruption of viral DNA synthesis. Most of the antiviral agents are activated by their phosphorylation by virus-specific thymidine kinase. The more specific activation by viral thymidine kinase, the less toxicity the agent will possess.

The commonly used agents are idoxuridine (IDU), vidarabine, trifluorothymidine, acyclovir, ganciclovir and foscarnet. But the most commonly used agent is acyclovir.

Acyclovir

Acyclovir is an acyclic nucleoside analog of guanosine. It has excellent antiviral activity against herpes virus. It is the only antiviral agent that can be administered intravenously, orally and topically.

Mechanism of Action

Mechanism of action has got selectivity for cells infected with HSV. It is due to two herpes specific enzymes, which are thymidine kinase and DNA polymerase. Acyclovir is selectively phosphorylated by herpes thymidine kinase to a monophosphate form. Cellular enzymes then convert acyclovir monophosphate to acyclovir diphosphate and acyclovir triphosphate. This compound has a greater affinity for viral DNA polymerase than for cellular DNA polymerase.

It is a relatively safe drug. It is not effective against adenovirus, but effective against both herpes simplex and herpes zoster. Oral acyclovir is a useful alternative for patients suffering from topical ocular toxicity of trifluridine or IDU and can lower the incidence of herpetic keratitis. Oral or intravenous acyclovir is effective for therapy for herpes zoster ophthalmicus (HZO). Cytomegalovirus (CMV) is relatively insensitive to acyclovir.

Acyclovir is used as 3% ointment applied five times daily. Oral dose is 1 g/day in five divided doses for 10 days.

Indications for Topical Use

- Patients with primary herpetic keratitis, dendritic keratitis
- Herpes zoster ophthalmicus
- Herpetic keratitis and blepharitis.

Indications for Systemic Use

- Herpes simplex virus (HSV) or HZO in immunosuppressed patients
- Patients undergone keratoplasty for herpetic keratitis
- Acute retinal necrosis.

Ganciclovir

Ganciclovir is structurally related to acyclovir. The active form of this drug inhibits viral replication. It is a triphosphate like acyclovir. It is given intravenously because of its poor absorption from the gastrointestinal tract. The dose is 5 mg/kg IV in constant rate over a period of 1 hour and it has to be repeated every 12 hours. Its use in patients with renal impairment may cause toxicity. It is used in the treatment of CMV retinitis.

Idoxuridine

Idoxuridine is an analog of thymidine, which is metabolized by the normal enzymatic pathways of pyrimidine. It is used as 1% solution in herpetic keratitis.

Side Effects

Superficial punctate keratopathy, indolent ulceration, delayed epithelial healing and superficial stromal opacification. Since safer drugs are now available, its use is now limited.

Vidarabine

Vidarabine is useful for HSV epithelial keratitis in patients who are allergic to IDU and trifluridine. It is used as 3% topical ointment.

Trifluorothymidine

Trifluorothymidine is a drug of choice for the HSV keratitis. Mostly active in virus-infected cells, but slightly affects the metabolism of normal cells also. Topical preparation is 1% solution.

Foscarnet

Foscarnet can halt the progression of CMV retinitis in more than 80% of immunocompromised patients and appears to be as effective as ganciclovir.

Indications

- Acyclovir-resistant HSV and HZO infections
- Ganciclovir-resistant CMV retinitis
- CMV retinitis is most commonly seen in HIV patients.

Dose: 60 mg/kg body weight IV at constant rate 8 hourly for 2–3 weeks.

NSAIDs IN OPHTHALMOLOGY

Common non-steroidal anti-inflammatory drugs (NSAIDs) in use are given below:

1. Bromfenac (0.09% bd) for 2–3 weeks following surgery:
   a. Prescription of postoperative inflammation and pain following cataract surgery.
2. Nepafenac (0.1% bd dosage):
   a. Prescription of postoperative pain and inflammation following cataract surgery.
   b. For macular edema in diabetic retinopathy and wet age-related macular degeneration (ARMD).
3. Diclofenac (0.1%):
   a. Inhibition of perioperative miosis during cataract surgery.
   b. Treatment of postoperative inflammation in cataract surgery, squint surgery.
   c. Management of pain, photophobia following excimer photorefractive keratectomy (PRK) surgery, laser-assisted in situ keratomileusis (LASIK), argon laser trabeculoplasty.
   d. In seasonal allergic conjunctivitis.
4. Flurbiprofen (0.03%):
   a. Inhibition of intraoperative miosis.
   b. Management of pseudophakic cystoid macular edema (CME).
5. Ketorolac (0.5%):
   a. Treatment of postoperative inflammation following ocular surgery.
   b. Treatment of postoperative CME.
   c. In seasonal allergic conjunctivitis.
   d. Inflamed pterygium.

Contraindications

If hypersensitivity to any ingredients:

1. In dendritic keratitis, flurbiprofen is avoided.
2. In patients with known hemostatic defects or who are receiving medications, which prolong bleeding time.
3. Intraocular use during surgical procedures.
4. Cross-sensitivity to acetylsalicylic acid and other NSAIDs.

Diclofenac and Nepafenac are contraindicated in the following situations:

1. Patients in whom attacks of asthma, urticaria or acute rhinitis are precipitated by acetylsalicylic acid or by other drugs with prostaglandin-inhibiting activity.
2. Intraocular use during surgery.

Ketorolac is inhibited during pregnancy, labor, delivery or in mothers who are breastfeeding.

Adverse Reactions

1. Foreign body (FB) sensation, redness, eye pain, pruritus, burning, stinging.
2. In diclofenac, blurred vision soon after instillation of drops.
3. Punctate keratitis or corneal disorders.
4. Urticaria, eczema, rash, cough, rhinitis, etc. are noted.

Ketorolac

- Superficial punctate keratitis, eye pain, lid edema
- Transient blurring of vision may occur on instillation of eyedrops.

Nepafenac

- Eyelid crusting, FB sensation, dry eye
- Iritis, keratitis, corneal deposits, allergic conjunctivitis, headache, nausea, dry mouth.

STEROIDS IN OPHTHALMOLOGY

Steroids were first introduced in ocular therapy by Gordon and McLean.

Mechanism of Action

1. Has action on nearly every aspect of the immune system.
2. Inhibits migration of neutrophils into the extracellular space and their adherence to the vascular endothelium at the site of injury.
3. Inhibits macrophage access to the site of inflammation.
4. Interferes with lymphocyte activity.
5. Decreases the number of T lymphocytes.
6. Inhibits histamine release.
7. Inhibits phospholipase A_2, which prevents biosynthesis of arachidonic acid and subsequent formation of prostacyclin, thromboxane A, prostaglandins and leukotrienes.
8. Decreases capillary permeability, fibroblast proliferation and quality of collagen deposition, thereby influencing tissue regeneration and repair.

Bioavailability of Topical Steroids

1. Acetate and alcohol derivatives are more lipophilic or fat soluble; so they penetrate intact cornea better than the water-soluble phosphates.
2. Phosphates and hydrochlorides are more water soluble. So they are available as drops.

Therapeutic Principles

1. Specific type and location of inflammation determines whether topical or periocular or systemic route is needed.
2. First dose should be given as early as possible and should be a high dose to suppress the inflammatory response.
3. Long-term, high-dose therapy should not be discontinued abruptly; it should be reduced over time.
4. Short-term, low-dosage topical steroids does not produce significant side effects.

Systemic Effects of Corticosteroid Therapy

- Adrenal insufficiency
- Cushing's syndrome
- Peptic ulceration
- Osteoporosis
- Hypertension
- Muscle weakness/atrophy
- Inhibition of growth
- Dermatomyositis
- Activation of infection
- Mood changes
- Delay in wound healing.

Indications

Eyelids

- Allergic blepharitis
- Contact dermatitis
- Herpes zoster dermatoblepharitis
- Chemical burns
- Neonatal hemangioma.

Conjunctiva

- Allergic conjunctivitis
- Vernal conjunctivitis
- Herpes zoster conjunctivitis
- Chemical burns
- Mucocutaneous conjunctival lesions.

Cornea

- Immune reaction after keratoplasty
- Herpes zoster keratitis
- Disciform keratitis
- Marginal keratitis
- Superficial punctate keratitis
- Chemical burns
- Acne rosacea keratitis
- Interstitial keratitis.

Uvea

- Anterior uveitis
- Posterior uveitis
- Sympathetic ophthalmia.

Sclera

- Scleritis
- Episcleritis.

Retina

- Retinal vasculitis
- Retinochoroiditis.

Optic Nerve

- Optic neuritis
- Temporal arteritis.

Globe

- Endophthalmitis
- Hemorrhagic glaucoma.

Orbit

- Pseudotumor
- Graves ophthalmopathy.

Extraocular Muscles

Ocular myasthenia gravis.

Ocular Side Effects of Corticosteroids

- Posterior subcapsular cataract
- Ocular hypertension or glaucoma
- Secondary ocular infection
- Retardation of corneal epithelial healing
- Keratitis
- Corneal thinning or melting
- Scleral thinning
- Uveitis
- Mydriasis
- Ptosis
- Transient ocular discomfort.

Absolute Contraindications

- Peptic ulcer
- Osteoporosis
- Psychosis.

Caution

- Diabetes mellitus
- Infectious diseases, especially active tuberculosis (TB)
- Chronic renal failure
- Congestive cardiac failure
- Hypertension
- Glaucoma.

Drug Interactions

- Barbiturates
- Phenylbutazone
- Phenytoin
- Anticoagulants.

COMMON ANTIGLAUCOMA MEDICINES

Common antiglaucoma drugs can be grouped as follows (common drugs used in the treatment of eye diseases are enlisted in Table 32.1):

TABLE 32.1: Common drugs

Name	Derivative	Formulation	Concentration (%)
Prednisolone	Acetate	Suspension	0.125
Prednisolone	Acetate	Suspension	1.0
Prednisolone	Sodium phosphate	Solution	0.125
Dexamethasone	Alcohol	Suspension	0.1
Dexamethasone	Sodium phosphate	Solution	0.1
Dexamethasone	Sodium phosphate	Ointment	0.05
Loteprednol	Etabonate	Suspension	0.5
Loteprednol	Etabonate	Suspension	0.2
Rimexolone	Etabonate	Suspension	0.5
Fluorometholone	Alcohol	Ointment	0.2
Fluorometholone	Acetate	Suspension	1.0
Fluorometholone	Acetate	Suspension	0.1
Medrysone	Alcohol	Suspension	1.0

1. Carbonic anhydrase inhibitors, e.g. acetazolamide.
2. Hyperosmotic agents, e.g. mannitol, glycerol.
3. Beta blockers, e.g. timolol maleate.
4. Parasympathomimetic drugs, e.g. pilocarpine.
5. Prostaglandin analog, e.g. latanoprost.
6. Adrenergic agonist.

Newer classification is:

1. Drugs increasing the aqueous outflow.
2. Drugs reducing aqueous production.

Carbonic Anhydrase Inhibitors

Carbonic anhydrase inhibitors belong to the sulfonamide group. The drugs in this group are:

1. Acetazolamide—most commonly used drug systemically to bring down intraocular pressure (IOP).
2. Methazolamide (mostly used as topical application).
3. Ethoxzolamide (mostly used as topical application).
4. Dorzolamide (mostly used as topical application).

Mechanism of Action

Carbonic anhydrase inhibitors decrease aqueous production by inhibiting the carbonic anhydrase enzyme. Carbonic anhydrase inhibitors contain free sulfonamide, which competes with the bicarbonate ion in binding to the enzyme carbonic anhydrase. This blocks the bicarbonate synthesis and the sodium movement is directly linked to bicarbonate synthesis. Thus aqueous production is decreased.

Acetazolamide

Dose: Action starts 2 hours after administration and lasts for 6 hours. 250 mg qid.

Indications: For quick reduction of high IOP in an attack of acute congestive glaucoma, preoperatively in trabeculectomy or cataract surgery, as an interim measure when IOP is not controlled by topical medications alone and there is a delay for surgery and in cystoid macular edema with pigment epithelial detachment (PED).

Side effects: Metabolic acidosis and hypokalemia leading to fatigue, malaise; paresthesia gastrointestinal tract (GIT) disturbances; renal calculi; thrombocytopenia, aplastic anemia and Stevens-Johnson (SJ) syndrome (hence the drug should be given with caution in people with allergy to sulfa drugs).

Contraindicated in severe renal or hepatic impairment; renal calculi, in metabolic acidosis and sulfonamide hypersensitivity.

Topical Carbonic Anhydrase Inhibitors

- Dorzolamide: 2% drops
- Brinzolamide: 1% drops
- Acetazolamide drops.

They are administered two to three times daily and they reduce IOP by reducing aqueous production.

Side effects of topical carbonic anhydrase (CA) inhibitors include burning, stinging, superficial punctate keratitis, etc.

Hyperosmotic Agents

Hyperosmotic agents are used systemically for immediate control of IOP.

Mechanism of Action

Hyperosmotic agents increase plasma osmolarity and draw fluid from the eye, mainly vitreous, thus decreasing the vitreous volume and reducing the IOP. The available drugs are mannitol, glycerin and isosorbide.

Drugs in Clinical Use

Mannitol: Available as 5%–25% solution. Dosage is 1–2 g/kg body weight given as a fast drip in 20–30 minutes.

Indications: Acute congestive attacks, preoperatively and intraoperatively to bring down the increased IOP quickly.

In any case of primary or secondary glaucoma, when acetazolamide and topical medications are not able to control the high IOP.

Adverse reactions: Systemic hypertension, vomiting, congestive cardiac failure, pulmonary edema and confusion.

Contraindicated: In oliguria and anuria. To be used with caution in hypertensive and cardiac patients.

Glycerine: A drink given with 50% glycerine flavored with lime juice, at the dose of 1–2 g/kg body weight.

Side effects: Nausea and vomiting, it can elevate blood sugar levels in diabetic patients since glycerine is metabolized to glucose.

Isosorbide: Available as 45% flavored solution and dose is 1–2 g/kg of body weight.

Beta Blockers

Topical β-adrenergic antagonists are the most frequently used hypotensive agents. These agents do not produce any unwanted side effects like intense miosis and myopic shift like parasympathomimetic drugs.

Mechanism of Action

Fluorophotometric studies indicate that beta blockers reduce the aqueous humor formation by antagonizing the effect of circulating catecholamines on the β2 receptors in the ciliary epithelium. Inhibition of β activation results in inactivation of chloride pump consequently reducing the aqueous production and IOP.

Timolol Maleate

Timolol is a non-selective adrenergic antagonist. It reduces the IOP in normal and glaucomatous eyes without changing pupillary size, accommodation and visual acuity. It binds to melanin, but not metabolized by ocular tissues.

Dosage: About 0.25% or 0.5% drops twice daily.

Pharmacodynamics: It penetrates eye rapidly and IOP begins to fall in 30–60 minutes; the duration of action lasts up to 24–48 hours.

Short-term escape and long-term drift: After initial administration of the drug, 90% of the patients respond well and IOP falls by 40%. But this effect diminishes over days or few weeks. This is known as 'short-term escape'. It is probably due to possible increase in the number of β receptors in ciliary process.

After the initial adjustment process, most patients maintain a reduction in IOP for month to years. Then 10%–20% of patients show some loss of drug effect known as 'long-term drift', possibly due to a time-dependent decrease in sensitivity to adrenergic antagonists.

Side Effects

- Stinging and burning sensations in eye
- Dryness of eyes
- Allergic blepharoconjunctivitis (levobunolol)
- Corneal hypoesthesia
- Blurred vision
- Superficial punctate keratitis
- Conjunctival hyperemia
- Hypotony.

Systemic side effects: Systemic absorption of drugs (non-selective beta blockers) can cause the following:

- Bronchospasm in asthmatics
- Bradycardia
- Accentuation of heart block and congestive heart failure (CHF) in elderly. So, Timolol maleate should be avoided in patients with bronchial asthma, heart block or heart failure.

Other Beta Blockers

- Betaxolol (selective β1 blocker): Safer in asthmatics, 0.5% bd dosage
- Levobunolol (non-selective β1 and β2 blockers) 0.5% od dosage
- Carteolol (β1 + β2 + intrinsic sympathomimetic activity) 1%–2% od dosage. It causes less bradycardia and so safer in patients with heart block.

Parasympathomimetic Drugs

Pharmacology

Parasympathomimetic agent directly act as cholinergic agonist with dominant action at both peripheral and central muscarinic sites acts on muscarinic acetylcholine receptor M3. The response of intraocular smooth muscle to pilocarpine is pupillary constriction, spasm of accommodation and reduction of IOP.

Preparations and Dose

The concentration and frequency of administration of pilocarpine is detailed in Table 32.2.

TABLE 32.2: Concentration and frequency of administration of pilocarpine

Generic name	Concentration (%)	Frequency
Pilocarpine hydrochloride solution	0.5, 1, 2, 4, 6	qid
Pilocarpine nitrate	0.5, 1, 2, 4, 6	qid
Pilocarpine gel	4	od (at bedtime)
Oral pilocarpine (Salagen)	5 mg, 7.5 mg tablets	

Duration of Action and Half-life

Ocular hypotensive effect last for 4–6 hours. Half-life is 0.76 hour (5 mg).

Pilocarpine

An alkaloid of plant origin derived from leaves of shrub of genus *Pilocarpus microphyllus.*

Therapeutic uses of topical pilocarpine: It is used for both open- and closed-angle glaucoma.

Open-angle glaucoma: In open-angle glaucoma, the cholinergic agents reduce the IOP by increasing the outflow facility. Pilocarpine stimulates the ciliary muscle, putting traction on the scleral spur and the trabecular meshwork, separating the trabecular sheets and the Schlemm's canal is kept open and the fluid outflow is improved.

Angle-closure glaucoma: Pilocarpine constricts the pupil, tighten the iris, decrease the volume of iris tissue at the angle and pull the iris periphery away from trabecular tissue. These changes open up the angle and reduce the IOP by allowing aqueous humor to reach the outflow channels. In acute angle closure, the pressure has to be brought down to 50 mm Hg for pilocarpine to act as the ischemic iris sphincter is unresponsive to pilocarpine.

Therapeutic use of oral pilocarpine: Oral pilocarpine improves the radiotherapy-induced dry eye symptoms and also in Sjögren's syndrome by increasing the aqueous tears production through the muscarinic secretagogue effect.

Diagnostic Uses

- Adie's pupil cholinergic hypersensitivity tested by using pilocarpine 0.0625%, 0.1%, 0.125% or 0.25%
- Neurogenic (III cranial nerve) and anticholinergic pupillary paralysis: In III nerve palsy, pilocarpine (0.5%–1%) act on the intact muscarinic receptors and cause pupillary constriction; helps to distinguish between the two.

Adverse Effects

Ocular side effects: As follows:

- Periocular pain
- Orbicularis muscle spasm and lid twitching
- Conjunctival hyperemia
- Allergic blepharoconjunctivitis
- Punctal stenosis
- Corneal vascularization and epithelial staining
- Atypical band keratopathy
- Iris hyperemia, pigment epithelial cyst formation
- Ciliary muscle spasm
- Postoperative iritis and posterior synechiae
- Anterior subcapsular cataract
- Retinal hole, retinal detachment, vitreous hemorrhage
- Pupillary block with secondary angle-closure glaucoma.

Systemic side effects: As follows:

- Headache, brow ache
- Marked salivation
- Profuse perspiration
- Nausea and vomiting
- Bronchospasm
- Pulmonary edema
- Systemic hypotension
- Bradycardia
- Generalized muscular weakness
- Increased tone and motility of GIT.

Contraindications

- Presence of cataract
- Patients younger than 40 years of age
- Neovascular and uveitic glaucoma
- History of retinal detachment
- Bronchial asthma.

Prostaglandin Analogs

Prostaglandin analogs are a class of drugs similar in structure and function to prostaglandins. Prostaglandin analogs are:

- Bimatoprost
- Latanoprost
- Travoprost
- Unoprostone.

Mechanism of Action

Prostaglandin analogs reduce IOP by increasing the removal of aqueous humor from the eye through the uveoscleral route.

Uses

In glaucoma treatment for reducing IOP (lower IOP by 20%–30%). It can be used as a first-line drug in the management of primary open-angle glaucoma.

Side Effects

- Blurred vision
- Dry eye
- Itching
- Burning
- Stinging
- Increased coloring of iris
- Increased growth of eyelashes
- Periocular skin pigmentation
- Allergic skin reactions
- Cystoid macular edema.

Contraindications

- Infections in eye
- Inflammation in eye
- Pregnancy
- Breastfeeding.

Adrenergic Agonists

Drugs

- Epinephrine
- Dipivefrin

- Apraclonidine
- Brimonidine.

Epinephrine: Direct action on both α- and β-adrenergic receptors.

Mechanism of action: Increases aqueous outflow. Available as 0.5%, 1% and 2% drops. Applied bd.

Dipivefrine: It is a prodrug of epinephrine. It is converted to epinephrine in the body after absorption. Mechanism of action is same as epinephrine.

Side effects: Are as follows:

- Itching, burning and hyperemia
- Tearing and punctal occlusion
- Adrenochrome deposits on palpebral conjunctiva
- Madarosis
- Epinephrine maculopathy.

Side effects are less with the prodrug dipivefrin.

Apraclonidine: It is an α-adrenergic agonist and reduces IOP by decreasing aqueous production. It is available as 1% and 2% drops.

Uses: It is mainly used for treating transient rise in IOP as in postlaser or postiridotomy spikes. It is also used for treating open-angle glaucoma.

Brimonodine 1% solution: It is an α-2 adrenergic agonist, which decreases aqueous production by the ciliary body as well as increase the uveoscleral outflow.

Dosage: Applied three times daily.

Side effects: Allergic conjunctivitis, drowsiness, hypotension.

Contraindicated in children below 2 years.

ANTIHISTAMINES AND MAST CELL STABILIZERS

Antihistamines and mast cell stabilizers are mainly indicated in seasonal and perennial allergic conjunctivitis. The commonly available drugs are:

1. Azelastine 0.05% drops bd:
    a. It is a H_1 histamine receptor blocker.
    b. Not to be used in children below 4 years and contact lens users.
2. Ketotifen 0.025% drops bd or tid:
    a. It is a selective H_1 receptor antagonistic.
    b. Not to be used in children below 3 years and pregnant and lactating mothers.
3. Olopatadine 0.1% drops od or bd:
    a. Selective H_1 receptor antagonist as well as mast cell suppressant.
    b. Not to be used in children below 3 years, and pregnant and lactating mothers.
4. Epinastine 0.05% drops od or bd:
    a. Selective H_1 receptor antagonist as well as mast cell suppressant.
5. Chlorpheniramine maleate 0.1% or 0.2% drops:
    a. H_1 receptor antagonist and α adrenergic agonist, used four times daily, usually used in combination with decongestants like phenylephrine or naphazoline.

Mast Cell Stabilizers

Sodium Cromoglycate

Dosage: About 2%–4% drops used bd or tid. It inhibits degranulation of sensitized mast cells.

Indications

Vernal keratoconjunctivitis and atopic allergic conjunctivitis.

MYDRIATICS, CYCLOPLEGICS AND MIOTICS

Atropine

Atropine is a naturally occurring alkaloid obtained from the plant belladonna. It is the strongest and longest lasting mydriatic and cycloplegic. Available as 1% ointment and drops.

Maximum mydriasis is obtained in 45 minutes and the mydriatic effect lasts for 7–10 days and the cycloplegia for 10–12 days. The action is slow to start and takes longer to wear off in pigmented eyes. So in pigmented eyes both actions can last up to 3 weeks.

Uses

1. In the treatment of uveitis and corneal ulcers.
2. For refraction in children below 7 years and in older children suspected to have latent hypermetropia and accommodative esotropia.
3. In the treatment of amblyopia by 'penalization'.

Side Effects

1. Irritation of the eyes and allergic reaction.
2. Photophobia and blurring of near vision due to its pharmacological action.
3. Risk of angle-closure glaucoma in persons with occludable angles.

Systemic side effects: As follows:

1. Dryness of mouth.
2. Pyrexia and flushing of the skin in infants. To be used with extreme caution in children below 2 years. To lessen systemic absorption and side effects only ointment should be used in children below 7 years. If at all drops have to be used, punctum should be closed with finger pressure for 1 minute and only a single drop be applied.
3. Frequent use in elderly males with prostatic hypertrophy can lead to acute urinary retention.
4. Delusions, confusion (atropine psychosis) and convulsions can occur as central nervous system (CNS) side effects with atropine overuse.

Homatropine

Homatropine is less potent and shorter acting than atropine. Available as 2% drops.

Mydriasis is obtained in 40–60 minutes and the effect lasts for up to 3 days. Cycloplegia may at times last longer, up to 1 week.

Cyclopentolate

Available as 0.5% and 1% drops. Mydriasis and cycloplegia are maximum after 30–45 minutes and lasts for 1 day.

Its cycloplegic action is stronger than that of homatropine and the duration of action is shorter. So it is ideal for doing refraction in children.

Tropicamide

Tropicamide is a non-selective muscarinic antagonist. Available as 1% solution and also in combination with phenylephrine.

Faster onset and shorter duration of mydriasis, and minimal cycloplegic action makes it an ideal drug for dilatation of the pupil for fundus examination and also for preoperative dilatation before cataract surgery.

For both purposes it is usually used in combination with phenylephrine to obtain maximum mydriasis.

Phenylephrine

Phenylephrine is a synthetic sympathomimetic drug, which acts primarily on α1 receptors.

Topical application leads to contraction of the dilator muscle and blanching of conjunctival blood vessels. Since the sphincter muscle is not affected and being a stronger muscle than dilator, the dilated pupil will constrict on throwing light into the eye. So the pupil will remain mobile and at the same time dilated, and this is supposed to prevent formation of posterior synechiae. Hence preferred by many ophthalmologists for treatment of uveitis and for use in the postoperative period.

Available as 2.5% and 10% drops, and also in combination with tropicamide.

Uses

1. For preoperative dilatation of pupil usually in combination with tropicamide.
2. Treatment of uveitis.
3. To improve vision in patients with cataract by mydriasis.
4. As a diagnostic test in Horner's syndrome.

Side Effects

- Allergic conjunctivitis
- Release of pigment granules into aqueous
- Rebound miosis and congestion.

Systemic side effects: As follows:

- Systolic hypertension and ventricular arrhythmias
- Hence to be used with caution in patients with hypertension and cardiac problems
- Blanching of skin.

ARTIFICIAL TEARS

Artificial tears are drops used to increase the lubrication and comfort of the eyes in various ocular surface disorders. They can be preservative-free or those with added preservatives like benzalkonium chloride and chlorobutanol. Since preservatives are toxic to the eyes, preservative-free tear substitutes are preferred, but they are costlier.

Indications

- Dry eye conditions
- Blepharitis and meibomianitis
- Irritant conjunctivitis
- Contact lens wearers
- Computer vision syndrome.

Commonly used polymers in artificial tears are methyl cellulose and its derivatives like hydroxyethyl cellulose, hydroxypropyl cellulose, carboxymethyl cellulose, polyvinyl alcohol or povidone. Viscoelastics like sodium hyaluronidase are also used as lubricating drops as 0.1% solution.

Artificial tears are water based and they enhance lubrication, retention time and stability of the tear film.

OCULAR VISCOELASTIC DEVICES

Ocular viscoelastic devices (OVDs) are used in anterior segment surgeries like cataract surgery, trabeculectomy, keratoplasty, etc.

Uses

1. To prevent collapse of the anterior chamber during surgical manipulations.
2. To protect the corneal endothelium.

Types

Based on their viscoelasticity and surface tension, they are divided into two groups.

Cohesive Viscoelastics

Cohesive viscoelastics adhere to each other and are excellent for space maintenance, shock absorption and they are easy to remove. But protection to the endothelium is less (e.g. sodium hyaluronate 4%).

Dispersive Viscoelastics

Dispersive viscoelastics have lower surface tension and less viscosity, and gives better protection to the endothelium (e.g. hydroxypropyl methylcellulose).

Side Effects

1. Increase in IOP if not completely removed from the eye at the end of the surgery.
2. Sometimes increases intraocular inflammation.

DYES USED IN OPHTHALMOLOGY

Fluorescein Sodium

Fluorescein sodium is a fluorescent vital dye with many clinical applications in ophthalmology. It is available as topical drops, dye impregnated strips and as 5%, 10% and 20% IV injection.

Uses

1. To assess the ocular surface integrity. Areas denuded of epithelium, stain a green color with this dye.
2. Seidel's test: To test for wound leak, this reddish-brown dye is put in the conjunctival sac. If there is a wound leak and aqueous is coming out that spot will show a green color.
3. To test the patency of the lacrimal drainage system, especially in children and uncooperative patients. A drop of dye put in the eye will give a green tinge to cotton tipped applicator introduced into the nasal cavity.
4. To do applanation tonometry.
5. In contact lens fitting to assess the clearing or touching of the corneal surface by evaluating the precorneal tear film colored with the dye.
6. To do fundus fluorescein angiogram.
7. Vitreous fluorometry: To assess the integrity of the blood retinal barrier, the amount of fluorescein in the vitreous is measured after giving 1–2 g dye in powder form.

Side Effects of Systemic Administration

1. Nausea and vomiting.
2. Temporary staining of skin and urine with the dye.
3. Yellow vision, if there is pooling of the dye in the edema fluid in the macula.
4. Allergic reactions like pruritus or anaphylactic reaction. It can stain soft contact lens.

Indocyanine Green

Indocyanine green is a water-soluble dye with peak absorption at 805 nm and maximal emission at 835 nm. Since the dye is protein bound it does not leak through choriocapillaris and gives better delineation of choroidal circulation. So it is mainly used for visualization of choroidal neovascular membranes in ARMD. The choroidal neovascular membranes (CNVMs) are better visualized with indocyanine green (ICG) angiography than fluorescein fundus angiography (FFA). The ICG angiogram is done with infrared light.

Rose Bengal

Rose Bengal is not a vital dye. It binds to damaged and devitalized epithelium. It is useful for identifying the virus-damaged epithelial cells in viral keratitis.

Lissamine Green

Lissamine green is usually available as impregnated strips and used for staining corneal surface.

Effects of Various Systemic Medications on the Eye

33

Girija Devi PS

EFFECTS OF DRUGS

Drugs Affecting Conjunctiva, Lids and Sclera

1. Tetracycline produces pigmented conjunctival inclusion cysts whereas minocycline produces bluish discoloration of sclera.
2. Sulfonamides produce lid edema, conjunctivitis and chemosis.
3. Chlorpromazine produces blue discoloration of lid and conjunctiva.
4. Gold deposits in conjunctiva are produced by gold salts.

Drugs Affecting Cornea

1. Chloroquine and hydroxychloroquine produce whorl-like epithelial opacities, whereas chlorpromazine produces pigmentation of endothelium and Descemet's membrane. Indomethacin produces stromal opacities or whorl-like epithelial opacities, while gold salts produce minute stromal gold deposits.
2. Amiodarone and atovaquone produce whorl-like epithelial opacities.
3. Isotretinoin produces corneal opacities and neovascularization.

Drugs Affecting Lens

1. Chlorpromazine and amiodarone cause anterior subcapsular cataract.
2. Corticosteroids produce posterior subcapsular cataract.
3. Gold salts produce anterior capsular or subcapsular gold deposits.

Drugs Affecting Retinal Function

Antineoplastic agents like tamoxifen produce refractile opacities in the posterior pole whereas chloroquine and hydroxychloroquine produce bull's eye maculopathy and color vision loss. Cardiac glycosides produce color vision disturbances and entoptic phenomena. Sildenafil produce color vision disturbance and retinal vascular occlusion. Indomethacin produce pigmentary changes, color vision loss and visual field defects.

Drugs Affecting Optic Nerve

Corticosteroids, tetracyclines, nitrofurantoin, nalidixic acid and vitamin A produce pseudotumor cerebri. All antituberculous drugs produce optic neuritis or retrobulbar neuritis except rifampicin. Tamoxifen and oral contraceptives can also produce optic neuritis.

SECTION 9

Neuro-ophthalmology

Diseases of the Optic Nerve

34

Anuja Sathar, Girija Devi PS

ANATOMY

The optic nerve extends from the optic disk to the optic chiasma. It is about 4.5–5.5 cm in length. It consists of about 1.2 million axons from the retinal ganglion cells. Optic nerve is divided into four parts:

1. Intraocular part or optic nerve head—1 mm long part, which is seen as optic disk.
2. Intraorbital part is the longest, measuring about 2.5–3 cm in length.
3. Intracanalicular portion—passes through optic canal and measures 10 mm.
4. Intracranial portion—measures about 10 mm and extends up to optic chiasma.

The optic nerves from both sides converge to join the anterolateral angles of optic chiasma at an angle of 60°. The optic nerve is covered by the meningeal sheaths as it leaves the eyeball. It does not have the capacity to regenerate as it is not covered by neurilemma. It is a sensory tract and contains oligodendrocytes, astrocytes and microglia differing from the peripheral nervous system, which contains Schwann cells. The subarachnoid and subdural spaces are continuous with those of the brain.

Blood Supply

Intraocular part is supplied by branches of central retinal artery (CRA), circle of Zinn, short and long posterior ciliary arteries and cilioretinal artery. Intraocular part consists of:

1. Surface layer supplied by retinal arterioles.
2. Prelaminar region by peripapillary choroidal plexus.
3. Laminar portion by posterior ciliary artery and circle of zinn.
4. Retrolaminar portion by CRA and pial plexus.

Intraorbital part is supplied by an axial system contributed by CRA and peripheral system by pial plexus.

Anatomy of Optic Nerve Head

Optic nerve head is the site of exit of axons of all retinal ganglion cells and is about 1.5 mm diameter. There are no photoreceptors in the disk and therefore it corresponds to the blind spot of marriotte which is an absolute scotoma in visual field.

Axoplasmic Flow

Consists of glycoproteins, intracellular organelles like smooth endoplasmic reticulum, mitochondria, neurotrophic factors, etc. Two types of transport are there—orthograde or anterograde, i.e. from retinal ganglion cells along optic nerve to lateral geniculate body (LGB) and retrograde transport from LGB to retinal ganglion cells. Orthograde transport consists of slow and rapid components. Rate of slow component is 0.5–1 mm/day and that of fast component is 200–1,000 mm/day.

CLINICAL FEATURES

Localization of optic nerve lesions can be reached by history, clinical signs like reduced visual acuity, pupillary reaction, color vision, visual field, fundus examination for optic disk changes, light brightness sensitivity, contrast sensitivity, etc. Imaging techniques like computed tomography (CT) scan, magnetic resonance imaging (MRI), fundus fluorescein angiography (FFA) and electrodiagnostic tests like visual evoked potential test (VEP) also help in arriving at a diagnosis.

DISEASES OF THE OPTIC NERVE

Optic nerve diseases can be grouped as follows:

- Papilledema
- Optic neuritis
- Ischemic optic neuropathy
- Optic atrophy
- Congenital anomalies
- Miscellaneous.

PAPILLEDEMA

Definition

Papilledema is a non-inflammatory passive congestion or swelling of optic disk invariably associated with raised intracranial pressure.

It is most often bilateral and can occur over hours, days or weeks. The term disk edema denotes swelling of the disk due to various pathological conditions that reflect diseases of brain, eye or optic nerve and can be active or passive.

Pathogenesis

Pathogenesis of papilledema is attributed to the mechanical obstruction of axoplasmic transport and vascular congestion due to compression of the central retinal vein. The slow component of the orthograde transport is affected first. According to Hayreh there occurs stasis of the axoplasm in the prelaminar portion of the optic disk due to alteration in the pressure gradient across the lamina cribrosa. This is affected by the tissue pressure inside the optic nerve and the intraocular pressure.

Etiology

Due to causes that increase intracranial tension:

- Intracranial mass lesion, e.g. tumor, hematoma and abscess
- Intracranial tumors, especially those in the posterior fossa and parieto-occipital region produce papilledema early except those in medulla oblongata and diffuse cerebral glioma
- Cerebral edema (trauma, infarction, hypoxic ischemic encephalopathy, etc.)
- Increased cerebrospinal fluid (CSF) production (choroid plexus papilloma)
- Decreased CSF absorption, e.g. decreased arachnoid granulation absorption after bacterial meningitis
- Intracranial hemorrhages—cerebral or subarachnoid the latter cause papilledema in hours
- Obstruction of venous flow, e.g. venous sinus thrombosis, jugular vein compression and neck surgery
- Systemic conditions like malignant hypertension, pregnancy-induced hypertension
- Blockage of ventricular system by congenital or acquired lesions
- Idiopathic intracranial hypertension (IIH) or pseudotumor cerebri.

Idiopathic Intracranial Hypertension

Idiopathic intracranial hypertension or pseudotumor cerebri occurs with signs and symptoms of raised intracranial pressure without any intracranial mass lesion.

Clinical features: The incidence is more in the third decade with preponderance for obese females. Other neurological signs are absent except for VI nerve palsy. Transient obscuration of vision is more common. Vision is otherwise normal with enlargement of blind spot on field charting.

Cerebrospinal fluid composition is normal and ventricles are small or normal on imaging.

Causes: Use of drugs like high dose of vitamin A (> 100,000 U/day) nalidixic acid, oral contraceptives, tetracyclines, use or sudden withdrawal of steroids, hormonal imbalance, etc. are implicated.

Though the exact cause is unknown, it is postulated to be due to defective CSF absorption across arachnoid granulations into the dural venous sinuses.

Treatment: It includes weight reduction and measures to reduce intracranial pressure like Acetazolamide, Furosemide, etc.

Surgical treatment includes optic nerve sheath fenestration or by lumboperitoneal or ventriculoperitoneal shunt.

Clinical Features

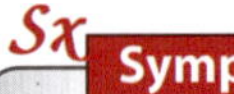

It include both systemic and ocular features.

Systemic Features

1. Headache, which is more in the morning associated with nausea.
2. Projectile vomiting.
3. Diplopia due to non-specific paresis of VI nerve due to increased intracranial pressure, which appears as a false localizing sign.
4. Focal neurological deficits may occur depending on the lesion.

Ocular Features

Ocular features include transient obscuration of vision, which may be unilateral or bilateral blackouts lasting for seconds often associated with orthostatic changes. The optic nerve functions, like visual acuity, color vision and pupillary reactions are normal unless there is optic atrophy. Visual fields show enlargement of blind spot.

Signs

The appearance of papilledema depends on the stage of the disease process in which the eye is examined. Papilledema may be classified into various stages as given below.

Early Stage

Blurring of disk margin, hyperemic disk and loss of venous pulsation. About 20% of normal population does not have spontaneous venous pulsations. The blurring of the disk margin is the first to appear and starts in the superior and inferior margins and extends into the nasal and temporal margins (Fig. 34.1). The margins will not appear clear even with any lens of the ophthalmoscope.

Established

Established papilledema shows venous engorgement, edema of the disk, obliteration of cup, flame-shaped hemorrhages and cotton wool spots (Fig. 34.2). Retina is displaced from disk with enlargement of blind spot (Fig. 34.3). Patons lines, which are radial retinal lines cascading from the disk may also be seen. Fundus fluorescein angiogram shows dilated disk capillaries followed by increasing hyperfluorescence with vertical pooling of the dye beyond the disk margin.

Vintage or Chronic

Acute and hemorrhagic components resolve, disk become gray and pale due to pressure-induced axonal damage and may be swollen to resemble a champagne cork (Fig. 34.4). Milky gray color of disk, loss of optic cup, hard exudates in superficial optic disk (pseudodrusen) and optociliary shunt vessels (retinochoroidal collaterals) may be seen. Peripheral vision may be lost in chronic cases where it is frequently accompanied by concentric contraction of visual field.

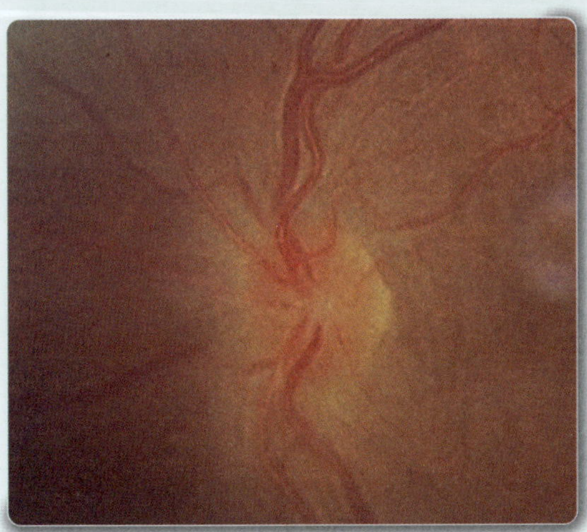

FIGURE 34.1: Early papilledema

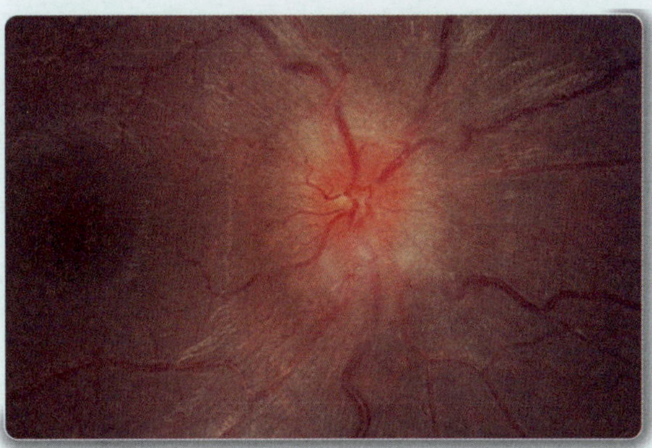

FIGURE 34.2: Established papilledema

Postpapilledema Optic Atrophy

Postpapilledema optic atrophy occurs weeks to months later. Disk is atrophic, dirty gray, with indistinct margins and sheathing of retinal vessels. Visual acuity is severely impaired.

If timely relief of intracranial pressure before optic atrophy starts is done, a normal disk returns when the papilledema disappears. Chronic cases lead onto pale disk with gliosis.

A disk edema (Table 34.1) of about 2D–6D (difference in the focusing of blood vessels on the surface of the disk and adjacent retina) will be seen. Papilledema is usually bilateral, but can be unequal. Sometimes, it is more on the side of the lesion in anterior and middle cranial fossa tumors. Unilateral papilledema suggests optic nerve pathology

TABLE 34.1: Causes of disk edema

Unilateral	Bilateral
Optic neuritis—papillitis, neuroretinitis	Papilledema—increased ICT
Anterior ischemic optic neuropathy (AION)	Systemic diseases—malignant hypertension (refer Fig. 34.6)
Papillophlebitis	Anemia, hypoxia, blood dyscrasias
Orbital causes—tumors, cellulitis	Carotid-cavernous fistula
Ocular causes—uveitis, hypotony venous occlusion	Compressive thyroid ophthalmopathy Cavernous sinus thrombosis
Foster-Kennedy syndrome	Pseudopapilledema—optic disk drusen hypermetropia

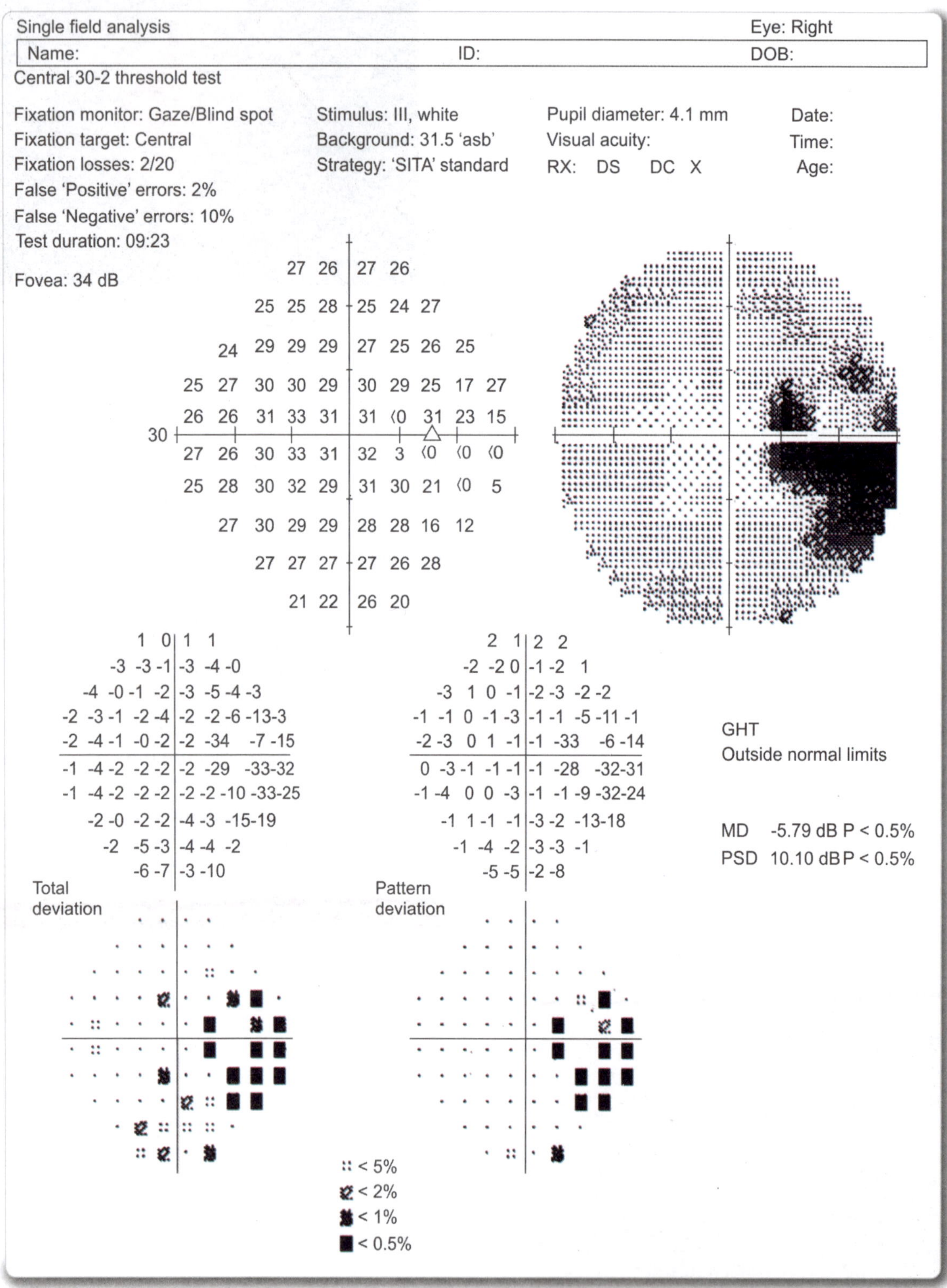

FIGURE 34.3: Enlargement of physiological blind spot in papilledema

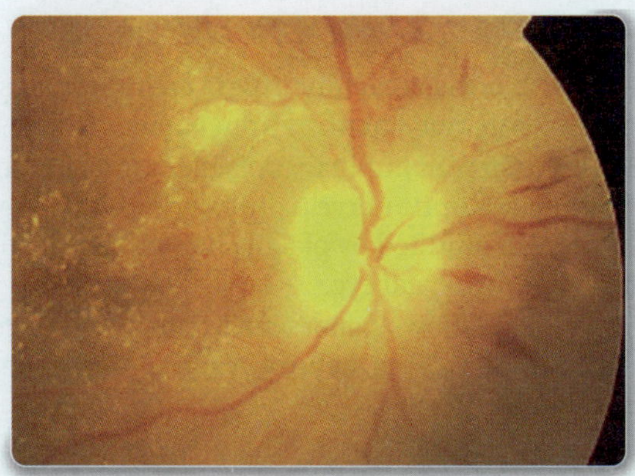

FIGURE 34.4: Chronic papilledema

such as optic nerve glioma or nerve sheath meningioma. Unilateral papilledema with optic atrophy on the other side often indicates opposite olfactory groove meningioma, frontal lobe tumors, sellar or suprasellar tumors or other basofrontal intracranial space occupying lesions. It is known as **'Foster-Kennedy syndrome'.**

Papilledema may lead to diagnostic difficulties in different stages. It should be differentiated from optic neuropathies and structural abnormalities of optic disk such as pseudopapilledema. When disk edema is found on fundoscopy, further evaluation is warranted with CT/MRI of brain and/or spine. Differential diagnosis is by techniques such as optical coherence tomography (OCT), FFA (Fig. 34.5) and B-scan.

Treatment

Depends on the underlying cause. Surgical management will be required in case of CNS tumors. Meanwhile intracranial tension (ICT) can be kept low with acetazolamide and diuretics like furosemide. The patient has to be closely watched for repeated visual field charting and fundus examination for the commencement of optic atrophy.

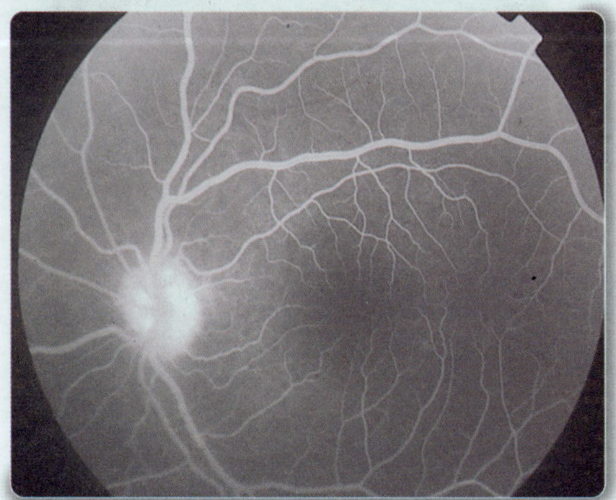

FIGURE 34.5: Fundus fluorescein angiogram showing disk hyperfluorescence in papilledema

OPTIC NEURITIS

Optic neuritis is the term used for inflammation of the optic nerve.

Etiology

The various etiological factors of optic neuritis can be classified as:

1. Demyelinating—multiple sclerosis, neuromyelitis optica (Devics disease). Multiple sclerosis is the most common etiological condition. About 15%–20% of patients with multiple sclerosis present with optic neuritis and 30%–40% of multiple sclerosis patients develop optic neuritis at some course of the disease.
2. Parainfectious—following viral infections like measles, mumps, chickenpox, whooping cough and immunization.
3. Infectious—sinus related especially acute ethmoiditis, cat scratch fever, syphilis, Lyme disease, cryptococcal meningitis in patients with acquired immunodeficiency syndrome (AIDS) and herpes zoster.
4. Non-infectious—sarcoidosis, autoimmune diseases like systemic lupus erythematosis (SLE), polyarteritis nodosa (PAN) and other vasculitis.
5. Drugs like ethambutol.
6. Hereditary (Leber's).
7. Idiopathic—the basic cause of optic neuritis is often unknown.

Ophthalmoscopic Classification

Papillitis is the type that presents with the typical fundus changes. It is the most common type in children. The ophthalmoscopic findings include hyperemia, blurring of disk margins, edema of optic disk, which is not more than 2D–3D, peripapillary flame-shaped hemorrhages, mild tortuosity of retinal veins and associated fine vitreous cells (Fig. 34.6).

Retrobulbar neuritis (RBN) is the most common type and may be associated with multiple sclerosis. In this, the optic nerve head is normal. The common saying is that neither the ophthalmologist nor the patient sees anything (Fig. 34.7).

Neuroretinitis is involvement of optic disk and surrounding retina with macular edema giving a macular star figure composed of lipid exudates. It is rare in multiple sclerosis (Fig. 34.8).

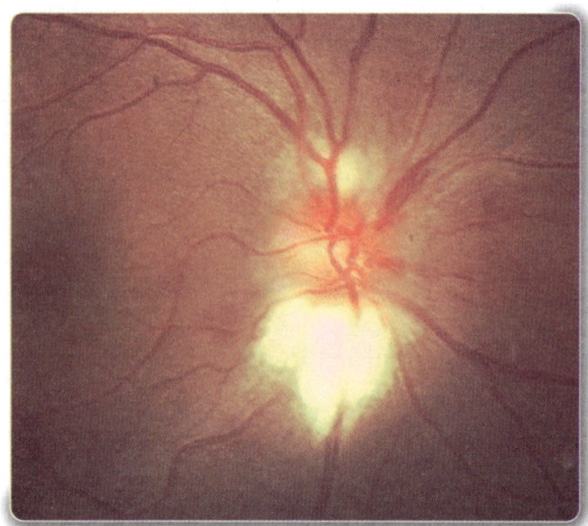

FIGURE 34.6: Optic neuritis-papillitis

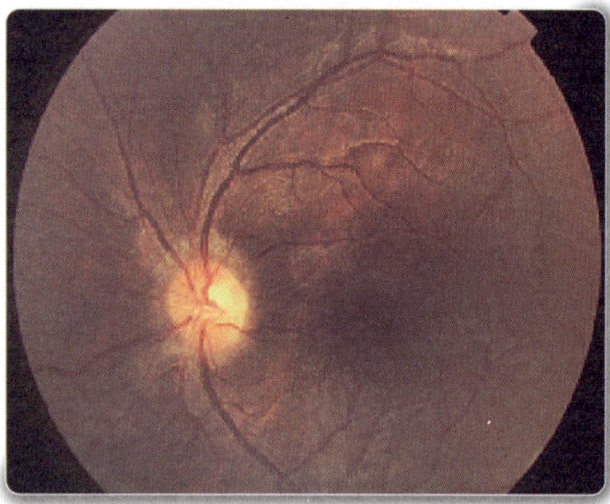

FIGURE 34.7: Retrobulbar neuritis

Clinical Features

Sx **Symptoms**

Optic neuritis presents with the triad of visual loss, ipsilateral eye pain and defective color vision. Vision loss may occur rapidly within 1 hour (29%) or over a period of 3–7 days (23%). Ipsilateral eye pain occurs in 53%–93% and is increased with eye movements. Decreased color vision occurs in 94%.

Triad of visual loss, ipsilateral eye pain and defective color vision. Other visual symptoms include phosphenes, which are glowing sensations produced by inadequate stimuli and Uhthoff's phenomenon. In this phenomenon, there is blurring of vision with exertion and elevation of body temperature.

Signs

1. Decrease in visual acuity: This is an important sign to differentiate optic neuritis from papilledema.
2. Relative afferent pupillary defect or Marcus Gunn pupil indicates optic nerve pathology in the affected eye. It can be quantified by placing neutral density filter in front of the normal eye.
3. Visual field shows generalized reduction in sensitivity, central scotoma, centrocecal scotoma or nerve fiber bundle defects.
4. Color dyschromatopsia, which is best identified by Farnsworth-Munsell 100-hue testing in which color desaturation is noted.
5. Optic disk: In two-third of the cases optic disk are normal (RBN). In one-third cases swollen optic disk with hemorrhages and mild elevation may be seen. The disk edema is never more than 2D–3D in contrast to papilledema.
6. Loss of contrast sensitivity is seen in 98%. This persist even after visual improvement and accounts for defective vision complained by patient in later stages.
7. Pulfrich phenomenon measures reduced stereoacuity. The affected optic nerve transmission is slow and hence this disparity in time caused by the difference in latency between eyes is interpreted as disparity in space that results in stereo illusion.

Investigations

1. Visual evoked potential—increase in latency of P100 over 118 ms or an interocular difference of more than 9 ms signifies optic nerve dysfunction (Fig. 34.9).
2. Pattern electroretinography (ERG).

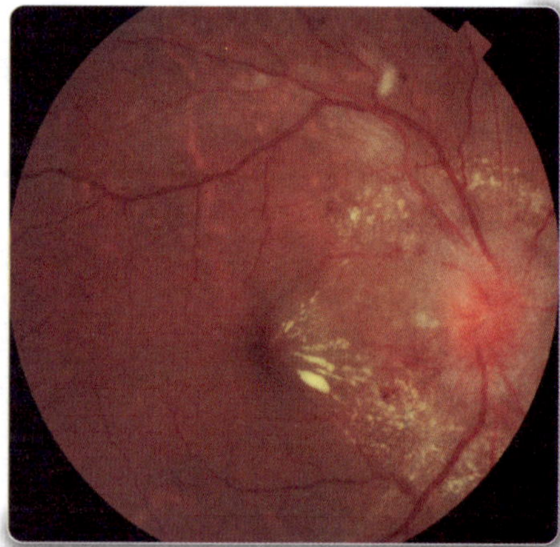

FIGURE 34.8: Neuroretinitis

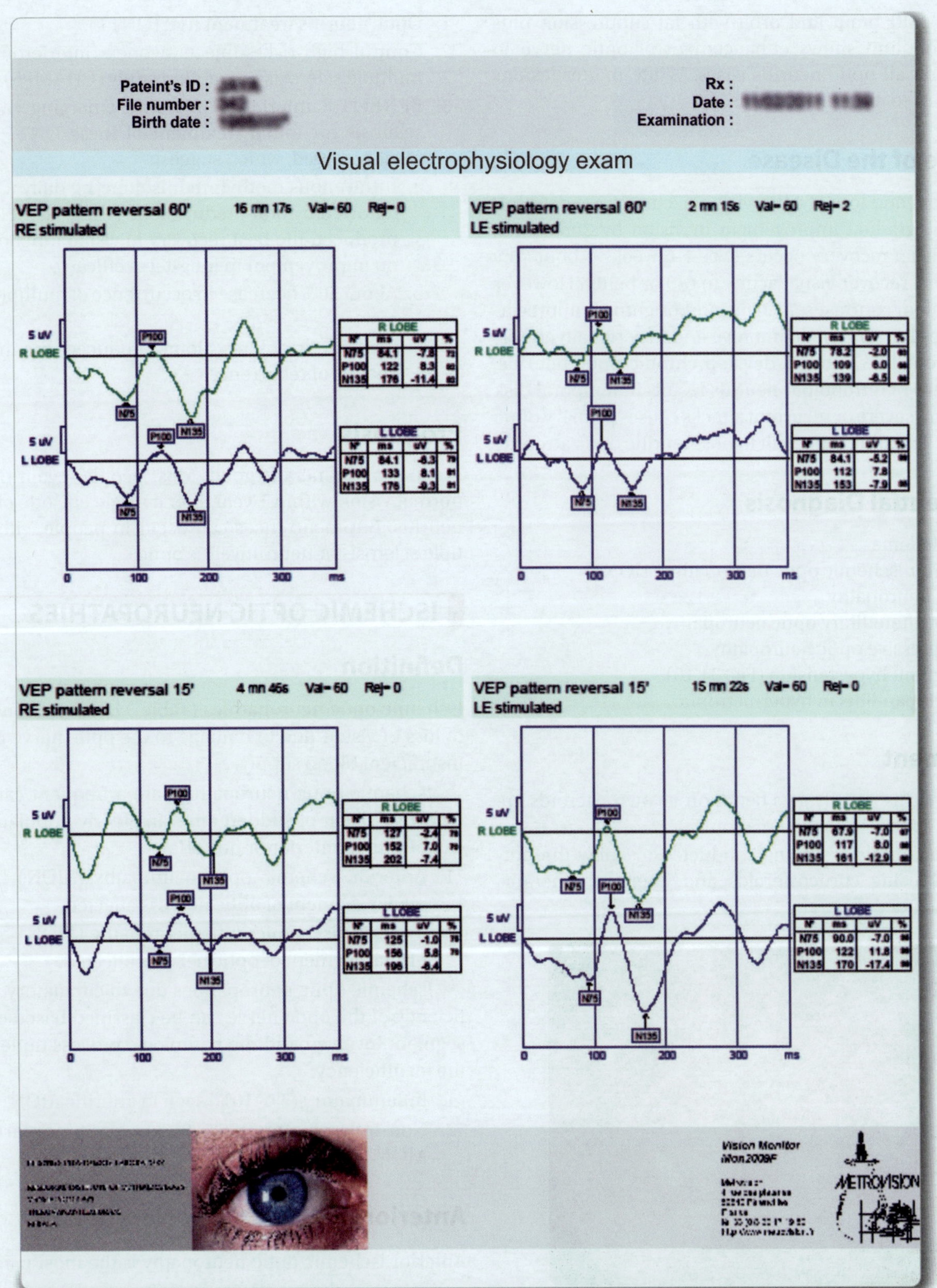

FIGURE 34.9: Prolonged latency and decreased amplitude of P100 wave in right eye (RE) indicating optic neuritis (VEP, visually evoked potential)

3. The MRI brain and orbit with fat suppression plus gadolinium shows enhancement of optic nerve in nearly all optic neuritis cases. White matter lesions points to multiple sclerosis.

Course of the Disease

Vision loss and loss of color vision occurs in 2–4 days followed by gradual improvement in vision by 2nd or 3rd week. Visual recovery occurs over 4–6 weeks. About 75% of patients recover visual acuity to 6/9 or better. However color vision, contrast sensitivity and brightness appreciation takes longer time to improve and may remain abnormal. About 10% patients develop chronic optic neuritis. Mild cases of retrobulbar neuritis results in temporal disk pallor and severe or recurrent attacks causes primary optic atrophy. Papillitis can result in postneuritic optic atrophy.

Differential Diagnosis

- Papilledema
- Anterior ischemic optic neuropathy (AION)
- Toxic neuropathy
- Leber's hereditary optic neuropathy
- Compressive optic neuropathy
- Malignant hypertension (Fig. 34.10)
- Pseudopapillitis in hypermetropia.

Treatment

Optic neuritis usually gets better on its own. Steroids are given to control the inflammation.

Various trials are being conducted to know the outcome of using corticosteroids and interferon therapy. These include:

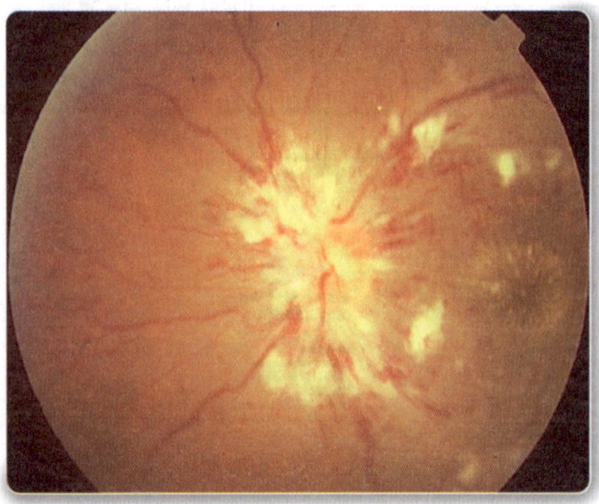

FIGURE 34.10: Disk edema in malignant hypertension

1. Optic neuritis treatment trial (ONTT).
2. Control high-risk subjects avonex (interferon ß 1a) multiple sclerosis prevention study (CHAMPS).
3. BENEFIT-ß interferon in newly emerging multiple sclerosis for initial treatment of these ONTT is the most accepted, which suggest:
   a. Intravenous methylprednisolone 1 g daily × 3 days followed by oral prednisolone (1 mg/kg × 11 days) produced the best recovery in visual function, but no improvement in long-term efficacy.
   b. About 50% decrease in occurrence of multiple sclerosis.
   c. Oral prednisolone alone produced the highest chance of recurrence.

Prognosis

Prognosis is generally good. Most people regain near to normal vision within 1 year after a single episode of optic neuritis. But recurrences can occur in people with multiple sclerosis or neuromyelitis optica.

ISCHEMIC OPTIC NEUROPATHIES

Definition

Ischemic optic neuropathies (Table 34.2) are a condition of loss of vision due to damage to the optic nerve due to insufficient blood supply.

Ischemic optic neuropathies are a frequent cause of defective vision of sudden onset in elderly population. It can be either anterior or posterior:

1. Anterior ischemic optic neuropathy (AION)—intraocular segment of optic nerve is affected.
2. Posterior ischemic optic neuropathy (PION)—intraorbital segment of optic nerve is affected.

Ischemic optic neuropathies due to circulatory insufficiency of the optic nerve can be classified based on the segment involved and the pathologic process underlying the insufficiency:

1. Inflammatory (5%–10%) seen in arteritic AION.
2. Non-inflammatory (90%–95%) seen in non-arteritic AION.

Anterior Ischemic Optic Neuropathy

Anterior ischemic optic neuropathy is the most common optic neuropathy in patients over 50 years, the cause being ischemic damage to optic nerve head (Figs 34.11A and B).

TABLE 34.2: Ischemic optic neuropathy—differentiating features		
Features	**Arteritic AION***	**Non-arteritic AION**
Age and sex	70–80, females > males	55–70, females > males
Visual dysfunction	Severe loss Transient obscurations	Minimal to severe
Second eye involvement	90% in day or week	40% month to year
Optic disk	Pallid disk edema	Hyperemia > pallid edema, often segmental
Systemic features	Headache, scalp tenderness, polymyalgia, fever, malaise, jaw claudication, thickened and palpable temporal arteries	Hypertension in 50%, diabetes, shock, massive blood loss, severe anemia
ESR†	50–120 mm/h	Up to 40 mm/h
Response to steroids	Systemic symptoms improve, reduces chance of second eye involvement	None
Visual prognosis	Very poor	Poor

*AION, anterior ischemic optic neuropathy; †ESR, erythrocyte sedimentation rate.

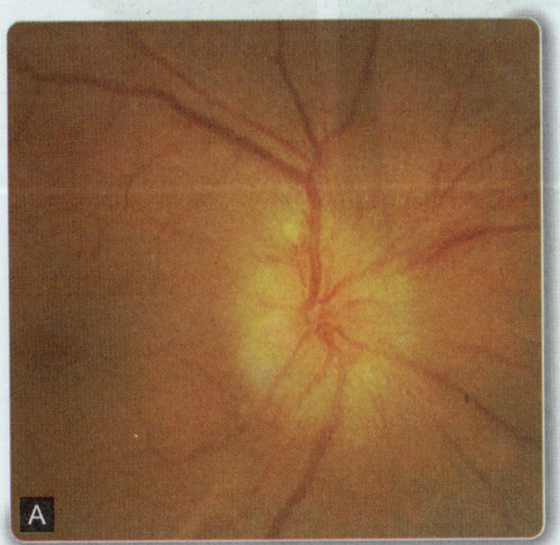
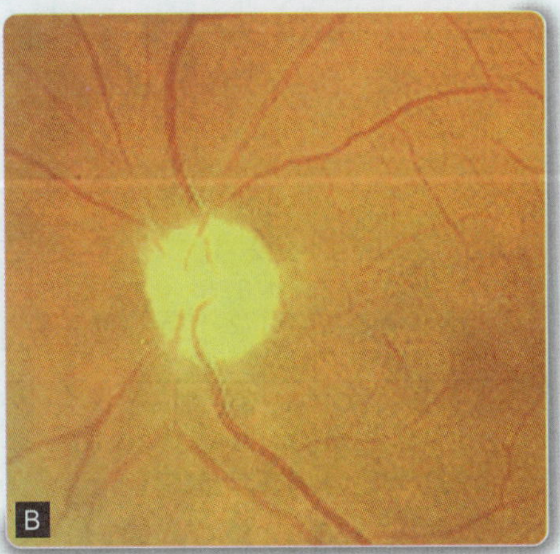

FIGURES 34.11A and B: Fundus in case of arteritic anterior ischemic optic neuropathy (AION) showing pallid disk edema in right eye (RE) and optic atrophy in left eye (LE).

Sx **Symptoms**

Painless mono-ocular visual loss developing over hours to days. Other symptoms of arteritic AION includes headache, neck pain, polymyalgia rheumatica, etc.

Signs

1. Decreased visual acuity.
2. Visual field defects (most common is altitudinal field defects) (Fig. 34.12).
3. Relative afferent pupillary defect (RAPD).
4. Fundus shows optic disk edema, which can be pallid edema or diffuse hyperemia, peripapillary flame-shaped hemorrhages and retinal arteriolar narrowing.

Arteritic AION

Arteritic AION accounts for 5%–10% cases of AION and giant cell arteritis (GCA) is the cause for this condition. The GCA mainly affects large and medium-sized arteries particularly the superficial temporal, ophthalmic, posterior ciliary and proximal vertebral arteries. It typically affects the older patients (over 70 years) and is more common in females.

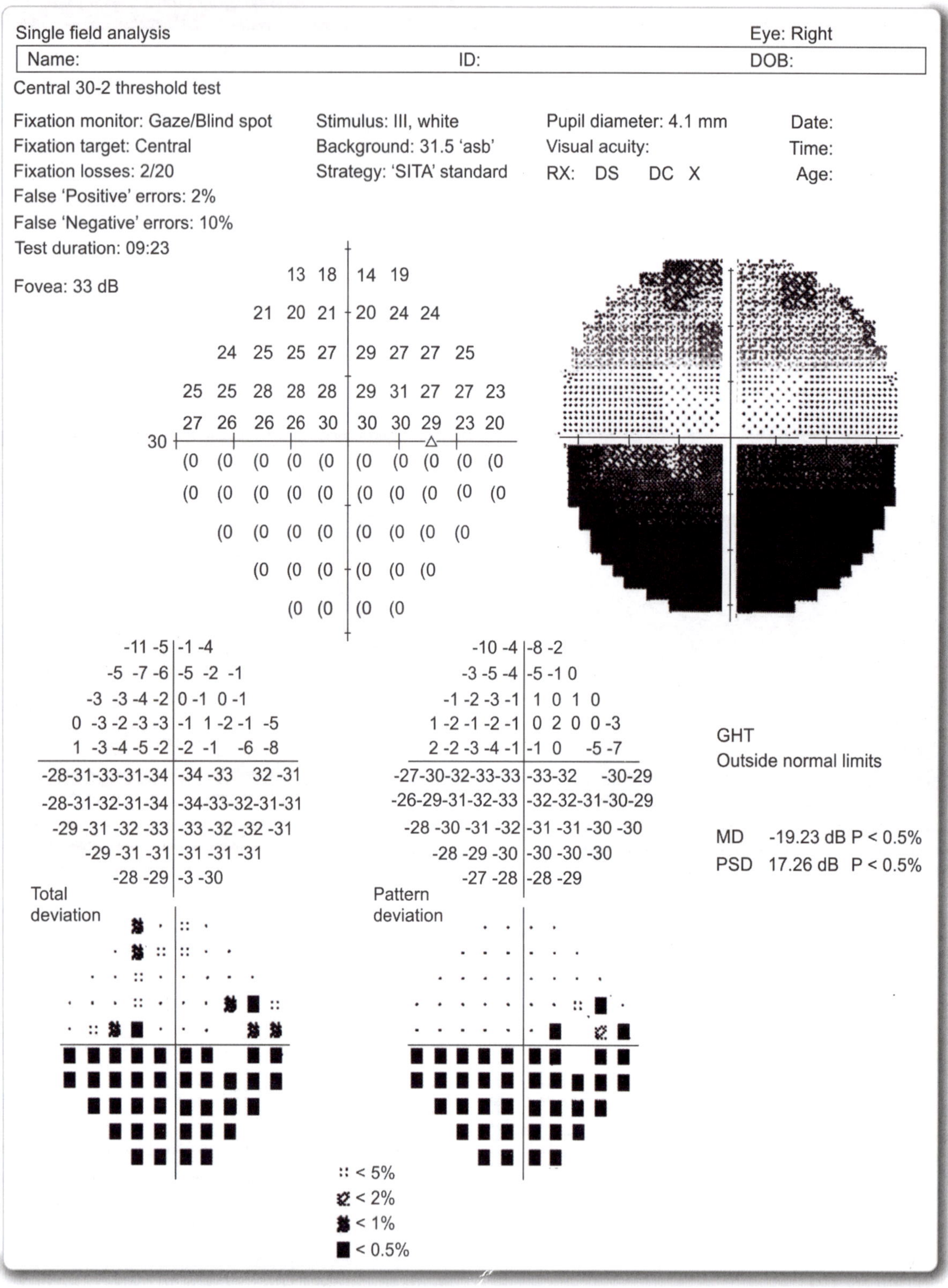

FIGURE 34.12: Inferior altitudinal field defect in AION

Sx Symptoms

It can be general/ophthalmic.

General: It includes scalp tenderness, headache, jaw claudication, polymyalgia rheumatica, neck pain, fever, weight loss, night sweats and malaise. However, no symptoms are seen in 20% people (occult GCA).

Ophthalmic: It includes transient loss of vision several weeks prior to occurrence of AION. Sudden loss of vision often less than 6/60 can occur.

Signs: It can be general/ophthalmic.

General examination: The superficial temporal artery will be thickened, tender and nodular with loss of pulsations.

Ophthalmic signs: It include decrease in vision, visual field defects, RAPD, fundus showing optic disk edema, cotton wool spots and peripapillary pallor. A chalky white optic disk is particularly suggestive of GCA.

Investigation: It includes the following:

1. Blood: Erythrocyte sedimentation rate (ESR) is usually very high or may be normal (occult GCA) in less than 20%.
2. C-reactive protein (CRP) is raised.
3. Platelet count is elevated.
4. FFA: Shows delayed choroidal filling.
5. Temporal artery biopsy: 2.5 cm of superficial temporal artery is taken from temple and examined prior to or within 3 days of starting systemic steroids. It shows granulomatous inflammation with infiltration of lymphocytes, plasma cells, multinuclear giant cells and macrophages along the entire thickness of vessel wall.

Treatment: Systemic steroids such as IV methyl prednisolone 1 g × 3–4 days followed by oral prednisolone 80 mg daily for 3 days, which is then reduced to 60 mg OD and 50 mg for 1 week each. The daily dose is reduced by 5 mg weekly till 10 mg is reached keeping a watch on ESR, CRP and the patient is maintained on 10 mg OD, and which is continued for 1–2 years.

In untreated cases contralateral eye involvement is 95%. Even in adequately treated cases 25% involvement of contralateral eye is noted and in corticosteroid withdrawal, 7% show risk of recurrent or chronic AION.

Prognosis: The disease has a very poor visual prognosis as the visual loss is usually permanent.

Non-arteritic AION

Non-arteritic AION (NAAION) is the most common optic neuropathy in elderly affecting the 55–70 year age group due to compromise in the disk microcirculation due to structural crowding of the disk (small disk at risk). Predisposing conditions include systemic hypertension, diabetes mellitus, hypercholesterolemia, collagen vascular disease and antiphospholipid antibody syndrome.

Sx Symptoms

Sudden painless monocular visual loss usually noticed on awakening.

TABLE 34.3: Clinical features of optic neuritis, papilledema, AION

Features	Optic neuritis	Papilledema	Ischemic optic neuropathy
Symptoms			
Visual	Rapid loss of central vision. Painful ocular movements	Transient obscurations, headache nausea, vomiting	Acute field defect, usually altitudinal
Laterality	Unilateral, may alternate in multiple sclerosis. Bilateral more in children	Bilateral	Unilateral in acute stage, second eye involved subsequently
Signs			
Pupil	RAPD present	Normal unless optic atrophy occurs	RAPD present
Acuity	Decreased	Normal	Variable. Severe loss common.
Fundus	Disk edema less than 2D, few hemorrhages, few vitreous cells in papillitis. Normal in retrobulbar.	Disk edema up to 6D–8D, hemorrhages, clear vitreous	Pallid disk edema, which may be segmental, few hemorrhages
Visual prognosis	Usually good with return to near normal	Good unless there is optic atrophy	Poor

Signs: Decrease in vision not severe, usually not more than 6/60, impaired color vision and visual field defects usually of inferior altitudinal type are seen. Fundus shows disk edema with peripapillary hemorrhages.

Investigations: Blood glucose, fasting lipid profile, FFA—no delayed choroidal filling, localized disk hyperfluorescence.

Management: There is no definite treatment for NAAION. Aspirin is given to reduce the systemic vascular events. However, it does not prevent involvement of the contralateral eye.

Posterior Ischemic Optic Neuropathy

Posterior ischemic optic neuropathy occurs due to ischemia of the optic nerve caused by involvement of the pial vessels, which supplies the intraorbital portion of the optic nerve.

The symptoms include loss of vision and RAPD can be elicited. However, ophthalmoscopic examination shows normal fundus.

Pseudo-Foster Kennedy syndrome is seen in AION in which there is optic atrophy in one eye and disk edema in the fellow eye when the second eye is involved.

OPTIC ATROPHY

Optic atrophy represents permanent loss of retinal ganglion cell axons in association with retinal ganglion death and clinically presents as pale optic disk on fundus examination. It is a finding of the optic disk due to degeneration of optic nerve fibers.

Classification

1. Primary optic atrophy (simple optic atrophy).
2. Secondary optic atrophy (following disk edema).

Primary Optic Atrophy

Primary optic atrophy (Box 34.1) is caused by injury to the retinal ganglion cells or its axons from the retrolaminar optic nerve to LGB. There is loss of optic nerve fibers with minimal changes in the optic nerve head anatomy. Lesions anterior to the optic chiasma results in unilateral optic atrophy and those involving the optic chiasma and optic tract results in bilateral optic atrophy.

BOX 34.1: Causes of primary atrophy

- Retrobulbar neuritis—multiple sclerosis
- Hereditary optic neuropathies
- Toxic and nutritional optic neuropathies
- Compression of the optic nerve by tumors and aneurysms
- Traumatic optic neuropathy
- Tabes dorsalis

Sx Symptoms

Loss of vision, usually of long duration, which initially started as a sudden loss of vision.

Signs: Decreased visual acuity, RAPD, visual field loss. Fundus examination shows chalky white disk pallor with margins sharply outlined and shallow cupping due to degeneration of nerve fibers (Fig. 34.13). There is also a reduction in the number of small vessels that cross disk margin. Surrounding retina is normal. Kestenbaum capillary index is less than six. Histopathology shows absence of glial reaction on disk surface and within the nerve the axons are replaced by glial cells.

Secondary Optic Atrophy (Postneuritic Optic Atrophy)

Secondary optic atrophy occurs as a consequence of severe disk edema or inflammation of the optic nerve head reflecting the disorganized disk surface (Fig. 34.14). The various causes include chronic papilledema, AION and papillitis. In contrast to primary optic atrophy, which affects a normal disk it affects a previously swollen disk.

Sx Symptoms

Vary according to the cause.

Signs: Optic disk is slightly raised and is white or dirty gray in color, the margins of the disk are blurred and irregular

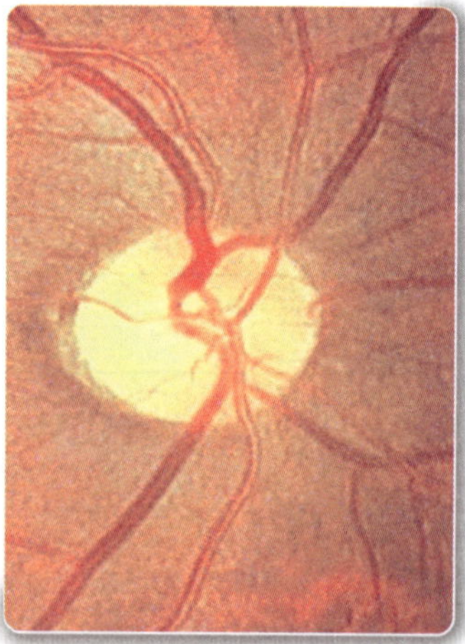

FIGURE 34.13: Primary optic atrophy with sharp optic disk margins, shallow cupping and normal vessels

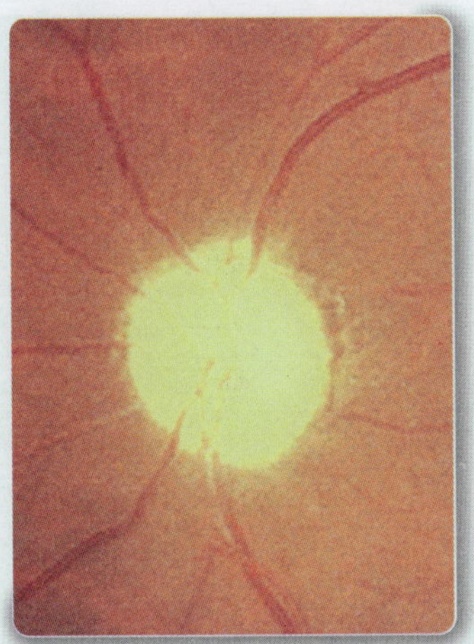

FIGURE 34.14: Secondary optic atrophy with ill-defined disk margins, cup filled by gliosis and narrowed vessels

due to gliosis, physiological cup is obliterated, peripapillary sheathing and narrowing of blood vessels are seen.

Two other forms of optic atrophy also have been described based on ophthalmoscopic findings.

Consecutive Optic Atrophy

Consecutive optic atrophy occurs as a consequence of degenerating or inflammatory lesions in the retina and choroid, e.g. retinal pigmentary dystrophy like retinitis pigmentosa, pathological myopia, occlusion of central retinal artery, etc. The disk is waxy yellow in appearance, the edges are irregular and blurred and retinal vessels attenuated.

Glaucomatous Optic Atrophy

Glaucomatous optic atrophy is due to long standing raised intraocular pressure damaging the optic nerve head. Fundus examination shows deep wide cupping of optic disk and nasal shift of vessels (Fig. 34.15).

Treatment: Once total optic atrophy has started, the prognosis for vision is guarded. Identification and control of causative factor should be done as early as possible.

CONGENITAL ANOMALIES

Tilted disk occurs due to oblique insertion of optic nerve into the eyeball. Commonly associated with myopia, astigmatism, inferior crescent and superotemporal field changes.

Optic Disk Drusen

They are hyaline bodies embedded deep in the optic nerve head giving appearance of disk edema, therefore the condition is known as pseudopapilledema (Fig. 34.16). The disk shows lumpy margins with anomalous branching of blood vessels. They autofluorescence with fluorescein angiography and can be readily identified with ultrasound or CT scan. They become larger and move anteriorly with time. They are sometimes inherited with an autosomal dominant trait.

Optic Disk Pit

Appears as an oval or round-shaped crater like depression, usually in the temporal optic disk (Fig. 34.17). It is a rare and usually unilateral condition. The optic disk is larger than in the fellow eye. Histologically, it is due to an outward herniation of rudimentary neuroectodermal tissue into a depression within the nerve substance. These may be associated with intracranial malformations.

It may be asymptomatic or present with variable field defects in correlation with the morphology of the pit. The most common defect being an arcuate scotoma, which is paracentral in location and connected to an enlarged blind spot. About 45% of optic disk pits are associated with serous detachment of the macula. The subretinal fluid forming the detachment has been postulated to arise from either the CSF from the subarachnoid space or from the vitreous gaining access through a defect in the edge of the disk. The appearance is similar to that of central serous retinopathy and therefore warrants careful disk examination in such cases.

Treatment: It is by photocoagulation at the temporal disk margin to block the flow of subretinal fluid into the macular region. Vitrectomy with internal gas tamponade to displace the subretinal fluid from beneath the macula is considered in unresponsive cases.

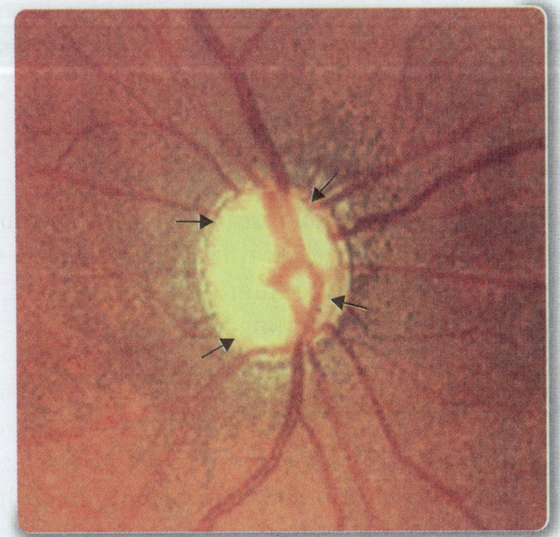

FIGURE 34.15: Glaucomatous optic atrophy (black arrows show the edge of the cup)

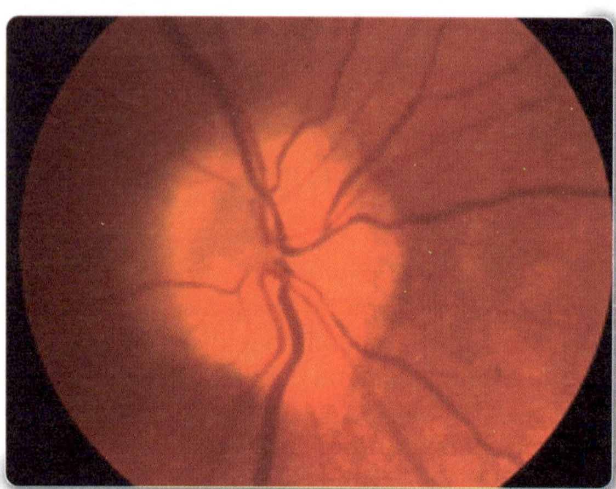

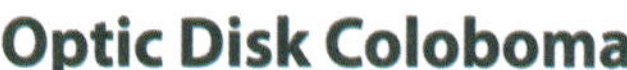

FIGURE 34.16: Optic disk drusen

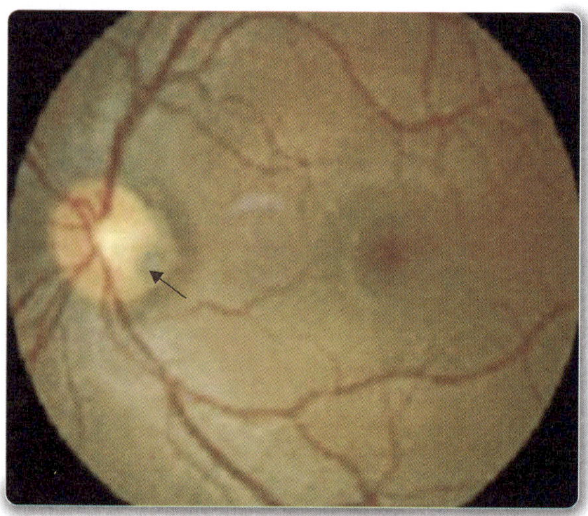

FIGURE 34.17: Optic disk pit

Optic Disk Coloboma

Optic disk coloboma is a rare condition due to incomplete closure of the embryonic fissure. It may manifest as extensive involvement of optic disk and peripapillary region or as an inferior crescent. In the extensive form, the disk is large and excavated showing the sclera and the inner side of the optic nerve sheath and the original disk tissue is confined to a small superior wedge.

Another variant of coloboma is morning glory anomaly, which may be isolated or with neurological abnormalities (Fig. 34.18). There is a funnel-shaped excavation of disk, with central glial tissue due to persistent hyaloid remnants. The disk has an elevated rim with chorioretinal pigmentary disturbances. The appearance of the disk resembles that of a morning glory flower with vessels emerging radially like spokes of a wheel. Associated serous retinal detachment occurs in about 30% cases.

Bergmeister Papillae

Remnants of hyaloid vessels form a persistent fibrous tissue like structure on the disk. It may also extent a short distance onto vitreous or the anterior end may be attached to posterior lens capsule forming Mittendorf dot.

Optic Nerve Hypoplasia

The disk is small with small tortuous blood vessels surrounded by yellowish-mottled peripapillary halo due to concentric chorioretinal atrophy, corresponding to the size of the original disk known as double ring sign (Fig. 34.19). It is unilateral or bilateral and as the number of optic nerve fibers are diminished, visual acuity is usually less. The condition is associated with other ocular abnormalities like microphthalmos, strabismus, nystagmus, etc. and neurological malformations like basal encephalocoele, agenesis of corpus callosum, absence of septum pellucidum and hypopituitarism.

Medullated Nerve Fibers

Normally the myelination of the optic nerve stops at the lamina cribrosa. Occasionally, the myelination follows the optic nerve fibers and may extend into the nerve fiber layer of the retina. They appear as whitish patches with feathery margins, which may or may not obscure the retinal blood vessels (Fig. 34.20). Visual field charting shows enlargement of blind spot. It is usually permanent, but disappears with demyelinating conditions and optic atrophy.

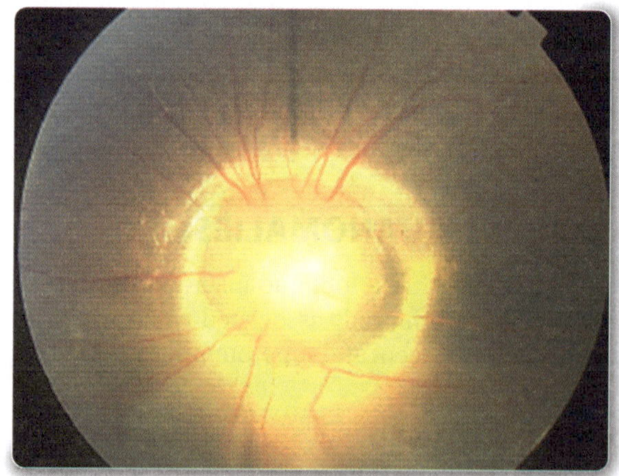

FIGURE 34.18: Morning glory anomaly with serous RD

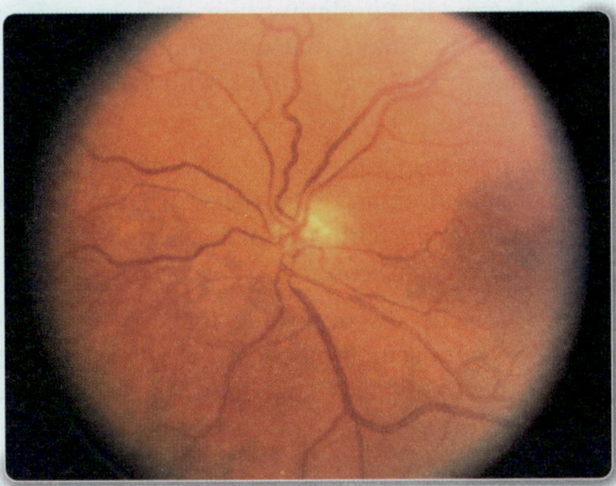

FIGURE 34.19: Optic nerve hypoplasia

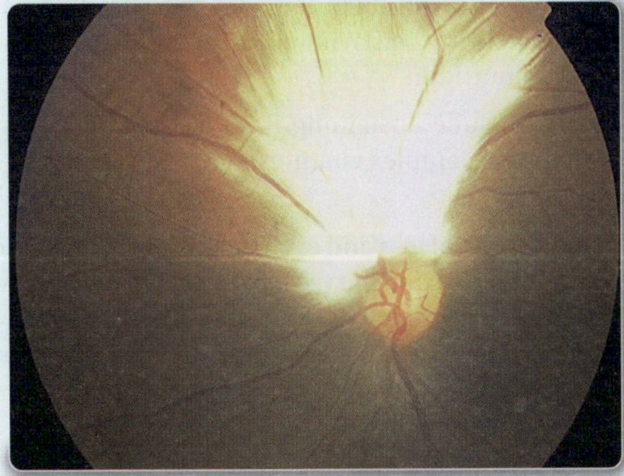

FIGURE 34.20: Medullated nerve fibers

Hereditary Optic Neuropathies

The hereditary optic neuropathies consist of a group of disorders in which the optic nerve dysfunction is either isolated or is a part of a systemic disease and direct inheritance is clinically or genetically proven.

The most common of these disorders are autosomal dominant optic atrophy (Kjer's disease) and maternally inherited Leber's hereditary optic neuropathy. The most common hereditary optic neuropathy with systemic involvement is Wolfram syndrome.

Inheritance patterns of hereditary optic neuropathies include autosomal dominant, autosomal recessive and maternal (mitochondrial). They manifest as symmetric, bilateral, painless central visual loss as the papillomacular bundle is involved resulting in central or cecocentral scotomas, which may be progressive. The pathology is thought to lie in the ganglion cell and its axon in which mitochondrial functions form an important part.

Leber's Hereditary Optic Neuropathy

Leber's hereditary optic neuropathy is a maternally inherited optic neuropathy with bilateral sequential painless subacute vision loss. About 80%–90% affecting young adult males, but can affect women and subjects of any age. Age of onset usually occurs between 15 and 30 years. It is one of the first diseases to be linked to mitochondrial mutations. Transmission of the disease is through an unaffected female to all offsprings, but manifests in males, females being unaffected. The most common specific mitochondrial DNA mutations occur at positions 11,778, 3,460 and 14,484. In some cases, minor neurological abnormalities may be seen referred to as Leber's plus. Some patients can also have cardiac conduction defects.

Clinical features: Painless central visual loss occurs in one eye followed by the involvement of the second eye weeks or months later. Color vision is affected early. Vision loss is central. Visual acuity is worse than 6/60 in each eye though it can range from 6/6 to no perception of light. Pupillary light reflexes are initially normal.

In acute phase of visual loss, there may be hyperemia of the optic nerve head, dilation and tortuosity of vessels, hemorrhages and circumpapillary telangiectasia microangiopathy. The characteristic abnormality has been described as a triad of circumpapillary telangiectasia, swelling of the nerve fiber layer around the disk and absence of leakage on fluorescein angiography. Optic atrophy develops later with pallor on temporal side progressing to whole of the disk.

Blood testing for mitochondrial DNA shows point mutations at the specified sites. Differential diagnosis includes infiltrative, compressive and toxic neuropathies.

Treatment: It includes therapies, which increase mitochondrial energy production like mitochondrial cocktail containing coenzyme Q, vitamin E and vitamin B, but with not much benefit. Avoidance of agents such as ethanol and tobacco, which might stress mitochondrial energy production, is recommended.

Prognosis: It is guarded, especially for 11,778 mutations than others and visual loss is irreversible. Genetic counseling should be done.

Kjer Autosomal Dominant Inherited Optic Atrophy

Kjer autosomal dominant inherited optic atrophy is the most common hereditary optic atrophy. Visual symptoms, which are bilateral, occur in the first or second decade of life and acuity may vary from 6/6 to 6/60. Color vision abnormalities more of tritanopic deficiency, mild optic atrophy and positive family history occurs when the gene is localized to chromosome 3q. Visual loss may progress, but remain stable after teens and recovery does not occur. Neurological imaging should be done to rule out compressive lesions.

Recessive Optic Neuropathy

Recessive optic neuropathy may be isolated or more commonly associated with other systemic disorders. These include Friedreich's ataxia, spinocerebellar ataxia, Behr syndrome, Charcot-Marie-Tooth disease, Wolfram syndrome, etc. Wolfram syndrome is also known as DIDMOAD syndrome (diabetes insipidus, diabetes mellitus, optic atrophy and deafness) in which early onset optic atrophy occurs along with endocrine and neurological abnormalities.

Toxic and Nutritional Optic Neuropathy

Toxic and nutritional optic neuropathy may be considered together because they have a common mechanism and share many clinical features.

Progressive bilateral visual loss associated with defective color vision and central or centrocecal scotoma usually occurs. Initially optic nerve is normal, but later on develops pallor.

Nutritional deficiency

Causes: Deficiency of thiamine and B_{12}, protein deprivation, use of tobacco and alcohol and lack of natural antioxidants and exercise.

One has to keep a high index of suspicion in patients with bilateral progressive symmetric visual loss and a detailed social history should be taken. In dietary deprivation onset of visual loss is usually about 4 months from deprivation. In pernicious anemia, which is an autoimmune disorder, malabsorption of vitamin B_{12} causes its deficiency. Patients present with other clinical features of the disease. Treatment is with hydroxocobalamin and chance of visual recovery is good.

Toxic optic neuropathy

Toxic optic neuropathy is often referred to as chronic retrobulbar neuritis. Features may be similar to nutritional deficiency, but magnitude of visual loss is variable depending on the toxic agent and may even result in blindness. Binocular visual loss occurs due to systemic medications or toxins. Ethambutol is the most common medication and methanol is the most common toxin.

Tobacco-induced optic neuropathy

Smoking can cause or contribute to optic neuropathy. Pipe smokers are more at risk than other forms of tobacco use. Cyanide in tobacco is the suspected etiological agent and other factors like undernutrition, low serum B_{12} and associated alcohol intake may contribute. Pathologically there is ganglion cell degeneration with vacuolation and Nissl body degeneration.

Clinical features: It include progressive binocular loss of central vision and color vision defects. Fundus shows a normal disk or mild temporal pallor, visual fields show central or centrocecal scotoma.

Treatment: It is by discontinuing tobacco and alcohol along with intramuscular injections of hydroxocobalamin and improvement of diet. Visual improvement is slow and prognosis depends upon the extent of damage.

Ethyl alcohol

Causes: optic neuropathy similar to that mentioned above either alone or in combination with tobacco. Associated peripheral neuritis and avitaminosis may be seen due to chronic malnutrition.

Treatment: Include abstaining from alcohol and supplementation of B complex vitamins.

Methyl alcohol

Acute severe visual loss and even death may occur by consumption of the toxin. The use of ethyl alcohol along with it decreases the toxicity, as it competes with alcohol dehydrogenase enzyme. The neurotoxic metabolite formic acid acts on the central nervous system by inhibiting cytochrome oxidase.

Sx Symptoms

Occur in 12–18 hours with headache, nausea, vomiting and acute severe visual loss. Optic disk is at first swollen with peripapillary edema. Atrophy occurs in 1–2 months with cupping. Improvement can occur if intervened early. Coma and death can occur due to format accumulation.

Diagnosis: It is by serum methanol levels > 20 mg/dL.

Treatment: It is by correcting metabolic acidosis, hemodialysis and use of ethyl alcohol as competitive drug. Permanent damage occurs if treatment is delayed and can result in total or partial blindness.

Ethylene glycol

Ethylene glycol is used as antifreeze in automobiles, results in similar picture, but associated with renal failure and oxalate crystals.

Ethambutol

Ethambutol is an antituberculous drug, which may cause retrobulbar neuritis associated with reduced visual acuity, dyschromatopsia and central scotoma. Frequent ophthalmic examination should be done while on therapy, however a dose < 15 mg/kg/day is considered to be safe. Prompt discontinuation of the drug helps in recovery and reversal of symptoms to some extent. Other antituberculous drugs like isoniazid (INH) and streptomycin can also produce optic atrophy.

Chloroquine
Chloroquine is an antimalarial drug, which can produce ocular side effects like keratopathy, myopathy, retinopathy and optic neuropathy and is dose related. Patients with lupus erythematosus who need prolonged course of treatment are more susceptible. Visual field testing with colored targets especially red, within the central 10° will show field defects and impaired color vision indicates early toxicity.

Quinine
Quinine is also an antimalarial drug and it produces optic neuropathy and atrophy following contracture and narrowing of retinal vessels with pale edematous retina resembling central retinal artery occlusion.

Amiodarone
Amiodarone is an antiarrhythmic drug and the toxicity is not dose or duration dependent. It may present with bilateral subacute vision loss with disk edema and should be differentiated from non-arteritic AION. Resolution of the disk edema is slow and occurs months after discontinuing the drug.

Other drug
Other medications include isoniazid, chloramphenicol, penicillamine, sulfonamides, *Digitalis,* chlorpropamide, tolbutamide, oral contraceptives, etc.

Treatment of toxic neuropathy is stopping the medication or substance abuse and replacing the dietary deficiency. Although not completely reversible, visual prognosis is good unless optic atrophy has occurred.

MISCELLANEOUS

Traumatic Optic Neuropathy

Optic nerve injury may be due to trauma to head, orbit or eyeball.

Types

Traumatic optic neuropathy can be classified into direct or indirect.

Direct traumatic optic neuropathy: It occurs due to laceration by bone fragments or from avulsion of the optic nerve from the eyeball.

Indirect type: It is more common and often occurs in frontal head trauma a few inches above the orbital rim (sweet spot) due to shearing forces on the nerve and its blood vessels, most often at its intracanalicular portion.

Clinical Features

Visual loss is sudden and often severe. External evidence of injury need not be present. An afferent pupillary defect is always present, but the optic disk appears normal in the acute stage. Optic disk becomes atrophic within 4–8 weeks of injury.

Suspected cases need imaging of brain and orbit to assess intracranial injuries intraorbital fragments, hematoma, optic canal or other sphenoidal fractures.

Treatment

High dose corticosteroid treatment preferably methyl prednisolone in 30 mg/kg loading dose followed by 5.4 mg/kg/day for 3 days has been used based on National Acute Spinal Cord Injury Study (NASCIS). It may have some benefit if administered within 8 hours as in acute spinal injury. Steroids reduce the edema and tissue damage from ischemia and have an antioxidant effect. Surgical decompression of the optic canal by transethmoidal route may be tried if there is no improvement within 1–2 days, but the results are variable. There is no effective treatment for direct contusion and avulsion.

Diabetic Papillopathy

Denotes optic disk swelling in patient with both insulin-dependent diabetes mellitus (IDDM) and non-insulin-dependent diabetes mellitus (NIDDM). It may be a form of AION. Patients may be asymptomatic or have monocular or binocular subacute or chronic mild blurring of vision. The finding of RAPD is variable and visual field shows enlargement of blind spot. Optic disk shows hyperemia with edema and dilatation of surface microvasculature. These surface telangiectasias may resemble neovascularization of the disk (NVD), but shows a characteristic radial pattern (Fig. 34.21). FFA shows leakage within the disk substance in contrast to NVD, which shows leakage into the vitreous cavity. Associated diabetic retinopathy may be present in 60%–80% of patients.

Bilateral diabetic papillopathy needs investigations to rule out papilledema. Brain and orbital imaging are negative. The condition may resolve spontaneously over 2–10 months to normal or result in optic atrophy. Good control of blood sugar is recommended with adequate treatment of coexisting diabetic retinopathy.

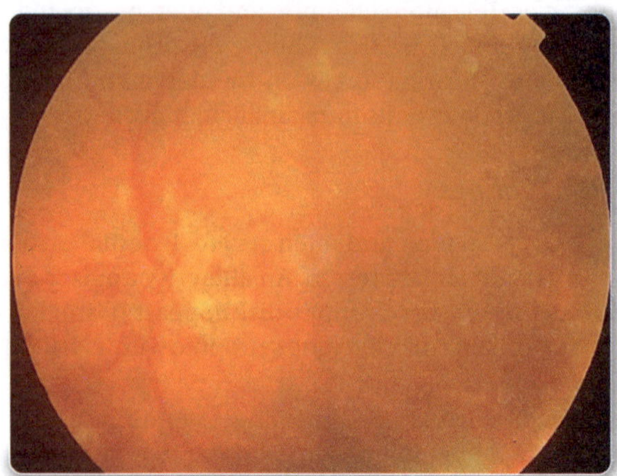

FIGURE 34.21: Diabetic papillopathy

Compressive and Infiltrative Neuropathy

Pressure on the optic nerve by orbital or anterior cranial fossa space occupying lesions causes compression on the optic nerve and optic atrophy. Infiltrative lesions include optic nerve tumors like glioma and optic nerve sheath meningioma, which are discussed along with orbital diseases.

Clinical features include visual loss, RAPD and disk edema initially, which may lead onto optic atrophy.

Graves' Optic Neuropathy

Graves' optic neuropathy occurs due to compression of the optic nerve at the orbital apex by the swollen extraocular muscles. It may be unilateral or bilateral and associated with reduced eye movements, but without significant proptosis. Optic nerve dysfunction results in gradual visual loss, dyschromatopsia, decreased contrast sensitivity and loss of peripheral vision. Visual field may be normal or shows central scotoma or arcuate nerve bundle defect. History of thyroid dysfunction associated with other signs of thyroid eye disease like lid retraction, conjunctival congestion may be present. RAPD may be present if optic neuropathy is asymmetric. The optic disk is commonly normal, but may be edematous. Optic atrophy is present in chronic cases.

Thyroid function may be normal, subnormal or above normal. Orbital imaging shows enlarged extraocular muscles and crowding at orbital apex.

Management: Includes decompression of the orbital soft tissue. Systemic corticosteroids or radiotherapy provides rapid, but temporary improvement in vision. If symptoms persists or recur on tapering doses, surgical decompression of the orbit should be done. Visual recovery depends on the extent of optic nerve damage.

Pupillary Anomalies

35

Girija Devi PS

The pathways for the pupillary reflexes and the different pupillary reflexes are already been described.

ABNORMALITIES OF THE PUPILLARY REFLEXES

Abnormalities in the pupillary reaction can occur in various disorders affecting the afferent or efferent pathway. Abnormalities in the pupillary reflexes can be classified into:

1. Physiological changes in pupil, e.g. anisocoria.
2. The changes in pupillary reaction in lesions of visual pathway are as follows:
   a. Absolute afferent pupillary defect.
   b. Relative afferent pupillary defect.
   c. Wernicke's hemianopic pupillary reaction.
3. Horner's syndrome.
4. Argyll Robertson pupil.
5. Adie's pupil.
6. Effects of drugs.

Physiological Changes in Pupil

Normally the pupil is 3–4 mm in size and equal in size in both eyes and reacts equally to light and convergence. The pupil tends to be smaller in children and in old people (senile miosis).

The pupil tends to be larger in myopia and in conditions of nervous excitement, but the pupillary reactions are unimpaired.

Anisocoria

Anisocoria is a difference in the size of the pupil of two eyes. This is usually pathological due to involvement of either the afferent or efferent pathway of one eye. Rarely, it can occur in normal people.

Hippus

Hippus is a spasmodic, rhythmic, but irregular oscillatory reaction of the pupil when light is thrown into the eye. The pupil constricts, then dilates slightly and constricts again and these changes in the pupil are repeated. It is independent of the illumination or eye movements. It is normal, but pathological hippus can occur associated with trauma, renal diseases, cirrhosis, etc. It is an abnormality of the nervous centers controlling the pupillary reaction.

Pupillary Abnormalities in Lesions of the Visual Pathway

Absolute Afferent Pupillary Defect

Absolute afferent pupillary defect occurs in lesions of the optic nerve when the vision is completely lost (i.e. vision is no PL). Both pupils are equal in size when there is no light stimulation, but in diffuse light as in normal conditions of ocular examination, the affected pupil is slightly larger due to the direct light reaction in the uninvolved eye. When light is shown into the involved eye, direct light reflex in that eye as well as consensual reaction in the other eye are both absent. When light is thrown into the other eye with normal vision, both eyes react normally, i.e. direct light reflex in the uninvolved eye and consensual in the blind eye are present equally. This is the absolute afferent papillary defect. On looking at a near object both pupils constrict normally.

Relative Afferent Pupillary Defect

Relative afferent pupillary defect (RAPD) occurs in an incomplete involvement of the optic nerve or severe retinal disease (where large areas of retina are damaged as in central retinal vein occlusion). The patient is partially blind in one eye. The pupillary reactions are sluggish when the affected eye is stimulated and reactions are normal when the uninvolved eye is stimulated. This unequal reaction (Marcus Gunn pupil) is best demonstrated by the swinging flashlight. Light is first thrown into the unaffected eye and then into the affected eye, this is repeated in quick succession and the reaction of the pupils is noted. The pupil of the involved eye seems to dilate when light is thrown into that eye. This is because the weak constriction of the affected eye is overtaken by the dilatation of both pupils produced by removing the light from the normal eye.

Relative afferent pupillary defect can be demonstrated only if there is a marked disparity in the involvement of both optic nerves or if one is normal and the other is uninvolved. Either if both optic nerves are involved or there is bilateral diffuse retinal damage, RAPD cannot be demonstrated. In such a situation both pupils will be sluggish in reaction.

Wernicke's Hemianopic Pupillary Reaction

Wernicke's hemianopic pupillary reaction is demonstrated in optic tract lesions. On stimulation of one half of the retina the pupillary reaction will be brisk and in stimulation of the other half the reaction will be sluggish. It is not possible to demonstrate this abnormality with diffuse illumination like that of a torch light, since both sides of the retina will be stimulated simultaneously. The spot beam of the slit lamp has to be used to demonstrate this pupillary abnormality.

Pupils in Lesions of Optic Radiations and Occipital Cortex

In blindness due to involvement of the visual pathway beyond the proximal part of the optic tract the pupils are uninvolved since the pupillary pathway separate from the visual pathway at this point.

Abnormal Pupillary Reactions

Large Pupil

Application of mydriatics: Very large immobile pupils are usually due to the application of mydriatics, sometime by mistake due to use of some misplaced eyedrops or touching eyes with fingers contaminated with atropine ointment. In this case pupils are completely immobile and there is paralysis of accommodation also. In unilateral cases, the light reaction in the other eye, both direct and consensual will be normal and consensual reaction will be absent in the involved eye showing an abnormality affecting the efferent pathway of pupillary reflex.

III nerve palsy: Large pupils can occur in III nerve palsy. Accommodation also will be affected (ophthalmoplegia interna). By the application of pilocarpine III nerve palsy can be differentiated from atropinization. In III nerve palsy the pupil will constrict to pilocarpine if the lesion is proximal to the ciliary ganglion and dilates further with atropine. If the dilatation is due to atropinization, pilocarpine will not have any effect.

Sympathetic irritation: Large pupil can occur in irritation of the cervical sympathetic. Such a pupil will constrict to stimulation with light. Eventually the pupil will become miotic, if paralysis of the sympathetic supply develops.

Acute rise intraocular pressure (IOP): It can cause an increase in the size of the pupil.

Increase in intracranial pressure: It can lead to dilatation of the pupil and this is a warning sign in head injury. The dilated non-reacting pupil **(Hutchinson's pupil)** is a warning sign for cerebral decompression on the same side.

Small Pupil

Miotics: Abnormally small pupils can be due to the use of miotics like pilocarpine drops for the treatment of glaucoma or use of morphine. Small sluggishly reacting often irregular pupil is a sign of **iridocyclitis**.

Bilateral small pupils can occur due to **irritation of the III nerve** as in pontine hemorrhage. It can also occur in **paralysis of the sympathetic** supply to the pupil.

Argyll Robertson Pupil

Argyll Robertson pupil (AR pupil) is characteristically seen in neurosyphilis due to involvement of the central decussation in the midbrain. Both eyes are involved, but asymmetrically. Characteristic features of AR pupil:

1. Pupils are small (spinal miosis) and irregular.
2. They do not react to light, but the contraction to convergence is retained (light—near dissociation).
3. Pupils show poor dilation to atropine.

Unilateral AR pupil is seen in lesions of the ciliary ganglion.

Tonic Pupil of Adie

Tonic pupil of Adie's is also called Adie's syndrome or Holmes-Adie syndrome. It is a condition of unknown cause and presumed to be of viral etiology that produces inflammation and damage to the area of brain controlling pupillary constriction. It is often unilateral. Young people are affected more and the condition is more common in women.

The affected pupil is larger in size. The light and near reflex appears to be absent, but careful examination will show that they are present and a sluggish reaction appears after a long latent period. The Adie's pupil constricts with 1/8% pilocarpine due to denervation cholinergic supersensitivity, but normal pupil does not.

This condition is often associated with diminished deep tendon reflexes (Holmes-Adie pupil). In long standing cases the pupil may finally become smaller (little old Adie).

Differential Diagnosis from AR Pupil

The AR pupil is small, but Adie's pupil is large. Adie's pupil dilates well with atropine, but AR pupil does not.

Horner's Syndrome (Oculosympathetic Palsy)

Horner's syndrome occurs due to lesion of the sympathetic supply to the pupil:

1. It can be due to involvement of the first order neuron as in:
   a. Brainstem disease.
   b. Syringomyelia.
   c. Lateral medullary syndrome.
   d. Spinal cord tumors.
2. Due to involvement of the second order neuron as in:
   a. Carotid artery aneurysms.
   b. Lesions and injuries at the neck.
3. Due to involvement of the third order neuron as in:
   a. Internal carotid artery dissection.
   b. Nasopharyngeal tumors.
   c. Cavernous sinus tumors.

Clinical Features

There will be:

1. Mild ptosis (1–2 mm) due to weakness of the Muller's muscle.
2. Mild enophthalmos.
3. Narrow palpebral fissure due to ptosis and slight elevation of the lower lid.
4. Miosis.
5. Normal reactions to light and near.
6. The iris may have a lighter color in long standing cases.
7. There may be associated decreased sweating of the face in lesions below the superior cervical ganglion.

Ptosis in Horner's syndrome is associated with miosis, while ptosis in III nerve palsy is associated with dilated pupil.

Pharmacological Tests

Cocaine drop test: Cocaine 4% will not have any action on the Horner's pupil, but dilate a normal pupil and confirm the diagnosis of Horner's syndrome. Cocaine blocks the reuptake of noradrenaline at the sympathetic nerve endings. In Horner's syndrome there is no noradrenaline secreted at the sympathetic nerve endings and hence cocaine has no action. But cocaine, being a narcotic drug is not freely available.

Apraclonidine: Application of α-agonist apraclonidine in both eyes leads to increased dilation in affected pupil due to hypersensitivity (opposite to cocaine test).

Adrenaline 1:1,000: In preganglionic lesions both pupils will not dilate because adrenaline is rapidly destroyed by monoamine oxidase. In postganglionic lesions, dilator pupillae muscle shows denervation hypersensitivity to adrenaline. So it dilates maximally in Horner's syndrome.

Action of Drugs on the Pupil

Mydriatics

Drugs, which dilate the pupil are called mydriatics. Most of these drugs produce paralysis of the ciliary muscle also (cycloplegia) and hence called cycloplegics.

Atropine: It is the strongest mydriatic cycloplegic drug. It is a parasympatholytic drug, which abolishes the action of acetylcholine at the nerve endings which supply the sphincter pupillae and ciliary muscle.

Miotics

Drugs, which constrict the pupil are called miotics. All of these drugs causes contraction of the ciliary muscle also and result in a condition of partial or complete sustained accommodation (ciliary spasm). This will result in blurring of distant vision especially in children and young adults who have good power of accommodation.

Pilocarpine: It is a cholinergic drug, which acts at the myoneural junction and supplement the action of acetylcholine.

The anticholinesterase group of miotics, e.g. physostigmine abolishes the action of anticholinesterase enzyme and the acetylcholine liberated at the myoneural junction has sustained effect.

Sympathomimetic Drugs

Sympathomimetic drugs like adrenaline and phenylephrine directly stimulates the myoneural junction at the dilator muscle and produce mydriasis. The eyes dilated with adrenaline and phenylephrine will show reaction to light since the action of the sphincter pupillae is unimpaired and it is a stronger muscle than dilator pupillae.

Sympatholytic Drugs

Sympatholytic drugs like ergotamine have effect on pupils on systemic administration, but they are not clinically used topically.

Nystagmus

36

Anuja Sathar, Girija Devi PS

Nystagmus (in Greek nystagmus means 'to nod') is the repetitive, rhythmic, involuntary to and for oscillations of the eyes. It is most commonly horizontal, but can also be vertical, torsional or mixture of all the three. Movements which are not rhythmic and regular are called 'nystagmoid movements'.

CAUSES

Lesions affecting the structures in maintaining normal ocular posture can result in nystagmus like:

1. Visual pathway.
2. Vestibular apparatus.
3. Midbrain.
4. Cerebellum.
5. Semicircular canals.

FEATURES

1. May be jerky or pendular: Movements are equal in both directions in pendular nystagmus, while it has a slow and fast component in jerky nystagmus, the direction of which is denoted by the direction of the fast component.
2. Rapid/slow: Rate or frequency of nystagmus is inversely proportional to the amplitude.
3. Latent/manifest: Latent, when it appears only in closure of the other eye.
4. Fine/coarse: Depending on the amplitude of excursion. Alexander's law states that, "amplitude is greatest in the direction of fast component."
5. Null zone: It is a position in jerk nystagmus when nystagmus is not evident. Patients with null zone assume head posture, so that eyes are in null zone.

TYPES

Physiological Nystagmus

End Positional Nystagmus

Fine, low amplitudinal jerk nystagmus at extreme gaze, equal in amplitude in both gazes, but more evident in abducting than adducting eye. It stops with three or four beats and has no symptoms.

Optokinetic Nystagmus

Optokinetic nystagmus is a physiological jerk nystagmus induced by moving repetitive stimuli like stripes of an optokinetic drum or looking out of a moving vehicle. There is a slow pursuit movement in which the eyes follow the target followed by fast saccadic movements in opposite direction due to refixation. It can be used to test visual acuity in infants and malingering persons.

Physiological Vestibular Nystagmus

Physiological vestibular nystagmus is a jerk nystagmus caused by stimulating the vestibular apparatus with caloric stimuli. When cold water is poured into one ear, the patient will develop jerk nystagmus to opposite side and when warm water is poured, jerk nystagmus to same side occurs. The mnemonic cold-opposite, warm-same (COWS) indicates the direction of nystagmus.

Sensory Nystagmus

Sensory nystagmus is also known as sensory deprivation or ocular nystagmus.

It is due to severe deprivation of vision early in life and usually appears within first 6 months of life. It is of horizontal and pendular type, and is dampened by convergence. Common causes include Leber's congenital amaurosis, congenital cataract, aniridia, albinism and achromatopsia.

Miners' nystagmus is seen in coal mine workers and is of rotary type. It is due to difficulty in fixation in coal mines due to dim illumination. Increase in illumination improves the condition.

Motor Nystagmus

Congenital Motor Nystagmus

Congenital motor nystagmus may be isolated or occurs with strabismus or developmental delay. It is a horizontal jerk nystagmus, which occurs early in life and is uniplanar, i.e. remains horizontal in all fields of gaze. It may be dampened by convergence or extreme eye positions and is absent during sleep. Oscillopsia is not seen. Head posture in order to get eyes into null zone and head nodding may be seen.

Spasmus Nutans

Usually appears within first 2 years of life with a triad of intermittent binocular horizontal pendular nystagmus, head nodding and torticollis. It may be sometimes asymmetric or monocular. It usually disappears spontaneously in 3 years. Other neurological abnormalities may be absent except strabismus or amblyopia. Lack of resolution of symptoms or development of new symptoms suggests further evaluation like electroretinography (ERG) or neuroimaging.

Monocular Nystagmus of Childhood

Small amplitude vertical or elliptical nystagmus occurs in one eye due to poor vision known as Heimann-Bielschowsky phenomenon. Lesions of optic nerve or chiasmal glioma should be ruled out.

Nystagmus Blockage Syndrome

Fixating eye in the adducted position causes decrease of nystagmus in this condition, so that esotropia dampens the nystagmus.

Latent Nystagmus

Latent nystagmus is a horizontal jerk nystagmus that appears in monocular viewing with fast phase toward the viewing eye. Latent nystagmus is often associated with dissociated vertical deviation or congenital esotropia. Manifest latent nystagmus occurs with characters of latent nystagmus in which small amount of esotropia or microtropia behaves similar to that of occluded eye.

Gaze-evoked Nystagmus

Gaze-evoked nystagmus occurs with fast phase and increased amplitude in the direction of gaze, because of inability to maintain fixation in extremes of gaze. It is due to damage of the neural integrator for horizontal or vertical gaze. When asymmetric, ipsilateral brainstem or cerebellar lesions should be considered. Metabolic or toxic factors like anticonvulsants, sedatives, alcohol and Wernicke's encephalopathy also cause similar nystagmus.

Downbeat Nystagmus

Downbeat nystagmus is a present in primary position and increased by down gaze. Structural lesions at the cervicomedullary junction usually an Arnold-Chiari malformation is the most common etiology.

Upbeat Nystagmus

Upbeat nystagmus occurs with fast phase upwards. Lesions in the brainstem and anterior cerebellar vermis including demyelination, stroke and drug toxicity or tobacco may cause this type of nystagmus.

Periodic Alternating Nystagmus

Periodic alternating nystagmus (PAN) is a horizontal nystagmus that oscillates in direction, amplitude and frequency. It occurs for about 1–2 minutes in one direction and then reverses the direction repeatedly. Periodic head turn and oscillopsia may be seen. Common causes include demyelination, stroke, Arnold-Chiari malformation or bilateral visual loss.

See-saw Nystagmus

See-saw nystagmus is a pendular and torsional nystagmus in which one eye rises and intorts, while the other eye falls and extorts resembling a see saw. It is due to parachiasmal or third ventricular lesions.

Vestibular Nystagmus

Vestibular nystagmus may be central or peripheral vestibular type and is horizontal jerk and rotational type.

Central vestibular type occurs due to demyelination, tumors or vascular accidents. Peripheral type occurs due to lesions of the labyrinth or VIII cranial nerve and is associated with vertigo, tinnitus and deafness.

Convergence Retraction Nystagmus

In this type, repetitive convergence associated with retraction of globe on attempted upgaze or by viewing an optokinetic strip moved downwards; occurs in both the eyes. It occurs most commonly due to lesions in the dorsal midbrain region like pinealoma or abnormalities involving the aqueduct of Sylvius and is known as Sylvian aqueduct syndrome or Parinaud's syndrome. Other features include defective convergence, light near dissociation, vertical nystagmus, defective vertical gaze, lid retraction, etc.

MANAGEMENT

A proper evaluation including history, detailed ocular examination and neuroimaging in needed cases should be done.

Non-surgical Methods

Non-surgical methods of treatment include optical devices like spectacles, contact lens, prisms and correction of amblyopia. Medical treatment includes use of baclofen (in PAN), clonazepam, barbiturates, etc.

Surgical Methods

Surgical methods include:

1. Shifting the null position to primary position by modified Kestenbaum procedure.
2. Bimedial recession is to induce convergence.
3. Faden or supramaximal recession of horizontal recti—to reduce amplitude of nystagmus.

NYSTAGMOID MOVEMENTS

Nystagmoid movements are abnormalities of ocular movement, which resemble nystagmus.

Ocular Flutter

Ocular flutter is seen in cerebellar diseases and characterized by horizontal oscillations, which are intermittent and occurs when there is change of gaze.

Opsoclonus

Opsoclonus is similar to ocular flutter, but is multiplanar and of large amplitude, and may be associated with the myoclonus of face, arms and legs. It is seen in patients with metastatic neuroblastoma, encephalitis, demyelination, etc.

Ocular Bobbing

Characterized by fast conjugate downward movements with a slow updrift to primary position; occurs in pontine lesions and metabolic encephalopathy.

Neuro-ophthalmologic Features of ICSOLs

37

Girija Devi PS

The visual pathway (Fig. 37.1) runs a long course from the optic disk to the occipital cortex and neurological problems can affect any part of this long path, and can produce a variety of problems depending on the site of the lesion.

SYMPTOMS AND SIGNS

Symptoms and signs produced by intracranial space occupying lesions (ICSOLs), especially intracranial tumors can be divided into:

1. Non-localizing.
2. Falsely localizing.
3. Those that are truly localizing.

NON-LOCALIZING

Headache

Headache is a common complaint of patients visiting the medical or ophthalmology outpatient department (OPD), but an intracranial problem has to be suspected if:

1. The headache is constantly present in early morning.
2. The headaches wake up the patient from sleep at night.

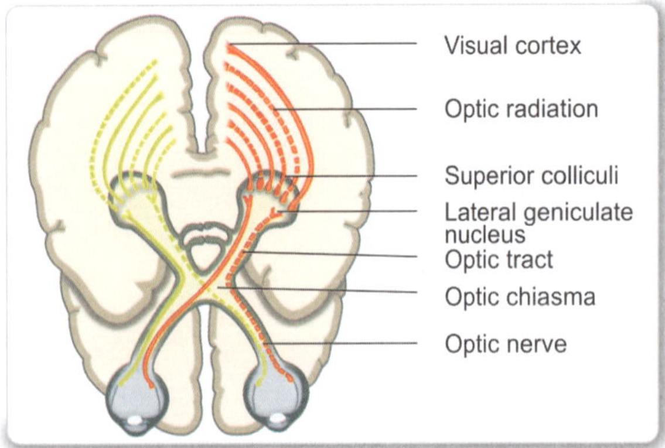

FIGURE 37.1: Visual pathway

3. Headache is intense and prolonged, and the patient is incapacitated by it.
4. Nausea or vomiting is associated with headache.
5. Recent onset of severe headache.

Patients whose history gives these characteristic features should undergo further neurological and radiological evaluation for ICSOL. Localized pain on the head may be felt in the case of meningeal tumors and malignant tumors that invade the bone meninges.

More the increase in intracranial tension (ICT), the changes in the intracranial pressure and effect of changes in pressure by traction or displacement of pain-sensitive intracranial structures is the cause of headache in intracranial tumors.

Papilledema

Disk swelling is caused by increased intracranial tension. The increase in intracranial pressure may be due to:

1. Increase in intracranial tissue volume due to the tumor.
2. Obstruction to the flow of cerebrospinal fluid (CSF) or cerebral venous flow.
3. Diffuse or local cerebral edema.
4. Increased production of CSF in excess of the rate at which it is absorbed.

Infratentorial tumors produce papilledema more frequently than supratentorial tumors and the mechanism is usually obstruction of the aqueduct of Sylvius. There is a greater tendency for papilledema to occur in rapidly growing tumors like meningiomas.

Seizures

When seizures develop for the first time in a person above 20 years of age, an intracranial lesion has to be suspected. When the seizures are associated with forced turning of the head and eyes, the cause for the seizure is usually located in the hemisphere opposite to the direction of the head and eye movements.

VI Nerve Palsy

Due to its long subarachnoid course, one or both VI nerves may be involved in cases of increased intracranial pressure due to its compression between the pons and basilar artery or by stretching on the sharp edge of the petrous bone. The involvement is usually incomplete and tends to recover, if the ICT is brought down.

FALSELY LOCALIZING

Falsely localizing sign is a sign that cause confusion in diagnosis by suggesting an abnormality at a site away from the actual site of the mass lesion. They are of less practical importance now and that magnetic resonance imaging (MRI) and computed tomography (CT) scans are able to locate the problem accurately. Most false localizing signs occur late in the course of ICT. Increased intracranial pressure, brain movement and hydrocephalus are the important causes for the development of false localizing signs. Some false localizing signs are given below.

Visual Field Defects

Bitemporal hemianopia is seen in chiasmal lesions. Posterior fossa tumors can cause bitemporal hemianopia by producing hydrocephalus with dilatation of the third ventricle and pressure on the optic chiasma.

Visual Hallucinations

Formed visual hallucinations are seen in temporal lobe lesions and unformed visual hallucinations in occipital lobe lesions. But both unformed and formed visual hallucinations can sometime occur in frontal lobe tumors.

Cranial Nerve Involvement

Cranial nerve involvement is a common false localizing sign.

Olfactory nerve: Bilateral anosmia is a common false localizing sign. It often has no significance because it is frequently seen unassociated with any intracranial tumor, due to some local pathology.

III nerve palsy: It is usually a localizing sign when it occurs on the same side as an intracranial tumor. Partial or total involvement on the opposite side can occur as a falsely localizing sign.

IV nerve paresis: It can occur in benign intracranial hypertension. Sometime it may be a decompensation of a congenital trochlear nerve palsy that has occurred when the patient became ill.

Trigeminal nerve dysfunction: Decreased corneal sensation can occur as a falsely localizing sign in posterior fossa tumors by stretching and compression of the sensory root of the trigeminal by a shift of the brainstem.

TRUE LOCALIZING

Tumors of the Orbit

Gaze-evoked amaurosis: There will be a transient loss of vision of one eye when looking in a particular direction. It is often due to a compression of the optic nerve or the blood vessels supplying the optic nerve on looking in that direction. This will be relieved by removal of the mass.

Proptosis: Most orbital tumors produce proptosis, but in the early stages, it will be minimal or present only in certain circumstances like stooping down.

Enophthalmos: Most causes of enophthalmos are not related to orbital tumor. A scirrhous carcinoma of the breast can metastasize into the orbit and result in a fibrotic reaction in the orbit leading to progressive enophthalmos. It can be a specific sign of metastatic breast carcinoma.

Optic disk swelling: Orbital tumor is the most common cause of unilateral optic disk swelling without significant visual loss. Even in patients without visual loss, testing for color vision may show defects and field changes can be elicited like enlargement of the blind spot or peripheral field constriction.

Opticociliary shunt vessels: They are communicating vessels between retinal and choroidal circulation seen on the optic disk. They can appear as a congenital anomaly, but most commonly appear as the result of chronic compression of optic nerve and obstruction of central retinal vein. In many cases of orbital tumors, the clinical triad of ipsilateral visual loss, disk edema (optic atrophy) and opticociliary shunt vessels is seen.

Choroidal folds: In the presence of papilledema, choroidal folds appearing as linear folds radiating from the optic disk (in the case of intraconal lesion) and curvilinear folds (in the case of extraconal lesion) is pathognomonic of orbital tumors.

Limitation of ocular movement: This can be paretic due to involvement of ocular motor nerves or mechanical restriction due to mass lesion.

Syndrome of the floor of the orbit: The tumor of the floor of the orbit may complain of severe pain on the same side cheek or anesthesia in the area of nerve supply of the infraorbital nerve—the numb cheek syndrome.

Tumors Involving the Superior Orbital Fissure and Cavernous Sinus

They produce ocular motor palsies especially involving the III nerve and optic nerve, and this may be combined with Horner's syndrome due to involvement of the sympathetic supply, and also involvement of the first and occasionally the second division of trigeminal nerve. III nerve palsy with a pupil smaller than that of the normal eye on the other side denotes involvement of the sympathetic.

Tumors in the Suprasellar Area

The most common tumors in this area are pituitary adenoma, craniopharyngioma and glioma.

Anterior Chiasmal Syndrome

Anterior chiasmal syndrome is a compression involving the intracranial portion of the optic nerve. What differentiates lesion of the intracranial portion of the optic nerve from that of the orbital portion is the demonstration of the damage to the crossed inferior nasal fibers from the other eye that loop anteriorly into the posterior end of the optic nerve before turning back into the optic chiasma. There will be slowly progressive loss of vision with a normal optic disk. But the involvement of the optic nerve is revealed by the afferent pupillary defect, color vision defects and visual field changes. The fields will show a superior temporal field defect in the normal eye, which cannot be explained by any retinal pathology. This is due to involvement of the loop of inferior nasal fibers from the other eye. This is called the anterior chiasmal syndrome, which is a misnomer, since damage is not to the involvement of the chiasma, but the distal end of the optic nerve.

The crossed and uncrossed fibers are separated at the level of the distal end of the optic nerve, and a small lesion here can involve either the crossed or uncrossed fibers alone, resulting in a unilateral hemianopic field defect-the junctional scotoma of Traquair (Fig. 37.2).

Syndrome of Optic Chiasma

Lesions of optic chiasma are characterized by a bitemporal hemianopia due to involvement of the crossing nasal fibers. The visual field may be symmetrical or asymmetrical depending on the level of pressure effect, but it will not cross the vertical midline. These patients will also have see-saw nystagmus. This is due to damage to the rostral mesencephalon, possibly to the interstitial nucleus of Cajal and not due to the chiasma itself. Bitemporal hemianopia can occur as a false localizing sign as mentioned earlier.

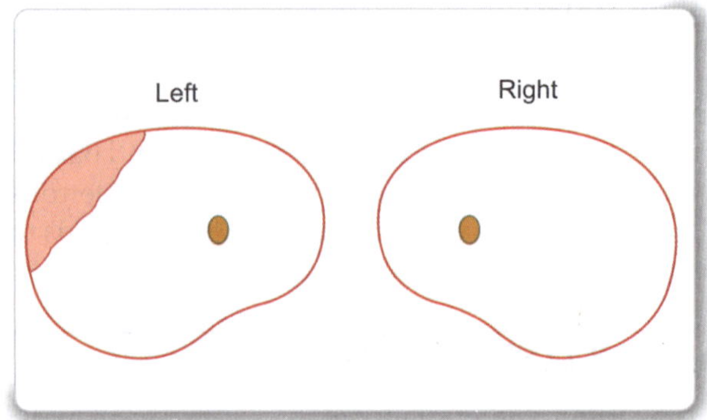

FIGURE 37.2: Junctional scotoma of Traquair

Suprasellar Lesion

Lesions in the suprasellar region can damage the hypothalamus and pituitary, and present as several different syndromes. Lesions involving hypothalamus can produce diabetes insipidus, hyperthermia and disturbance of appetite.

Froelich's Syndrome

Froelich's syndrome is characterized by arrest of social development and obesity. Usual cause is craniopharyngioma.

Russell Syndrome

Russell syndrome or diencephalic syndrome is caused by tumors in the optic chiasma and anterior hypothalamus like glioma, ependymoma epidermoid cyst, etc. The principal features are emaciation, normal linear growth, alert appearance with increased vigor and euphoria. Visual problems are not seen in all patients. Involvement of the distal portion of the optic nerve can cause decrease in vision and optic atrophy. Nystagmus is present in majority of the patients and it may be vertical, horizontal or torsional.

The diagnosis of diencephalic syndrome is confirmed by CT scan and MRI. These lesions are very sensitive to radiotherapy. On treatment, these children gain weight, recover subcutaneous fat and resume normal growth and development. The elevated growth hormone levels also come back to normal.

Syndromes of Pituitary Dysfunction

The optic nerve and the chiasma lie above the diaphragma sellae, the fold of dura mater, which forms the roof of the sella turcica, which contain the pituitary gland.

So, a visual field defect in a patient with pituitary tumor means suprasellar extension. Laterally expanding pituitary tumor can affect the cavernous sinus and affect the III, IV and VI cranial nerves.

The chromophobe adenoma is the commonest pituitary tumor to produce neuro-ophthalmological changes. Acidophil adenomas do not extent beyond the sella and the basophil adenomas are also small, and rarely involve the chiasma.

The visual symptoms have a gradual progression and may not be noticed until it is fairly advanced. The field defects can vary depending on the anatomical relationship of the chiasma and the pituitary mass. If the chiasma is central, both upper temporal fields are affected first and then lower temporal fields are affected. The involvement of both eyes will be asymmetrical, since the growth of the tumor will vary. The defects can be relative and may be demonstrated only with red objects. The visual acuity will be normal. In some patients the picture of 'anterior chiasmal syndrome' may be produced and rarely field defects may be confined to one eye only. All there variations depend on the direction of growth of the tumor. When the macular fibers are involved there will be drop in visual acuity.

Optic Atrophy

Optic atrophy will be seen in 50% of cases showing field defects. The appearance of optic atrophy denotes poor visual prognosis. The visual recovery after management of the pituitary tumor will be rare.

Lateral expansion of the tumor can lead to involvement of the ocular motor nerves. The paresis can lead to diplopia. The involvement of the ocular motor nerves leads to a see-saw nystagmus. The diagnosis is confirmed by MRI and CT scan and by the associated endocrinological abnormalities.

Treatment: It is by surgery through a transsphenoidal approach and by radiotherapy or stereotactic radiotherapy in which radiation is applied to the tumor alone, without affecting the surrounding tissues.

Pituitary Apoplexy

A rare disorder caused by the hemorrhage in the pituitary tumor. It can occur in persons with normal pituitary gland also.

The patient presents with severe headache, visual loss, ophthalmoplegia and decreased sensation over distribution of the first and second division of the trigeminal.

Treatment: Systemic steroids. Sometimes surgery may be needed to prevent blindness and other complications.

Lesions of the Optic Tract

Optic tract can be damaged by lesions of the suprasellar area as well as the temporal lobe. Complete optic tract lesions are characterized by the following:

1. Complete homonymous hemianopia.
2. An afferent pupillary defect without any loss of visual acuity or color vision in the eye, ipsilateral to the hemianopia.
3. Normal optic head initially and finally, hemianopia optic nerve and nerve fiber layer atrophy.

Lesions of Lateral Geniculate Body

The field defects are typical. Wedge shaped horizontal homonymous sectoranopia that may be symmetrical or asymmetrical in both eyes are produced by lesions of the lateral geniculate body. Similar field defects can occur in lesions of optic radiations also, but lesions of the optic radiation does not produce any change in the optic disk. In lesions of the lateral geniculate body, homonymous hemianopic optic atrophy will occur. The common lesions here are astrocytomas or metastatic tumors in the deep temporal lobe involving the lateral geniculate body.

Ocular Symptoms of Frontal Lobe Lesions

They may be severe, but rarely localizing. Papilledema may occur in 50% of cases, it can be bilateral or unilateral or asymmetric involvement.

Foster Kennedy Syndrome

Typically seen in meningiomas of the olfactory groove or sphenoid ridge. It can occur in frontal lobe tumors also. There will be papilledema in one eye due to increased ICT and optic atrophy in the other eye due to direct compression of the optic nerve.

Progressive visual loss will occur either due to chronic papilledema or by compression of the intracranial portion of the optic nerve or the optic chiasma. The visual field defects can vary (Fig. 37.3). It can be central scotoma, arcuate scotoma or even nasal or temporal hemianopic field defects. The field defects can be due to chronic papilledema or due to compression of the optic chiasma or optic tract.

Ocular Motor Abnormalities

Ocular motor abnormalities can also occur. The frontal eye fields in the prefrontal cortex control the initiation of saccadic eye movements to the opposite side. Patients with frontal lobe tumors may be unable to initiate saccadic eye movements in one or more directions depending on the pressure effects of the tumor. Conjugate deviation of the eyes and sometimes the head may be seen during or immediately after an attack of seizure. Since patients with

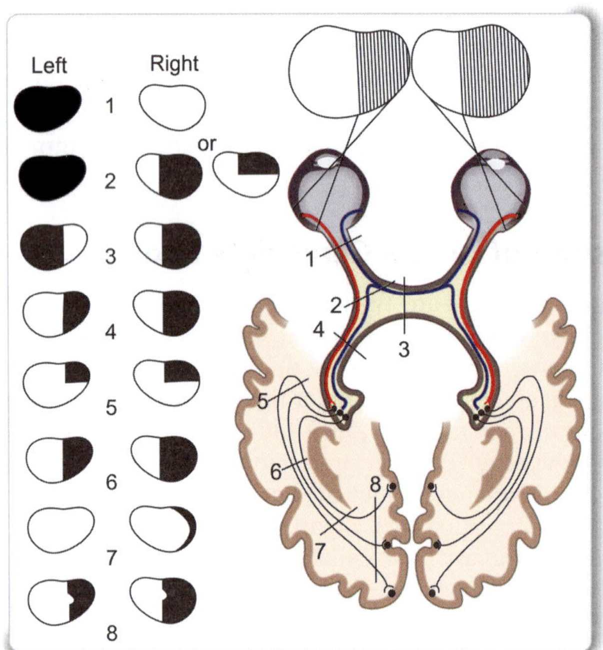

FIGURE 37.3: Field defects in lesions at various sites along the course of the visual pathway (for details of 1–8 points, refers the end of the Chapter)

frontal lobe tumor may have behavioral abnormalities they may not cooperate with testing of ocular movements. VI nerve palsy may occur unilaterally or bilaterally due to raised ICT. III and IV nerve palsy also may rarely occur due to extension of the tumor into the subarachnoid space or from herniation of the incus.

Nystagmus is rare in frontal lobe tumors, but true vestibular nystagmus can occur as a false localizing sign due to the effect of increased intracranial pressure on central vestibular structures.

Inability to voluntarily close the eyelids may occur in bilateral frontal tumor even through reflux closure is retained.

Tumors of the Olfactory Groove

Tumors of the olfactory groove produce signs and symptoms similar to frontal lobe tumors. But they develop in a neurologically and visually 'silent' area and hence they produce symptoms only when they assume considerable size. The most frequent symptom is anosmia, which is often overlooked, since the most common cause for anosmia is chronic rhinitis. Anosmia can be the only symptom for several years.

The most common visual symptom is loss of central vision. The visual loss is slowly progressive and it can be due to papilledema due to increased ICT or due to direct compression of the optic nerve and chiasma. Since both mechanisms can act, the clinical picture can be a combination of optic atrophy in one eye and papilledema in the other eye. This is called the Foster Kennedy syndrome. It is a triad that includes anosmia also. But there can be variation in clinical picture with bilateral papilledema or optic atrophy, which is unilateral or bilateral.

Diagnosis: It is confirmed by imaging techniques.

Treatment: Surgical excision, radiotherapy is also given postoperatively, if it is a neuroblastoma.

Lesions of the Temporal Lobe

The temporal lobe is a common site of intracranial tumors. The majority of them are gliomas.

Seizures: It occur frequently in temporal lobe tumors. Temporal lobe epilepsy is often associated with alteration in mood and the patient may show head and eye movements, away from the side of the lesion.

Visual hallucinations: It may precede a particular form of temporal lobe seizure, the 'uncinate fits'. The visual hallucinations in temporal lobe lesions are formed and complex, but they occur much less frequently than olfactory or gustatory hallucinations.

Papilledema: It may occur and this can lead to postneuritic optic atrophy. Optic atrophy can also occur due to forward extension of the tumor leading to invasion of the optic chiasma or optic tract.

Visual field defects: It occurs frequently. Homonymous field defects are more common than quadrantanopia. The field defects are congruous in pure temporal lobe lesion. If the field defects are incongruous, it is usually due to involvement of the optic tract and the larger defect will be seen in the visual field of the eye, ipsilateral to the lesion. The field defects are usually produced by damage to the optic radiation and do not affect visual acuity.

Lesions of the Parietal Lobe

Tumors of the parietal lobe are rare.

Visual field defects: It consists of a homonymous contra lateral inferior quadrantanopia (pie on the floor) field defect because of the involvement of the superior fibers of the optic radiation, which proceed through the parietal lobe. The hemianopia is frequently congruous.

Visual hallucinations: It may occur in parietal lobe tumors and such hallucinations are generally unformed.

Associated features: They are abnormal color discrimination, difficulty in recognizing familiar face (prosopagnosia), difficulty in identifying one's own fingers (finger agnosia), acalculia and agraphia.

Occipital Lobe Lesions

Apart from the ocular symptoms and signs the occipital lobe is a neurologically silent area. Visual field defects are seen in 95% of occipital lobe lesions. They are contralateral to the side of the lesion, congruous hemianopia or quadrantanopia or hemianopic scotomas, usually with macular sparing. Many patients, even with complete homonymous hemianopia are unaware of the field defects.

Unformed visual hallucinations occur. Damage to the tip of the occipital lobe as in a head injury will give rise to congruous homonymous macular defects. The anterior most part of the calcarine cortex corresponds to the extreme temporal monocular field. The lesion in the area can give rise to a unilateral temporal field defect on the opposite side called temporal crescent.

Alexia (the inability to read) and agraphia (the inability to write) may be produced by lesions of the ungulate gyrus of the dominant hemisphere. Alexia may occur without agraphia. The clinical picture will consist of a right homonymous hemianopia with alexia.

Lesions of inferior occipitotemporal area can produce a variety of clinical pictures. Bilateral involvement can lead to visual agnosia (the inability to recognize object by sight) and also prosopagnosia. Color vision is also represented in this area. Lesions here can cause contralateral hemiachromatopsia.

Therefore, in occipital lobe involvement it is important to test the ability to read and write, and also to test for visual fields using colored objects.

The availability of the neuroimaging techniques have brought down the importance of the clinical signs in lesions of the central nervous system, but their assessment is still important to decide on the type of investigative procedures to order and to decide on the mode of management, and subsequent follow-up (refer Fig. 37.3):

1. Lesion involving the optic nerve—ipsilateral blindness.
2. Lesion through the junction of the optic nerve and chiasma—ipsilateral blindness and contralateral hemianopia or superior quadrantanopia (Traquair junctional scotoma) due to involvement of the inferior nasal fibers looping into the terminal portion of the optic nerve before turning back to continue into the optic tract.
3. Bitemporal hemianopia due lesions affecting the optic chiasma.
4. Homonymous hemianopia due to lesions of the optic tract.
5. Quadrantic homonymous defect due to lesions of the optic tract.
6. Homonymous hemianopia in lesions of optic radiations.
7. Contralateral temporal crescent in anterior lesions of occipital cortex involving the monocular temporal field.
8. Homonymous hemianopia with macular sparing in lesions of occipital cortex.

Oculomotor Nerves

38

Girija Devi PS

The movements of the eyes are controlled by seven muscles, four recti muscles (medial, lateral, superior and inferior recti), two oblique muscles (superior and inferior oblique) and the levator palpebrae superioris.

Three oculomotor nerves (III or oculomotor, IV or trochlear and the VI or abducent nerve) supply these muscles. III nerve supply the medial, superior and inferior recti, inferior oblique and the levator palpebrae superioris. VI nerve supply the lateral rectus and IV nerve supply the superior oblique. The III nerve supply the internal musculature, the ciliary muscle and the sphincter pupillae, but the dilator pupillae is supplied by the sympathetic.

The coordinate movements of the two eyes are made possible by intermediate centers linking the nuclei of both sides. The connection to the vestibular apparatus help to maintain equilibrium and the links to the cerebral cortex helps the voluntary movements of the eye.

OCULAR MOTOR NERVES (III, IV AND VI)

Applied Anatomy

III and IV Nerves

The III and IV nerve nuclei are situated near the midline in the floor of the aqueduct of Sylvius beneath the superior colliculus. The levator palpebre superioris (LPS) is supplied bilaterally from both nuclei. The other muscles are supplied by the ipsilateral nuclei. The Edinger-Westphal nucleus in the III nerve nucleus supplies the sphincter pupillae and ciliary muscle (Fig. 38.1).

III NERVE

Course and Relations

Fascicular Portion

Fascicular portion of the nerve appears within the brainstem. The fibers pass through the medial longitudinal fasciculus (MLF) and the red nucleus to emerge from the sulcus oculomotorius on the medial aspect of the basis pedunculi (Fig. 38.2).

Course in the Posterior Cranial Fossa

The oculomotor nerve passes downward and forward in the cisterna interpeduncularis between the posterior cerebral and superior cerebellar arteries. The cisterna interpeduncularis contains the cerebral peduncles and the circle of Willis (Fig. 38.3).

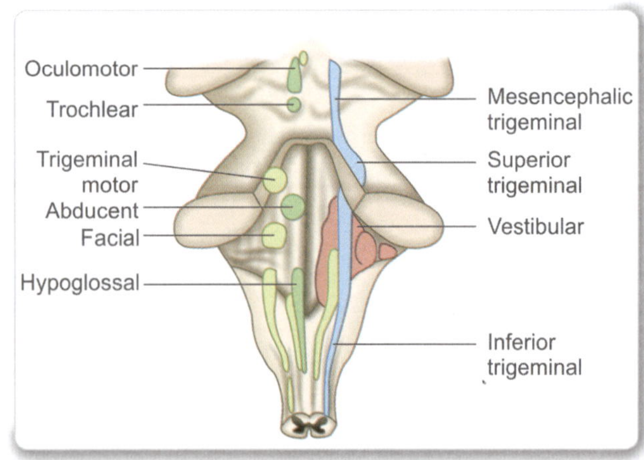

FIGURE 38.1: Nuclei of oculomotor nerves

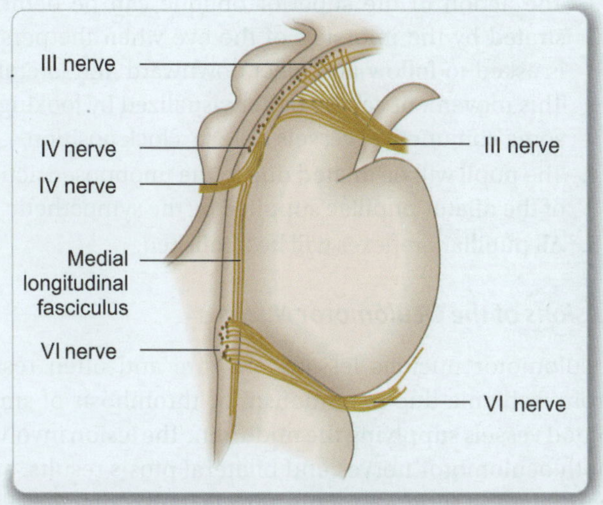

FIGURE 38.2: Nuclei and fascicular portion of oculomotor nerves

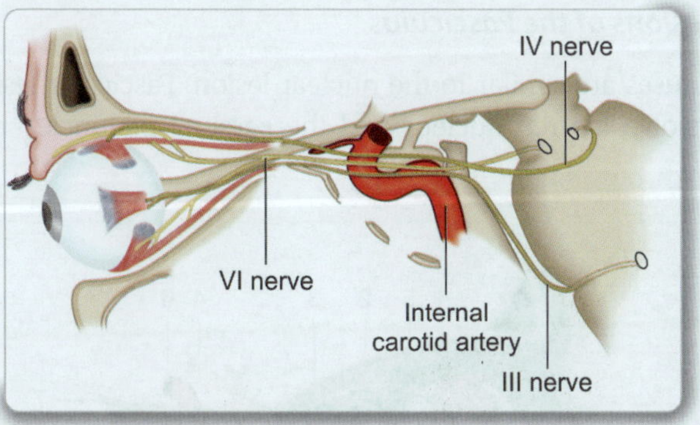

FIGURE 38.3: Course of oculomotor nerve

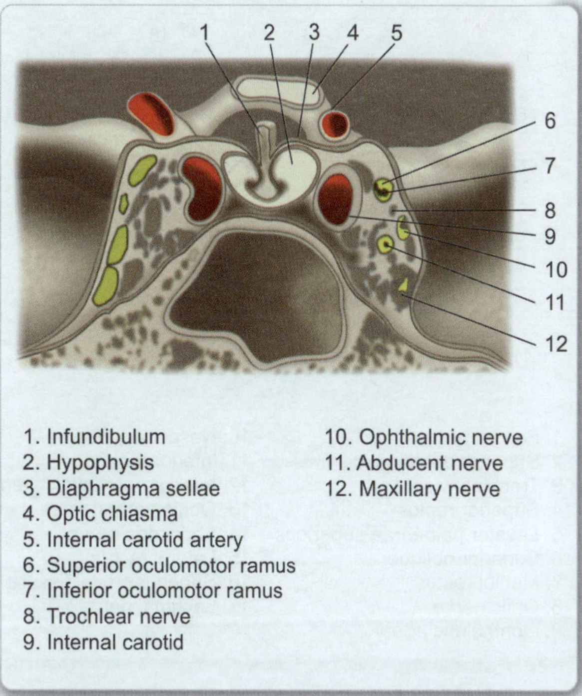

FIGURE 38.4: Arrangement of nerves in the cavernous sinus

Course in the Middle Cranial Fossa

The oculomotor nerve passes into the middle cranial fossa and lies lateral to the pituitary fossa above the cavernous sinus. There it pierces the dura mater midway between the anterior and posterior clinoid processes and reaches the lateral wall of the cavernous sinus. In the lateral wall of the cavernous sinus, the trochlear and the first and second divisions of the V nerve are inferolateral to it and the VI nerve and the internal carotid artery lies within the cavernous sinus below and medial to III nerve. The III nerve divides into the superior and inferior division just before it enters the orbit through the superior orbital fissure within the two heads of the lateral rectus muscle within the annular tendon. The IV, frontal and lacrimal nerves pass through the superior orbital fissure above the annular tendon (Figs 38.4 and 38.5).

In the Orbit

The superior division passes into the orbit above the optic nerve behind the nasociliary nerve and divide to supply the superior rectus and the LPS.

The inferior division immediately divides into three branches; branches to the inferior rectus, medial rectus and the inferior oblique. The branch to the inferior oblique is long and runs along the floor of the orbit and it gives the short branch to the ciliary ganglion, which carries the nerve supply to the sphincter pupillae and the ciliary muscle (Figs 38.6A and B).

Pupillary Fibers

Within the subarachnoid space, pupillary fibers are located superficially in the superior portion of the nerve. Within the cavernous sinus and the orbit, the pupillary fibers are in the inferior division of the nerve.

Lesions

Lesions of the Oculomotor Nerve

Complete paralysis of the oculomotor nerve results in:

1. Ptosis due to paralysis of LPS.
2. The eye will be abducted due to the action of the lateral rectus, but other movements will be absent.

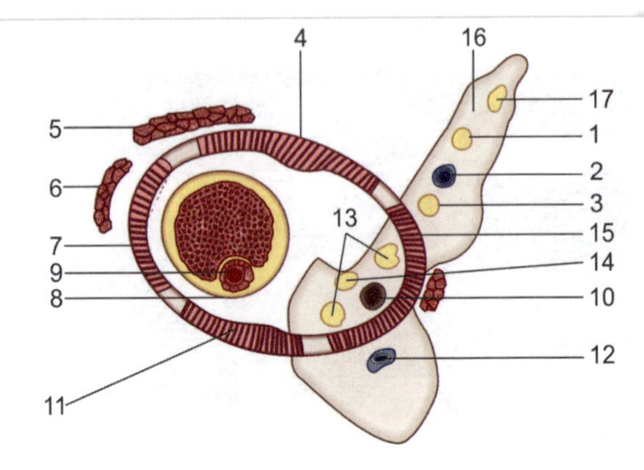

FIGURE 38.5: Anatomy of superior orbital fissure

3. The action of the superior oblique can be demonstrated by the intorsion of the eye when the person is asked to follow an object downward and laterally. This movement can be better visualized by looking at some conjunctival vessels at 12 O' clock position.
4. The pupil will be dilated due to the unopposed action of the dilator pupillae supplied by the sympathetic.
5. All pupillary reflexes will be abolished.

Lesions of the Oculomotor Nucleus

Oculomotor nucleus lesions are rare and often result from ischemia due to embolism or thrombosis of small blood vessels supplying the midbrain. The lesion involves both oculomotor nerves and bilateral ptosis results, and contralateral superior rectus muscle is also affected (Figs 38.7A to C).

Lesions of the Fasciculus

Causes are similar to the nuclear lesion. Fascicular lesions involve the red nucleus and the cerebral peduncle—both

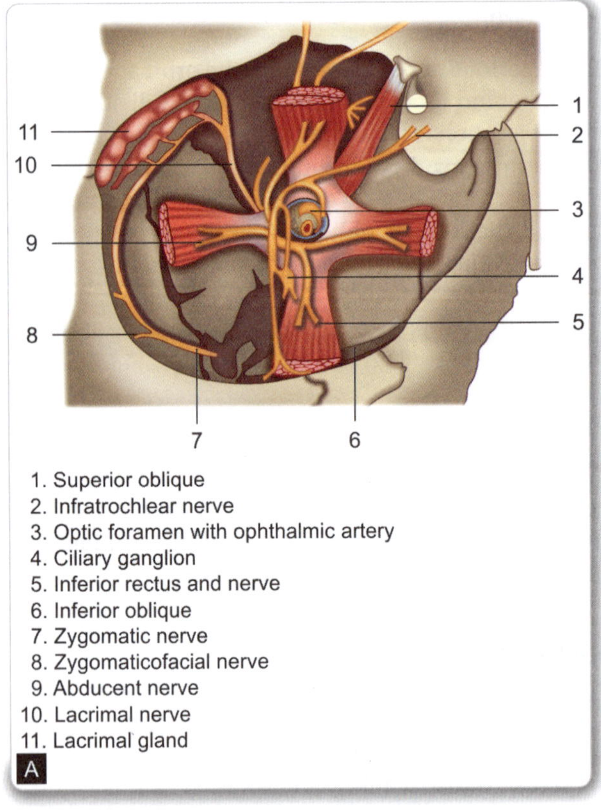

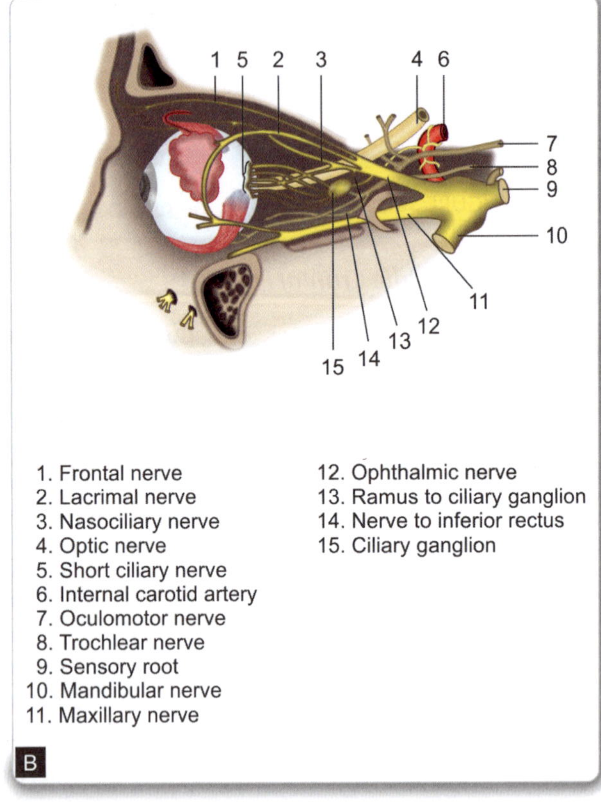

FIGURES 38.6A and B: Nerves in the orbit. **A.** Arrangement of nerves in the orbit; **B.** Course of oculomotor nerves in orbit—lateral view.

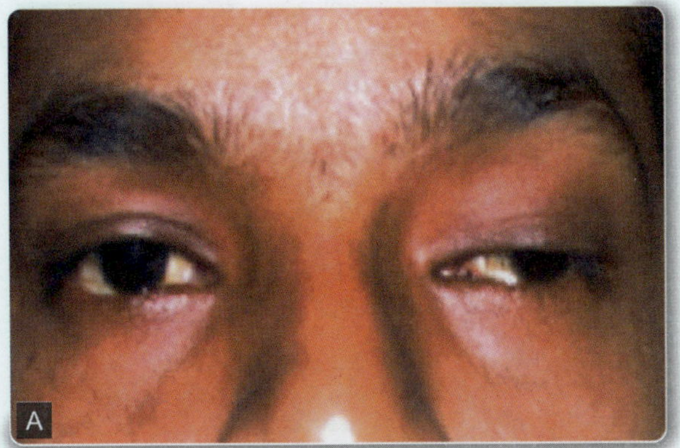

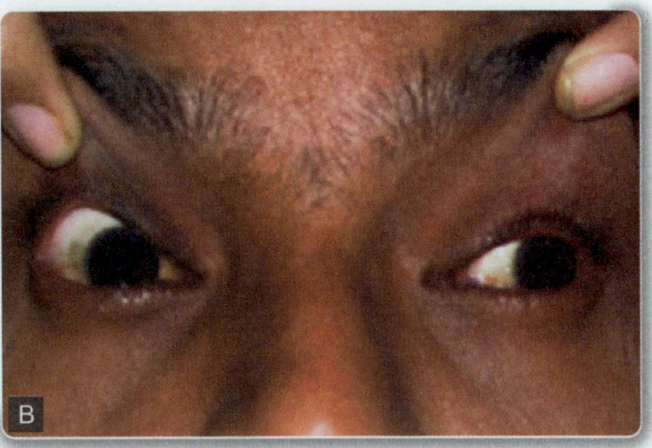

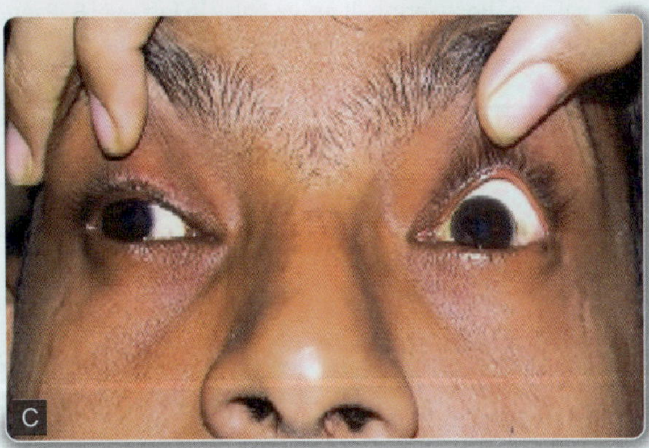

FIGURES 38.7A to C: Features of III nerve palsy. **A.** Pupil sparing III nerve palsy of left eye; **B.** Eye divergent on elevating the lids; **C.** Adduction restricted on looking to right.

structures being in close proximity. This can result in several syndromes.

Benedikt's syndrome: It is characterized by ipsilateral III nerve palsy and contralateral hemitremor due to involvement of the red nucleus and hemiplegia.

Weber's syndrome: Ipsilateral III nerve palsy and contralateral hemiplegia and upper motor neuron (UMN) facial palsy. It involves the fasciculus as it passes through the cerebral peduncle.

Nothnagel's syndrome: Ipsilateral III nerve palsy and contralateral cerebellar ataxia caused by involvement of the fasciculus and the superior cerebellar peduncle.

Lesions in the Basilar Part

Basilar part is the commonest site of involvement of III nerve. The important causes are aneurysm of the posterior communicating artery or head injury resulting in extradural or subdural hematoma. The nerve is pressed against the tentorial edge resulting in irritation followed by paralysis. This results in initial miosis followed by mydriasis and total III nerve palsy.

Lesions of the Intracavernous Part

The commonest cause for lesions of III nerve in this area are diabetes (involvement of vasa nervorum with sparing of the pupil) pituitary lesions, aneurysm of the internal carotid artery, caroticocavernous fistula and idiopathic granulomatous inflammation called Tolosa-Hunt syndrome. Along with the III nerve, IV, V and VI nerves are also involved.

Intraorbital Part

The superior or inferior divisions may be involved or nerve supply to individual muscles may be affected. Lesions of the inferior division involve the pupil also. The causes are usually trauma or vascular accidents.

Aberrant regeneration of the III nerve can occur following traumatic and aneurysmal lesions. Due to damage to the endoneurial nerve sheaths, misdirection of the regenerating nerve fibers can occur, leading to bizarre ocular movements. Elevation of the eyelids on attempted abduction or depression can occur. This is called **pseudo-Graefe phenomenon** (Figs 38.8A and B).

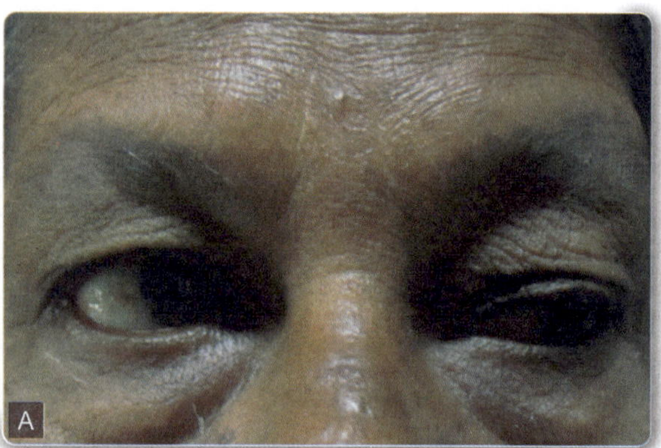
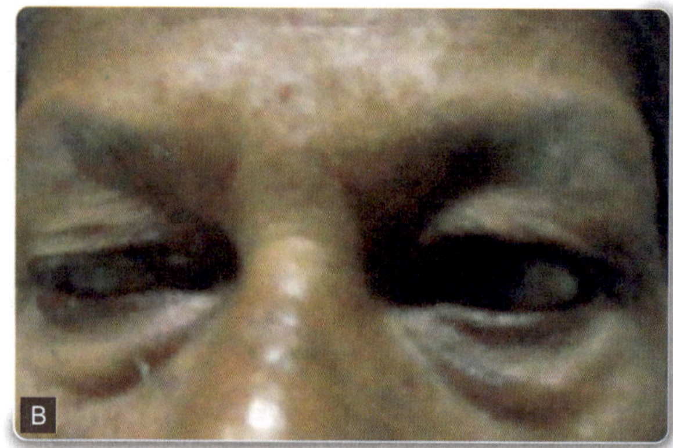

FIGURES 38.8A and B: Recovering III nerve palsy. **A.** Recovering III nerve palsy in left eye; **B.** Pseudo-Graefe phenomenon (lid retraction on adduction).

TROCHLEAR OR IV NERVE

Practical Anatomy

Nucleus of the IV nerve is caudal to and continuous with that of the III nerve.

This nerve has many anatomical peculiarities. This is the most slender cranial nerve and the only cranial nerve with emergence from the dorsal aspect of the brain and has the longest intracranial course. The IV nerve nucleus supplies the contralateral superior oblique muscle.

The IV nerve, after leaving the brainstem on the dorsal surface below the inferior colliculus curves laterally around the brainstem; and runs forward beneath the free edge of the tentorium. After passing between the posterior cerebral artery and the superior cerebellar artery, in company with the III nerve, it pierces the dura and enters the cavernous sinus. On the lateral wall of the cavernous sinus, it is placed below the III nerve and above the first division of the V nerve. It passes into the orbit above the annulus of Zinn and runs upward and medially and supplies the superior oblique muscle.

Paralysis of IV nerve results in superior oblique paralysis and also results in limitation of depression of the eye in adduction and causes vertical diplopia. The diplopia is more in looking downward and the patient experiences more difficulty in climbing down stairs. To overcome diplopia, the head will be tilted to the opposite side and face turned to the opposite side and the chin is depressed.

Lesions

Lesions of the Nucleus and Fascicle

Causes of lesions of the nucleus and fascicle include medulloblastoma, multiple sclerosis and brainstem arteriovenous (AV) malformation. Superior oblique paresis in such cases is often obscured by conjugate or internuclear gaze defects. Both unilateral and bilateral superior oblique paresis can be associated with Parinaud's dorsal midbrain syndrome, pineal tumors, aqueduct stenosis and hydrocephalus.

Lesions of the Trochlear Nerve in the Subarachnoid Space

Trauma, tentorial meningioma, pinealoma and encephalitis can cause trochlear nerve paresis in the subarachnoid space.

Lesions in the Cavernous Sinus

Lesions in the cavernous sinus will be associated with III nerve palsy and involvement of first division of trigeminal. Causes can be ischemia due to diabetes or hypertension and cavernous sinus diseases (Fig. 38.9).

Lesions in the Orbit

The damage to the nerve from damage to the trochlea or the superior oblique muscle is impossible to differentiate. Trauma or surgery, or orbital inflammation may be the cause.

Treatment

Treatment in persistent cases:

1. Occlusion of the affected eye to avoid diplopia.
2. Use of vertical prisms to overcome diplopia.
3. Surgery:
    - Weaken its antagonist: Ipsilateral inferior oblique muscle
    - Weaken its yoke muscle: Contralateral inferior rectus muscle.

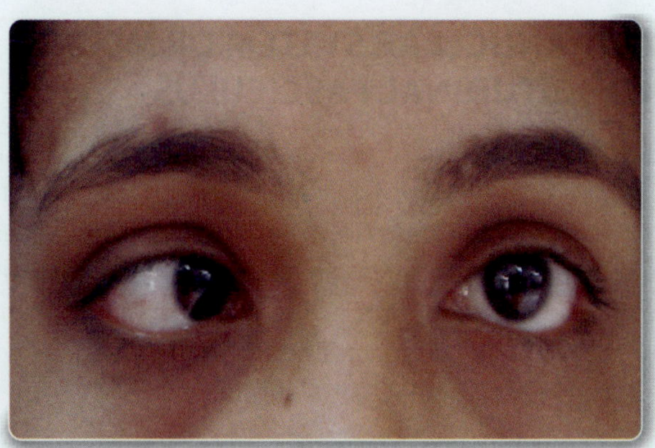

FIGURE 38.9: Nerve palsy in right eye

VI NERVE (ABDUCENT NERVE)

Practical Anatomy

The nucleus of the VI nerve is in the pons close to the midline, closely related to the horizontal gaze center in the paramedian pontine reticular formation (PPRF) (Fig. 38.10). The fasciculus of the VII nerve curves around the abducent nucleus and produces an elevation in the floor of the IV ventricle called facial colliculus. So a nuclear lesion of VI nerve will involve the VII nerve also and an isolated VI nerve palsy can never be a nuclear lesion.

The fasciculus pass forwards through the whole length of the pons and pass lateral to the pyramid, and leave the brainstem at the pontomedullary junction. It has a long course at the base of the skull before it enters the cavernous sinus. In this course, it is crossed by the inferior cerebellar artery and angles over the tip of the petrous bone where it can get compressed by an increase in intracranial tension (ICT).

In the cavernous sinus, it passes below the III and IV nerve and the first division of the V nerve. Unlike the other nerves, which are in the lateral wall of the sinus and hence in a relatively protected position, VI nerve runs through the sinus close to the internal carotid artery. In the cavernous sinus, the VI nerve is joined by the sympathetic branches from the carotid plexus, which is involved in Horner's syndrome. It enters the orbit through the annulus of Zinn and passes laterally to innervate the lateral rectus muscle.

Paralysis of VI Nerve

Paralysis of VI nerve results in paralysis of the lateral rectus muscle and results in convergent squint and homonymous diplopia, which is worse on looking toward the affected side. There will be compensatory head turn toward the paralyzed side to minimize diplopia.

Lesions

Lesions of the Nucleus of the VI Nerve

There will be weakness of abduction of the ipsilateral side, failure of horizontal gaze toward the side of the lesion (due to involvement of the horizontal gaze center in the PPRF) as well as lower motor neuron (LMN) facial palsy due to involvement of the facial fasciculus.

Mobius syndrome (congenital bulbar paralysis): There is bilateral VI nerve palsy and facial nerve palsy giving a mask-like facies and incomplete closure of the eyelids. It is sometimes associated with deafness and many congenital anomalies.

Lesions of the Fasciculus

Foville's syndrome: It is due to vascular causes or tumors involving the dorsal pons. It is characterized by the involvement of V–VIII nerve and central sympathetic fibers involvement (to produce central Horner's syndrome).

Millard-Gubler syndrome: It is due to lesions of the VI nerve as it passes through the pyramidal tract. The cause can be vascular accidents, demyelination or tumors. It consists of ipsilateral VI nerve palsy and contralateral hemiplegia.

Lesions of the Basilar Part

Acoustic neuroma can involve the VI nerve at pontomedullary junction. It will be associated with hearing loss (due to involvement of VIII nerve) and corneal anesthesia (due to involvement of V nerve).

Raised intracranial pressure (ICP) can stretch the VI nerve over the petrous bone and cause VI nerve palsy and this can be a false localizing sign in tumors or benign intracranial hypertension.

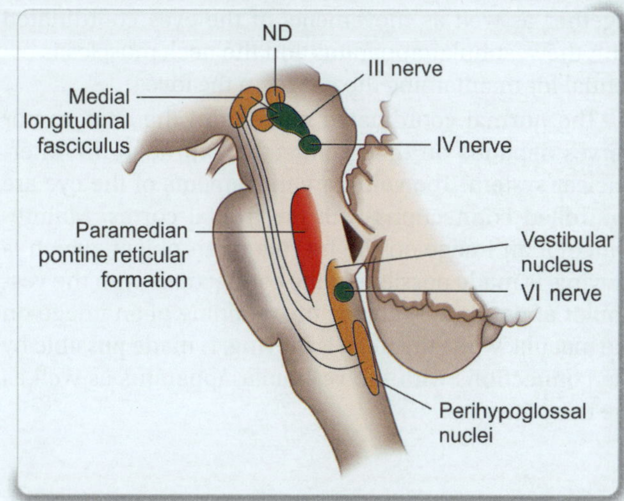

FIGURE 38.10: Arrangement of nuclei of III–VI nuclei in brain

Gradenigo's syndrome: Mastoiditis and spread of infection to petrous bone to cause VI nerve palsy with facial palsy and defective hearing. Involvement of the V nerve nucleus will cause trigeminal neuralgia.

Lesions in the Cavernous Sinus

Lesions will be involved along with the other nerves in the cavernous sinus.

Lesions Within the Orbit

Isolated involvement in the orbit is rare. In fractures and tumors of the orbit other oculomotor nerves will also be involved.

Management of VI Nerve Palsy

The underlying causes may be investigated and treated, if possible.

Surgical treatment is undertaken only after waiting for 6–12 months for natural improvement. Meanwhile occlusion of the affected eye may be done to avoid diplopia. Surgical correction is undertaken only, if no more further improvement is occurring. Surgery includes weakening of the ipsilateral medial rectus muscle combined with strengthening of the ipsilateral lateral rectus also.

SUPRANUCLEAR PATHWAYS FOR OCULOMOTOR CONTROL

It is important to maintain the image of the object of interest on the fovea for good vision. But the object may be moving or the observer himself/herself or his/her head may be moving. Coordinated movements of the both eyes together as well as movements of the eyes coordinated with the vestibular apparatus and the neck muscles is essential for maintaining the image on the fovea.

The normal coordinated function of the oculomotor nerves depends on their connections through the internuclear system. The voluntary movements of the eye are controlled connections with the frontal cortex. Maintenance of an image on the macula of an object, which is moving, is made possible by the connections with the vestibular apparatus. Similarly, the retaining of an image on the macula, while the head is moving, is made possible by the connections with the vestibular apparatus as well as the neck muscles.

INTRANUCLEAR SYSTEM OR MEDIAL LONGITUDINAL FASCICULUS

Intranuclear system or medial longitudinal fasciculus (MLF) is a fiber tract, which extends from the nuclei of the III nerve at the midbrain downward up to the spinal cord. The major part of these fibers comes from the vestibular nuclei. The most important fibers connecting the three oculomotor nuclei connect the ipsilateral VI nucleus with the contralateral medial rectus subnucleus.

Paramedian Pontine Reticular Formation

Paramedian pontine reticular formation extends from the IV nuclei up to the VI nerve nuclei and horizontal gaze center is controlled by the fibers in this PPRF. A horizontal gaze center is postulated to exist in the pons close to the VI nerve nucleus. Lesions involving the horizontal gaze center result in paralysis of conjugate gaze to the same side, while paralysis of the VI nerve produce absence of abduction in the ipsilateral eye only.

The afferent fibers of PPRF include those from vestibular nuclei and the superior colliculus. It is also connected to the frontal eye field, the pretectal nucleus and the spinal cord. The important connections of PPRF related to ocular mobility are generated from the horizontal gaze center. Fibers from the horizontal gaze center connect to the ipsilateral VI nerve to abduct the ipsilateral eye. From the PPRF, fibers cross the midline at the level of the pons and pass to the contralateral III nerve nucleus to connect to the medial rectus subnucleus. Stimulation of the PPRF on one side causes conjugate deviation of the eye to the same side. A lesion involving the PPRF causes horizontal gaze palsy to the direction of the lesion.

Intranuclear Ophthalmoplegia

This lesion results from a lesion involving the medial longitudinal fasciculus. In this condition, the gaze toward the side of the lesion will be normal, on attempted gaze toward the opposite side, there will be defective adduction of the eye on the same side. But the eye will be moving inward to maintain normal convergence.

Migraine

39

Anuja Sathar, Girija Devi PS

Migraine (in Greek 'hemi' meaning half and 'kranion' meaning skull) is a recurrent typically unilateral episodic throbbing or pulsating headache lasting from 4 to 72 hours, associated with nausea, vomiting, mood disturbances, photophobia or fatigue, the symptoms generally aggravated by routine activity. A family history may be seen.

PREDISPOSING FACTORS

There are a number of trigger factors for migraine, the factors will vary for each individual:

1. Common foods that trigger attack of migraine include aged meat, aged cheese, banana, monosodium glutamate, chocolate, wine, beer, nitrite containing beverages, etc.
2. Strong odors, bright lights, flickering lights, loud noises, sleep deprivation, fatigue, stress, etc. also trigger migraine.
3. Approximately 10% of people who suffer from migraine perceive an aura, which may be transient visual, sensory, language or motor disturbances.
4. About 75% of adult patients are women, although migraine occurs with equal frequency in prepubertal boys and girls. Migrainous attacks usually decrease during pregnancy, but may become frequent in some cases.
5. Migraine may be exacerbated by menstruation, puberty and oral contraceptive pill indicating hormonal involvement.

ETIOPATHOGENESIS

Most supported theory is that of hyperexcitability of the cerebral cortex and/or abnormal control of pain neurons in the trigeminal nucleus of the brainstem. Migraine is a neurovascular disorder. The interaction of trigeminal nerve, autonomic system and blood vessels is referred to as the trigeminovascular system. Serotonin receptors are mainly responsible for triggering the neural origin of migraine. The aura symptoms of migraine are likely to be due to cortical spreading depression.

Pain in migraine is limited to pain sensitive structures in brain, dura and cranial blood vessels by activation of cells of trigeminal nucleus caudalis in medulla, resulting in release of vasoactive neuropeptides at the vascular terminations of the above area.

CLASSIFICATION

International Headache Society (IHS) classifies migrainous headache in a document called International Classification of Headache Disorder-2 (ICHD-2) into seven subclasses, which include further subdivisions:

1. **Common migraine or headache without aura:** Constitutes 80% of cases and may be associated with nausea, vomiting or mood changes, and with no neurological features. Acute frontotemporal pulsatile headache occurs, which improves after sleep or vomiting.
2. **Classic migraine or migraine with aura:** Seen in 10% and the headache is heralded by visual aura, usually lasting for about 20–30 minutes. Visual disturbance include photopsia, dazzling zigzag lines or scintillating scotoma often known as fortification spectra or teichopsia. Fully reversible unilateral sensory symptoms like paresthesias or feeling of pins and needles may also occur. The headache phase begins within 60 minutes of the end of the aura, but can be delayed. The severity and frequency of headaches varies between migraineurs. In acephalgic migraine, aura occurs without headache. Classic migraine includes:
   a. Familial hemiplegic migraine.
   b. Sporadic hemiplegic migraine. In both a and b full recovery of motor weakness is delayed after the migrainous attack.
   c. Basilar type migraine (Bickerstaff) in which there is vertigo, tinnitus, hearing impairment, difficulty in speaking or paresthesia associated

with migrainous aura. Symptoms and signs are bilateral and more common in the young.
3. **Childhood periodic syndromes:** These are migraine precursors like cyclical vomiting, abdominal migraine and occasional attacks of vertigo.
4. **Retinal migraine:** It involves migraine with unilateral visual disturbances or temporary blindness similar to amaurosis fugax.
5. **Complicated migraine:** It includes headache or aura that is unusually long or frequent or associated with seizure or brain lesions.
6. **Probable migraine:** It has migrainous characteristics, but not certain due to medication overuse.
7. **Chronic migraine:** Fulfills criteria for migraine, but occurs after a greater time interval, 15 days to 3 months.

Ophthalmoplegic Migraine

Ophthalmoplegic migraine or isolated oculomotor nerve palsy is not a true migraine and hence removed from ICHD-2. It usually occurs in childhood and is transient and recurrent, the III nerve being the frequently involved.

Evaluation of a Patient with Migraine

A detailed evaluation with history, systemic and ocular examination including refraction should be done. Typical history and normal neurologic examination usually excludes any intracranial abnormality. Neuroimaging is warranted if:

- Headache or aura is always on same side
- Headache precedes aura
- Neurological and visual defects persists after aura resolves
- Atypical aura.

Treatment

Treatment involves a multimodal approach.

General Measures

General measures include avoidance of migraine triggers, lifestyle alterations, stress management and correction of refractive errors, if any. A migraine diary can also be maintained.

Prophylaxis

Prophylaxis is in the form of preventive drugs. The goals of preventive therapy are to reduce the frequency, painfulness and/or duration of migraine and to increase the effectiveness of abortive therapy. Preventive drugs are prescribed for frequent migraineurs and are considered effective, if they reduce the frequency or severity of migraine attacks by at least 50%. These include beta blockers, such as propranolol, atenolol, calcium channel blockers like flunarizine, amlodipine, anticonvulsants like sodium valproate, tricyclic antidepressants like amitriptyline, low-dose aspirin, etc.

Treatment of Acute Attack

1. Migraine of mild-to-moderate intensity may be relieved by sleep or by simple analgesics.
2. Severe attacks need specific treatment with any one of the drugs like ergotamine 2 mg or dihydroergotamine 4 mg, sumatriptan orally or as nasal spray, butorphanol nasal spray, etc. with analgesics and antiemetics.
3. Constant use of these drugs should be avoided to prevent medication overuse headache, leading to refractory headaches.

Cluster Headache

1. Cluster headache is a form of trigeminal autonomic cephalalgia most frequently seen in men in their 30s and 40s. It is precipitated, usually by alcohol or nitroglycerin.
2. Unilateral stabbing oculotemporal headache occurs associated with ipsilateral tearing, rhinorrhea and droopy eyelids. It recurs once or twice daily for several weeks, followed by headache free interval for months to years.

Treatment

Attacks are relieved by oxygen, sumatriptan, calcium channel blockers or steroids.

Section 10

Systemic Diseases and the Eye

Diabetes Mellitus

40

Girija Devi PS

The eye is the mirror that reflects the health of a person. Peter Mayer Latham, an English clinician, rightly said more than a century ago to his students, "If you desire to make pathological knowledge the ground work of your credit and usefulness through life, do not pass by without making a special study of diseases of the eye. Here you see almost all diseases in miniature; and from the peculiar structure of the eye, you see them as though, through a glass; and you learn many of the little wonderful details in the nature of the morbid processes, but for the observation of them in the eye, would not have been known at all."

So, whenever one sees some abnormality in the eye, that may be warning sign of some serious systemic disorder, e.g. some microaneurysms and hemorrhages in retina, show the presence of diabetes in that patient. Similarly, when some systemic problem is suspected, a careful examination of the eye will confirm diagnosis, e.g. Kayser-Fleischer (KF) ring in Wilson's disease.

Diabetes mellitus (DM) is one of the leading causes of blindness all over the world. In the developed countries such as United States, it is the most common cause of blindness in people between 50 and 65 years of age. In developing countries like India, diabetes is gaining prominence in the causes of blindness.

Even though diabetic retinopathy (DR) is the cause of blindness due to diabetes in the majority of patients, diabetes can affect vision in a variety of ways:

1. Changes in refraction—occur depending on the level of blood sugar; increase in blood sugar producing myopia and a rapid decrease in blood sugar from high levels leading to a hypermetropic shift.
2. Increased risk of developing glaucoma, retinal vascular occlusions and ischemic optic neuropathy.
3. Increased risk of developing iridocyclitis, especially postoperatively after cataract surgery.
4. Increased risk of ocular infections.
5. Ocular motor nerve palsies due to involvement of vasa nervorum of the VI and III nerves.
6. Early onset of age-related cataract or true diabetic cataract in uncontrolled diabetes.

DIABETIC RETINOPATHY

Diabetic retinopathy (DR) can affect both insulin dependent (type I) and non-insulin-dependent (type II) diabetes, but type I is more commonly affected.

Influencing Factors

Factors influencing the development of retinopathy in diabetic patients are detailed below.

Duration of Diabetes

Duration of diabetes is the most important single factor influencing the development of retinopathy. Unfortunately people have no control over this factor. People who get diabetes at a younger age are at greater risk of developing DR, because of their longer life expectancy after the onset of diabetes. The signs of retinopathy start appearing 3–5 years after the onset of diabetes. Its prevalence increases gradually as the diabetic age increases and in patients who had diabetes for 25 years or longer, 100% of them will have some changes of retinopathy on fundus examination.

Control of Diabetes

Intensive metabolic control of diabetes delay the onset of retinopathy as well slows down its progression. Fluctuations in the blood sugar level, both hyper as well as hypoglycemia are harmful. Multidose insulin regime is ideal for maintaining blood sugar level at normal levels round the clock. The early detection of diabetes is also important. If diabetes goes undetected, its control will not be taking place and the patient will be going in for an earlier onset of retinopathy.

Puberty and Pregnancy

The hormonal changes that occur at puberty (in children who develop DM at a young age) and at the time of pregnancy will cause a rapid deterioration of DR.

Other General Conditions

Other general conditions that adversely affect the circulation like hypertension, hyperlipidemia, smoking, obesity and diabetic nephropathy are factors that accelerate the progression of diabetic retinopathy.

Pathogenesis

Diabetic retinopathy is a microangiopathy affecting mainly the small caliber vessels such as capillaries, precapillary arterioles and postcapillary venules. There is thickening of the basement membrane of the capillaries and loss of pericytes that line the basement membrane.

At the same time there are hematological changes also, like sluggishness of circulation due to increased rouleaux formation of red blood cells (RBCs) and increased aggregation of the platelets.

These intravascular as well as intramural factors lead to occlusion of the precapillary arterioles leading to closure of large areas of capillary bed and tissue hypoxia. The damage to the vessel walls and tissue hypoxia lead to breakdown of the blood-retinal barrier—leading to accumulation of fluid in the retina, especially in the macular area, which has a high metabolic requirement (macular edema). The tissue hypoxia leads to development of shunt vessels across areas of capillary occlusion (capillary dropout) connecting arterioles and venules called **intraretinal microvascular abnormalities (IRMA)**. The tissue hypoxia leads to release of vascular endothelial growth factors (VEGF), which stimulate growth of new vessels at the disk (NVD) or along the major blood vessels [neovascularization of the disk (NVD)].

The loss of pericytes and hypoxia lead to globular protrusions on the capillary vessel walls called microaneurysms. They are most common at the macular area. The microaneurysms leak plasma of the blood until they become thrombosed after a few weeks. The new vessels are also friable and bleed easily, and they lead to preretinal and vitreous hemorrhages.

The lipids and lipoproteins in the fluid that exude from the vessels into the tissue can accumulate as 'hard exudates' in the outer plexiform layer, mainly at the macula and the area around the disk. The blood cells can also leak from the damaged vessels and can appear as intraretinal hemorrhages.

The changes in DR are concentrated at the macula and the area surrounding the optic disk (posterior pole). This is because this is the most metabolically active area of the retina and hence the main effect of the hypoxic damage caused by DR is seen in this area (Fig. 40.1).

Classification

1. Proliferative diabetic retinopathy (PDR) (Table 40.1):
   a. Mild to moderate.
   b. High risk.
   c. Advanced diabetic eye disease (ADED).
2. Non-proliferative diabetic retinopathy (NPDR) (Figs 40.2A and B, Table 40.2):
   a. Mild.
   b. Moderate.
   c. Severe:
      i. Mild NPDR: The retina shows only few hemorrhages and microaneurysms.

TABLE 40.1: Additional changes seen in proliferative diabetic retinopathy

Changes	Features
Preretinal neovascularization	Hallmark of proliferative diabetic retinopathy (PDR); most often occurs on and near the optic disk [neovascularization of the disk (NVD)] or near the major retinal vessels [neovascularization elsewhere (NVE)].
Preretinal and vitreous hemorrhages	Preretinal hemorrhages appear as pockets of blood within the potential space between the retina and the posterior hyaloid face. As the blood pools within this space, they may appear boat shaped. Hemorrhage into the vitreous may appear as a diffuse haze or as clumps of blood clots within the gel.
Fibrovascular tissue proliferation (FVP)	Fibrovascular tissue proliferation is usually seen associated with the neovascular complex and also may appear avascular when the vessels have already regressed.
Tractional retinal detachment (RD) (due to traction of vitreous scarring)	Traction RDs usually appear tented up, immobile and concave compared to rhegmatogenous RDs.
Rubeosis iridis	Neovascularization of the iris that can occlude the angle of the anterior chamber; this entails the risk of acute secondary angle-closure glaucoma.

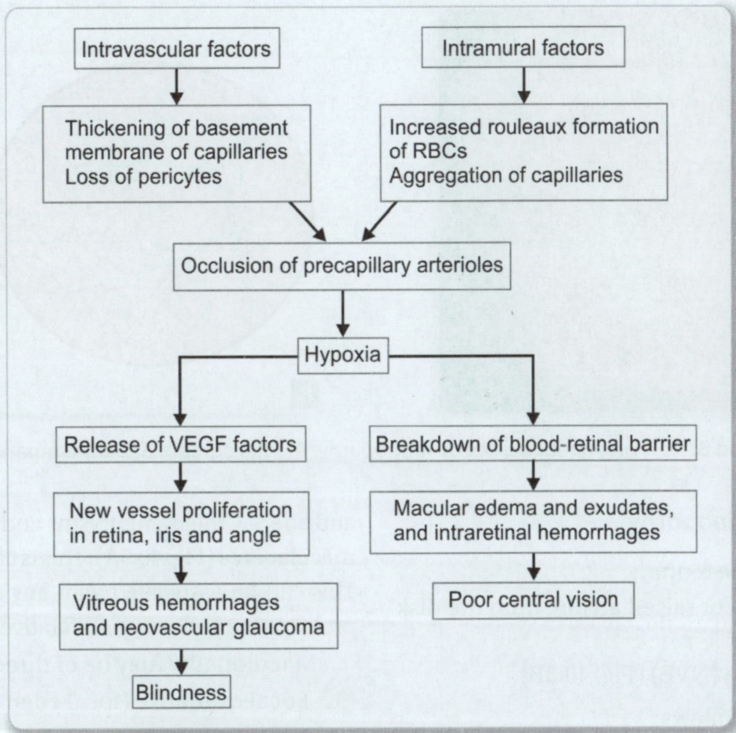

FIGURE 40.1: Pathogenesis of diabetic retinopathy (RBCs, red blood cells; VEGF, vascular endothelial growth factor)

ii. Moderate NPDR: There will be extensive hemorrhages, microaneurysms and hard exudates involving up to three quadrants. Few cotton-wool spots may be present. Venous beading, if present, will involve not more than one quadrant.

iii. Severe NPDR: Severe hemorrhages will be present in all four quadrants, venous abnormalities like venous beading, loops, etc. will be present in two or more quadrants and IRMA will be present in at least one quadrant.

TABLE 40.2: Abnormalities in non-proliferative diabetic retinopathy

Abnormalities	Features
Microaneurysms	Earliest clinical sign of diabetic retinopathy (DR). Secondary to capillary wall outpouching due to pericyte loss. Appear as small red dots in the superficial retinal layers. Fibrin and red blood cell (RBC) accumulate in the microaneurysm and lead to their thrombosis. Rupture produces blot/flame hemorrhages.
Intraretinal hemorrhages	Dot and blot hemorrhages occur as microaneurysms rupture in the deeper layers of the retina such as the inner nuclear and outer plexiform layers. Flame-shaped hemorrhages are less common. Occur in the more superficial nerve fiber layer.
Lipid deposits in the retina (hard exudates)	Caused by the breakdown of the blood-retinal barrier, allowing leakage of serum proteins, lipids and protein from the vessels. These are mostly found in the outer plexiform layer.
Retinal edema	Caused by the breakdown of the blood-retinal barrier. Mostly involves the macula.
Venous beading	Frequently adjacent to areas of non-perfusion. Reflects increasing retinal ischemia. Important predictor of progression to proliferative diabetic retinopathy (PDR).
Cotton-wool spots (soft exudates)	Results from nerve fiber layer infarction from occlusion of precapillary arterioles. Frequently bordered by microaneurysms and vascular hyperpermeability.
Intraretinal microvascular anomalies	These are remodeled capillary beds without proliferative changes. Collateral vessels that do not leak on fluorescein angiography. Usually can be found on the borders of the non-perfused retina.

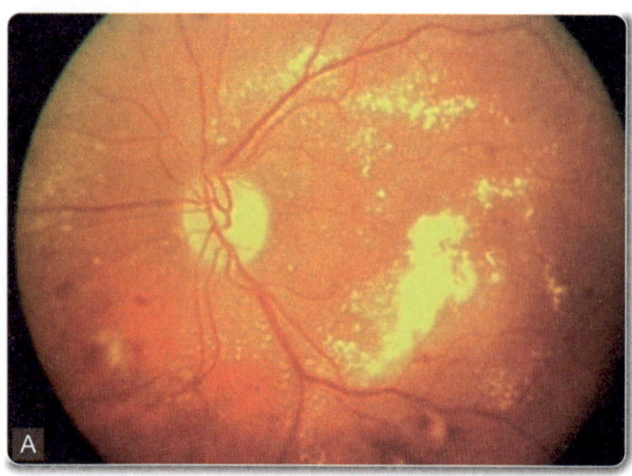

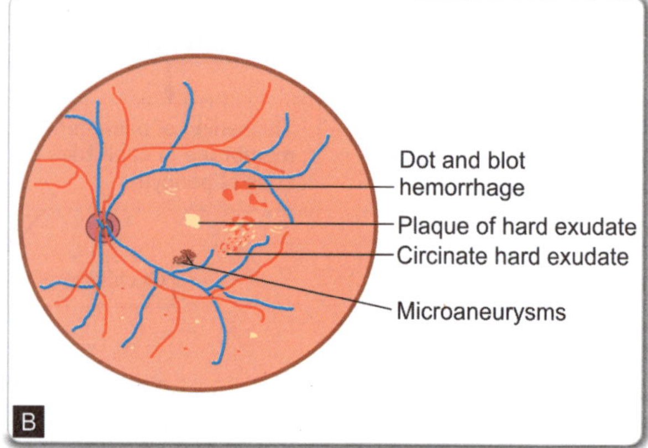

FIGURES 40.2A and B: Non-proliferative diabetic retinopathy. **A.** Photograph; **B.** Diagrammatic representation.

Proliferative Diabetic Retinopathy

There are new vessels on the retina:

1. Either flat on the retina or raised arising from the disk (NVD) (Fig. 40.3A).
2. Elsewhere on the retina (NVE) (Fig. 40.3B).

High-risk PDR: These are as follows:

1. The NVD involving more than one third of the disk.
2. The NVD with preretinal or vitreous hemorrhage (Fig. 40.4).
3. The NVE greater than one half of the disk area in size with preretinal or vitreous hemorrhage.

Maculopathy

Macula is the area enclosed by the superior and inferior temporal vascular arcades, and it is the most important part for clear detailed vision. In DR, the macula is specifically involved, and edema, microaneurysms and exudates can appear in the macular area (Fig. 40.5A). This is called diabetic maculopathy. This can be associated with any stage of retinopathy—both proliferative and non-proliferative.

Maculopathy may be of three types:

1. Focal exudative (focal edema) (Fig. 40.5B).
2. Diffuse exudative (macula is diffusely thickened) (Fig. 40.5C).
3. Ischemic (no edema, but only capillary closure and ischemia).
4. Mixed (both ischemic and edematous areas coexist).

Clinically Significant Macular Edema

Changes in the macula can be mild with minimal involvement of vision or it can be moderate to severe with significant impairment of vision.

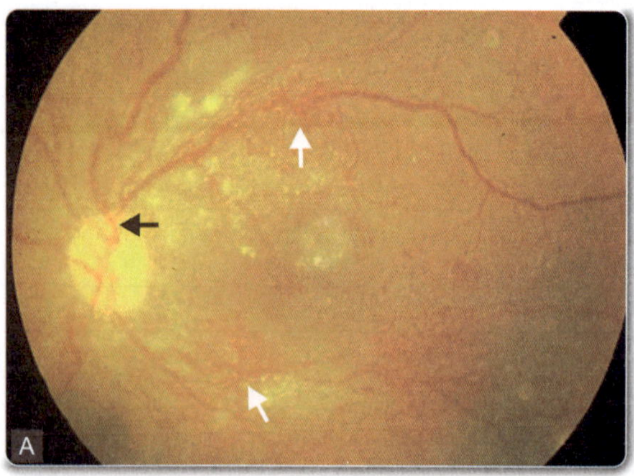

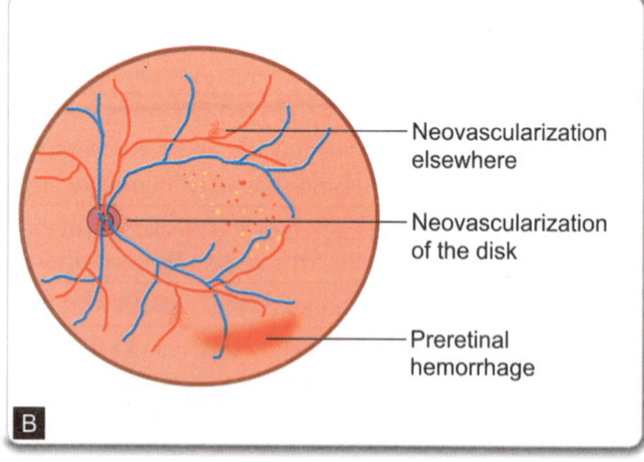

FIGURES 40.3A and B: Proliferative diabetic retinopathy (PDR). **A.** PDR with neovascularization of the disk (NVD) (black arrow) and neovascularization elsewhere (NVE) (white arrows); **B.** Diagrammatic representation.

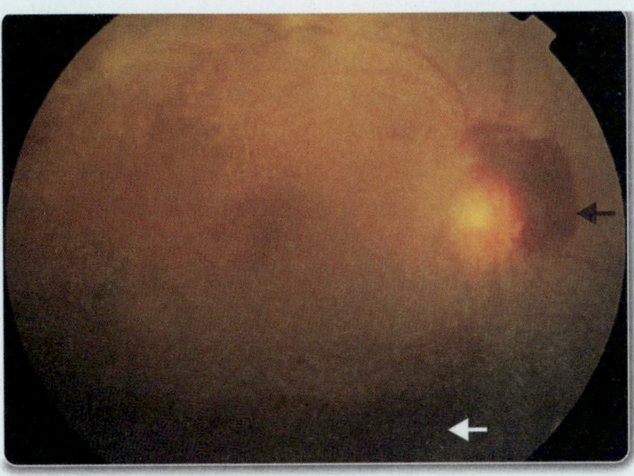

FIGURE 40.4: Proliferative diabetic retinopathy with vitreous hemorrhage (white arrow) and preretinal hemorrhage over the disk (black arrow).

A person is said to be having clinically significant macular edema (CSME) if:

1. There is retinal edema within 500 microns from the center of the fovea.
2. Hard exudates within the 500 microns from the center of the fovea with adjacent retinal edema (which may be outside the 500 micron diameter area).
3. Retinal edema 1 disk diameter area (1,500 micron) or larger, any part of which is within 1 disk diameter from the center of the fovea.

Patients with CSME require laser photocoagulation, but laser treatment will not benefit ischemic maculopathy. In fact it will aggravate the ischemia and so laser photocoagulation should be done with extreme caution in the mixed type of maculopathy.

ADVANCED DIABETIC EYE DISEASE

Patients with PDR can have recurrent vitreous hemorrhages from the new vessels. Initially these hemorrhages may get absorbed spontaneously, but recurrent hemorrhages or persistent vitreous hemorrhage can lead to fibrous tissue proliferation into the vitreous. Contraction of these fibrous bands will lead to tractional retinal detachment (TRD),

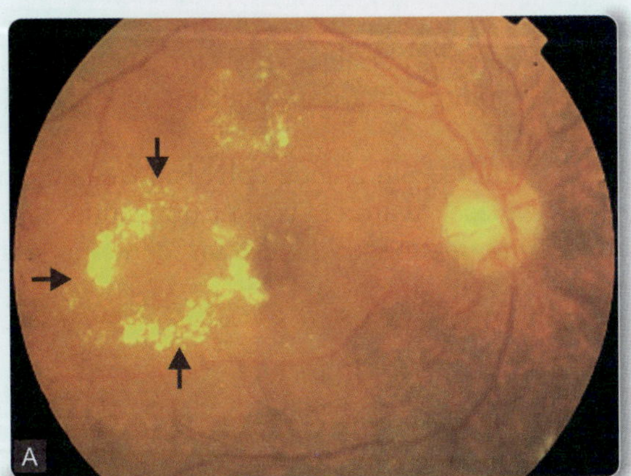

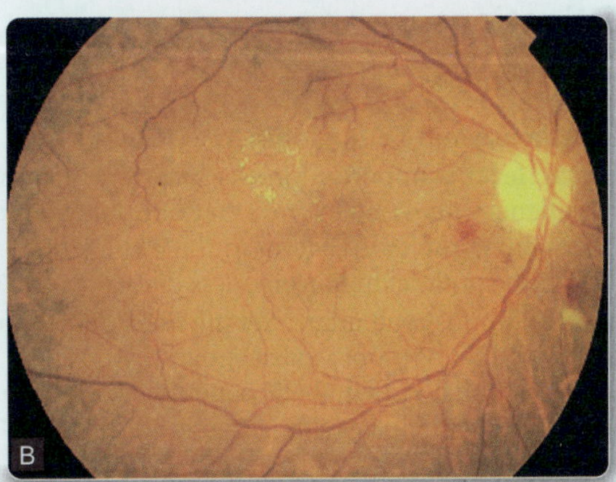

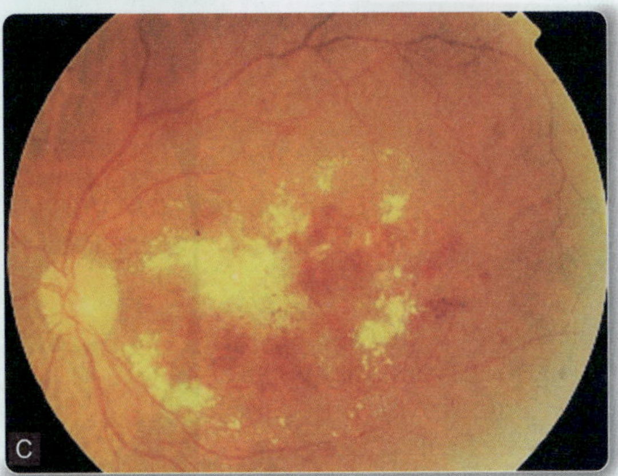

FIGURES 40.5A to C: Non-proliferative diabetic retinopathy (NPDR). A. Circinate pattern of hard exudates with central microvascular abnormalities; B. Mild NPDR with early maculopathy; C. NPDR with severe clinically significant macular edema.

which usually develops in the posterior pole. Patients with these advanced DR changes with considerable loss of vision are said to have advanced diabetic eye disease (ADED) (Fig. 40.6). Persistent macular edema will lead to cystic degeneration and considerable drop in vision. The VEGF can involve the iris also and lead to neovascularization of the iris, and angle leading to secondary angle-closure glaucoma.

Differential Diagnosis

A differential diagnosis must exclude other vascular retinal diseases, which can produce vascular leakage and/or occlusion.

These include:

- Branch retinal vein occlusion
- Central retinal vein occlusion
- Ocular ischemic syndrome
- Hemoglobinopathies
- Sickle cell disease
- Radiation retinopathy.

Investigations

Laboratory Studies

Fasting glucose and hemoglobin A1c (HbA1c)

The HbA1c level is important in the long-term follow-up care of patients with diabetes and DR. Controlling diabetes and maintaining the HbA1c level in the 6%–7% range are the goals in the optimal management of diabetes and DR.

Detailed fundus evaluation after pupillary dilatation using direct ophthalmoscopy, indirect ophthalmoscopy and 78D lens is essential in all diabetic patients at least once in a year. Patients having no DR changes or mild NPDR with no maculopathy can be followed up at yearly or 6-month intervals. Patients with moderate DR, but no maculopathy needs close follow-up at 3-month intervals. All patients with severe NPDR with or without CSME and all PDR cases need further evaluation to decide further management and must be referred to a center with facilities for it.

Fundus Fluorescein Angiography

Fundus fluorescein angiography (FFA) (Fig. 40.7A) is done using a fundus camera and 20% of sodium fluorescein intravenous injection. Sodium fluorescein is a vital dye, which preferentially absorbs light at 490 m and emits light at 530 m. When injected intravenously, it binds to the proteins in the blood. The choroidal vessels are freely permeable and allow the fluorescein bound to proteins to pass into the extravascular spaces in the choroid, but not the retinal vessels.

In the retina there is an outer blood-retinal barrier between the retinal pigment epithelial cells, which prevent passage of any fluid and also fluorescein from the choroid into the retina. The inner blood-retinal barrier formed by the tight functions of the cells of the capillary walls do not allow any free or protein bound fluorescein to escape. So the fluorescein will be confined to the lumen of the retinal vessels in a normal retina. If there is any abnormal permeability of the vessels as in diabetic retinopathy, the fluorescein-stained fluid can be seen leaking from the microaneurysms, abnormal capillaries and new vessels, and can be seen accumulating in the extracellular spaces of retina (Figs 40.7B and C).

The equipment for fundus angiogram consists of:

1. A fundus camera with suitable lenses to visualize the retina.
2. Appropriate filters (blue filters for the camera flash for allowing only the light rays to which fluorescein is sensitive to enter and yellow-green filter in the path of the emitting light, which allows only the yellow-green light emitted by the fluorescein to reach the viewer's eye).
3. The recording computer or photographic film.

The FFA will clearly show microaneurysms and new vessels, which may not be visible on fundus examination. The areas of macular edema or ischemia as well as areas of capillary dropout or occlusion will be clearly visualized.

Fundus fluorescein angiography is a valuable tool to decide when laser treatment is to be done, the extent and area requiring treatment and also for follow-up to assess the response to treatment.

Optical Coherence Tomography

Optical coherence tomography (OCT) is a retinal scan, which gives high resolution optical cross section of the

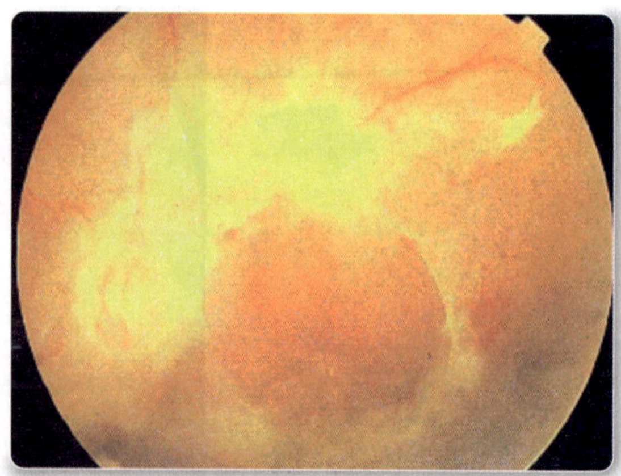

FIGURE 40.6: Advanced diabetic eye disease (ADED) with fibrovascular proliferation and tractional retinal detachment (RD)

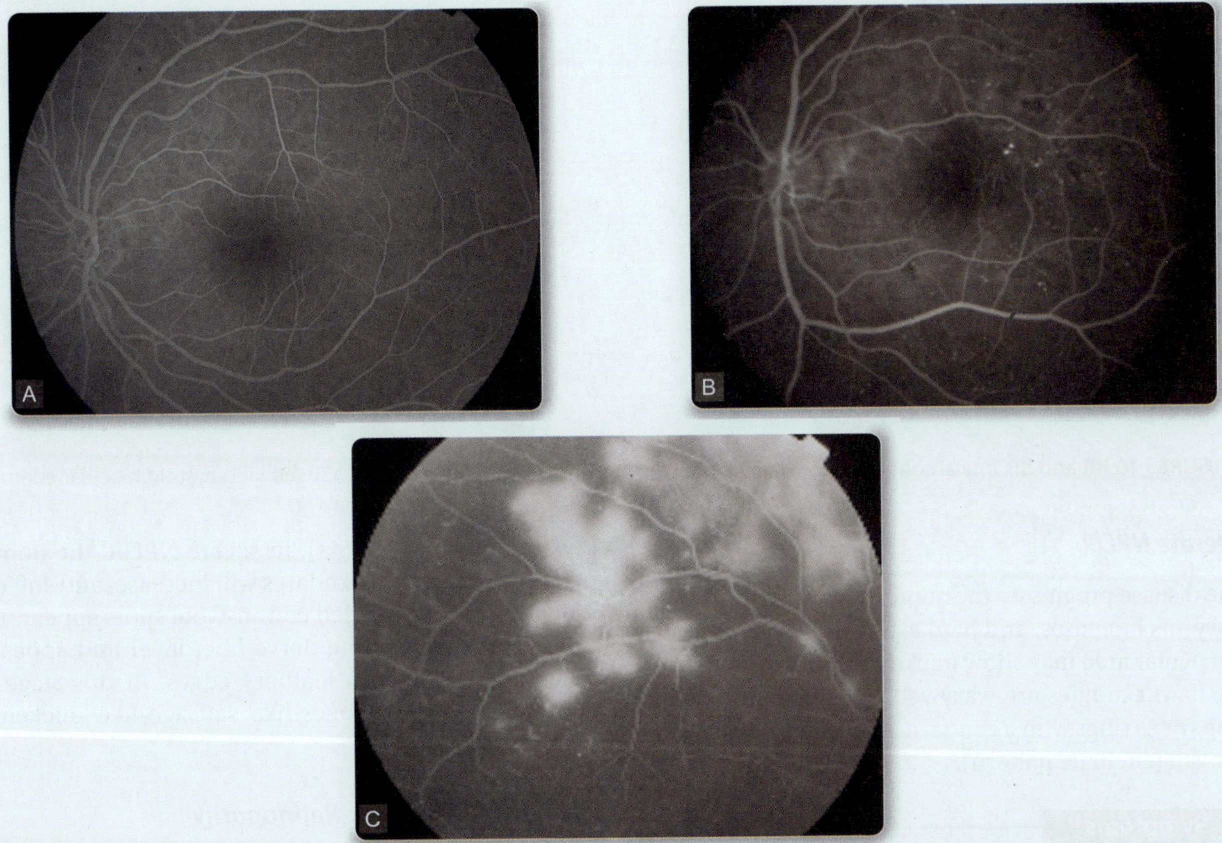

FIGURES 40.7A to C: Fundus fluorescein angiography (FFA). **A.** Normal FFA; **B.** FFA showing microaneurysms seen as globular spots (black arrows); **C.** FFA showing diffuse hyperfluorescent areas denoting leaking new vessels.

retina. It helps to assess the macular edema and the macular thickness, and helps us follow-up to assess the response to treatment (Figs 40.8A and B).

B-scan Ultrasonography

B-scan ultrasonography can be used to evaluate the status of the retina if the media is obstructed by vitreous hemorrhage or cataract.

Slit Lamp Examination and Gonioscopy

In all cases of severe NPDR and PDR, periodic slit lamp examination and gonioscopy is essential to rule out development of any iris or angle neovascularization.

Clinical Features

Advanced Diabetic Eye Disease

Fibrous tissue will also appear along with the new vessels and they tend to contract as the new vessels regress. The traction exerted on the retina by these fibrous bands will lead to tractional RD. These traction can lead to retinal hole formation also, and combined tractional and rhegmatogenous RD can also appear.

The VEGF that has stimulated the growth of the new vessels in the retina can stimulate new vessel growth on the iris and the angle of anterior chamber also. This neovascularization at the angle can lead to secondary angle -closure glaucoma and a painful blind eye.

The ADED with tractional RD and neovascular glaucoma lead to severe permanent loss of vision in patients with diabetes.

CLINICAL FEATURES AND SIGNS OF DIABETIC RETINOPATHY

Signs

Mild NPDR

Initially a few fine small globular microaneurysms and small dot and bolt hemorrhages appear in the macular area and around the disk.

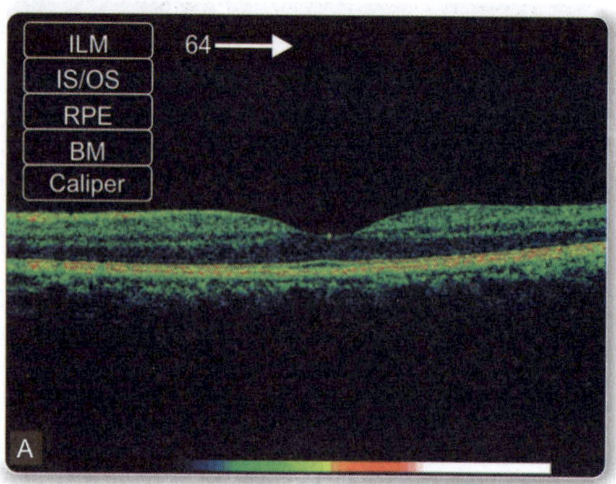

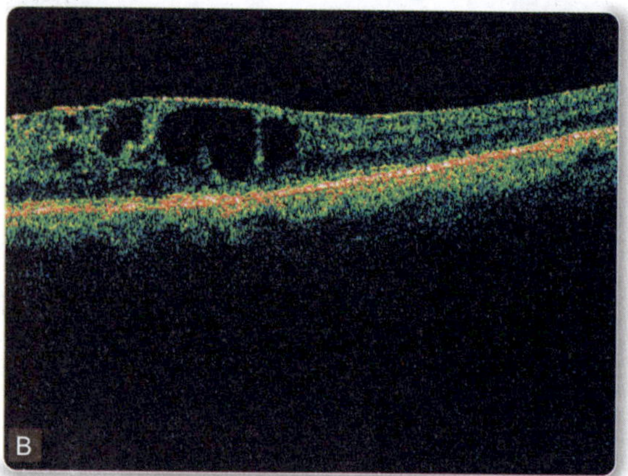

FIGURES 40.8A and B: Optical coherence tomography (OCT). **A.** Normal OCT of macula; **B.** OCT showing cystoid macular edema.

Moderate NPDR

As the disease progresses the number of hemorrhages and aneurysms increases, and hard exudates begin to appear. The macular area may show thickening due to edema and these hard exudates are waxy yellow lesions arranged in clumps or as rings with a central area of edema and micro-organism (circinate pattern).

Sx Symptoms

In the early stages of DR, there will be hardly any visual problems. When macular edema develops there will be gradual deterioration of central vision and difficulty in reading small print even with presbyopic correction. This is the stage at which a patient usually reports for an eye checkup.

If there is no significant macular edema the patient may feel the problem only when the new vessels have already developed and the patient has a vitreous hemorrhage. If the bleeding is small, the complaint of the patient is that there is sudden appearance of black spots floating before the eye. If the bleeding is massive, there will be 'sudden loss of vision'. A preretinal hemorrhage at the macula can also cause sudden drop in vision.

Severe NPDR

With time the number and size of hard exudates increase, and plaques of hard exudates may appear at the fovea, permanently destroying central vision. The retinal edema will be initially localized to a small area of the macula (usually in the central area of circinate exudates), but as disease progresses the whole of the macula will be involved and large cystic spaces will appear at macula (cystoid macular edema). In severe NPDR, the number of hemorrhages and exudates will increase, and soft exudates or otherwise called cotton-wool spots appear. They are microinfarcts of the nerve fiber layer and appear as pale white areas with feathery edges. At this stage the veins also show changes-like sausage-like thickening, beading, looping, etc.

Proliferative Diabetic Retinopathy

With the appearance of fine new vessels at the disk or along the course of the major vessels the disease reaches the proliferative stage. The vessels may be flat on the retina or float freely into the vitreous. Bleeding from these vessels appears as boat-shaped preretinal hemorrhages or as small clumps of intragel hemorrhages in the vitreous. If this bleeding is massive, there will be complete loss of view of the fundus and the vision will be reduced to this hand movement (HM) or perception of light (PL). These hemorrhages may gradually absorb and the vision may improve over a few weeks or months, or it may remain status quo.

MANAGEMENT OF DIABETIC RETINOPATHY

There is no scientifically proven medical treatment for DR.

Glucose Control

The landmark Diabetes Control and Complications Trial has taught us that intensive glucose control can decrease the incidence and progression of DR. All diabetics [non-insulin-dependent diabetes mellitus (NIDDM) and insulin-dependent diabetes mellitus (IDDM)] should strive to maintain glycosylated hemoglobin levels of less than

7% to prevent or at the very least to minimize or delay the long-term complications of DM, including DR.

Treatment

The treatment modalities available for DR today are:

- Laser photocoagulation
- Intravitreal injections:
  - Triamcinolone acetonide
  - Anti-VEGF agents.
- Vitrectomy.

Laser Photocoagulation

The indications are CSME and PDR.

In CSME laser photocoagulation is done as focal treatment directed at the microaneurysms and leaking capillaries. In diffuse macular edema grid treatment is done to the area of macular edema excluding the central 500 micron area at the fovea. The aim is closure of the leaking microaneurysms and stimulates the retinal pigment epithelium for reabsorption of the edema fluid. This will help to stabilize the vision. The spot size is 50–100 micron, at duration of 0.1 second and at sufficient power to create a just visible burn.

When the macula edema is due to vitreomacular traction as demonstrated by OCT, the management is surgical. Pars plana vitrectomy is employed to relieve the traction and there by lessen the edema.

Panretinal photocoagulation (PRP) done in PDR. Settings are 300–500 micron spot size at duration of 0.1 second and the power is selected to create a distinct yellow burn on the retina. About 2,000–3,000 burns are created excluding the macular area within the vascular arcade and starting 2D away from the superior, nasal and inferior margins of the disk and extending up to the equator. The PRP burns leave permanent pigmented scars on the retina (Fig. 40.9A).

The exact mechanism by which PRP works is not entirely understood. One theory is that destroying the hypoxic retina presumably decreases the production of vasoproliferative factors such as VEGF, which in turn reduces the rate of neovascularization (Fig. 40.9B). Another theory is that PRP allows increased diffusion of oxygen from the choroid, supplementing retinal circulation.

Intravitreal Injections

Intravitreal injections are the latest in the armamentarium in the fight against DR.

Triamcinolone acetonide: 0.1 mL of 4 mg/1 mL solution is given as intravitreal injection to decrease persistent macular edema (preservative free).

Anti-VEGF: Factors such as ranibizumab, bevacizumab, etc. cause regression of new vessels and can prevent recurrent vitreous hemorrhage. They will also reduce macular edema. Repeated injections are often required.

Vitrectomy

Vitrectomy is indicated in:

1. Persistent vitreous hemorrhage, which fails to clear spontaneously.
2. Tractional RD threatening or involving the macula.
3. Combined tractional and rhegmatogenous RD.
4. Preretinal hemorrhages in front of the macula.

The purpose of surgery is to remove the blood to permit evaluation and possible treatment of the posterior

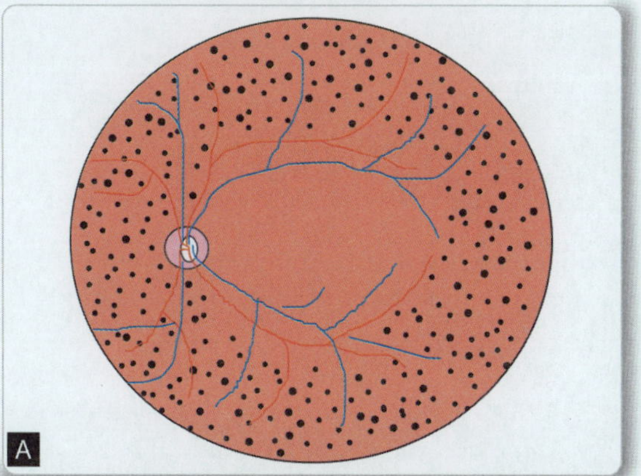

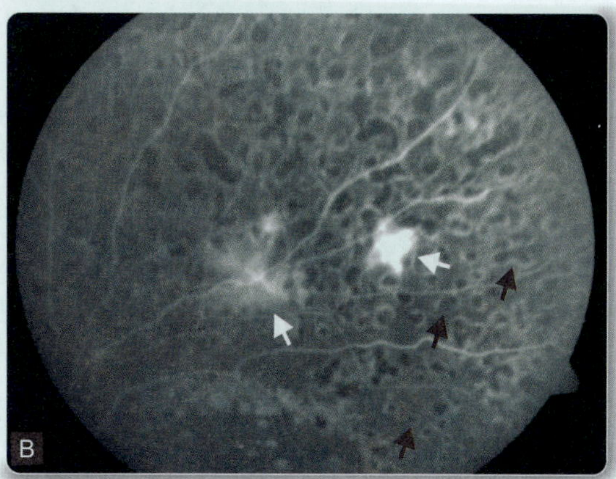

FIGURES 40.9A and B: Pattern of laser burns in panretinal photocoagulation (PRP). **A.** Diagrammatic representation; **B.** PRP burns (black arrows) around an area of NVE (white arrows).

pole, to release tractional forces that pull on the retina, to repair a retinal detachment and to remove the scaffolding into which the neovascular complexes may grow. Laser photocoagulation through indirect delivery systems or through the EndoProbe can be performed as an adjunctive procedure during surgery to initiate or continue laser treatment.

Prognosis

The damage that is produced by DR is irreversible. The purpose of all modalities of treatment is to contain the damages, to arrest or delay the worsening of DR to conserve as much residual vision as possible.

Hence, the importance of diabetic patients undergoing yearly detailed retinal examination even if there is no visual problems. Therefore all type II diabetics should undergo ophthalmologic examination upon diagnosis of the disorder and type I diabetics should undergo ophthalmologic examination within 5 years of the diagnosis. Even those who had undergone laser treatment should have lifelong regular follow-up. Pregnant patients should be examined once every trimester since the risk of rapid progression of retinopathy is high during pregnancy.

It is very important that DR is detected early before significant damage to retina and vision has occurred.

Failure to perform regular ophthalmologic screening examinations in patients with DM is a negligent omission that exposes patients to the risk of blindness.

Patient Education

One of the most important aspects in the management of DR is patient education. Inform patients that they play an integral role in their own eye care. Emphasize the following facts:

1. Excellent glucose control is beneficial in any stage of DR. It delays the onset and slows down the progression of the diabetic complications in the eye.
2. Other systemic problems such as hypertension, renal disease and hyperlipidemia may contribute to the progression of the retinopathy and should be addressed promptly.
3. Smoking may play a role in further compromising oxygen delivery to the retina. Therefore, all efforts should be made to quit smoking.
4. Visual symptoms (e.g. changes in vision, redness and pain) could be manifestations of disease progression and should be reported immediately.
5. Diabetes mellitus in general and DR in particular are progressive conditions such that regular follow-up care with a physician and ophthalmologist is crucial to detect any changes that may benefit from treatment.

41 Hypertension

Girija Devi PS

The high lateral pressure exerted on the vessel walls in hypertension can damage the vessel walls and can cause breakdown of the inner blood-retinal barrier (BRB). This produces a specific retinopathy called hypertensive retinopathy.

The vascular damage caused by hypertension can contribute to many ocular problems like:

- Retinal arteriosclerosis
- Increased incidence of central retinal artery (CRA) occlusion
- Increased incidence of central retinal vein (CRV) occlusion
- Retinal artery macroaneurysm
- Anterior ischemic optic neuropathy
- Choroidal vascular occlusion
- Exudative retinal detachment (RD) (in toxemia of pregnancy and hypertension secondary to renal problems)
- Oculomotor nerve palsies.

HYPERTENSIVE RETINOPATHY

Hypertensive retinopathy is produced by damage to the retinal arterioles caused by the high lateral pressure exerted on the vessel walls in uncontrolled hypertension.

Pathophysiology

The damage produced to the retinal arterioles by sustained hypertension depends on pre-existing **involutional fibrosis,** which is a normal change that occurs in the vessel walls as age advances. In young people, the vessel walls are unprotected by involutional fibrosis and they respond to elevation of blood pressure (BP) by narrowing. The vessels become narrow, straightened and show acute-angled branching. More often, there will be focal arterial narrowing, involving only a small segment.

In older people, in whom the vessels are more rigid due to involutional fibrosis, the narrowing will be less evident. The inner BRB is also disrupted with increased vascular permeability, leading to retinal edema and hemorrhages.

Sustained hypertension leads to structural changes in the vessel walls; hyalinization of the intima and endothelial proliferation as well as hypertrophy of the media. This is called **arteriosclerosis**. This usually manifests as a loss of transparency of the vessel walls and arteriovenous (AV) crossing changes at areas, where arteries and veins cross each other. Normally, the retinal vessels are transparent and what we see is the blood column in the vessels with a light reflex running along the center of the blood column.

The loss of transparency leads to:

- Broadening and softening of the light reflex from the retinal arteries
- Copper wire arteries (where the reflex occupying most of the width of the arteries)
- Finally, silver wire arteries (where the arteries appear as white lines) (Figs 41.1A and B).

Grades of Hypertensive Retinopathy

The grades of hypertensive retinopathy are as follows:

- Grade I: Generalized arteriolar constriction
- Grade II: Grade I + localized constrictions and AV crossing changes
- Grade III: Grade II + cotton-wool spots and hemorrhages
- Grade IV: All the above + papilledema.

Clinical Features

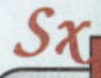

Symptoms

Hypertensive retinopathy does not usually produce any symptoms. There may be complaints of headache and slight blurring of vision, when there is an acute rise in BP and development of disk edema.

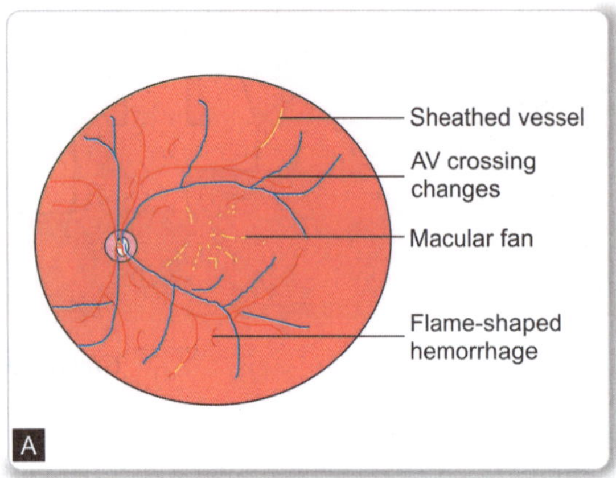

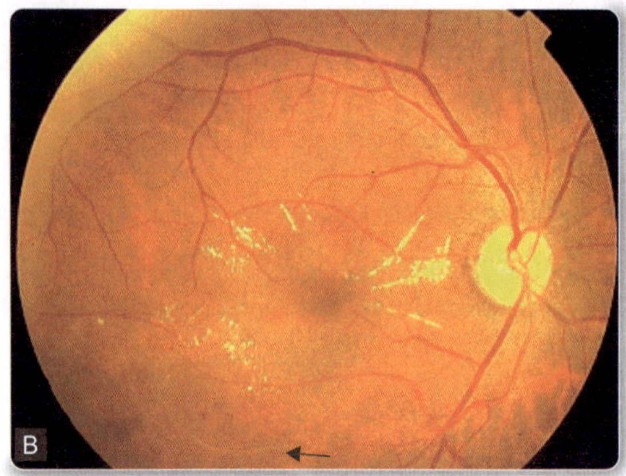

FIGURES 41.1A and B: Hypertensive retinopathy. **A.** Diagrammatic representation; **B.** Photograph showing grade III hypertensive retinopathy with macular star and silver wire artery (black arrow) (AV, arteriovenous).

Signs

On examination of the fundus in young people, the earliest changes are generalized narrowing of the arteries with straightening and acute-angled branching. Generalized narrowing is often difficult to assess, but segmental narrowing, if present, is often diagnostic of hypertensive retinopathy.

In sustained hypertension, the vessel walls develop structural changes of arteriosclerosis, which lead to appearance of copper wire and silver wire arteries and AV crossing changes. This can be a tapering of the veins on either side of the crossings **(Gunn sign)** or engorgement of the veins distal to AV crossings **(Bonnet's sign)**.

The breakdown of BRB leads to grade III stage of hypertensive retinopathy with retinal edema and accumulation of hard exudates as radiating lines around the center of the fovea. This is called macular star or macular fan if it forms an incomplete ring (Fig. 41.2). Thus, the pattern of arrangement of hard exudates differs from that of diabetic retinopathy (DR). The retinal hemorrhages in hypertensive retinopathy are mainly in the superficial nerve fiber layer and are 'flame shaped' unlike the deep 'dot and blot' hemorrhages in DR. Occlusion of the preretinal arterioles lead to nerve fiber layer infarcts, which appear as multiple cotton-wool spots at the posterior pole. Cotton-wool spots are seen only in severe non-proliferative diabetic retinopathy (NPDR) and not in the early stages.

In malignant hypertension when there is an acute rise in BP (the diastolic pressure 140 mm Hg or above) in young people, with arteries undefended by involutionary

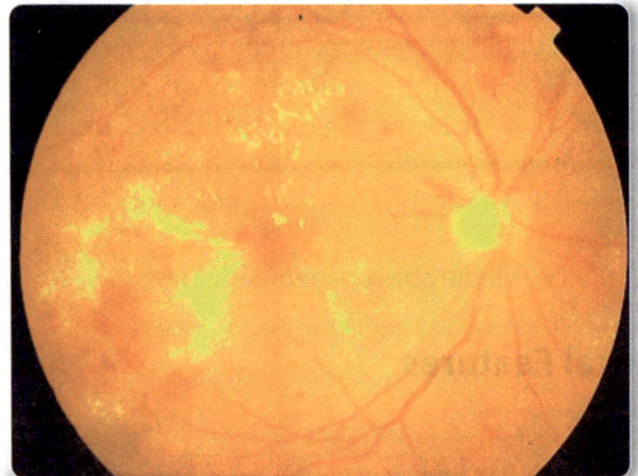

FIGURE 41.2: Severe grade III hypertensive retinopathy with macular fan

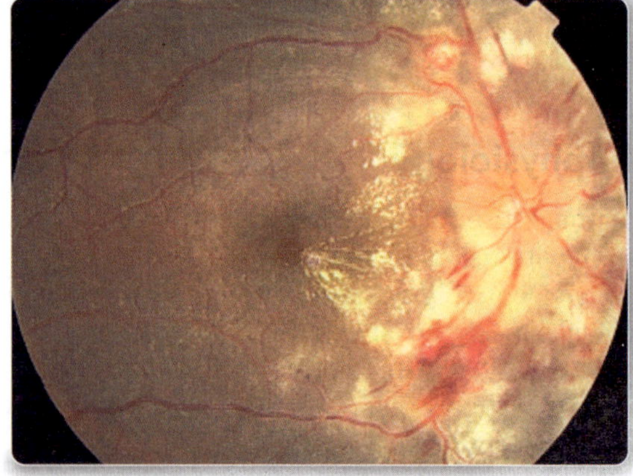

FIGURE 41.3: Grade IV hypertensive retinopathy with disk edema

TABLE 41.1: Comparison of diabetic retinopathy and hypertensive retinopathy	
Diabetic retinopathy	**Hypertensive retinopathy**
Symptoms are mainly visual	Minimal symptoms, headache, if there is sudden increase in BP*
Severity is related to duration and control of diabetes	No relation to duration of disease, mainly related to increase in BP
Changes not reversible	Reversible, if BP is brought under control
Changes are mainly in capillaries and veins	Retinal arteries are mainly affected
Hard exudates arranged as circinates, cluster or as plaques	Arranged as macular star or as fan pattern
Hemorrhages are mostly dot and blot	Flame-shaped hemorrhages
Cotton-wool spots seen in severe NPDR† only	Cotton-wool spots can be an early feature
Microaneurysms, new vessels and vitreous hemorrhages are characteristic features	Rare in hypertensive retinopathy

*BP, blood pressure; †NPDR, non-proliferative diabetic retinopathy.

sclerosis, there will be disk edema with extensive retinal edema, e.g. as in toxemia of pregnancy or renal problem complicated by hypertension (Fig. 41.3). If the high BP is not controlled, hard exudates will also appear in the form of macular star or fan.

Appearance of malignant hypertension is a grave warning sign and if BP is not immediately brought under control, there is a grave risk to life as well as vision.

Treatment

Treatment is adequate control of hypertension. There is no specific ocular treatment. If BP is brought under control and maintained at normal level, the retinal changes will also reverse, unlike in diabetic retinopathy, where the damage is irreversible (Table 41.1). The prognosis for vision is usually good if the BP is maintained at normal levels with medicines.

Blood Disorders

42

Girija Devi PS

SEVERE ANEMIA

Changes in the fundus correlates most closely with the degree of anemia, rather than the cause of anemia.

The retinal veins will be tortuous and the tortuosity is related to the severity of the anemia. Hemorrhages with characteristic white centers called **Roth's spots** will appear. They represent fibrin thrombi occluding ruptured blood vessels. Flame-shaped hemorrhages and cotton-wool spots may also be seen.

Optic neuropathy is characteristically seen in pernicious anemia. If not promptly corrected with vitamin B_{12} injections, it can result in optic atrophy. This optic neuropathy is the effect of deficiency of vitamin B_{12} on neuronal functions, rather than the effect of anemia.

Pathogenesis

The exact mechanism for the retinal changes is the hypoxia caused by the low hemoglobin (Hb) levels. The changes are observed when the Hb level falls below 7 g/dL. The retinal changes disappear when the anemia gets corrected.

LEUKEMIA

Ocular changes are more common in acute, than chronic leukemia. The ocular changes are of two types:

1. The retinopathy produced by the anemia, and increased white blood cells (WBC) count and hyperviscosity.
2. The infiltration of ocular tissues except the avascular structures like the cornea and lens.

Retinopathy

The hemorrhages can be superficial and deep, and are seen throughout the fundus, but more in the posterior pole. White centered hemorrhages like Roth's spots are seen and are caused by the accumulation of WBCs. Hyperviscosity will produce tortuosity of the veins and retinal infarcts, which appear as cotton-wool spots. Pale, broad, fuzzy whitish lines along vessels are seen and they strongly suggest the presence of leukemia.

Infiltration

Diffuse infiltration of the choroids or nodules on the retina can occur. Disk edema can occur due to direct invasion of the nerve or secondary to increased intracranial pressure (ICP).

BLEEDING DISORDERS

Hemorrhagic Disorders

Hemorrhagic disorders like hemophilia and von Willebrand's disease can cause bleeding in both intraocular and extraocular tissues. This is often precipitated by mild trauma or ocular surgery. The extraocular hemorrhages can be mild as subconjunctival (s/c) hemorrhages or severe orbital hemorrhages leading to acute proptosis. Intraocular hemorrhages can be retinal or preretinal hemorrhages or can be massive vitreous hemorrhages, leading to sudden loss of vision.

Hyperviscosity Syndrome

Increased blood viscosity can be due to increased circulating immunoglobulins as in Waldenström's macroglobulinemia and multiple myeloma or due to increased cellular components as in leukemias, polycythemia and the myeloproliferative disorders.

Hyperviscosity leads to decreased microvascular circulation. It affects both central and peripheral retinal circulation. Fluorescein angiogram showed increased circulation time. There will be engorgement of both arteries and veins and venous tortuosity, and retinal hemorrhages and a picture resembling 'venous stasis retinopathy' will appear.

RETICULOENDOTHELIOSIS

The condition called 'histiocytosis X' includes three syndromes:

- Eosinophilic granuloma
- Hand-Schüller-Christian disease
- Letterer-Siwe disease.

Eosinophilic Granuloma

Eosinophilic granuloma causes benign, localized bone lesions in children and young adults. If it involves the orbit it can cause proptosis.

X-ray: Shows sharply demarcated, radiolucent punched-out lesions.

Hand-Schüller-Christian Disease

Hand-Schüller-Christian disease has a classical triad of bony lesions, exophthalmos and diabetes insipidus.

Treatment: In both conditions it is by radiations, steroids or by excision of the lesions.

Letterer-Siwe Disease

Letterer-Siwe disease is the rarest and most severe form, and runs a rapidly progressive and fatal course in infants and children. Lesions can involve the choroid, retina or anterior uveal tract. When anterior uvea is involved, recurrent hyphema can occur.

Treatment: Steroids are usually used for treatment.

AIDS and the Eye

43

Girija Devi PS

INFECTION BY HUMAN IMMUNODEFICIENCY VIRUS

Human immunodeficiency virus (HIV) infection is the most feared infectious disease of today. Nearly 14,000 new HIV infections are reported to be occurring globally every day and the majorities are in developing countries. The trend of transmission is shifting from the high-risk groups (commercial sex workers, drug abusers, multiple sexual partners and homosexuals) to heterosexual transmission.

The first HIV infection in India was identified in Chennai in a commercial sex worker in 1986. Currently there are about 2.5 million HIV-infected people in India. About 40%–45% of HIV-infected persons have some ophthalmic manifestations, but are more commonly seen in the late stages.

With the advent of the three-drug therapy, **highly active antiretroviral therapy (HAART), AIDS-related-blinding** posterior segment conditions and even anterior segment problems have decreased in severity, and the life expectancy of the patients have also increased. At the same time, 'HAART-led immune recovery' acts like a 'double-edged sword'. The immune recovery leads to immune-mediated inflammatory response to dormant antigens and lead to several problems mainly dermatologic, but the eye can also be involved as in immune recovery uveitis.

Anterior Segment Lesions

Anterior segment lesions due to HIV diseases are:

1. Infections:
   - Herpes zoster ophthalmicus (HZO)
   - Herpes simplex keratitis
   - Cytomegalovirus (CMV) keratitis
   - Molluscum contagiosum
   - Bacterial keratitis
   - Microsporidial keratitis
   - Toxoplasma uveitis
   - Fungal infections.
2. Ocular adnexal infections:
   - Preseptal cellulitis
   - Lid abscess.
3. Neoplasms:
   - Kaposi's sarcoma (KS)
   - Squamous cell carcinoma.
4. Other manifestations:
   - Keratoconjunctivitis sicca (KCS)
   - Conjunctival microvasculopathy
   - Non-specific conjunctivitis
   - Trichomegaly.
5. Iatrogenic and post-treatment manifestations:
   - Immune recovery uveitis
   - Drug-induced uveitis
   - Stevens-Johnson syndrome.

Posterior Segment Manifestations

1. Microvasculopathy.
2. Opportunistic infections:
   - Cytomegalovirus retinitis
   - Necrotizing herpetic retinopathy
   - Toxoplasmosis
   - Pneumocystis choroiditis
   - Cryptococcal choroiditis
   - Ocular tuberculosis
   - Ocular syphilis.
3. Neuro-ophthalmologic abnormalities:
   - Papilledema
   - Papillitis
   - Retrobulbar neuritis
   - Optic atrophy
   - Oculomotor nerve palsies.

ANTERIOR SEGMENT LESIONS

Infections

Herpes Zoster Ophthalmicus

There is a high incidence of HZO in HIV patients. The infection is likely to be severe and prolonged. It may be associated with generalized and neurological manifestations. The postherpetic neuralgia tends to be more severe and prolonged. *Any young person below 45 years developing HZO has to be investigated for underlying HIV infection.*

Treatment: The treatment also has to be very aggressive with IV Acyclovir (10 mg/kg body weight 8 hourly for 7 day) followed by oral therapy 800 mg five times a day for 3–6 weeks.

Herpes Simplex Virus Infection

Both herpes simplex virus (HSV)-1 as well as HSV-2 infection occurs in AIDS patients. Herpetic keratitis will be more severe and painful with recurrent dendritic keratitis. It is usually accompanied by iritis, secondary glaucoma and tends to recur frequently. Both HSV and HZO may be present simultaneously. The HSV stromal keratitis is less frequent, probably due to the immunosuppressed state.

Cytomegalovirus Keratitis

Cytomegalovirus retinitis is the commonest AIDS-related opportunistic infection. Rarely, it can involve the anterior segment also, leading to keratitis and iritis.

Molluscum Contagiosum

In HIV positive people, lesions are produced by molluscum on lids as well as the conjunctiva, they are larger in size, often confluent, bilateral and resistant to treatment. They often recur after treatment.

Treatment: It is by excision and curettage, cryotherapy or cauterization with phenol or trichloroacetic acid.

Bacterial Keratitis

Bacterial keratitis is often caused by the normal flora of the conjunctival sac; often multiple pathogens are involved and run a higher risk of perforation.

Microsporidial Keratitis

Microsporidia is an intracellular spore-bearing protozoan parasite that usually produces gastrointestinal (GI) problems. In AIDS patients, it can cause bilateral superficial punctate epithelial keratitis.

Toxoplasmosis

Toxoplasma usually produces anterior uveitis secondary to retinochoroiditis, but in AIDS patients, it can cause a primary anterior uveitis without retinal lesions. This inflammation requires antitoxoplasma therapy combined with steroids.

Fungal Keratitis

Acquired immunodeficiency syndrome patients can develop fungal keratitis without preceding trauma or steroid therapy.

Ocular Adnexal Infections

There is a higher incidence of preseptal cellulitis in AIDS patients, compared to normal people. Similarly, eyelid abscesses are also more common. Both are caused by *Staphylococcus aureus.*

Neoplasms

Kaposi's Sarcoma

Kaposi's sarcoma is a vascular mesenchymal tumor arising from the skin of the eyelids or from the conjunctiva. It is rarely seen in India, possibly because the probable causative organism, human herpesvirus-8 is rare in India. It can be the initial manifestation of AIDS. The tumor appears as multiple red nodules. The most common site is the inferior fornix.

Histologically, Kaposi's sarcoma consists of complex vascular spaces without endothelium and malignant spindle cells of vascular channels. It will not be invading the eye and treatment is required only if it is cosmetically unappealing.

Treatment: It includes surgical excision, cryotherapy and radiation. HAART may cause regression of KS.

Squamous Cell Carcinoma

Squamous cell carcinoma of conjunctiva is the third common neoplasm associated with AIDS.

Treatment: It is by surgical excision. HAART therapy may cause regression of these lesions.

Cutaneous and Conjunctival Lymphoma

Cutaneous and conjunctival lymphoma are a higher grade of malignancy than the previous two malignancies described; and second common neoplasm associated with AIDS.

Other Manifestations

Keratoconjunctivitis Sicca

Due to lymphocytic infiltration of the lacrimal gland, KCS can occur in 20%–40% of AIDS patients. They will aggravate viral or bacterial infections.

Management: Lubricants and punctal occlusion in severe cases.

Conjunctivitis

A non-specific, chronic, culture negative conjunctivitis may occur. Some rare organisms may be the etiological agents.

Conjunctival Microvasculopathy

Segmental vascular dilatations, microaneurysms, etc. occur. This may be associated with retinal microvasculopathy. The exact cause is unknown. It is probably due to deposition of abnormal immune complexes or coagulopathy. This condition requires no treatment.

Iatrogenic and Post-treatment Manifestations

Immune Recovery Uveitis

As the CD4 count rises with HAART, a uveitis with vision drop can develop probably as an inflammatory response to some pre-existing antigen. Treatment with anti-inflammatory drugs will control this inflammation and prevent vision loss.

Drug-induced Uveitis

As a toxic effect of drugs, i.e. Rifabutin and Cidofovir, an anterior uveitis can develop.

Stevens-Johnson Syndrome

Any of the many drugs used by AIDS patients can produce a Stevens-Johnson syndrome. The pre-existing KCS will aggravate the ocular problem.

POSTERIOR SEGMENT MANIFESTATIONS

Microvasculopathy

Microvasculopathy is the most common ocular manifestation of AIDS. It manifests as cotton-wool spots. They are asymptomatic and do not require any treatment.

Posterior Segment Opportunistic Infections

Posterior segment opportunistic infections are associated with disseminated infections. They occur as necrotizing uveitis or as unifocal or multifocal choroiditis.

Cytomegalovirus Retinitis

Cytomegalovirus retinitis the most common ocular opportunistic infection in AIDS. Its incidence has come down with HAART. But it is still the most common opportunistic infection. It can be unilateral or bilateral and manifests in patients with CD4 count less than 50/uL. The classical picture is called **cottage cheese with ketchup retinopathy**. White areas of retinal necrosis appear at the posterior pole with hemorrhages at the advancing edge as they spread over the retina (Fig. 43.1). As the areas heal, pigment proliferation and gliosis will appear. Retinal holes can appear in the affected areas leading to rhegmatogenous retinal detachment (RD).

Treatment: Ganciclovir and its prodrug Valganciclovir, Foscarnet, Cidofovir, etc. Ganciclovir can be given as a retinal implant.

Necrotizing Herpetic Retinopathy

Necrotizing herpetic retinopathy can appear in two forms. *Acute retinal necrosis (ARN) or progressive outer retinal neurosis (PORN)* ARN usually occurs in relatively healthy patients, while PORN develops in severely immune-compromised patients. In ARN, multiple areas of retinal necrosis appear with vitritis, which later become confluent. In PORN, multiple patches appear with minimal vitritis. Even with treatment, there will be severe visual loss.

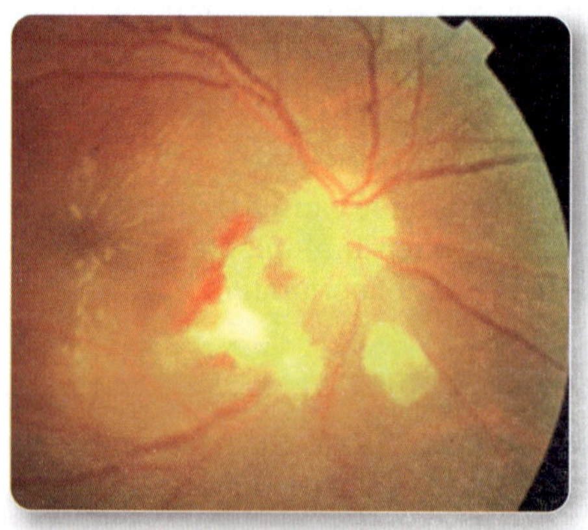

FIGURE 43.1: Cytomegalovirus retinitis

Treatment: Intravenous Acyclovir, Famciclovir 500 mg bid orally for 3 months. Systemic steroids are later added.

Toxoplasmosis

Toxoplasmosis in AIDS patients is often bilateral multifocal severe inflammation with intense vitritis. It is differentiated from CMV retinitis by the fewer number of hemorrhages in toxoplasmosis.

Pneumocystic and Cryptococcal Choroiditis

Pneumocystic and cryptococcal choroiditis can occur in AIDS patients as opportunistic infection. They are often bilateral multifocal lesions.

Ocular Tuberculosis

Ocular tuberculosis is a rare infection in AIDS even though pulmonary tuberculosis is the commonest systemic opportunistic infection in AIDS. It may appear as a solitary tuberculosis granuloma or multiple military tubercles of the choroid. It may be associated with exudative RD.

Treatment: It includes long-term systemic antituberculosis (anti-TB) therapy.

Ocular Syphilis

Ocular syphilis may manifest as iritis, neuroretinitis, retinal vasculitis, retrobulbar neuritis and necrotizing retinitis. It may develop when CD4+ counts are more than 200/uL and this will differentiate it from CMV retinitis.

Neuro-ophthalmologic Manifestations

Neuro-ophthalmologic manifestations indicate involvement of the brain or the meninges by infections or lymphoma. They occur only in 6% of HIV patients. This can manifest as:

1. Optic nerve involvement such as optic neuritis, retrobulbar neuritis, papilledema and optic atrophy.
2. Ocular motor nerve palsies.
3. Pupillary anomalies especially in patients with neurosyphilis.

Eye and Acquired Connective Tissue Disorders

44

Girija Devi PS

The various rheumatoid diseases, otherwise called 'acquired diseases of connective tissue' affect the eye to various extents. Autoimmunity plays an important role in the pathogenesis of most of these diseases.

RHEUMATOID ARTHRITIS

Rheumatoid arthritis (RA) is the most common inflammatory articular disease. It affects mostly women in childbearing age. The women:men ratio is 3:1. All joints are involved, but it typically involves the small joints of the hand and feet. About 80% of patients with RA are positive for rheumatoid factor. Detection of anti-cyclic citrullinated peptide (anti-CCP) antibodies is a more recent test and patients with 'anti-CCP antibodies' tend to have severe illness.

Ocular Manifestations

1. Keratoconjunctivitis sicca (KCS) is a common ocular association of RA.
2. Scleritis and episcleritis are the most common systemic associations of RA. Scleritis can be the necrotizing or non-necrotizing type:
    a. Sclerosing keratitis: There is infiltration and opacification of the peripheral cornea in a tongue-shaped fashion adjacent to an area of scleritis. This can lead to permanent corneal scarring and vascularization.
    b. Sclerokeratitis or acute stromal keratitis: Deep stromal infiltration of the cornea followed by vascularization and scarring can occur associated with non-necrotizing scleritis. The area of infiltration is not continuous with the scleritis patch, as in sclerosing keratitis.
3. Peripheral corneal infiltration:
    a. Peripheral corneal thinning (contact lens cornea): There is gradual corneal thinning in a ring-shaped fashion in the corneal periphery leaving the epithelium intact. The picture resembles a contact lens placed on the cornea.
    b. Acute corneal melting: There will be complete loss of corneal tissue in an area of peripheral corneal thinning. This can occur without any evidence of inflammation or may be associated with scleritis at the corresponding limbus.
4. Anterior chamber uveitis can occur associated with the corneal and scleral inflammation.

SPONDYLOARTHROPATHIES

Earlier called seronegative arthropathies, with the term 'seronegative' referring to a negative rheumatoid factor. That term is now less commonly used. This group is linked with human leukocyte antigen B27 (HLA-B27) and includes:

1. Both juvenile and adult form of ankylosing spondylitis.
2. Reactive arthritis.
3. Reiter's syndrome.
4. Undifferentiated spondyloarthropathy.
5. Spondyloarthropathies associated with psoriasis.
6. Spondyloarthropathies associated with inflammatory bowel diseases.

Of all these conditions, undifferentiated spondyloarthropathy is the most common, followed by ankylosing spondylitis. All these conditions have the potential to develop HLA-B27-associated acute anterior uveitis. Reiter's syndrome and psoriatic arthritis can develop bilateral conjunctivitis.

JUVENILE IDIOPATHIC ARTHRITIS

Previously called 'juvenile rheumatoid arthritis'; the term 'rheumatoid' is now not used, since this condition has no relationship to adult-onset rheumatoid arthritis.

The ophthalmologic involvement is chronic anterior uveitis with minimal symptoms. It is usually detected on routine eye checkup of children with juvenile idiopathic arthritis (JIA). The inflammation is usually mild-to-moderate and lasts for few months. In one fourth of this group, the inflammation will be severe, responds poorly to treatment and end up with complications like band keratopathy, cataract and secondary glaucoma.

SYSTEMIC LUPUS ERYTHEMATOSUS

Systemic lupus erythematosus (SLE) is an autoimmune disease with genetic predisposition and the patients exhibit a variety of antibodies. Women in second and third decade are more affected than men.

A positive antinuclear antibody (ANA) test is the best diagnostic test, since SLE can involve multiple organs and thus have a variety of manifestations. About 3%–29% of patients can develop a variety of eye manifestations. These include:

1. Discoid lesions can develop on the skin of the eyelids.
2. Dry eye problem due to secondary Sjögren's syndrome.
3. Inflammatory vasculopathy can involve the retinal and choroidal circulation leading to vascular occlusions, hemorrhages, soft exudates and neovascularization.
4. Hypertensive retinopathy.
5. Anterior and intermediate uveitis.
6. Optic neuropathy.
7. Oculomotor palsies.
8. Visual hallucinations, field defects and cortical blindness.

ANTIPHOSPHOLIPID ANTIBODY SYNDROME

The syndrome can occur in association with SLE and other rheumatic disease and it can be caused by some drugs and infections also. When it occurs unassociated with these conditions it is called primary antiphospholipid syndrome (APS).

It causes arterial and venous thrombosis in retina as well as choroid. Vascular occlusions can lead to ischemic optic neuropathy. Cerebrovascular accidents can also cause visual symptoms.

Management

1. Diagnosed by tests for antiphospholipid antibodies.
2. These patients require anticoagulant therapy and this can lead to intraocular and extraocular hemorrhages.

SCLERODERMA

Scleroderma disease leads to fibrous replacement of the dermis and vasospasm.

The thickening and contracture of the skin can involve the lids and can result in blepharophimosis and sometimes, corneal exposure. KCS and vascular abnormalities can occur on the conjunctiva. Renal involvement can lead to hypertensive retinopathy.

SJÖGREN'S SYNDROME

Primary Sjögren syndrome is dry eye without any specific connective tissue disease.

Secondary Sjögren syndrome is dry eye and dry mouth in association with a definite connective tissue disease. The dry eye and dry mouth is due to inflammatory cellular infiltrate of the lacrimal and salivary glands, and salivary gland biopsy can confirm this. These patients usually have anti-SSA and anti-SSB autoantibodies.

Treatment

Treatment is with tear substitutes. Severe cases will require topical and systemic immunosuppressive therapy like cyclosporin A.

POLYMYOSITIS AND DERMATOMYOSITIS

Polymyositis and dermatomyositis are characterized by pain and weakness of skeletal muscle groups starting from the proximal muscle groups. In dermatomyositis, there will be skin lesions also. Erythematous rashes will appear on the eyelids (heliotrope rash), face, chest and extensor surfaces. The disease can be confirmed by skeletal muscle biopsy and by abnormal electromyography and abnormal levels of skeletal muscle enzymes. Apart from the heliotrope rash, ophthalmoplegia can rarely occur due to ocular muscle involvement.

RELAPSING POLYCHONDRITIS

Relapsing polychondritis is characterized by recurrent inflammation of the cartilage of the nose, ear lobe, cardiovascular system and the laryngotracheobronchial system. It can occur alone or in association with other autoimmune diseases like SLE or systemic vasculitis like Wegener's granulomatosis.

The ocular manifestations are conjunctivitis, scleritis and vasculitis involving the uvea and retina.

VASCULITIS

Vasculitis can be:

1. Primary, where the primary pathology is inflammation of the vessel walls.

2. Secondary, where vascular inflammation occurs as part of other autoimmune disorders or due to factors like infections, neoplasm, etc.

Primary vasculitis can be classified based on the size of the vessel involved:

1. Large-vessel vasculitis:
   - Giant cell arteritis
   - Takayasu arteritis.
2. Medium-sized vessel vasculitis:
   - Polyarteritis nodosa (PAN)
   - Kawasaki disease.
3. Small-vessel vasculitis:
   - Wegener's granulomatosis
   - Churg-Strauss syndrome
   - Microscopic polyangiitis
   - Essential cryoglobulinemic vasculitis
   - Behcet's syndrome.

Large-vessel Vasculitis

Giant Cell (Temporal) Arteritis

Giant cell arteritis is a granulomatous necrotizing arteritis, which involve arteries that have good quality of elastic tissue in the media and adventitia, like the superficial temporal, ophthalmic and posterior ciliary arteries. The intracranial arteries, which have very little elastic tissue, are not usually affected.

Clinical features: It affects elderly people in the seventh or eighth decade. When it involves the superficial temporal artery, the patients present with severe headache, scalp tenderness and pain on mastication (jaw claudication).

The superficial temporal artery is thickened, nodular and tender with absent pulsation in advanced stages.

There may be sudden loss of vision due to involvement of the ophthalmic artery without any symptoms of temporal arteritis.

Investigation are as follows:

- Erythrocyte sedimentation rate (ESR) will be very high
- High levels of C-reactive proteins
- Temporal artery biopsy will confirm the diagnosis.

Treatment includes systemic steroids.

Takayasu Arteritis

Takayasu arteritis is common in Japan and Far East. It affects particularly aorta and its branches. Inflammation of the vessel walls leads to their obliteration and ischemia of the areas supplied by it or leads to aneurysms. In the eye it can lead to amaurosis fugax or sudden loss of vision due to non-perfusion. It can lead to arteriovenous (AV) anastomosis, peripheral retinal non-perfusion, retinal and iris neovascularization and vitreous hemorrhages.

Treatment: Systemic steroids help to suppress the arterial inflammation.

Medium-vessel Vasculitis

Polyarteritis Nodosa

The disease is characterized by segmental necrotizing inflammation of medium-sized arteries. The problems depend on the organs affected. Central nervous system (CNS) involvement can lead to mononeuritis multiplex—involvement of unrelated peripheral nerves. Renal involvement can lead to hypertension and hypertensive retinopathy. Retinal and choroidal vasculitis can occur, leading to visual impairment and exudative retinal detachment (RD). Cranial nerve palsies can occur; Cogan's syndrome characterized by interstitial keratitis, hearing loss, tinnitus and vertigo may be associated with PAN.

Treatment: Systemic steroids or a combination of systemic steroids and cyclophosphamide.

Small-vessel Vasculitis

Wegener's Granulomatosis

Wegener's granulomatosis consists of necrotizing granulomatous inflammation of the upper respiratory tract (involving the sinuses and esophagus), of the lower respiratory tract and focal segmental glomerulonephritis.

If there is renal involvement, the disease can be fatal, unless treated promptly with immunosuppressants.

Ocular involvement occurs in more than 50% of cases and it can be the presenting feature. It can be scleritis with peripheral keratitis, orbital pseudotumors and retinal vasculitis.

Investigations: The presence of the disease is confirmed by the demonstration of cytoplasmic antineutrophil cytoplasmic antibody (c-ANCA) and autoantibodies to proteinase 3.

Treatment: Immunosuppressant drugs like cyclophosphamide and methotrexate.

Churg-Strauss Syndrome

Churg-Strauss syndrome presents with asthma, eosinophilia, vasculitis, transient pulmonary infiltration and neuropathy.

Ophthalmic manifestations are conjunctival granuloma, uveitis, retinal vasculitis, vascular occlusions and cranial nerve palsies.

Behcet's Syndrome

Behcet's syndrome was initially considered to be a triad of oral ulcers, genital ulcers and hypopyon uveitis. It is now considered to be multisystem vasculitis of unknown etiology. Therefore, its clinical manifestations also vary depending on the organ involved. It is particularly common in Japan and Far East.

The most common clinical feature is oral ulceration. The common ocular lesions are uveitis and retinal vasculitis. The skin involvement includes erythema nodosum, pyoderma, pathergy (pustular response to skin injury) and dermatographism (urticarial wheal occurs on stroking the skin). Some patients also show polyarteritis, vasculitis leading to major vessel thrombosis, aneurysm, etc. CNS involvement is also seen.

Many circulating immune complexes and high ESR with C-reactive proteins are demonstrated. HLA-B51 is also common in patients in some countries.

The diagnosis is based on the clinical criteria that include oral ulcers and any two of the following—uveitis, genital ulcers, skin involvement or pathergy.

Treatment: Corticosteroids and immunosuppressants like azathioprine or cyclosporine.

Ocular Changes in Inborn Errors of Metabolism

45

Girija Devi PS

There are a few hundreds of errors of metabolism caused by inherited genetic mutation and new diseases are continuously added to the list.

Of these, 50% of conditions affect eye and more than one part of the eye is affected. The cornea and retina are the most commonly involved structures. In spite of the common involvement of the eye, only a few conditions namely, albinism, Fabry's disease and Wilson's disease have distinctly characteristic eye changes, which will confirm the diagnosis. In most of the other conditions, the ocular lesion will give a clue to the differential diagnosis of etiology and further examination and investigations are required to confirm the diagnosis.

The common ocular abnormalities and the inborn errors of metabolism associated with it are listed below:

- **Corneal clouding:**
  - Mucopolysaccharidosis (MPS) except MPS II or (Hunter's syndrome)
  - Gangliosidosis
  - Mannosidosis
  - Mucolipidosis
  - Cystinosis.
- **Corneal pigmentation:**
  - Alkaptonuria.
- **Arcus senilis-like ring in cornea:**
  - Familial hyperlipoproteinemia type II and III
  - Osteogenesis imperfecta.
- **Kayser–Fleischer (KF) ring (Figs 45.1A and B):**
  - Wilson's disease.
- **Cataract:**
  - Galactosemia
  - Wilson's disease
  - Homocystinuria
  - Lowe's syndrome
  - Myotonic dystrophy
  - Pseudohypoparathyroidism
  - Weill-Marchesani syndrome.
- **Subluxation of lens:**
  - Marfan's syndrome
  - Ehlers-Danlos syndrome
  - Homocystinuria
  - Sulfite oxidase deficiency
  - Weill-Marchesani syndrome.
- **Vitreous opacities:**
  - Hereditary amyloidosis.
- **Retinitis pigmentosa:**
  - Abetalipoproteinemia
  - Mucopolysaccharidosis
  - Refsum's syndrome.
- **Cherry-red spot:**
  - GM1 gangliosidosis
  - GM2 gangliosidosis, especially Tay-Sachs disease
  - Niemann-Pick disease.
- **Retinal detachment:**
  - Ehlers–Danlos syndrome
  - Homocystinuria
  - Marfan's syndrome.
- **Angioid streaks:**
  - Pseudoxanthoma elasticum.
- **Optic atrophy:**
  - Homocystinuria
  - Krabbe's disease
  - Metachromatic leukodystrophy (late infantile and juvenile).
- **Retinal depigmentation:**
  - Albinism
  - Cystinosis with nephropathy.
- **Depigmentation of iris:**
  - Albinism
  - Phenylketonuria.
- **Discoloration of sclera:**
  - Alkaptonuria
  - Cystinosis

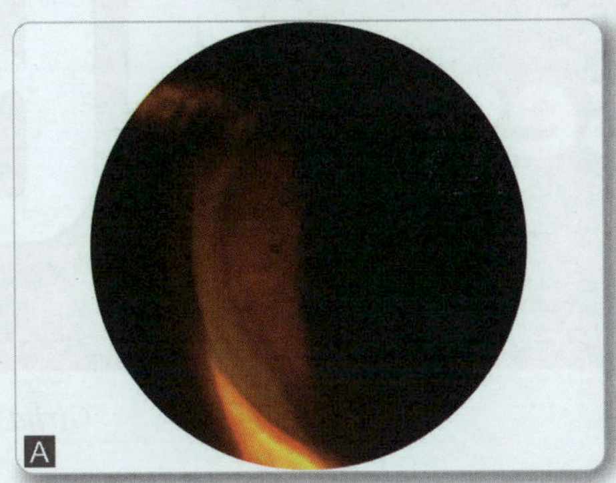
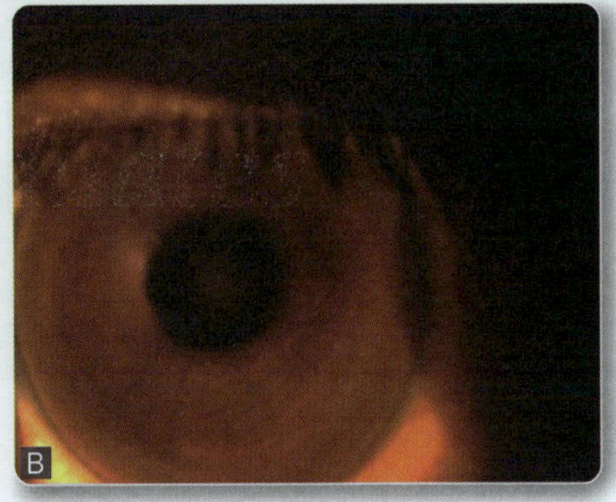

FIGURES 45.1A and B: Kayser-Fleischer (KF) ring

- Ehlers–Danlos syndrome
- Osteogenesis imperfecta.
- **Vascular deformities of conjunctiva:**
  - Fabry's disease
  - Sickle cell disease.
- **Jaundice:**
  - Hereditary hemolytic anemia
  - Hereditary hyperbilirubinemia.
- **Xanthelasma of lids:**
  - Familial hyperlipoproteinemia.
- **Ptosis and ophthalmoplegia:**
  - Abetalipoproteinemia
  - Hyperkinetic periodic paralysis
  - Tangier disease.

Endocrine Diseases 46

Girija Devi PS

Thyrotoxicosis and diabetes mellitus are the most common endocrine disorders that involve the eye.

THYROID EYE DISEASE OR GRAVES' DISEASE

1. Thyroid eye disease (TED) or Graves' disease is the commonest cause of both bilateral and unilateral proptosis.
2. Patient with proptosis may be euthyroid, hypo- or hyper-thyroid.

It is an autoimmune disorder where IgG antibodies are produced against the thyroid as well as the extraocular tissues. Women are more affected than men and the disease usually manifests in the third or fourth decade of life. The eye changes do not always correlate with the thyroid status. The patient may be hyperthyroid, euthyroid or hypothyroid. When TED occurs unassociated with hyperthyroidism, it is called ophthalmic Graves' disease.

Pathogenesis

There is accumulation of glycosaminoglycans and consequently osmotic imbibition of water in the extraocular muscles. The muscles become enlarged and swollen, and subsequently the muscle fibers degenerative and fibrosis occurs leading to restrictive myopathy. There is cellular infiltration as well as glycosaminoglycan, and fluid accumulation in the orbital fat and lacrimal gland. All these changes increase the orbital volume leading to proptosis and the soft-tissue changes.

The clinical features can be divided into:

1. Soft-tissue changes.
2. Lid abnormalities.
3. Proptosis.
4. Ocular motility problems.
5. Optic neuropathy.

Soft-tissue Involvement

There is lid and periorbital swelling. There will be conjunctival and episcleral congestion, especially in the interpalpebral area at the insertion of the medial and lateral rectus muscle.

The fluid retention leads to chemosis of the conjunctiva and in severe forms, horizontal folds of conjunctiva will be hanging out through closed lids (Fig. 46.1).

Lid Changes

There is retraction of both upper and lower lids. Normally, the upper lid covers 2 mm of the cornea at the upper limbus. In TED, the lid margin may be seen at the limbus or an area of sclera will be visible above the upper limbus.

This lid retraction in looking straight is called Dalrymple's sign (Fig. 46.2A).

On looking down, the lid lags behind the eyeball during the downward motion and more sclera will be bared on downward movement of the eye. This is called von Graefe's sign (Fig. 46.2B).

The staring look of the eye is called Kocher's sign.

The blinking rate is decreased. The cause for these lid abnormalities is sympathetic overstimulation of

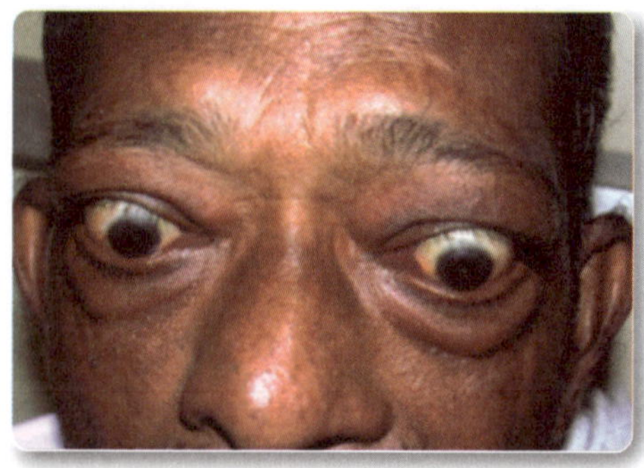

FIGURE 46.1: Advanced thyroid exophthalmos with soft-tissue changes

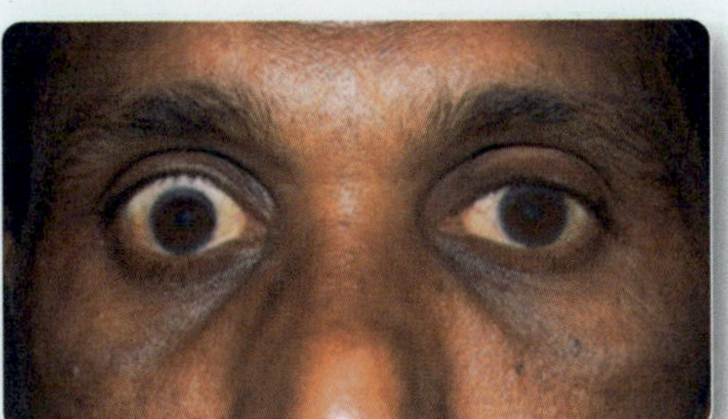

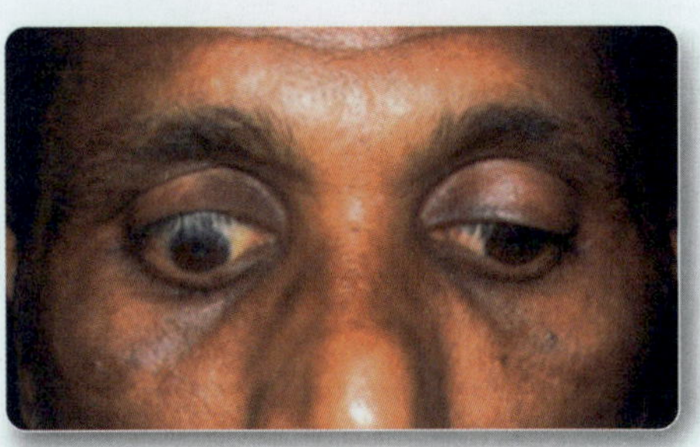

FIGURES 46.2A and B: Lid changes. **A.** Lid retraction more in right eye. Normally upper lid covers 2 mm of upper limbus; **B.** Lid lag on looking down.

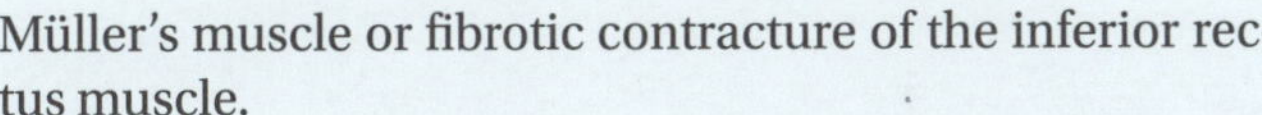

Müller's muscle or fibrotic contracture of the inferior rectus muscle.

Proptosis

Proptosis is axial and it can be unilateral or bilateral. Severe proptosis can lead to exposure keratopathy.

Ocular Mobility Problems

Initially there is mechanical restriction of ocular movements due to the swelling of the muscles and the increase in the orbital contents. Later there is fibrosis of the muscles. The inferior rectus is the muscle commonly affected first leading to mechanical restriction of elevation of the eye. The medial rectus will be affected leading to defective adduction. Depression and abduction can be involved subsequently, and in later stages all motility will be severely restricted.

Optic Neuropathy

The increased tissue volume in the orbit can lead to compression of the optic nerve or its blood supply. This will lead to decrease in visual acuity. The visual field changes can be a central or centrocecal scotoma and later peripheral constriction of the visual field can occur.

If orbital tissue pressure is not relieved at this stage with medical or surgical measures, optic atrophy can occur.

Sx Symptoms

Symptoms in the initial stages are usually mild. The cosmetic problem due to the puffiness of the lids and proptosis may be the main complaint. If motility is affected, the patient can develop diplopia. In the advanced stages marked pain and redness can occur if cornea is involved, and the vision can be affected due to corneal involvement or optic neuropathy.

Visual loss in TED can be due to the optic nerve involvement due to compressive optic neuropathy or vascular occlusion, the exposure keratopathy or corneal ulceration.

Management

In the mild cases, lubricants can be given to prevent cornea from getting dry. Diuretics may help to reduce the orbital volume. So sleeping with the head end of the bed elevated, can be tried. When there is marked tissue changes, systemic steroids will reduce the cellular infiltration and fluid retention in the orbit. If steroids fail to give the desired effect, low dose radiation or azathioprine can be tried.

Orbital Decompression

Orbital decompression is indicated if medical management fails and optic neuropathy is progressing.

Two-wall Decompression

Part of the floor and medial wall of the orbit is removed, sparing the orbital margins. The orbital tissue can occupy the space in the maxillary antrum and ethmoidal sinuses. This will decrease the orbital pressure and proptosis.

Three-wall Decompression

Here part of the lateral wall is also removed. This is done when two-wall decompressions do not give improvement.

Lateral tarsorrhaphy is done where there is exposure keratitis.

Injection of Botulinum Toxin

In persistent diplopia, injection of botulinum toxin into the involved muscle or recession of the involved muscles is done to achieve binocular single vision in primary gaze.

Treatment for thyrotoxicosis should also be given if the patient is hyperthyroid. The dose of thyroid hormone should be carefully adjusted to avoid hypothyroidism, which may aggravate the ocular problems.

HYPOTHYROIDISM

Ptosis and edema of the lids, and periorbital edema can occur in hypothyroidism.

Hypothyroidism in children can be associated with cataract formation.

Parathyroid Involvement

Hyperparathyroidism leads to hypercalcemia and this can result in calcium deposits on the corneal surface as band keratopathy. Hypoparathyroidism can lead to cataract.

Pituitary Gland

Suprasellar tumors can cause papilledema. Tumors of the pituitary gland (anterior lobe) can cause temporal pallor, optic atrophy and ophthalmoplegia.

Ocular Manifestations of Systemic Infections

47

Girija Devi PS

Systemic infections can spread to the eye through bloodstream bacteremia, which can be transient or recurrent and prolonged.

Non-specific features of ocular spread include cotton-wool spots, retinal hemorrhages and Roth's spots (white-centered hemorrhages).

ENDOGENOUS ENDOPHTHALMITIS

The bacteremia may have occurred before the clinical presentation of endophthalmitis. 75% of endophthalmitis show positive bacterial cultures at the onset of clinical signs. But endophthalmitis develops in less than 1% of patients who develop bacteremia. The most common source of infection in endogenous endophthalmitis is endocarditis, liver abscess or urinary tract infection. *Staphylococcus aureus* is the commonest pathogen with *Escherichia coli* coming second.

In children less than 3 years, preseptal cellulitis is the commonest manifestation of bacteremia. *Haemophilus influenzae* was the commonest pathogen before the introduction of influenza vaccine. Now, streptococci and pneumococci are the commonest causative agents.

Uveitis: Endogenous infection may be causative factor behind many of the idiopathic uveitis. As molecular diagnostic tests like polymerase chain reaction (PCR) become cheaper and widely used, many cases of idiopathic uveitis may prove to be of bacterial origin.

SPECIFIC INFECTIONS WITH OCULAR MANIFESTATIONS

Bacterial Infections

Tuberculosis

About 50% of cases of ocular tuberculosis are present without any evidence of systemic involvement. In a study conducted in India, only 1.4% of cases of systemic tuberculosis have ocular manifestations.

Healed or active unifocal, or multifocal choroiditis is the commonest ocular manifestation seen in 80% of cases.

A chronic granulomatous uveitis comes second followed by retinal vasculitis (Eales' disease).

In human immunodeficiency virus (HIV) infected people, extrapulmonary tuberculosis is a special problem.

Diagnosis: Ocular tuberculosis cannot be distinguished from sarcoidosis or mycotic infections by clinical examination alone. A positive result in Mantoux test is not of much significance in countries like India, where the prevalence of tuberculosis is high. A presumptive diagnosis can be made from the evidence of pulmonary or extrapulmonary tuberculosis (like lymph node involvement), history of treatment for tuberculosis or history of contact with infected persons.

Anterior chamber or vitreous tap for PCR test for tuberculosis deoxyribonucleic acid (DNA) will confirm the diagnosis.

A therapeutic trial test of antituberculosis drugs can be given and a positive response will confirm diagnosis.

Treatment: Antituberculosis regimen. Most extrapulmonary lesions including ocular infection is treated with the same drugs and for the same duration as in pulmonary tuberculosis.

With increase in the number of acquired immunodeficiency syndrome (AIDS) patients, tuberculosis infection is also currently increasing in prevalence and any granulomatous infection of the uveal tract or retinal vasculitis should give the suspicion of tuberculosis as well as HIV infection.

Leprosy

Ocular involvement in leprosy can be due to:

1. Primary infection of the eye.
2. Secondary involvement due to impaired action of VII and V nerve.

Primary infection involves the anterior segment of the eye. The ocular involvement usually occurs where leprosy relapses despite treatment or when left untreated.

Lesions produced are prominent corneal nerves, conjunctivitis, superficial punctuate keratitis, scleral nodules and chronic uveitis. Granulomatous uveitis can occur probably as an antigen-antibody reaction. Rarely interstitial keratitis and lepromatous pannus can occur.

Involvement of the VII nerve can lead to paralysis of orbicularis oculi, ectropion, lagophthalmos and exposure keratitis. Corneal anesthesia due to involvement of V nerve can lead to neurotrophic keratitis. Uveitis and corneal ulcer are the causes of blindness in leprosy. Patients presenting with granulomatous uveitis, or orbiculous paresis or prominent corneal nerves have to be examined for any hypoanesthetic patches or thickened peripheral nerves. Simultaneously all patients with leprosy should be periodically examined by an ophthalmologist for development of corneal anesthesia or any other ocular problem. Early detection and treatment of the systemic condition or the ocular problem can prevent blindness due to leprosy.

Treatment: For systemic diseases, it is treated with dapsone.

Treatment of the ocular problem is an general lines of management. Tarsorrhaphy will be required in patients with VII and V nerve involvement to limit ocular damage.

Syphilis

Syphilis infection is caused by *Treponema pallidum*, can occur as a congenital form transmitted from the mother transplacentally or as an acquired form as a sexually transmitted disease.

Its incidence had come down with the introduction of antibiotics to treat the infection, but recently its incidence is increasing in the AIDS patients.

Congenital syphilis

Congenital syphilis occurs by the transplacental spread from the infected mother. The spread occurs almost invariably in the primary and secondary stages of the disease, but rarely in tertiary stage.

The manifestations in the infant can be divided into early congenital syphilis and late congenital syphilis.

Early congenital syphilis: These signs may not appear until several days after birth. If serological tests are not done both for the mother and the baby at the time of birth the newborn may be considered as normal. Serological tests will be negative at the time of delivery if infection is acquired in the third trimester of pregnancy.

A generalized rash may appear—usually vesicular or bullous. Rhinitis (also called snuffler) osteochondritis with pathologic fractures, jaundice, anorexia and hepatosplenomegaly will appear. Chorioretinitis is the ocular manifestation that will appear in the first few months of life.

Late congenital syphilis: After 2nd year of age, the child is described to have late congenital syphilis. The typical features of this condition are Hutchinson's triad, which comprises of interstitial keratitis, deafness and Hutchinson's teeth (deformities of the upper incisions). But the occurrence of all three in the same patient is sometimes rare. Bilateral interstitial keratitis, considered to be the classic sign of congenital syphilis occur in 10% of patients. A pigmentary retinitis and glaucoma can occur secondary to syphilitic uveitis.

Acquired syphilis

Ocular manifestations can occur in all the three stages of the illness.

Primary syphilis: Chancres can develop on the eyelids and conjunctiva.

Secondary syphilis: Anterior uveitis is the commonest finding in the secondary syphilis. The generalized rash of the secondary syphilis can involve the skin of the eyelids, and the conjunctiva leading to blepharitis and conjunctivitis. Episcleritis, scleritis, chorioretinitis and perivasculitis of the retina are rare manifestations.

Tertiary syphilis: Gumma can occur on the eyelids. Unilateral interstitial keratitis can develop. Neurosyphilis will lead to the classical Argyll Robertson (AR) pupil and ocular motor nerve palsies.

Recurrent inflammation of the uveal tract—both anterior and posterior uveitis, neuroretinitis, retinal vasculitis as well as scleritis and episcleritis can occur. Optic atrophy can occur late in the course of meningovascular syphilis. Optic atrophy and AR pupil are pathognomonic of tertiary syphilis.

Fungal Infections

Candidiasis

Disseminated candidiasis can occur in patients:

1. On immunosuppressive therapy.
2. With indwelling central venous catheters.
3. On long-term antibiotic therapy.
4. Dialysis.
5. Burns.
6. Convalescing after major surgical procedures.

In this high-risk group, any sudden drop in vision should arouse suspicion of candidal endophthalmitis.

Clinical features: Multiple raised white fluffy cotton-ball lesions of chorioretinal inflammation will appear with vitreous haze. The lesions will rapidly extend into vitreous, but hemorrhages are less common. Lesions may resemble 'head light in the fog'. The lesser number or lack of hemorrhages differentiates it from cytomegalovirus retinitis. Hypopyon uveitis may rarely occur.

Diagnosis is confirmed by a vitreous aspirate.

Treatment: If fungal elements are identified, intravitreal amphotericin B is indicated. Amphotericin B and flucytosine should be given intravenous (IV) for 6–10 weeks combined with repeated intravitreal injections and topical amphotericin B drops. Vitrectomy is indicated in patients with considerable visual loss and dense vitreous infiltration. Removal of the indwelling catheters if possible may help for resolution of the condition.

Mucormycosis

Mucormycosis is the infection caused by the fungi belonging to the order mucorales. Mucorales reach the body by inhalation of the spores. Clinical manifestations typically occur in people with diabetic ketoacidosis.

Mucormycosis is characterized by invasion of arteries, rapid tissue destruction and often fatal course. It usually produces a rhinocerebral infection. The infection starts in the nose with pain and blood-stained discharge, and nasal mucosa will show necrotic turbinates. This will appear as 'black eschar.' The spread of infection into the orbit leads to orbital cellulitis. It produces rapid fall in vision due to involvement of the optic nerve, complete ophthalmoplegia, fixed dilated pupil and infraorbital anesthesia. Infection can spread to cavernous sinus and thrombosis of the internal carotid artery can occur. Infection will spread to meninges and the brain through the cribriform plate.

In any diabetic patient presenting with orbital cellulitis, mucormycosis has to be suspected. Tissue necrosis due to occlusion of the arteries leading to 'black eschar' in the nose is a valuable clue to diagnosis.

Treatment: Unless promptly diagnosed and treated, the infection if fatal. The steps are:

1. Correction of diabetic ketoacidosis.
2. Surgical debridement of devitalized tissue and drainage of sinuses.
3. Amphotericin B 1–1.5 mg/kg/day as IV infusion.

Prognosis: Prompt diagnosis and medical and surgical management is needed to save the life of the patient.

Miscellaneous Systemic Diseases Affecting the Eye

48

Girija Devi PS

The important miscellaneous systemic diseases with significant involvement of the eyes are:

- Sarcoidosis
- Multiple sclerosis
- Myasthenia gravis
- Myotonic dystrophy
- Neurofibromatosis (NF)
- Sturge-Weber syndrome
- Tuberous sclerosis
- von Hippel-Lindau syndrome
- Cicatricial pemphigoid (refer Chapter 14 Conjunctiva)
- Stevens-Johnson syndrome (refer Chapter 14 Conjunctiva)
- Rosacea.

SARCOIDOSIS

Sarcoidosis is a granulomatous inflammation characterized by the presence of non-caseating epithelioid granuloma. It affects almost all organs, but particularly affects lungs, thoracic lymph nodes, skin and eyes.

There are two peaks of incidence between 20 and 40 years, and between 50 and 60 years.

Etiology

Sarcoidosis results from an impaired cell-mediated immunity although the trigger for the inflammatory response is known.

The disease was once considered to be rare in India, but with improvement in the facilities for investigation, this disease is now found to be more prevalent in India, than expected before.

Pathology

The sarcoid nodule is a non-caseating epithelioid granuloma. It consists of a central core of tightly packed epithelioid cells, macrophages and multinucleated giant cells, surrounded by a layer of lymphocytes, monocytes and fibroblasts. The epithelioid cells fuse to join Langhans' giant cells. These granulomas may degenerate centrally and it may disappear without any sign of its presence or it may undergo an obliterative fibrosis.

Clinical Features

Half of the cases are present with respiratory symptoms. In one fourth of patients, the disease is diagnosed by an abnormality in the chest X-ray or some other abnormality in investigations. In the eye, the uveal tissue and retina are preferentially affected:

1. Granulomatous anterior uveitis is the commonest ocular manifestation. This usually affects older patients with chronic pulmonary involvement. The inflammation can be chronic, persisting for months or years and can cause severe visual loss due to secondary glaucoma, complicated cataract or cystoid macular edema.
2. An acute non-granulomatous anterior uveitis can occur in younger patients with acute onset sarcoidosis. This inflammation can be controlled with treatment.
3. Intermediate uveitis is a rare manifestation. It is characterized with snow ball peripheral vitreous opacities and periphlebitis affecting the peripheral vessels. Sarcoidosis has to be ruled out in any patient with intermediate uveitis.
4. Posterior uveitis occurs in 25% of cases of sarcoidosis. It is characterized by:
   a. Choroidal granulomas, which can be small and multiple or a single large swelling.
   b. Retinal granulomas, rare small white lesions.
   c. Optic disk granulomas.
5. Retinal periphlebitis: The perivenous exudates are typically described as 'candle wax drippings' (Figs 48.1A and B).
6. Heerfordt's disease (uveoparotid fever): It is characterized by fever, parotid gland enlargement and uveitis. This is a rare presentation of sarcoidosis.

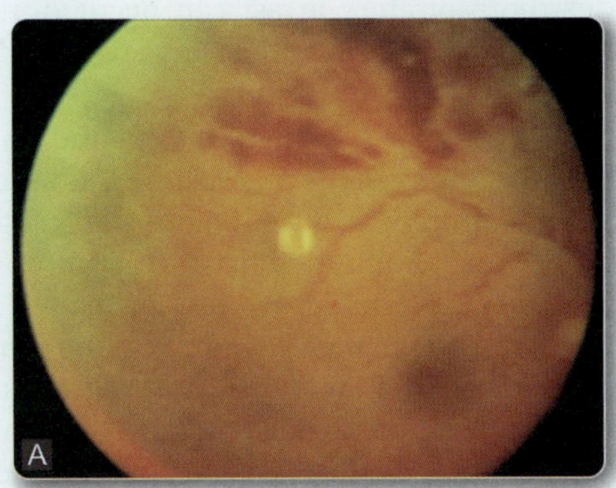

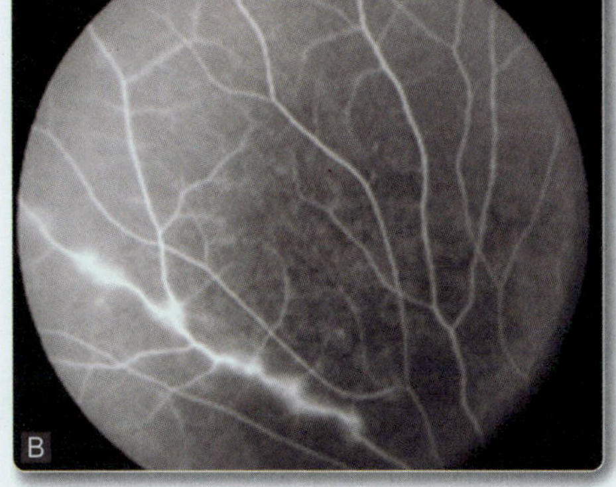

FIGURES 48.1A and B: Retinal periphlebitis. **A.** Clinical photograph; **B.** Fundus fluorescein angiogram of the same eye.

7. Dermatological changes like erythema nodosum and lupus pernio (indurated purple-blue lesions) can affect the skin of the lids.
8. The VII nerve palsy can occur as part of the central nervous system (CNS) involvement.

Diagnostic Tests

1. Chest X-ray is the most useful diagnostic test. The characteristic change is hilar lymphadenopathy.
2. Angiotensin-converting enzyme (ACE): Elevated ACE levels are seen in sarcoidosis, but it is not specific for sarcoidosis.
3. Hypercalcemia is found in 5%–18% of patients with sarcoidosis.
4. Gallium scans of head, neck and thorax. Increased gallium uptake is seen in lungs, lacrimal and parotid glands.
5. Kveim test is an intradermal test using a suspension of spleen tissue obtained from a confirmed case of sarcoidosis. After 6–8 weeks, biopsy from the injection site will show a sarcoid granuloma.
6. Biopsy: Diagnosis can be confirmed by a biopsy from a skin nodule, or hilar or any affected lymph node.

Treatment

Systemic Steroids

For ocular lesions, topical as well as subtenon injection of steroids is given.

MULTIPLE SCLEROSIS

Multiple sclerosis is a demyelinating disease affecting the white matter in the CNS. The neurological manifestations will vary depending on the site of lesions in the CNS.

Clinical Features

Demyelination of the optic nerve fibers can lead to optic neuritis or retrobulbar neuritis with sudden loss of vision. One or both eyes can be involved simultaneously or one after the other. Retrobulbar neuritis is more common than optic neuritis.

The vision may improve spontaneously or on administration of systemic steroids, but it can recur and can lead to permanent partial or complete blindness.

Internuclear ophthalmoplegia, nystagmus and oculomotor palsies are rare manifestations.

Diagnosis

Diagnosis is done by magnetic resonance imaging (MRI) scan. Acute demyelinating plaques can be demonstrated in the periventricular area or corpus callosum.

Treatment

Intravenous (IV) methylprednisolone for 3–5 days followed by tapering dose of oral steroids.

MYASTHENIA GRAVIS

Myasthenia gravis is an autoimmune disorder in which antibodies produced block the acetylcholine receptors (AChR) at the postsynaptic neuromuscular junction of the striated muscles. The smooth muscles are unaffected. The disease is characterized by fluctuating muscle weakness and fatigability on repeated use of a muscle (Fig. 48.2).

Classification of myasthenia gravis by the Myasthenia Gravis Foundation of America:

1. *Class I:* Any eye muscle weakness, possibly ptosis, no other evidence of muscle weakness.

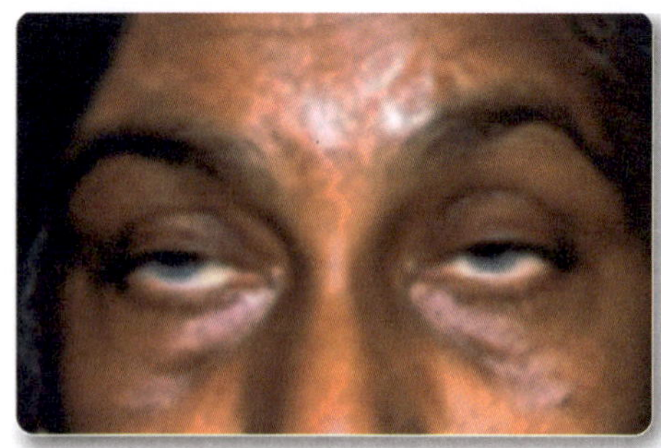

FIGURE 48.2: Myasthenia gravis—with ptosis and defective elevation of the eyes

2. *Class II:* Eye muscle weakness of any severity + mild weakness of other muscles.
3. Class III: Eye muscle weakness of any severity + moderate weakness of any other muscles.
4. Class IV: Eye muscle weakness of any severity + severe weakness of other muscles.
5. *Class V:* Intubation needed to maintain airway.

Clinical Features

The muscles become progressively weaker on usage of that muscle and recovers to some extent after a period of rest. Eyelids and ocular muscles are particularly affected. This can lead to ptosis (often asymmetrical and worse toward the end of the day) and eye muscle weakness leading to diplopia. The diplopia is also intermittent and often manifest or worse towards the evening.

Myasthenia may be associated with other autoimmune diseases like:

1. Thyroid disease (Graves' disease or Hashimoto's thyroiditis).
2. Diabetes mellitus.
3. Rheumatoid arthritis.
4. Demyelinating CNS diseases.

Pathophysiology

Autoantibodies against AChR are produced by plasma cells. Myasthenia is closely associated with thymoma.

Diagnosis

Diagnosis can be confirmed by the following test.

Edrophonium Test

Edrophonium or Tensilon is an anticholinesterase drug, which increases the concentration of acetylcholine at myoneural junction and thus increases muscle activity.

Since cardiorespiratory arrest can occur during this test, all resuscitation measures should be ready, while doing this test.

The ptosis and muscle strength may be measured before the test. To counteract the muscarinic actions of edrophonium, 3 mg atropine is given before starting the test. At first, 2 mg of edrophonium is given. If an improvement in the muscle action is noted, the test is stopped here. If no improvement is seen after giving 2 mg, the remaining 8 mg is given after 1 minute. Ptosis and muscle strength are measured. If there is a decrease in ptosis and improvement in muscle strength, the test is positive and a diagnosis of myasthenia is confirmed.

Treatment

Medical: Anticholinesterase drugs like neostigmine; immunosuppressants like steroids.

Surgery: Thymectomy—in patients with thymoma or thymus hyperplasia.

Prognosis: Myasthenia gravis is not usually a progressive disease and with treatment the patients can lead a fairly normal life.

MYOTONIC DYSTROPHY

Myotonic dystrophy is a dominantly inherited condition, which manifests between third and sixth decades. It is characterized by delayed muscle relaxation after a muscle action comes to an end. It starts with difficulty in walking and weakness of hands. There will be difficulty in releasing a grip. This is followed by muscle wasting, facial wasting due to muscle wasting and slurring of speech due to involvement of the tongue.

The characteristic ophthalmic manifestation is the appearance of polychromatic iridescent crystals in the lens cortex, which progress to posterior subcapsular (PSC) cataract and finally complete cortical opacification. These crystals are composed of whorls of plasmalemma from the lens fibers. Rare features are ptosis and external ophthalmoplegia.

PHAKOMATOSES

Phakomatoses include a group of hereditary diseases characterized by tumorous growths in different organs.

These include:

1. Tuberous sclerosis (Bourneville disease).
2. Neurofibromatosis (von Recklinghausen's disease)—autosomal dominant.
3. Angiomatosis retinae (von Hippel-Lindau syndrome).

Other conditions included later:

1. Ataxia-telangiectasia (Louis-Bar syndrome)—autosomal recessive.
2. Sturge-Weber syndrome—no definite hereditary influence.
3. Wyburn-Mason syndrome.

Tuberous Sclerosis

Bourneville first described this disease and hence the name Bourneville syndrome. One third is familial cases whereas two thirds are sporadic. Genetic studies have shown that parents of many of the sporadic cases are gene carriers of the disease.

Ophthalmologic Features

The classic feature is **retinal hamartomas**. The lesions can be single or multiple, small or large and usually appear at the posterior pole. The smaller lesions are flat, gray white translucent non-calcified masses near the optic disk. The larger lesions are calcified elevated mulberry-like opaque white lesions two or more disk diameters in size and appear on or close to the optic disk. These lesions are astrocytic hamartomas.

Central Nervous System Involvement

Similar hamartomas develop in CNS, in the basal ganglion, brainstem or cerebellum and can be detected radiographically (calcified lesions) or by computed tomography (CT) scan. They give rise to seizures and mental retardation.

Cutaneous Involvement

The skin lesions are **adenoma sebaceum**—a brown papular rash seen on the face and chin. The name is a misnomer since the lesions are angiofibromatous and usually appear by 2 years of age. Hypopigmented macules called **ash-leaf spots** are seen in 50% of affected persons. They have a characteristic shape; rounded at one end and tapered at the other, and hence the name. They are best detected by ultraviolet (UV) light.

Visceral Involvement

Hamartomas can develop in various organs, especially kidney and heart, and lead to renal failure or cardiac failure and early death.

Neurofibromatosis

Neurofibromatosis (NF) is the most common phakomatosis. It is an autosomally dominant inherited disorder resulting in hamartomas affecting the skin, eyes and CNS. It is classified as two types:

1. Neurofibromatosis type 1 (NF-1), which is the peripheral variant.
2. Neurofibromatosis type 2 (NF-2) is the central variant.

Neurofibromatosis Type 1 (von Recklinghausen's Disease)

The characteristic features of NF-1 are given below.

Cutaneous lesions: It includes:

1. *Café au lait spots:* These are hyperpigmented macules, is a diagnostic characteristic. Six or more café au lait spots larger than 1.5 m in diameter are generally considered diagnostic of NF-1. They appear in the 1st year of life and increases in number and size throughout the growth period of childhood.
2. *Axillary freckles:* They appear around 10 years of age.

Fibroma mollusca: They are fleshy pedunculated soft nodules seen all over the body. They appear around puberty and increase in number throughout life (Fig. 48.3).

Plexiform neurofibromas: They are soft fleshy 'bag of worm' swellings with pigmentation. They may appear in early childhood and can occur anywhere on the body. They consist of markedly enlarged peripheral nerves with thickened perineural sheath and hypertrophy of the surrounding subcutaneous tissues (Figs 48.4A and B).

Involvement: Intracranial and spinal cord gliomas and meningiomas can occur with various neurological deficits and paralysis. They are less common in NF-1 than NF-2, but can occur in both types. Optic nerve gliomas are common in NF-1.

Skeletal involvement: Progressive kyphoscoliosis can occur. Defects in the bony walls of the orbit can occur leading to spheno-orbital encephalocele.

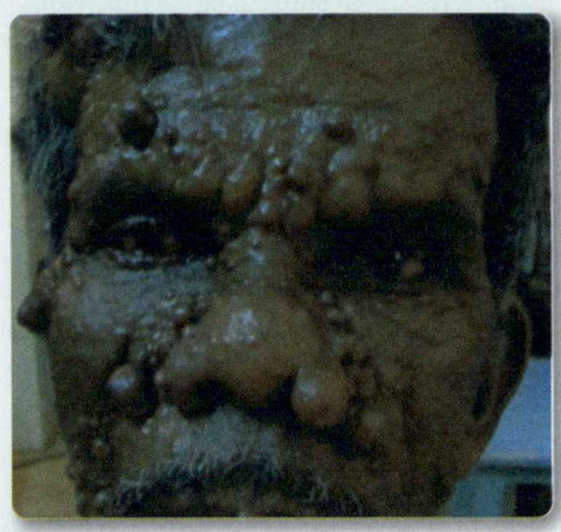

FIGURE 48.3: Fibroma molluscum in neurofibromatosis

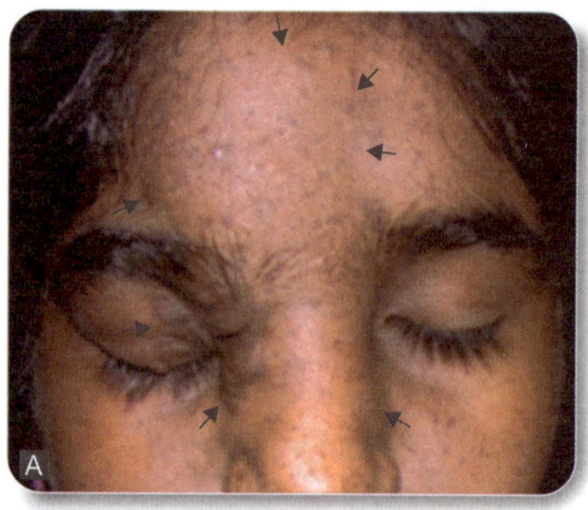

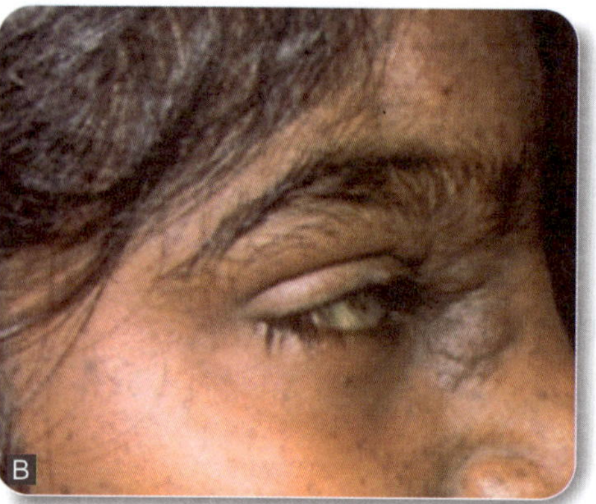

FIGURES 48.4A and B: Plexiform neurofibromatosis. **A.** Frontal view; **B.** Lateral view.

Visceral: Neurofibromatous hamartomas in gastrointestinal tract (GIT) can occur leading to intestinal obstruction. Pheochromocytomas are 10 times more frequent in patients with NF than general population.

Neurofibromatosis Type 2

Neurofibromatosis type 2 is characterized by multiple schwannomas and meningiomas. Common involvement is the VIII nerve. About 90% of patients show bilateral acoustic schwannomas. Other cranial nerves and spinal cord may show meningiomas.

Eye involvement is usually due to involvement of the ocular motor nerves, VII or V nerve by the tumors. These patients may also develop a posterior subcapsular cataract at a young age.

Ophthalmic Involvement

1. Plexiform neurofibromas can involve the eyelids and face leading to swellings of the lids and surrounding tissue with ptosis, amblyopia and disfigurement. Surgery is often unsuccessful because they tend to recur.
2. Lisch nodules are seen in 95% of patients. They are smooth light brown nodules on the iris and appear in early childhood. They are hamartomatous lesions (Fig. 48.5).
3. Prominent corneal nerves are seen.
4. Conjunctival hamartomas can occur.
5. Optic nerve gliomas can occur leading to proptosis.
6. Neurofibromas in the orbit can lead to meningoencephalocele and pulsating exophthalmos.

Angiomatosis Retinae

Angiomatosis retinae is a rare disorder with autosomal dominant inheritance characterized by retinal and CNS vascular hamartomas. They also tend to develop renal cell carcinoma and pheochromocytoma. These hamartomas are mesodermal in origin unlike NF or tuberous sclerosis, which are ectodermal in origin.

If the patient has only retinal lesions it is called von Hippel disease and to be called von Hippel-Lindau syndrome, both retinal and CNS lesions should be present.

Ophthalmic Features

The typical ocular lesion is a globular red retinal mass with prominent afferent and efferent retinal vessels. These lesions are capillary hemangioblastomas and can give use to massive subretinal and intraretinal exudation. Macular exudation can lead to considerable drop in vision. Intraocular bleeding can also occur and can lead to proliferative vitreoretinopathy and tractional retinal detachment. Unless treated at an early stage these hemangioblastomas can end in blindness.

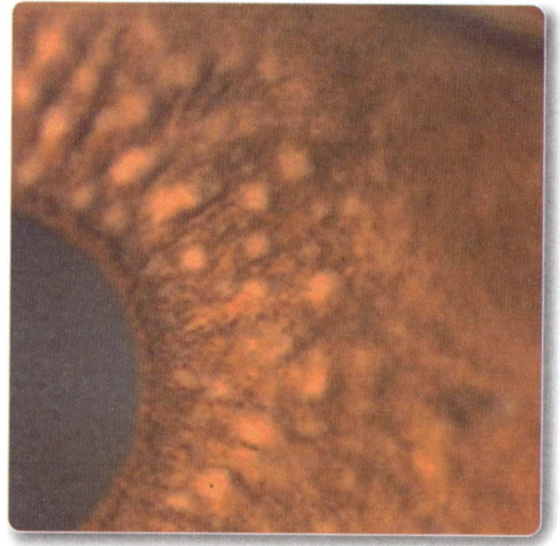

FIGURE 48.5: Lisch nodules on the iris

Lesions in CNS

The characteristic manifestation is a cerebellar hemangioblastoma, which can be solid or cystic. They can lead to cerebellar dysfunction ataxia, slurred speech, cerebellar signs and nystagmus.

Management

Occlusion of the feeder vessels by argon laser is successful in treating small- and medium-sized tumors. The lesions can also be treated directly with laser after occlusion of the feeder vessels. In large tumors with large arterioles supplying them, occlusion of the arterioles with laser is often impossible or the effect will be temporary.

Cryotherapy

Cryotherapy or irradiation may be successful in larger lesions.

Visual Prognosis

Visual prognosis is poor in eye with large untreated angiomas. Cerebellar hemangioblastomas or renal cell carcinomas may shorten the life expectancy also.

Sturge-Weber Syndrome

Sturge-Weber syndrome is a dermato-oculo-neural syndrome. Incomplete forms are more common than the complete form (Fig. 48.6).

Cutaneous Involvement

The facial hemangioma often called nevus flammeus is seen in the area of distribution of the first and second divisions of the trigeminal nerve. It consists of cutaneous telangiectatic capillaries. It is present at birth, but the depth of color and nodularity increase with age. Often there is a facial hemihypertrophy also.

Involvement of CNS

A leptomeningeal hemangioma can occur on the same side as the facial hemangioma. Progressive calcification can occur in a pattern of double contour lines mostly in the occipital and temporal lobes leading to the sign called the 'railroad track' sign. These lesions can lead to seizures and mental retardation and various neurological defects can rarely occur.

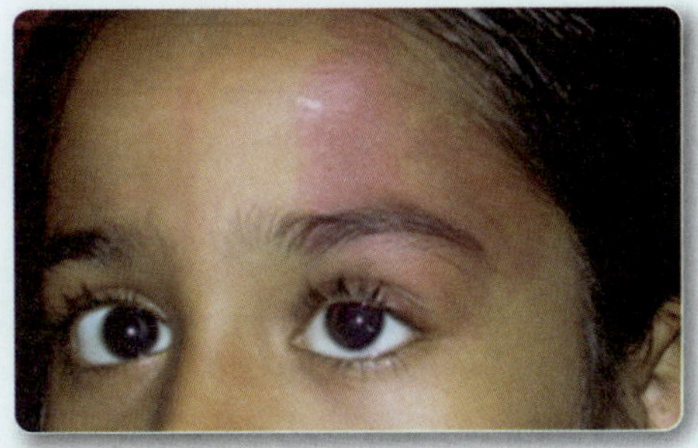

FIGURE 48.6: Sturge-Weber syndrome

Ophthalmic Involvement

A diffuse choroidal hemangioma on the same side as the facial hemangioma. It is usually diffuse, flat and generally involves more than half of the choroid. It enlarges slowly and can lead to serous retinal detachment, field defects and cystoid degeneration of the macula.

Developmental glaucoma can develop early in life. Cause of this glaucoma is angle abnormalities or elevated episcleral venous pressure. This glaucoma is resistant to medical management and often requires surgery. All patients with nevus flammeus has to be evaluated for the presence of glaucoma.

Ataxia-telangiectasia

Ataxia-telangiectasia is a rare disorder with autosomal recessive inheritance. It is characterized with progressive cerebellar ataxia and telangiectasia, which involve the conjunctiva, malar area, ears, palate and neck. These telangiectasias appear within 3–7 years of age and with increasing age, extend to the neck and hands. Cerebellar ataxia appears before telangiectasia and progresses with age.

Wyburn-Mason Syndrome

Wyburn-Mason syndrome is a condition characterized by arteriovenous communications of the retina as well as brain.

Ophthalmic Involvement

The retinal arteriovenous communication appears as a large mass of dilated vessels that resemble a tumor. Visual loss can occur due to retinal and vitreous hemorrhage. Rubeosis iridis and neovascular glaucoma have also been reported. Rarely spontaneous thrombosis of the arteriovenous communication with regression can also occur.

Involvement of CNS

The intracranial arteriovenous anastomosis can lead to subarachnoid hemorrhage and death.

Treatment

Occlusion of the feeder vessels may be successful in smaller lesions. In larger lesions it may fail or can lead to massive intraocular hemorrhage due to rupture of the vessel.

ROSACEA

Rosacea is a chronic condition affecting the central face—cheeks, nose forehead and chin; typically seen in Europeans. The involved areas are erythematous, thickened and show telangiectatic vessels and red papules. There will be some burning and irritation of the affected areas. The triggering factors are exposure to sunlight, emotional stress, some spicy foods, certain cosmetics and alcohol consumption, etc.

Ocular rosacea is one of the four subtypes. These patients have dry gritty eyes and eyelids with itching, burning and stinging sensations. The eyes will be congested and are easily susceptible to infections.

Diagnosis: It is by clinical features of the facial lesions.

Treatment: There is no clinical cure for this condition:

1. Avoid the triggering factors like sunlight, spicy foods, emotional stress, etc. Oral antibiotics like doxycycline may help in some cases.
2. Warm compresses and artificial tears will give some relief to the eye problems.

SECTION 11

Community Ophthalmology

National Program for Control of Blindness and its Activities

49

Girija Devi PS, Rajeevan P, Simon George

National Program for Control of Blindness (NPCB) was launched in India in 1976 as a 100% centrally sponsored scheme with the goal to reduce the prevalence of blindness from 1.4% to 0.3%.

OBJECTIVES OF NPCB

Objectives of NPCB include:

1. To reduce the backlog of blindness through identification and treatment of blind.
2. To develop eye care facilities in every district.
3. To develop human resources for providing eye care services.
4. To improve quality of service delivery.
5. To secure participation of voluntary organizations in eye care.

ACTIVITIES OF NPCB

There is a decentralized implementation of the program via the District Health Societies and District Blindness Control Society (DBCS). The main activities undertaken include:

1. Reduction in the backlog of blind persons by active screening of population above 50 years, organizing screening eye camps and transporting operable cases to eye care facilities.
2. Free cataract surgery.
3. School eye screening program.
4. Training of ophthalmic surgeons.
5. Involvement and support to voluntary organizations.

The core diseases tackled via NPCB include:

- Cataract
- Focal trachoma
- Refractive errors
- Low vision.

The issues that are being addressed with renewed emphasis under the present 11th Five Year (2007–2012) plan period via the NPCB include:

1. Diabetic retinopathy.
2. Glaucoma.
3. Childhood blindness like congenital cataract, squint, amblyopia and strabismus.

The implementation of the NPCB was decentralized in 1994–1995 with formation of the State and District Health Societies.

State Health Society

Members

1. Chairman: State Mission Director/Secretary.
2. Vice Chairman: Director Health Services.
3. Member Secretary: Joint/Deputy Director (from the state cadre).

Functions

1. To coordinate and monitor the activities of all the District Health Societies.
2. To conduct regular review meeting with districts in coordination with center.
3. To procure equipments and drugs required using Government of India Funds.
4. To receive and monitor use of funds, equipments and material from the government and other agencies.
5. To involve voluntary organization and private practitioners providing free/subsidized eye care services in district and identity non-government organizations (NGOs) facilities that can be considered for non-recurring grants under NPCB.
6. To promote eye donation through various media, and monitor the districts for collection and utilization of

eyes collected by eye donation centers and eye banks and directly identify NGOs facilities that can be considered for grants under NPCB.

District Health Society

Members

Maximum of 15 members, consisting not more than eight ex-officio members and seven other members, as detailed below:

1. Chairman: District Collector/District Mission Director.
2. Vice-Chairman: Chief Medical and Health Officer/ District Health Officer.
3. Member Secretary: Officer of the level of Deputy Chief Medical Officer (CMO) preferably an ophthalmologist may be designated as District Program Manager who would also be the Member Secretary of the Society.
4. Technical Advisor: Chief Ophthalmic Surgeon of District Hospital. In districts where medical colleges are located, Head of the Department of Ophthalmology may be designated as Technical Advisor to the Society.
5. Other members: Medical Superintendent/Civil Surgeon of District Hospital/District Education Officer/ Indian Medical Association (IMA), District chapter of All India Ophthalmological Society (AIOS)/representatives from NGOs engaged in eye care services District Mass media/Information, Education and Communication (IEC) officer/prominent practicing eye surgeons.

Note: There should be at least one woman and one SC/ST member in the District Health Society.

The membership of non-officials should be of 1 year only and renewable as per the general body decisions for further period. The ex-officio members shall be members as long as they hold the office by virtue of which they are members. The term of other members shall be for the period notified by the Chairman of the society.

The primary purpose of the District Health Society is to plan, implement and monitor blindness control activities in the district as per pattern of assistance approved for the NPCB.

Important Functions

Important functions of the District Health Society are:

1. To assess the magnitude and spread of blindness in the district by means of active case finding village wise, to be recorded and maintained in blind registers.
2. To organize screening camps for identifying those requiring cataract surgery and other blinding disorders, organize transportation and conduct of free medical or surgical services including cataract surgery for the poor in government facilities or NGOs supporting the program.
3. To plan and organize training of community level workers, teachers and ophthalmic assistants/nurses involved in eye care services.
4. To procure drugs and consumable including micro-surgical instruments required in the government facilities.
5. To receive and monitor use of funds, equipments and materials from the government and other agencies/ donors.
6. To involve voluntary and private hospitals providing free/subsidized eye care services in the district and identify NGOs facilities that can be considered for non-recurring grants under the program.
7. To organize screening of school children for detection of refractive errors and other eye problems, and provide free glasses to poor children.
8. To promote eye donation through various media and monitor collection, and utilization of eyes collected by eye donation centers and eye banks.

Eye Camps

Eye camps are conducted to reach out to needy patients and help restore their vision. They help to detect causes of blindness like cataract, glaucoma and refractive errors. Health education of the community is also possible during these camps.

Conduct of an Eye Camp

1. The camp should be conducted in an area, which:
   a. Is accessible to the people.
   b. Has adequate population for check-up.
   A large school building or community hall is the usual convenient venue for conducting a camp. Two rooms with electricity connection and length at least 7 meters are needed for the camp.
2. The camp coordinator should coordinate with the local social service provider/sponsor to decide a convenient date and time for the camp:
   a. The date should be fixed at least a month in advance to give sufficient time for planning.
   b. There should be no important activity in that area at the time of the camp that would affect the patient turnout in the camp.

3. Proper planning is essential for the success of a camp:
   a. Visual, audio and paper publicity measures help in improving the turnout.
   b. Adequate furniture for seating is required.
   c. Volunteers have a big role in venue arrangements and in assisting the medical team.
   d. The accounts have to be properly kept by the organizer.
   e. Transportation facilities may be provided.

ROLE OF NGOs IN NPCB

The 11th Five Year (2007–2012) Plan has devised schemes for voluntary organizations to help develop eye care infrastructure and to provide appropriate eye care services to reduce the prevalence of blindness. For availing these schemes, a voluntary organization/NGO should meet the following requirements:

1. Should be registered under the Indian Societies Registration Act, 1860) or a charitable public trust registered under any law for the time being in force.
2. Track record of having experience in providing health services preferably eye care services over a minimum period of 3 years.
3. Properly constituted managing body with its powers, duties, and responsibilities clearly defined and laid down.
4. Services open to all without distinction of caste, religion or language.
5. Having available well-trained staff, infrastructure and the required managerial expertize to organize and carry out various activities under the scheme.
6. Agreeing to abide by the guidelines and norms of the program.

The following grants are available to NGOs:

1. Non-recurring grant-in-aid (up to maximum ₹30.00 lakh) given via the District Health Societies (NPCB) for strengthening/expansion of Eye Care Units in rural/tribal areas.
2. Non-recurring grant-in-aid for eye banks (up to maximum ₹15.00 lakh).
3. Non-recurring grant-in-aid for Eye Donation Centers (EDCs) (up to maximum ₹1.00 lakh).
4. Non-recurring grant-in-aid of ₹50,000 for setting up or strengthening vision centers.
5. Financial assistance (recurring) will be provided for the following:
   a. Up to a maximum of ₹750 (rupees seven hundred and fifty only) for each free cataract operation.
   b. ₹1,000 (rupees one thousand only) per case for management of diseases like diabetic retinopathy, glaucoma (surgery and laser intervention), squint, retinopathy of prematurity and low vision aids.
   c. ₹1,500 per pair of eyes collected to eye banks toward honorarium for staff and for purchasing consumables like preservation media, etc.
   d. ₹1,000 per pair of eyes to eye donation centers.

Non-government organizations are playing a crucial role in India in providing eye care facilities in remote areas by organizing eye camps. They also provide quality eye care including eye surgeries especially cataract surgery by involving the private institutions also, by availing the financial assistance given under the NPCB.

Vision 2020

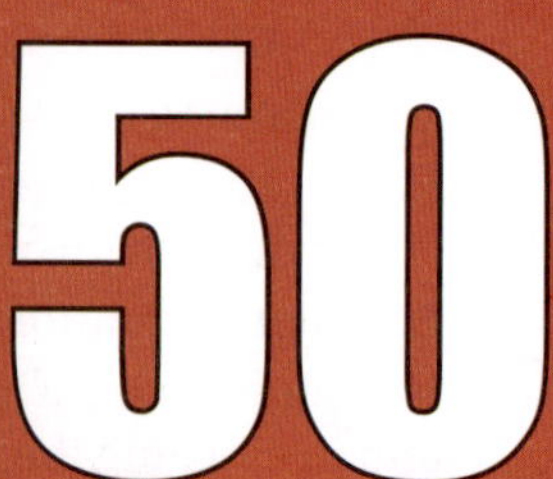

Girija Devi PS, Simon George

Vision 2020 is the global initiative for the elimination of avoidable blindness, launched in 1999, jointly by the World Health Organization (WHO) and the International Agency for the Prevention of Blindness (IAPB) with an international membership of non-government organization (NGO), professional associations, eye care institutions and corporations.

VISION 2020

Principles

Basic principle of vision 2020 is based on the right to sight for each human being. The goal is to eliminate avoidable blindness by year 2020 (Fig. 50.1).

Components

Components of vision 2020 are illustrated in Figure 50.2.

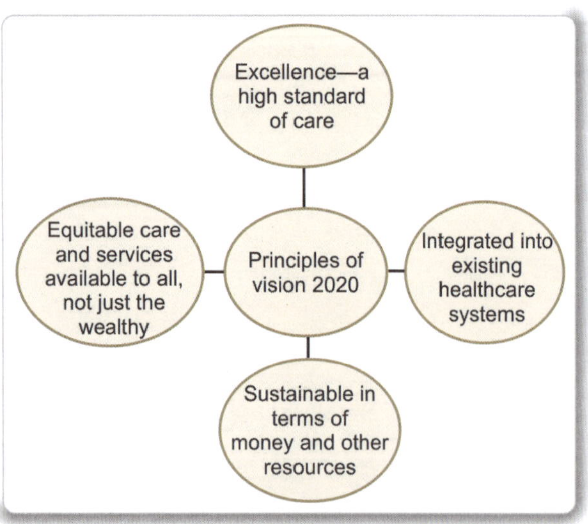

FIGURE 50.1: Principles of vision 2020

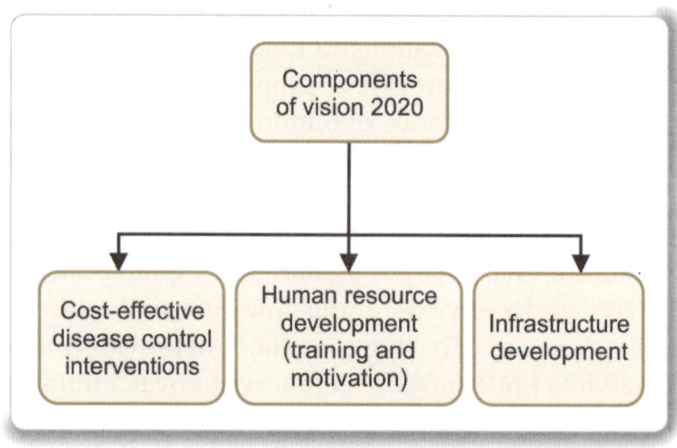

FIGURE 50.2: Components of vision 2020

Vision 2020—International Efforts

Globally, five conditions have been identified for immediate attention (Fig. 50.3).

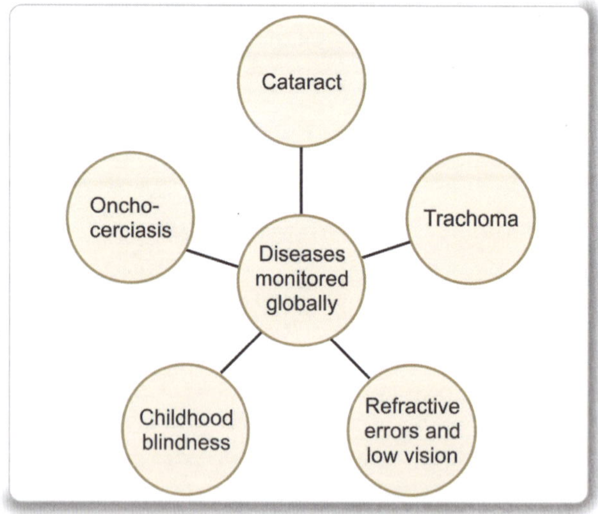

FIGURE 50.3: Five diseases given top priority

Vision 2020 in India

India was the 1st country in the world to launch the National Program for Control of Blindness (NPCB) in 1976. A decentralized approach is adopted with District Blindness Control Societies (DBCs) being set up for identifying blind persons and providing treatment facilities.

The target diseases identified for Vision 2020 in India include:

- Cataract
- Childhood blindness
- Refractive error and low vision
- Corneal blindness
- Diabetic retinopathy
- Glaucoma
- Trachoma (focal) can be controlled by the implementation of SAFE strategy:
  - S: Surgery for entropion and trichiasis
  - A: Antibiotic treatment (tetracycline eye ointment twice daily × 6 week in adults)
  - F: Facial cleanliness
  - E: Environmental improvement (personal hygiene and community sanitation).

Causes of Blindness 51

Girija Devi PS, Rajeevan P

According to the 10th revision of the World Health Organization's (WHO's) International Statistical Classification of Diseases, Injuries and Causes of Death, blindness is defined as best corrected visual acuity of less than 3/60 or corresponding visual field defect less than 10°, in the better eye.

In North America and most of Europe, legal blindness is defined as best corrected visual acuity (vision) of 20/200 (6/60) or less in the better eye. About 65% of people with visual impairment (partially blind) are above the age of 50 years, whereas 82% of the totally blind are above 50 years. So, the majority of people who are visually disabled are elderly.

According to the 2010 WHO report, roughly 284 million people are visually impaired of which 39 million are blind worldwide. The most common causes of blindness around the world are shown in Figure 50.1.

The top three causes of blindness in the 2010 estimate were—cataract, glaucoma and age-related macular degeneration.

However, there is a difference in the causes of blindness in developed and developing countries. Cataract (47.9%) remains the leading cause of visual impairment in all areas of the world except for developed countries.

In the third world countries (85% of the world's blindness is seen here), the principal causes include cataract, infections (like trachoma, onchocerciasis and leprosy), glaucoma and ocular injury. In developed nations, the leading causes of blindness include ocular complications of diabetes, macular degeneration and traumatic causes.

Other causes of blindness in the world include vitamin A deficiency, retinopathy of prematurity, blood vessel diseases involving the retina or optic nerve including ocular inflammatory diseases, retinitis pigmentosa, primary or secondary malignancies of the eye, congenital abnormalities, hereditary diseases of the eye and chemical poisoning from toxic agents such as methanol.

BLINDNESS IN INDIA

Blindness is a major public health problem in India. India is the first country in the world to launch a 100% government-funded program for control and prevention of blindness—National Program for Control of Blindness (NPCB).

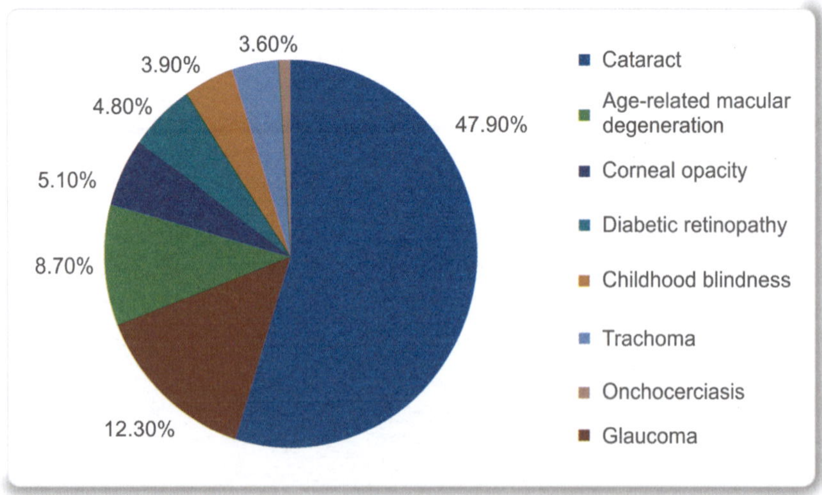

FIGURE 51.1: Common causes of blindness

TABLE 51.1: Levels of prevention of blindness

Level of prevention	Methods
Primary	Government-funded National Program for Prevention of Blindness in each country
	Blindness control programs with both private/non-government organization involvement
	Avoid injuries to eye by using protective goggles during work
	Health education, school eye health programs
	Good nutrition to avoid vitamin A deficiency; breastfeeding of infants
	Regular exercise, good blood sugar control and weight reduction to reduce chances of developing diabetes retinopathy
Secondary	Early identification and treatment of glaucoma
	Yearly fundus examination of diabetic patients
	Medical and surgical treatment of diabetic retinopathy
	Surgical treatment of cataract
	Vitamin A supplementation in vitamin A deficient patients
	Prompt and complete treatment of eye infections, which can cause blindness
	Proper treatment of eye injuries
Tertiary	Rehabilitation of the blind using visual aids, text-reading software and Braille books

The prevalence of blindness in India is 1%. The target of Vision 2020 program is to bring it down to 0.3% by the year 2020. Cataract is the major cause for blindness and it contributes to 55% of the total blindness.

PREVENTION OF BLINDNESS

Above 80%–90% of the blindness is preventable through a combination of education and access to good medical care. The WHO coordinates the international efforts to reduce visual impairments by:

- Developing policies/strategies/guidelines for management of diabetic retinopathy, glaucoma, age-related macular degeneration, etc. to prevent blindness
- Providing technical assistance to member states and partners
- Monitoring and evaluating programs to strengthen health systems
- Coordinating international partnerships.

The International Agency for the Prevention of Blindness was formed in 1975 with the encouragement of the World Health Organization to achieve the global initiative 'Vision 2020: The Right to Sight.'

In 2009, the World Health Assembly approved the 2009–2013 action plans, for the prevention of avoidable blindness and visual impairment, a roadmap for member states, WHO Secretariat and International partners.

These preventive measures have helped in the control of blindness in the world.

BLINDNESS IN INDIA—THE CHANGING SCENARIO

Even though India is one of the developing countries, with the effective implementation of many national programs, many common causes for blindness seen in developing countries is on decline in India. At the same time, there is an increase in the prevalence of many conditions common in developed countries.

With vitamin A supplementation program for mothers and preschool children, blindness due to vitamin A deficiency has come down. Trachoma control program was started in India in 1963 and it was included in the NPCB, which started in 1976. The effective implementation of this program has decreased the level of blindness due to trachoma also. Blindness (Table 51.1) due to cataract was above 80% two decades back and now it has come down to around 55%.

At the same time, with the increase in life expectancy and increase in the incidence of diabetes, blindness due to diabetic retinopathy is on the increase. Similarly, age-related macular degeneration, which was common only in Western countries, is also increasing in India. With improvements in facilities for babies born prematurely are encouraged, more preterm babies are surviving and hence there is an increase in visual impairment due to retinopathy of prematurity (ROP). Vision 2020 program is targeting these conditions also.

Low Vision Aids

52

Girija Devi PS, Rajeevan P, Sheeba CS

DEFINITION

Definition of low vision: It was previously defined as vision less than 6/60 in the better eye or field less than 20° in the better eye.

Current definition: Low vision is the level of visual function that prevents a person from performing customary visual activities with standard or conventional spectacle correction.

A person with low vision is one who, because of the irreversible disorder of the visual system, cannot perform customary visual tasks without special vision enhancing devices.

For patients with end-stage macular diseases in the past were told as 'nothing more can be done'. Now the approach to visual rehabilitation is, "since nothing more can be done either medically or surgically, you have another option, which is to be evaluated for visual aids."

Low vision aids (LVAs) are optical devices [i.e. convex lenses, telescopes and electronic devices such as closed-circuit television (CCTV), reading machines or large print computers] that enhance visual performance by magnification of the image.

Low vision devices are non-optical devices that complement low vision in simplifying visual tasks and these include lighting, large print, reading stands and electronic reader scans with voice output. The factors that determine acceptance of a LVA are skill and experience of examiner, personality and outlook on life of patient, and type of adjustment the patient has made to visual impairment. The categories of visual impairment and level of visual acuity are give in Table 52.1.

CAUSES OF LOW VISION

In general, irreversible damage to ocular media or visual pathway due to any disease entity may result in low vision.

TABLE 52.1: Visual impairment

Category of visual impairment	Level of visual acuity
Low vision	
1	Less than 6 /18–6/60
2	Less than 6/60–3/60
Blindness	
3	Less than 3/60–1/60
	Visual field between 5° and 10°
4	Less than 1/60 to light perception or visual field less than 5°
5	No light perception

Common Conditions Causing Low Vision

In Children

Albinism, optic neuropathy, trauma and congenital malformations.

In Young Adults

Late-onset congenital malformations, ocular injuries, retinitis pigmentosa (RP).

In Old Age

- Age-related macular degenerations, diabetic retinopathy, glaucoma
- Patients with different macular diseases are among the most responsive to LVAs.

LOW VISION DEVICES

A LVA refers to an optical device, which improves or enhances residual vision by magnifying the image of the object at the retinal level.

Here are some optical and non-optical aids, which may help in enhancing the visual performance.

Optical Low Vision Aids

Optical low vision aids are based on the fact that with sufficient magnification, the normal retina surrounding the damaged central retina can be used for central vision. The measure of visual acuity varies with extent of involvement of central retina. The visual acuity is maximum at the fovea where there are maximum numbers of cones and decreases rapidly toward the periphery.

Types of optical LVAs:

1. Magnifying spectacles.
2. Hand magnifiers.
3. Stand magnifiers.
4. Telescopes.
5. Closed-circuit television.

Basic features of optical LVAs:

1. Power in diopter is variable.
2. Focus may be fixed or variable.
3. Illumination—may be self-illuminated or not.
4. It may be monocular or binocular.
5. It may be unifocal, bifocal or trifocal.

Magnifying Spectacles

Magnifying spectacles are the most commonly prescribed LVAs and suitable for near and intermediate distance (Fig. 52.1):

1. Binocular spectacles prescribed usually vary in power from +4D to +12D.
2. Monocular spectacles consist of standard aspheric lenses from +4D to +20D.

Advantages: As follows:

1. Cosmetically acceptable.
2. Easy to use.
3. Both hands are free to hold the reading material.
4. Less expensive.

Disadvantage: Due to short focal length of high plus lenses, the patient has to hold the print close to the eye.

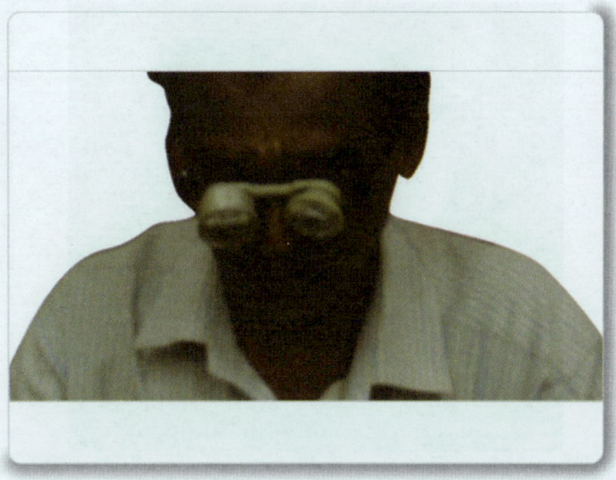

FIGURE 52.1: Magnifying spectacles

Handheld Magnifiers

Handheld magnifiers help patients with near vision problem and they can be used along with distance and reading spectacles (Fig. 52.2).

Indication: Used for spot or short-time task in patients with visual field reduced to 10°.

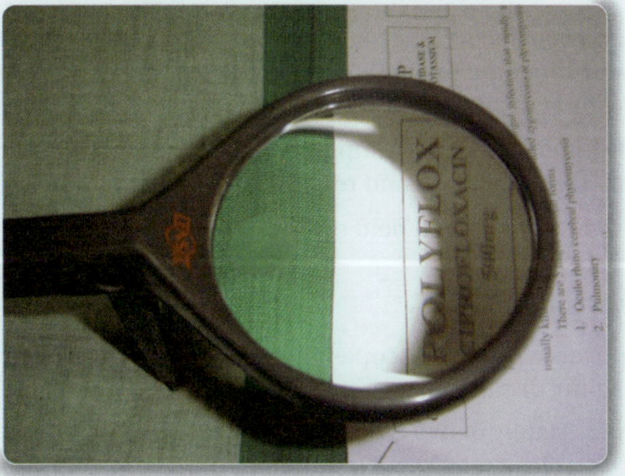

FIGURE 52.2: Handheld magnifiers

Type and design: These are available from +4D to + 40D.

Instructions for use: The patient should be shown how to put the magnifier flat on the reading surface to begin with and raise it until the image is clear.

Advantages: It has three advantages:

1. Easy to manipulate.
2. Accommodation is not required.
3. Working distance is more.

Disadvantages: These are as follows:

1. Not useful in the absence of manual dexterity.
2. Reduced field of vision.

Stand-mounted Magnifiers

Types and designs: Available in two forms—prefocused and focusable. These range in power from +4D to +60D (Fig. 52.3).

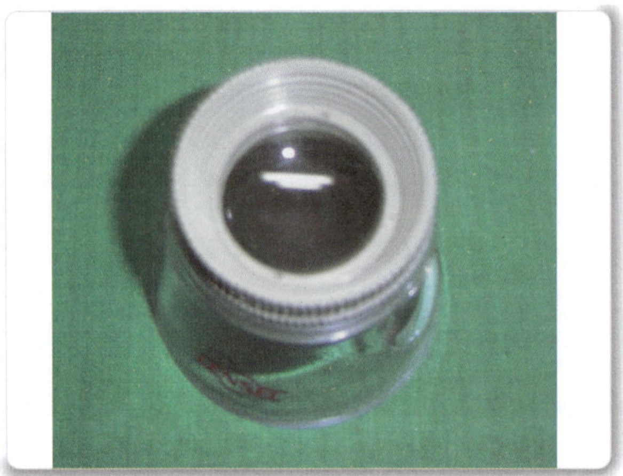

FIGURE 52.3: Stand-mounted magnifier

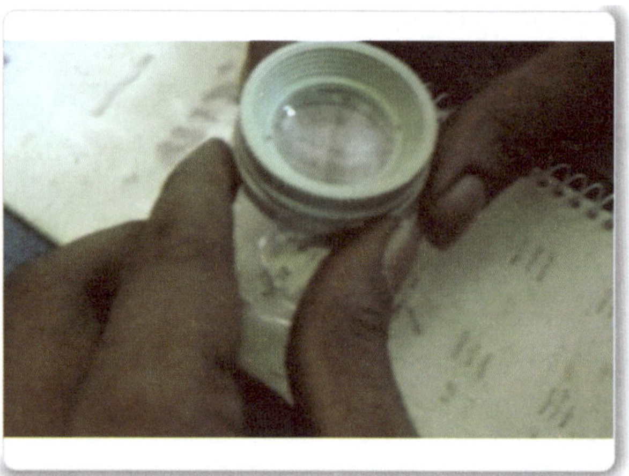

FIGURE 52.4: Using stand-mounted magnifier

Instructions for use: The patient should be taught to place the stand-mounted magnifier flat on the reading material and to look at the image through the reading glasses (Fig. 52.4).

Advantage: They are simple for a patient to use because they are prefocused and rest on a rigid mount.

Disadvantage: Small field of vision.

Telescopes

Optical system telescopes are the optical aids used to magnify distant objects.

Types: Mainly of two types:

1. Galilean telescope: It produces upright magnified virtual image.
2. Kepler telescope: It produces magnified inverted image.

Designs: Based on designs:

1. Uniocular/binocular.
2. Handheld/spectacle mounted.

The maximum useful power for handheld telescope is 8X and for spectacle type is 4X.

Indications: It is indicated in:

1. Sedentary distance viewing.
2. Handheld telescopes are suitable for distance spotting such as bus signs.

Limitations: Main limitations are:

1. Limitation of field of view.
2. Ring scotoma.
3. Decrease in depth of focus.

Closed-circuit Television

The camera picks up the reading material, magnifies it and displays on the TV screen. This provides electronic magnification up to 60X (Figs 52.5 and 52.6).

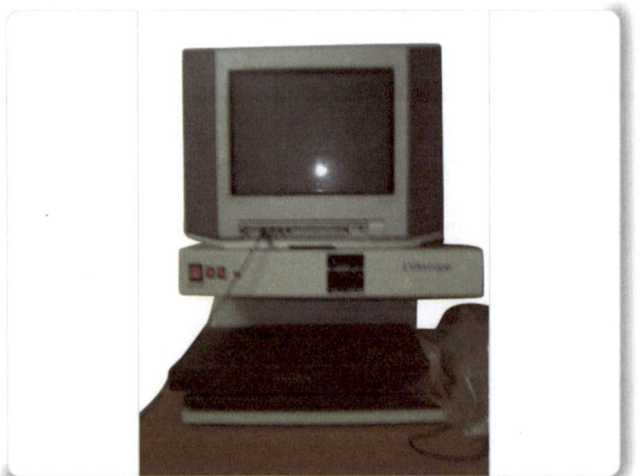

FIGURE 52.5: Closed-circuit television (CCTV)

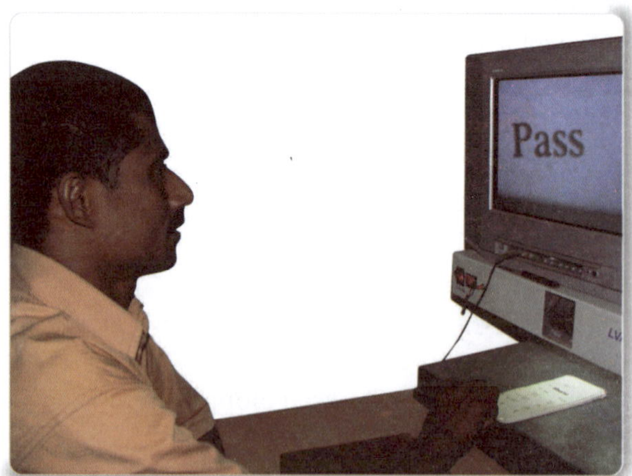

FIGURE 52.6: Reading using CCTV

Advantage: It provides a distortion free, brighter magnified image with enhanced contrast on a larger screen. White letters on black screen helps in improvement of image clarity.

Limitation: A CCTV is expensive.

Non-optical Devices

Non-optical devices are aids other than lenses that may supplement lenses:

1. Approach magnification: The partially sighted patients should be encouraged to move as close as possible to the screen, while watching TV.
2. Lighting: Maximum illumination should fall on the reading material.
3. Contrast enhancement: Reading is aided by use of a typoscope as a line guide.
4. Increasing size of the object to be viewed, e.g. large print books.
5. Personal items, e.g. bold, digital display thermometer.
6. Auditory aids such as talking clocks, computers with speech synthesizer.
7. Electronic devices like text reader, LVA scope.
8. Fiber-tipped pen with black ink provides best contrast, while writing.
9. White cane: It is a walking stick, which is white in color with red tip, used by blind people all over the world. The characteristic colors of the stick denotes that the person using it is blind. This helps others to give necessary assistance, for example, help the person to cross the road or at least get out of the way of a person walking with a white cane.

Uses of appropriate optical and non-optical devices help to improve the quality of life of visually challenged individuals and help them to lead a dignified life with less dependence on others for routine daily activities. Now low vision clinics are run in most of the major eye hospitals and visually impaired people should be encouraged to seek the help of these clinics.

SECTION 12

Multiple Choice Questions

Multiple Choice Questions

53

Girija Devi PS

1. The crystalline lens is embryologically derived from
   a. Neuroectoderm b. Surface ectoderm
   c. Paraxial mesoderm d. Endoderm
2. The Schwalbe's line is the termination of
   a. Bowman's membrane
   b. Endothelium
   c. Trabecular meshwork
   d. Descemet's membrane
3. Which part of the human lens contains Y sutures?
   a. Embryonic nucleus b. Fetal nucleus
   c. Posterior cortex d. Adult nucleus
4. Which of the following statement is wrong?
   a. Lacrimal nerve passes above the tendinous ring in SOF
   b. Trochlear nerve passes above the tendinous ring in SOF
   c. Inferior ophthalmic vein passes through the tendinous ring
   d. Abducens nerve passes through the tendinous ring
5. Which of the following is a wrong statement?
   a. IO arise from the floor of the orbit
   b. SO tendon passes through the trochlea
   c. Orbital axes meet at 900 to each other
   d. Infraorbital foramen has infraorbital nerve and vessels
6. Optic canal transmits all except
   a. Optic nerve b. Ophthalmic artery
   c. Ophthalmic vein d. Sympathetic plexus
7. The outer blood retinal barrier is formed by
   a. Vascular endothelium
   b. Müller cells
   c. Rods and cones
   d. Retinal pigment epithelium
8. The choroid is supplied by
   a. Long posterior ciliary
   b. Short posterior ciliary arteries
   c. Lacrimal artery
   d. Anterior ciliary artery
9. Ophthalmic artery is a branch of
   a. Internal carotid artery
   b. External carotid artery
   c. Ethmoidal artery
   d. Lacrimal artery
10. Medial wall of orbit consists of all bones except
    a. Maxillary b. Lacrimal
    c. Ethmoid d. Palatine
11. The accessory lacrimal glands seen in the fornix are
    a. Glands of Krause b. Glands of Wolfring
    c. Henle's glands d. Moll's glands
12. The mucin layer of tear film is secreted by
    a. Conjunctival epithelium
    b. Goblet cells
    c. Zeis' gland
    d. Moll's gland
13. The multinucleated giant cells seen in trachoma are called
    a. Herbert cells b. HP bodies
    c. Langhans' cells d. Leber cells
14. Shield ulcer is seen in
    a. Neurotrophic keratopathy
    b. Trachoma
    c. VKC
    d. Herpetic keratitis
15. Which is not a mast cell stabilizer?
    a. Olopatadine b. Ketotifen
    c. Sodium cromoglicate d. Naphazoline

Note: IO, inferior oblique; SO, superior oblique; SOF, superior orbital fissure; VKC, vernal keratoconjunctivitis.

16. SAFE strategy is recommended for the control of
    a. Trachoma b. Glaucoma
    c. Diabetic retinopathy d. Cataract
17. Which organism is associated with Bitot's spots?
    a. *Corynebacterium xerosis*
    b. *Propionibacterium acnes*
    c. *Chlamydia*
    d. *Staphylococcus*
18. Which dye is not used in ocular surface staining?
    a. Fluorescein b. Rose Bengal
    c. Trypan blue d. Lissamine
19. Cobblestone papillae occurs in
    a. Trachoma b. Acute conjunctivitis
    c. Spring catarrh d. Ophthalmia nodosa
20. HP bodies in trachoma are
    a. Intracytoplasmic b. Intranuclear
    c. Intramitochondrial d. Transmembrane
21. D-shaped pupil is seen in
    a. Ectopia lentis b. Iridodialysis
    c. Sphincter tear d. Iridoschisis
22. Which is not true in VKC?
    a. Shield ulcer
    b. Pseudogerontoxon
    c. Sodium cromoglicate may be used
    d. Steroids are contraindicated
23. All of the following are neural crest derivatives except
    a. Stromal keratocytes b. Ciliary muscles
    c. Ciliary epithelium d. Corneal endothelium
24. Regarding phlycten, which is not true?
    a. May be seen as a limbal nodule
    b. Pain and photophobia
    c. May be associated with TB
    d. Antibiotics are used to treat this
25. Mechanism of action of excimer laser is
    a. Photodisruption b. Photocoagulation
    c. Photoablation d. Photochemical reaction
26. Which is not true about dry eye?
    a. Schirmer's test is used to diagnose it
    b. Tear substitutes is used to treat it
    c. SJS does not produce it
    d. Topical cyclosporine is used to treat it
27. Conjunctivitis is seen in all except
    a. Coxsackie B24 b. Adenovirus
    c. Enterovirus 70 d. CMV
28. Argyrosis results from application of
    a. Silver salts b. Gold salts
    c. Lead d. Copper salts
29. Which syndrome is associated with epibulbar dermoids?
    a. Goldenhar syndrome
    b. Sturge-Weber syndrome
    c. Treacher Collins syndrome
    d. Apert syndrome
30. The causative organism of Parinaud's oculoglandular syndrome is
    a. *Brucella* b. *Borrelia*
    c. *Bartonella* d. *Treponema*
31. What is the refractive index of cornea?
    a. 1.32 b. 1.34
    c. 1.376 d. 1.486
32. Palisades of Vogt are seen in
    a. Corneal stroma b. Corneal endothelium
    c. Bowman's membrane d. Limbus
33. Prominent corneal nerves occur in all except
    a. Keratoconus b. Neurofibromatosis
    c. Congenital glaucoma d. Macular dystrophy
34. The efferent for corneal sensation is
    a. V CN b. VII CN
    c. III CN d. VI CN
35. Most common organism causing corneal ulcer in contact lens wearers is
    a. Pneumococci b. *Acanthamoeba*
    c. Streptococci d. *Pseudomonas*
36. Recurrent corneal erosions are commonly produced by
    a. Cricket ball injury
    b. Chemical injury
    c. Blunt injury
    d. Finger nail injury
37. Corneal ulcer with overhanging edge is
    a. Mooren's ulcer b. Pneumococcal ulcer
    c. Shield ulcer d. *Pseudomonas* ulcer
38. Intrastromal rings are used in the treatment of
    a. Keratoconus b. Glaucoma
    c. RD d. Strabismus
39. In herpes zoster, which is not true?
    a. May involve ophthalmic division of V nerve
    b. Should arouse the suspicion of HIV if seen in young

Note: SAFE, surgery for trichiasis, antibiotics, facial cleanliness and environmental improvement; TB, tuberculosis; SJS, Stevens-Johnson syndrome; CMV, cytomegalovirus; CN, cranial nerve; RD, retinal detachment; HIV, human immunodeficiency virus.

c. Can produce nummular keratitis
d. Can produce acute corneal necrosis

40. Regarding herpes simplex keratitis, which statement is false?
a. Dendritic ulcer
b. Corneal sensation is normal
c. Acyclovir ointment is used for treatment
d. It can produce nummular keratitis

41. Föster-Fuchs' spots are seen in
a. Pathological myopia b. Hypermetropia
c. Aphakia d. Astigmatism

42. Excellent prognosis in penetrating keratoplasty is described in
a. Keratoconus
b. Chemical injuries
c. Therapeutic graft
d. Vascularized corneal scar

43. KF ring is seen at level of
a. Descemet's membrane
b. Endothelium
c. Lens capsule
d. Bowman's membrane

44. Regarding *Acanthamoeba* keratitis, which is not true?
a. Can occur after swimming
b. Severe pain
c. Propamidine isethionate is used
d. Chocolate agar is the culture medium

45. Vitamin used for collagen cross linking is
a. B1 b. B2
c. B6 d. B12

46. Neuroparalytic keratitis occurs in lesions of
a. III CN b. V CN
c. VII CN d. IV CN

47. Which is not true regarding keratoplasty?
a. M-K medium is a storage medium
b. Stromal rejection is the most severe form of graft rejection
c. Cryopreservation of cornea can be done
d. Graft size in keratoconus is small

48. Which statement is not true about peripheral ulcerative keratitis?
a. May be due to allergy to staphylococcal proteins
b. Connective tissue disorders can cause it
c. May be the first presentation of connective tissue disorder
d. Topical steroids are contraindicated

49. Which systemic condition is often associated with superior limbic keratoconjunctivitis?
a. Peripheral neuropathy
b. Diabetes
c. Pituitary adenoma
d. Thyroid disease

50. Stocker's line is seen in
a. Keratoconus b. Pellucid degeneration
c. Pterygium d. Mucopolysaccharidosis

51. Which treatment modality cannot be used in keratoconus?
a. Lamellar keratoplasty
b. Scleral contact lenses
c. Collagen cross linking
d. LASIK

52. An ulcer occurring in a corneal opacity is
a. Phlyctenular b. Catarrhal
c. Neurotrophic d. Atheromatous

53. Salmon patches in cornea are seen in
a. TB b. *Onchocerca*
c. Viral Keratitis d. Syphilis

54. Chronic serpiginous ulcer of cornea is
a. Pneumococcal ulcer b. *Acanthamoeba ulcer*
c. Shield ulcer d. Mooren's ulcer

55. What is the percentage of acyclovir eye ointment?
a. 3.5% b. 3.75%
c. 3% d. 2.5%

56. The foci of infection in herpes zoster ophthalmicus is
a. Ciliary ganglion b. Gasserian ganglion
c. Spinal ganglion d. Cervical ganglion

57. Sectoral iris atrophy is characteristic of
a. Acute angle-closure glaucoma
b. Herpes zoster iridocyclitis
c. Herpes simplex iritis
d. Fuchs' uveitis

58. Among the following, which is an indication for oral acyclovir?
a. Dendritic ulcer
b. Punctate epithelial keratitis
c. Neurotrophic ulcer
d. Herpes zoster iridocyclitis

Note: KF, Kayser-Fleischer; M-K, McCarey-Kaufman; LASIK, laser-assisted in situ keratomileusis.

59. Which is not an antifungal?
   a. Natamycin b. Ketoconazole
   c. Idoxuridine d. Nystatin

60. A tissue adhesive that can be used in small corneal perforations is
   a. Fibrin glue b. Thrombin glue
   c. Cyanoacrylate glue d. Membrane glue

61. Which of the following is false?
   a. Endothelium—specular microscopy
   b. Corneal curvature—keratometry
   c. Corneal epithelium—topography
   d. Corneal thickness—pachymetry

62. All of the following organisms can penetrate the intact corneal epithelium except
   a. *Neisseria gonorrhoeae*
   b. *Corynebacterium diphtheriae*
   c. *Listeria*
   d. *Pseudomonas*

63. Sclera is thinnest at
   a. Limbus
   b. Equator
   c. Just behind recti muscle insertions
   d. Lamina cribrosa

64. T-sign in ultrasound B scan is suggestive of
   a. Choroidal melanoma b. Optic neuritis
   c. Posterior scleritis d. Foreign body

65. Which is not true?
   a. Scleromalacia perforans is an anterior scleritis without inflammation
   b. Seen more in women
   c. Seen with longstanding seropositive rheumatoid arthritis
   d. Painful scleral thinning

66. In a patient presenting with scleritis, on examination has an ulcer/granuloma nose, the most appropriate investigation of choice is
   a. ANA b. ANCA
   c. VDRL d. ELISA for HIV

67. Which is not true regarding Behçet's disease?
   a. Mouth ulcers are universal
   b. Hypopyon
   c. Ophthalmic involvement is a minor criterion
   d. Retinal exudation

68. A 25 year-old-male was complaining of decreased vision in right eye for the last 1 year. On examination both eyes were white, right eye shows stellate KP, posterior subcapsular cataract, mild anterior chamber cells and flare. The diagnosis is
   a. Fuchs' heterochromic iridocyclitis
   b. Behçet's disease
   c. Traumatic iridocyclitis
   d. TB uveitis

69. Candle wax dripping type of vasculitis is a feature of
   a. Behçet's disease b. TB uveitis
   c. Traumatic uveitis d. Sarcoidosis

70. Which is not true?
   a. Keratic precipitates are cellular deposits on endothelium
   b. Seen in a triangular fashion in inferior cornea called Arlt's triangle
   c. Stellate KPs are seen in Fuchs' uveitis
   d. Mutton fat KPs are a feature of non-granulomatous uveitis

71. Which is a correct statement?
   a. Busacca nodules are seen in pupillary margin
   b. Koeppe's nodules are at collarette
   c. Stellate KPs are seen in Fuchs' uveitis
   d. Cells in the anterior chamber come from iris vessels

72. Which is not true about Reiter's syndrome?
   a. Causes conjunctivitis, in third decade, in males
   b. Conjunctivitis follows arthritis and precedes urethritis
   c. Arthritis typically affects knee and ankle
   d. They may have HLA association

73. Head light in fog appearance is a feature of
   a. Toxoplasmosis b. Toxocariasis
   c. *Acanthamoeba* d. Herpes zoster

74. Which is not true regarding sympathetic ophthalmitis?
   a. Blurring of near vision is the first symptom
   b. Dalen-Fuchs' nodules are seen
   c. Bilateral granulomatous uveitis
   d. Earliest sign is keratic precipitates

75. In juvenile rheumatoid arthritis, which is not true?
   a. White eye uveitis
   b. Non-granulomatous bilateral uveitis
   c. Polyarticular form is commonly associated with uveitis
   d. Band keratopathy

Note: ANA, American Nurses Association; ANCA, antineutrophil cytoplasmic antibody; VDRL, Venereal Disease Research Laboratory; ELISA, enzyme-linked immunosorbent assay; KP, keratic precipitate; HLA, human leukocyte antigen.

76. All are features of complicated cataract except
   a. Polychromatic luster
   b. Bread crumb appearance
   c. Posterior subcapsular cataract
   d. Nuclear cataract

77. Iris Bombe is caused by
   a. Posterior uveitis   b. Seclusio pupillae
   c. Occlusio pupillae   d. Blunt trauma

78. Which is false about sarcoidosis?
   a. c/c granulomatous uveitis
   b. Retinal periphlebitis
   c. Retinal granuloma
   d. Optic neuritis is very common

79. Following are true about Vogt-Koyanagi-Harada syndrome except
   a. c/c granulomatous iridocyclitis
   b. Multifocal choroiditis
   c. Multifocal detachment
   d. Unilateral disease

80. In toxoplasmosis, which is not true?
   a. Congenital toxoplasmosis may have B/L or U/L macular chorioretinal scar
   b. Chorioretinitis, convulsions and calcifications are seen in congenital toxoplasmosis
   c. Toxoplasmosis retinal lesions may have 'head light in fog' appearance
   d. AIDS patients usually do not develop toxoplasmosis

81. All are true in viral uveitis except
   a. May be associated with keratitis
   b. May be associated with iris atrophy
   c. May produce hyphema
   d. Usually caused by adenovirus

82. Regarding Posner-Schlossman syndrome, which is true?
   a. Uveitis with glaucoma
   b. Posterior synechiae
   c. Severe uveitis
   d. Causes blindness

83. The chief type of protein in human lens is
   a. Alpha crystallins   b. Albuminoids
   c. Beta crystallins   d. Gamma crystallins

84. The weight of human lens at birth is around
   a. 30 mg   b. 65 mg
   c. 90 mg   d. 150 mg

85. One of the following can occur with cardiac conduction defects, premature baldness and tonic relaxation of skeletal muscles
   a. Snowflake cataract
   b. Microspherophakia
   c. Christmas tree cataract
   d. Sunflower cataract

86. Bilateral inferior lens subluxation is typically seen in
   a. Marfan's syndrome   b. Homocystinuria
   c. Hyperinsulinemia   d. Ocular trauma

87. Which of the statements regarding endophthalmitis is not correct?
   a. Acute postoperative endophthalmitis is usually caused by *Staphylococcus epidermidis*
   b. Postoperative endophthalmitis presents with severe pain, lid edema, chemosis within 1 or 2 days after surgery
   c. Fungal endophthalmitis presents typically within 2 days after surgery
   d. The drug of choice for fungal endophthalmitis is intravitreal amphotericin

88. In congenital cataract, which is not true?
   a. Congenital cataract larger than 3 mm should be operated early
   b. Maternal malnutrition produce cataract
   c. Hypocalcemia produce it
   d. Cataract in congenital rubella is usually non-progressive

89. The energy used in phacoemulsification is
   a. Ultrasound   b. Laser
   c. Electrical energy   d. None of the above

90. Foldable intraocular lenses (IOLs) are made of all except
   a. Silicon   b. Collamer
   c. Hydrogel   d. PMMA

91. Which is true in Marfan's syndrome?
   a. Lens subluxation is present in majority of patients at birth
   b. Lens subluxated inferiorly
   c. Marfan's do not develop glaucoma
   d. Retinal detachment is common in Marfan's syndrome

92. Which is not true?
   a. Lens subluxation occur in chalcosis
   b. Siderosis produce retinal degeneration

Note: c/c, chronic; B/L, bilateral; U/L, unilateral; AIDS, acquired immunodeficiency syndrome; PMMA, polymethyl methacrylate.

c. Homocystinuria produces lens subluxation
d. Trauma causes snowflake cataract

93. Pigment ring seen in the lens after blunt trauma
a. Scheie's ring b. Vossius ring
c. Coat's ring d. Campbell's ring

94. Oil droplet cataract is seen in
a. Diabetes b. Galactosemia
c. Wilson's disease d. Myotonic dystrophy

95. 'Riders' are seen in
a. Rosette cataract b. Brunescent cataract
c. Sunflower cataract d. Zonular cataract

96. Atopic dermatitis produces
a. Shield cataract b. Polar cataract
c. Microphakia d. Blue dot cataract

97. What is the percentage of ophthalmic preparation of povidone iodine for topical use?
a. 1% b. 5%
c. 10% d. 0.5%

98. Which is the dye used for staining anterior capsule during cataract surgery?
a. Alcian blue b. Toluidine blue
c. Trypan blue d. Triamcinolone blue

99. The best optical rehabilitation after removal of cataract is
a. Aphakic glasses b. Contact lens
c. IOL d. Monovision

100. All are types of posterior capsular opacification except
a. Elschnig's pearls b. Sommering's ring
c. Capsular fibrosis d. Mittendorf's dots

101. Most common organism implicated is delayed onset postoperative endophthalmitis is
a. Coagulase negative staphylococci
b. *Haemophilus*
c. *Aspergillus*
d. *Propionibacterium acnes*

102. The most common side effect associated with carbonic anhydrate inhibitor therapy is
a. Nausea b. Alkalosis
c. Paresthesia d. Nervousness

103. Parenteral steroid causes mainly causes
a. Cataract b. Glaucoma
c. Papilledema d. Ptosis

104. Which of the following antiglaucoma medications can cause drowsiness?
a. Latanoprost b. Timolol
c. Brimonidine d. Dorzolamide

105. Which one of the antiglaucoma medications causes retinal breaks and RD?
a. Beta blockers b. Pilocarpine
c. Brimonidine d. Prostaglandins

106. Which one of the following has neuroprotective action?
a. Timolol b. Pilocarpine
c. Brimonidine d. Prostaglandins

107. Which is not true in acute congestive glaucoma?
a. Shallow AC
b. Miotic pupil
c. Circumcorneal congestion
d. Corneal edema

108. Glaucomflecken is a feature of
a. Angle-closure glaucoma
b. POAG
c. Pigmentary glaucoma
d. Traumatic glaucoma

109. Which is not true regarding laser iridotomy?
a. Nd:YAG laser is used
b. Wavelength of the laser used is 532 nm
c. Prophylactically done in the other eye in acute congestive glaucoma
d. Used in pupillary block glaucoma

110. A child born with congenital glaucoma will have all except
a. Hazy cornea b. Haab's striae
c. Hypermetropia d. Myopia

111. Molteno implant is
a. An IOL
b. Implant for RD surgery
c. Intravitreal implant
d. Glaucoma drainage device

112. In lens induced glaucoma, the treatment of choice is
a. Trabeculectomy
b. Trabeculectomy with cataract surgery
c. Cataract surgery
d. Topical antiglaucoma medication

Note: AC, anterior chamber; POAG, primary open angle glaucoma; Nd:YAG, neodymium-doped yttrium aluminum garnet.

113. In POAG, which is not true?
a. Optic disk changes
b. Field changes
c. Pilocarpine is a very useful drug
d. Trabeculectomy in late stages

114. Intumescent lens produces
a. Phacolytic glaucoma
b. Phacotopic glaucoma
c. Phacomorphic glaucoma
d. Phacoanaphylactic glaucoma

115. The drug, which should not be used in acute attack of PACG is
a. Mannitol b. Pilocarpine
c. Acetazolamide d. Atropine

116. Phacolytic glaucoma is produced by
a. Intumescent lens b. Hypermature cataract
c. Brown cataract d. Black cataract

117. Which is not true?
a. Timolol act by decreasing aqueous humor production
b. Acetazolamide acts by decreasing aqueous humor production
c. Pilocarpine acts by decreasing aqueous humor production
d. Brimonidine acts by decreasing aqueous humor production

118. Angle recession glaucoma occurs in
a. Lens induced glaucoma
b. Steroid use
c. Iris tumors
d. Blunt trauma

119. Mechanism of action of latanoprost is
a. Decrease aqueous humor production
b. Increases the drainage through trabecular meshwork
c. Increases the uveoscleral outflow
d. When used in combination with pilocarpine, acceleration effect

120. Adverse effects of topical beta blockers include all except
a. Bradycardia
b. Dyslipidemia
c. Masks the symptoms of hypoglycemia
d. Bronchodilatation

121. Which is not true regarding pigmentary glaucoma?
a. Seen in young b. Myopic
c. Male d. Female

122. Krukenberg spindle is a characteristic feature of
a. Pigmentary glaucoma
b. Pseudoexfoliation glaucoma
c. POAG
d. PACG

123. In POAG, which is not seen?
a. Vertical cupping b. Bayoneting sign
c. Laminar dot sign d. Macular edema

124. Aniridia may be associated with
a. Mutation in *PAX6* gene
b. Wilms tumor
c. Stem cell deficiency
d. All the above

125. Treatment of congenital glaucoma is
a. Acetazolamide b. Timolol
c. Trabeculectomy d. Trabeculotomy

126. The magnification obtained with a direct ophthalmoscope is
a. 5 times b. 10 times
c. 15 times d. 20 times

127. Which drug can cause macular toxicity when given intravitreally?
a. Gentamicin b. Vancomycin
c. Dexamethasone d. Ceftazidime

128. Which is not true regarding hypertension and eye?
a. Can produce superficial retinal hemorrhages
b. Hard exudates
c. Soft exudates
d. Cannot produce disk edema

129. Hypertensive retinopathy classification is
a. Keith-Wagner-Barker classification
b. Airlie house classification
c. McCallum's classification
d. Reese-Ellsworth classification

130. Which is not a feature of hypertensive retinopathy?
a. Salus sign b. Gunn's sign
c. Bonnet sign d. Elschnig/Siegrist spot

131. Which is not true regarding diabetic retinopathy?
a. Main risk factor is duration of diabetes
b. Strict control of hyperglycemia delays the onset of DR

Note: PACG, primary angle closure glaucoma; DR, diabetic retinopathy.

c. DR patients are likely to have nephropathy
d. Comorbidities like HTN, dyslipidemia have no bearing on the onset of DR

132. Exudative retinal detachment is produced by all except
a. Anemia b. PIH
c. Uremia d. Leukemia

133. All are true regarding enucleation in retinoblastoma except
a. Minimum manipulation
b. Longest possible optic nerve should be cut
c. Bleeding may be a problem
d. Should be done in all stages

134. All are associations of retinitis pigmentosa except
a. Keratoconus
b. Drusen of optic nerve head
c. Myopia
d. Hypermetropia

135. Which is not true regarding central retinal artery occlusion?
a. Ophthalmic emergency
b. Causes cherry red spot
c. Usually reversible
d. Vasculitis can cause it

136. All are true regarding central retinal vein occlusion except
a. RAPD and markedly decreased vision are features Ischemic CRVO
b. Posterior pole of fundus will be full of hemorrhages in Ischemic CRVO
c. Non-ischemic CRVO may get converted Ischemic CRVO
d. Non-ischemic CRVO cannot produce macular edema

137. Risk factors for ROP include
a. Prematurity
b. Low birth weight < 1.5 kg
c. Supplemental oxygen
d. All the above

138. Which among the following is an acquired cause of cherry red spot at the macula?
a. Commotio retinae b. Niemann-Pick
c. Tay-Sachs d. Gangliosidosis

139. Which is the laser most commonly used for retinal photocoagulation?
a. Nd:YAG
b. Argon
c. Frequency doubled Nd:YAG
d. Krypton red

140. Sildenafil citrate can produce
a. Glaucoma
b. Cataract
c. Uveitis
d. Ischemic optic neuropathy

141. Knudson's hypothesis is for
a. Retinoblastoma
b. Retinocytoma
c. Choroidal melanoma
d. None of the above

142. Which is not a feature of retinoblastoma?
a. May present as squint
b. May be associated with pineal gland tumor
c. Second tumors are most common in soft tissues
d. Indirect ophthalmoscopy is a must

143. Retinal degeneration most often leading to RD is
a. Lattice degeneration
b. Snail track degeneration
c. Paving stone degeneration
d. White without pressure

144. Which of the retinal break is most likely to lead to rhegmatogenous RD?
a. Retinal hole b. Operculated hole
c. Macular hole d. Horseshoe tear

145. Refractive error most commonly associated with rhegmatogenous RD is
a. Hypermetropia b. Myopia
c. Astigmatism d. Presbyopia

146. Risk factors for retinal detachment are all except
a. Family history of RD b. RD in the other eye
c. Marfan's syndrome d. High hypermetropia

147. Retinal detachment surgery may use all except
a. Silicone band, tyre, sponge
b. Silicone oil
c. Perfluoropropane (C3F8) gas
d. Hydroxypropyl methylcellulose

148. Antiangiogenic drug used for intravitreal injection include all the following except
a. Bevacizumab b. Ranibizumab
c. Pegaptanib d. Thiotepa

149. EOG is typically diagnostic in
a. Best disease b. RP
c. CRVO d. CRAO

Note: HTN, hypertension; PIH, pregnancy-induced hypertension; RAPD, relative afferent pupillary defect; CRVO, central retinal vein occlusion; ROP, retinopathy of prematurity; RP, retinitis pigmentosa; CRAO, central retinal artery occlusion.

150. The earliest change in diabetic retinopathy is
a. Hard exudates b. Soft exudates
c. Microaneurysms d. IRMA

151. Metastasis into the orbit may present with all the following except
a. Proptosis b. Enophthalmos
c. Diplopia d. Severe pain

152. Uhthoff's symptom in optic neuritis is
a. Electric shock like sensation with neck flexion
b. Ability to see moving objects but not stationary ones
c. Decrease in vision with increase in body temperature
d. Inability to distinguish face

153. In idiopathic intracranial hypertension, which is not true
a. Bilateral disk edema
b. Steroids may produce this
c. CT scan brain shows dilated ventricles
d. Middle aged obese lady

154. In drusen of the optic nerve head, which is not true?
a. Disk will appear edematous
b. Autofluorescence in blue filter
c. Anomalous branching of vessels
d. Disk is small

155. The type of optic atrophy seen following retrobulbar neuritis is
a. Consecutive b. Primary
c. Secondary d. Cavernous

156. Altitudinal field defects are typically seen in
a. AION b. CRAO
c. Optic neuritis d. Glaucoma

157. In one and a half syndrome, which is not true?
a. Lesions affecting MLF and PPRF on the same side
b. Loss of horizontal eye movements of the same side
c. No adduction in the contralateral eye
d. No abduction in contralateral eye

158. A patient who had carcinoma lung (right) underwent lobectomy now complains of ptosis of the right eye, the other sign that you will look for is
a. Miosis b. Mydriasis
c. Strabismus d. Nystagmus

159. A patient who had headache, detected to have a BP of 200/120 mm Hg got admitted and was put on antihypertensives and his/her BP next day is 140/80 mm Hg, but the patient now complains of sudden decrease in vision in right eye, the most possible cause is
a. CRAO
b. CRVO
c. Optic neuritis
d. Infarction to optic nerve head

160. Which is not true regarding myasthenia?
a. May have unilateral ptosis
b. May have bilateral ptosis
c. May mimic INO
d. Ocular involvement is a late sign

161. Which is not true?
a. Myasthenia-neostigmine test is diagnostic
b. Improved response in EMG on repetitive stimulation
c. Thymectomy is a treatment option
d. Plasmapheresis is also a treatment option

162. Canaliculitis is produced by
a. *Pneumococcus* b. *Staphylococcus*
c. *Pseudomonas* d. *Actinomyces*

163. Nasolacrimal duct opens into
a. Inferior meatus b. Middle meatus
c. Superior meatus d. Maxillary antrum

164. In DCR, lacrimal sac is anastomosed to
a. Inferior meatus b. Middle meatus
c. Superior meatus d. Maxillary antrum

165. Which is not true in orbital cellulitis?
a. Painful eye movements
b. Mixed infection from respiratory pathogens
c. Spreads from sinuses
d. Spontaneous resolution is common

166. In cavernous sinus thrombosis, the earliest sign is
a. Lateral rectus palsy
b. III nerve palsy
c. Decreased corneal sensation
d. Papilledema

167. Recurrent chalazion in elderly signify
a. Sarcoidosis
b. TB
c. Meibomian carcinoma
d. Refractive error

168. Recurrent chalazion in children means
a. Sarcoidosis
b. TB

Note: IRMA, intraretinal microvascular abnormalities; CT, computed tomography; AION, anterior ischemic optic neuropathy; BP, blood pressure; MLF, medial longitudinal fasciculus; PPRF, paramedium pontine reticular formation; DCR, dacryocystorhinostomy; INO, internuclear ophthalmoplegia; EMG, electromyogram.

c. Meibomian carcinoma
d. Refractive error

169. Which is not true about basal cell carcinoma?
a. 90% BCC is located in head and neck region
b. 90% of malignant eyelid tumors
c. Tumors of medial canthus has best prognosis
d. Lower eyelid is mostly involved

170. Which is not true about squamous cell carcinoma?
a. 5%–10% of eyelid malignancy
b. Better prognosis compared to BCC
c. Arise de novo or from precancerous lesion
d. Intradermal keratin pearls in histology is diagnostic

171. All are features of congenital ptosis except
a. Severe ptosis
b. Absent upper lid crease
c. Poor levator function
d. Aponeurosis repair is treatment

172. Indian file appearance (palisading) is a feature of
a. Basal cell carcinoma
b. Squamous cell carcinoma
c. Sebaceous gland carcinoma
d. Malignant melanoma

173. Which is not a feature of capillary hemangioma of orbit?
a. Appears by 6 months
b. Grows for 6 years
c. Majority disappear by 7 years
d. Majority persist up to late teens

174. Which is not true about rhabdomyosarcoma?
a. Sudden onset of proptosis
b. Highly malignant
c. Arise from muscle fibers
d. Usually in upper nasal orbit

175. In pseudotumor of the orbit, all are true except
a. CT may show a mass lesion
b. Ultrasound may show a muscle thickening including the tendon
c. May cause decrease in vision
d. Antibiotics are the treatment of choice

176. Arden index is related to
a. ERG b. EOG
c. VEP d. Perimetry

177. A patient who has suffered orbital fracture complains of vomiting the ideal approach is
a. Reduce orbital fracture
b. Give antiemetics
c. Order for CT brain
d. Admit and put the patient on a course of IV antibiotics before reducing the fracture

178. Blepharophimosis syndrome has all the following except
a. Ptosis b. Telecanthus
c. Epicanthus inversus d. Entropion

179. Which is not true regarding chalazion?
a. Chalazion is a acute granulomatous inflammation of the meibomian gland
b. There are 30–40 glands in upper tarsus and 20–30 in lower tarsus
c. Associated with rosacea and seborrheic dermatitis
d. I and C is the treatment

180. Which is not true?
a. Kaposi's sarcoma is a vascular tumor
b. May appear as a small hematoma
c. Low dose chemotherapy is usually effective
d. May be seen in advanced cases of AIDS, but may be the only manifestation

181. What is true about blowout fracture of the orbit?
a. Always contents migrate into antrum
b. Diplopia on lateral gaze
c. Anesthesia of lower molar teeth
d. Medial wall fractures are less common than that of inferior wall

182. Choroidal neovascular membrane is seen in all except
a. ARMD b. High myopia
c. Angioid streaks d. Retinal detachment

183. Infrequent blinking in thyroid ophthalmopathy is
a. Stellwag's sign b. Dalrymple's sign
c. von Graefe's sign d. Mobius sign

184. Chocolate cysts are a feature of
a. Lymphangioma
b. Capillary hemangioma
c. Cavernous hemangioma
d. Orbital varix

185. Goldenhar syndrome has all the following except
a. Limbal dermoid b. Preauricular ear tag
c. Renal anomalies d. Vertebral anomalies

Note: BCC, basal cell carcinoma; ERG, electroretinography; EOG, electro-oculogram; VEP, visual evoked potential; I and C, incision and curettage; ARMD, age-related macular degeneration.

186. A patient with ptosis presents with retraction of ptotic eyelid on chewing. This represents
    a. Oculomotor nerve palsy
    b. Abducens nerve palsy
    c. Marcus Gunn jaw winking syndrome
    d. III nerve misdirection syndrome
187. Majority of cases of myopia are
    a. Axial b. Index
    c. Curvatural d. Positional
188. Most common cause of low vision in children is
    a. Refractive error b. Cataract
    c. Corneal opacity d. Strabismus
189. Amblyopia in children is most commonly caused by
    a. Hypermetropia b. Myopia
    c. Astigmatism d. Corneal opacity
190. Regarding use of botulinum toxin in strabismus, all are true except
    a. Used for chemodenervation
    b. Injection is to paralyzed muscle
    c. Blocks acetylcholine release
    d. Used when surgery is contraindicated
191. All are features of paralytic squint except
    a. Diplopia
    b. Abnormal head posture may be seen
    c. Early surgery is not needed
    d. Primary deviation = secondary deviation
192. All are true in the management of squint except
    a. Measure the degree of squint by prisms
    b. Refractive error if any should be corrected before surgery
    c. Amblyopia should be corrected before surgery
    d. Amblyopia correction is done only after surgery
193. All are features of amblyopia except
    a. Decreased visual acuity—loss of two or more lines in Snellen's chart
    b. Crowding phenomenon
    c. Normal eye anatomically
    d. RAPD
194. All are true about esotropia, except
    a. Surgery is the treatment of choice in congenital esotropia
    b. Congenital esotropia usually do not have high hypermetropia
    c. Cross fixation is a feature of congenital esotropia
    d. Surgery is usually required in accommodative esotropia
195. Mobius syndrome includes all except
    a. Esotropia
    b. Exotropia
    c. Facial diplegia
    d. Hypoplasia of 6 and 7 nucleus
196. All are true regarding Brown's syndrome except
    a. Superior oblique tendon sheath syndrome
    b. Defective elevation in adduction
    c. Systemic steroids may be indicated
    d. Abnormal head posture
197. About childhood squints, all are true except
    a. May be due to retinoblastoma
    b. Macular diseases like toxoplasmosis may cause it
    c. Refractive error should be ruled out
    d. All of them require surgery
198. All are features of congenital nystagmus except
    a. Horizontal nystagmus
    b. Sleep aggravates it
    c. Horizontal nystagmus even on vertical gaze
    d. Fixation decreases it
199. All are true about myasthenia except
    a. Usually starts in eye muscles
    b. 20% remain ocular
    c. Pupil is almost always involved
    d. Neostigmine test is used to diagnose it
200. All are used to check visual acuity in children except
    a. VEP
    b. Teller acuity cards
    c. Cardiff acuity cards
    d. Perimetry

ANSWERS

1. b
2. a
3. a
4. c
5. c
6. c
7. d
8. b
9. a
10. d
11. a
12. b
13. d
14. c
15. d
16. a
17. a
18. c
19. c
20. a
21. d
22. d
23. c
24. d
25. d
26. c
27. d
28. a
29. a
30. c
31. c
32. d
33. d
34. b
35. d
36. d
37. a
38. a
39. d
40. b
41. a
42. a
43. a
44. d
45. b
46. c
47. b
48. d
49. d
50. c
51. d
52. d
53. d
54. d
55. c
56. b
57. b
58. d
59. c
60. c
61. c
62. d
63. c
64. c
65. d
66. b
67. c
68. a
69. d
70. d
71. c
72. b
73. a
74. d
75. c
76. d
77. b
78. d
79. d
80. d
81. d
82. a
83. c
84. b
85. c
86. b
87. c
88. d
89. a
90. d
91. d
92. d
93. b
94. b
95. d
96. a
97. b
98. c
99. c
100. d
101. d
102. c
103. a
104. c
105. b
106. c
107. b
108. a
109. b
110. c
111. d
112. c
113. c
114. c
115. d
116. b
117. c
118. d
119. c
120. d
121. d
122. a
123. d
124. d
125. d
126. c
127. a
128. d
129. a
130. d
131. d
132. d
133. d
134. d
135. c
136. d
137. d
138. a
139. c
140. d
141. a
142. c
143. a
144. d
145. b
146. d
147. d
148. d
149. a
150. c
151. d
152. c
153. c
154. d
155. b
156. a
157. d
158. a
159. d
160. d
161. b
162. d
163. a
164. b
165. d
166. a
167. c
168. d
169. c
170. b
171. d
172. a
173. d
174. c
175. d
176. b
177. c
178. d
179. a
180. c
181. d
182. d
183. a
184. a
185. c
186. c
187. a
188. a
189. a
190. b
191. d
192. d
193. d
194. d
195. b
196. c
197. d
198. b
199. c
200. d

Index

Page numbers followed by *f* refer to figure and *t* refer to table

A

B

D

E

F

G

H

K

L

M

P

Q

R

S

T

X

Y

Z